Pediatric Respiratory Diseases

Pablo Bertrand • Ignacio Sánchez
Editors

Pediatric Respiratory Diseases

A Comprehensive Textbook

EDICIONES UC

Springer

Editors
Pablo Bertrand
Pontificia Universidad Católica de Chile
Santiago
Chile

Ignacio Sánchez
Pontificia Universidad Católica de Chile
Santiago
Chile

Translation from the Spanish language edition: "Enfermedades Respiratorias del Niño - Segunda edición" by Pablo Bertrand and Ignacio Sánchez. Original Publication ISBN 978-956-14-1945-2.

ISBN 978-3-030-26960-9 ISBN 978-3-030-26961-6 (eBook)
https://doi.org/10.1007/978-3-030-26961-6

This Springer imprint is published by the registered company Springer Nature Switzerland AG
The registered company address is: Gewerbestrasse 11, 6330 Cham, Switzerland

We acknowledge the support/assistance of Ms. Mirta Guerra in the translation of the chapters of this book to English.

Contents

Contributors

Verónica Aguerre Hospital Garrahan, Buenos Aires, Argentina

Viviana Aguirre Camposano Department of Pediatrics, School of Medicine, University of Santiago, Santiago, Chile

Ofelia Álvarez Clinical Pediatrics, University of Miami, Coral Gables, FL, USA

Lidia Amarales Osorio Ministry of Health, Santiago, Chile

Claudia Astudillo Maggio Pediatrics, Respiratory Diseases, Hospital Josefina Martínez, Puente Alto, Chile

Pontificia Universidad Católica de Chile, Santiago, Chile

Luis Avendaño Carvajal Faculty of Medicine, Universidad de Chile, Santiago, Chile

Patricio Barañao Garces Respiratory Kinesiotherapy, Hospital Josefina Martínez, Puente Alto, Chile

Pontificia Universidad Católica de Chile, Santiago, Chile

Salesa Barja Yáñez Pontificia Universidad Católica de Chile, Santiago, Chile

Andrea Beckhaus Faccin Department of Pediatrics, School of Medicine, Pontificia Universidad Católica de Chile, Santiago, Chile

Constanza Beltrán Morales Department of Otorhinolaryngology, School of Medicine, Universidad de los Andes, Santiago, Chile

Katalina Bertrán Salinas Department of Pediatrics, Hospital Clínico Universidad Católica de Chile, Santiago, Chile

Pablo Bertrand Department of Pediatrics, School of Medicine, Pontificia Universidad Católica de Chile, Santiago, Chile

Arturo Borzutzky Schachter Department of Pediatrics School of Medicine, Pontificia Universidad Católica de Chile, Santiago, Chile

María Lina Boza Costagliola Pediatrics, Respiratory diseases, University of Chile, Santiago, Chile

Pablo Brockmann Veloso Department of Pediatrics, School of Medicine, Pontificia Universidad Católica de Chile, Santiago, Chile

Raúl Bustos Betanzo Pediatrics, Intensive Care at Clínica Sanatorio Alemán, Concepción, Chile

Andrew Bush Faculty of Medicine, Imperial College of London, London, UK

Mario Calvo Gil Department of Pediatrics, School of Medicine, Universidad Austral, Valdivia, Chile

Mauricio Campos Daziano Pontificia Universidad Católica de Chile, Santiago, Chile

Juan Andrés Carrasco Orellana Department of Pediatrics, School of Medicine, Universidad del Desarrollo, Santiago, Chile

Carlos Casar Collazo Department of Pediatrics, Hospital Roberto del Río, Santiago, Chile

Claudio Castaños Hospital Garrahan, Buenos Aires, Argentina

Andrés Castillo Moya Department of Pediatrics, School of Medicine, Pontificia Universidad Católica de Chile, Santiago, Chile

José Antonio Castro-Rodríguez Department of Pediatrics, School of Medicine, Pontificia Universidad Católica de Chile, Santiago, Chile

Solange Caussade Larraín Department of Pediatrics, School of Medicine, Pontificia Universidad Católica de Chile, Santiago, Chile

Bernardita Chateau Infante Department of Pediatrics, Clínica Los Andes, Santiago, Chile

Lilien Chertkoff Hospital Garrahan, Buenos Aires, Argentina

Alejandro Colom Pediatric Pulmonology, Hospital Ricardo Gutiérrez, Buenos Aires, Argentina

Ida Concha Murray Department of Pediatrics, School of Medicine, Pontificia Universidad Católica de Chile, Santiago, Chile

Ilse Contreras Estay Department of Pediatrics, Hospital Padre Hurtado, Santiago, Chile

Mara Cvejic Division of Sleep Medicine, School of Medicine, Stanford University, Redwood City, CA, USA

Jacques de Blic Université Paris Descartes, Hôpital Necker Enfants Malades, Paris, France

Raúl Escobar Henríquez Department of Pediatrics, School of Medicine, Pontificia Universidad Católica de Chile, Santiago, Chile

Jorge Fabres Biggs Department of Pediatrics, School of Medicine, Pontificia Universidad Católica de Chile, Santiago, Chile

Albert Faro Washington University in St. Louis School of Medicine, St. Louis, MO, USA

Gerardo Ferrero Respiratory Kinesiology and Physiatry, Hospital Rehabilitación Respiratoria Maria Ferrer, Buenos Aires, Argentina

Marcela Ferrés Garrido Department of Pediatrics, School of Medicine, Pontificia Universidad Católica de Chile, Santiago, Chile

Gilberto Fischer Pediatric Pulmonology, Federal University of Health Sciences of Porto Alegre, Porto Alegre, Brazil

Carlos Flores Berríos Department of Pediatrics, Hospital de Ovalle, Ovalle, Chile

Ximena Fonseca Arrieta Otorhinolaryngology, Pontificia Universidad Católica de Chile, Santiago, Chile

Claudia Fuentes Saez Pediatrics, Respiratory Diseases, Hospital Regional de Concepción, Concepción, Chile

Juan Cristóbal Gana Ansaldo Pontificia Universidad Católica de Chile, Santiago, Chile

Cristián García Bruce Pediatric Radiology, School of Medicine, Pontificia Universidad Católica de Chile, Santiago, Chile

Guido Girardi Briere Faculty of Medicine, Universidad de Chile, Santiago, Chile

Verónica Giubergia Hospital Garrahan, Buenos Aires, Argentina

Aviv Goldbart Ben Gurion University of Negev, Beersheba, Israel

Sergio González Bombardiere Pathological Anatomy, Pontificia Universidad Católica de Chile, Santiago, Chile

Álvaro González Morandé Pediatrics, Neonatology, Pontificia Universidad Católica de Chile, Santiago, Chile

David Gozal Department of Pediatrics, The University of Chicago, Chicago, IL, USA

Luis Gravina Hospital Garrahan, Buenos Aires, Argentina

María Elena Guarda Barros Department of Pediatrics, Hospital Roberto del Río, Santiago, Chile

Christian Guilleminault Division of Sleep Medicine, School of Medicine, Stanford University, Redwood City, CA, USA

Carolina Gvirtzman Department of Pediatrics, Hospital Garrahan, Buenos Aires, Argentina

Gonzalo Hidalgo Soler Respiratory Kinesiology, Faculty of Medicine, Universidad de Chile, Santiago, Chile

Nils Linus Holmgren Palmen Department of Pediatrics, Clínica Alemana and Universidad del Desarrollo, Santiago, Chile

Fernando Iñiguez Osmer Department of Pediatrics, Hospital de Puerto Montt, Puerto Montt, Chile

María Francisca Jaime Méndez Pontificia Universidad Católica de Chile, Santiago, Chile

Javier Kattan Said Department of Pediatrics, School of Medicine, Pontificia Universidad Católica de Chile, Santiago, Chile

Carlos Kofman Department of Pediatric Pulmonology, Hospital Ricardo Gutiérrez, Buenos Aires, Argentina

Ricardo Kogan Alterman Department of Pediatrics, Faculty of Medicine, Universidad de Chile, Santiago, Chile

Marcelo Laufer Pediatrics, Infectious Diseases, Nicklaus Children's Hospital, Miami, FL, USA

Agustín León Cortés Pediatrics, Respiratory Diseases, Clínica Santa María, Providencia, Chile

Marcela Linares Paserini Department of Pediatrics, Clínica Indisa, Santiago, Chile

Alejandro Lozano Department of Allergy and Immunology, Faculty of Medicine, Universidad Católica de Córdoba, Córdoba, Argentina

Julio Maggiolo Massone Department of Pediatrics, Hospital Exequiel González Cortés, San Miguel, Chile

Mireya Mendez Raggi Pediatrics, Respiratory Diseases, Hospital Josefina Martínez, Puente Alto, Chile

Pontificia Universidad Católica de Chile, Santiago, Chile

Cecilia Méndez Rivera Pediatrics, Immunology and Rheumatology, Pontificia Universidad Católica de Chile, Santiago, Chile

Carlos Mendoza Fox Department of Pediatrics, Hospital Nacional Hipólito Unanue, Lima, Peru

Pamela Morales Matamala Department of Pediatrics School of Medicine, Pontificia Universidad Católica de Chile, Santiago, Chile

Ana Moya Isamitt School of Health, Duoc UC, Santiago, Chile

Ana Moya Olivares Department of Pediatrics, School of Medicine, Pontificia Universidad Católica de Chile, Santiago, Chile

Gabriela Muñoz Gómez Faculty of Medicine, Universidad de Chile, Santiago, Chile

Harlan Muntz Health Sciences Center, Universidad de Utah, Salt Lake City, UT, USA

Pamela Navarrete Contreras Department of Pediatrics, Hospital de Los Ángeles, Los Ángeles, Chile

María Angélica Oyarzún Pontificia Universidad Católica de Chile, Santiago, Chile

María Angélica Palomino Montenegro Faculty of Medicine, Universidad de Chile, Santiago, Chile

Rodrigo Parra Rojas Pediatric Radiology, School of Medicine, Pontificia Universidad Católica de Chile, Santiago, Chile

Anand Patel Washington University in St. Louis School of Medicine, St. Louis, MO, USA

Juan Carlos Pattillo Silva Pediatric Surgery, Pontificia Universidad Católica de Chile, Santiago, Chile

Anamaría Peña Donati Pontificia Universidad Católica de, Santiago, Chile

Miriam Pérez Cleveland Clinic Children's Hospital, Cleveland, OH, USA

José Luis Pérez Sánchez Department of Pediatrics, Universidad Austral de Chile, Osorno, Chile

Cecilia Perret Pérez Department of Pediatrics, School of Medicine, Pontificia Universidad Católica de Chile, Santiago, Chile

Giovanni Piedimonte The Cleveland Clinic at Cleveland, Cleveland, OH, USA

María Ester Pizarro Gamboa Pediatrics, Respiratory Diseases, Associate Asociado, School of Medicine, Pontificia Universidad Católica de Chile, Santiago, Chile

Christian Poets Department of Neonatology, University Children's Hospital Tübingen, Alemania, Tübingen, Germany

Francisco Prado Atlagic Department of Pediatrics, Hospital Clínico San Borja Arriarán, Santiago, Chile

María José Prieto Correa Respiratory Kinesiology, Academic at UMCE, UNAB, Santiago, Chile

Homero Puppo Gallardo Respiratory Kinesiology, Faculty of Medicine, Universidad de Chile, Santiago, Chile

Felix Ratjen The Hospital for Sick Children, University of Toronto, Toronto, ON, Canada

Pamela Salinas Flores Pediatric Service, Clínica Las Lilas, Providencia, Chile

José San Martín Prieto Pontificia Universidad Católica de Chile, Santiago, Chile

Ignacio Sánchez Department of Pediatrics, School of Medicine, Pontificia Universidad Católica de Chile, Santiago, Chile

Óscar Sans Capdevila Departament of Pediatric Neurology, Hospital Sant Joan de Déu, Barcelona, Spain

Ricardo Saranz Department of Allergy and Immunology, Faculty of Medicine, Universidad Católica de Córdoba, Córdoba, Argentina

Manuel Soto Martínez Department of Pediatrics, School of Medicine, University of Costa Rica, San José, Costa Rica

Manuel Soto Quirós Department of Pediatrics, Hospital San José, San José, Costa Rica

Asher Tal Ben Gurion University of Negev, Beersheba, Israel

Eduardo Talesnik Guendelman Pediatrics, Immunology and Rheumatology, Pontificia Universidad Católica de Chile, Santiago, Chile

José Luis Tapia Illanes Department of Pediatrics, School of Medicine, Pontificia Universidad Católica de Chile, Santiago, Chile

Alejandro Teper Faculty of Medicine, Universidad de Buenos Aires and Division of Pediatric Pulmonology, Hospital Ricardo Gutiérrez, Buenos Aires, Argentina

Rodrigo Torres Castro Respiratory Kinesiology, Faculty of Medicine, Universidad de Chile, Santiago, Chile

Alberto Toso Milos Department of Pediatrics, Pontificia Universidad Católica de Chile, Santiago, Chile

Paulina Toso Milos Department of Pediatrics, Pontificia Universidad Católica de Chile, Santiago, Chile

Carlos Ubilla Pérez Faculty of Medicine, Universidad de Chile, Santiago, Chile

Patricio Varela Balbontín Pediatric Surgery, Hospital Luis Calvo Mackenna, Universidad de Chile, Santiago, Chile

Rodrigo Vásquez-De Kartzow Department of Pediatrics, Faculty of Medicine, Universidad de Chile, Santiago, Chile

Luis Enrique Vega-Briceño Faculty of Medicine, Universidad del Desarrollo, Santiago, Chile

José Vuletin Solís Pediatric Surgery, Pontificia Universidad Católica de Chile, Santiago, Chile

María Angélica Wietstruck Pediatrics, Oncology, Pontificia Universidad Católica de Chile, Santiago, Chile

Alejandra Zamorano Wittwer Department of Pediatrics, School of Medicine, Pontificia Universidad Católica de Chile, Santiago, Chile

Daniel Zenteno Araos Department of Pediatrics, Universidad de Concepción, Concepción, Chile

Sergio Zúñiga Rocha Pediatric Surgery, Pontificia Universidad Católica de Chile, Santiago, Chile

1 History of Specialist Training in Respiratory Diseases

Ignacio Sánchez

Contents

Introduction

Mortality caused by pediatric respiratory diseases continues to represent a challenge for doctors and health systems worldwide, although the prevalence and incidence of different diseases vary greatly among countries and regions. While the specific requirements of suitable attention vary, the aspiration is to have common standards for clinical management, besides training specialists in pediatric respiratory diseases in order to provide the best possible care to children with these types of illnesses. It is desirable that future specialists know of global issues, besides having a standpoint on respiratory health. An updated and published plan of study describes the content of specialist training, and advances are being made in updating the full curriculum. Efforts to improve training in pediatric respiratory medicine benefit from exchanges among those who work in this field. Considering this, those who develop standards and structures for formal training can learn from others practicing medicine in places where the specialty has a long tradition. Because there has been a long-standing exchange of researchers and students between different countries, it is important to invite the international pediatric respiratory community to report on the state of the specialty in different areas around the world so that current training standards and potential future developments can be advanced.

The Situation in South America

Pediatric respiratory diseases are among the main causes of morbidity in South America. Viral and bacterial infections of the upper respiratory airway, pneumonia, and obstructive diseases of the lower airway are the major reasons for consultation with pediatricians and hospitalization of children. The South American countries that have facilitated access to data about training programs in pediatric respiratory diseases are Argentina, Brazil, Chile, and Peru. Training programs have

I. Sánchez (✉)
Department of Pediatrics, School of Medicine, Pontificia Universidad Católica de Chile, Santiago, Chile

P. Bertrand, I. Sánchez (eds.), *Pediatric Respiratory Diseases*,
https://doi.org/10.1007/978-3-030-26961-6_1

existed in these countries since the late 1970s, with 2–10 programs per country, each of which has trained between 10 and more than 100 specialists. The main reason to start these programs has been to create schools and achieve advances in medical training, as well as building on and disseminating knowledge acquired by academics overseas at medical schools in North America, Europe, and Australia. After completing their studies, these academics have returned home to work in public and university hospitals. In these settings, they have developed training programs at a local level that have had clear objectives and university certification, which are officially recognized. To enter any of these programs in pediatric respiratory medicine and to apply for studies in subspecialization, candidates must complete 3 years of training in the specialty of pediatrics. In most cases, these are 2-year programs with an optional third year, which is mainly focused on clinical and basic research.

The objectives and content of all existing programs include a broad and detailed review of basic sciences: anatomy, physiology, physiopathology, biochemistry, and molecular genetics; a complete review of the various respiratory diseases that affect the upper and lower respiratory tract; restrictive pathologies; bronchial and pulmonary deformations; and obstructive and genetic diseases. Students should also measure and analyze pulmonary function in children of all ages and learn about their potential applications in research. The programs have a wide range of techniques and methods like: spirometry, plethysmography, histamine bronchial challenge test, exercise challenge test, measurement of exhaled nitric oxide, polygraphy, sweat test and assessment of ciliary function among others. At some centers, pulmonary function tests include assessment of pulmonary mechanics and of the volume and function of airways through rapid thoracoabdominal compression. Rotations during training in the specialty include basic hospital admission services, intensive and intermediate units, neonatology, ambulatory attention, the lung function laboratory, the bronchoscopy unit, and rotational units such as pathological anatomy, immunology, radiology, and otorhinolaryngology. Research is usually offered in an optional rotation period that allows students to participate in a wide range of research projects and in the development of a research line---in particular, during the training period. This is especially useful for those who voluntarily take a third year of training. This part is crucial to define specific interests in the pediatric respiratory specialty, knowing that the chosen project can be the basis of future academic activities. Mixed-content programs have been developed in recent years, such as those that combine intensive child care, neonatology, and specific research areas. More in-depth studies have also been strengthened in sleep medicine, invasive procedures, and diseases such as cystic fibrosis and others.

The professors in these programs are full-time university academics, most of whom have worked overseas to perfect their knowledge and have experience in basic, clinical, and epidemiological research. Several of them have taken academic positions and have received recognition of great renown. They participate with residents in journal clubs in order to critically analyze the most recent scientific publications and asses medical evidence for treatment.

At the end of the program, scholarship recipients must complete a written exam and an oral exam before an examination committee. The majority of schools require that as part of completing their program, students publish a scientific manuscript or article that may summarize a research project that the student has participated in and that may have been presented previously at a scientific meeting.

Research conducted in South America and published in international scientific journals has approached themes such as asthma, pediatric lung function, cystic fibrosis, bronchopulmonary dysplasia, and infectious respiratory diseases---in particular, infection by the syncytial virus and bronchiolitis obliterans caused by an adenovirus. Noninvasive ventilation for patients with chronic respiratory diseases has received considerable interest in recent years. While there have been fewer publications at the regional level in relation to these subjects, in comparison with the numbers published in developed countries, these publications have been the result of significant efforts at different South American centers and the work of different universities.

Specialists in South America have historically joined societies focused on respiratory diseases with pediatric chapters. In recent years, pediatric respiratory societies have been created at the local level, including the Latin American Pediatric Respiratory Society. For 25 years, this organization has held meetings every 3 years, with the participation of 1000 pediatricians and specialists in the region. These encounters have encouraged discussion of clinical cases and their treatment, besides the multicenter and multidisciplinary planning of clinical and basic research protocols.

The development of pediatric respiratory medicine in South America is based on international networks and agreements between academics and former students from training programs in North America, Europe, and Australia. These contacts and exchanges have been of great importance in achieving harmonic development. Ongoing training also keeps academics up to date on research projects and medical issues. A permanent challenge is to strengthen collaborative research and academic exchange to promote ongoing upgrading and training. South American centers can offer interesting areas for academic exchange and research with centers in North America, Europe, and Australia because they have highly trained specialists, excellent students, and a wide range of patients with a variety of pathological entities. An ongoing challenge for specialists in our region is to continue improving our programs to cover a wide variety of pathologies in pediatric respiratory medicine. The aim is to involve current and future specialists in creative and innovative basic and clinical research to transfer knowledge "from the laboratory to the patient," thus achieving ongoing improvement in patient care.

The longest-standing programs in the world, with more than 40 years of experience, are in Australia and the USA. Despite this vast educational experience and the great reputations of many centers in the USA in clinical experience and research, there is major concern about the increasing lack of new applicants in this training area, which threatens the future of this specialty in this region. Similarly, there is a longstanding training program in Canada, although there is a lack of experts. Some of the training centers in Australia do not regularly receive funding, which limits the future development of the specialty. However, the fact that there is only one body of national authority for the USA and one for Canada can make it easier to deal with the deficiencies in their respective programs and the needs of the society. In the other regions of the world, although they present different situations, the principal challenge is to achieve a consensus to harmonize training and flexibility in different countries, both during and after the training period. It may be easier to establish research networks than to achieve a consensus about the best and most appropriate training. Ongoing exchange among specialists is fundamental to support the development of the specialty at regional and national levels. A successful initiative in one region can be expected to facilitate the development of harmonized training in other regions. Consequently, the European pediatric project HERMES (Harmonised Education in Respiratory Medicine for European Specialists) can serve as a positive example of how to develop the pediatric respiratory specialty in a region where national governments are responsible for developing specialties.

Respiratory diseases are among the most important challenges for pediatricians, as well as for health systems and societies in general, whether the focus is on infectious diseases, as it is in developing countries, or on allergic respiratory disorders and respiratory problems caused by increasing pollution, as is the case in developed countries. The respiratory pediatric community continues to collaborate and exchange knowledge in the interest of young patients and their families. Student exchange programs between low-, medium-, and high-income countries can improve training and the transfer of competencies, besides promoting greater global awareness of pediatric respiratory diseases. The positive attitude of specialists and their respective societies toward the goal of improving the care of pediatric respiratory diseases is reflected in this book, which demonstrates worldwide support to increase the harmonization of content in training and programs related to this specialty.

Sources

Cockcroft DW, Wensley D. Respirology manpower in Canada—a report for the Canadian Thoracic Society Education Committee. Can Respir J. 2000;7:451–5.

Chernick V, Mellins RB. Pediatric pulmonology: a developmental history in North America. Pediatr Res. 2004;55:514–20.

Fok AO, Wong GW. What have we learnt from ISAAC phase III in the Asia–Pacific rim? Curr Opin Allergy Clin Immunol. 2009;9:116–22.

Freed GL, Dunham KM, Switalski KE, Jones MD Jr, McGuinness GA. Pediatric fellows: perspectives on training and future scope of practice. Pediatrics. 2009;123:S31–7.

Gappa M, Ferkot T, Kovesi T, Landau L, McColley S, Sanchez I, Tal A, Wong GHGK, Zar H. Paediatric respiratory medicine: an international perspective. Pediatr Pulmonol. 2010;45:14–24.

Gappa M, Noel JL, Severin T, et al. Paediatric HERMES: a European syllabus in paediatric respiratory medicine. Breathe. 2009a;5:237–47.

Gappa M, Paton J, Baraldi E, et al. Paediatric HERMES: update of the European training syllabus for paediatric respiratory medicine. Eur Respir J. 2009b;33:464–5.

Mellins RB, Zar HJ. Training pediatric pulmonologists for the future: academic is a state of mind not just a location. Pediatr Pulmonol Suppl. 2004;26:9–11.

Taussig L. Pediatric pulmonology. In: Pearson H, editor. History of the American Board of Pediatrics. Chapel Hill: American Board of Pediatrics; 2008. p. 163–7.

Zach M. Pediatric respiratory training in Europe: political, educational and historical perspective. Breathe. 2009;5:374–83.

Development of the Respiratory System

2

Fernando Iñiguez Osmer
and Ignacio Sánchez

Contents

Introduction

Events in fetal and early postnatal life influence the respiratory health of the child and even of the adult. Alveolar development occurs mainly postnatally, and injuries that can affect the fetus or newborn undoubtedly have an impact on this process. Preterm newborns are often submitted to artificial ventilation and oxygen administration. These therapies can save their lives, but they can also cause lung damage.

To have a better understanding of how the lung functions in newborns, it is necessary to explain the normal development of the fetal lung. Three things must take place for the newborn to adapt to the extrauterine environment: lung fluid must be absorbed, the lungs must be filled with air, and an adequate gas exchange surface must be present.

Stages in Lung Development

Lung development is a series of closely interrelated events. Several stages have been described in the development of the prenatal human lung on

F. Iñiguez Osmer
Department of Pediatrics, Hospital de Puerto Montt, Puerto Montt, Chile

I. Sánchez (✉)
Department of Pediatrics, School of Medicine, Pontificia Universidad Católica de Chile, Santiago, Chile

P. Bertrand, I. Sánchez (eds.), *Pediatric Respiratory Diseases*,
https://doi.org/10.1007/978-3-030-26961-6_2

Table 2.1 Stages of lung development

Stage	Postnatal or gestational age	Main events
Embryonic	3–7 weeks	Development of main airway Appearance of pulmonary circulation
Pseudoglandular	7–17 weeks	Development of conduction airway until terminal bronchi (preacinar) Differentiation of epithelial cells Vascular growth in parallel with airway growth; appearance of lung arteries and veins
Canalicular	17–27 weeks	Acinus formation Growth of the capillary bed (angiogenesis) Epithelial differentiation; surfactant appears
Saccular	28–36 weeks	Formation of transient air space Gas exchange area increases Elastic fiber accumulation in places where future secondary septa will be
Alveolar	36 weeks–3 years	Appearance of secondary septa; formation of alveoli
Microvascular maturation	0–3 years	Thinning of the intra-alveolar wall; fusion of the capillary double layer into a single layer
Active hyperplasia	0–3 years	Number of alveoli increases; discrete changes in size
Hypertrophy	3–21 years	Size of alveoli increases; cellular growth is greater than body growth

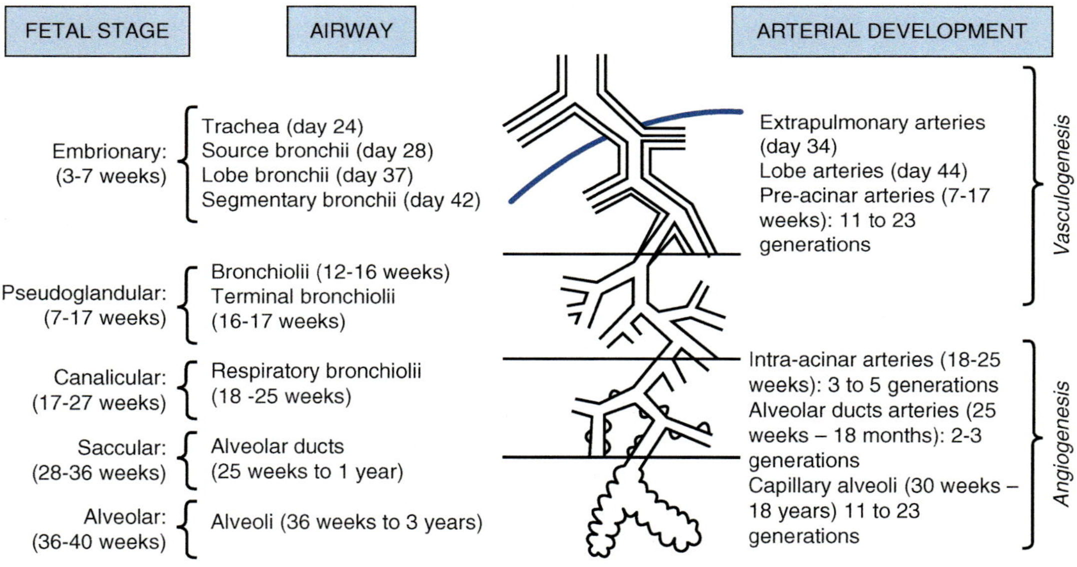

Fig. 2.1 Stages of lung development: airway and lung vessels

the basis of its morphology (Table 2.1). Figure 2.1 illustrates the relationship between the airway and lung vasculature development.

The Embryonic Stage (Weeks 3–7) At days 24–26 of gestation, a lung bud emerges from the epithelial cells of the endoderm in the primitive anterior intestine, taking the shape of a ventral diverticula, which penetrates the surrounding mesenchyme. After this, it grows by dichotomous division downward to form the proximal structures of the tracheobronchial tree. The epithelial cells of the entire respiratory tree, from the central airway to the pneumocytes, derive from this bud, while the cartilage, smooth muscle, connective, and vasculature lung tissue originate from the mesenchyme. Division into two main branches occurs around day 33, with the lung buds lying on either side of the future esophagus. The surrounding mesoderm regulates the branching of the tracheobronchial tree. The lobular bronchi begin their formation by day 37 and by the end of this stage (day 42) the 19 pulmonary segments can be distinguished. The mesenchyme surrounding the lung buds has cells that stain positively for epithelial cell marker (CD31), indicating the origin of future capillaries. By day 34, a network of capillaries has formed around each future main bronchus. In the upper part, this plexus communicates with the aortic sac via the pulmonary arteries, and the lower part communicates with the venous sinus (the future left atrium) through the pulmonary veins. At this point, circulating blood cells are evident. The first pulmonary vessels form de novo from the underlying mesenchyme through the process of vasculogenesis—cellular differentiation forming unique epithelial cells, which are organized into capillary tubes. These capillaries coalesce, forming small blood vessels throughout the airway.

The Pseudoglandular Stage (Weeks 7–17) The main airway develops during this period through successive dichotomous divisions. The name of this stage reflects the glandular histological aspect of bronchioles that end in the stroma as glands. During this period the most rapid division of the intersegmental airway can be seen. The bronchial wall cells develop from the mesenchyme, giving rise to cartilage, smooth bronchial muscle, and submucosal glands. By the end of this stage the definitive number of terminal bronchioles has been established. The pseudostratified columnar epithelium is replaced progressively by tall columnar cells in the proximal airway and cuboidal cells toward the periphery. The latter, rich in glycogen, are immature type II epithelial cells.

The vasculature branches out following the airway. As each new bud penetrates the mesenchyme, a new capillary plexus surrounds it like a halo, joining the pre-existing venous and arterial vessels. Vasculogenesis continues until week 17, at which point all of the preauricular airways and their respective veins and arteries have formed, with little undifferentiated mesenchyme remaining between these structures.

The Canalicular Stage (Weeks 17–27) The terminal bronchioles split to form respiratory bronchioles and alveolar ducts in the form of sacs, which constitute acinar structures. The thinning of the epithelium progresses with the approximation of the capillaries that lie just below it. The cuboidal epithelium differentiates and the alveolar ducts are lined with type II alveolar cells (pneumocytes), from which type I pneumocytes come, which line the distal sacs, thinning out as they approach the capillaries. Toward week 24, the alveolar–capillary barrier has been formed, which has a similar thickness to that in adults (0.2 μm), and the area available for gas exchange allows some extreme preterm newborns to survive. The metabolic machinery of type II pneumocytes increases in preparation for synthesis of surfactant, and toward week 24, surfactant proteins can be observed in the form of lamellar bodies in the cytoplasm. Toward the end of this stage the periphery of the lung is composed of transitory saccules with fine walls, which have formed as a result of the decrease in the number of mesenchyme cells.

At this stage, capillaries are formed by angiogenesis (sprouting of blood vessels from pre-existing vessels) and the dividing cells are more commonly found in the capillary tubes than in the undifferentiated mesenchyme.

The Saccular Stage (Weeks 28–36) The division of the peripheral airways continues in this period. Each terminal bronchiole gives rise to three generations of respiratory bronchioles, each of which gives rise to a generation of transitory ducts, which in turn generate three sacs that flow into the terminal saccules. In this way, the size of the peripheral airway increases and the surface for gas exchange increases as the walls continue to thin out (the primary septa). In preparation for the alveolar stage, elastic fibers are deposited at the points where secondary septa will emerge.

Type II pneumocytes increase the number of lamellar bodies and the differentiation into type I pneumocytes continues.

The arteries that feed the alveolar ducts develop from week 25 to 18 months after birth. The alveolus and small pre- and postcapillary vessels appear at week 30.

The Alveolar Stage (Week 36 to 2–3 Years) The onset of this stage is defined by the appearance of small prominences on both sides of the saccular walls where the elastic fibers are deposited. These grow perpendicularly to the airspace, incompletely dividing the sacs into smaller units (alveoli), which form to a lesser extent in the respiratory bronchioles and transitory ducts. These secondary septa consist of a double capillary loop separated by a sheath of connective tissue. At this point, there is a marked proliferation of all cell types. The mesenchyme cells proliferate, depositing the necessary cellular matrix. Type I and II pneumocytes increase in number to delineate the alveolar walls, where approximately 85–90% of the surface will be coated with type I pneumocytes.

As new alveoli form, new capillaries are also created by angiogenesis and increase the size of the proximal veins and arteries, thus accommodating the increased flow and volume of blood to the growing capillary bed. These processes imply an increase in the net gas exchange surface and preparation of the cells of the airway that will respond to the extrauterine environment.

Postnatal Growth Most of the development of the pulmonary parenchyma occurs after birth. The alveolus forms rapidly in the first months of life, with maturation of the transitional ducts and alveolar sacs. The alveolar stage lasts for up to 2–3 years, with increases in the number and size of the alveoli. The epithelial cells in the secondary septa undergo massive growth, followed by apoptosis (programmed cell death without inflammation), which remodels the irrigation of the septa from a double capillary loop to the definitive morphology of a single loop, in a process termed microvascular maturation. This phenomenon begins at birth and continues for approximately 3 years. Alveolar multiplication continues for at least 2–3 months after birth, while the alveolar surface size continues to increase even after adolescence. A study that measured the caliber of the small airway and alveoli in maximum extension in 53 children and youth aged 6–22 years and in 59 adults aged 23–80 years reported that the size of the small bronchioles and alveoli increased significantly with age and size until the age of 22 years, at which point there were no differences.

It is estimated that at birth there are 20–50 million alveoli, while in the developed lung of an adult there are 300–500 million, with approximately 170 alveoli/mm^3. The gas exchange surface is estimated to be 2.8 m^2 at birth, 32 m^2 at 8 years of age, and 75 m^2 in adulthood. Males have larger lungs than do females, which results in a larger number of alveoli and a larger alveolar surface in comparison with females of the same age and stature. The dimensions of the alveoli and the number of alveoli per unit of area do not differ between the sexes.

Development of Bronchial Circulation

The second circulatory system of the human lung is the bronchial system, through which oxygen and nutrients are supplied to the walls of the airways and large pulmonary vessels. In adults, the bronchial arteries reach the peripheral alveolar ducts. They do not appear at the same time as the pulmonary circulation, given that it begins around week 8 with one or two vessels that emerge from the dorsal aorta and are directed to the lung, as the cartilaginous plaques of the bronchi extend to the periphery as the airway grows and the components of their walls differentiate. These vessels, which are smaller than the nearby pulmonary vessels, form a network through the airway wall under the epithelium and on the outer wall. Several small bronchial veins of the airway drain into the pulmonary veins, while the larger bronchial veins in the hilum drain into the cardinal veins and right atrium.

Respiratory Mechanics

It is estimated that the functional residual capacity (FRC) of term newborns of either sex is around 21 ml/kg and the total distensibility (compliance) of the respiratory system (CRS) is 5 ml/cm H_2O. This is mainly provided by the lungs, given that the thoracic wall at this age is very compliant, in contrast to a later stage in childhood when the distensibility decreases. The total resistance of the respiratory system can reach up to 70 cm H_2O/l/s, the major part of which is given by the bronchial tree. It is estimated that the distensibility of a newborn is one twelfth of that of an adult, while the resistance is 15 times that in an adult. In the first breath, a thoracic pressure of −70 cm H_2Oc can be generated.

The current volume of a term newborn is 6–8 ml/kg, and the minute volume is around 0.6 l. The anatomical dead space approximates half the current volume, which translates into a level of alveolar ventilation of 0.3 l/min. Oxygen consumption is within the range of 20–30 ml/min.

There are several anatomical and functional differences between the infant and adult respiratory systems, which are summarized in Table 2.2.

Lung Weight/Body Weight and Lung Volume/Body Weight Ratios

The pulmonary development status can be verified in a perinatal autopsy. One of the elements to consider is the lung weight/body weight ratio (LW/BW). According to an autopsy study, the LW/BW between 17 and 27 weeks is 2.98–3.15% and then decreases to 2.55% between 28 and 36 weeks, the average at 40 weeks being 1.79%. The tenth percentile is 2.24% between 20 and 23 weeks, 2.59% between 24 and 27 weeks, 2.27% between 28 and 36 weeks, and 1.24% beyond 37 weeks. These reference values (percentile 10) are useful for detecting milder degrees of pulmonary hypoplasia than the values that Wigglesworth proposed in 1981 of 1.2% as the lower limit of normality for premature newborns >28 weeks and 1.5% for those under this gestational age.

The increase in pulmonary liquid can result in overestimation of lung growth on the basis of weight, while lung volume is not affected by intra-alveolar pulmonary liquid. In 2013, De Paepe reported reference values according to gestational age for the lung volume/body weight index. The lungs were inflated to a standardized pressure and submerged in water to determine

Table 2.2 Anatomical and functional differences in babies

Anatomical differences	Functional differences
Upper airway:	Hering–Breuer deflation reflex present in newborns and babies
Proportionally larger tongue	Babies have greater chest wall distensibility than preschoolers
Small nostrils	Lung distensibility increases with age
Nasal breathing during the first 3 months of life	Resistance decreases with growth (greater diameter of the airway)
Larynx shaped like a cone; the cricoid is the smaller area	Greater reactivity of the airway
Central and inferior airway:	Weaker elastic retraction opposing contraction (less stable airway)
Scarce cartilage at birth, which will develop during the following years	
Airway poor in collagen and elastin at birth	
The thickness of the wall corresponds to 30% of the airway (15% in the adult)	
Poorer tracheal mucociliary clearance	
Smooth muscle is present during early stages	
Greater number of mucus glands per surface unit	
Inefficient collateral ventilation	
Compliant chest wall (newborn)	
Ribs oriented horizontally	
Sternal ossification starting in week 22	
Progressive development of muscle mass during childhood	

their volume, which increases by 11 times between weeks 16 and 41, while in the same period the body weight increases by 16 times. The index remains constant at around 33–34 ml/kg between week 16 and 31 weeks of gestational age and then decreases to 23.4 ml/kg at the end of gestation. According to the authors, this index can also serve to detect more subtle degrees of pulmonary hypoplasia (premature rupture of membranes, chromosomic anomalies), in which this index can be normal.

Genetic Control of Lung Development

Lung development is a highly organized process in which the interactions between the mesenchyme and epithelia control and coordinate the temporal and spatial expression of multiple regulatory factors that are necessary for appropriate formation and growth of the lung. Diverse endogenous and exogenous factors can alter this delicate balance, which can result in disorders related to growth, maturation, or function of the tissues in formation. A series of controlling factors have been identified for each lung development stage, consisting mainly of transcription and growth factors (and their respective receptors), extracellular matrix molecules, integrin, intercellular adhesion molecules, and others. As a whole, these factors interact throughout the distal proximal axis of the respiratory system, locally influencing numerous genes that control modeling of the endotherm and the morphogenesis of the lung branches, left–right asymmetry, vascularization, and the response to mechanical forces.

Growth factors are diffusible proteins that act at a short distance from their production site, inducing various cellular activities through biochemical signals, promoting cellular proliferation, and mediating tissue interactions during embryogenesis and in postnatal life. In organogenesis, these molecules provide information for the appropriate feedback response among the different germ layers. Growth factors define the cellular signaling centers that control the behavior of neighboring cells, forming gradients in a structure under development. In the developing lungs, they define branching patterns and control the sizes of the airway and its cells, among other functions. In general, growth factors, whose signals are mediated by tyrosine kinase–type receptors, promote cell differentiation and multiplication (fibroblast, epidermal, vascular endothelial, and platelet-derived growth factors). There are growth factors that act through serine/threonine–type receptors (transforming growth factor 1 and morphogenetic bone protein 4), which oppose the previously mentioned factors. These signals achieve equilibrium when the lungs are developed in such a way that they can preserve cellular activities and lung structure and function. Table 2.3 shows growth factors and their functions at different developmental stages.

Table 2.3 Growth factors and their roles in growth and lung development

Transforming growth factor beta: lung healing after injuries and extracellular matrix production; cellular proliferation inhibition; appearance of secondary septa
Epidermal growth factor: ramification, differentiation, and proliferation of the airway epithelium
Keratinocyte growth factor: macrophage differentiation
Fibroblast growth factors (FGFs; a 23-subgroup family): location of organs that originate at the primitive intestine; budding and ramification (FGFs 9 and 10); alveolar development, type II cell differentiation, and surfactant protein C induction (FGFs 2 and 7); creation of tracheal cartilage rings (FGFs 10 and 18)
Bone morphogenic protein: formation and control of dorsal and ventral branches; angiogenesis and vasculogenesis
Platelet-derived growth factor: alveolar development
Granulocyte–macrophage colony–stimulating factor: macrophage differentiation
Vascular endothelial growth factor: angiogenesis, vasculogenesis, and lymphangiogenesis
Insulin-like growth factor: Airway proliferation may facilitate the effect of other growth factors; Fetal endothelial cell tropism
Sonic hedgehog (SHH): suppression of FGF 10 expression, preventing ramification in unsuitable places
Retinoic acid: FGF 10 induction and endoderm differentiation
MicroRNA, noncodifying: development of epithelial cells

Factors That Influence Lung Development

For normal lung development to take place, fetal respiratory movement (FRM) is fundamental, besides adequate intrathoracic space, sufficient intra- and extrapulmonary fluid, and good irrigation. Aspects of maternal health such as nutrition, smoking, endocrine factors, pregnancy-related factors (e.g., gestational diabetes and hypertensive syndrome), and unrelated health factors also influence fetal development (Fig. 2.2).

Developmental Anomalies Abnormalities can occur at any of the stages of lung development, caused by maternal–fetal factors (e.g., oligohydramnios), genetic factors (e.g., a deficit of protein B in the surfactant), or developmental anomalies (Table 2.4). Table 2.5 lists factors that adversely affect lung development in both the pre- and postnatal periods.

Fetal Respiration and Pulmonary Fluid Pulmonary fluid is produced by the epithelial cells of the lung, especially in the distal airway. The pulmonary fluid flows toward the amniotic fluid or is swallowed. The fluid is poor in proteins (<0.03 g/100 ml) and bicarbonate, but it is rich in chlorine (>150 mEq/l). The velocity of pulmonary fluid production increases as gestation progresses. Its presence in the airways exerts mild positive pressure in relation to amniotic fluid pressure and prevents collapse. Toward the end of the gestation, the fetal airway contains approximately 40 ml of pulmonary fluid, which is rapidly exchanged. A balance between production and drainage appears crucial for lung development.

FRM has been observed from as early as week 11. Toward the end of gestation, movements are present a third of the time and increase in periods of fetal activity, and the diaphragm is the main muscle involved. There is a circadian rhythm to FRM, with movements decreasing in the hours prior to

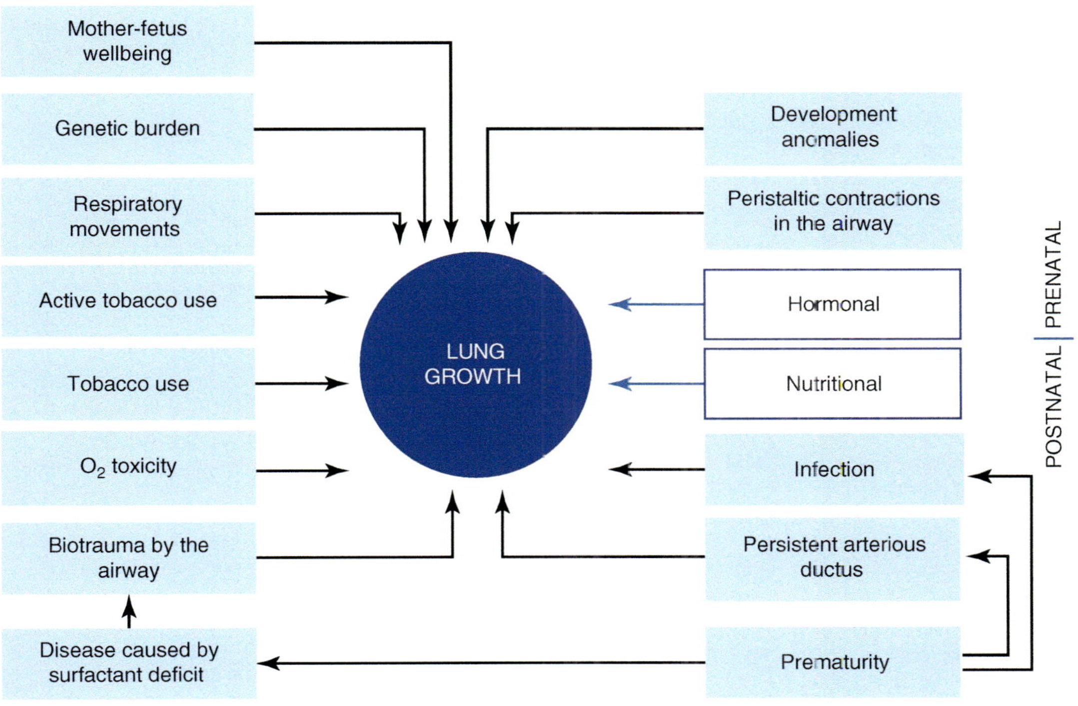

Fig. 2.2 Prenatal and postnatal factors that influence lung development. Nutritional and hormonal factors are active during the prenatal and postnatal periods. Infections can also act during the prenatal period

Table 2.4 Stages of lung development during which certain congenital malformations related to abnormal lung development appear

Embryonic stage	Pseudoglandular stage	Canalicular stage	Saccular and alveolar stages
Lung, tracheal, or laryngeal agenesis Laryngeal or tracheal stenosis Tracheomalacia and bronchomalacia Bronchial malformations Ectopic lobes Horseshoe lung Congenital lung cysts (including bronchogenic cysts) Tracheoesophageal fistula	Cystic adenomatoid malformation Lung hypoplasia Congenital lung lymphangiectasia Congenital diaphragmatic hernia Pulmonary sequestration	Lung hypoplasia Acinar dysplasia	Lung hypoplasia Acinar dysplasia Alveolar capillary dysplasia

Table 2.5 Factors that adversely affect lung development

Prenatal factors	Postnatal factors
Intrathoracic space reduction	Prematurity
Diaphragm alterations	Drugs: tobacco smoke, steroids
Diaphragmatic agenesis: poor development of septum transversum	
Posterolateral hernia (Bochdalek): failure of pleuroperitoneal canal to seal	
Anterior or Morgagni hernia: lack of development of the retrosternal septum transversum	
Eventration: failure of primitive muscle cell migration	
Cystic adenomatoid malformation:	
Type 0: acinar dysplasia	
Type 1: multiple large cysts or a dominant one	
Type II: multiple small cysts	
Type III: solid mass	
Type IV: peripheral cysts	
Pulmonary sequestration:	
Intralobar	
Extralobar	
Congenital lobar emphysema	
Pleural effusion	
Idiopathic	
Chylothorax	
Immune or nonimmune generalized hydrops	
Chromosome abnormalities, congenital heart disease, diaphragmatic hernia associated with the antenatal period	
Newborn transient tachypnea, persistent lung hypertension, meconium aspiration syndrome, heart failure associated with the postnatal period	
Trauma: nasogastric tube injuring the hypopharynx, erosion of the inferior vena cava toward the pleural space through a total parenteral feeding tube	
Bone disorders:	
Asphyxiating thoracic dystrophy (Jeune syndrome)	
Ellis–van Creveld syndrome	
Saldino–Noonan syndrome (short ribs syndrome type I)	
Majewski syndrome (short ribs syndrome type II)	
Diastrophic dysplasia	
Thanatophoric dwarfism	
Osteogenesis imperfecta	

Table 2.5 (continued)

Prenatal factors	Postnatal factors
Achondrogenesis	
Hypophosphatasia	
Campomelic dysplasia	
Jarcho–Levin syndrome	
Reduction of fetal respiratory movement	
Neurological anomalies: Werdnig–Hoffmann syndrome, congenital muscular dystrophy	
Imperfections in the anterior abdominal wall: omphalocele, gastroschisis	
Drugs: tobacco	
Amniotic fluid reduction (oligohydramnios)	
Reduced production: nephropathies (e.g., Potter)	
Amniotic fluid leak: premature rupture of membranes	
Invasive procedures: amniocentesis	

midnight and increasing between 4 a.m. and 6 a.m. FRM increases after maternal feeding (hyperglycemia) and also in situations of hypercapnia, acidosis, or temperature rise, and before administration of indomethacin, caffeine, or theophylline. FRM is depressed in the context of hypoxia (a global depressor of fetal activity), hypoglycemia, administration of prostaglandin E_2, intrauterine infection, maternal smoking, consumption of alcohol, or use of sedatives such as diazepam or morphine. FRM is fundamental to maintenance of adequate lung volume. In periods of apnea, the pharynx collapses and the larynx offers resistance to the escape of liquid, with maintenance of the pressure gradient. The upper airway dilates and the diaphragm contracts in the inspiration phase, allowing fluid to enter, which contributes to lung expansion.

The physical forces referred to as stretching or distension are in fact better described as a variety of different mechanical forces, such as stress (force per unit of area), elongation (lengthening of a structure), restoring force (when the structure returns to its original length), surface tension (differences between intracellular adhesion and cytoskeletal contractility), and prestress (isometric tension that balances intra- and extracellular elongation tension). These different mechanical forces within and between cells, tissues, and organs are as important as genes and chemical signals in controlling lung development.

Several methods have been developed to study the role of physical forces in pulmonary development and epithelial differentiation. Pulmonary subdistension occurs in cases of congenital diaphragmatic hernia, drainage of pulmonary fluid, or abolition of FRM (in the medullar or phrenic section), which causes the lungs to be small (hypoplasia) and favors the type II epithelial phenotype at the cost of type I, while pulmonary overdistension (tracheal ligation) promotes lung growth (hyperplasia) and favors the type I epithelial phenotype at the expense of type II.

Toward the end of gestation, the volume of pulmonary fluid and its rate of production decrease. The expression of sodium channels and the sodium–potassium ATPase pump in the epithelium increase at this stage. These changes in ion transport in the pulmonary epithelial cells in late gestation reflect the change from a pattern of chlorosecretion to one of sodium absorption near birth, thus preparing the lung for postnatal adaptation.

Peristaltic Contractions Studies with animals have highlighted the importance of spontaneous peristaltic contractions that occur in the airway. Peristaltic waves originate in the trachea, propagated by the bronchial tree, and pump lung fluid distally. When the tubes relax, the flow reverses. The frequency is 2–3 per minute in the fetal pig lung at the pseudoglandular and canalicular stages, while it is 10–12 per minute in the rabbit lung at the saccular stage. The intraluminal pressure measured in the trachea of fetal rabbits is

2.3 cm H_2O. It is highly probable that the expansion of the most peripheral buds is favored by this phenomenon, which facilitates its growth toward the surrounding mesenchyme.

Peristaltic waves of smooth muscle emanate from certain pacemaker areas in the proximal airway before being transmitted to the distal area. Study of peristaltic wave frequency in embryonic lung cultures has shown that acceleration of the frequency with cholinergic agents or fibroblast growth factor (FGF)-10 stimulates pulmonary growth, while inhibition of the frequency reduces growth. Other studies have shown that there are spontaneous intercellular calcium waves that are propagated throughout the air just before the peristaltic contractibility wave. These waves depend on intra- and extracellular calcium and the integrity of intercellular bonds. These oscillations stimulate lung development by regulating growth through muscular peristalsis.

Steroids Prenatal administration of steroids accelerates lung growth by several mechanisms; among them, steroids favor lung maturation, with an increase in the volumetric density of the air spaces and increased maturation of epithelial cells. Early thinning of the double capillary loop is promoted during the saccular and alveolar stages, but the final number of secondary septa decreases and, with this, so does the final number of alveoli. Type II pneumocytes increase in number and functionality with increased levels of messenger RNA for the surfactant proteins. Other effects include increased transcription of the genes responsible for growth and maturation, as well as increased levels of antioxidant enzymes. When administered postnatally, steroids accelerate the maturation of developing lung tissue, shortening the time in which the double loop is present, which is vital for the development of secondary septa. In this way, septation is shortened and the total number of alveoli that can develop is limited.

When premature birth is imminent, antenatal steroids can affect respiratory mechanics. A prospective study compared the CRS of premature newborns (32 weeks of gestation, <3 days of life, prior to administration of surfactants, if required) who had received steroids more than a week before birth and that of infants who had received steroids 1–7 days before birth. CRS was measured in 28 patients by use of the single-breath occlusion technique. Infants born more than a week after administration of steroids had significantly lower CRS values, in terms of both the absolute value and the value normalized for weight, than infants born between 1 and 7 days after steroid administration (1.52 ml/cm H_2O versus 2.12 ml/cm H_2O, and 0.98 ml/cm H_2O/kg versus 1.41 ml/cm H_2O/kg, respectively). A lower CRS value may reflect dissipation of the beneficial effects of antenatal steroids on lung function when birth occurs more than 7 days after steroid administration.

Nutrition Fetal malnourishment appears to decrease lung volume but not airway maturation. Studies with animals have shown that a decrease in fetal nutrition alters the development of secondary septa, with a reduced exchange area, but without affecting alveolar size. It has been argued that less elastin is deposited in the saccular and alveolar stages. In addition to the fact that malnourished infants have less muscular mass, they have a greater tendency to experience bronchial collapse during respiratory infections. Studies in adults who were the children of mothers who suffered a famine in 1944–1945 have indicated the importance of adequate intrauterine nutrition for pulmonary development. Subjects exposed to maternal malnutrition between the second and third trimesters of gestation had a higher incidence of airway obstructive diseases in adulthood, without alterations in the level of immunoglobulin E or in lung function tests.

Conclusion

Lung development is a highly coordinated and complex process, about which much remains unknown. Future developments will provide use of concrete tools to help newborns afflicted with bronchopulmonary dysplasia or other congenital conditions in which normal lung development is altered.

Sources

Baguma-Nibasheka M, Gugic D, Saraga-Babic M, Kablar B. Role of skeletal muscle in lung development. Histhol Histopathol. 2012;27:817–26.

Copland I, Post M. Lung development and fetal lung growth. Pediatr Respir Rev. 2004;5(Suppl A):S259–64.

De Paepe M, Shapiro S, Hansen K, Gündogan F. Postmortem lung volume/body weight standards for term and preterm infants. Pediatr Pulmonol. 2014;49(1):60–6.

Gibson A. Perinatal corticosteroids and the developing lung. Pediatr Respir Rev. 2002;3:70–6.

Greenough A. Factors adversely affecting lung growth. Pediatr Respir Rev. 2000;1:314–20.

Hislop A. Developmental biology of the pulmonary circulation. Pediatr Respir Rev. 2005;6:35–43.

Hulskamp G, Pillow J, Dinger J, Stocks J. Lung function tests in neonates and infants with chronic lung disease of infancy: functional residual capacity. Pediatr Pulmonol. 2006;41:1–22.

Iñiguez F, Sánchez I. Desarrollo pulmonar. Neumología Pediátrica. 2008;3:148–55.

Katz C, Bentur L, Elias N. Clinical implications of lung fluid balance in the perinatal period. J Perinatol. 2011;31:230–5.

Lopuhaa C, Roseboom T, Osmond C, et al. Atopy, lung function, and obstructive airways disease after prenatal exposure to famine. Thorax. 2000;55:555–61.

McEvoy C, Schilling D, Spitale P, Peters D, O'Malley J, Durand M. Decreased respiratory compliance in infants less than or equal to 32 weeks' gestation, delivered more than 7 days after antenatal steroid therapy. Pediatrics. 2008;121:e1032–8.

Roth-Kleiner M, Post M. Similarities and dissimilarities of branching and septation during lung development. Pediatr Pulmonol. 2005;40:113–34.

Schittny J, Miserocchi G, Sparrow M. Spontaneous peristaltic airway contractions propel lung liquid through the bronchial tree of intact and fetal lung explants. Am J Respir Cell Mol Biol. 2000;23:11–8.

Waburton D, El-Hashash A, Carraro G, et al. Lung organogenesis. Curr Top Dev Biol. 2010,90:73–158.

Wilson S, Olven R, Walters D. Developmental regulation of lumenal lung fluid and electrolyte transport. Respir Physiol Neurobiol. 2007;159:247–55.

Zeman K, Bennet W. Growth of the small airways and alveoli from childhood to the adult lung measured by aerosol-derived airway morphology. J Appl Physiol. 2006;100:956–71.

Physiological Basis of the Respiratory System

3

Pablo Bertrand and Ignacio Sánchez

Contents

Respiratory Mechanics

Respiratory system mechanics analyzes the forces and resistances that determine the movement of gases between the lungs and the exterior. Airflows from the region of greater pressure to that of lesser pressure as a result of the changes in the thorax, but it must overcome the elastic resistance of the respiratory system (the lungs and rib cage) and frictional resistance to airflow, which is known as airway resistance.

The respiratory system contains the lungs within the rib cage. The two structures adhere to each other through pleural surface contact. The lungs have a natural tendency to reduce their volume and the rib cage has a natural tendency to increase its volume; thus, between them, they create negative subatmospheric pressure at the level of the pleural space. The lung behaves like elastic because of its structure and the presence of an extensive liquid interface that reduces the force of surface tension, which is very important for production of the elastic recoil pressure of the lungs. Because of this, all of the 300 million alveoli tend to retract. The sum of this force exercised throughout the lung determines the resistance to dilation. Surface tension depends on lung volume. Surface tension values are low at small volumes

P. Bertrand (✉) · I. Sánchez
Department of Pediatrics, School of Medicine, Pontificia Universidad Católica de Chile, Santiago, Chile
e-mail: pbertrand@med.puc.cl

P. Bertrand, I. Sánchez (eds.), *Pediatric Respiratory Diseases*, https://doi.org/10.1007/978-3-030-26961-6_3

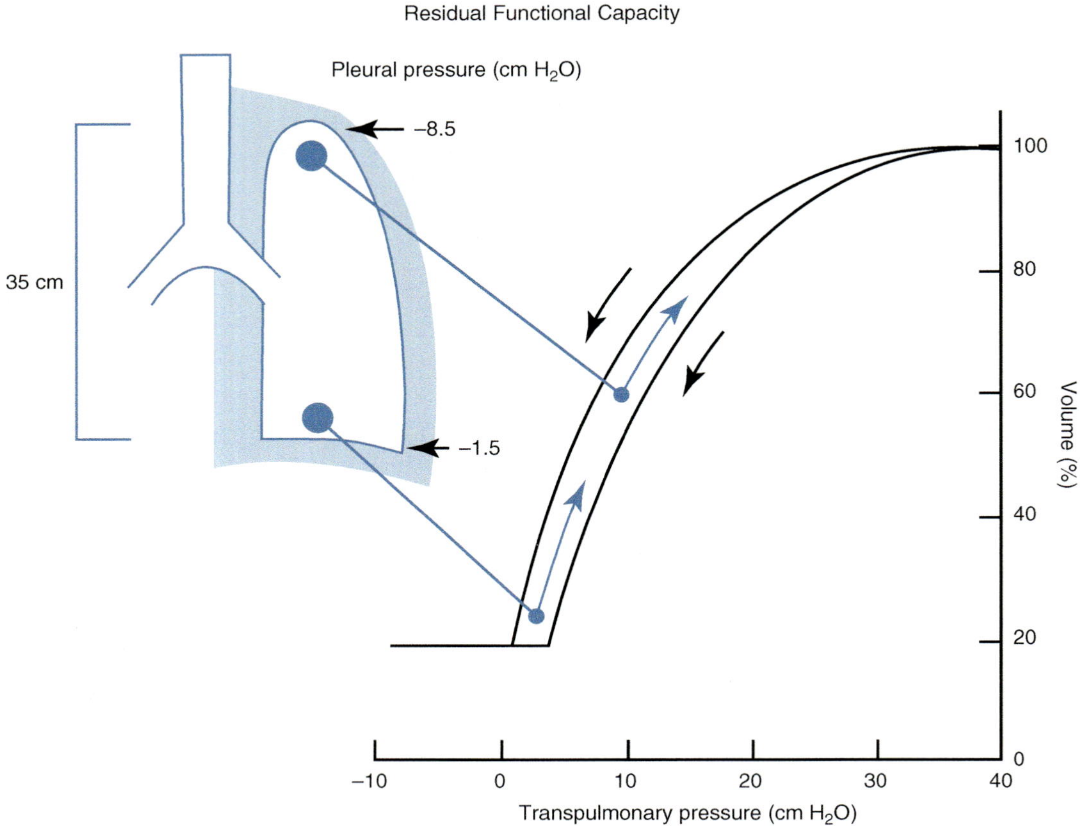

Fig. 3.1 Changes in distensibility (the change in volume divided by the change in pressure) (ΔV/ΔP) according to the lung zone (standing position)

and high at large volumes. At the alveolar level, the surfactant is responsible for reducing surface tension and avoiding alveolar collapse at small volumes. The respiratory system follows Hook's law: "The greater the muscular force or pressure applied to the lungs, the greater the change in the volume obtained." The relation between the volume that is reached and the pressure that is used is known as lung compliance, which is defined as the change in volume determined by the changes in pressure at zero airflow. It is expressed as the coefficient ∅V/∅P, measured in milliliters per centimeter of H_2O. The measurement that considers the flow and resistance of the airway to the change in volume determined by changes in pressure is termed dynamic pulmonary compliance. Compliance varies according to the different lung volumes in which it is measured, as well as the area, considered with the patient in a standing position. Compliance is lower if lung volume is greater, as occurs in the apex, and it is greater if lung volume is lower, as occurs in the base (Fig. 3.1). In other words, close to total lung volume, the elastic is more difficult to extend, while the opposite is true at residual volume. To determine if a lung has normal elastic properties, compliance must be corrected for the residual functional capacity (RFC), which is called specific compliance, a value that changes little with age. The factors that decrease pulmonary compliance are pulmonary edema, alveolar collapse, inflammation, pulmonary hyperflow, and pulmonary fibrosis. A factor that increases compliance is structural destruction of the parenchyma.

Airway Resistance

According to pressure measurements done throughout the intrathoracic airway, airway resistance decreases as the airway gets smaller. Therefore, the greatest airflow resistance is in the trachea and large bronchi, and the smallest airflow resistance is in the small bronchioles. The small airway (<2 mm in diameter) represents only 20% of the total resistance because transversal resistance in this area adds a significant diameter in comparison with that of the central airway. Moreover, the flow is laminar at the level of the small airway; thus, diseases that affect this area theoretically increase the resistance very little. Consequently, this area is termed the "quiet zone."

The causes of increased airway resistance are:

1. Constriction of the bronchial and bronchiolar smooth muscles
2. Inflammation or edema of the bronchial or bronchiolar wall
3. Obstruction of the lumen due to exudate, mucus, or foreign bodies
4. Fibrosis of the bronchial wall
5. External compression of the airways
6. The diameter of the airway, which is subject to the lung volume

The last factor has a significant influence on airway resistance, given that the tensor action of the tissue maintains the caliber of the airway and at large lung volumes the diameter of the airway tends to increase, while at low volumes the diameter decreases and resistance increases. At low lung volumes, where the airway does not have structural rigidity and its permeability depends on the elastic support of the surrounding tissue (peripheral airway), the airway can collapse.

Under any condition that decreases pulmonary compliance, optimal breathing occurs at low tidal volumes (TVs) to reduce the respiratory work in distending rigid lungs. Compensation is achieved by increasing the respiration rate to obtain adequate alveolar ventilation (VA). Under any condition that increases airway resistance, the respiratory rate will optimally decrease to obtain slower and less turbulent airflows and reduced respiratory work. In this scenario, the compensation to achieve adequate VA is an increased TV, but the displacement of the equal pressure point to the proximal airway causes pulmonary hyperinflation, such that the lungs are at maximum volume. In this case, lung compliance is reduced and the TV therefore cannot increase.

Lung compliance and airway resistance can be determined only by invasive tests in specialized laboratories, because of which simpler procedures have been developed to ascertain the mechanical characteristics of the lungs and chest. To analyze ventilation function it is possible to measure the volume of gas that can be moved with maximum respiratory force, which is expressed adequately with the vital capacity (VC) and the velocity with which this volume is exhaled, known as spirometry. This pulmonary function test depends on airway resistance and the elastic resistance of the lungs and chest. During much of the maneuver of forced expiration, the maximum airflow is fixed, such that increased effort does not result in increased flow, and it is only at very high lung volumes of over 75% of the VC that the flow is effort dependent. Forced respiratory flow is determined by the alveolar pressure and dynamic compression of the intrathoracic airways. Alveolar pressure is determined by the elastic rebound pressure of the lung tissue and positive intrapleural pressure produced by the rib cage muscles, which can be summarized in the following manner:

$$\text{Alveolar pressure} = \text{Elastic rebound pressure} + \text{Intrapleural pressure}$$

Intrathoracic airways are subjected to intrapleural pressure, which is transmitted through the parenchyma surrounding them. During normal respiration, the pressure in the lumen is greater than the pressure in all of the intrathoracic airway, so the airway remains permeable. However, in the forced expiration maneuver, the existing positive pressure in the airway is less than or equal to the pressure exerted from outside the airway, which is termed the equal pressure point. At

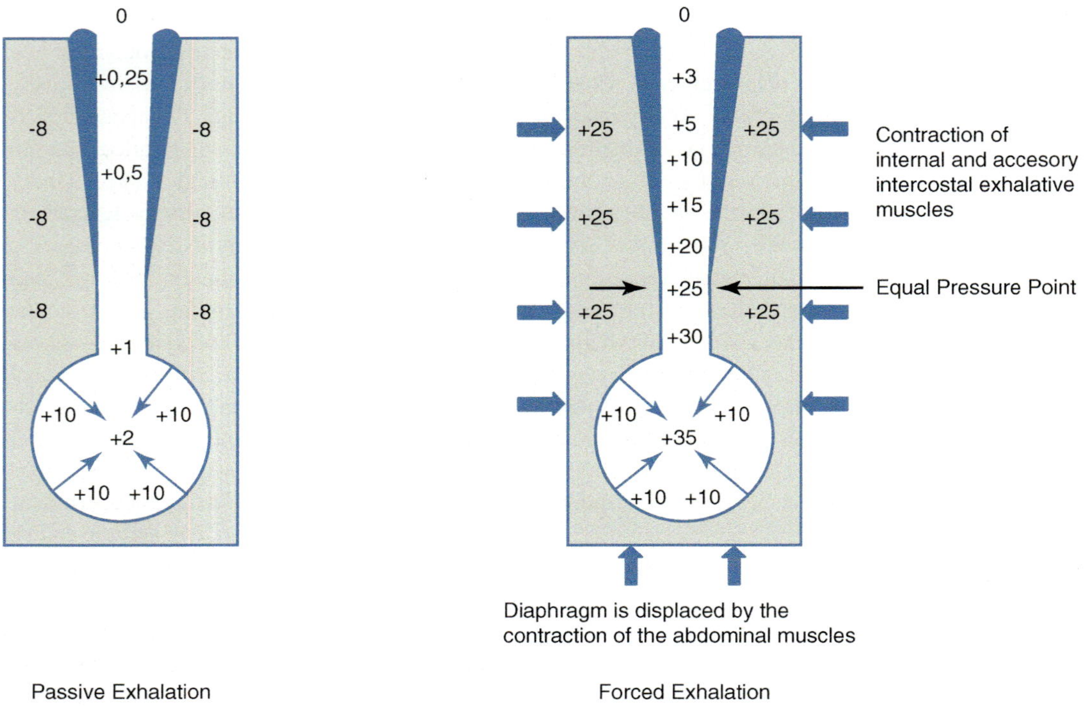

Fig. 3.2 Equal pressure point

this point the nonrigid airway collapses, provoking a valve effect that maintains critical lung volume, which is termed the residual volume (Fig. 3.2). At any lung volume below 75% of the VC, a pressure point equal to collapse appears in all of the airway, which determines a fixed airflow that cannot increase beyond an equal increase in pleural pressure. The location of this point varies with the lung volume: at high volumes it is located at the second to third bronchial generation, and with lower volumes it moves toward the small distal airway.

Pulmonary Ventilation

Pulmonary ventilation is a cyclical process of inspiration and expiration through which alveolar air is renovated in each respiratory cycle through the airway. The airway is composed of a series of ramifications that are divided dichotomously, resulting in 23 generations at the alveolar level. The conduction airway extends from the trachea to the terminal bronchioles (generation 16), and the transition and respiratory airway extends from the respiratory bronchioles (generation 17) to the alveoli (generation 23). Of the total air inhaled, 70% is involved in gas exchange and the remaining 30% remains in the anatomical dead space of the airway.

Inspiration is produced by active contraction of the diaphragm and external intercostal muscles, which determines a tridimensional increase in the rib cage (Fig. 3.3), with a decrease in thoracic pressure to create a gradient that permits air from the mouth and nose to reach the alveoli. The degree to which these muscles participate in inspiration varies depending on the patient's age and physical position. Respiration with the diaphragm predominates in the first years of life, mainly because at this stage of life the child frequently lies in a supine position, but also because of the low level of resistance by the abdominal cavity to displace the diaphragm. As the child

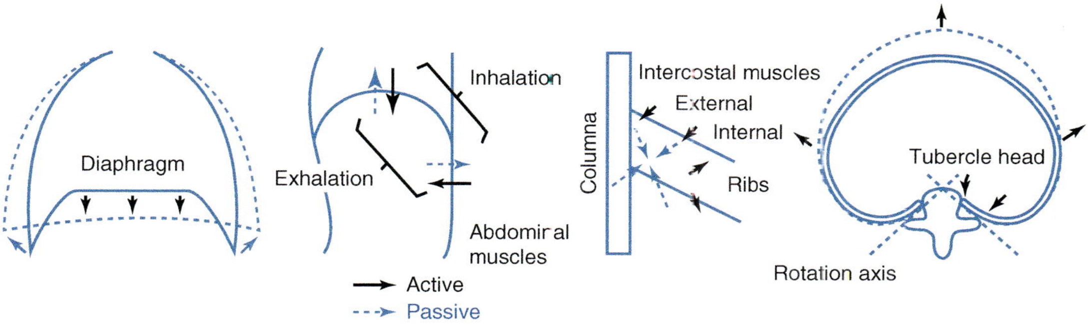

Fig. 3.3 Action mechanism of respiratory muscles

grows, the external intercostal muscles start to become more important and are responsible for equivalent breathing work during adolescence when the patient is in a standing position, and this set of muscles is predominant when the patient is in a sitting position, when increased abdominal pressure reduces diaphragmatic displacement. In adolescence, respiration in a supine position continues to be largely diaphragmatic and involves approximately 70% of the volume change in each respiratory cycle. The supine position is slightly more advantageous in the context of respiratory difficulty, especially in the case of newborns and infants. The accessory inspirational muscles, such as the scalene and sternocleidomastoid muscles, are used only in forced inspiration, and their participation in upper airway obstruction is evident. With conditions that produce pulmonary hyperinflation, such as asthma or bronchiolitis, the inspiratory muscles are shortened, which reduces their efficiency when they are contracted. In this situation, the flattening of the diaphragm also conditions the retraction of the free costal edge, which is considered a marker of respiratory difficulty.

Expiration is passive under normal conditions of quiet respiration, and it is determined by the elastic force of the lungs and rib cage, and by relaxation of the inspiratory muscle. In contrast, during exercise or in the context of airway obstruction, expiration is active, using the musculature of the abdominal wall and the internal intercostal muscles to facilitate pulmonary action.

Alterations in Pulmonary Ventilation

Pulmonary ventilation is altered by excess (hyperventilation) or by deficit (hypoventilation) and can be understood as the result of the volume of each respiratory cycle, or TV, and the number of times it occurs in 1 minute, or the respiratory frequency (RF). In this way, the 1-minute exchange volume, or VA (which is summarized in the equation below), provides the best clinical estimation of hypoventilation or hyperventilation:

$$VA = VC \times RF$$

Uniform and adequate chest movement in quiet breathing mobilizes about 5–6 ml/k of air in every cycle. This is the TV, and in an adolescent male it is approximately 500 ml. This expansion is greater in a crisis of adolescent panic, but it is reduced by poor thoracic–abdominal dynamics due to diaphragmatic paralysis or muscular fatigue. There is inherent variability in a child's respiratory rate, and it is influenced by stress, pain, and other factors. Clinical integration of the chest expansion and RF is what matters from a physiological perspective. The compensation that occurs in the context of an increased breathing rate or an increased TV results in adequate, insufficient, or excessive VA, which in every case depends on the minute volume that fills the physiological dead space (PDS). The increased respiratory rate in a subject compared with the same proportional increase in TV in the same subject at another moment yields less VA in the former situation because there is more ventilation of the

PDS. The diagnosis of hyperventilation or hypoventilation is closely related to the measurement of the partial pressure of carbon dioxide ($PaCO_2$), given that the level of this gas is one of the most important regulators of VA. A condition is defined as hyperventilation when the $PaCO_2$ falls below 40 mmHg (respiratory alkalosis) and as hypoventilation when the $PaCO_2$ goes above 40 mmHg (respiratory acidosis).

Alveolar Hypoventilation

Hypoventilation is a condition in which the quantity of air that is circulating does not meet the needs of the organism. The quantity of oxygen that enters the organism is smaller, which causes a decrease in the partial pressure of oxygen in arterial blood (PaO_2). At the same time, the smaller quantity of air that is circulating does not succeed in removing all of the CO_2 produced in the organism, which increases the partial pressure of CO_2 in venous blood ($PvCO_2$) and in the alveolus ($PACO_2$), in turn causing a reduction in the blood pH. The combination of these two changes is termed respiratory acidosis. A child who is hypoventilating and breathing environmental air will always suffer from hypoxemia and hypercapnia; administration of oxygen will improve the hypoxemia but not the hypercapnia. The causes of hypoventilation are an alteration in the central nervous system (brain contusion, stroke, etc.), an alteration in nerve conduction (phrenic paralysis, Guillain–Barré syndrome, etc.), muscular dysfunction (myopathy, myasthenia gravis), an alteration in the rib cage (costovertebral malformations, kyphoscoliosis), and airway obstruction (severe laryngitis, foreign body inhalation, asthma crisis, etc.).

Alveolar Hyperventilation

Hyperventilation is a condition in which the quantity of air circulating is excessive for the requirements of the organism. Thus, the circulating air removes more CO_2, and so the $PaCO_2$ in the arterial flow decreases, which raises the pH level in the blood. This is termed respiratory alkalosis. The partial pressure of O_2 increases marginally at the alveolar level in such a way that the hemoglobin saturation of the arterial blood does not increase, given that this part of the hemoglobin disassociation curve is flat. Hyperventilation is caused by anxiety, pain, lesions in the central nervous system, intoxication with medication, increased metabolism, and a compensation mechanism in the context of hypoxemia or metabolic acidosis.

Pulmonary Circulation

The pulmonary circulation begins in the pulmonary artery, which receives venous blood from the right ventricle and then successively branches, together with the respiratory paths, until it reaches the terminal bronchioles, providing the capillary bed located in the alveolar walls. This network contains 280 billion capillaries, which supply approximately 300 million alveoli, with a potential gaseous exchange of between 50 and 100 m^2—an area comparable to half a tennis court.

The pulmonary blood circulation is at a much lower pressure than that of the blood in the circulatory system and is very closely related to the alveolar pressure.

With a deep inhalation, the alveolar vessels tend to collapse with the increase in alveolar pressure, while the extra-alveolar vessels tend to expand because of the radial traction of the surrounding parenchyma. With a deep exhalation, the alveolar vessels do not collapse, because of alveolar pressure, while the extra-alveolar vessels do collapse because of the lack of radial traction. Figure 3.4 shows that the optimal vascular pulmonary resistance is in the center of the curve, near the RFC.

It is important to consider that the pulmonary circulation also has the capacity to maintain and even reduce vascular pulmonary resistance when the pulmonary circulation pressure increases, which occurs through the recruitment mechanism, through which it is possible to circulate the blood through capillaries that are normally closed or open, but without a flow of blood and distension, through which the capillary segments widen, changing tridimensionally from flat to more circular (Fig. 3.5).

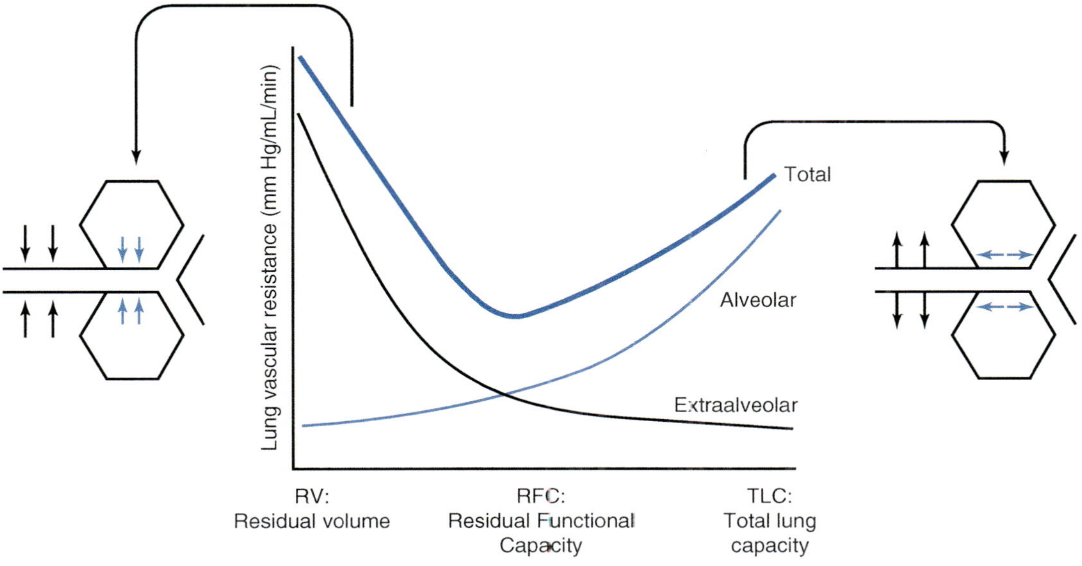

Fig. 3.4 Pulmonary vascular resistance according to the lung zone (in a standing individual)

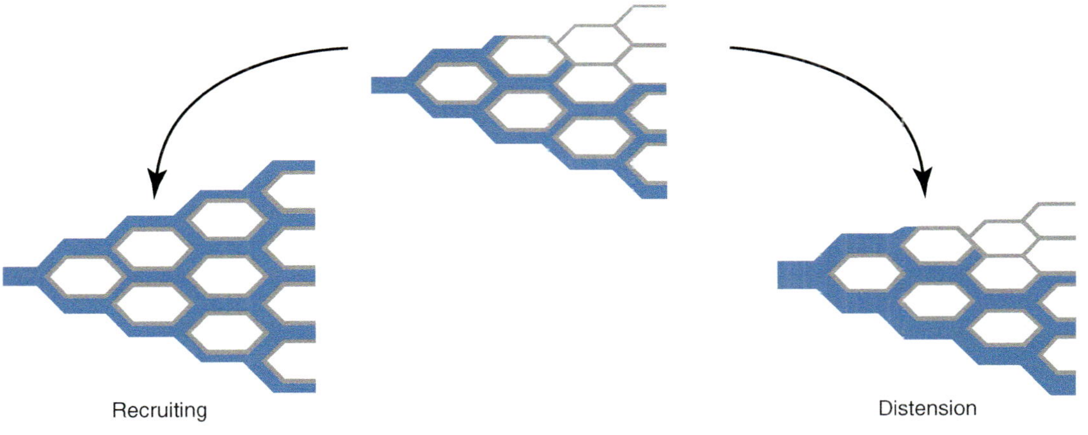

Fig. 3.5 Pulmonary circulation, recruitment, and vascular distention

The Ventilation/Perfusion Ratio

The efficacy of pulmonary gas exchange depends on uniform distribution of the inhaled air and blood flow (Q) that circulates in the pulmonary vascular bed. The VA in a young adult is 4 l/min and the blood flow is 5 l/min. The ventilation/perfusion (V/Q) ratio of the entire pulmonary system is thus 4/5 = 0.8. Ventilation and perfusion are not homogeneously distributed throughout the lungs. These values vary according to the areas established in a standing individual, favoring better ventilation at the bases because the apices are more distenced (more negative intrapleural pressure at the apices) and also favoring more perfusion at the base because of the effect of gravity. However, the result in the bases is that the V/Q ratio is 0.6. In effect, there is proportionally more perfusion acting as shunt areas (with shunting from right to left). The result in the apices is a V/Q ratio of 3, in which the ventilation acting as alveolar dead space is proportionally greater (Fig. 3.6).

These phenomena, which occur in normal children because of gravity, can be accentuated

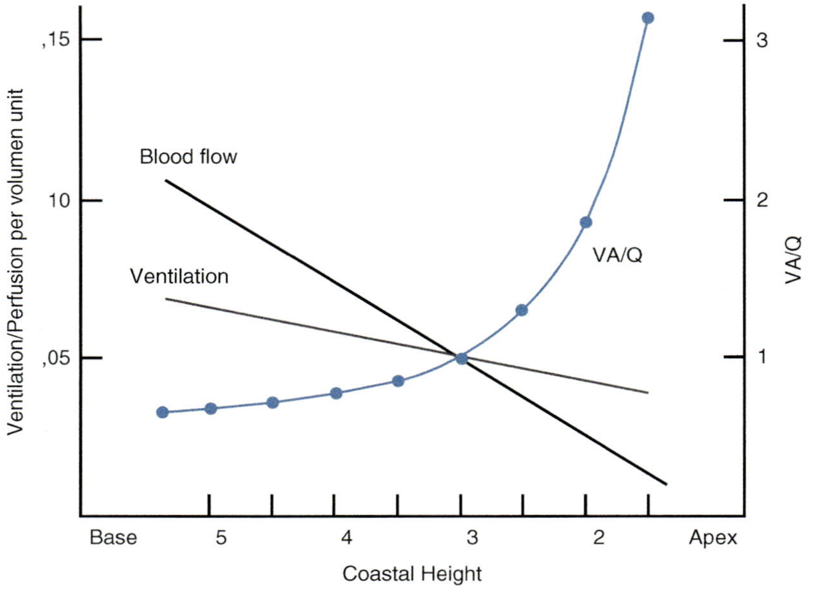

Fig. 3.6 Ventilation/perfusion ratio according to the lung zone (in a standing individual)

in cases of illness. An alteration in the V/Q ratio is the most common physiopathological disorder in pediatric respiratory diseases. The clinically significant aspect in this alteration is the decrease in the PaO_2, given that well-ventilated areas do not improve the low blood PaO_2 from poorly ventilated areas, because the hemoglobin saturation in the former is almost 100%. In contrast, the well-ventilated areas do improve the $PaCO_2$ in poorly ventilated areas, easily compensating for the decreased elimination of CO_2 in hypoventilated areas. For these reasons, alterations in the V/Q ratio always lead to arterial hypoxemia—whether it is due to irregular ventilation with uniform blood flow or irregular blood flow with regular ventilation—and, in contrast, its influence on the $PaCO_2$ is variable, given that this parameter depends more on the efficacy of the total VA.

Alveolar areas that do have exchange because of nil or insufficient vascular perfusion are not used in gaseous exchange and constitute dead alveolar space. The PDS is the sum of the anatomical dead space in the airways and the alveolar dead space, which is normally 30% of the total pulmonary volume. The PDS is calculated on the basis of simultaneous measurements of the partial pressure of CO_2 in blood ($PaCO_2$) and in exhaled air ($PeCO_2$), according to a simplified Bohr equation:

$$PDS = \left(PaCO_2 * PeCO_2\right) / PaCO_2$$

Respiratory Gases in the Blood

According to Dalton's law of partial pressure, the pressure exerted by each gas in a mixture of gases is independent of the other gases, and the total pressure of a mixture of gases is equal to the sum of each gas separately. Atmospheric air contains 20.93% oxygen, 0.04% carbon dioxide, and 79.03% nitrogen, with a pressure of 760 mmHg at sea level (barometric pressure). The partial pressure of O_2 in inhaled air (PIO_2) is consequently 20.93% of 760 mmHg, or 159.1 mmHg. When air is inhaled, it is saturated with water vapor, which evaporates from the surface of the nasal tissue and is diluted in the air occupying the airways and the lungs. The gaseous mixture that reaches the alveoli is termed alveolar air and now contains the gases from inhaled air: O_2, N_2, and CO_2, as well as water vapor. The partial water vapor pressure is a saturated mix in the function of temperature, such that at 37 °C it is 47 mmHg'. The total pressure of the gases in alveolar air is equal to the barometric pressure, and as 47 mmHg of this pressure is necessarily water vapor, the pressure of the other gases has to be equal to the barometric pressure minus 47 mmHg.

In a normal male at rest and breathing normally, the $PACO_2$ is around 40 mmHg. In contrast, the partial pressure of O_2 in alveolar air (PAO_2) depends on the $PACO_2$ (given that the partial pressure of N_2 and water vapor do not vary). This relationship is expressed in the alveolar air equation:

$$PAO_2 = \left(FIO_2 * \left(Patmos - PH_2O\right)\right) - \left(PaCO_2 / R\right)$$

where FIO_2 is the inhaled O_2 fraction, Patmos is the local atmospheric pressure, PH_2O is the water vapor pressure in the airway and its value is 47 mmHg, and R is the normal respiratory quotient and its value is 0.8.

$$R : \text{normal respiratory quotient} = 0.8$$

The $PACO_2$ can be estimated from the $PaCO_2$ at the arterial level, which can be measured. Resolving the alveolar air equation for a person with a $PaCO_2$ of 40 mmHg at sea level yields a PAO_2 of 109 mmHg during breathing of an FIO_2 of 21%. Oxygen in the lungs diffuses from alveolar air into the blood because venous blood arriving in the lungs has a lower mixed venous oxygen tension than the PAO_2. As the blood passes through the lung capillaries, it never reaches a complete equilibrium with the alveolar air, and so the PaO_2 of the blood that leaves the lung capillaries is slightly lower than the PAO_2; in normal circumstances, this difference is not greater than 1 mmHg. However, before this arterialized blood reaches the arteries systematically, it mixes with a small quantity of venous blood that has not passed through the lung capillaries, which comes from anastomosis with the bronchial system, from venoarterial shunts or hypoventilated alveoli. This mixture determines a decrease in the PaO_2 of 9 mmHg. In this way, a PAO_2 of 109 mmHg, which is normal at sea level, determines a PaO_2 of 100 mmHg. Because the primary purpose of respiration is to maintain a normal PaO_2 and a normal $PaCO_2$, knowledge of the partial pressures of these gases in arterial blood allows us to assess the degree of sufficiency of the total respiratory function. These determinations are indispensable in pulmonary function studies and are now routine examinations in the treatment of serious respiratory problems.

The oxygen hemoglobin saturation is related closely to the arterial oxygen content, given that the fraction of dissolved oxygen in the blood is negligible because of the low solubility coefficient. The oxygen saturation depends on the partial pressure of oxygen and the characteristics of the hemoglobin disassociation curve, which is influenced by factors such as the type of hemoglobin (fetal, adult, abnormal), pH, $PaCO_2$, temperature, and 2,3-diphosphoglycerate content. The hemoglobin disassociation curve has an inflection point, below which small decreases in the PaO_2 correlate with substantial decreases in the hemoglobin saturation and consequently the arterial O_2 content. Above the inflection point, the slope is flattened and small increases in hemoglobin saturation correlate with a pronounced increase in the PaO_2. The decrease in the PaO_2 from 100 mmHg to 70 mmHg has only a minimal effect on hemoglobin saturation. In contrast, an increase in hemoglobin saturation above 93% is associated with proportionally greater increases in the PaO_2 (Fig. 3.7).

Because of the characteristics of fetal Hb, the newborn dissociation curve shifts to the left. This means that at a determined hemoglobin saturation level, the PaO_2 is lower than the O_2 tension in an older child. Hemoglobin saturation at 80% is reached in a newborn at a PaO_2 of 30 mmHg, and in an older child at a PaO_2 of over 50 mmHg.

The transport of CO_2 is totally different from that of oxygen because of the differences in their chemical properties. CO_2 moves through the bloodstream in a dissolved form, combining with proteins and transformed into bicarbonate. CO_2 is 20 times as soluble as O_2; thus, up to 10% of the total CO_2 is dissolved in the bloodstream. Moreover, CO_2 combines easily with proteins in the plasma in an enzyme-independent reaction, and so another 10% moves through the bloodstream bonded to proteins, the most abundant being carboxyhemoglobin. The most efficient CO_2 transport mechanism is conversion into bicarbon-

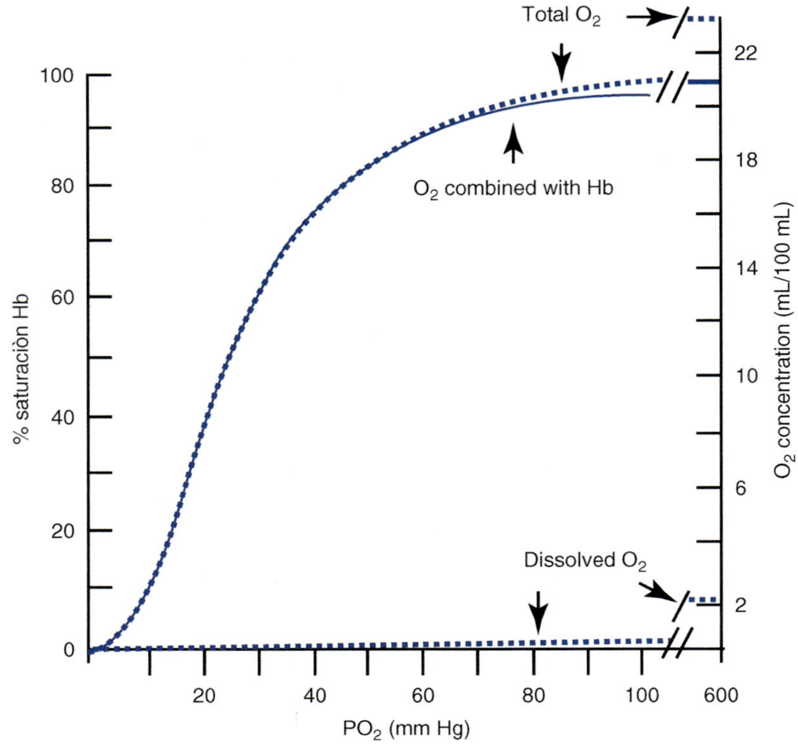

Fig. 3.7 Hemoglobin dissociation curve

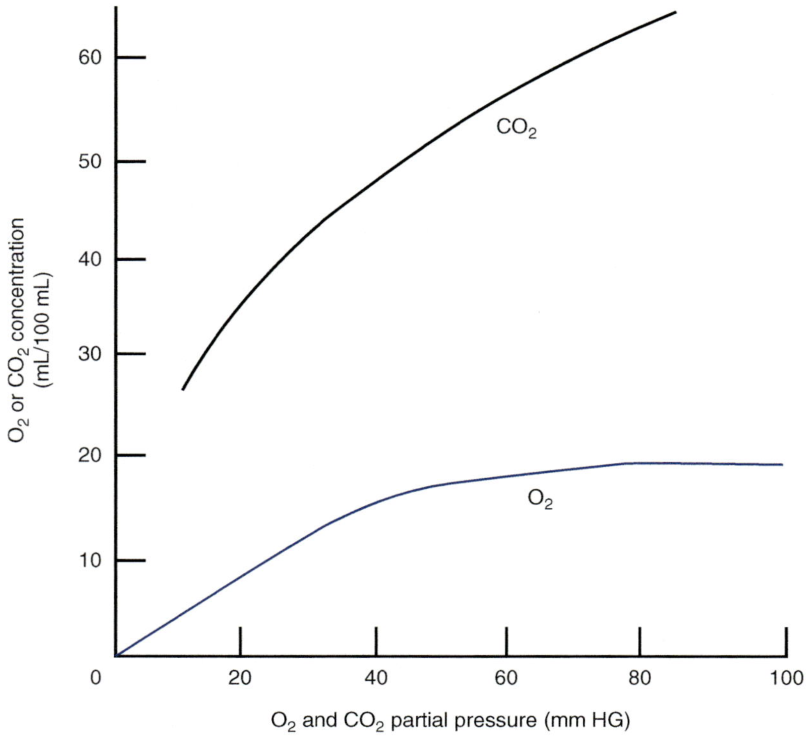

Fig. 3.8 Comparative concentration curves for CO_2 and O_2

ate, which involves 80% of the total. This reaction is highly efficient because of the presence of the carbonic anhydrase enzyme found in erythrocytes. The CO_2 blood concentration curve is much more pronounced, which determines that the changes in the partial pressure of CO_2 are proportional to the changes in the CO_2 blood content (Fig. 3.8).

Sources

Berger AJ. Control of breathing. In: Murray JF, Nadel JA, editors. Textbook of respiratory medicine. 3rd ed. Filadelfia, PA: Saunders; 2000. p. 179–96.

Decramer M. The respiratory muscles. In: Fishman AP, et al., editors. Pulmonary diseases and disorders. 3rd ed. New York: McGraw-Hill; 1998. p. 63–71.

Griese M. Pulmonary surfactant in health and human lung diseases: state of the art. Eur Respir J. 1999;13:1455–76.

Levitzky MG. Pulmonary physiology. 8th ed. New York: McGraw-Hill; 2013.

Lumb A. Nunn's applied respiratory physiology. 7th ed. London: Elsevier; 2010.

Moyle J. Uses and abuses of pulse oximetry. Arch Dis Child. 1996;74:77–80.

Murray JF. The normal lung. 2nd ed. Filadelfia, PA: Saunders; 1986. p. 108–17, 339–358.

Sly P, Collins RA. Applied clinical respiratory physiology. In: Taussig L, Landau L, Le Souëf P, Martinez F, Morgan W, Sly P, editors. Pediatric respiratory medicine. 2nd ed. St. Louis: Mosby; 2008. p. 73–88.

Sola A, Chow L, Rodrigo M. Oximetría de pulso en la asistencia neonatal en 2005. Revisión de los conocimientos actuales. An Pediatr (Barc). 2005;62:266–81.

West JB. Ventilation/blood flow and gas exchange. 5th ed. Oxford: Blackwell; 1990. p. 25–9.

West JP. Respiratory physiology: the essentials. 9th ed. Philadelphia: Lippincott Williams & Wilkins; 2012.

West JP. Pulmonary pathophysiology: the essentials. 8th ed. Philadelphia: Lippincott Williams & Wilkins; 2013.

Clinical History and Physical Examination of the Respiratory System

4

Pablo Bertrand

Contents

Anamnesis

The clinical diagnosis of a respiratory disease begins with an interview to gather information pertinent to the clinical situation, which is then supplemented with a physical examination. In this interaction with the family and the patient, it is important, when appropriate, to develop a bond before proposing a deeper study plan and treatment that is realistic and in line with the family's expectations.

In the interview, the doctor must question all caregivers who can provide information, including the patient, if he or she is old enough. The doctor should ask about the main reasons for the consultation and proceed to characterize the manifestations and what repercussions they may have on the patient's daily activities such as playing, eating, or sleeping. During the interview it is important to ask open-ended questions that allow the parents to provide a broader description of the symptoms, which often reveal other hidden reasons for the consultation. Likewise, the doctor must supplement the interview with closed-ended and specific questions in relation to the symptoms, in order to precisely evaluate their relative importance, as well as any other relevant information.

The symptom or set of symptoms that have prompted the respiratory consultation are not always those most relevant to the child's health, but they show quite well the main concerns of the family. Thus, if in the course of the interview, very relevant symptoms appear that require consideration of the reason for the consultation, it is advisable to address the doubts that led the family to seek medical help in the first place.

Most respiratory symptoms are apparent in a regular patient interview, but it is always useful to look for symptoms that are not mentioned and are relevant to respiratory diseases. It is suggested to inquire about the following: cough, sneezing, coryza, fever, epistaxis, nasal pruritus, sputum, odynophagia, dysphagia, gagging, snoring, noisy

P. Bertrand (✉)
Department of Pediatrics, School of Medicine, Pontificia Universidad Católica de Chile, Santiago, Chile
e-mail: pbertrand@med.puc.cl

P. Bertrand, I. Sánchez (eds.), *Pediatric Respiratory Diseases*, https://doi.org/10.1007/978-3-030-26961-6_4

breathing, dysphonia, wheezing, dyspnea, chest pain, hemoptysis, tachypnea, apnea, and cyanosis.

The duration of the respiratory symptoms makes it possible to characterize, in a simple way, those diseases that have less than a 4-week duration as an acute course, and those that exceed this period as a chronic course. This definition is extended to consider an intermediate subacute period of between 4 weeks and 3 months in adolescent children and young adults. If the symptoms are clearly discontinuous, with documented intervals of general well-being, the disease is recurrent. It is important to clarify this distinction for the parents, who often perceive that their child has a chronic disease, without realizing that the symptoms are actually intermittent.

When characterizing the symptoms, it is useful to describe the intensity with which they occur and the functional repercussion they involve. For example, an episode of cyanosis in a breastfed baby is just as serious for both the parents and the doctor because it implies an episode severe enough to completely compromise respiratory function. As a counterpart, parents can seek attention if the child has a persistent cough, which in the vast majority of cases will be attributable to a benign and self-limited cause. A set of symptoms and their frequency over time will be very valuable to classify a disease from mild to severe and from controlled to uncontrolled, as happens with asthma.

Part of the symptom characterization is the exploration of triggers and ways to alleviate the patient's condition. This is useful information in relation to daily activities, which are very clear for the caregiver, such as feeding, exercise, sleep, etc.

Feeding can be a triggering and/or worsening factor, from reporting of choking and cyanosis during swallowing of food to a persistent cough that worsens during feeding. When the voice acquires a wet tone it is suggestive of faulty swallowing, but a hoarse voice can also suggest glottic inflammation caused by intermittent tracheal aspiration. It is relevant to determine if the symptoms appear before, during, or after feeding, besides determining if their appearance changes according to the consistency of the food.

Exercise is a common triggering factor for cough, shortness of breath, and wheezing in many patients with hyperreactivity, especially during exercise in cold areas. Besides this, exercise increases cough in those who have persistent bronchorrhea and in those who have a running nose or sputum caused by a common respiratory infection; however, in the former patients the symptoms appear during exercise, while in the latter patients they appear later. Exercise may be good to quantify the importance of functional compromise in advanced diseases. In this case, the doctor should ask about dyspnea during minimal or little effort. The characteristics of the cough, as well as the strength of the voice, can also be considered, which will directly reflect inhalation and/or exhalation weakness. Playing, laughing, and crying in infants are considered the equivalent of exercise in older children. In newborns and young infants, feeding is an exercise that shows how tolerant the child is, considering how long he or she takes to finish feeding.

The child's sleep provides information about several symptoms. This happens mainly because of the supine decubitus position, but also because of the alternance between active and passive periods that every child has. Parents of newborns and young infants, whose children sleep often, may seek urgent medical care if there is apnea or if there is irregular or rapid breathing. In contrast, the parents of schoolchildren or adolescents who snore and present apneas many times consider this a normal finding, although it may reflect an obstruction of the superior airway. If there is a cough when the child goes to bed, it is possible that there are secretions in the posterior area of the pharynx or gastroesophageal reflux, but if there is no cough it is still relevant if there is no cough, it is still relevant to consider a possible diagnosis of a habit cough or psychogenic cough. If an infant has tachypnea or difficulty during breathing in the supine position, it can suggest diaphragmatic muscular weakness. This sign when the infant is sitting suggests chest muscular weakness. For the parents, an increase in respiratory frequency may not be clear, but they will describe "agitated" and "different" breathing. Clinical variations in symptoms between day and night may be evident in the clinical history, but they are not always caused by the child's position.

Sometimes, the explanation will lie in the air that the child breathes in the room while sleeping (e.g., the presence of contaminant heating, allergen exposure, etc.). Respiratory diseases tend to be related to environmental factors, and so a detailed description of the place where the patient lives in is very important. Most of the symptoms may worsen or persist when there is exposure to allergens or irritating inhaled agents such as those caused by industrial pollution or household pollution due to tobacco smoke, or contaminant heating involving burning of wood or paraffin. At the same time, there must be careful identification of seasonal and/or geographical changes that affect the symptoms, in order to discover possible triggers such as those related to the weather, altitude, etc. Respiratory symptoms that can be caused by respiratory infections—such as cough, fever, a running nose, or sputum, among others—make it necessary to ask about family members or people in usual contact with the patient who may also be affected. At this stage it is very important to note the order in which the different symptoms have appeared in the different patients.

The longer-term general history provides a good summary of the health condition of the child. Information from the pregnancy and the perinatal period is very important in relation to its consequences—for example, if the mother or the fetus suffered from infections or metabolic disorders, or if they were exposed to toxic agents such as nicotine. A stridor appearing during the first year of life may be caused by multiple factors, and knowing about the sequence of the events, and aggravating and alleviating circumstances, is the basis of a good diagnosis. The events that happened within this period—for example, neonatal asphyxia or recurrent seizures—may determine the persistent respiratory problems that the child may have afterward, such as a cough, sputum, choking, and wheezing. Growth during the first months of life is a good indicator of the health of an infant. If there is a lack of growth related to respiratory symptoms, this points to greater systemic compromise due to the disease.

There are many respiratory diseases that have a Mendelian genetic component (cystic fibrosis, alpha-1 antitrypsin deficiency, Duchenne's dystrophy, chronic granulomatous disease, etc.), caused by a mutation (Prader–Willi syndrome or cri du chat) or that are multigenic (asthma). This forces us to investigate the family history for at least two generations of every origin, with special attention to blood relationships and information about any infant deaths in the family. It is advisable to document the health of the direct family, including both parents and siblings.

Physical Examination

Inspection

Simple observation of the child during the interview and during the physical examination provides a lot of information. The first thing that must be observed is the respiratory pattern; this includes the respiratory frequency and rhythm, and the work of breathing. The respiratory frequency is a measurement taken routinely and must be interpreted as part of the physical examination. Because of the inherent variability that the rhythm of the respiratory cycle presents—which is heavily influenced by the state of alertness, besides the presence of pain or crying—it is important to measure a full minute of it instead of estimating it on the basis of a 30-second measurement. This is more important in newborns, in whom the presence of periodic breathing is common. There are reference tables for the respiratory frequency range and average at different ages, and these are very useful for global approximation of the breathing of a child (Table 4.1). Auscultation will corroborate the inspection or can be used to evaluate very superficial breathing. An increase in the respiratory frequency or tachypnea is nonspecific and appears in normal conditions such as crying, pain, fear, or as compensation for losses caused by anemia or hypoxemia, as well as conditions of reduced distensibility in the respiratory system and metabolic alterations. A reduction in the respiratory frequency or bradypnea is less common and difficult to perceive. It happens as a manifestation of central neurological or metabolic alterations. The respiratory rhythm varies greatly during the first months of life. In newborns, especially premature newborns, breathing is irregular, and they normally present a percentage of periodic breathing (apneas lasting <6 seconds in three bursts or more with alternate breathings separated by <20 seconds). After this period, the presence of periodic breathing is abnormal. Cheyne–Stokes respiration (cycles of increasing and decreasing work, separated by absence of breathing) is always an abnormal and infrequent finding in children with intracranial hypertension or heart failure. Biot's respiration (irregular and variable work cycles with absence of breathing) is a common finding and is characteristic of severe brain damage. Kussmaul's breathing, or acidotic breathing, is fast breathing along with an increase in chest incursion, which is very characteristic of metabolic alterations (Fig. 4.1.). Absence of breathing with flow stopping is called apnea and is always serious, no matter what context it appears in. Normal breathing work is reflected in synchronized chest and abdominal expansion, as exhalation takes place as a passive phenomenon at rest. Increased breathing work is reflected in the use of accessory muscles and chest wall retraction (Fig. 4.2). The infant may also present nasal flaring and sometimes an increase in the work when he or she goes to bed (orthopnea). The presence of paradoxical movement (thoracoabdominal asynchrony during inhalation) is a sign of severe and imminent compromise in relation to muscular fatigue in a child with respiratory distress, but it may also appear during sleep in schoolchildren or adolescents with obstructive sleep apnea, or sleep paralysis caused by medications used in surgery or endotracheal intubation. Subcostal retraction is easily visible in newborns, especially premature newborns, who have greater chest lung compliance than older children. Suprasternal retraction during inhalation is a sign of upper airway obstruction and is usually accompanied by hoarseness and stridor.

Table 4.1 Respiratory rates in children by age

	Respiratory rate (percentile)								
Age	1	5	10	25	50	75	90	95	99
0 to <3 months	20	25	27	30	35	40	47	51	60
3 to <6 months	20	23	25	27	31	36	42	46	55
6 to <9 months	20	22	24	26	29	33	38	42	51
10 to <12 months	20	21	23	25	28	31	36	39	46
12 to <18 months	20	20	22	24	26	29	33	36	42
18 to <24 months	19	20	21	23	25	28	31	34	40
2 to <3 years	18	20	20	22	24	27	30	32	38
3 to <4 years	18	20	20	21	24	25	28	30	34
4 to <6 years	18	19	20	20	23	24	27	28	32
6 to <8 years	17	18	20	20	22	24	26	28	31
8 to <12 years	16	18	18	20	20	23	24	26	29
12 to <15 years	14	16	16	18	20	22	24	24	28
15 to <16 years	13	16	16	18	20	20	23	24	28

Modified from O'Leary et al. (2015)

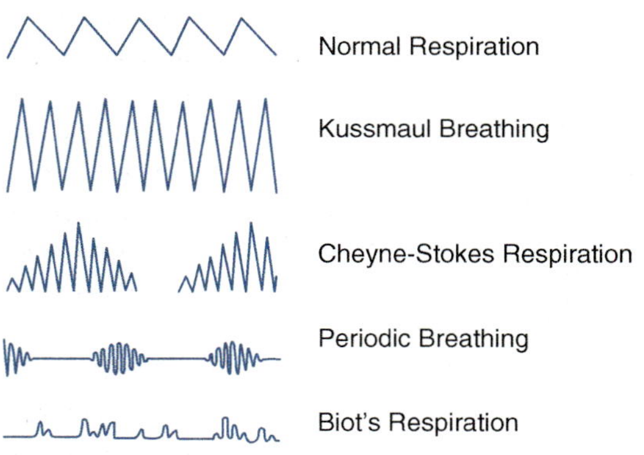

Fig. 4.1 Respiratory rhythm

Asymmetry in chest expansion is difficult to perceive in infants, but it can be noticeable in older children who have pain and who manage not to move the affected side with greater flexion

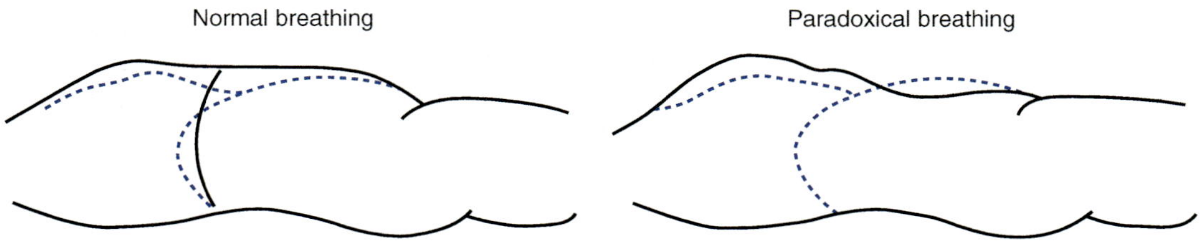

Fig. 4.2 Breathing synchronization

of the trunk. Evidence of the use of abdominal muscles at exhalation is a reflection of active breathing secondary to respiratory distress. In infants this mechanism may appear with glottic closure at the end of exhalation, which can be heard and is called a breathing grunt. In an infant with diaphragmatic paralysis, inhalation will cause a noticeable sinking of the abdomen when the infant is in the decubitus supine position, and there will also be asymmetry on the nonaffected side, which will sink when the infant is in the lateral decubitus position.

Chest dimensions may differ in different geographical zones and in different races. The chest undergoes a change from the newborn period, when it tends to be round, toward the school stage, when it acquires a flattened ovoid configuration when considered from the anteroposterior angle. A barrel-shaped chest in a teenager is a sign of chronic obstructive lung disease, which, in infants with severe bronchopulmonary dysplasia, manifests as a dove-shaped chest (Fig. 4.3).

A head and neck examination is useful to complement the respiratory diagnosis. Extremely obvious and characteristic findings in the facies of a child may determine the presence of craniofacial syndromes, as happens in Down syndrome, Apert syndrome, Crouzon syndrome, and CHARGE syndrome, among others. Usually, medial facial dysplasia in these children causes respiratory distress in the upper airway. The presence of purple skin under the lower eyelid, the finding of a fold in the skin of this zone (the Dennie–Morgan line), a transverse nasal crease under the bony section that is visible to the naked eye, or edema of the nasal mucosa, dry secretions, or abundant and aqueous rhinorrhea that unites the nasal septum and the turbinate (nasal bridges) on anterior rhinoscopy are all findings that are suggestive of allergic rhinitis. It is extremely useful to observe the nasal mucosa in a routine examination, because it can show purulent discharges, blood, polyps, and even foreign bodies. In allergic children, the presence of serum fluid can be confirmed by observation of the tympanum. With this technique the sequelae of recent infections can be controlled, such as when there is a perforation of the membrane or when there are plaques of tympanosclerosis. Inspection of the pharynx may show isolated malformations such as a palatine fissure or findings that are part of a syndrome such as macroglossia in a child with Beckwith–Wiedemann syndrome.

Opening of the oral cavity in a simple examination gives a hint if the airway is in a difficult condition (according to the Mallampati index), and it also reveals the proportion that the amygdules occupy; they are frequently increased in size in children who snore at night. Skin alterations are extremely relevant in respiratory diseases. For example, the presence of keratosis pilaris, pityriasis alba plaques, or eczema are all signs of atopic dermatitis. Pigmentation changes, light brown spots, and vascular tumors such as hemangiomas are indicators of diseases that may compromise the respiratory system. The most relevant skin sign that reflects respiratory compromise is cyanosis. When cyanosis appears, it means that the hemoglobin level is reduced (>5 g/dl) in the skin capillaries (distal cyanosis) or in the tongue and mucosal capillaries (central cyanosis). It tends to be an indicator of hypoxemia because of the presence of reduced hemoglobin, but it is clearly a poor indicator of hypoxemia when there is anemia, because in this situation a hemoglobin reduction large enough for cyanosis to become clinically evident rarely occurs.

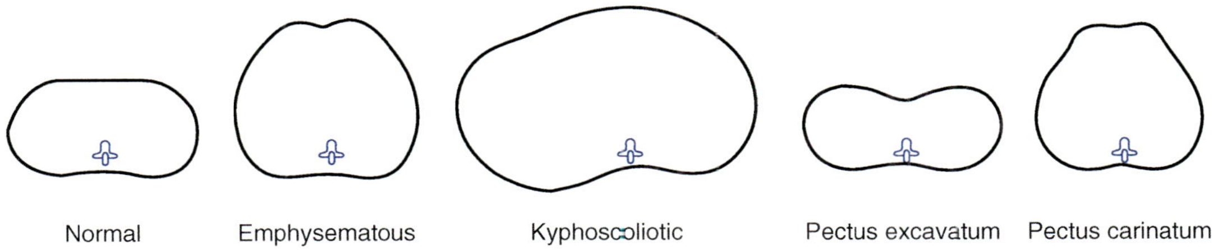

Fig. 4.3 Thoracic configuration

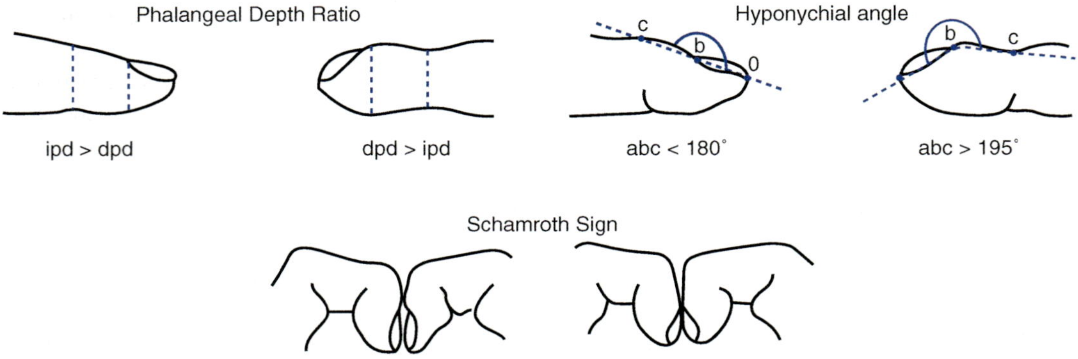

Fig. 4.4 Nail clubbing

The presence of digital clubbing is a nonspecific indicator of chronic lung disease, which is characteristic of cystic fibrosis, although it is also present in heart and gastrointestinal disease. It appears as a focal increase in the connective tissue in the distal phalanges of the feet and hands (Fig. 4.4).

The rest of the examination may contribute to the diagnosis of respiratory disease and is part of a good evaluation. Findings in the heart, abdominal, and limb examinations are especially important.

Palpation

Chest palpation is done at the same time as the inspection, and it follows a sequence that starts in the cervical area and ends in the abdominal area. At the neck it is important to notice any increase in volume or the presence of masses caused by adenopathies, growth of the thyroid gland, or hemangiomas and lymphangiomas. All of these structures may partially or totally occlude the upper airway and cause noisy breathing, stridor, and tracheal cough.

Anomalous positioning of the trachea may indicate related intrachest malformations. Palpation and soft pressure in the cricoid area can be used to trigger a cough in order to evaluate it. Chest palpation helps to find deformities, asymmetries of the costal structure, and areas where there is pain. Besides this, it is possible to perceive vibrations created by the voice when the child speaks out loud cries, in the case of infants. This technique is instinctively used by mothers to describe the presence of secretions in the lower airway, but the perception of "wet" vibrations in chest palpation does not necessarily have a localization. If air or fluid has entered the pleura, the transmission of these vibrations is reduced.

Percussion

The chest can be percussed because of its resonance, which is a consequence of its air capacity. Percussion in this area maintains the vibration, which is not softened, so the vibration resounds, and this is called "tympanic." When percussion is done in solid tissue, the vibration propagates quickly and is rapidly deafened, and this is called "dull." Percussion is done using the index finger over the distal phalange of the middle finger of the other hand, making equal and symmetrical movements, and then making comparisons. This technique shows the maximum lung excursion in the posterior wall of the chest, as well as the areas that should have a tympanic sound but where—because of fluid in the pleural space, or because of some peripheral consolidation in the lung parenchyma—a dull sound can be heard instead. When the sound of the chest is not symmetrical and increased, a pneumothorax must be considered.

Auscultation

The auscultation technique yields variable results depending on the conditions in which it is done. In order to improve sound perception, the child must be calm and the environment must be quiet. Therefore, it is not unwise to start the auscultation when the baby is in the arms of the mother, before he or she starts crying out of fear. If the patient cooperates, it is desirable to have the patient sitting with his or her back straight in order to have the sound flowing normally. The number of areas that are evaluated during auscultation are variable, but at least three areas per side, anterior and posterior, should be considered. The breathing that shows more sound is deep breathing through the open mouth, with which the airflow is increased. Among infants, distraction and, in many situations, play can achieve this objective, although sometimes this includes only those sounds that are produced by sighing during crying. It is advisable to avoid the appearance of "artifact" sounds caused by forced breathing or affected by the phonation of the child.

The auscultation technique is based on bilateral comparison of sounds, but it also uses the intensity with which the patient may produce the sounds in different situations. In this way, it is possible to describe respiratory sounds as symmetrical or asymmetrical and as increased or reduced, according to the situation.

The respiratory sounds we hear during auscultation in the respiratory examination are caused by turbulence in the air in the central airway. The tracheal breathing sound is normally heard symmetrically above the jugular notch during the whole respiratory cycle. The tracheal sound has a wide spectrum (0–2000 Hz) and is enriched by the resonance of the area. The tracheal sound increases in intensity proportionally to the circulating flow, especially at high frequencies. In this way, when there is a narrowing at this level, the sound increases with the speed, which even allows us to perceive it at distance. Normal lung sounds can be heard on the surface of the chest and are well represented during inhalation but cannot be heard during exhalation. The lung sound has a lower frequency than the tracheal sound (0–500 Hz) because of the filtration—particularly in relation to the higher frequencies—that happens when air enters the lungs. The lung sound is produced in the primary and segmental bronchi during inhalation, and in the trachea during exhalation; therefore, it is affected by the convergence of the flow in the airway bifurcations. The lung sound of a child in the compared areas of the chest can be heard as being quite symmetrical but not precisely symmetrical, as there may be differences in the auscultation of both hemithoraxes. Sound transmission is very useful in abnormal situations. When passing through the airway, respiratory sounds are usually filtered, but in the presence of consolidation, their transmission improves and it is possible to hear a tracheal sound in lung areas (a tubular breath sound) and transmission of vocal sounds in a similar way (bronchophony), even during whispering (aphonic pectoriloquy). The terminology used to describe respiratory sounds has been reviewed recently, and an effort has been made to create universal terminology (Table 4.2). Adventitious breath sounds are extra sounds that occur besides the normal sounds specified for the respiratory disease.

Wheezing

Wheezing is a musical and continuous sound (lasting >250 milliseconds) that is produced when the airway vibrates in a narrowing area.

Table 4.2 Classification of breath sounds

Sounds
Breath sounds
Normal breath sounds
Laryngotracheal sounds
Lung murmur
Abnormal breath sounds
Noisy breathing
Tubular breathing
Decreased or absent lung murmur
Transmitted voice sounds
Normal sounds
Bronchophony
Egophony
Adventitious breath sounds
Continuous sounds
Rhonchi
Wheezing
Stridor
Discontinuous sounds
Crackles
Pleural rubs

The frequency of this oscillation depends on the vibrating mass around this airway but not on the diameter of the airway. Diffuse narrowing of the airway causes different wheezes with different or polyphonic tones. In turn, narrowing of the central airway creates wheezing in a similar or monophonic tone. Wheezing during exhalation shows narrowing of the airway and flow limitation, and these are the hallmarks of asthma and bronchiolitis. Wheezing shows frequencies close to 600 Hz, and some authors use the term rhonchus to refer to those frequencies close to 200 Hz, although they are also called low-tone wheezing.

Crackles

Crackles are discontinuous cracking sounds (lasting <20 milliseconds) due to the passage of air through the secretions of the airway, caused by sudden equalization of the gas pressure. Crackles can be fine or thick, depending on how long the sound lasts and its frequency. Fine crackles during the end of exhalation are common in active lung diseases. Fine crackles cannot be heard in the mouth, whereas thick crackles are transmitted through the airway and can be heard in the mouth.

Stridor

A stridor is a musical and continuous sound that is produced by vibration of the phonation system: the larynx, vocal cords, and adjacent tissues, as well as narrowing of the tracheal extrathoracic area. The sound can be heard with no instruments, mainly during inhalation, but as the obstruction continues, it may be audible throughout the respiratory cycle. The resonance spectrum of a stridor is very wide (200–1000 Hz), and it has a high intensity.

Grunting

A grunt is a musical and continuous sound caused by vibration of the vocal cords when they are closed forcibly and abruptly. In a similar way, snoring comes from vibration of the soft tissues in the pharynx, which causes a mixture of continuous and discontinuous low-tone sounds throughout the breathing cycle.

Pleural Friction Rub

A pleural friction rub is the only sound that is caused not by airflow but by the cuff of structures that are not smooth and are inflamed. It sounds like a discontinuous sound and it occurs in a symmetrical way during inhalation and exhalation.

Sources

Bohadana A, Izbicki G, Kraman S. Fundamentals of lung auscultation. N Engl J Med. 2014;370:744.

Brown MA, Von Mutius E, Morgan WJ. Clinical assessment and diagnostic approach to common problems. In: Taussig L, Landau L, editors. Pediatric respiratory medicine. 2nd ed. Philadelphia: Mosby; 2008. p. 125–8.

Finder JD, Noyes BE, Orenstein DM. Pulmonary disorders. In: Zitelli-Davis BJ, Davis HW, editors. Atlas of pediatric physical diagnosis. 3rd ed. St. Louis: Mosby; 1997. p. 467–86.

Fleming S, Thompson M, Stevens R, et al. Normal ranges of heart rate and respiratory rate in children from birth to 18 years of age: a systematic review of observational studies. Lancet. 2011;377:1011–8.

Gagliardi L, Rusconi F. Respiratory rate and body mass in the first three years of life. The Working Party on Respiratory Rate. Arch Dis Child. 1997;76:15.

Gilmartin JJ, Gibson GJ. Mechanisms of paradoxical rib cage motion in patients with chronic obstructive pulmonary disease. Am Rev Respir Dis. 1986;134:683–8.

O'Leary F, Hayen A, Lockie F, et al. Defining normal ranges and centiles for heart and respiratory rates in infants and children: a cross-sectional study of patients attending an Australian tertiary hospital paediatric emergency department. Arch Dis Child. 2015;100:733–7.

Yernault JC, Bohadana AB. Chest percussion. Eur Respir J. 1995;8:1756–9.

Physiological Evolution of Sleep

5

Mara Cvejic and Christian Guilleminault

Contents

Introduction

Education on sleep has become a priority for many communities, social services, medical institutions, and government and educational bodies. Parallel to this, sleep disorders have become an important problem for doctors and patients alike. A study of the prevalence of neurological problems in Europe ranked sleep disorders third in terms of prevalence and impact, after headaches and anxiety disorders. The study estimated that the costs secondary to sleep disorders were over US $35 billion in 2010—more than the costs associated with epilepsy and multiple sclerosis put together.

Children are particularly affected by respiratory disorders and alterations in normal sleep architecture. In itself, the total time spent sleeping does not correlate directly with academic performance. The

M. Cvejic · C. Guilleminault (✉)
Division of Sleep Medicine, School of Medicine, Stanford University, Redwood City, CA, USA
e-mail: MCvejic@watsonclinic.com; cguil@stanford.edu

P. Bertrand, I. Sánchez (eds.), *Pediatric Respiratory Diseases*,
https://doi.org/10.1007/978-3-030-26961-6_5

physiological mechanisms underlying these associations remain unclear. It is thought that intermittent hypoxemia decreases brain blood flow to specific areas, and alterations in the architecture of sleep contribute significantly.

Given that there are no clear algorithms of study, doctors should use clinical tools to diagnose and treat patients with sleep disorders. There are few doctors specializing in sleep medicine or centers that can provide more in-depth studies. Consequently, there are long waiting lists for sleep studies in several countries. Waiting lists in the USA for polysomnography are 3–6 weeks long, while in Canada there are waiting lists of more than a year to get into a tertiary center capable of diagnosing sleep disorders with methods that are accepted as standard today. Consequently, it is critical that the treating physician—whether he or she is a neurologist, pediatrician, bronchopulmonary specialist, or child psychiatrist—is informed as to how to diagnose these very prevalent disorders, which leave many sequelae. In current pediatric practice, we need to know where patients with suspicion of sleep disorders should be referred to. Education on healthy and safe sleep should be an important theme in the training of pediatricians and doctors who work with children. Despite this evident need, studies show that education on sleep occupies less than 4.4 hours in total in the average training of a pediatric resident in the USA.

There is a high prevalence of sleep disorders, comparable to that of bronchial asthma. It is estimated that 12% of children experience daily problems associated with sleep, while 76% have occasional problems. Certain populations have a greater risk of developing sleep-related problems, such as children with Down syndrome, neuromuscular diseases, craniofacial alterations, epilepsy, intracranial tumors, and late development.

History and Anamnesis

The first step in diagnosing a possible sleep disorder is to study and understand the child in wakefulness. An example of this is the low yield of the symptom of snoring to predict obstructive sleep apnea in a child, in contrast to what happens in adults. Questions should be directed at academic performance, daytime sleepiness, naps, sleep routines and hygiene, eating habits, attentional conflicts, and hyperactivity. Children often present symptoms and problems of concentration, disruptive behavior, and lack of concentration in school and at home, rather than evident somnolence (unlike adults). There are numerous questionnaires that investigate these symptoms, such as the Pediatric Daytime Sleepiness Scale (PDSS), which is a tool with broad support for application by parents who have noted drowsiness and tiredness in their children.

The investigation into sleep hygiene and symptoms suggestive of insomnia should be presented in a directed way in an anamnesis. The use of televisions, radios, cell phones, computers, and various portable devices is associated with poor sleep and numerous sleep disorders. Special attention should be given to questions regarding the number of hours these devices are used for. The family context should also be explored; the working routines of the parents and the family composition themselves imply an implicit adaptation of the children's sleeping habits.

Age and Development

Given that sleep disorders in children can manifest themselves in a number of ways, search and screening tools should be adapted specifically to age groups and the type of sleep disorder being considered. The first step in developing these kinds of tools is to define what is normal at each age level. In the following sections, we summarize the main characteristics of sleep at different ages.

The Fetal Stage

It has been possible to obtain information about sleep at the early stages of life. Apart from what can be observed in premature newborns, noninvasive techniques have been used to study neurophysiological waves at the fetal stage to allow for the study of sleep in children before their birth.

Prechtl defined four stages of fetal sleep as measured by ultrasound:

1. Regular and slow heart rate, twitching, absence of eye movements
2. Irregular heart rate, eye movements, occasional body movement
3. Regular and rapid heart rate, eye movements, absence of body movements
4. Irregular and rapid heart rate, eye movements, continuous body movements

Premature Newborns

Premature newborns have more complex sleeping patterns in parallel with development. Active and quiet sleep can be distinguished between 33 and 34 weeks of gestational age, with greater reactivity evident around 35–36 weeks.

Movements, blinking, smiles, and nonspecific facial movements can be observed during active sleep. Jerking and twitching occur at the onset of sleep, which should not be interpreted as pathological. This sleep is not equivalent to REM in older children. While there are common phenomena, studies in newborn rats have found that lesions in the nuclei of the anterior raphe result in either the absence of rapid eye movement (REM) at the adult stage or no alteration, depending on the gestational age when the lesions occur. Given the above, it is unclear if REM sleep emerges subsequently as an independent stage per se. Non-REM (NREM) or slow-wave sleep is not present in newborns. It develops between the second and sixth weeks after birth, parallel to the appearance of greater brain voltages. Quiet sleep in newborns is equivalent to NREM.

The development of the sleep/wakefulness cycle in the brain includes the mesencephalic reticular formation, the posterior hypothalamus, and the medullary magnocellular nucleus. These structures are present at birth and, over the course of the first year of life, they mature concomitantly with their myelination, which begins with the posterior structures and proceeds anteriorly through the cerebral cortex.

There is evidence from animal models that somatostatin promotes the development of REM sleep. It is detectable in human at 120 days of gestation. This hormone reaches its maximum concentration at birth, whereupon it decreases progressively until it reaches 15–30% of its initial concentration in adulthood. However, because numerous neurotransmitters have been identified in different species of mammals, it is not clear which of these is responsible for the development and differentiation of sleep in humans. Among the neurotransmitters involved in the sleep/wakefulness cycle are glutamate, glycine, and γ-aminobutyric acid (GABA).

An electroencephalography (EEG) study of newborns should include at least 16 channels. The reading is highly complex and distinctly different from one for an adult, in terms of both voltage and EEG morphology. A premature patient can demonstrate periods of bursts of delta activity, followed by more than 25 μV of amplitude. This has classically been called an alternating trace pattern.

The *tracé discontinue* refers to a discontinuous pattern of alternating bursts of activity and intervals of apparent inactivity, which can be seen in premature newborns of less than 32 weeks of gestational age. This pattern has an amplitude of less than 25 μV and is transformed into quiet sleep at 36 weeks. At around 36 weeks the pattern termed "continuous slow-wave sleep" emerges, which predominates by 36 weeks (Table 5.1).

Bilateral synchrony has bimodal development; it is initially synchronic (until 30 weeks of gestational age), then becomes 25% asynchronic at up to 35 weeks, and then becomes synchronic again at 40 weeks. The symmetry is considered normal if the ratio of the interhemispheric amplitude is no greater than 2:1.

Newborns

There are many sleep-related situations in the neonatal period that can be stressful for parents or caregivers. The normal sleep patterns at this age should be explained to them, with screening to identify postpartum depression among mothers. One of the most common questions relates to the impression of inversion of the sleep–wakefulness cycle between night and day.

Table 5.1 Description of sleep patterns of newborns and premature newborns

Type of pattern	Description	State	Gestational age
Tracé alternant	Interburst intervals >25 μV	Alert	34–37 weeks
Tracé discontinue	Interburst intervals < 25 μV	Quiet	32–36 weeks
Slow-wave sleep	High-amplitude delta and theta waves	Quiet	36–45 weeks
Activité moyenne	Low voltage, irregular, continuous	Wakeful, active	>36 weeks
Sleep spindles	12–14 Hz, central	Quiet	44–49 weeks
Delta bursts	0.3–1.5 Hz, high-amplitude waves (50–250 μV), occipitotemporal, asynchronous	Quiet	29–33 weeks

At birth, babies have a very basic and initial circadian rhythm that is sensitive to changes in light in relation to melatonin secretion. Although parents may not note a significant difference in the distribution of hours of sleep between day and night, it has been demonstrated that there is a tendency from the first days of life for the baby to sleep more during night hours. It is estimated that term newborns sleep on average for 16 hours a day. Newborns present a polycyclic pattern that ranges between 1 and 4 hours, with the need for feeding between the cycles. The alternation between the sleep stages is shorter in newborns—on average, 50–60 minutes—in contrast to the 90-minute alternation in adults.

It is estimated that 50% of newborn sleep is REM and that REM sleep latency is shorter in newborns than in adults.

A sleep anamnesis of a newborn should include:

1. Gestational age and neonatal complications
2. Complications of the birth
3. Admissions to neonatological care
4. Presence of apnea or family history of any apparent life-threatening events (ALTEs; events that put the infant's life at risk, in the eyes of the observer) or sudden death syndrome
5. Environment for sleeping: where, how much, and how the baby sleeps; shared bed, exposure to smoking
6. Safe environment for sleeping: separate and strong crib, absence of stuffed animals or pillows, sleeping on her or his back, avoidance of soft surfaces to avoid the risk of suffocation
7. Sleeping position: the baby should sleep on his or her back; recommendations followed to prevent sudden death of the baby

Newborns with apnea represent a special and unique population. There are several risk factors that facilitate the development of apnea, one of which is premature birth. The gestational age marks the presence of "premature apnea," such that 7% have it at 34–35 weeks of gestational age, 15% at 32–33 weeks, 54% at 30–31 weeks, and almost 100% of newborns at less than 29 weeks. Although premature apnea is considered a self-limiting condition, it is treated to avoid possible neurocognitive consequences associated with desaturations. The underlying physiological mechanism of this phenomenon is not completely understood, and it is supposed that it is based on the immaturity of the respiratory center. In all cases of persistent apnea, the possibility of conditions such as hemorrhages, infections, intracranial lesions, gastroesophageal reflux, convulsions, and metabolic and electrolytic alterations should be considered.

One theory is that premature babies are particularly sensitive to inhibitory neurotransmitters such as GABA, adenosine, serotonin, and other prostaglandins. Adenosine is one of the key targets of treatment with methylxanthine. There is evidence that adenosine facilitates the release of GABA, leading to respiratory depression in the newborn. More recent studies have shown the presence of prostaglandins that induce the formation of proinflammatory mediators such as interleukin beta 1.

The experience of newborn admissions to neonatological care raises questions about the stressful effect that intensive services can have on sleep. The overstimulation of arousals and awakenings by sounds, and the attention related to continuous monitoring, raise concerns. There have been few studies on this issue, but simple interventions such as the use of music have been shown to reduce parental stress and improve newborn sleep stages.

Long-term follow-up has shown that newborns who have had efficient sleep are more attentive between 4 and 18 months of age than those who did not sleep efficiently at the newborn stage.

Infants

Infancy is a period of significant changes for the normal sleep pattern, and questions should be directed in particular to the following aspects:

1. Number and duration of naps: In total, these should not exceed 3–4 hours.
2. Total time spent sleeping: Nocturnal sleep around 9–10 hours, total time 12–13 hours.
3. Sleep routine and rituals: Incipient routines and rituals generally already exist at this age.
4. Presence of colic, diseases, and the use of medications.
5. Gastroesophageal reflux: This condition, which is often physiological, has been associated with an increase in arousals, although it is sometimes associated with apnea.
6. Details of any ALTEs.
7. Psychomotor development: Nonacquisition of the different stages in psychomotor development can involve concomitant problems related to sleep. This should be investigated to determine the presence of hypotony, which can affect the occurrence of hypoventilation.
8. Use of pacifiers and bottles: The American Academy of Pediatrics currently recommends the use of pacifiers to avoid sudden infant death.
9. Parents' attention and routines: In many cases, parents sleep with their infant as a result of sleep problems. Parents respond in different ways to their infant's crying and needs. Some actions can interrupt the infant's sleep, such as using a baby bottle as a pacifier, but can also help the baby go back to sleep once he or she has woken up.

At 3–4 months of age, the infant develops more consistent sleeping blocks, which can be a source of relief to the parents, who will say the baby now "sleeps the whole night through." During the first 6 months of life, melatonin secretion matures concomitantly, with a strong correlation between melatonin levels and sleep/wakefulness cycles. This correlation is not observed in children who have lost their vision. The aberrant sleep patterns of blind infants tend to improve with use of exogenous melatonin.

Nap taking begins to decrease at 6 months of age, and the majority of infants continue with two naps in the second semester of life. Most infants immediately begin with REM sleep or with significantly shorter REM latency than adults. The REM cycles get longer with the passing months. The time passed in REM sleep decreases progressively from 50% of the total sleep time in small infants to less than 30% as they reach the age of 1 year.

The response of infants to arousals matures rapidly in the first 9 months of life. The response to hypoxia with arousals decreases toward week 9, because of which responses to microawakenings gradually shift from subcortical to cortical responses.

One theory for infant sudden death is a failure to adapt an arousal response to particular stimuli or a toxic substance. It is especially important with infants to prepare guidelines to prevent sudden death: the baby should sleep on his or her back, the bed should not be shared, and exposure to cigarette smoke should be avoided. A low socioeconomic level and prematurity have also been identified as risk factors for infant sudden death. The reticular formation of the brain stem is involved in balancing inhibitory and excitatory impulses that collect sensorial, somatic, and chemical/mechanical receptor–sourced information. The progression of microawakenings in response to stimuli, such as tactile stimuli and an increase in CO_2, have demonstrated an ascending spinal, subcortical, and cortical pattern. Waking begins with small subtle movements, following by swaying, and culminating in eye opening and full awakening, with the shift to wakefulness. These microawakenings occur in both active and quiet sleep.

Preschool Children and Older Infants (1–3 Years of Age)

The sleeping habits of small preschool children is biphasic, with sleep concentrated in the night and two naps during the day. The sleep/wakefulness cycle gradually consolidates, and by the age of 3 years the child usually has only one nap during the day. By the age of 6 years, naps have become abnormal and suggest a sleep-specific disorder. REM sleep decreases gradually at this stage, reaching 30% after the age of 1 year. By 9–11 years of age, the REM/NREM ratio is similar to that in adults. EEG spectral analysis can show the changes over time during this period.

Parallel to the decrease in REM sleep, the total sleeping time decreases from 16–18 hours to ≤9 hours at the postpuberty stage. The average number of hours of sleep at the preschool stage is 10 hours.

Between 20% and 30% of older infants and preschool children remain awake during the night, which constitutes a common reason for medical consultation. It is considered that intervention is appropriate for awakenings when the family routine is disrupted and the parents are forced to take actions such as staying with the child or forcing the child to return to his or her room. However, as actigraphy studies have shown, most preschool children wake up twice a night without their parents realizing it. In most cases, the children go back to sleep and do not alter the family's sleep routine. The data from EEG studies of children between 6 and 11 years of age who experience 1–3 three small awakenings per night suggest that the sleep of preschool children is more fragmented than we might think.

Another aspect that implies complex interaction of several factors is the initiation of sleep. In general, by 2–3 years of age, children are adapted to the routines and rituals of the family with respect to sleep. The use of audiovisual media, extended working hours of parents, or bedroom sharing with siblings can result in alteration of the time for going to sleep.

Nocturnal fears and nightmares are characteristic of this age and can often disrupt sleep.

A sleep anamnesis at this age should include the following points:

1. Sleep rituals and hygiene
2. Switching from a crib to a bed at around 2.5–3 years of age
3. Naps: their number and duration
4. Symptoms of attention deficit, misbehavior, hyperactivity, bad moods, changes in regular patterns in daycare or school
5. Nightmares or nocturnal fears
6. Shared bed, sleep space environment, use of a pacifier
7. Enuresis (which generally should not occur beyond 6 years of age)
8. Drowsiness and problems in waking up
9. Use of electronic devices (e.g., television, radio, cell phone, computer, tablet, or electronic game)
10. Allergies, dermatitis, asthma
11. Snoring

Respiratory sleep disorders begin to increase at this age.

Schoolchildren and Neuronal Plasticity

Slow-sleep-wave activity can be mapped with EEG spectral analysis, showing cortical development. Slow-wave activity in preschool children is predominant in the occipital lobes and moves progressively to the parietal and occipital regions during adolescence. The role of naps in this maturation process is not clear, but it appears that they play an important role in consolidating learning and memory. Naps remain important in the schedules of many daycare centers and schools. In this respect, a study indicated that the use of naps resulted in a 10% improvement in learning of visual–spatial tasks by preschool children. The concomitant polysomnography record in this study showed the presence of a larger number of sleep spindles among the children, which would improve their learning.

The impact of sleep on memory is one the main concerns at this vulnerable stage of neurocognitive development. Memory development is influenced by a series of molecular factors and signals. One of the processes of memory is consolidation, which is favored by repairing sleep. It is assumed that there are regenerative processes during sleep, distributed into two stages, the first occurring immediately at the beginning of sleep, characterized by signals and protein synthesis in the hippocampus, and a second stage 4 hours later. The kinase that facilitates these processes is altered when individuals lose sleep or change their sleep schedule.

Adenosine inhibits the hippocampus, which reduces neuronal plasticity. The oscillating theta rhythm in the hippocampus can be shown both in REM sleep and in wakefulness during the execution of neurocognitive learning and memory tasks. It was initially believed that REM sleep was responsible for memory consolidation, but in the 1980s it was shown that slow-wave NREM sleep affects memory consolidation. The increase in slow-wave NREM sleep and the density of sleep spindles subsequent to training and learning has been demonstrated in studies with human and with animal models. A "dual hypothesis" is currently proposed and assumes that NREM sleep is responsible for declarative memory consolidation in the hippocampus, while REM sleep tends to regulate functional (procedural) and emotion-related memory. However, this vision is possibly too simplistic and cannot explain a series of much more complex interactions.

Nevertheless, it has been clearly demonstrated that sleep deprivation affects memory and changes the cytoarchitecture of the hippocampus. Considering how both REM and NREM sleep decrease over the course of one's life, the preschool and early school stages should be when more effort is made to protect neuronal homeostasis and the consolidation of memory in the hippocampus.

Attention deficit–hyperactivity disorder (ADHD) has been linked directly to sleep disorders, especially at the preschool and school stages, where it is also more evident to teachers. Treatment of this syndrome can alter the normal sleep of the child. Changes have been evidenced in slow-wave and REM sleep in children with ADHD in a manner similar to what was described above in relation to memory consolidation. The frontal brain activity of children with ADHD is slow during wakefulness and presents an anteroposterior imbalance in slow-wave activity during sleep. In particular, alterations have been found in the frontal circuits associated with control of emotions and memory regulation in children with ADHD. These circuits change over time and cease to be as important in adulthood, which could explain the lower prevalence of ADHD in adults than in children. This change with age could also explain why children show more hyperactive symptoms in response to poor sleep, while adults show more drowsiness.

Adolescents

The sleep patterns of adolescents are very similar to those of adults and, on average, adolescents sleep for 8–9.5 hours per night, 25% of which is REM sleep. Neuronal pruning continues, and it is supposed that this is the main mechanism producing changes in the sleep architecture seen in this population. In particular, there is a shift in the sleep phases at this age; thus, adolescents go to sleep later and wake up later. The normal phenomenon does not change the total number of hours of sleep. Distinct chronotypes can be distinguished at this age, and common complaints from parents and teachers are difficulty in waking up adolescents and their morning drowsiness. The idea of starting school at a later hour for adolescents than for preadolescents has been discussed in some parts of the USA and Canada.

An anamnesis at this age should include:

1. School performance: drowsiness can change performance and behavior in school
2. Depression and psychiatric illnesses
3. Hours slept
4. Daytime drowsiness: sleeping in classes or while doing tasks
5. Dental history: bruxism or cavities
6. Consumption of coffee, cola, energy drinks, or sports supplements
7. Headaches, blows, or falls

The interaction between sleep, puberty, and hormones is complex. Even when adolescents are not tired, they experience changes in melatonin secretion that invariably lead to a shift in the hours of the sleep phase. It is believed that this is linked to sexual hormonal development in adolescents. Endocrine changes during sleep follow fixed patterns specific to each hormone. Growth hormone is secreted in the first hours of sleep, reaching its maximum exactly an hour after the rise in prolactin. Follicle-stimulating hormone (FSH) and luteinizing hormone (LH) also follow fixed patterns, and their release is delayed in adolescence. In contrast, the time when cortisol is released does not change during adolescence, and its maximum release is always kept for dawn at the end of sleep.

The maturation of the cerebral cortex in adolescents is not explained simply by an EEG phenomenon or change. One of the maturational mechanisms of the cerebral cortex is sleep spindles, which change with age and increase in frequency toward the frontal area. A lower frequency of spindles in children shows better neurocognitive performance, while the reverse has been demonstrated in adults, with a higher frequency of sleep spindles indicating better neurocognitive performance.

The cyclic alternating pattern (CAP) is an EEG and polysomnography pattern for assessing sleep stability. CAP alterations are associated with conditions such as Asperger syndrome and poor cognitive performance.

Risk Factors and Academic Performance

It should be kept in mind that there is a series of risks in relation to adolescents; an examining physician should ask about these and should be vigilant when dealing with an adolescent patient with a sleep disorder. Risky sexual behavior, eating habits, abrupt changes in mood, and use of medications or other drugs should immediately be associated with base diseases or mental health compromise. It is during adolescence that diseases such as depression, bipolar disorder, and (less commonly) Kleine–Levin syndrome appear. The latter is characterized by hypersomnia, hallucinations, hyperphagia, and hypersexuality. The syndrome is episodic and tends to resolve 5–10 years after its appearance.

Anxiety, mood, and depression disorders are often associated with sleep disorders. Adolescents who get less sleep (an average of 6.75 hours) than normal (an average of 8.25 hours) have been reported to have more mood disorders. Adolescents who are defined as "night persons" are more often reported as having symptoms of anxiety than those defined as "daytime" persons.

Mood disorders can result from even brief periods of sleep deprivation. It has been shown that patients with anxiety disorders in adolescence often had early sleep problems in childhood, including before the age of 4 years. One study found that adolescents with obsessive–compulsive disorder had shorter hours of sleep, reduced NREM sleep, and less REM latency than control subjects. Another study found more sleep fragmentation, microawakenings, and decreased slow-wave sleep among adolescents with anxiety disorders than among control subjects. In particular, adolescent males with depression have demonstrated decreased latency in REM sleep, an increase in the N1 sleep stage, a larger number of microawakenings, and decreased short-wave sleep.

Academic performance correlates significantly in many studies with sleep-related problems. Treatment of these problems has been shown to improve poor academic performance. A study of first graders found that students who had undergone surgical treatment had improved their grades. Similar results from other studies suggest that good school performance is associated with regular long hours, while daytime drowsiness is associated with lower grades.

Specific Sleep-Associated Symptoms

There is a long list of symptoms that are understood as physiological and normal in sleep. Among the most common are the following:

1. Benign childhood myoclonus, which refers to local or diffuse twitching in otherwise healthy children (with normal EEG readings) that stops immediately upon the child waking up.
2. Movements at the beginning of sleep, related to small tremors in the transition between wakefulness and sleep.
3. Somniloquy or sleep-talking, which occurs particularly during NREM sleep.
4. Nonepileptic nocturnal psychogenic con vulsions.
5. Sandifer syndrome, which is nocturnal waking with rigidity and movement of extremities, associated with the presence of gastroesophageal reflux.
6. Sleep paralysis, which generally occurs during the transition from sleep to wakefulness. Paralysis that occurs at the beginning of sleep is termed hypnagogic, and that which occurs upon waking is termed hypnopompic. While sleep paralysis is benign in most cases, it is associated with epilepsy in a small percentage of cases.
7. *Jactatio capitis*, which is rhythmic head movement that is sometimes accompanied by similar body movement. This is typically found in patients with Down syndrome or neurocognitive disabilities.
8. Parasomnias, which occur in up to 80% of children between 2 and 6 years of age. This commonly occurs during NREM sleep and is distinguished among types of parasomnia by the frequency of disorders of the "arousal" or awakening type. The latter tend to be benign and are associated with premature birth and difficulties during pregnancy or birth.
9. Confusional arousal, which can emerge from deep NREM sleep and has an autonomic component ranging from the very simple to the complex.
10. Somnambulism or sleepwalking, which can occur at any age but is most common in adolescents. Episodes occur during NREM sleep, with general rhythmic activity of 2–7 Hz. An autonomic component is generally absent.
11. Nocturnal terror, which is one of the most common reasons for medical referral, owing to the dramatic nature of these episodes. The child awakens in an agitated state, screaming in terror, and parents often report an inconsolable cry. Diagnosis is generally possible with polysomnography or a video EEG. Seizures, which are the differential diagnosis, frequently occur during stages 1 and 2, while most parasomnias occur during stage 3. Children do not remember nocturnal terrors from one day to another.
12. Nightmares, which are disagreeable dreams, typically in childhood. They occur in the early hours of dawn during REM sleep, and a memory of this type of dream almost always remains the following day.
13. Bruxism, which is the habit of moving and grinding one's teeth. It is most common among children between 7 and 10 years of age. It rarely continues beyond adolescence, except in association with stress or obstructive sleep apnea.

Sources

Curzi-Dascalova L, Challamel M-J. Neurophysiologic basis of sleep development. In: Loughlin GM, Caroll JL, Marcus CL, editors. Sleep and breathing in children, a developmental approach. New York: Marcel Dekker; 2000. p. 3–37.

Anders TF, Keener M. Developmental course of nighttime sleep–wake patterns in full-term and premature infants during the first year of life. Sleep. 1985;8:173–92.

Drake C, Nickel C, Burduvali E, Roth T, Jefferson C, Pietro B. The pediatric daytime sleepiness scale (PDSS): sleep habits and school outcomes in middle-school children. Sleep. 2003;26(4):455–8.

Espezel H, Jan JE, O'Donnell ME, Milner R. The use of melatonin to treat sleep wake–rhythm disorders in children who are visually impaired. J Vis Impair Blind. 1996;90:43–50.

Fallone G, Owens JA, Deane J. Sleepiness in children and adolescents: clinical implications. Sleep Med Rev. 2002;6(4):287–306.

Franco P, Kato I, Richardson HL, Yang JS, Montemitro E, Horne RS. Arousal from sleep mechanisms in infants. Sleep Med. 2010;11:603–14.

Fricke-Oerkermann L, Pluck J, Schredl M, Heinz K, Mitschke A, Wiater A, Lehmkuhl G. Prevalence and course of sleep problems in childhood. Sleep. 2007;30(10):1371–7.

Geva R, Yaron H, Kuint J. Neonatal sleep predicts attention orienting and distractibility. J Atten Disord. 2016;20(2):138–50.

Herlenius E. An inflammatory pathway to apnea and autonomic dysregulation. Resp Physiol Neurobiol. 2011;178:449–57.

Husain AM. Review of neonatal EEG. Am J End Technol. 2005;45:12–35.

Loewy J, Steart K, Dassler AM, Telsey A, Homel P. The effects of music therapy on vital signs, feeding, and sleep in premature infants. Pediatrics. 2013;131:902–18.

Martin RJ, Abu Shaweesh JM, Baird TM. Apnea of prematurity. Paediatr Respir Rev. 2004;5(Suppl 1):S377–82.

Mindell JA, Bartle A, Ahn Y, Ramamurthy MB, Huong HT, Kohyama J, Li AM, Ruangdaraganon N, Sekartini R, Teng A, Goh DY. Sleep education in pediatric residency programs: a cross-cultural look. BMC Res Notes. 2013;6:130.

Prechtl H. F. (1985). Ultrasound studies of human fetal behaviour. Early. Hum. Dev. 12 91–98 10.1016/0378-3782(85)90173-2.

Sadeh A. Maturation of normal sleep pattern from childhood through adolescence. In: Loughlin GM, Caroll JL, Marcus CL, editors. Sleep and breathing in children, a developmental approach. New York: Marcel Dekker; 2000. p. 3–37.

Tzischinsky O, Shlitner A, Lavie P. The association between the nocturnal sleep gate and nocturnal onset of urinary 6-sulfatoxymelatonin. J Biol Rhythm. 1993;8:199–209.

Zhao J, Gonzalez F, Mu D. Apnea of prematurity: from cause to treatment. Eur J Pediatr. 2011;170:1097–105.

Immunological Defense Mechanisms of the Respiratory System

6

Arturo Borzutzky Schachter
and Pamela Morales Matamala

Contents

Organization of the Respiratory Immune System

The lung can be divided into two functional areas: the airways and the lung parenchyma. In each of these areas there are different cellular populations that take part in the immune response.

In the airway, which is the conduit area, the epithelium is mainly composed of hair cells and secretory (goblet) cells, which, together with secretory immunoglobulin A (sIgA) produced locally, provoke mucociliary elimination of inhaled antigens. In the mucosa there are macrophages, dendritic cells, plasma cells, and T lymphocytes, which are explained in more detail in later sections of this chapter. In the airway there are resident dendritic cells that specialize in immune monitoring similarly to what happens in the gastrointestinal tract. Epithelial T lymphocytes in the mucosa are mainly T CD8+ lymphocytes, and the T lymphocytes in the lamina propria are T CD4+ lymphocytes. The predominant cellular population in the lamina propria consists of mastocytes and plasma cells, which secrete IgA. In the airway mucosa there are also areas of lymphoid tissue, associated with the bronchus, which is similar to amygdalar tissue and Peyer's patches in the intestine. This tissue is considered to play an important role during childhood, characterized by great

A. Borzutzky Schachter (✉) · P. Morales Matamala
Department of Pediatrics School of Medicine,
Pontificia Universidad Católica de Chile,
Santiago, Chile
e-mail: arturobor@med.puc.cl

P. Bertrand, I. Sánchez (eds.), *Pediatric Respiratory Diseases*,
https://doi.org/10.1007/978-3-030-26961-6_6

immune activity, before reducing its function and devolving during adulthood. These zones of lymphoid tissue associated with mucosa are located mainly in the nasal mucosa (nasal-associated lymphoid tissue (NALT)) and in the bronchial mucosa (bronchus-associated lymphoid tissue (BALT)). In contrast to the lymph nodes, this tissue is not encapsulated and does not have afferent lymph vessels. It is in direct contact with the epithelial mucosa and reacts to antigens that cross the epithelial barrier. Given its location, it can respond quickly to upper and lower respiratory tract infections.

In the lung parenchyma, where gas exchange occurs, 90% of the cellular population of the alveoli corresponds to alveolar macrophages. There are also small populations of T lymphocytes, B lymphocytes, and dendritic cells, but there are no plasma cells as there are in the airway. In the lung parenchyma vascular bed there is a large population of T lymphocytes, many of which are anergic, and their contribution to the defense and regulation of lung immunity is still unclear. This anergic cellular immunity might contribute to a decrease in the local inflammatory response, decreasing possible tissue damage in the event of activation caused by antigens.

Immune Induction in the Lung

The respiratory mucosa, especially in the upper airway, is constantly exposed to nonpathogenic environmental antigens, including various vegetable and animal proteins. It is essential for the respiratory system to be inert against nonpathogenic antigens, otherwise it would collapse in a continuous inflammatory process. As a mucosal protection mechanism, it constantly activates a tolerogenic response, apart from a low-grade type 2 helper T cell (T_h2) response, to stop activation of the T_h1 inflammatory response. This discrimination of cellular responses is permanently regulated by the local dendritic cells. The inhibitory response of the airway is reinforced by the inhibitory activity of the alveolar macrophages.

Innate Immunity

As in other systems covered in epithelium, the first line of defense in the respiratory system is composed of epithelial cells of the airway.

Innate immunity responds to two kinds of stimuli: molecules derived from exogenous microorganisms and molecules produced as a result of tissue damage.

There are receptors that specifically recognize a narrow variety of molecular patterns, called pattern recognition receptors (PRRs). These are classified according to the types of molecule they recognize.

Pathogen-Associated Molecular Patterns We know that pathogenic molecules derived from viruses and bacteria are recognized by PRRs. Among these molecules are lipopeptides, liposaccharides, viral RNA, viral DNA, and flagellin.

Damage-Associated Molecular Patterns Several molecules associated with tissue damage can activate PRRs. Among these are proteins, transcription factors, RNA, DNA, matrix components (hyaluronic acid and fibronectin), and fibrinogen.

Tissue Damage and Recognition of Infection Recognition patterns are coded in the toll-like receptors (TLRs) expressed on the surfaces of cells and vesicles, and in intracytoplasmic nucleotide-binding oligomerization domain (NOD)–like receptors (NLRs). Also, retinoic acid receptors induced by NRA helicase (retinoic acid–inducible gene I (RIG-I)–like helicase (RLH)) have been described, among other receptors.

Each of these receptors can detect different molecules. There are 10 types of TLR, 20 types of NLR, and one type of RLH.

Toll-Like Receptors These can be divided into those that have an antibacterial response (TLR1, TLR2, TLR4, TLR5, TLR6, and TLR9) and those that have an antiviral response (TLR3, TLR7, and TLR8), although some viral proteins activate TLR4. The most-studied receptors are TLR2 and

Table 6.1 Innate immune receptors and ligands in respiratory system cells

Receptor	Ligands
TLR1	Bacterial lipoproteins
TLR2	Lipopeptides, lipoteichoic acid
TLR3	Double-stranded RNA
TLR4	Lipopolysaccharides
TLR5	Flagellin
TLR6	Lipopeptides
TLR7/TLR8	Imidazoquinolines, single-stranded RNA
TLR9	Unmethylated CpG DNA
TLR10	Unknown
NOD-like receptor	Ligands
NOD1, NOD2	Peptidoglycan derivatives

NOD nucleotide-binding oligomerization domain, *TLR* toll-like receptor

TLR4, and it is widely known that they respond to the molecules of the bacterial wall (lipopeptides and lipopolysaccharides). TLR4 responds mainly to lipopolysaccharides present in Gram-negative bacteria, pathogen-associated molecular patterns (PAMPs) such as pneumolysin in *Streptococcus pneumoniae*, and the proteins of respiratory syncytial virus (RSV). TLR2 is heterodimerized with TLR1 and TLR6, and recognizes lipoproteins and lipoteichoic acid in Gram-positive bacteria. TLR5 recognizes flagellin in *Legionella pneumophila*, *Pseudomonas aeruginosa*, and *Klebsiella* spp. TLRs can distinguish between human and bacterial DNA (Table 6.1).

NOD-Like Receptors Twenty types of these receptors have been identified. They are involved in detection of bacterial pathogens. Two NLR types—NOD1 and NOD2—recognize bacterial peptidoglycan from Gram-positive bacteria and activate nuclear factor (NF)-κB, which generates an increase in interleukin (IL)-1. This is an important way of controlling intracellular bacteria such as *L. pneumophila*.

Many types of cell participate in the innate immune response of the respiratory system.

Epithelial Cells Type 2 alveolar cells express TL2 and TL4, contributing to the response to lipopolysaccharides and bacterial peptidoglycans.

The epithelial cells of the airway express TLR1–TLR10, and their stimulation increases the production of various proinflammatory cytokines.

Neutrophils Neutrophils are recruited rapidly by the production of proinflammatory mediators such as B4 leukotriene, C5a, and IL-8. Pathogens are then phagocytized. Neutrophils have a short half-life; after their apoptosis, they trigger an anti-inflammatory response and restore the normal architecture of the epithelium.

Macrophages and Monocytes There are macrophages in the interstice and the alveolus. Alveolar macrophages are located in the surfactant in the air–lung tissue interface, and this location allows them to be the first barrier of defense against inhaled pathogens and environmental toxins. They are involved in phagocytic activity, starting an inflammatory cascade and participating as antigen-presenting cells before being replaced by monocytes.

Dendritic Cells Dendritic cells play a fundamental role in the interface between the innate immune response and the adaptive immune response. They have the ability to capture antigens and, through damage-associated molecular pattern (DAMP) stimulation, they migrate toward the lymph node and present the antigens to activate T cells.

Adaptive Immunity

For many years, our understanding of cellular immunity in the lungs has been simplified, divided only into T_h1 and T_h2 responses; however, it is now understood that there are other kinds of cellular response, forming a system that is more diverse and complex. T_h1 immunity (mediated by T CD4+ lymphocytes, which secrete cytokines such as interferon (IFN)-γ, IL-6, and IL-12) is fundamental in defense against environmental pathogens, both bacterial and viral. In particular, it plays a fundamental role in defense against intracellular bacteria such as *Mycobacterium tuberculosis*. The T_h2 response is mediated by T CD4 lymphocytes, which secrete mainly IL-4, IL-5, and IL-13. Its main function is defense against helminths, but it also takes part in defense against viral pathogens and in immune system regulation. T_h2 immunity is possibly better known for its pathogenic role; it is central to generation of allergic responses mediated by IgE, which can trigger asthma and allergic rhinitis, as in excessive immune responses to some respiratory viruses such as RSV.

Our understanding of the T_h1–T_h2 balance has been modified since the discovery of the T_h17 immune response, which is essential for defense against extracellular bacteria and plays an important role in diverse inflammatory illnesses. Differentiation of T lymphocytes into T_h17 lymphocytes is provoked by the combination of IL-6, IL-1β, and IL-23. Once the response has been activated, large amounts of IL-17 are produced. This cytokine participates in the mobilization of neutrophils and plays an essential role in the elimination of pathogens in the airway. It has been observed that there is an inhibitory interaction between the different responses: T_h1 cytokines inhibit T_h2 and T_h17 responses, and T_h2 cytokines inhibit T_h1 and T_h17 responses. The inflammatory response provoked by T_h17 can participate in the pathogenesis of bronchial asthma. There is a relationship between the production of T_h17 cells and regulator T cells; when T cell production is inhibited by IL-6, the differentiation into T_h17 increases. Once the levels of proinflammatory cytokines increase, the regulator T cell population starts to grow to re-establish the basal state.

Regulatory T lymphocytes (Tregs) play a fundamental role in the regulation of the peripheral immune response of T lymphocytes; other mediators also participate: IL-10, transforming growth factor (TGF)-β, and nitrous oxide. Tregs have a fundamental function in the regular postviral inflammatory response (helping to avoid sequelae of postviral infections) and in modulation of tolerance of aeroallergens to avoid allergic illnesses.

Immune Responses to Respiratory Infections

Infection of the respiratory system initiates a cascade of events that end in activation of the cellular immune response in the lung (Fig. 6.1). The initial respiratory infection provokes the production of inflammatory mediators in the epithelial cells, which activate the innate immune system. The dendritic cells of the upper airway detect the presence of pathogens via TLRs. The combination of the presence of proinflammatory mediators and the activation of dendritic cells increases the expression of type I and type II major histocompatibility complex, initiating the production of costimulatory molecules and cytokines required for induction of the response mediated by T cells. The dendritic cells migrate to the lymph nodes and activate virgin or naïve T cells, initiating the adaptive immune response. When the virgin T CD4+ and CD8+ lymphocytes activate, these present clonal expansion and differentiation from effector T lymphocytes into some helper T cell types (T_h1, T_h2, or T_h17), depending on the cytokine environment at the moment of activation. The T cells present three antiviral action mechanisms: (1) lithic mechanisms associated with T CD8+ lymphocytes, which provoke the lysis of infected cells; (2) induction by T cells of tumor necrosis factor (TNF) in the infected cells, causing their apoptosis; and (3) production of proinflammatory factors by cells that attract other cells of the immune system.

It has been observed that in influenza virus infection, the cytolytic response of the T CD8+ lymphocytes is very important, and they also contribute to viral elimination and recovery. In viral infections, T CD8+ lymphocytes produce IL-10, which takes part in the regulation of the immune response, and they also produce IFN-γ. The production of these two cytokines decreases when viral clearance occurs. For production of IL-10 to occur in the lung tissue, IL-2 (produced by T CD4+ lymphocytes) and IL-27 (produced by mononuclear cells and neutrophils) must be present. Some viruses such as RSV trigger an

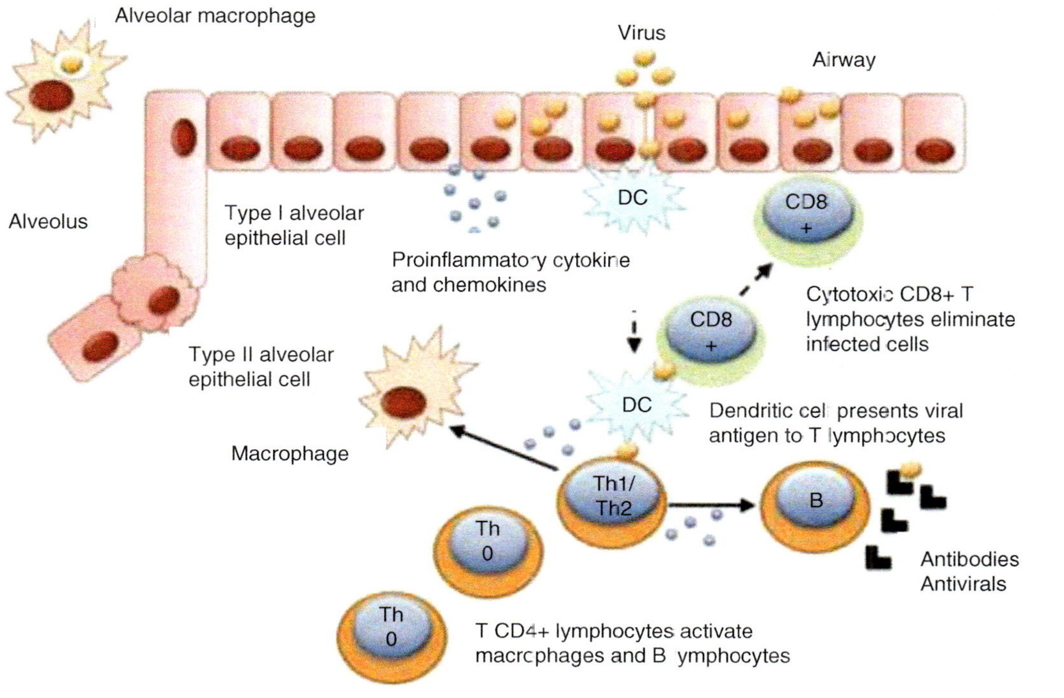

Fig. 6.1 Activation of the cellular immune response in the airway

exacerbated T_h2-type response, which can trigger bronchial hyperreactivity and eventually lead to development of bronchial asthma. This T_h2 response is mediated not only by T CD4+ lymphocytes but also by T_h2 cytokines such as IL-13, which can be secreted by innate type 2 lymphoid cells and by natural killer T cells (NKTs). In addition to the regulation mediated by CD4+ and CD8+ T lymphocytes, the modulation of the immune response involves the participation of Tregs (which produce thousands of regulatory interleukins such as IL-10 and TGF-β1) and expression of inhibitory molecules such as cytotoxic T-lymphocyte-associated protein (CTLA)-4.

Regarding bacterial infections, which normally occur after viral infections as superinfections, the first line of defense is generally composed of alveolar macrophages, which are capable of limiting the spread of the bacterial infection and orchestrating the recruitment and activation of other immune cells to control bacterial growth. In the case of extracellular bacteria such as *S. pneumoniae*, an inflammatory response is triggered, mediated mainly by massive infiltration of neutrophils and, secondarily, by a late response of the adaptive immunity normally orchestrated by T_h1 and T_h17 cells, in turn activating macrophages and B lymphocytes, which produce specific antibodies against the invading microorganism.

Immunology of Acute Alveolar Damage and Tissue Repair

Acute alveolar damage can originate from multiple causes such as trauma, infections, allergies, cancer, and chemical injury. When there is damage, an inflammatory cascade is generated in the lung, and if there an imbalance in this cascade, an exacerbated inflammatory response occurs, which provokes increased injury and exacerbates the illness. This is mainly due to deregulation in the recruitment of leukocytes and to their exaggerated activation, with inappropriate expression of proinflammatory cytokines and lipid mediators, and uncontrolled activation of platelets and the coagulation cascade. All of this is initiated and perpetuated by the presence of antigens, which activate the innate immunity receptors in the alveolar epithelium. The hypoxia that is generated, which is secondary to the acute alveolar damage, is also proinflammatory and contributes to the production of greater epithelial and endothelial damage.

After episodes of acute injury comes tissue repair, in which immune elements also participate. This process is essential for epithelial integrity and lung homeostasis. After lung injury, repairing factors are liberated, including epidermal and fibroblast growth factors, cytokines, and prostaglandins, which coordinate the repair process through matrix proteins, metalloproteinases, and integrins. An important role of Tregs is that they decrease fibrosis in the repair; TNF-α reduces cellular proliferation after the injury and alveolar macrophages attenuate alveolar damage, secreting an IL-1 receptor antagonist. However, exacerbated tissue repair can contribute to pathologies such as lung fibrosis and asthma.

The Microbiome

For many years it was thought that lung tissue was sterile. However, research in recent years has shown that a bacterial population is present, which consists of the respiratory microbiome; the presence of viruses and fungi is still being studied. The microbiome is defined by the presence of microorganisms organized at a particular time and in a specific location. The microbiome in the airway mucosa is separated from the host by the epithelium, as is also the case in the intestine, skin, and genitourinary system.

Lungs in healthy humans without infections have been tested, and the following populations have been identified through molecular biology: Proteobacteria, Firmicutes, Bacteroidetes, and Actinobacteria. This microbiome differs from the one found in the upper airways, where *Streptococcus*, *Prevotella*, *Fusobacterium*, and *Veillonella* can be found, with small populations of *Haemophilus* and *Neisseria*. The presence of these bacteria in small numbers in asymptomatic patients has no significant clinical implications.

The microbiome is considered symbiotic and is associated with cell growth; tissue repair after injury; maintenance of barrier function; and induction, development, and modulation of the immune response. Quantitative alterations in the microbiome of the airway have been described, such as obstructive lung diseases, asthma, and cystic fibrosis. A potential therapeutic mechanism is administration of probiotic supplements. However, more studies are necessary for us to completely understand the role of the airway and lung parenchyma microbiomes in the immune homeostasis of these organs.

Sources

Beck JM. ABCs of the lung microbiome. Ann Am Thorac Soc. 2014;11 Suppl 1:S3–6.

Braciale TJ, Sun J, Kim TS. Regulating the adaptive immune response to respiratory virus infection. Nat Rev Immunol. 2012;12(4):295–305.

Crosby LM, Waters CM. Epithelial repair mechanisms in the lung. Am J Physiol Lung Cell Mol Physiol. 2010;298(6):L715–31.

Chaudhuri N, Sabroe I. Basic science of the innate immune system and the lung. Paediatr Respir Rev. 2008;9(4):236–42.

Heier I, Malmstrom K, Pelkonen AS, et al. Bronchial response pattern of antigen presenting cells and regulatory T cells in children less than 2 years of age. Thorax. 2008;63(8):703–9.

Herold S, Gabrielli NM, Vadasz I. Novel concepts of acute lung injury and alveolar–capillary barrier dysfunction. Am J Physiol Lung Cell Mol Physiol. 2013;305(10):L665–81.

Holt PG, Strickland DH, Wikstrom ME, Jahnsen FL. Regulation of immunological homeostasis in the respiratory tract. Nat Rev Immunol. 2008;8(2):142–52.

Kim EY, Battaile JT, Patel AC, et al. Persistent activation of an innate immune response translates respiratory viral infection into chronic lung disease. Nat Med. 2008;14(6):633–40.

Lukacs NW, Moore ML, Rudd BD, et al. Differential immune responses and pulmonary pathophysiology are induced by two different strains of respiratory syncytial virus. Am J Pathol. 2006;169(3):977–86.

Neish AS. Mucosal immunity and the microbiome. Ann Am Thorac Soc. 2014;11 Suppl 1:S28–32.

Strickland DH, Thepen T, Kees UR, Kraal G, Holt PG. Regulation of T-cell function in lung tissue by pulmonary alveolar macrophages. Immunology. 1993;80(2):266–72.

Suzuki T, Chow CW, Downey GP. Role of innate immune cells and their products in lung immunopathology. Int J Biochem Cell Biol. 2008;40(6–7):1348–61.

Woodland DL, Randall TD. Anatomical features of antiviral immunity in the respiratory tract. Semin Immunol. 2004;16(3):163–70.

New Frontiers in Research on the Respiratory System

7

Andrew Bush and Luis Enrique Vega-Briceño

Contents

A. Bush (✉)
Faculty of Medicine, Imperial College of London, London, UK
e-mail: a.bush@imperial.ac.uk

L. E. Vega-Briceño
Faculty of Medicine, Universidad del Desarrollo, Santiago, Chile
e-mail: levega@udd.cl

P. Bertrand, I. Sánchez (eds.), *Pediatric Respiratory Diseases*,
https://doi.org/10.1007/978-3-030-26961-6_7

Cystic Fibrosis as a Model for Dealing with Chronic Lung Disease

The old biomedical paradigm was the diagnosis of cystic fibrosis in a child with chronic lung disease (CLD) and malnutrition. Cystic fibrosis is increasingly being diagnosed by neonatal screening based on blood samples taken by heel puncture or from cord blood. There are different protocols for this, which are dependent on combinations of immunoreactive trypsin (IRT), pancreatic polypeptide, and polymerase chain reaction (PCR) for several cystic fibrosis genes. All early detection programs for cystic fibrosis have the following characteristics in common: they detect the majority of newborns with this disease, but they also do not detect the disease in a small minority of newborns who may even have severe phenotypes.

There is a guiding consensus on handling of cystic fibrosis that has been identified early through neonatal screening. For example, in the randomized, controlled Infant Study of Inhaled Saline (ISIS), preschool children with cystic fibrosis were treated with hypertonic saline solution (HSS), the use of which improved the lung clearance index (LCI). While there are diverse opinions about the prophylactic role of antibiotics for newborns, there is universal concurrence that the use of prophylactic cephalosporin is contraindicated owing to the greater risk of infection by *Pseudomonas aeruginosa*, although the role of prophylactic flucloxacillin remains a matter of debate. The clinical evolution of these children following diagnosis by screening is even more controversial. AREST-CF (the Australian Respiratory Early Surveillance Team for Cystic Fibrosis) showed that while the nutritional state of these children may be very good, the forced expiratory volume in 0.5 seconds ($FEV_{0.5}$) diminishes over 2 years. In fact, high-resolution computed tomography (HRCT) reveals the presence of bronchiectasis, trapped air, and other abnormal structures at 1 year of age. In contrast, the LCFC (London Cystic Fibrosis Collaboration) showed that the $FEV_{0.5}$ was decreased at the time of diagnosis but was normalized by the age of 1 year and remained normal until subjects were 2 years old. The pulmonary clearance rate decreased throughout the study period, although most of the infants had levels in the normal range. The structural changes detected by HRCT were so minor at 1 year of age that they could not be assessed in a reproducible manner using the Brodie score. As in the AREST-CF study group, the nutritional condition of the subjects remained normal throughout the study.

There are consequences of early neonatal detection and favorable clinical evolution. Firstly, it is important to consider the possibility that there are children with late-manifestation cystic fibrosis (without pancreatic disease) and other atypical forms. Secondly, we are diagnosing a "new" generation of cystic fibrosis patients who have never been sick and who increasingly see themselves as persons with non-neonatal detection, which can have implications for their subsequent treatment. It is increasingly necessary to adapt treatment and protocols to attend to persons who are healthy, not sick, changing the therapeutic load without risking the loss of benefits provided by the aggressive therapy of the past. We need to explore innovative modes of attention, including telemedicine. Finally, the good results reported by the LCFC group imply that the number of patients (small children) needed for randomized, controlled clinical trials would be prohibitively large, and such trials would be virtually impossible. It is probable that clinical trial that evaluate new therapies have to be postponed until after the patient is 2 years old, which is a critical time in terms of pulmonary development. The variables of clinical trials will be increasingly more difficult to establish even with older children.

The implications in terms of treatment indicate that the old paradigm was "reactive" and responded to the complications of cystic fibrosis. The new paradigm begins with novel treatment strategies for the current objectives—management of infection, inflammation, and mucus clearance—as well as "modern" prescriptions for novel objectives (perhaps the most interesting of all). A last aspect is the greater risk of toxicity or the adverse effects of using medications in the context of increased longevity.

Novel Strategies for Current Objectives

These include the development of new mucolytic agents, antibiotics, and delivery devices. Inhaled mannitol is defined as auxiliary in mucus clearance in patients with cystic fibrosis for whom suppression subtractive hybridization (SSH) and DNase are not effective, although the need to inhale multiple capsules could limit adherence to its use. New nebulized antibiotics include liposomal amikacin and ciprofloxacin. The use of nebulized amikacin poses a dilemma. It is so useful for treating atopic infection by mycobacterium that there is a strong argument in favor of limiting its use to this indication. On the other hand, there are commercial considerations that argue for its availability for treating airway infections by *P. aeruginosa*, arguing that its use once a day (or perhaps once a week) would be beneficial for many patients with cystic fibrosis. This dilemma has not yet been resolved.

Nebulized therapy has historically not been used that extensively. Although there are powder forms of tobramycin and colomycin, it has been shown that they are not superior to traditional nebulized formulations. The technology of nebulized medications has greatly reduced the time required to administer drugs. The most interesting development in relation to cystic fibrosis has been initiatives to treat the consequences of CFTR mutation, thus attacking the fundamental disease instead of waiting for clinical manifestation of the problem.

Gene Therapy

This is the simplest of treatments in conceptual terms: a defective gene is replaced by a normal gene and the cystic fibrosis is cured (or at least decreased) independently of the mutation. There have been numerous studies with single or multiple doses and using a variety of vectors, including an adenovirus, adeno-associated viruses, liposomes, and nanoparticles. These studies have focused on determining whether gene transfer is feasible rather than on the clinical benefits for patients. Two issues are the optimal vector and variables to employ. A recent double-blind, randomized trial included 130 patients who received 12 monthly doses of a nebulized gene–liposomal complex or a saline solution placebo at 0.9%. The first response to evaluate is the relative change in the FEV_1, with responses of secondary efficacy in the LCI, on HRCT, and on the Cystic Fibrosis Questionnaire—Revised (CFQ-R). Subgroups have been submitted to more detailed molecular and physiological studies of the nose and lower airway. The results promise to be interesting. Another even more sophisticated strategy is repair of the abnormal CFTR gene. It should be remembered that gene repair is a normal physiological process. At present, gene manipulation with appropriate primers is still in the future.

Small Molecules

Genetic mutations in cystic fibrosis can be divided into six classes (Table 7.1). Increasing attention has been directed at specific therapies for small-molecule mutations. This has been spurred by multimillion-dollar investments by the US-based Cystic Fibrosis Foundation in high-yield robotic detection to discover novel compounds. In fact, the first of these treatments comes from the observation that aminoglycosides can inhibit premature detention codons (class 1 mutations) without interfering with natural detention codons, leading to the formation of functional CFTR. This was followed by testing of the orally active compound PTC_{124} (Ataluren™), which has proved to be effective for other genetic conditions (for example, the rat model of Duchenne muscular dystrophy). Phase 2 studies showed very diverse effects in different populations, attributed to the probability of different effects of messenger RNA decay, mediated by "nonsense" sequences or the position or nature of "early termination" codons. A phase 3 trial did not meet the primary response for the group as a whole, but in an analysis of planned subgroups of patients who did not use nebulized tobramycin, the FEV_1 was significantly higher than that of patients who received the placebo. The argument

Table 7.1 Types of CFTR mutations, their consequences, and potential treatments

Type and consequences	Examples of mutations	Potential therapies
1. No CFTR synthesis	G542X, W1282X, R553X, 3950delT	PTC_{124}
2. Abnormal CFTR retained in the endoplasmic reticulum and damaged	ΔF508	VX-809 VX-700 Other
3. CFTR reaches the cell membrane but does not open correctly	G551D, 9 other known gating mutations	VX-770
4. CFTR reaches the cell membrane but the channel properties are abnormal	R1117H, R334W	VX-770
5. Decreased CFTR synthesis	3120+1G>A	
6. Unstable CFTR in the cell membrane (rapid replacement)	N287Y, 120del23, 4326delTC, 4279insA	

is that those who used tobramycin could have received the benefit of inhibition of "early stop" codons. New clinical trials of better compounds will probably be developed in the future.

The most dramatic molecular success has been observed with VX-770 (ivacaftor; Kalydeco) for class 3 mutations. It was approved initially for the mutation G551D, and its approval was then broadened to include eight of another nine known class 3 mutations. A large-scale, double-blind, randomized, placebo-controlled trial was conducted in children aged over 12 years and adults with at least one G551D mutation. The study showed an improvement of absolute FEV_1 of 12% with concomitant improvements in weight and quality of life associated with cystic fibrosis, as well as in the timing of the first pulmonary exacerbation. Surprisingly, the chloride level in sweat fell by close to 50% toward the doubtful diagnostic range (60–80 mEq/l). Other studies have subsequently shown similar benefits in children 6–11 years old and in children with a normal FEV_1 (≥90% of the predicted value). There is currently a tendency to broaden the use of VX-770 to prevent pathological complications in very small children. Other proposed indications include the class 4 mutation R117H, the channel conductance of which decreases by 20%, with a 75% reduction in the probability of channel opening. The high cost of this medication is questionable, given the slight mutation, never mind the fact that patients effectively lose a significant level of pulmonary function in adult life. Theoretically, VX-770 can also be used to strengthen class 5 mutations and to "rescue" DF508, which has a residual gate defect.

VX-809 (lumacaftor) has been studied in class 2 mutations—in particular, DF508. These studies have shown small improvements in chloride levels in sweat, but when lumacaftor is combined with ivacaftor, the changes are less notable than those seen with VX-770, and it is improbable that VX-809, used by itself or in association with VX-770, serves to undo the dysfunction of the residual damper of "recovered" CFTR DF508 and is sufficient to provide real clinical benefit. This is because CFTR folding has multiple phases. Formation of functional CFTR requires contact between the domains and cotranslational and post-translational folding. Consequently, it is likely that more than one compound is required to correct class 2 mutations. Small-molecule therapy for DF508 is currently being developed.

Introduction to Complex Mutations

The problem of correcting class 3 mutations has been resolved easily, but a more sophisticated strategy could be required for other more complex anomalies. One model is that CFTR function can be described as an equation: CTFR function = (quantity of CFTR) × (probability of opening) × (protein conductance). Hypothetically, independently of the mutation, VX-770 can be used to improve the probability of opening and possibly conductance, while specific strategies are required to raise the quantities of CFTR in the epithelium. A new era of specific and multiple molecular manipulations has begun. The effects of VX-770 on sweat chloride are notable, although it is not clear if this finding is significant. There is only a weak correlation between sweat chloride and change in pulmonary function. We know that the sweat test provides one of the best diagnoses in medicine, but this does not mean that chloride transport is related to chronic lung disease. In fact, there are reasons to suppose that it is not.

A major challenge for the community with cystic fibrosis is control of the costs of these new molecules. VX-770 currently costs US$330,000 per patient per year. It is not clear how it has become so expensive. It is calculated that use of VX-770 raises the cost of treating cystic fibrosis in the UK by 50%, driven by the 5% of the population with this disease. If patients need to take two or more newly discovered molecules, the cost can be frightening. There are no easy answers. Without public and private investment, these medications would not have been discovered, no country anywhere in the world—whatever its political system is—has unlimited resources for health care.

The Challenge: How Can We Know It Works?

In the past, mortality was an inevitable outcome of cystic fibrosis. Subsequently, improvements in the FEV_1 were accepted as a reasonable substitute for mortality, although the relationship between the FEV_1 and mortality is increasingly uncertain. However, the FEV_1 is currently so good and the decline curves are so flat that measurement is becoming less useful as a variable for clinical assessment. The US CF Gene Therapy Consortium has used an innovative strategy to address this problem on the basis of the observation that substitute markers improved during an intervention with demonstrated efficacy (intravenous antibiotics) for pulmonary exacerbations in 44 cystic fibrosis patients. The improvements were evidenced by symptoms, the FEV_1, the LCI, HRCT (showing thickening of the airway wall, air entrapment, and large mucosal buffers) and markers of inflammation in serum (interleukin (IL)-6, C-reactive protein (CRP), and calprotectin). However, what can be considered more direct measures of airway inflammation (sputum and mucus rheology, exhalation condensate) have not changed. The study would have been more important if it had been considered ethical to recruit a control group to establish the natural variability among the events in these measurements.

The Problem: Delicate Secondary Effects Associated with Longevity

Historically, cystic fibrosis was a childhood disease, with patients rarely surviving into adulthood. Consequently, the long-term toxicity of medications did not need to be balanced against their short-term benefits. However, patients now have life expectancies of several decades, and so it is necessary to consider the question of long-term accumulation of toxicity.

Selection of Resistant Organisms

The use of antibiotics has provided major benefits for cystic fibrosis patients, but there has been a cost in terms of selecting new organisms and selecting for antibiotic resistance in organisms that are known and common in this disease. A study compared a historical cohort of 520 patients with a comparable contemporary cohort and found an increase in *P. aeruginosa* resistant to tobramycin, amikacin, and other drugs, and a higher percentage of isolation of methicillin-resistant *Staphylococcus aureus* (MRSA), *Stenotrophomonas maltophilia*, and *Achromobacter*. It is evident that we cannot stop using antibiotics, but this information emphasizes the need for responsible antibiotic management and use.

Allergies to Antibiotics

It is inevitable that the more antibiotics are used, the more allergy to antibiotics becomes a factor. Allergy to antibiotics is common with cystic fibrosis and although desensitization is possible, it must be repeated with each application, which is time consuming and poses potential risks. This is not an argument against the use of antibiotics; rather, it is a reminder that they need to be used responsibly.

Chronic Renal Insufficiency

Chronic renal insufficiency (CRI) has been well described and is usually the consequence of treatment with aminoglycosides indicated at the same time as other nephrotoxic drugs—in particular, nonsteroidal anti-inflammatory drugs—and dehydration owing to excessive sweating or gastroenteritis. Nevertheless, CRI is a growing problem. The cause is controversial. One study has pointed to the glomerular filtration rate (GFR) with respect to the number of intravenous antibiotic treatments received (in some cases, >100). Another study identified nebulized aminoglycosides, and a third study found that the GFR is higher in persons who require insulin. Whatever the explanation is, it is clear that a medication that is administered for many decades needs to be carefully monitored.

Cystic fibrosis has set the pattern in this changing paradigm, but other diseases will certainly follow. For example, it is probable that primary ciliary dyskinesia (PCD) is on the cusp of similar advances, considering the rapid expansion of knowledge of multiple genetic mutations that cause diseases and their consequences, for example, such as nonsense mutations that can be sensitive to PTC_{124}. It is clear that we need to expand our therapeutic horizons in the coming years. The challenge is to overlook therapies without losing the benefits of the aggressive regimens that have accomplished so much to improve the prognosis of cystic fibrosis in the past. There is a real danger of complacency; in the case of children who have been diagnosed but have never been sick, it can be difficult to get them to adhere to treatment, which could be especially important if unexpected complications emerge. We need to maintain clarity between the double risk of imposing a large therapeutic load on persons who are asymptomatic but have this disease and thinking that the problem of cystic fibrosis is resolved.

Chronic Lung Disease Crises or Attacks: Lessons for a Long-Term Response

"Exacerbation" is a not-very-convincing term that describes acute deterioration in the symptoms of a chronic lung disease. The definition is often circular: "I know this is an exacerbation because I have received treatment (prednisone for asthma, intravenous antibiotics for cystic fibrosis), and I have received this treatment because it is an exacerbation." The term "exacerbation" implies something relatively benign—a minor inconvenience that is completely reversible. The purpose of the following section is to suggest that this is an error and that the term "pulmonary attack" is preferable. A pulmonary attack is an emergency that could lead to irreparable harm and must therefore be addressed, necessitating a response focused on determination of the cause and measures to prevent it from occurring again.

Pulmonary Attacks in Cystic Fibrosis

These are common (so-called pulmonary exacerbations—a term that will not be employed here) and have been used increasingly in randomized, controlled therapeutic trials. In fact, in a study of airway clearance in cystic fibrosis, positive pressure techniques were superior to external oscillation of the thoracic wall in decreasing pulmonary attacks, but there was no change in spirometry findings. Pulmonary attacks in the context of cystic fibrosis are far from benign.

Several studies have concluded that these patients cannot recover a basal spirometry level after completing adequate treatment in response to a pulmonary attack. Another study showed that at 3 months after treatment, 24 of 104 cystic fibrosis patients (23.1%) had not recovered even 95% of their maximum FEV_1 from 6 months earlier. Pulmonary attacks in cystic fibrosis are associated with a more rapid rate of FEV_1 reduction. A study of 8490 patients from the Cystic Fibrosis Foundation Patient Registry reported that 60% had no exacerbations, 23% had one per year, 10% had two per year, and 7% had at least three per year. Even one exacerbation per year in children is associated with accelerated rates of FEV_1 decline, while in adults, accelerated decline is observed only in those with at least three exacerbations per year.

Pulmonary attacks with cystic fibrosis are associated with a higher rate of mortality. In a three-year prospective cohort study involving 446 adult patients, 140 subjects had one exacerbation per year at most, 160 had one or two exacerbations per year, and 146 had more than two exacerbations per year. In this work, the exacerbations were defined as an indication for oral or intravenous antibiotics. There was a higher probability of more frequent exacerbations in women, individuals with low pulmonary function, and diabetics. Individuals with more than two exacerbations per year had a higher probability of having a reduction of more than 5% per year in the FEV_1 and a higher probability of death or of receiving a transplant.

Not surprisingly, those with a high risk of not achieving a complete recovery had a more pronounced decline in the FEV_1, with respect to the baseline value, during the exacerbation, which provides more evidence of inflammation (a higher CRP level at the time of hospitalization and a higher white blood cell count at the end of treatment). However, the absence of these risk factors should not be considered satisfactory. Given the evidence above, are we making optimal use of conventional treatments? For example, would use of more antibiotics be more helpful than intensive use of anti-inflammatories? In terms of the duration of treatment with antibiotics, there is no evidence to guide the doctor. However, in a study that was an extension of work on antibiotics, which analyzed the evolution of spirometry in 95 cystic fibrosis patients who had received antibiotics intravenously for at least 4 days (mean 12.6 days, median 13, standard deviation 3.2), the average time to reach the maximum FEV_1 was 8.7 days and, in practice, everyone reached a FEV_1 peak within 13 days of treatment. These data indicate that 2 weeks of treatment with intravenous antibiotics does not result in an improved response to pulmonary attacks in cystic fibrosis.

There have been several studies on the use of anti-inflammatory medication for short-term treatment of pulmonary attacks in cystic fibrosis. Studies of steroids (prednisolone 2 mg/kg up to a maximum of 60 mg for 5 days and methylprednisolone in pulses) indicate that the benefits do not exceed the potential secondary effects. An initial trial of DNase (which has certain putative anti-inflammatory effects) showed no benefits of application during exacerbation.

There is a tacit supposition that pulmonary attacks in cystic fibrosis involve a general change rather than a focused change. This notion has been challenged by a recent report featuring fluorodeoxyglucose–positron emission tomography (FDG-PET), which detected inflammation and infection, and HRCT in 20 cystic fibrosis patients 14–54 years of age. FDG-PET showed active focal spots, which were more pronounced during pulmonary attacks in cystic fibrosis and, in contrast to the HRCT findings, the changes were sensitive to intravenous antibiotics, at least in this study. We may need biomarkers of local signals of the disease. Unfortunately, the level of exposure to radiation with the current technique is prohibitively high.

Pulmonary Attacks in Asthma

There is less evidence of long-term effects of pulmonary attacks in children with asthma. Asthma attacks are significant causes of morbidity and a reduction in the quality of life. Observational studies suggest that exacerbations are associated at some level with a more rapid decline in spirometry readings, but it is not clear if this is related to low adherence associated with exacerbations independent of the accelerated decline in lung function, due possibly to nonuse of medications. In an original study based on a controlled trial, 7165 adults and children with asthma were randomly assigned to receive either a low dose of budesonide or a placebo by inhalation. Despite the large size of the study, only a minority of patients experienced exacerbations (190 in the placebo group and 115 in the budesonide group). There was an accelerated decline in spirometry values among both children and adults who were taking the placebo and experienced an exacerbation, but not in the group that received budesonide (−2.43% in placebo recipients without exacerbations versus −6.44% in placebo recipients with exacerbations, $p < 0.001$; and −1.72% in budesonide recipients without exacerbations versus −2.48% in budesonide recipients with exacerbations, p value not significant). This study did not establish whether the exacerbations caused the decline in spirometry values or whether the accelerated decline and the exacerbations were part of an underlying phenotype, but subsequent analysis of the data suggested that budesonide lessened the effects of the exacerbations. Inhaled steroids can have more long-term benefits than has been thought.

It is important to understand that pulmonary attacks in asthma and control of asthma at the basal level should not be treated in a similar manner, even though they can coexist in the same subject; in fact, poor control of asthma is an important risk factor for the development of acute attacks. The new antibiotics appear to be good, particularly for reducing acute infectious attacks, but they have a much smaller effect on basal control of asthma. This might be surprising, considering that acute attacks are almost invariably due to viral infection. Although there are certainly interactions between viral infection and inflammation of the airway by eosinophils, controlling basal eosinophilic inflammation reduces exacerbations, as can be clearly seen with the use of omalizumab to prevent seasonal outbreaks of acute asthma among children returning to school.

Like a heart attack, a pulmonary attack requires a focused response and a detailed assessment to prevent a reoccurrence. Protocols have been recommended for asthma and cystic fibrosis. The general theme in the context of asthma has been To achieve what it is suggested by the guidelines. We use a detailed protocol with a nursing guide indicating that in at least half of the patients with severe asthma, we need to consider adherence to medication (including use of the appropriate drug and correct use of the device employed), the environment (allergens and exposure to cigarette smoke), and educational as well as psychological problems. We need to understand that pulmonary attacks are not benign, and we also need to focus on other diseases (PCD and bronchiectasis) and work to prevent their recurrence. An important scientific focus is the mechanisms of pulmonary attacks in the different diseases and factors for prediction and optimal management.

Genetically Associated Diseases and Their Close Systemic Relationship: Ciliopathy

Until now, ciliary bronchopulmonary disease has been limited to PCD. It is now clear that aspects of ciliary function extend to the systems of practically all organs, and pediatric bronchopulmonary specialists need to be familiar with these manifestations. There are three types of cilia (Table 7.2): primary (which, disconcertingly, are not really abnormal in PCD), nodal, and mobile. The cilium structure is very complex, with at least 1000 polypeptides. The process of elaboration and assembly is also complex and involves multiple stages coded by genes that do not by themselves have a role in ciliary structure. Functional genomic detection using RNA interference recently found 36 positive cilium assembly modulators and 13 negative ones. Consequently, the genetics of ciliopathy is clearly complex, which should be registered during assessment of diagnostic paths in PCD. It can be argued that there is at least one additional level of complexity. The cilia function not in isolation but, rather, in a complex extracellular environment of periciliary mucus and fluid. At least in

Table 7.2 Different types of cilia

Type	Description
Primary	They have a 9+0 axoneme structure (generally with no pair of central microtubule singlets) There is a primary cilium in every tubular epithelial cell and in many others They participate in numerous chemosensory and mechanosensory functions, linking with key metabolic pathways such as Hippo, Sonic Hedgehog, canonical and noncanonical wnt, pdgf, and mtor The structure varies along the axoneme (they may have regions with central singles) They play an important role in reabsorption of water in the kidney
Nodal	They are structurally of the primary type and are the only known primary mobile cilia
Motile	They have the classic 9+2 axoneme structure (9 outer doublets, 2 central microtubule singlets) They move mucus along epithelial surfaces or drive unicellular organisms through liquids

theory, a PCD phenotype should be produced, even if the cilia are completely normal in cases where the genes that regulate the extraciliary environment mutate.

An important aspect of ciliary function is intraflagellar transport, which is evidenced by the movements of A and B "cumulus" of different sizes, ascending and descending, respectively, in the cilia. The physiological function of this process is not clear, but it is probably related to ciliary growth and nutrition. Mutations in A and B genes result in thick and short cilia. This process is related to the key cilium signaling paths and clinical syndromes such as Jeune asphyxiating thoracic dystrophy and Sensenbrenner and other syndromes.

There is growing interest in the regulatory role of primary cilia. For example, a layer of primary cilia can be detected in the smooth musculature of the airway by immunofluorescence and confocal microscopy and by transmission and scanning electron microscopy. They are enriched by mechanical–chemical sensors, polycystins, and the epidermal growth factor receptor, and have roles in healing injuries and in cellular migration.

Research into this disease has experienced a resurgence, led by the European Respiratory Society (ERS) task force and the North American group. The most important recent advances have been in diagnostics and genetics, with the discovery of more PCD genes. Unfortunately, there have not been comparable advances in therapies, the management of which is not evidence based; rather, it is generally based on protocols for cystic fibrosis. Table 7.3 shows the current standard diagnostic criteria for PCD. However, these criteria are currently under review by the ERS task force. In particular, novel techniques such as immunofluorescence and electron microscopic tomography are available for challenging cases.

The first prerequisite in a contemporary response to PCD is to establish the probability of a diagnosis of PCD. In the case of a child with a low-risk history, a nasal nitric oxide test and measurement of the ciliary beat frequency is all that is required to rule out PCD, whereas in a child with a high-risk history, broader examinations are necessary. Obviously, more sophisticated tests are not necessary if the child fulfills the classical diagnostic criteria (Table 7.3),

Chronic rhinitis can make it impossible to harvest enough cells for a first measurement. In such cases, it may be possible to culture epithelial cells, with new growth of cultured cilia and determination of ciliary beat patterns and morphology. Immunofluorescence can be used in diagnosing PCD to show misplaced ciliary proteins. This test has the advantage that it captures many mutations that carry misplaced proteins. Moreover, the necessary equipment is much simpler and less costly than that used for ciliary beat frequency testing. It is likely to have broader applications in the future.

PCD primary ciliary dyskinesia

A growing number of PCD genes have been discovered, and it is probable that in the future there will be therapies for specific mutations, such as PTC_{124}. The diagnosis is certain if two mutations known to produce disease in trans are detected. However, as with cystic fibrosis, not finding two mutations does not exclude PCD. The genetics of PCD is also much more complex,

Table 7.3 Diagnostic criteria for primary ciliary dyskinesia (PCD)

Clear diagnosis	Probable diagnosis	Improbable diagnosis
Clinical phenotype + low nNO[a] + CBF or pattern anomaly + EM[b] anomalies or Two known diseases that produce mutations in trans or A specific disease that produces abnormalities on EM (e.g., ODA abnormalities)	Clinical phenotype + low nNO, regardless of EM and CBF findings; test repetition is mandatory	Normal nNO + abnormal CBF or EM findings; it is necessary to exclude secondary changes

CBF ciliary beat frequency, *EM* electron microscopy, *nNO* nasal nitric oxide, *ODA* outer dynein arm

[a]nNO should be interpreted with caution unless the patient is old enough to use the breath hold technique

[b]Functional structural abnormalities may appear in freshly harvested epithelial cells or after in vitro ciliary culturing

involving multiple loci in the karyotype and large, complex genes with multiple mutations. The general problem of genetics is evidently distinguishing causal mutations from harmless polymorphisms. For example, of the close to 2000 described CFTR mutations, fewer than 150 are currently known to cause disease. Consequently, there is a real danger in PCD that genetic searches will aggravate existing diagnostic confusion.

Conventional electron microscopy is viewed by some as the reference standard. This is clearly a mistake, given that many patients with PCD have a normal ultrastructure. More sophisticated techniques will change this in the future. Sophisticated tomography, which requires highly qualified personnel and is very time consuming, can detect subtle anomalies that are overlooked by electron microscopy. Clearly, the range of novel testing has allowed for confirmation of the diagnosis of PCD in patients whose condition would otherwise have remained a diagnostic puzzle. As with cystic fibrosis, there are atypical cases of PCD that resist a definitive diagnosis. These children should be kept under strict follow-up, and any manifestation of the disease should be dealt with aggressively. Diagnostic uncertainty should never lead to therapeutic paralysis.

Table 7.4 summarizes the manifestations of ciliopathy. The most obvious question is why the bronchopulmonary system of children should be linked to obscure genetic syndromes. There are several reasons. Firstly, we need to encourage colleagues in other disciplines (especially cardiology, neurology, and nephrology) to consider PCD. No place can be more dangerous than specialist care for a patient with a problem the specialist does not recognize. We should be aware of the possibility of another pathology in the PCD patients, such as retinitis pigmentosa. There has not been any recommendation for routine detection of patients with PCD—for example, echo-

Table 7.4 Summary of pulmonary and systemic manifestations of ciliopathy

Manifestations of ciliopathy	
Respiratory manifestations	
Upper airway (PCD)	Rhinosinusitis, chronic secretory otitis media and impaired hearing, nasal polyps (rarely in children)
Lower airway (PCD)	Recurrent lower respiratory infections, bronchiectasis, respiratory failure
Chest wall (ciliopathy)	Small thoracic cavity, anomalies of the ribs
Sleep disorder (ciliopathy)	Central apnea, obstructive sleep apnea, obesity
Control of breathing (ciliopathy)	Abnormal pattern of breathing
Systemic manifestations	
Cardiovascular	Complex congenital heart disease (especially with laterality disorders), cardiomyopathy
Renal	Polycystic kidney, nephronophthisis, renal dysplasia, glomerulonephritis
Hepatic	Congenital fibrocystic disease
Ocular	Retinitis pigmentosa, photophobia, keratoconus, hyperopia, nystagmus, reduced pupillary response, cone dystrophy, strabismus, cataracts, astigmatism, epicanthal folds
Neurological	Hydrocephalus, development delay, ataxia, cerebellar disease, hypotonia or hypertonia, oculomotor apraxia, diseases of the brain stem, sensorineural hearing loss, hypoplasia of the corpus callosum, Dandy–Walker malformation, posterior encephalocele
Musculoskeletal	Polydactyly, brachydactyly, syndactyly, facial abnormalities including midface hypoplasia, short ribs, hypoplasic iliac crests, trident acetabulum, rhizomelic limb shortening, nail dysplasia, brachycephaly
Genitourinary	Sperm without motility (only in 50% of men with PCD), ectopic pregnancy (PCD), hypogonadism, instability of the urinary detrusor, hydrometrocolpos
Others	Anosmia, insulin resistance, diabetes, nasal abnormalities, frontal alopecia, large ears, narrow nasolabial groove, alterations of teeth, intestinal malrotation

cardiography or ophthalmoscopy when PCD is diagnosed—but we should not require guidelines in order to be clinically alert. Finally, without doubt, there are more associations with ciliopathy to be discovered. This is another fruitful area for bronchopulmonary specialists.

Ciliopathies make up a spectrum of congenital, hepatorenal, bronchial, and multisystem syndromes, in which renal compromise is common. Depending on whether the genetic defect leads to dysfunction or nonfunction, complete absence results in different syndromes, such as Meckel–Gruber syndrome, while there are aberrant results with late-onset adult polycystic kidney disease. There is a marked heterogeneity in these syndromes; overlap syndromes are common, and different manifestations of genetic mutations can appear among members of the same family. The same phenotype can be caused by very disparate genes. The bronchopulmonary specialist should be alert to the possibility of ciliopathy among patients with heterotaxy syndromes. The disposition of the organs is determined by nodal cilia during embryogenesis. Classic Kartagener syndrome is characterized by complete specular imaging, but isolated abdominal and thoracic imaging has been described, as well as isomeric sequences. These are associated with complex congenital heart disease. Specialists should always keep PCD in mind during consultations about these children. They normally present defects in the outer dynein arm (DNAH1 and DNAI5 mutations). Congenital heart defects without lateral disorders are part of other nonmobile ciliopathies.

The possibility of bronchiectasis should be considered in patients with renal disease, as well as in those with hepatic cysts, which can be the first manifestation of renal disease. Renal ciliopathies include juvenile and adult polycystic kidney disease, nephronophthisis, and renal dysplasia syndromes. It is interesting to note that polycystin 1, the mutated gene in polycystic kidney disease, is expressed in the airway. Even patients with renal disease unassociated with ciliopathies have a higher than expected prevalence of bronchiectasis.

The associated deformities of the thoracic wall and pulmonary hypoplasia can be part of the specialty of bronchopulmonary medicine. The ciliopathies include asphyxiating thoracic dystrophy (Jeune syndrome) and Mainzer–Saldino syndrome, in which genetic mutations can affect intraflagellar transport. Retinitis pigmentosa is itself a ciliopathy and is also found in families in which PCD occurs. This area of research is at an early stage. There are many more discoveries to be made about these complex and multisystem disorders. Pediatric bronchopulmonary specialists should advise their colleagues in other specialties with respect to the manifestations of ciliopathy in their patients and keep in mind the possibility of manifestations of PCD in nonrespiratory examinations.

Learning from Follow-Up Studies on Chronic Lung Diseases

We have learned much about childhood wheezing and allergies from numerous neonatal cohort studies. Recent scientific developments have made phenotyping more effective, using unsupervised mathematical techniques that overcome researcher bias and combining neonatal cohorts. This has the effect of greatly increasing the power of studies. This has been Medall's focus and undoubtedly will increase our knowledge of diseases that include childhood wheezing.

Beyond Tucson: Patterns of Wheezing in Preschool Children

The Tucson study did a great service by discovering four wheezing patterns: absence of wheezing, early transitory wheezing (at 0–3 years of age), persistent wheezing (at 0–6 years of age), and wheezing with late manifestations (at 3–6 years of age). These were "self-fulfilling," given that the children were assessed at the ages of 3 years and 6 years and no other phenotypes could be detected. ALSPAC (the Avon Longitudinal Study of Parents and Children), which gathered information from subjects at 6, 18, 30, 42, 54, 69, and 81 months of age, employed mathematical analysis (to overcome researcher bias) to define six phenotypes: "early nontransitory," "intermittent appearance," "persistent," "early prolonged," "late," and "never/infrequent". These phenotypes were confirmed by similar studies in Southampton and the Netherlands, thus strengthening the evidence that they represent real entities. This further supported genetic studies. Locus 17q21 (which contains, among other things, ORMDL3) was a novel and solid discovery in recent asthma genome-wide association studies. When the six wheezing phenotypes were genotyped, only "children with persistent wheezing" had a persistent single-nucleotide polymorphism (SNP) at this locus. Moreover, in follow-up studies, these wheezing phenotypes predicted abnormal developments in spirometry. Children with persistent intermediate or late manifestations had a comparatively lower FEV_1 in adolescence. Finally, a study that combined the ALSPAC, KOALA (Child, Parents and Health: Lifestyle and Genetic Constitution), and PIAMA (Prevention and Incidence of Asthma and Mite Allergy) cohorts explored whether early transitory wheezing is associated with genes of chronic obstructive pulmonary disease (COPD). The results were not completely consistent for the three cohorts, but the data did indicate a genuine association for at least some genes, supporting the follow-up results of the 1964 Aberdeen neonatal cohort, in which children with what was termed "wheezing bronchitis" (but probably could be termed "early transitory wheezing") experienced an accelerated decline in spirometry in middle age, predisposing them to COPD. Considered together, these novel phenotypes are closely related to the clinical reality, and these correlations require further exploration.

Atopy has traditionally been considered a "yes/no" condition on the basis of the presence or absence of a 3-mm burr with a skin prick test and a blood IgE level of >0.34, but these limits are arbitrary and reinforce the belief in grouping children with a weak positive skin prick test for a milk allergy with children with strong positive tests for multiple aeroallergens. The Manchester study reported that there was—as expected—a broad range of sensitivities to airborne allergens, determined by either the skin prick or IgE tests. There were good dose–response relationships between the degree of allergic sensitization and allergic rhinitis and rhinoconjunctivitis. It was proposed that atopy be assessed by the sum of diameters or IgE values for airborne and food-based allergens. A classification strategy was later employed to divide atopy into phenotypes that employed wheezing phenotypes. Five types of atopy were defined: nonlatent atopic vulnerability, atopic vulnerability not from household dust mites, atopic vulnerability from household dust mites, late multiple atopic vulnerability, and early multiple atopic vulnerability. Early multiple atopy was the only condition that predicted asthma, which is consistent with the results of other studies, effectively indicating the importance of the early appearance of atopy.

Improved Phenotyping

We have reached a point where combination of phenotypes is possible. The Manchester group has taken the lead, combining its five "atopies" with four w-heezing phenotypes (absence of wheezing, transitory wheezing, late-appearance wheezing, and persistent wheezing). They showed that persistent wheezing combined with early multiple atopy is the only combination that predicts progressive worsening of airflow obstruction in childhood. This type of work can make an important contribution to predictive indices of asthma, which will be needed when we finally discover therapeutic strategies to prevent the progression from episodic viral wheezing to asthma. Current indices have good negative predictive values, but the positive predictive values are only a little better than a toss of the coin. This probably reflects the crude way in which we have assessed parameters such as atopy.

The Microenvironment of the Airway and Development of Respiratory Diseases: The Microbiome

It has long been believed that the airway below the larynx is sterile, despite the large quantities of air that we inhale daily and the fact that the air is laden with microorganisms, allergens, and contaminants. One reason this myth persists over time has been the excessive confidence we have in conventional microbiology based on cultures, which is able to detect only about 1% of total bacteria. A battery of increasingly sophisticated molecular tools has been developed, resulting in the detection of bacterial DNA, which has revealed that human beings have more than ten times as many bacterial cells as eukaryote cells. An early bronchoscopy study highlighted that there is an abundant lower flora; it identified 5054 bacterial 16S ribosomal RNA (rRNA) sequences from 43 adults and children, which represented more than 70% of the species that were present. The bronchial tree is not sterile and contains on average 2100 bacterial genomes per square centimeter of the sampled surface. The number of proteobacteria is significantly higher in children with asthma than in healthy children, while Bacteroidetes—in particular, *Prevotella* species—are more common in healthy children than in asthmatic children. This and other original works have highlighted the scientific importance of the microbiome and have promoted a new vision of inflammatory diseases. Moreover, it is clear that there is a high degree of interaction between the airway and the intestinal microbiome.

The Importance of the Microbiome in Healthy Children

A major part of the work on lung development has been done in animals, and significant insights into early stages of human lung development have been gained. One study investigated the development of allergic inflammation induced by intraperitoneal ovalbumin in three groups of rats: rats bred normally, germ-free rats, and germ-free rats that had been reconstituted with bacterial flora from normal rats. The germ-free rats had more pronounced type 2 helper T cell (T_h2) responses, evidenced by having more IL-4$^+$ or IL-5$^+$ CD4+ cells in the broncoalveolar lavage, without differences in IL-10$^+$ or in interferon (IFN)-γ^+ cells. They also had a more pronounced IgE response to intranasal provocation. It was concluded that exposure to a mixture of bacterial species can have a more powerful inhibiting effect on the allergic response than exposure to *Bifidobacterium* alone. It was also shown that germ-free rats had lower IgA levels in the broncoalveolar lavage, larger numbers of basophils, and smaller numbers of alveolar macrophages and plasmacytoid dendritic cells, while the number of regulatory T lymphocytes (Tregs) was not affected. It was concluded that commensal bacteria are important for the normal maturation of immune cells.

Another study using an ovalbumin model of murine allergic airway disease showed that previous exposure to *Escherichia coli* precluded the possibility of airway eosinophilia, which probably requires signaling through TLR4 but does not function via T_h1 or Treg mechanisms. The authors concluded that the effect occurred via dendritic and T cells, although this was not confirmed. Infection of murine models with *Helicobacter* provoked by ovalbumin or household dust mite allergens prevented eosinophilia and T_h2 and T_h17 infiltration. Neonatal infection altered the maturation of dendritic cells and induced inhibitory Tregs. The researchers showed that the mechanism of the effects of *Helicobacter* functions via Tregs. Adoptive protector Tregs were observed, and there was no depletion of Tregs in a rat model. Finally, in another study that used rats with ovalbumin provocation, allergic airway disease was inhibited by viable and dead *Streptococcus pneumoniae*. The study demonstrated inhibition of a T_h2-specific antigen response and pulmonary and peripheral eosinophils, hyperplasia of calciform cells, and hyperactivity of the airways. The probable mechanisms included Treg induction, less T cell proliferation, and release of T_h2 cytokines. The effects were reversed by anti-CD25. In summary, there is clearly an important interaction between airway infection and immune response, which we have recently begun to understand. We also need to demonstrate the complexities of fungi and viruses, which have been found in large quantities with molecular techniques.

It should not be supposed that bacteria are benign in normal immune development. In

COPSAC (the Copenhagen Prospective Study on Asthma in Childhood), early isolation of *S. pneumoniae*, *Moraxella catarrhalis*, *Haemophilus influenzae*, or a combination of these organisms from the nasopharynx was closely associated with persistent wheezing, acute exacerbations of severe wheezing, and hospitalization due to wheezing. The blood eosinophil and total IgE counts at the age of 4 years were found to be significantly higher in children colonized with these organisms in the neonatal phase, but there was no effect on specific IgE. The incidence of asthma and acute bronchodilator response were significantly higher in children colonized at the age of 5 years. Colonization was associated with an inflammatory response in the nasal coating fluid, of a mixed $T_h1/T_h2/T_h17$ type. It remains to be determined whether this is a cause or a consequence of colonization.

There is increasingly convincing evidence that early exposure to both good and bad microbes is important for children. The place and mode of release have been demonstrated to affect the long-term results, and the probable mechanism functions through early bacterial exposure. Two meta-analyses have shown greater risk of atopic disease, including food allergies, in newborns delivered by cesarean section. Notably, the intestinal flora of newborns delivered by cesarean section was different from that of other newborns. Vaginal flora was reduced in newborns delivered by cesarean section. Another research group collected fecal samples from 1167 participants when they were 1 month old, took blood samples for specific IgE when the participants were 2 years old and again when they were 6–7 years old, and gathered data through questionnaires repeatedly applied from the birth of the participants until they were 7 years old. The study found that isolation of *Clostridium difficile* at 1 month of age was associated with wheezing and eczema throughout the follow-up period. Children of atopic parents who were born vaginally at home had lower prevalence rates of eczema and asthma.

There are major unknown areas. However, the data do have implications for the use of antibiotics in preschool children. It is interesting to speculate whether there is an airway equivalent to antibiotic-associated diarrhea. The use of antibiotics has the potential to alter the microbiome of the airway and modulate the immune response over the long term. This is obviously not an argument against the use of antibiotics for life-threatening diseases for children, but it is another potent argument against the use of antibiotics for more trivial self-limiting problems.

The Microbiome in Early Wheezing Disorders

There is evidence that environmental microbial diversity has a positive effect on the risk of asthma. It has been known for many years that the children of Friesen farmers in the Netherlands have a very low prevalence of atopic diseases. GABRIELA (the Multidisciplinary Study to Identify the Genetic and Environmental Causes of Asthma in the European Community [GABRIEL] Advanced Study) and PARSIFAL (the Prevention of Allergy-Risk Factors for Sensitization in Children Related to Farming and Anthroposophic Lifestyle study) joined forces and showed that the diversity of bacteria and fungi in the environment was greater in children living on farms and this was associated with better responses to asthma and atopy. The presence of Gram-negative environmental bacilli such as *Staphylococcus* spp. and *Listeria monocytogenes*, and fungi such as *Eurotium* and *Penicillium*, was protective. There are still many unanswered questions. It is not clear if diversity is causal of better responses or a marker of something else that is really responsible. The mechanism by which the environment affects the flora of the lower airway is not clear.

Another group pyrosequenced amplifications of the polymorphic bacterial rRNA gene 16S from oropharyngeal samples collected from 24 infants in tropical Ecuador with noninfectious early-appearance wheezing and 24 healthy controls (average age 10.2 months). The researchers found pathogens much more often in the wheezing infants than in the controls (for example, species of *Haemophilus* and *Staphylococcus*), while species of *Veillonella* were less common in subjects with wheezing. The important things to note about this study were that (1) the results were confounded by treatment with antibiotics or inhaled steroids, and (2) the results implied that throat samples can be helpful in understanding the microbiota of the lower airway. As repeated bronchoscopy is never possible in children, whereas collection of repeated throat samples is possible, it will be an immense advance if this is confirmed.

These results are challenging, and it is interesting to speculate that asthma is an infectious disease or at least has a major contributing component of airway infection. Will we treat asthma with antibiotics someday? Before ruling out this idea as too absurd, we should remember that we treat duodenal ulcers with antibiotics directed at *Helicobacter pylori*. We should also remember that the first reports of findings of spirochetes in the duodenal mucosa were received with sarcasm.

The Microbiome and Cystic Fibrosis

Life used to be simple. The pathogens involved in cystic fibrosis were *S. aureus*, *H. influenzae*, *P. aeruginosa*, *Burkholderia cepacia*, and occasionally Gram-negative bacteria. Recent studies have challenged this view. Conventional culturing shows that there are large numbers and a high degree of diversity of obligate and facultative anaerobes in cystic fibrosis sputum. Molecular techniques have shown that there is a true fauna of bacteria in the cystic fibrosis airway, as well as a diversity of fungi and viruses. It is increasingly clear that the relationships in this diverse community are complex. A microorganism can inhibit the growth of a pathogen. Just because a microorganism is present does not mean that it is doing harm; the opposite could be true.

A longitudinal study of adult patients with cystic fibrosis found that bacterial communities were stable over time but, surprisingly, individuals with similar clinical evolutions had very different communities. The perturbations in the community in response to administration of antibiotics was evident but transitory. Multiple courses of antibiotics and a low level of pulmonary functioning were associated with less diversity. However, it could not be established whether the lower level of diversity was caused by the treatment or was a function of the underlying pathology. There is only limited information about early changes in the microbiome of patients with cystic fibrosis. The best study included just seven infants, who were studied over a 2-year period. Their intestinal and respiratory microbiota were investigated using fecal and oropharyngeal samples, respectively. *Veillonella* and *Streptococcus* were the main species found and, in general, the trajectories of the microbiome in the intestine and respiratory tract were comparable. Breastfeeding and the intestinal microbiome affected the respiratory tract. Diversity increased over time in the respiratory and gastrointestinal tracts. Diversity in the gastrointestinal tract was greater with breastfeeding than with formula feeding, while diversity in the respiratory tract increased more with formula feeding. Finally, a solid food diet increased diversity in the respiratory tract, whereas it had the opposite effect in the gastrointestinal tract.

Where do these complex data leave us in clinical terms? It would be easy to reach therapeutic paralysis as a result of this great mass of highly indigestible and undigested data. This new paradigm means that antibiotics can be beneficial, harmful, or neutral. John LiPuma has argued convincingly that while we attempt to figure out the implications of these new findings, we should not lose sight of strategies that have clearly been beneficial in the past. Current antibiotic policies should continue being implemented, and if the patient does not respond well, new molecular technologies can be applied to try to detect microorganisms can be applied to try to detect microorganisms not detected and not covered by current treatment. However, it should also be kept in mind that we do not currently have a base of evidence to interpret the information we receive from these new technologies.

Is Clinical Pediatric Pneumology Dead?

Enormous scientific advances have been made since the last edition of this book; does the increasing sophistication of laboratory techniques therefore mean that we no longer need our clinical skills? On the contrary: broad experience in the range of normality and the manifestations of disease are even more necessary. For example, the complete variety of increasingly sophisticated tests for PCD cannot be applied to all children who have a cough and intermittent rhinitis. Clinical skills are necessary to establish (1) who should be tested first and (2) who should continue on to sophisticated tests such as tomography, even when the diagnosis of PCD has been ruled out. In this sense, these are interesting times with great opportunities for young researchers, but we also need clinicians with discernment and experience for the near future.

Sources

Alton EW, Boyd AC, Cheng SH, Cunningham S, Davies JC, Gill DR, Griesenbach U, Higgins T, Hyde SC, Innes JA, Murray GD, Porteous DJ. A randomised, double-blind, placebo-controlled phase IIB clinical trial of repeated application of gene therapy in patients with cystic fibrosis. Thorax. 2013;68:1075–7.

Bilton D, Bellon G, Charlton B, Cooper P, De Boeck K, Flume PA, Fox HG, Gallagher CG, Geller DE, Haarman EG, Hebestreit HU, Kolbe J, Lapey A, Robinson P, Wu J, Zuckerman JB, Aitken ML; CF301 and CF302 Investigators. Pooled analysis of two large randomized phase III inhaled mannitol studies in cystic fibrosis J Cyst Fibros 2013; 12: 367–376.

Boyle MP, Bell SC, Konstan MW, McColley SA, Rowe SM, Rietschel E, Huang X, Waltz D, Patel NR, Rodman D, VX09-809-102 Study Group. A CFTR corrector (lumacaftor) and a CFTR potentiator (ivacaftor) for treatment of patients with cystic fibrosis who have a phe508del CFTR mutation: a phase 2 randomised controlled trial. Lancet Respir Med. 2014;2:527–38.

Clancy JP, Dupont L, Konstan MW, Billings J, Fustik S, Goss CH, Lymp J, Minic P, Quittner AL, Rubenstein RC, Young KR, Saiman L, Burns JL, Govan JR, Ramsey B, Gupta R, Arikace Study Group. Phase II studies of nebulized Arikace in CF patients with *Pseudomonas aeruginosa* infection. Thorax. 2013;68:818–25.

Davies J, Sheridan H, Bell N, Cunningham S, Davis SD, Elborn JS, Milla CE, Starner TD, Weiner DJ, Lee PS, Ratjen F. Assessment of clinical response to ivacaftor with lung clearance index in cystic fibrosis patients with a G551D-CFTR mutation and preserved spirometry: a randomised controlled trial. Lancet Respir Med. 2013;1:630–8.

Ege MJ, Mayer M, Normand AC, Genuneit J, Cookson WO, Braun-Fahrlander C, Heederik D, Piarroux R, von Mutius E, GABRIELA Transregio 22 Study Group. Exposure to environmental microorganisms and childhood asthma. N Engl J Med. 2011;364:701–9.

Horsley AR, Davies JC, Gray RD, et al. Changes in physiological, functional and structural markers of cystic fibrosis lung disease with treatment of a pulmonary exacerbation. Thorax. 2013;68:532–9.

Kerkhof M, Boezen HM, Granell R, Wijga AH, Brunekreef B, Smit HA, de Jongste JC, Thijs C, Mommers M, Penders J, Henderson J, Koppelman GH, Postma DS. Transient early wheeze and lung function in early childhood associated with chronic obstructive pulmonary disease genes. J Allergy Clin Immunol. 2014;133:68–76.

Knowles MR, Daniels LA, Davis SD, Zariwala MA, Leight MW. Primary ciliary dyskinesia: recent advances in diagnostics, genetics and characterization of clinical disease. Am J Respir Crit Care Med. 2013;188:913–22.

Konstan MW, Geller DE, Minić P, Brockhaus F, Zhang J, Angyalosi G. Tobramycin inhalation powder for *P. aeruginosa* infection in cystic fibrosis: the EVOLVE trial. Pediatr Pulmonol. 2011;46:230–8.

Kuehni CE, Frischer T, Strippoli MP. Factors influencing age at diagnosis of primary ciliary dyskinesia in European children. Eur Respir J. 2010;36:1248–58.

Lazic N, Roberts G, Custovic A, Belgrave D, Bishop CM, Winn J, Curtin JA, Hasan Arshad S, Simpson A. Multiple atopy phenotypes and their associations with asthma: similar findings from two birth cohorts. Allergy. 2013;68:764–70.

Lim MT, Wallis C, Price JF, Carr SB, Chavasse RJ, Shankar A, Seddon P, Balfour-Lynn IM. Diagnosis of cystic fibrosis in London and south east England before and after the introduction of newborn screening. Arch Dis Child. 2014;99:197–202.

Lodge CL, Lowe AJ, Allen KJ, et al. Childhood wheeze phenotypes show less than expected growth in FEV_1 across adolescence. Am J Respir Crit Care Med. 2014;189:1351–8.

Ooi CY, Dupuis A, Ellis L, Jarvi K, Martin S, Ray PN, Steele L, Kortan P, Gonska T, Dorfman R, Solomon M, Zielenski J, Corey M, Tullis E, Durie P. Does extensive genotyping and nasal potential difference testing clarify the diagnosis of cystic fibrosis among patients with single organ manifestations of cystic fibrosis? Thorax. 2014;69:254–60.

Pillarisetti N, Williamson E, Linnane B et al; Australian Respiratory Early Surveillance Team for Cystic Fibrosis (AREST CF). Infection, inflammation, and lung function decline in infants with cystic fibrosis. Am J Respir Crit Care Med 2011;184: 75–81.

Rosenfeld M, Ratjen F, Brumback L, Daniel S, Rowbotham R, McNamara S, Johnson R, Kronmal R, Davis SD, ISIS Study Group. Inhaled hypertonic saline in infants and children younger than 6 years with cystic fibrosis: the ISIS randomized controlled trial. JAMA. 2012;307:2269–77.

Sanders DB, Bittner RC, Rosenfeld M, Redding GJ, Goss CH. Pulmonary exacerbations are associated with sub-

sequent FEV_1 decline in both adults and children with cystic fibrosis. Pediatr Pulmonol. 2011;46:393–400.
Serisier DJ, Bilton D, De Soyza A, Thompson PJ, Kolbe J, Greville HW, Cipolla D, Bruinenberg P, Gonda I, ORBIT-2 Investigators. Inhaled, dual release liposomal ciprofloxacin in non-cystic fibrosis bronchiectasis (ORBIT-2): a randomised, double-blind, placebo-controlled trial. Thorax. 2013;68:812–7.
Sermet-Gaudelus I, Mayell SJ, Southern KW, European Cystic Fibrosis Society (ECFS), Neonatal Screening Working Group. Guidelines on the early management of infants diagnosed with cystic fibrosis following newborn screening. J Cyst Fibros. 2010;9:323–9.
Stressmann FA, Rogers GB, van der Gast CJ, et al. Long-term cultivation-independent microbial diversity analysis demonstrates that bacterial communities infecting the adult cystic fibrosis lung show stability and resilience. Thorax. 2012;67:867–73.
Thia LP, Calder A, Stocks J, Bush A et al., on behalf of the London Cystic Fibrosis Collaboration (LCFC). Original article: is chest CT useful in newborn screened infants with cystic fibrosis at 1 year of age? Thorax 2014;69: 320–327.
Van Nimwegen FA, Penders J, Stobberingh EE, et al. Mode and place of delivery, gastrointestinal microbiota, and their influence on asthma and atopy. J Allergy Clin Immunol. 2011;128:948–55.
Vernooij-van Langen AMM, Loeber JG, Elvers B, et al. Novel strategies in newborn screening for cystic fibrosis: a prospective controlled study. Thorax. 2012;67:289–95.
Vson Linstow ML, Schonning K, Hoegh AM, Sevelsted A, Vissing NH, Bisgaard H. Neonatal airway colonization is associated with troublesome lung symptoms in infants. Am J Respir Crit Care Med. 2013;188:1041–2.
Ware SM, Gubay-Aygun M, Hildebrandt F. Spectrum of clinical diseases caused by disorders of primary cilia. Proc Am Thorac Soc. 2011;8:444–502.

Evaluation of Pulmonary Function in Infants and Preschool Children

8

Alejandro Teper, Carlos Kofman, and Alejandro Colom

Contents

Pulmonary Function in Infants

The respiratory system undergoes extraordinary changes in the first 2 years of life, in terms of its growth and functional development. Knowledge of the mechanical properties of the lungs in the first years of life was limited until the development of sophisticated equipment to measure respiratory function that was adapted for use with small children. Since then, it has been possible to understand the inherent aspects of normal respiratory function, as well as the effects of diverse pre- and postnatal injuries, besides treatments. It has been possible to determine physiopathological mechanisms, therapeutic mechanisms, and certain prognostics in children with distinct pathologies.

Although there are centers around the world that study pulmonary function, the application of

A. Teper
Faculty of Medicine, Universidad de Buenos Aires and Department of Pediatric Pulmonology, Hospital Ricardo Gutiérrez, Buenos Aires, Argentina

C. Kofman · A. Colom (✉)
Department of Pediatric Pulmonology, Hospital Ricardo Gutiérrez, Buenos Aires, Argentina

P. Bertrand, I. Sánchez (eds.), *Pediatric Respiratory Diseases*,
https://doi.org/10.1007/978-3-030-26961-6_8

Table 8.1 Indications to perform functional respiratory studies in small children

Cystic fibrosis
Neonatal chronic lung disease
Postinfectious bronchiolitis obliterans
Recurrent bronchial obstruction that does not respond to the usual treatments
Central airway obstruction
Epidemiological and research studies

the results to medical care has not been generalized for various reasons: (1) some of the physiological principles on which the methods are based are still not sufficiently understood; (2) the instruments for measurement are complex and costly; (3) the procedures are lengthy and require sedation of the patient; and (4) there is no standardized form of these methods. However, in certain clinical situations it is appropriate to measure pulmonary function in the first years of life (Table 8.1).

Measurement Conditions

Infants who are to be assessed through a functional respiratory study should fast for the previous 4 hours and be examined to rule out certain conditions in which the procedure is not advised, such as fever or the presence of secretions in the upper airway. The patient's height and weight should be measured and the results should be compared with theoretical values. Prior to the procedure, 50–75 mg/kg of chloral hydrate is administered orally to induce a relaxed sleep, which in most cases lasts for 90–120 minutes. It is considered high-risk to administer this medication to patients with severe upper airway obstruction or those with some degree of hepatic, renal, or cardiac insufficiency.

The patient should be in a supine position during the study, with his or her head held straight in hyperextension. Small movements and flexing of the neck can alter the results and thus should be avoided. Arterial oxygen saturation and the heart rate are monitored continuously with an oximeter.

Methods

Measurement of Forced Expiratory Flow

Understandably, small children cannot perform maximum forced exhalations based on their total lung capacity for evaluation of the caliber of the peripheral airways. Different methods are used to prompt infants and small children to exhale forcibly. Deflation techniques, rapid thoracic compression at the tidal volume (RC-RTC), and rapid thoracoabdominal compression: RTC with preinsufflation are used to determine the magnitude of bronchial obstruction and variations in obstruction after administration of a bronchodilator or a bronchoconstrictor agent.

The deflation technique was the first to be developed, but it is no longer used, because it requires heavy sedation and intubation of the patient. Consequently, in this chapter, we discuss the other two methods.

Rapid Thoracoabdominal Compression Technique at Current Volume

Adler et al. (1978) and Taussig et al. (1982) described the rapid thoracoabdominal compression technique for determining the bronchial caliber in infants. It has been used to describe the normal growth and development of the airways in infancy, on the basis of which equations have been developed to establish the magnitude of bronchial obstruction, using a standard deviation score as a function of the sex and size of the subject. With this, the observed alterations in the functional response to the treatments applied in the respiratory clinic can be identified and evaluated.

The technique employs an inflatable vest inside another inextensible vest around the child's chest and stomach, which goes from the armpits to the pubis, with the child's arms outside both jackets. A reserve air tank connected to the inflatable jacket transmits air at the end of the inhalation, with sufficient pressure to produce rapid thoracoabdominal compression (Fig. 8.1). Expiratory flows are registered during forced

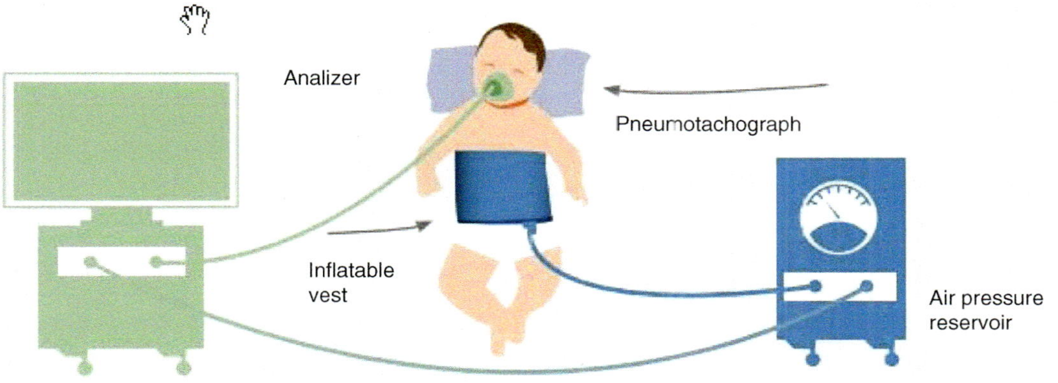

Fig. 8.1 Equipment used for rapid thoracoabdominal compression at tidal volume (calculation of the maximum flow at the functional residual capacity (VmaxFRC))

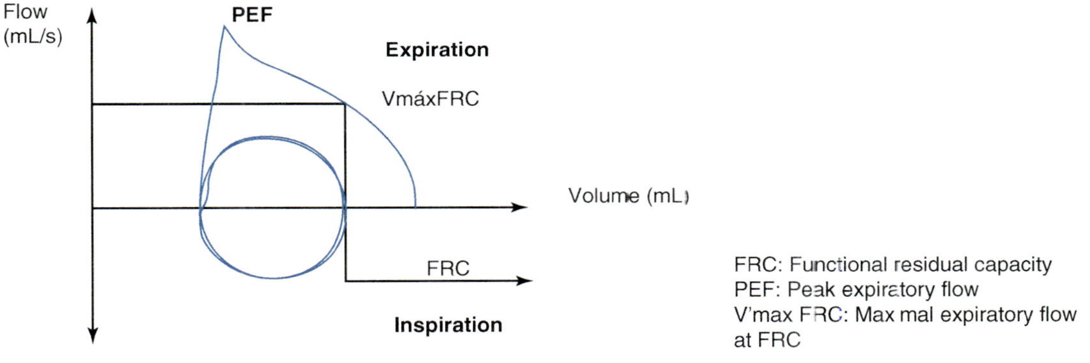

Fig. 8.2 Partial forced flow/volume curve

exhalation by a pneumotachograph equipped with a facial mask, which hermetically covers the nose and mouth of the patient. The resulting flow/volume curve is graphed in real time on a computer screen. The curve characteristically presents a rapid rise in the expiratory flow until the peak expiratory flow (PEF) is reached, and then it gradually descends to a point below the one established as the functional residual capacity (FRC). The flow obtained at this point is termed VFRC. To determine the limitation in airflow, the maneuver is progressively repeated with more pressure on the jacket, ranging between +20 and +100 cm of water. The maximum flow at the FRC (VmaxFRC), which correlates with the airway caliber, is determined by applying the pressure that yields the highest VFRC values (Fig. 8.2).

While the highest pressures have no limit in relation to airflow in healthy infants, this is not the case in patients with bronchial obstruction, where much less pressure is required. Abrupt falls in airflow are attributed to glottic or pharyngeal closure, and they can be corrected according to the correct location in the neck. At least three acceptable and reproducible curves are obtained with maximum FRC values that do not vary by more than 10%, and VmaxFRC is the average of the three values. The curves obtained with this method are "partial," given that they are based not on the total pulmonary capacity but, rather, on the end of the inspiration at the current volume.

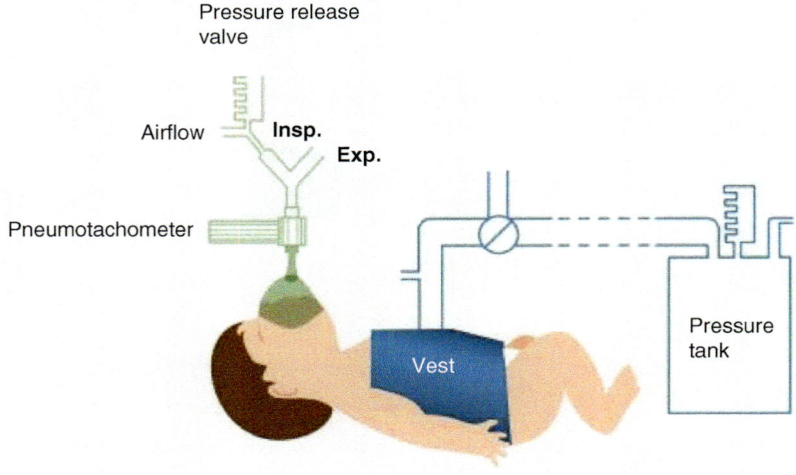

Fig. 8.3 Rapid thoracoabdominal compression with previous insufflation

Rapid Thoracoabdominal Compression Technique at a Volume with Previous Insufflation

A modification of the technique described above has recently been developed to obtain, in a noninvasive way, better forced expiratory curves. The equipment used is similar to that used for the other technique, with the addition of an insufflation system to take the patient close to his or her total pulmonary capacity immediately before the thoracoabdominal compression (Fig. 8.3).

The insufflation system consists of an external source of air, valves to automatically occlude the airway or a Y connector for manual insufflation, and a safety valve to control the insufflation pressure. The jacket reaches maximum pressure in 70–100 milliseconds. Given that there is a small delay between insufflation and compression, it is a common practice to activate the compression 10–100 milliseconds before releasing the occlusion of the airway. One of the main discrepancies among users has been the application of different insufflation pressures to reach higher volumes. However, there is a consensus in the application of 30 cm of water pressure for older infants and 20 cm of water pressure for newborns and premature babies. The inspiratory flow is established at 1.5 times the current flow. The real pressure at the level of the mouth is monitored in real time so that the operator can adjust the flows and optimize the pressure being administered. There are also disparate criteria in the ventilation pattern before the forced expiration. The pulmonary insufflation rate depends on the lung volume and flow magnitude, while the volume reached for a standard pressure is directly proportional to the infant's level of respiratory compliance. Most authors suggest 2–5 successive insufflations until pressure and volume plateaus are reached.

The most relevant functional parameters are obtained on the basis of the "maximum" forced curve of volume/time and flow/volume (Fig. 8.4)—namely, the forced vital capacity (FVC), forced expiratory volume (FEV) in 0.5 seconds ($FEV_{0.5}$), and forced expiratory flow at 25–75% of FVC (FEF_{25-75}). Other parameters that can be considered are the expiratory flows at 50%, 75%, and 85% of FVC, and $FEV_{0.4}$ in small children. The parameters that are reported are those that are obtained on the basis of the "best curve," and at least two values that do not differ by more than 10% should be used, with the better value reported. Similarly, the results refer to theoretical values.

Analysis of Breathing at Current Volume

Analysis of the curves obtained during current breathing is useful for functional respiratory assessment of infants, given that they yield

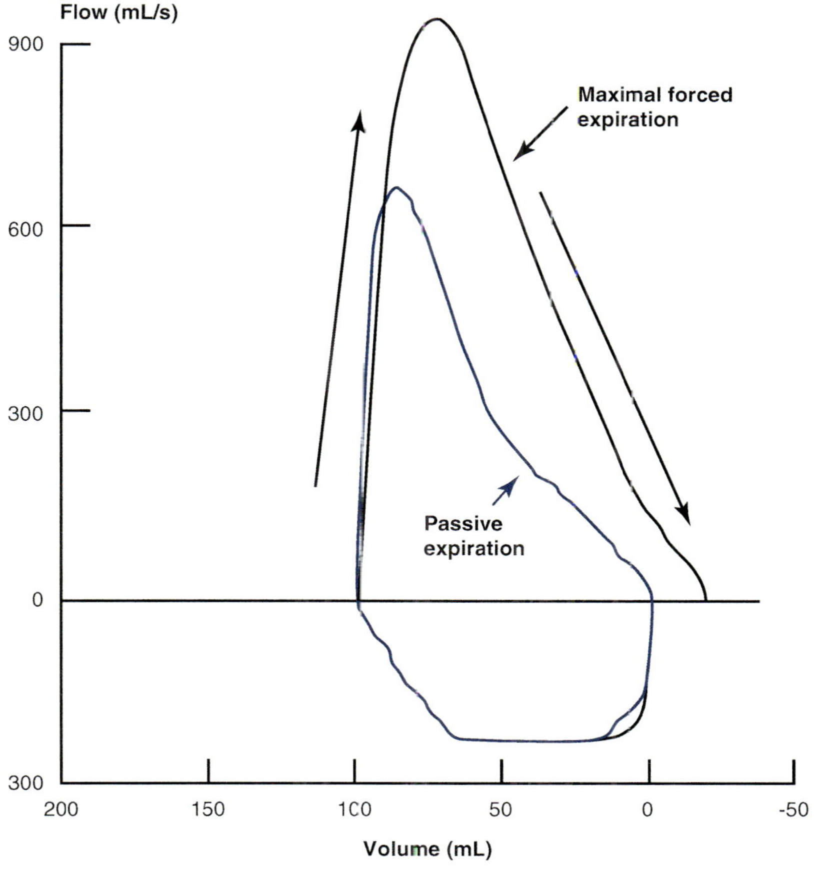

Fig. 8.4 Maximum forced flow/volume (F-V) loop obtained by rapid thoracoabdominal compression with previous insufflation

greater variability and lower levels of specificity. However, there are different parameters that can be obtained from observing the flow curves/tidal volumes that allow for establishment of obstructive and low-compliance patterns (Fig. 8.5).

Simply by the airtight mask being placed on the patient's face and attached to the pneumotachograph, the flow and volume signals are integrated to determine:

(a) Parameters that are altered in pulmonary elastic retraction disorders: the rate between the peak expiratory flow and current volume (PEF/Vc)
(b) Parameters that vary with obstructive pathologies: the percentages of volume and time to reach PEF

Some epidemiological studies have considered these measurements because of their technical simplicity in comparison with other methods.

Measurement of Respiratory Mechanics

Respiratory mechanics can be assessed by dynamic or passive methods. The respiratory cycle is not interrupted during measurements done with dynamic methods, whereas it is interrupted with use of passive methods. Body plethysmography and pressure/volume curves are dynamic methods. The main advantages of these methods are their greater sensitivity and specificity. Pressure/volume curves are particularly useful to optimize mechanical respiratory assistance in

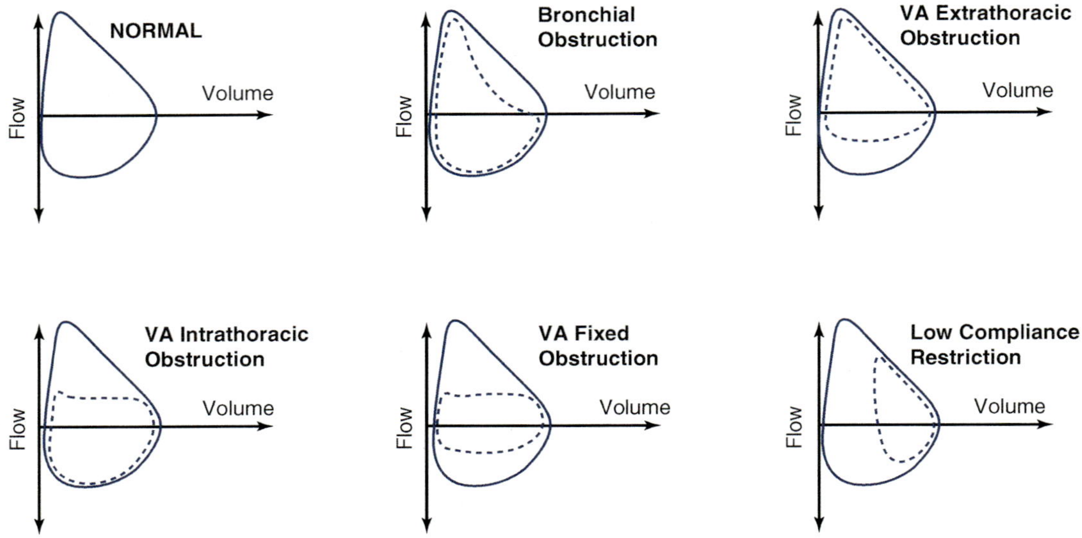

Fig. 8.5 Flow/volume loop patterns

ventilated patients. However, dynamic methods are not widely used, because they require sophisticated personnel and intubation of the patient.

Passive methods include single- and multiple-occlusion techniques, which assess changes in flow or volume in relation to changes in pressure at the level of the mouth during periods of relaxation of the respiratory muscles, triggered by the Hering–Breuer reflex in the occlusion of the airway at the end of the inspiration. The time constant of the respiratory system is thus determined on the basis of the slope of the flow/volume curve. The compliance and resistance of the respiratory system are then calculated. Passive methods are simple, rapid, and noninvasive, although they assess the entire respiratory system and not just the lungs.

Measurement of Lung Volume

FRC is defined as the volume of gas that remains in the lungs after a passive exhalation. It is the result of the balance between the force of elastic lung retraction and the expansive capacity of the rib cage. It is also the easiest method for obtaining precise and reproducible lung volume values when the patient is incapable of cooperating. The FRC is increased when air is trapped (obstructive pathologies), and it is lower in patients with restrictive pathologies. Consequently, determining the FRC allows us to differentiate these processes functionally. It also provides an objective parameter for following lung growth and development, although it does not provide information about the number or size of the alveoli.

The FRC can be quantified by two methods, which are discussed in the following sections.

Body Plethysmography

The principle of this technique is the same as that of plethysmography in older children and adults. The child is placed in a supine position in a hermetic box (plethysmograph) while breathing through a facial mask connected to a pneumotachograph. At the end of an inspiration current, the circuit is closed for 6–10 seconds, making the child breathe against the closed system. As the pressure in the lung decreases and its volume increases, the opposite occurs in the plethysmograph. The FRC is determined by applying Boyle's law (the product of pressure (P) and volume (V) are always constant in a closed system at a constant temperature: $P \times V = P' \times V'$). This technique measures all of the gas in the thoracic cavity, which is the areas that communicate with the airway and the areas that do not. As we saw before, the plethysmograph can also determine the airway resistance.

Multiple-Breath Washout

The multiple-breath washout (MBW) method is based on dilution of a marker gas to a known concentration in an unknown volume (the FRC) over multiple current breaths. This can be done in two ways:

- MBW using gases that are not involved in the gas exchange and are not absorbed into the blood flow or secreted by the tissues (helium or sulfur hexafluoride): The patient inhales a gas mixture with the gas marker until it reaches an equilibrium concentration (the same concentration for inhaling and exhaling). From this moment on, the patient begins to breathe environmental air (the washout principal phase) and the gas marker is lowered until it reaches a concentration lower than 2.5% of its initial concentration.
- Nitrogen MBW: The patient washes out the N_2 in his or her lungs by inhaling 100% O_2 in multiple breaths.

The child should be asleep (not necessarily sedated) in order to obtain a stable breathing pattern. An airtight facial mask is placed on the child's face, covering the mouth and nose. The mask is connected to the pneumotachograph and a mass spectrometer (or an ultrasonic transducer), which quantifies the concentration of the gases. The FRC is reported in millimeters as the average of three technically acceptable maneuvers with values that do not differ by more than 10%. There are different reference values for gas dilution methods using N_2 or He, as well as for the plethysmography method.

Lung Clearance Index

The Lung Clearance Index (LCI) can be determined with the gas dilution technique, which evaluates the distribution or degree of homogeneity of pulmonary ventilation. A high index indicates obstruction of the small airways. This reflects a nonhomogeneous ventilator pattern, which slows the N_2 (or marker gas) lavage at those zones with air trapping. This index is calculated by dividing the volume of exhaled volume (until the marker gas has been washed out and reaches a concentration of one fortieth of its initial concentration) by the FRC. A clearance index under 7.8 is considered normal regardless of the patient's sex, age, height, and weight. Its measurement is simple and noninvasive, and it has low variability and good reproducibility. The measurements are done three times, the FRC is noted, and the average lung clearance index of the three maneuvers is calculated. Because this method gives information about the peripheral airway (also called the "silent zones"), its clinical utility has been studied more extensively in patients with cystic fibrosis. It has been shown that this parameter is altered before the appearance of symptoms, making it possible to explore different therapeutic choices at an early stage. In the same way, the studies conducted in these patients have shown good correlation with the changes in high-resolution computerized tomography. Its usefulness in asthma and in chronic newborn lung diseases has been discussed, and it is still under investigation.

Study of the Diffusing Capacity of the Lung for Carbon Monoxide

Castillo et al. (2006) described determination of the diffusing capacity of the lung for carbon monoxide (DLCO), using the single-breath technique adapted for infants and small children. The test consists of placing the child (after sedation) in a supine position, breathing through a mask connected to a pneumotachograph and a mass spectrometer. As in the rapid thoracoabdominal compression technique at high volumes, the airway is insufflated at 20 cm of water pressure with a gaseous mixture (0.3% CO, 5% He, 21% O_2, and the rest N_2). The lungs remain insufflated for 6 seconds to diffuse the carbon, after which the child can exhale passively. The measurement principle is similar to that used to determine carbon monoxide diffusion in adults. The alveolar volume (AV) is determined by the gas dilution technique using He as the marker gas, and the diffusion capacity of the alveolar–capillary membrane is determined by measuring the concentration of exhaled carbon. The measurements are done three times and the AV and CO diffusion are noted. The value considered is the average of three technically acceptable measurements with values that do not differ from each other by more than 10%. Because anemia or polycythemia alter CO diffusion values, Hb must be determined beforehand in order to correct for altered carbon monoxide diffusion. With this method, the physiological shape of the surface that is available for gas exchange can be evaluated; therefore, alveolar growth and development can be studied without use of anatomopathological studies. Studies conducted in premature babies have shown a change in normal alveolar development. These children present an AV that is similar to that seen in term children, but they have a smaller area for gas exchange because the alveoli are larger and fewer in number. This technique may be useful in extremely premature patients to evaluate alveolar growth and development, as well as responses to different treatments. Besides this, the technique may be used to valuate children with lung hypoplasia, for follow-up of children treated with lung resections early in life, or in patients with necrotized parenchymal areas. Finally, this technique provides an objective parameter to establish a diagnosis and follow-up of interstitial diseases during the first years of life. However, commercial equipment to measure carbon monoxide diffusion in infants has not been developed yet, and its use is currently restricted to research practices.

Fraction of Exhaled Nitric Oxide

Measurement of the fraction of exhaled nitric oxide (FeNO) has recently emerged as a tool for evaluating, managing, and diagnosing asthma. Its determination is simple and it gives information about eosinophilic inflammation in the airway noninvasively. High nitric oxide levels are related to the increase of eosinophils in induced sputum, bronchoalveolar lavage, and bronchial biopsy materials. Atopic and asthmatic adults and children present high levels, which drop after anti-inflammatory treatment. Technically, determination of the fractional exhaled nitric oxide is done using a chemiluminescent analyzer. In infants it can be performed through the "current breathing technique" and the measurement can be done online (in real time) or offline (when the air is kept in a hermetic bag and is measured afterward). When the child is asleep (it can also be done during spontaneous sleep), the values for 1 minute are registered while the child breathes at his or her current breathing volume through a facial mask connected to a pneumotachograph and the fractional exhaled nitric oxide analyzer. It is reported as the average result of three technically accepted maneuvers with results that do not differ from each other by more than 10%. For this technique, the normal values considered are between 2 and 8 particles per billion (ppb).

Pulmonary Function in Preschool Children

Spirometry

Children aged 2–5 years present particular challenges for conducting pulmonary function tests, including lack of attention and cooperation, besides fear of the equipment that is used.

A variable to consider is the fact that preschool children exhale lung volumes faster than adults; therefore, evaluations of $FEV_{0.4}$, $FEV_{0.5}$, and $FEV_{0.75}$ are more important. Besides this, because of the smaller volumes that these subjects move, the equipment should include minimum dead space.

In the past, it was thought that children were incapable of acceptably carrying out the FVC maneuver and achieving maximum inspiration and expiration, because of lack of attention and concentration, besides low tolerance of frustration. This is why spirometry reference tables such as the Polgar and Knudson tables do not include measurements for children under 110 cm in height or under 6 years of age. Consequently, the reference values for small children have been extrapolated from those for older children.

However, the first spirometry studies of healthy 3- to 6-year-old children have been published in recent years. The measurement of pulmonary function takes into account the recommendations that (1) this should be done by an experienced technician, and (2) time should be taken prior to the procedure to explain what it involves and to demonstrate the maneuver.

There is no consensus about the benefits of using a nasal clip in open-circuit spirometry. It can depend on the experience of the technician who conducts the study, and its use can be decided for each individual patient to obtain the best FVC reading. The maneuvers are repeated until three acceptable curves have been obtained. The study should be brief, lasting no more than 15 minutes. Different interactive programs can be used with games on the spirometry screen to facilitate acquisition of adequate curves. If the patient cries during the study, there should be no further attempt, and the test should instead be done at another opportunity.

The maneuvers that are considered unacceptable are the ones in which:

- The maximum flow cannot be clearly identified.
- The expiratory effort stops abruptly at a point where it is less than 25% of the maximum flow.
- The expiratory flow lasts for less than 1 second.
- The child's inspiration is not greater than his or her current volume.
- There is a high degree of variability.

With these criteria, acceptable spirometry results are obtained in more than 80% of studied 3- to 6-year-old children, including both healthy children and those affected by different pathologies.

Forced Oscillation Technique

Advances have been made in the clinical study of pulmonary function using the forced oscillation technique (FOT), as described by Arthur DuBois in 1956. The necessary equipment to conduct this procedure is readily accessible and easy to use, and it requires a minimum of cooperation on the part of the patient. The child puts on the mouthpiece and the nasal clip, and breathes at his or her current volume for 17 seconds while holding his or her cheeks with both hands. The equipment creates a pulsating airflow at different oscillation frequencies, which may be measured in one maneuver, or each frequency can be studied in an individual maneuver. In this way, the resistance is measured and then calculated using a mathematical model of compliance. This technique measures the resistance of the entire respiratory system and provides information to ascertain if the resistance is increased in the central or peripheral airway. The bronchodilator response can be evaluated; if the resistance measured at 5 Hz falls by at least 30% of the basal value, the bronchodilator response is considered positive. The limitation of the forced oscillation technique is the difficulty in distinguishing between an obstructive pattern and a restrictive pattern. The main advantage of the technique is that it requires a minimum of cooperation from the patient; therefore, it can be used in patients while they sleep, with patients under mechanical ventilatory assistance, and also in children who are too young for acquisition of an acceptable result using the forced capacity maneuver. In the same way, it is a valid method to study patients with a collapsed airway, as can happen in cystic fibrosis or emphysema. In these cases, it is the ideal method to assess the bronchodilator response. In 2004, the European Respiratory Society published a standardization of the methodology, with recommendations for its clinical use, and stated that the diagnostic capacity of the method is equal to that of spirometry in patients with obstructive disorders.

Interrupter Resistance Technique

The interrupter resistance (Rint) technique allows noninvasive measurement of the resistance of the respiratory system while being normally breathing. Its main advantages are its simplicity, the need for minimal patient cooperation, and the fact that it requires only a small portable apparatus.

Among its principles are concepts that were first described in 1927, when it was proposed to estimate alveolar pressure by rapid occlusion of the airway during the respiratory cycle at rest, supposing that alveolar pressure will be equal to the pressure in the mouth.

The respiratory cycle is interrupted briefly (for <100 milliseconds) in the occlusion technique. The resistance (Rint) and pressure/flow rate are calculated from how the pressure rate changes in comparison with the flow evaluated in the respiratory airway before or after the occlusion (depending on the technique). While occlusion can be done during inspiration or expiration, both the American Thoracic Society and the European Respiratory Society recommend measurement during expiration.

Both entities have standardized norms to measure the mechanical properties of the respiratory system through occlusion techniques.

Hyperactivity Studies in Preschool Children

Forced oscillation and multiple occlusion are alternatives to spirometry to assess bronchial hyperactivity in preschool children. The two techniques used with uncooperative children—the transcutaneous oxygen pressure measurement and the tracheal auscultation method–merit certain attention. In this last test, the parameter to be determined is called PCwheeze, and it is defined as the concentration of bronchoconstrictor substance with which wheezing is heard in the trachea and lung fields. With the transcutaneous oxygen measurement method, the value in question is the concentration of methacholine that causes a 5% fall from the baseline value or an increase of 50% in the baseline heart frequency.

Sources

American Thoracic Society, European Respiratory Society. ATS/ERS statement: raised volume forced expirations in infants guidelines for current practice. Am J Respir Crit Care Med. 2005;172:1463–71.

Adler SM, Wohl MEB 1978 Flow-volume relationships at low lung volumes in healthy newborn infants. Pediatrics 61:636–40.

Aurora P, Gustafsson P, Bush A, Lindblad A, et al. Multiple breath inert gas washout as a measure of ventilation distribution in children with cystic fibrosis. Thorax. 2004;59(12):1068–73.

Balinotti J, Chakr V, Tiller C, Kimmel R, et al. Growth of lung parenchyma in infants and toddlers with chronic lung disease of infancy. Am J Respir Crit Care Med. 2010;181(10):1093–7.

Balinotti JE, Tiller CJ, Llapur CJ, Jones MH, et al. Growth of the lung parenchyma early in life. Am J Respir Crit Care Med. 2009;179(2):134–7.

Castillo A, Llapur CJ, Martinez T, Kisling J, et al. Measurement of single breath-hold carbon monoxide diffusing capacity in healthy infants and toddlers. Pediatr Pulmonol. 2006;41(6):544–50.

Delacourt C, Lorino H, Fuhrman C, Herve-Guillot M, Reinert P, Harf A, Housset B. Comparison of the forced oscillation technique and the interrupter technique for assessing airway obstruction and its reversibility in children. Am J Respir Crit Care Med. 2001;164(6):965–72.

Dubois AB, Botelho SY, Comroe JH Jr. A new method for measuring airway resistance in man using a body plethysmograph: values in normal subjects and in patients with respiratory disease. J Clin Invest. 1956 Mar;35(3):327–335.

Dubois AB, Brody AW, Lewis DH, Burgess BF Jr. Oscillation mechanics of lungs and chest in man. J Appl Physiol. 1956 May;8(6):587–594.

Hellinckx J, Cauberghs M, De Boeck K, Demedts M. Evaluation of impulse oscillation system: comparison with forced oscillation technique and body plethysmography. Eur Respir J. 2001;18(3):564–70.

Hoo AF, Dezateux C, Hanrahan JP, Cole TJ, Tepper RS, Stocks J. Sex-specific prediction equations for VmaxFRC in infancy: a multicenter collaborative study. Am J Respir Crit Care Med. 2002;165:1084–92.

Horsley AR, Gustafsson PM, Macleod KA, Saunders C, et al. Lung clearance index is a sensitive, repeatable and practical measure of airways disease in adults with cystic fibrosis. Thorax. 2008;63:135–40.

Jones MH, Castile R, Davis S, Kisling J, et al. Forced expiratory flows and volumes in infants: normative data and lung growth. Am J Respir Crit Care Med. 2000;161:353–9.

Morgan WJ, Geller DE, Tepper RS, et al. Partial expiratory flow–volume curves in infants and young children. Pediatr Pulmonol. 1988;5:232–43.

Nystad W, Samuelsen S, Nafstad P, Edvardsen E, Stensrud T, Jaakkola J. Feasibility of measuring lung function in preschool children. Thorax. 2002;57:1021–7.

Stam H, Van den Beek A, Grunberg K, Stijnen T, et al. Pulmonary diffusing capacity at reduced alveolar volumes in children. Pediatr Pulmonol. 1996;21:84–9.

Taussig LM, Landau LI, Godfrey S, Arad I. Determinants of forced expiratory flows in newborn infants. J Appl Physiol. 1982;53:1220–7.

Tepper RS, Morgan WJ, Cota K, et al. Expiratory flow limitation in infants with bronchopulmonary dysplasia. J Pediatr. 1986a;109:1040–6.

Tepper RS, Morgan WJ, Cota K, et al. Physiologic growth and development of the lung during the first year of life. Am Rev Respir Dis. 1986b;134:513–9.

Tepper RS, Reister T. Forced expiratory flows and lung volumes in normal infants. Pediatr Pulmonol. 1993;15:357–61.

9 Assessment of Pulmonary Function in Schoolchildren and Adolescents

Marcela Linares Paserini and Solange Caussade Larraín

Contents

Introduction

Assessment of pulmonary function is important in schoolchildren and adolescents with chronic or recurrent lung disease, especially in those with progressive lung damage. Several tests may aid understanding of lung function in this age group (Table 9.1). To obtain valid results, it is important to apply strict quality

M. Linares Paserini
Department of Pediatrics, Clínica Indisa, Santiago, Chile
e-mail: mlinares@manquehue.net

S. Caussade Larraín (✉)
Department of Pediatrics, School of Medicine, Pontificia Universidad Católica de Chile, Santiago, Chile

P. Bertrand, I. Sánchez (eds.), *Pediatric Respiratory Diseases*, https://doi.org/10.1007/978-3-030-26961-6_9

Table 9.1 Pulmonary function tests available in pediatrics

Test	Measured variables	Physiopathological diagnosis
Spirometry and flow/volume loop	Forced flows and volumes: Expiratory: PEF, FVC, $FEV_{0.5}$, $FEV_{0.75}$, FEV_1, FEV_6, FEV_1/FVC, FEF_{25}, FEF_{50}, FEF_{75}, FEF_{25-50} Inspiratory: FIF_{50}, FEF_{50}/FIF_{50}	Obstructive ventilatory alteration (with or without decreased FVC) Restrictive ventilatory alteration Bronchodilator response Fixed central airway obstruction Variable intra- or extrathoracic central airway obstruction
Measurement of static lung volumes: Plethysmography Nitrogen washout Helium dilution	Volumes and capacities not measurable with spirometry: FRC, RV, TLC	Restrictive lung disease Air trapping Hyperinflation
Bronchial challenge test Direct: methacholine, histamine Indirect: exercise, mannitol, adenosine	PC_{20} or Increased airway resistance	Presence and degree of bronchial hyperreactivity
Airway resistance Plethysmography Rint IOS	Specific resistance and airway conductance Airway resistance Fres, Rrs5, Rrs20, Xrs5, Zrs, reactance area	Increase in airway resistance Increase or decrease in compliance (IOS) Bronchodilator response Bronchial hyperreactivity
Diffusing capacity of the lung for carbon monoxide	DLCO	Alteration of the diffusing capacity of the alveolar–capillary membrane
Measurement of static pressures	MIP MEP Sniff nasal test Cough PEF	Strength of inspiratory muscles Strength of expiratory muscles Ability to mobilize secretions
Maximal voluntary ventilation	Maximum amount of air inhaled and exhaled within 1 minute	Thoracopulmonary capacity Resistance to fatigue, airway resistance, respiratory drive
6-Minute walk test	Distance traveled	Functional capacity to exercise Cardiac capacity, respiratory capacity, muscular function capacity

CO carbon monoxide, *DLCO* diffusing capacity of the lung for carbon monoxide, FEF_{25}, FEF_{50}, FEF_{75} forced expiratory flow at 25%, 50%, or 75% of FVC, FEF_{25-75} forced expiratory flow at 25–75% of FVC, $FEV_{0.5}$, $FEV_{0.75}$, FEV_1, FEV_6 forced expiratory volume in 0.5, 0.75, 1, or 6 seconds, FIF_{50} forced inspiratory flow at 50% of forced inspiratory capacity (FVC), *FRC* functional residual capacity, *Fres* resonance frequency, *FVC* forced vital capacity, *IOS* impulse oscillometry, *MEP* maximum expiratory pressure, *MIP* maximum inspiratory pressure, PC_{20} methacholine or histamine concentration that causes a 20% drop in FEV_1, *PEF* peak expiratory flow, *Rint* interrupter resistance, *Rrs5* resistance at 5 Hz, *Rrs20* resistance at 20 Hz, *RV* residual volume, *TLC* total lung capacity, *Xrs5* reactance at 5 Hz, *Zrs* respiratory impedance

control measures and interpret the results on the basis of internationally accepted standards. Better results are obtained if tests are conducted in an appropriate environment, without interference or distraction, and by personnel experienced in working with children. In some cases, training and use of incentive programs help to improve the performance. The respiratory laboratory should have a qualified doctor available who is responsible for supervising tests, managing emergency situations, and providing reports.

Spirometry and the Flow/Volume Curve

Spirometry measures lung volume and flow on the basis of forced expiration following maximum inspiration to reach the total lung capacity

Table 9.2 Definitions of lung volumes, flows, and capacities

Tidal volume (*TV*): volume of inspired and expired air during normal breathing
Inspiratory reserve volume (*IRV*): volume of air that enters the lungs when a deep inspiration is performed, above TV
Expiratory reserve volume (*ERV*): volume of air exhaled during a deep expiration after a normal expiration
Residual volume (*RV*): volume of air remaining in the lungs after a maximum expiration
Vital capacity (*VC*): sum of the maximum expired volume after a maximal inspiration
SVC: slow vital capacity
FVC: forced vital capacity
Inspiratory capacity (*IC*): maximum amount of air that can be inspired after normal expiration
Functional residual capacity (*FRC*): volume of air that remains in the lungs after normal expiration
Total lung capacity (*TLC*): maximum volume of air that the lungs can contain
RV/TLC ratio: percentage of RV in relation to TLC
Forced expiratory volume in a given time (FEV_t): volume of air expired during the FVC maneuver from TLC in a given time (e.g., 0.5, 0.75, 1, or 6 seconds)
FEV_1/*FVC ratio*: percentage of exhaled volume in 1 second in relation to FVC
Forced expiratory flow at 25–75% of FVC (FEF_{25-75}): slope of the spirometric volume/time curve between 25% and 75% of FVC
Forced expiratory flow at 25%, 50%, or 75% of FVC (FEF_{25}, FEF_{50}, FEF_{75}): forced expiratory flow when 25%, 50%, or 75% of FVC has been exhaled
Forced inspiratory flow at 50% of forced vital capacity (FVC) (FIF_{50}): forced inspiratory flow measured at the 50% point of the inspiratory part of the flow/volume curve
Peak expiratory flow (*PEF*): maximum flow velocity observed during the forced expiratory maneuver

(TLC). Table 9.2 lists lung volumes, flows, and capacities.

Spirometry is indicated to diagnose alterations in lung function in patients with respiratory symptoms and signs (pathologies that can directly or indirectly affect lung function) or with exposure to risk factors such as smoking, environmental contamination, radiotherapy, chemotherapy, or other drugs with known pulmonary toxicity. Spirometry is also indicated to assess anesthetic and surgical risks and the prognosis of patients with respiratory pathologies, to assess the response to different treatments (bronchodilators, inhaled corticosteroids, kinesiotherapy), and to control the advance of progressive pathologies such as neuromuscular diseases and cystic fibrosis.

The equipment used for spirometry should be calibrated daily.

The maneuver is performed with a maximum and rapid inspiration to reach the total pulmonary capacity, followed by a maximum expiratory effort 3–6 seconds in duration and/or a plateau of at least 1 second.

The test yields two graphic registers—the volume/time curve and the flow/volume curve—which should be analyzed to assess the acceptability of the examination. The volume/time curve (Fig. 9.1a) relates the volume of exhaled air to the time taken to exhale. It has an initial rapid increase and then reaches a plateau. The flow/volume curve (Fig. 9.1b) distinguishes between the inspiratory and expiratory phases. The inspiratory phase goes from the residual volume (RV) to TLC, constituting the lower part of the graph and forming a semicircle in which it is possible to measure the maximum inspiratory flow at 50% of forced vital capacity (FVC): (FIF_{50}). The expiratory phase has a triangular profile, with a rapid ascent from the total pulmonary capacity to the peak expiratory flow (PEF), and a slow descent with a constant slope until RV is reached. In the first part of the expiratory phase, in which pulmonary volume is high, the flow depends on effort, but after expiration of the first third of the vital capacity (VC), at the level of low pulmonary volumes, the flows are independent of effort. The shape of the flow/volume curve indicates the presence of fixed or variable obstruction of the central airway (Fig. 9.2). At least three curves that comply with international criteria for acceptability should be obtained, and at least two of these should be repeatable—that is, with variability of less than 5% in the forced vital

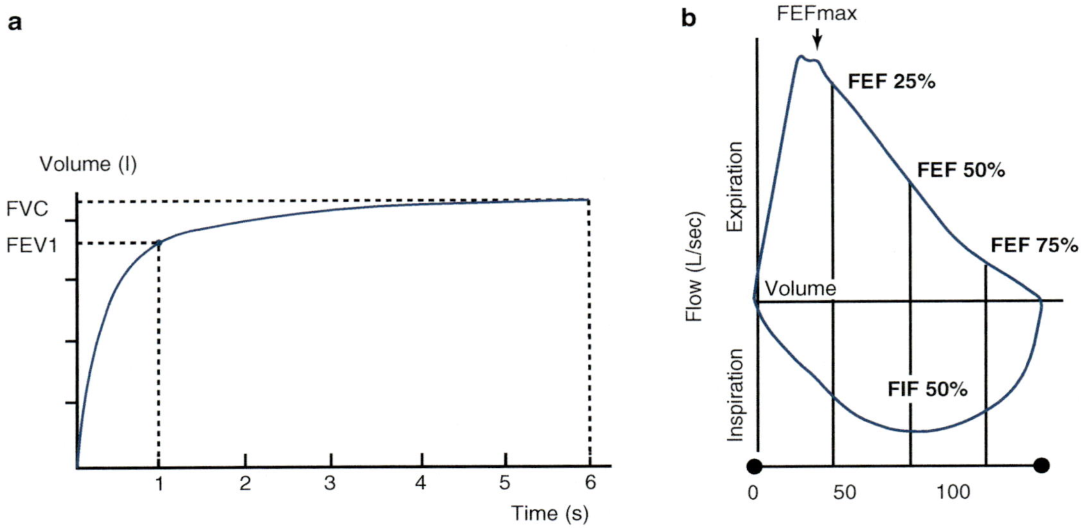

Fig. 9.1 Spirometric curves. **a** Volume/time curve showing the forced expiratory volume in 1 second (FEV1) and in 6 seconds (FEV6). **b** Flow/volume loop showing the forced expiratory flow (FEF) at 25% (FEF_{25}), 50% (FEF_{50}), and 75% (FEF_{75}) of the forced vital capacity (FVC), and the forced inspiratory flow (FIF) at 50% of the inspiratory loop. *FEFmax* maximum instantaneous flow achieved during a FVC maneuver

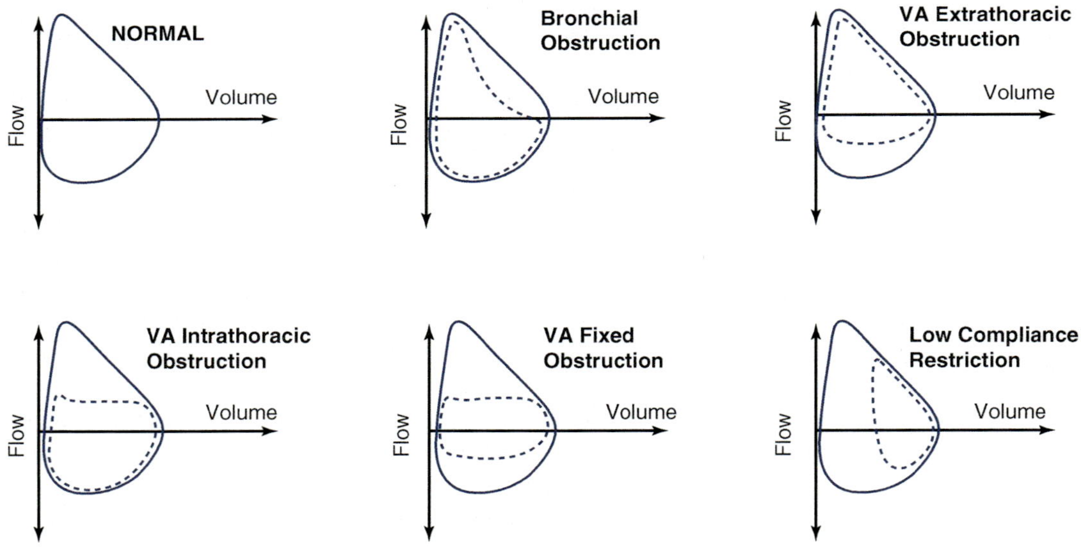

Fig. 9.2 Alterations in the flow/volume loop: forms of the loop that display pathophysiological changes in the airway and lungs. *Airway*: Extrathoracic airway Obstruction; Intrathoracic airway Obstruction; Fixed airway obstruction

capacity (FVC) and forced expiratory volume in 1 second (FEV_1). A numerical report should be produced for FVC, FEV_1, FEV_1/FVC, and forced expiratory flow at 25–75% of FVC ($FEF_{25–75}$).

The spirometry test is repeated 15 minutes after administration of 400 μg of salbutamol in an aerosol form to assess the response to the bronchodilator. Any increase of 12% in FEV_1 and/or 30% in $FEF_{25–75}$ is considered a significant response (provided that the postbronchodilatory FVC does not vary more than 10% from the basal value).

The reference values that are used should be registered in the report. Those most widely used at present are Knudson, NHANES III (National Health and Nutrition Examination Survey III), and Gutierrez. The Global Lung Function Initiative (GLI) has recently developed reference equations that address an age range from 3 to 90 years, with differences according to the ethnicity of the population. A spirometry reading is considered normal when the values are above P5 or within ±1.64 standard deviations (Z score) of the reference values.

Obstructive and restrictive alterations in ventilation, with or without a decrease in FVC, can be distinguished (Table 9.3).

The degree of severity of obstructive alterations is determined by FEV_1, and the severity of restrictive alterations is determined by FVC (Table 9.4).

Table 9.3 Types of alterations observed in spirometry

		Obstructive	
Parameter	Restrictive	With normal FVC	With decreased FVC
FVC	↓	Normal	↓
FEV_1	Normal or ↓	Normal or ↓	↓
FEV_1/FVC	Normal or ↑	↓	↓
FEF_{25-75}	Normal or ↓	Normal or ↓	↓

↑ increased, ↓ decreased, FEF_{25-75} forced expiratory flow at 25–75% of FVC, FEV_1 forced expiratory volume in 1 second, *FVC* forced vital capacity

Table 9.4 Degrees of severity in spirometry

Restrictive alteration	Obstructive alteration
Mild: 65% < FVC < LLN[a]	Minimum: FEF_{25-75} < LLN[b]
Moderate: 50% < FVC < 65%	Mild: FEV_1 > 65%[c]
Advanced: FVC < 50%	Moderate: 50% < FEV_1 < 65%
	Advanced: FEV_1 < 50%

FEF_{25-75} forced expiratory flow at 25–75% of FVC, FEV_1 forced expiratory volume in 1 second, *FVC* forced vital capacity, *LLN* lower limit of normal
[a]Percentage of the reference value
[b]Normal FVC, FEV_1, and FEV_1/FVC
[c]The FEV_1/FVC ratio must be less than LLN in cases with a normal FEV_1

Peak Expiratory Flow

The peak expiratory flow (PEF) documents lung function at different moments during the day and in the regular environment of the patient. It is used to determine bronchial ability, contributing to the diagnosis and treatment of asthma.

It can be used for self-control by the asthmatic patient for short periods—above all, when the patient and family have a limited perception of the symptoms.

What is termed the personal best value is recommended for interpretation of the results. This is the maximum value obtained from two readings per day during an asymptomatic 2-week period.

Although the major asthma guides advise the use of peak expiratory flow (PEF) for self-management, no improvement in asthma has been demonstrated in this case, and adherence is generally low.

Bronchial Provocation Tests

Bronchial provocation tests induce obstruction of the airway by using different stimuli to determine the presence and degree of bronchial reactivity. They are classified as (1) direct techniques, which act on the bronchial smooth muscle to provoke bronchoconstriction, using stimuli such as methacholine and histamine; and (2) indirect techniques, which cause release of mediators by mast cells, in turn triggering contraction of the bronchial smooth muscle, using stimuli such as exercise, cold air, adenosine, and mannitol. The most commonly used tests employ exercise and methacholine.

Increased bronchial reactivity is a distinctive characteristic of asthma, but reactivity is also present in other conditions such as atopy, bronchopulmonary dysplasia, cystic fibrosis, and exposure to pollen or contamination, because of which the results of the examination should be considered in the context of the individual patient.

The provocation test is contraindicated in patients with a base FEV_1 lower than 80% of the reference value. The methacholine test is contraindicated in pregnant patients, and exercise cannot be used in patients with heart disease (arrhythmia, hypertension, or aortic stenosis), physical incapacity (neuromuscular disease, orthopedic disease, or severe deformation), fever, chronic respiratory insufficiency, insulin-dependent diabetes, or uncontrolled epilepsy.

When the results of these examinations are being interpreted, it should be kept in mind that there are medications that reduce bronchial hyperreactivity, such as short- and long-acting bronchodilators. Antihistamines and antileukotrienes have the same effect on the exercise test. Inhaled corticoids attenuate the response of the airway when they are administered for more than 4 weeks. When the objective is to assess the degree of control over the disease and not to establish a diagnosis, the examinations can be conducted without these medications being stopped.

Provocation Test with Exercise

This test measures the response of the airway to exercise with pre-established intensity and characteristics. Hyperventilation experienced while exercising and breathing cold dry air causes dehydration and increases the osmolality of bronchial mucus, which triggers the release by mast cells of histamine, leukotrienes, and prostaglandins, in turn stimulating contraction of the bronchial smooth muscle. An environment with an absolute moisture content of less than 10 mg/l of air is recommended to increase the yield of the test. The report should include the moisture level and ambient temperature.

The exercise-induced provocation test is indicated to support the diagnosis of asthma in children with a compatible clinical picture and normal spirometry results. The test can be used to assess the response to maintenance treatment of asthmatic children and to assess bronchial hyperreactivity in athletes. It has a high degree of specificity (90%) and low sensitivity (50%) for diagnosing asthma.

The child runs for 6–8 minutes on a treadmill or a track while wearing a nose clip, with a requirement to reach a submaximal heart rate in the last 4–6 minutes of the run. FEV_1 is measured before the exercise and at 3, 5, 10, 15, and 30 minutes. The higher of two values is chosen for each measurement.

The exercise-induced test is considered positive when the maximum observed fall in FEV_1 is ≥10% of the baseline value (FEV_1 value at rest before the test). Inhaled salbutamol is administered to children who have positive responses or who present symptoms of bronchial obstruction.

False positive results can be due to vocal cord dysfunction, tracheobronchomalacia, use of propranolol, or suboptimal forced expiration. False negative results can be due to failure to achieve maximum ventilation, atmospheric conditions beyond the specified range, and use of medications that attenuate bronchial hyperreactivity.

Methacholine-Induced Bronchial Test

This test measures the response of the airway to different concentrations of nebulized methacholine, a cholinergic agonist that binds muscarinic receptors of the smooth muscles of the airways, provoking dose-dependent contraction.

The child should be free from acute respiratory infections for 3–4 weeks prior to the examination, otherwise a false positive result could be obtained.

The most widely used method is a modified version of the method described by Cockcroft et al., in which the patient is nebulized every 5 minutes, first with the diluent and then with increasing dilutions of methacholine. The concentrations of the latter are doubled with each successive nebulization, from 0.06 to 16 mg/ml. FEV_1 is measured at 60 and 90 seconds after each nebulization, with selection of the best determination. At the end of the examination, ipratropium bromide is administered together with fenoterol or inhaled salbutamol.

The level of response of the airway to methacholine is measured with the PC_{20} calculation, which is defined as the methacholine concentration that causes a 20% decrease in FEV_1 with respect to the FEV_1 value obtained with a diluent.

Table 9.5 Cutoff points used to establish the degree of bronchial hyperreactivity (BHR) in children under 15 years old

BHR degree	PC_{20}
Normal (no BHR)	>8 mg/ml
Limited	4–8 mg/ml
Mild	1–4 mg/ml
Moderate	0.25–1 mg/ml
Severe	<0.25 mg/ml

Arbitrary PC_{20} cutoff values have been established to determine the severity of bronchial hyperreactivity (Table 9.5).

The sensitivity and specificity of the methacholine test to diagnose asthma varies according to the PC_{20} value obtained. A PC_{20} value of less than 1 or 2 has high specificity for diagnosing asthma, similar to that of indirect tests such as the exercise-induced test. When the PC_{20} value is higher than 8 or 16, it is highly probable that the child does not have asthma, although it cannot be totally ruled out—above all, in athletes. The positive predictive value for diagnosing asthma increases as the PC_{20} decreases from scores between 4 and 16.

Static Lung Volume Measurement

This technique is used to determine the total lung volume and capacity (Fig. 9.3), through which the functional residual capacity can be measured, which is the sum of the reserve expiratory volume and RV. The latter is the volume that remains in the lungs after a forced maximum expiration, because of which it cannot be assessed with a spirometer. To calculate TLC, the functional residual capacity is added to IC, previously measured by spirometry.

Measurement of pulmonary volume is indicated for the study of restrictive pathologies, early assessment of airway obstruction in chronic pulmonary diseases such as cystic fibrosis, determination of the degree of air entrapment and hyperinflation, and determination of the existence of a restrictive limitation in patients with obstructive spirometry with reduced vital strength. TLC characteristically decreases with restrictive

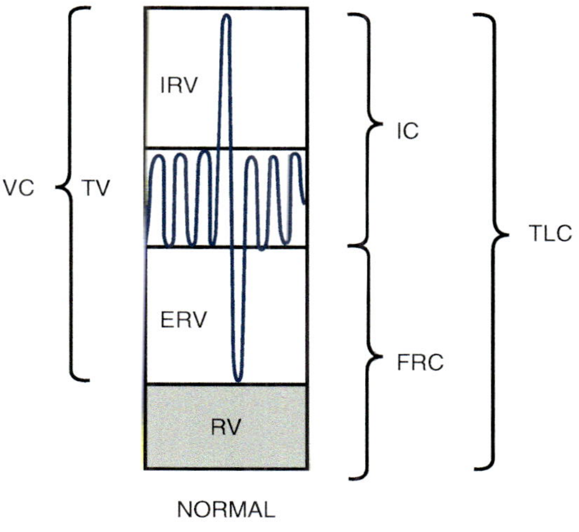

Fig. 9.3 Lung volumes and capacities. *ERV* expiratory reserve volume, *FRC* functional residual capacity, *IC* inspiratory capacity, *IRV* inspiratory reserve volume, *RV* residual volume, *TLC* total lung capacity, *TV* tidal voume, *VC* vital capacity

pathologies. In the case of chronic obstructive diseases, increases in RV and the RV/TLC ratio indicate air trapping. Moreover, an elevated CPT value confirms pulmonary hyperinflation (Fig. 9.4). Table 9.6 shows the percentage values used to interpret the results of the measurements.

The available techniques are a closed circuit with helium dilution, an open circuit or nitrogen wash, and plethysmography. The latter constitutes the gold standard in that it measures the total volume of thoracic gas, unlike other measures that only attempt to determine the quantity of gas that communicates with the airway.

There are national reference values for pulmonary volumes measured by plethysmography and nitrogen washout.

PC_{20} methacholine or histamine concentration that causes a 20% drop in the forced expiratory volume in 1 second (FEV_1)

Plethysmography

There are three types of plethysmography: flow, volume, and pressure; the last is the one that is most commonly used. Measurement of the func-

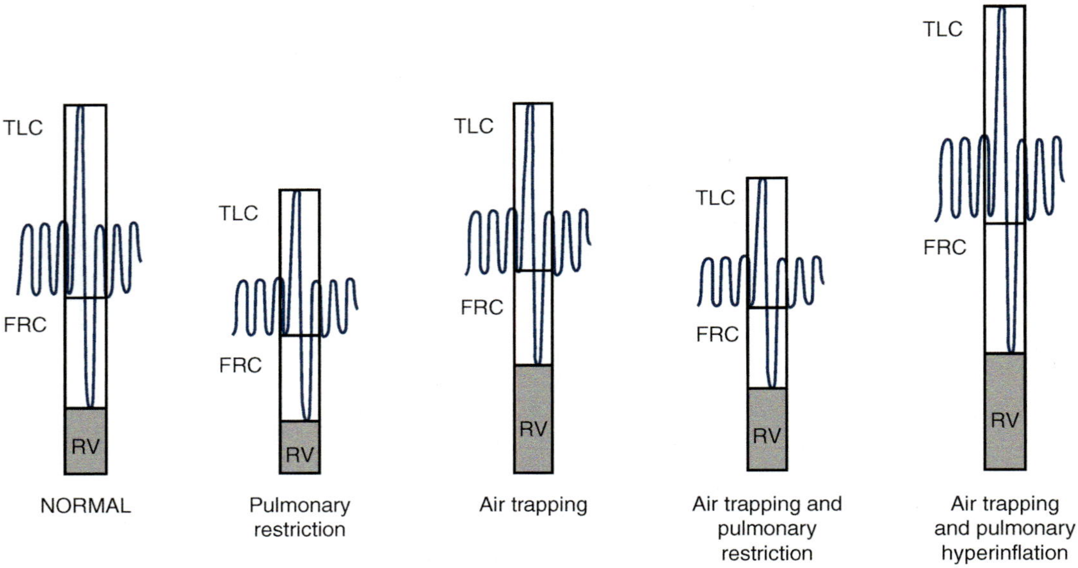

Fig. 9.4 Types of alterations in static lung volumes. *FRC* functional residual capacity, *RV* residual volume, *TLC* total lung capacity

Table 9.6 Percentage limits for static lung volumes

Parameter	Limit
TLC	Normal: 80–130% Pulmonary restriction: <80% Pulmonary hyperinflation: >130%
RV	Normal: ≤130% Air trapping: >130%
RV/TLC	Normal: ≤30% Air trapping: >30%

RV residual volume, *TLC* total lung capacity

tional residual capacity (FRC) is based on Boyle's law, which states that in an airtight system (in this case, the plethysmograph) at a constant temperature, the product of pressure multiplied by volume remains constant:

$$P_1 \times V_1 = P_2 \times V_2.$$

The patient sits in the plethysmograph box and is connected to a mouthpiece, which is blocked for 2–3 seconds, during which the patient must breathe at a high rate. This determines the compression and decompression of air trapped in the chest (FRC), which translates into pressure and volume in the plethysmograph box (Fig. 9.5). Variations at the level of the patient's mouth are equivalent to alveolar pressure. The pressure signals read by the transductors in the box are used to calculate the functional residual capacity on the basis of Boyle's law.

As well as measuring the total volume of intrathoracic gas, this method has the advantage of being rapid and reproducible. Its disadvantages are that it requires a high degree of cooperation and it is costly.

Helium Dilution

A closed-circuit system is used for this measurement, employing a spirometer containing a known concentration of inert helium in a known volume (Fig. 9.6). The patient is connected to the spirometer mouthpiece and breathes at the current volume until the helium concentration in the system is in equilibrium. The formula to calculate the functional residual capacity (FRC) is:

$$\text{CRF} = \frac{\left(\%\text{H}_{\text{initial}} - \%\text{H}_{\text{final}}\right)}{\%\text{H}_{\text{final}}} \times \text{volume}$$

Nitrogen Wash

The patient is connected through an open circuit to the mouthpiece of the equipment, breathing oxygen at 100% of the current volume. In this way, the intrapulmonary gas is "washed" with the volume and concentration of nitrogen being registered with each exhalation. The test ends when the concentration of nitrogen remains constant or falls below 5% in successive exhalations. To calculate the functional residual capacity, the volume of total exhaled gas and the final concentration of nitrogen are related to the initial nitrogen concentration in the intrapulmonary gas, which is assumed to be 80% (Fig. 9.7).

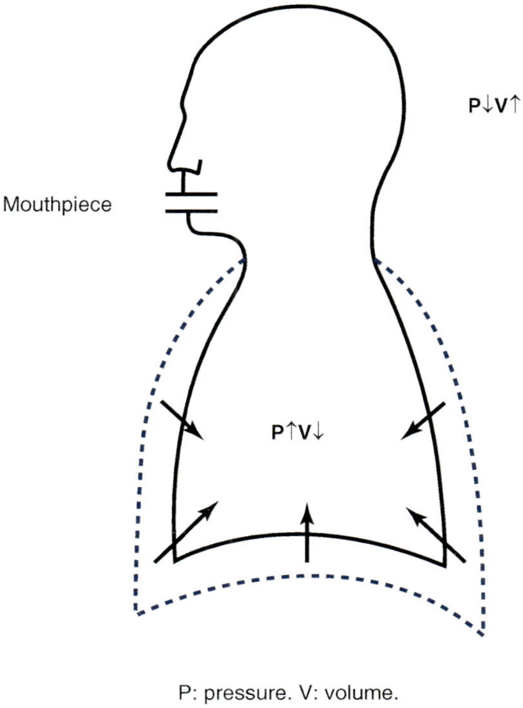

Fig. 9.5 Lung volumes: plethysmography. Boyle's law states that in a hermetically closed box, at a constant temperature, the pressure/volume (PV) relation remains constant. Increasing the chest volume increases the cabin pressure and decreases the volume, and vice versa. The calculation of the functional residual capacity (FRC) considers pressure changes inside the cabin and in the patient's mouth

Lung Carbon Monoxide Diffusion

The test for the diffusing capacity of the lung for carbon monoxide (DLCO) measures the capacity to transfer inhaled carbon monoxide to the erythrocytes of the pulmonary capillary blood. This phenomenon depends on the pulmonary volume, ventilation/perfusion ratio, surface and thickness of the alveolar membrane, capillary volume, concentration, properties of hemoglobin, and carbon monoxide affinity for hemoglobin. Because of the dependence on these multiple factors, it is termed a "transfer factor" in the European literature.

The main indications for this test in pediatrics are diseases that compromise the pulmonary interstitium, such as those secondary to immunological or rheumatic diseases, damage by drugs, radiotherapy, and checkups of patients who have received lung and hematopoietic cell transplants.

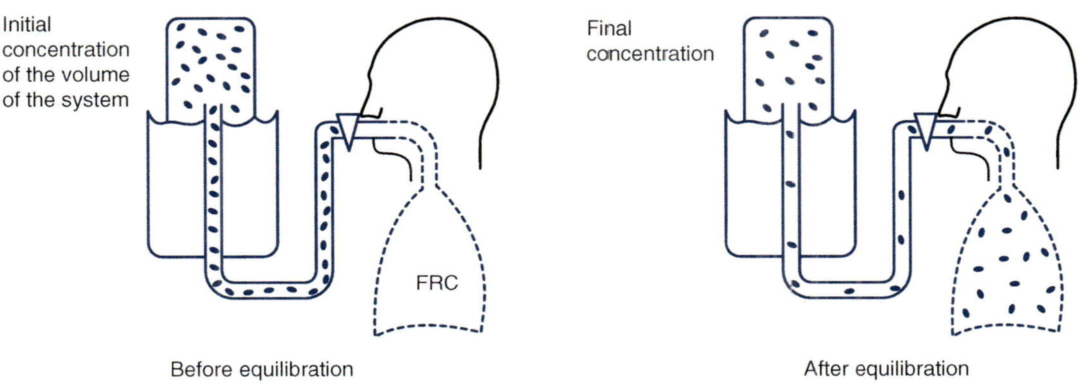

Fig. 9.6 Helium dilution technique. *FRC* functional residual capacity

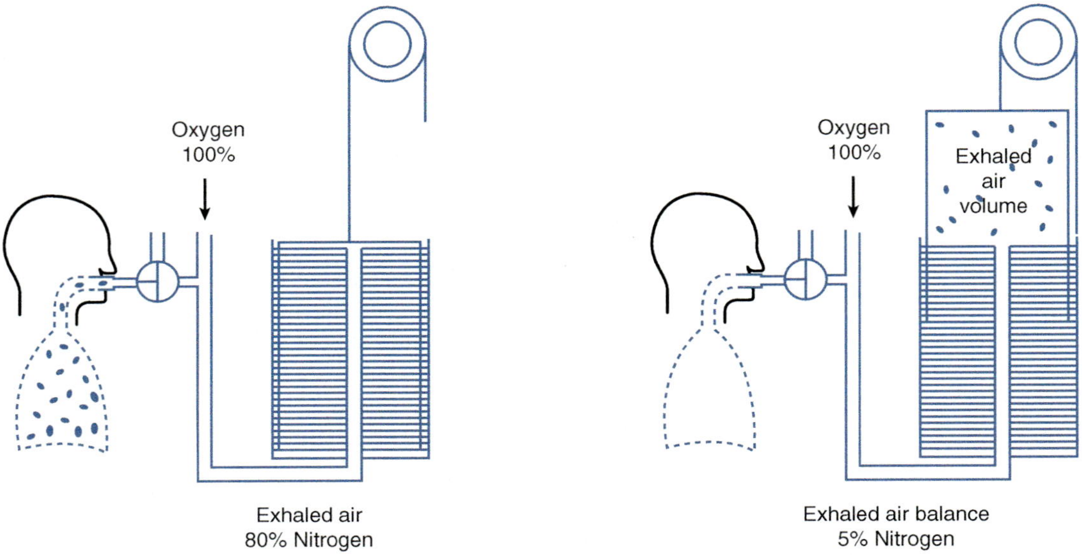

Fig. 9.7 Nitrogen washout technique

Because hemoglobin has high affinity for carbon, the partial pressure of this (carbon monoxide) in plasma can be considered zero when the concentration of carboxyhemoglobin is low. Thus, the carbon transfer capacity is the volume of carbon monoxide transferred per minute per millimeter of mercury of the partial alveolar pressure.

Because high levels of understanding and cooperation are required on the part of the patient, the procedure is usually not applied to children under 10 years of age. The single-breath method is the one most widely used. It consists of the subject exhaling until RV is reached, and then inhaling rapidly until more than 85% of FVC is reached, during which carbon is inhaled at 0.03%. The patient should remain in apnea for 10 seconds, during which the carbon is diffused. Finally, the patient should exhale slowly until RV is reached, at which point the final concentration of carbon is measured (Fig. 9.8). At least two acceptable measurements should be made, with a difference between them of 10% or less.

An inert gas (helium or methane) is included in the mixture of diffusion gases for calculation of the diffusing lung volume, which allows for adjustment of the values that are obtained. Adjustments should also be made in the case of patients with anemia or polycythemia, according to their hemoglobin values.

The complexity of the process of measuring carbon monoxide diffusion is reflected in discrepancies in results from different laboratories. Consequently, if no baseline values are available, the results obtained from each patient should be compared with one another.

Airway Resistance

Spirometry is usually employed to find limitations to airflow in patients with chronic obstructive disease. Since resistance is a contributing factor for obstruction, measurement of resistance can contribute additional information and more sensitivity for assessment of the response to bronchodilatory and bronchoconstriction agents such as methacholine. In pediatric practice the study is indicated mainly in patients with bronchial asthma, cystic fibrosis, or postinfectious bronchiolitis obliterans.

The methods used for assessing airway resistance are plethysmography (considered the gold standard), impulse oscillometry (IOS), and interrupter resistance (Rint). The latter two offer the

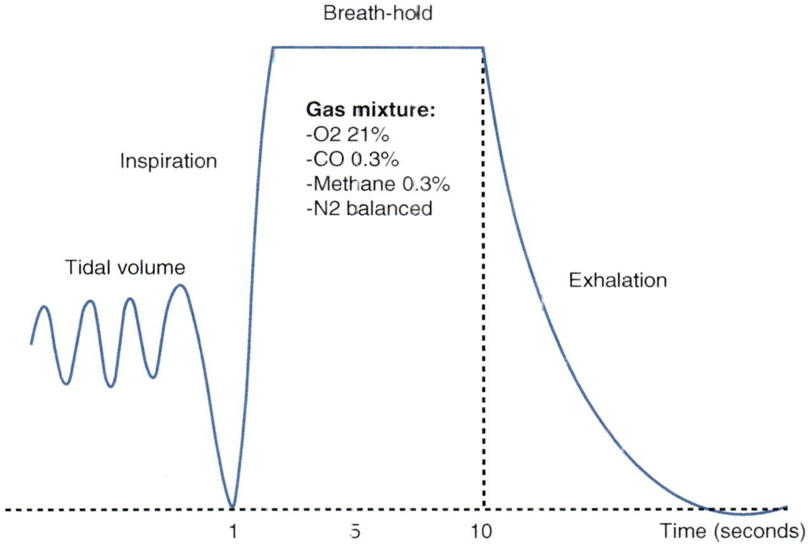

Fig. 9.8 Diffusing capacity of the lung for carbon monoxide (DLCO). *CO* carbon monoxide, *N2* nitrogen, *O2* oxygen

advantage that they can be used in children as young as 3 years old.

Exhaled Nitric Oxide Measurement

Although the relationship between airway inflammation and nitric oxide (NO) is not fully understood, there is evidence supporting the view that the measurement of NO exhaled (FeNO) from the lower respiratory tract is an indicator of eosinophilic inflammation. The main indication is assessment of the response to inhaled corticoid treatment for asthma.

The patient should be in a sitting position for the measurement, wearing nasal pincers to avoid measurement of nitric oxide from the upper airway. The mouthpiece is placed on the patient, and he/she inhales until TLC is reached. The subject should immediately exhale at a constant flow against the pressure exercised by the system, until at least a 2-second plateau in the concentration of nitric oxide is reached during an exhalation of at least 4 seconds. The results should be based on three repetitions of the procedure with no more than a 10% variation among them, or two repetitions with no more than a 5% variation.

There is also equipment to measure nasal nitric oxide, the production of which is greater than what is observed in the lower respiratory airway. The diagnostic value of nitric oxide concentrations has been demonstrated only for primary ciliary dyskinesia, in which the values are low.

Evaluation of Respiratory Muscle Strength

The failure of the respiratory pump is one of the main causes of complications and death among patients with neuromuscular diseases. However, the risk of respiratory insufficiency can be determined by assessing the strength of the respiratory muscles. Muscular weakness is sometimes difficult to detect clinically, which indicates the importance of objective measurements.

Sources

Anderson SD, Kippelen P. Assessment of EIB: what you need to know to optimize test results. Immunol Allergy Clin North Am. 2013;33:363–80.

American Thoracic Society, European Respiratory Society. ATS/ERS recommendations for standardized procedures for the online and offline measurement of exhaled lower respiratory nitric oxide and nasal nitric oxide, 2005. Am J Respir Crit Care Med. 2005;171:912–30.

Caussade S, Pulgar D, Vega-Briceño L, Viviani P, Díaz C, Contreras I, Sánchez I. Plethysmographic lung volumes in normal Chilean children and adolescents. Pediatr Pulmonol. 2008;43:866–73.

Criee CP, Sorichter S, Smith HJ, Kardos P, Merget R, Heise D, et al. Body plethysmography—its principles and clinical use. Respir Med. 2011;105:959–71.

Cockcroft DW, Davis BE. The bronchoprotective effect of inhaling methacholine by using total lung capacity inspirations has a marked influence on the interpretation of the test result. J Allergy Clin Immunol. 2006;117:1244–8.

Cockcroft DW, Davis BE, Todd DC, Smycniuk AJ. Methacholine challenge: comparison of two methods. Chest. 2005;127:839–44.

Cockcroft DW, Hurst TS, Gore BP. Importance of evaporative water losses during standardized nebulized inhalation provocation tests. Chest. 1989;96:505–8.

Cockcroft DW, Killian DN, Mellon JJ, Hargreave FE. Bronchial reactivity to inhaled histamine: a method and clinical survey. Clin Allergy. 1977;7:235–43.

Davies B, Cockcroft D. Past, present and future uses of methacholine testing. Expert Rev Respir Med. 2012;6:321–9.

Dweik RA, Boggs PB, Erzurum SC, et al. An official ATS clinical practice guideline: interpretation of exhaled nitric oxide levels (FeNO) for clinical applications. Am J Respir Crit Care Med. 2011;184(5):602–15.

Gutiérrez M, Rioseco F, Rojas A, Casanova D. Determinación de valores espirométricos en una población chilena normal mayor de 5 años, a nivel del mar. Rev Med Chile. 1996;124:1295–306.

Hankinson JL, Odencrantz JR, Fedan KB. Spirometric reference values from a sample of the general US population. Am J Respir Crit Care Med. 1999;159:179–87.

Kaminsky D. What does airway resistance tell us about lung function? Respir Care. 2012;57:85–96.

Lebowitz M, Quanjer P. ERS statement on peak expiratory flow. Eur Respir J. 1997;10:1s–83s.

Linares M, Sánchez I, Corrales R, Díaz A, Escobar A. Pruebas de función pulmonar en el niño. Rev Chil Pediatr. 2000;71(3):228–44.

McIntyre N, Crapo RO, Viegi G, Johnson DC, van der Grinten CPM, Brusasco V, et al. Standardization of the single breath determination of carbon monoxide uptake in the lung. Eur Respir J. 2005;26:720–35.

Miller M, Hankinson J, Brusasco V, Burgos F, Casaburi R, Coates A et al; ATS/ERS Task Force. Standardisation of spirometry. Eur Respir J. 2005;26:319–338.

Parsons J, Hallstarnd T, Mastronarde J, Kaminsky D, Rundell K, Hull J, et al. An official American Thoracic Society practice guideline: exercise-induced bronchoconstriction. Am J Respir Crit Care Med. 2013;187:1016–27.

Pellegrino R, Viegi G, Brusasco V, Crapo R, Burgos F, Casaburi R, et al. ATS/ERS task force: standardisation of lung function testing: interpretative Strategies for lung function tests. Eur Respir J. 2005;26:948–68.

Assessment of Respiratory Muscular Function in Patients with Neuromuscular Diseases

10

Solange Caussade Larraín

Contents

Introduction

The respiratory systems of patients with neuromuscular diseases (NMDs) are often compromised. The stage at which the compromise emerges depends on the base disease, the degree of muscular and neurological compromise, and the speed of its progression. The cause of respiratory alteration can originate in the lungs or in the respiratory pump (the rib cage and respiratory muscles). The function of the latter is to mobilize the air toward the alveoli, overcoming the elastic and resistive force of the lungs. It can be altered by central or mechanical causes or muscular fatigue. Its compromise is sometimes difficult to detect early on, indicating the importance of objective measurements. This chapter reviews the examinations that assess general respiratory function, force, and muscular fatigue.

S. Caussade Larraín (✉)
Department of Pediatrics, School of Medicine, Pontificia Universidad Católica de Chile, Santiago, Chile

P. Bertrand, I. Sánchez (eds.), *Pediatric Respiratory Diseases*,
https://doi.org/10.1007/978-3-030-26961-6_10

General Respiratory Muscle Assessment

These examinations are not specific to assessment of muscular function, although they provide useful information about the severity, functional consequences, and prognosis of NMDs.

Spirometry Flow/Volume Loops

A simple inspection of the flow/volume loops makes evident the presence of respiratory muscular weakness. In some cases, there is a decrease in the slope of the ascending phase and a delay in reaching the maximum expiratory flow (MEF). MEF can also be poorly defined. These findings reflect slow initial pulmonary emptying. At the end of expiration, there can be an abrupt drop just before the residual volume (RV) is reached, which is caused by expiratory muscular fatigue due to sustained effort (Fig. 10.1a). When there is greater muscular compromise, characteristically there is a more pronounced reduction in flows that depend on effort in the expiration and inspiration phases of the flow/volume loop (Fig. 10.1b).

An effective cough that efficiently removes secretions from the airway requires sufficient intrathoracic pressure to produce dynamic compression of the airway and respiratory flow at a high velocity. The expiratory flow/volume loop also serves to show the effect of coughing. In normal subjects, coughing appears as transitory flows that exceed the maximum flow achieved by a forced expiration, with spikes that rise above the loop. The absence of these spikes indicates respiratory muscular weakness and correlates very well with a maximum respiratory pressure of <40 cm H_2O (Fig. 10.1c).

Pulmonary Volume and Capacity

Spirometry Measurements: Volumes and Flows of Forced Expirations

The basic examination assesses respiratory mechanics and is used in patients with NMDs to establish the degree of respiratory muscular compromise through analysis of the shape of the inspiratory and expiratory flow/volume loops (described above) and their variables, the most useful being the forced vital capacity (FVC) test, which measures inspiratory and expiratory musculature at the time. A normal score indicates the absence of significant muscular compromise. However, it is not a sensitive indicator as it does not decrease until muscular force is highly compromised. It is mainly used to follow the evolution of patients as a marker of the risk of respiratory insufficiency and mortality. Thus, FVC of <1 liter predicts an 8% probability of 5-year survival in patients with Duchenne muscular dystrophy.

Another useful spirometry technique to identify diaphragmatic compromise is performance of the test with the patient first sitting or standing and then in the prone position. A 25% or greater decrease in FVC in the supine position indicates altered diaphragm functioning that is not able to overcome the gravitational force of the abdominal content. On the other hand, if the patient has an obstructive disease of the small intrathoracic airway (asthma, postviral damage, or other disease), measurements of forced expiratory flow (FEF) (e.g., FEF at 25–75% of FVC (FEF_{25-75}) and FEF at 50% of FVC (FEF_{50})) help to determine the presence of this associated compromise.

Measurement of Static Pulmonary Volume

The gold-standard method for performing these measurements is plethysmography. Measurement of the static pulmonary volume allows assessment of the balance between lung compliance, the rib cage, and the respiratory musculature. A characteristically restrictive pattern is observed in NMDs: diminished vital capacity, diminished total lung capacity (TLC), and RV proportional to this. The degree to which TLC decreases varies depending on the muscular impairment and is basically due to reduced inspiratory capacity (IC). Initially the RV remains in the normal range and increases with the appearance of significant compromise in the respiratory musculature at the cost of less expiratory reserve volume (ERV). In these cases, a higher RV/TLC ratio does not indicate the presence of trapped air (Fig. 10.2).

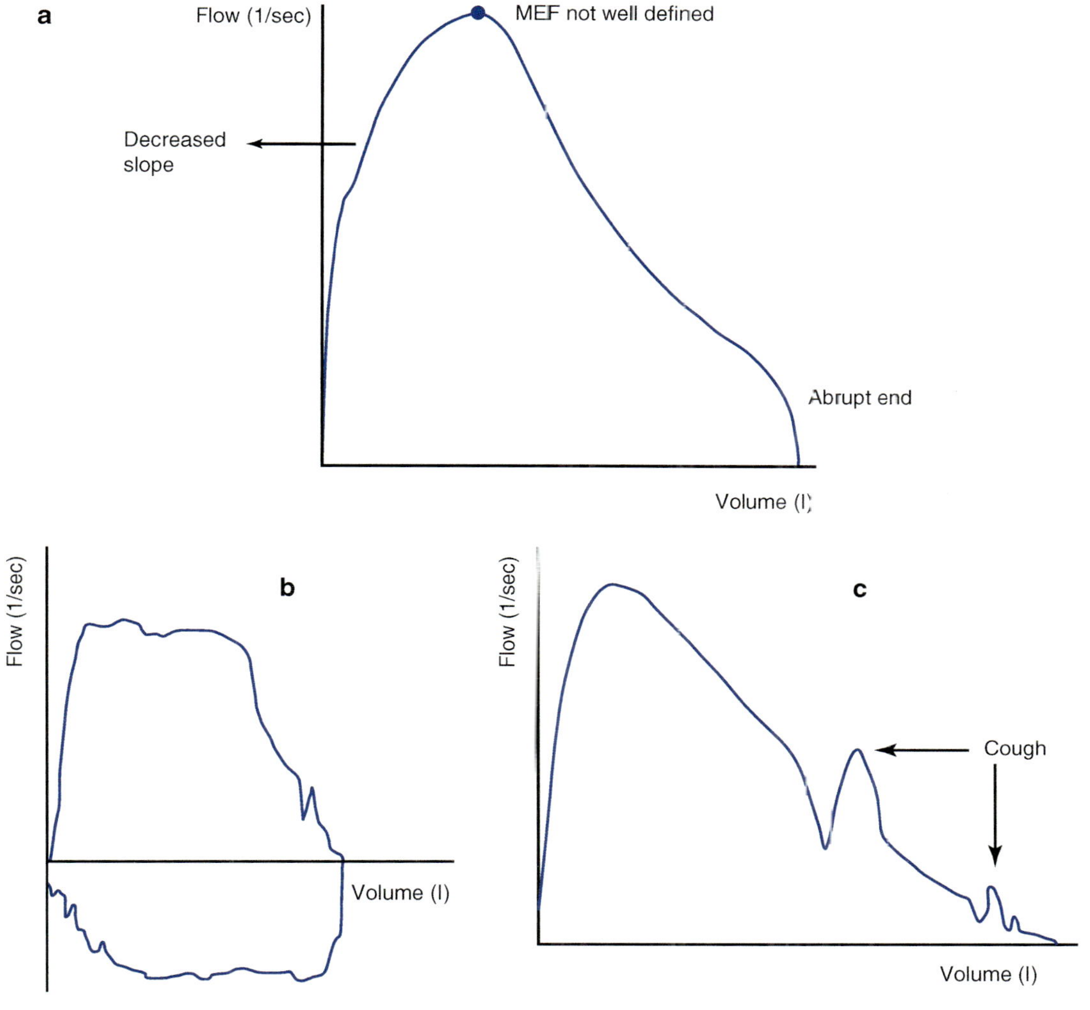

Fig. 10.1 Flow/volume curves. (**a**) Patient with mild to moderate expiratory muscular compromise. The initial slope of a slow ascent is observed. The maximum expiratory flow (MEF) does not show a defined peak. An abrupt end of the expiration is apparent. (**b**) Patient with moderate to severe muscular compromise. There is a flattening of the initial phase of the expiratory phase and of the inspiratory phase of the flow/volume loop. (**c**) Transient fluxes during the expiratory phase of the flow/volume curve, determined by coughing in a healthy subject. Its absence indicates expiratory muscle compromise

Maximum Voluntary Ventilation

The maximum voluntary ventilation (MVV) is a measurement (using a spirometer) of the volume of air that a subject can repeatedly move with maximum voluntary effort. It assesses the integration of several components of respiratory function: the musculature, chest and lung compliance, ventilation control mechanisms, and airway resistance. MVV can decrease as a result of a variety of neuromuscular, restrictive pulmonary, rib cage, and obstructive bronchial diseases. In the case of obstructive bronchial disease, the MVV maneuver exaggerates air trapping and limitation of airflow, and should be done with care. This maneuver relies heavily on the effort and cooperation of the patient, who must breathe deeply and rapidly for 12 seconds at a volume that is more than normal but less than the maximum capacity, the optimal volume being 30%. The graph of the maneuver should show a continuous and rhythmic trace, keeping the

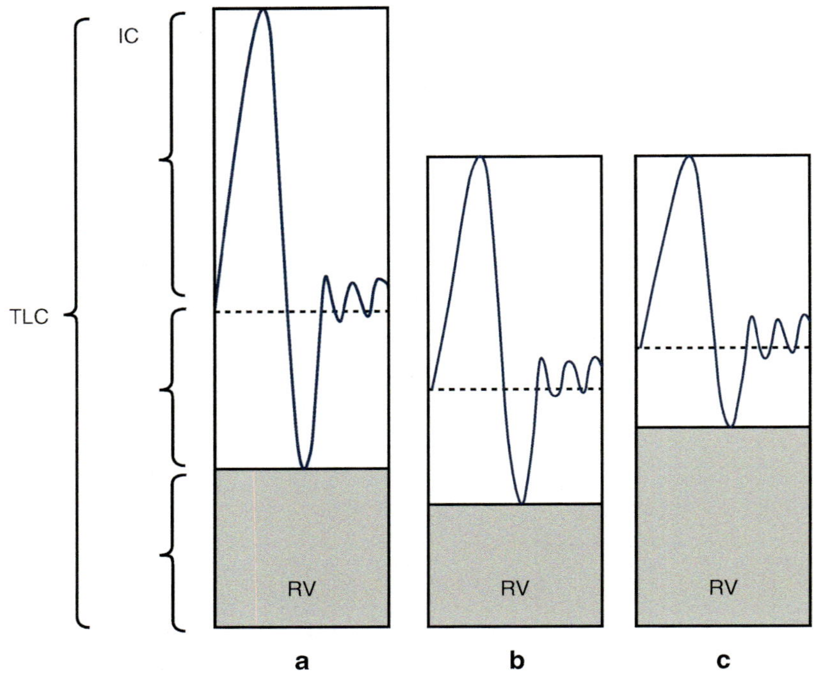

Fig. 10.2 Lung volumes. (**a**) Normal. (**b**) Restrictive lung disease, showing proportional decreases in all volumes. (**c**) Restrictive lung disease with air trapping, showing a proportional increase in the residual volume, due to the lower expiratory reserve volume and the decrease in inspiratory capacity

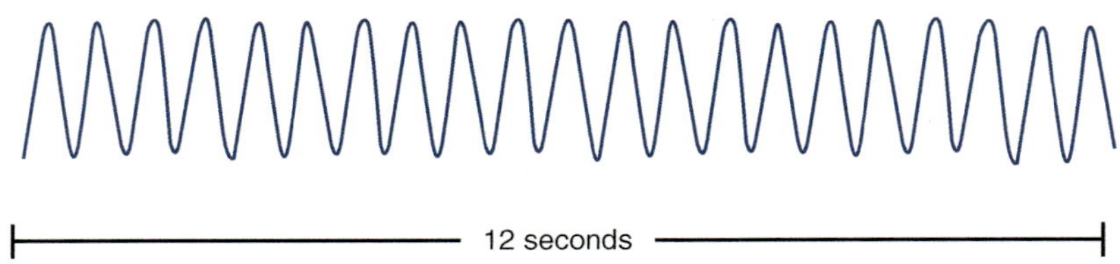

Fig. 10.3 Maximum voluntary ventilation measurement. The outline is homogeneous, with the end of expiration at a constant level

exhalation constant until the end (Fig. 10.3). At least two maneuvers should be obtained that do not differ by more than 10%. Because there is a good correlation between the forced expiratory volume in 1 second (FEV_1) and MVV in individuals without airway compromise, it is possible to assess whether the individual makes an adequate effort, using an indirect index: $FEV_1 \times 35$.

Arterial Gases and Saturometry

The main purpose of arterial gas measurement is detection of hypercapnia secondary to hypoventilation. This appears initially in patients with slow and progressive compromise during sleep; consequently, the sample should be taken upon awakening. Samples taken when patents are fully awake can underestimate the severity of the alteration of gaseous exchange.

In patients who have moderate to severe muscular compromise, continuous measurement of peripheral oxygen saturation (SpO_2) during sleep shows frequent falls due to apnea and/or central and/or obstructive hypopnea. This measurement correlates very well with the vital capacity. More details can be found in the chapter on pulse oximetry in this book. Polysomnography is the test of choice for diagnosing sleep disorders, with the capacity to register SpO_2 and transcutaneous CO_2 tension.

Ventilation Control: Measurement of Occlusion Pressure

Respiratory control depends on the partial pressures of carbon dioxide (pCO_2), and of oxygen (pO_2), the pH chemoreceptors in the neural centers and paths, and the motor action of the respiratory muscles. A progressive increase in pCO_2 is observed in patients with NMDs, which may be caused by alveolar hypoventilation and/or failure to control respiration. The latter has been described in myotonic dystrophy and other congenital myopathies. Measurement of occlusion pressure in the mouth in the first 100 milliseconds of inspiration ($P_{0.1}$) allows estimation of the response to CO_2 retention. This is the pressure generated in the airway by contraction of the inspiratory muscles when the airway is occluded at the end of an expiration at rest (the functional residual capacity (FRC)). FRC is the pressure generated in the first 100 milliseconds of inspiration, during which the conscious response does not interfere with the occlusion or the mechanical properties of the lung. However, it depends on the contractile state of the respiratory musculature and on the FRC variation in the subject. FRC can be measured in infants while they are sleeping and in older children when they are capable of breathing peacefully with a nasal clamp and a mouthpiece for at least 5 minutes, with occlusion occurring every minute until five acceptable measurements have been obtained.

The main purpose is assessment of respiratory control in stable patients with an increased respiratory load due to bronchopulmonary dysplasia, cystic fibrosis, bronchiolitis obliterans, or another cause. The normal value in adults is 1 cm H_2O, and under normal conditions of stability, $P_{0.1}$ increases by approximately 3 cm H_2O.

Functional Capacity: 6-Minute Walk Test

There are several ways to objectively study functional exercise capacity. The 6-minute walk test is considered the easiest to undertake, the easiest for the patient to tolerate, and the test that most reflects tolerance of regular activities. The test measures the distance the patient can cover when walking as rapidly as possible for 6 minutes. It assesses, in an integral manner, all of the systems involved in the exercise: pulmonary, cardiovascular, circulatory, blood, neuromuscular, muscular, and metabolic.

Because of their base condition, patients with NMDs have difficulty doing the test. The main purpose of the test in patients with chronic pulmonary disease is a checkup for respiratory rehabilitation.

The test requires a 30 m walkway with a smooth hard surface. A marker should be placed every 3 m, and turning points should be marked with a cone. The heart rate and SpO_2 are assessed before and after the exercise. When continuous monitoring is required, the patient should carry the equipment, which needs to be light enough not to hinder the patient's performance. The degree of basal and post-test dyspnea is measured on the modified Borg scale. If the patient requires continuous oxygen support, the system should not interfere with the walking circuit. Ongoing encouragement by the technician is important, drawing on the chronology and standard phrases. It has been observed that longer walk distances are achieved with encouragement.

There are several reasons for obtaining different results in the test performance. Factors that reduce the distance walked are smaller body size, obesity, failure to understand the technique, and a walkway of <30 m, given that this implies more turning. The most important factor in increasing the walk distance is the motivation of the patient.

The most reliable way to determine the clinical improvement of a patient on the basis of this test after some form of intervention is to conduct two or three pre- and post-treatment tests (thus ensuring the reproducibility of the test), using the same technician to ensure the same methodology.

In relation to Chilean reference values, we use those described by Gatica et al. (2002), which are described in greater detail in the chapter on respiratory rehabilitation in this book.

Muscular Strength

Muscular strength in the respiratory system is estimated as the pressure generated by muscular contraction. However, this relationship is complex and depends on the mechanical characteristics of the rib cage and the abdominal wall. Consequently, it is preferable to interpret the results of these measurements as a global index of respiratory musculature performance.

Static Pressures: Maximum Inspiratory and Expiratory Pressures

Tests that measure the maximum inspiratory pressure (MIP) and maximum expiratory pressure (MEP) are most commonly used to assess muscular strength, given that the MIP test is more sensitive than vital capacity measurements at the initial stage of the disease. The MIP is the maximum pressure generated during inhalation with the airway occluded and is based on RV. MEP is the maximum pressure generated during exhalation with the airway occluded and is based on TLC. Measurement of MIP assesses the functioning of the inspiratory musculature: the diaphragm and the external intercostal and accessory muscles (the scalenes and sternocleidomastoids). The abdominal and internal intercostal expiratory muscles are assessed with MEP.

These techniques measure the pressure generated by the respiratory muscles plus the pressure of the elastic retraction of the rib cage and the lungs. Consequently, it should be keep in mind that measurement of MIP on the basis of RV can increase the latter by up to −30 cm H_2O. Similarly, to measure MEP on the basis of TLC, the contribution can be up to +40 cm H_2O. Some specialists argue that, realistically, in MIP and MEP measurements in chronic respiratory failure (CRF)—that is, with elastic retraction at zero—the pressures measured in the mouth reflect only the pressure that is generated by muscular contraction.

For the measurement, a nasal clamp should be placed on the patient, and a cylindrical mouth piece is recommended. Although some authors have used scuba diving–type masks to obtain reference values, it is recommended that this be based on theoretical values for the same method used on the patient. The mouthpiece should have an escape 1 mm in diameter to avoid glottic closure and an artificially elevated MIP, and also to reduce the use of the mouth musculature during the maneuver for MEP.

The force should be maintained for a minimum of 1.5 seconds; at least five maneuvers should be conducted until at least two repeatable results are obtained (with a maximum variation of 10% between the two best values), and the better one should be chosen. A MIP value under −80 cm H_2O is of great value for ruling out diaphragmatic compromise.

The disadvantages of these measurements are their high degree of variability and the fact that they reflect the effect of learning. Consequently, it is advisable to do more than five maneuvers in patients who do not achieve an adequate technique, until two repeatable results are obtained. The analysis of the values obtained will be aided by inclusion of the FVC value, given that the pressures the patient can generate depend significantly on this. A MIP value of less than −25 cm H_2O suggests a risk of respiratory failure. This indicates the importance of serial measurements of pulmonary volumes and static pressure.

It is recommended to use the reference values provided by Szeinberg et al. with schoolchildren and adolescents. MIP and MEP values can be measured in infants when they cry, with the mask placed over the infant's mouth. The mouthpiece should have an escape to avoid glottic closure. The airway should be occluded at the end and at the beginning of the crying effort to measure MEP and MIP, respectively.

Nasal Sniff Test

Sniffing is a natural action, which many patients find easier than performing a maneuver for measuring static pressure. It is a reproducible method, validated in children, and used to assess global inspiratory muscular function. Measurement of MIP has the advantage of being an easily applied technique that avoids the problem of air loss through a mouthpiece, as often occurs in patients with neuromuscular illnesses. It consists of a short, rapid, voluntary inhalation through the nose and with the mouth closed, beginning after an exhalation at rest (FRC). One of the patient's nostrils is sealed with a rubber or sponge mold, into which a catheter is inserted. The patient breathes through the nostril that is not blocked. The catheter measures the nasopharyngeal pressure, which is a reasonable indicator of the intra-alveolar pressure. The values are generally lower than the MIP value because there is less shortening of the inspiratory musculature.

As with measurement of static pressure, a limitation is the dependence on effort. Most children over 4 years of age are capable of performing the maneuver adequately. There should be a 30-second lapse between maneuvers. If it is difficult to obtain reliable data in child subjects, it is recommended to make more than ten attempts, given the important effect of learning. The values tend to be underestimated in patients with intra- or extrathoracic airway obstruction.

Pressure values greater than −70 cm H_2O and −60 cm H_2O are considered acceptable for males and females, respectively.

Peak Cough Flow

Coughing is a basic defense mechanism to eliminate secretions from the airway. One or more coughing phases are affected in patients with NMDs: maximum inspiration, opening or closing of the glottis, keeping the glottis open or closed while increasing intrathoracic pressure, and opening the glottis together with forced expiration. Coughing can be assessed objectively by measuring the peak cough flow (PCF) or MEF generated while the subject is coughing. A nasal clamp is placed on the patient, who is asked to take a deep breath and then cough into the flow meter. The maneuver should be done at least five times, taking care to ensure that the mouthpiece remains well sealed. The normal MEF is above 300 l/min. A value of less than 160 l/min is associated with difficulty in eliminating secretions and a consequent risk of respiratory complications such as pneumonia, atelectasis, or respiratory insufficiency. If the reading is between 160 and 270 l/min, it is likely it will fall below 160 l/min in the context of a respiratory infection.

Invasive Methods: Transdiaphragmatic Pressure

These techniques are used especially in small children, in whom it is not possible to conduct the tests described above. The most commonly used of these techniques is measurement of transdiaphragmatic pressure (TDP), which specifically assesses the contraction of the diaphragm, unlike the aforementioned methods, which measure the synergetic action of several inspiratory and expiratory muscles. Transducers are placed on the stomach and esophagus to measure the gastric pressure (GP) and esophageal pressure (EP), respectively. Infants and small children should be sedated, with continuous monitoring of SpO_2. The most commonly used method is placement of a balloon catheter. The method used for calculating TDP is:

$$TDP = Ppl - AP$$

where:

$$\mathrm{TDP} = \mathrm{EP} - \mathrm{GP}$$

Ppl is the pleural pressure, which is measured in the esophagus, and AP is the abdominal pressure, which is measured in the stomach.

EP is generally negative. As the diaphragm is the only muscle that simultaneously determines a decrease in EP and an increase in GP when it contracts, its normal contraction results in increased TDP.

TDP has been measured by the nasal sniff test, with less variability observed than with the MIP technique. TPD is measured in infants in the inspiratory phase of crying, with values of ±60 cm H_2O being acceptable at 1 month of life, which is lower than what is registered by measurement of MIP during crying.

Another method to assess diaphragm function is electrical stimulation, the great advantage of which is that it does not require the cooperation of the patient. However, the stimulation is painful, and it is not easy to place the electrodes.

Muscular Fatigue

Muscular fatigue is defined as loss of capacity to generate force and/or contraction velocity, accompanied by recovery during muscle repose. The method to demonstrate the presence of muscular fatigue is serial measurements. Of the existing techniques, serial measurement of muscular tension, using an electrical or magnetic stimulus, is the most precise one, although it is technically complex and involves discomfort for the patient.

Ventilometry

Although it is not a specific marker of the presence of muscular fatigue, ventilometry has the advantage of being a simple and noninvasive method. It consists of measuring the ventilated volume in 1 minute, using a Wright respirometer. The total volume measured is related to the breathing rate per minute. A breathing rate associated with low tidal volumes may predict respiratory failure.

Tension/Time Index

Tension/time index (ITT) measurement contributes to determining the presence of diaphragmatic muscular fatigue. It is used in patients in the phase of suspension of ventilatory assistance and assessment prior to and after inspiratory muscular training. It measures the force generated by the diaphragm in each inspiration, establishing its relation to the maximum force that the same individual can reach, and the duration of inspiratory time with respect to the total time of the cycle. A value of <65% implies low resistance of the inspiratory musculature, even if MIP is normal. ITT is calculated as follows:

$$ITT = AI / MP \quad It / Tot\,T$$

where AI is the average inhalation pressure at tidal volume, MP is the maximum pressure, It is the inhalation time, and Tot T is the total inhalation time.

The It/Tot T ratio depends on the breathing rate and on the inhalation/exhalation relationship. The higher the It/Tot T ratio is, the greater the respiratory work is. The diaphragm does not benefit from the rest periods provided by the expiratory phase.

The calculation can use the maximum TDP or MIP.

Conclusion

There are now several methods used to precisely assess respiratory muscle function. The most widely used measure of static pressures is the maximum expiratory flow generated by coughing, which is a relatively simple and well tolerated technique. Of the general examinations, we highlight the usefulness of the graphic spirometry flow/volume loop, although their alterations appear late. In addition, the walk test contributes information about the functional capacity of the patient related to his or her quality of life.

One of the limiting factors in obtaining reliable results is the age of the patient, given that the techniques require a high level of cooperation. Moreover, it should always be keep in mind that these patients tire easily with performance of the tests, and sometimes they have problems coordinating movements or their muscular weakness is such that they cannot hold the nozzles. This highlights the importance of the technician being well trained and able to determine if a poor maneuver is due to the factors noted above, and if it will be acceptable for analysis.

New techniques of interest have been developed, such as inductance plethysmography—and, more recently, optoelectronic plethysmography—to assess thoracoabdominal respiratory patterns. Furthermore, ultrasonographic methods have emerged to assess diaphragmatic structure and dynamics, along with new tomographic technologies to measure regional ventilatory changes in patients with ventilatory assistance.

Sources

Allen J. Pulmonary complications of neuromuscular disease: a respiratory mechanics perspective. Paediatr Respir Rev. 2010;11:18–23.

American Thoracic Society/European Respiratory Society. ATS/ERS statement on respiratory muscle testing. Am J Respir Crit Care Med. 2002;166:518–624.

Bach JR, Ishikawa Y, Kim H. Prevention of pulmonary morbidity for patients with Duchenne muscular dystrophy. Chest. 1997;112:1024–8.

Birnkrant DJ, Bushby K, Amin RS, Bach JR, Benditt JO, Eagle M, Finder JD, Kalra MS, Kissel JT, Koumbourlis AC, Kravitz RM. The respiratory management of patients with Duchenne muscular dystrophy: a DMD care considerations working group specialty article. Pediatr Pulmonol. 2010;45:739–48.

Dohna-Schwake C, Ragette R, Teschler H, Voit T, Mellies U. Predictors of severe chest infections in pediatric neuromuscular disorders. Neuromuscul Dis. 2006;16:325–8.

Fauroux B. Respiratory muscle testing in children. Paediatr Respir Rev. 2003;4:243–9.

Fauroux B, Aubertin G. Measurement of maximal pressures and the sniff manoeuvre in children. Paediatr Respir Rev. 2007;8:90–3.

Fauroux B, Khirani S. Neuromuscular disease and respiratory physiology in children: putting lung function into perspective. Respirology. 2014;19:782–91.

Gatica D, Puppo H, Villarroel G, San Martin I, Lagos R, Montecino JJ, Lara C, Zenteno D. Valores de referencia del test de marcha de seis minutos en niños sanos. Rev Med Chil. 2012;140:1014–21.

Gauld LM, Boynton A. Relationship between peak cough flow and spirometry in Duchenne muscular dystrophy. Pediatr Pulmonol. 2005;39:457–60.

Lofaso F, Nicot F, Lejaille M, Falaize L, Louis A, Clement A, Raphael J-C, Orlikowsky D, Fauroux B. Sniff nasal inspiratory pressure: what is the optimal number of sniffs? Eur Respir J. 2006;27:980–2.

Masdeu MJ, Ferrer A. Función de los músculos respiratorios en enfermedades neuromusculares. Arch Bronconeumol. 2003;39:176–83.

Nicot F, Hart N, Forin V, Boule M, Clement A, Polket I, Lofaso F, Fauroux B. Respiratory muscle testing: a valuable tool for children with neuromuscular disorder. Am J Respir Crit Care Med. 2006;174:67–74.

Phillips MF, Quinlivan CM, Edwards RHT, Calverley PMA. Changes in spirometry over time as a prognostic marker in patients with Duchenne muscular dystrophy. Am J Respir Crit Care Med. 2001;164:2191–4.

Szeinberg A, Marcotte JE, Roizin H, Mindorff C, England S, Tabachnik et al. Normal values of maximal inspiratory and expiratory pressures with a portable apparatus in children, adolescents, and young adults. Pediatr Pulmonol 1987;3:255–8.

Tangsrud SE, Petersen IL, Lodrup Carlsen KC, Carlen KH. Lung function in children with Duchenne's muscular dystrophy. Respir Med. 2001;95:898–903.

Study of Images in Respiratory Diseases

11

Cristián García Bruce and Rodrigo Parra Rojas

Contents

Introduction

The radiologist should work closely with the clinician, not only to choose the best imaging study for every patient but also to meet one of our primary objectives: providing better care for our patients. We should not forget that the clinical aspects of every patient are fundamental to reaching a correct diagnosis.

Imaging methods that use ionizing radiation are not innocuous, and many of them are very costly, which should be considered when a study is requested. Imaging methods should not be misused and should be requested only when a direct benefit for the patient can be expected. Every time an examination is requested, it should be based on a diagnostic hypothesis, considering that the findings of the examination could determine the course of therapy.

Methods of Study

Chest X-Ray

There are numerous indications for a conventional chest x-ray in assessment of the chest and

C. García Bruce (✉) · R. Parra Rojas
Pediatric Radiology, School of Medicine, Pontificia Universidad Católica de Chile, Santiago, Chile
e-mail: cgarcia@med.puc.cl; rparra@med.puc.cl

P. Bertrand, I. Sánchez (eds.), *Pediatric Respiratory Diseases*,
https://doi.org/10.1007/978-3-030-26961-6_11

airway; among them are inflammatory diseases, tumors, deformations of the rib cage, heart disease, and trauma. If possible, anteroposterior (AP) and lateral projections should always be obtained for adequate assessment of thoracic structures. A chest x-ray of the patient lying on his or her side has traditionally been used to detect fluid in the pleural cavity, although it has progressively been replaced by ultrasound because the latter has greater sensitivity and the capacity to characterize the fluid. Fluoroscopy is useful to assess the dynamics of the chest, specifically in the study of diaphragm movement and in cases when there is suspicion that a foreign body is present in the airway.

Ultrasound

Chest ultrasonography is a highly useful technique, which complements x-rays. It was initially applied to detect pleural effusion, but in recent years its use in studying the chest has been greatly extended to include the study of other pleural lesions, juxtadiaphragmatic or juxtaparietal masses, neck masses, the mediastinum, pericardial diseases, diaphragm pathologies, etc. Color Doppler ultrasound is used to assess central catheters, vascular anatomy, vessel permeability, and vascular flow in thoracic masses. Echocardiography also has great value but is beyond the scope of this chapter.

Some of the advantages of ultrasound are that it is harmless (as it does not involve ionizing radiation), it does not require administration of a contrast medium or sedation, and it is a portable methodology that can be used at the patient's bedside. One of its main applications is assessment of the pleural space, because of its high sensitivity for detecting pleural effusion and its capacity to characterize pleural fluids. While both the exudate and transudate can be anecogenic, findings of echoes, partitions, and/or loculations generally indicate empyema. In the case of complete opacity of a hemithorax, pleural effusion can be easily distinguished from other expansive lesions or atelectasis.

Another common and important indication for ultrasound is assessment of diaphragm mobility, particularly following heart surgery. This is usually done at the patient's bedside in the intensive care unit. When there is unilateral diaphragm compromise, the affected side can be compared with the healthy side. The M mode also provides a spectral representation of diaphragmatic movement. Moreover, ultrasound can guide procedures such as pleural puncture or installation of central catheters. The main disadvantage of this technique is that it requires adequate equipment, with color Doppler and high-resolution transductors, as well as a trained operator.

We do not recommend this technique as an initial study for suspected pneumonia, as some authors have. A chest x-ray employs a very low dose of radiation and continues to be the gold standard in these cases. Doppler ultrasound can be applied to cases of suspected necrotizing pneumonia, but it is not used universally.

Computerized Tomography

The features of computerized tomography (CT) of the chest in children are quite different from those in adults. The lower percentage of adipose tissue and spontaneous movement of the patient reduce the quality of the image, making its interpretation more difficult. The introduction of helical and multislice or multidetector CT has increased the utility of the technique and broadened the indications for its use in assessing pediatric patients, because these techniques offer the possibility of optimizing intravenous contrast while reducing the study time and the need for sedation. In addition, these techniques significantly reduce the exposure of the patient to radiation while yielding images with submillimeter definition, thus significantly improving the quality of multiplane reconstructions and even permitting virtual navigation of the airway.

High-resolution CT assesses the lungs with excellent spatial resolution, providing precise anatomical detail of the parenchymal and airway.

It has a high yield in the assessment of diffuse pulmonary diseases. To obtain good spatial resolution, it requires a cut with a thickness of less than 3 mm (ideally 1 mm) with an interval of 5–10 mm, depending on the size of the patient. Reconstruction algorithms are techniques used to optimize CT performance, such as expiratory imaging while the patient is lying prone or laterally.

Expiratory imaging is extremely useful in patients with suspected abnormalities in fine airways and in patients with a history of repeated pulmonary infections. This technique shows areas with trapped air that are often not evident on conventional imaging. A practical method to obtain expiratory imaging in uncooperative children is to make axial cuts while they lie on their left or right side. If there is air trapping, the affected lung, lobe, or segment is hyperlucid when that side of the chest is in the dependent position. The same principle of gravity-dependent aeration can be used in prone cuts to obtain images with better expansion of the lower and inner lobes in their posterior or dependent aspect.

Expiratory imaging can also be useful to assess suspected tracheobronchomalacia, both as a primary condition and in association with other diseases. In this respect, CT provides an excellent anatomical demonstration of thorax structures and the airway. It often shows abnormalities that are poorly defined or not apparent on chest x-rays. CT can distinguish differences in density with 100 times the sensitivity of conventional radiography.

CT is used to assess different structures of the chest, including the chest wall, the mediastinum, the airway, vascular structures, and the pulmonary parenchyma. An intravenous contrast medium is usually not necessary to assess the pulmonary parenchyma but is used to study the mediastinum, vascular structures, masses, or congenital anomalies, or when looking for inflammation. CT should be used with strict criteria and caution, and only when it is strictly indicated, owing to the high dosage of radiation that its use entails.

Magnetic Resonance Imaging

The usefulness of magnetic resonance imagining (MRI) in chest pathologies lies basically in assessment of chest masses, given its excellent resolution for contrast and its multiplane capacity, as well as the possibility it offers for characterizing tissue. Another more recent and less defined practice is the use of studies triggered by the heartbeat (using electrocardiography), which can assess congenital heart disease and extracardiac vascular structures, with the great advantage of providing not just morphological information but also information on function and blood flow dynamics.

Although MRI has been used for evaluation of pulmonary the parenchyma, chest CT currently continues to be superior in this area. Advances in fetal MRI have been made in recent years with the development of ultrarapid sequencing, which reduces the examination time and the number of artifacts resulting from fetal movement. There are no known risks or harmful effects on either the mother or the fetus. It does not employ an intravenous contrast medium, nor does it require maternal sedation.

The indications have increased at some medical centers, but the examination is sometimes unnecessary and the findings do not contribute more than those of fetal ultrasound (which is the gold-standard technique) and do not necessarily modify the clinical evolution of the fetus, nor postnatal care.

Chest MRI should be limited to cases in which ultrasound findings are doubtful or inconclusive, or where it is desirable to assess the upper airway in the case of a fetal cervical mass. It is also used as an examination before an interventional procedure such as fetoscopy or fetal surgery. MRI provides excellent definition of fetal anatomy and can clarify doubts arising from ultrasound examinations.

Other Methods

Other methods that are less often used but can nevertheless be useful include nuclear medical studies (scintigraphy), angiography, and contrast studies of the upper digestive tract. This last test is particularly useful to detect extrinsic airway compression.

Evaluation of the Structures of the Chest

The Airways

There are currently only a few precise indications for simple radiography to assess the upper airway, including evaluation of nasopharyngeal adenoid tissue and the paranasal sinuses. One less common indication is acute obstruction of the upper airway; an x-ray can be performed when airway obstruction by a foreign body is suspected (Fig. 11.1). Radiography can also be useful in cases of suspected stenosis and/or tracheal compression, particularly in the context of suspected vascular rings, where a chest x-ray provides information about the position of the aortic arch. Considering the greater resolution of other methods, standard radiology has limited usefulness for studying the upper airway.

The standard radiography study should include anteroposterior and lateral projections. Lateral projections that show thickening of the epiglottis and the aryepiglottic folds suggest acute epiglottitis (Fig. 11.2), while increased thickness of the soft retropharyngeal and prevertebral tissue suggests inflammation at this level (a retropharyngeal abscess).

The upper airway can be evaluated precisely by CT, including tridimensional and multiplane reconstructions, especially in cases of acquired or congenital stenosis (Fig. 11.3) or extrinsic compression of the airway by vascular rings (Figs. 11.4 and 11.5). CT can characterize a cervical mass and its relationship to other structures—for example, in situations where the mass is compressing the airway. It is also the most sensitive method for detecting calcification.

CT is usually a good complement to fibroscopy in the study of a congenital stridor and subglottic hemangioma (Fig. 11.6). MRI is also useful in assessing cervical masses because of its contrast resolution, especially when a vascular component is suspected.

The Lung Parenchyma

Congenital Anomalies

Congenital bronchopulmonary anomalies are common and are composed of a heterogeneous

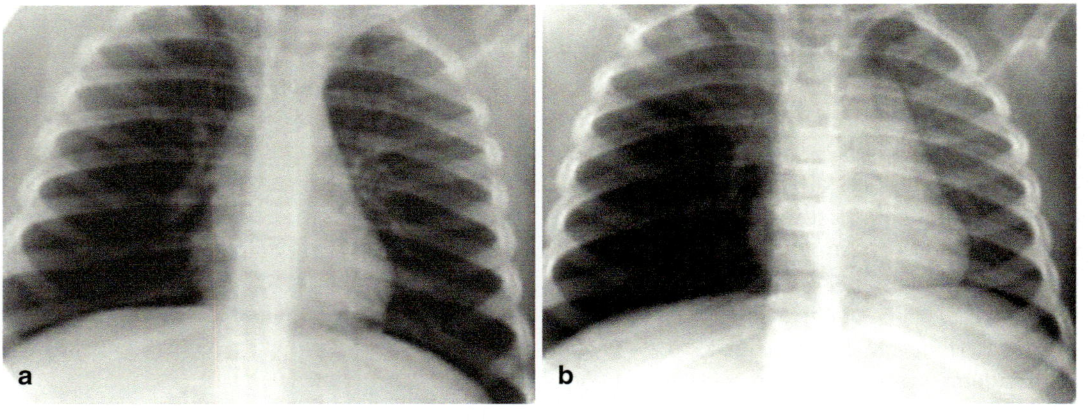

Fig. 11.1 Foreign bodies in the airway of a 14-month-old patient with a history of penetration syndrome. Chest x-rays obtained on inspiration (**a**) and expiration (**b**) show greater transparency in the right lung. On expiration, air trapping in the right lung is evident and is due to the valve mechanism, which determines a mass effect of that lung and displacement of the heart and mediastinum to the left. The air-trapping area excludes the right upper lobe, which is displaced cephalad (*arrow*). This is indicative of the presence of a foreign body in the right intermediate bronchus, which was confirmed by fiberoptic bronchoscopy. The foreign body (a peanut) was later extracted

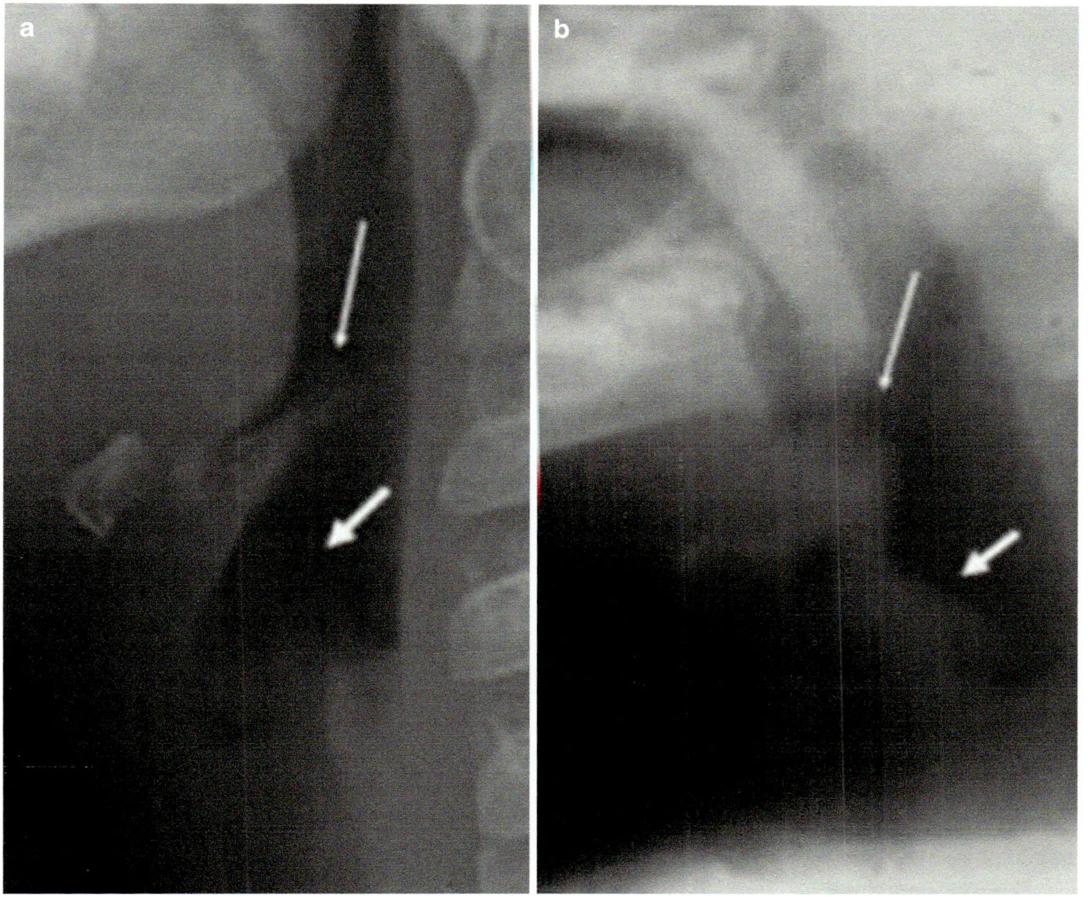

Fig. 11.2 Acute epiglottitis. (**a**) Lateral neck x-ray of a 3-year-old patient, showing the epiglottis (*thin arrow*) and the aryepiglottic folds (*thick arrow*), both of normal size and thickness. (**b**) X-ray of a 2-year-old patient with an acute stridor, showing significant thickening of the epiglottis (*thin arrow*) and of the aryepiglottic folds (*thick arrow*)

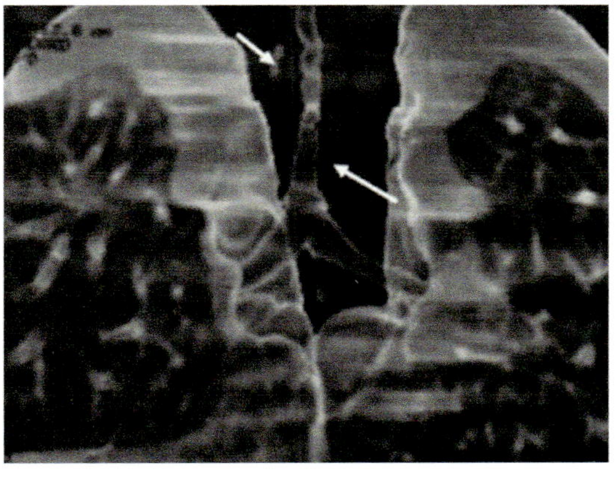

Fig. 11.3 Congenital tracheal stenosis in a 2-month-old patient with a congenital stridor. A multislice CT scan with three-dimensional reconstruction of the airway shows a long segment of tracheal stenosis (*arrows*)

group of anomalies that affect the pulmonary parenchyma, its vascularization, and the lower airway. More than one anomaly can coexist (hybrid forms), and their clinical presentation is variable. They have been classified in different ways by different authors—in particular, according to their anatomy and pathogeny.

A simple classification considers two types: (1) *focal malformations* (congenital pulmonary hyperinsufflation, bronchial atresia, simple intrapulmonary cysts, congenital pulmonary airway malformation (CPAM), pulmonary sequestration, and an irrigation system congenitally isolated from a normal lung segment); and (2) *a dysmorphic lung* (pulmonary aplasia–hypoplasia complex, lobar agenesis–hypoplasia).

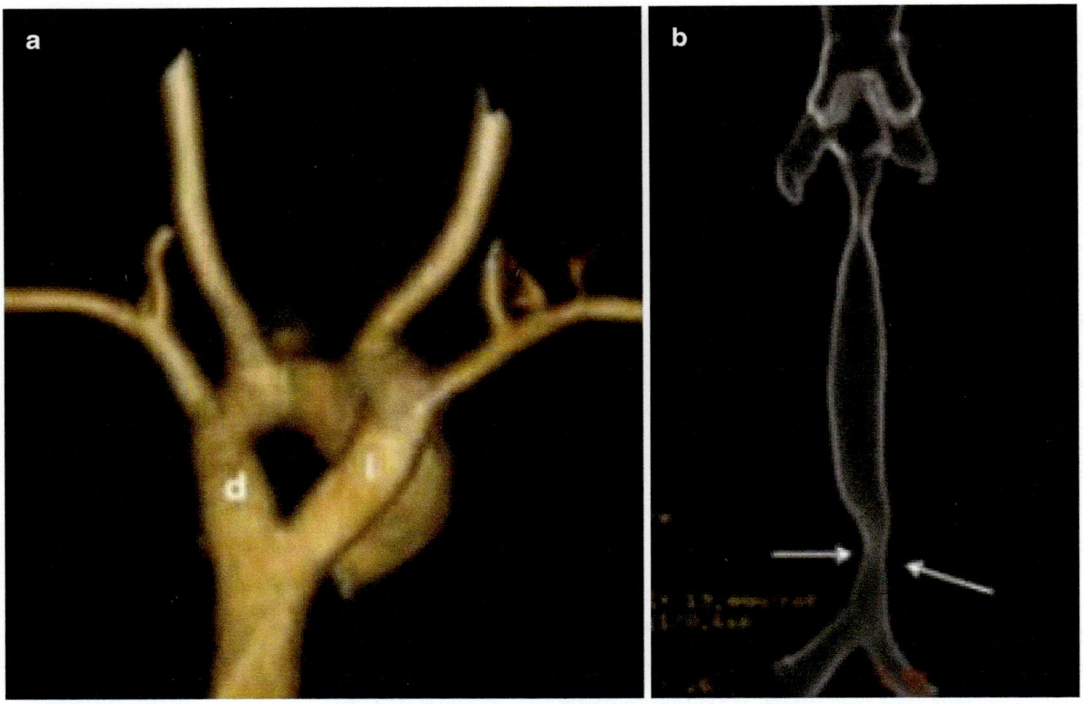

Fig. 11.4 Vascular ring in a 4-month-old patient with a congenital stridor, shown on multidetector helical CT scans with three-dimensional reconstruction. (**a**) An anteroposterior view shows a double aortic arch (d: right arch; i: left arch). (**b**) An anteroposterior view of the trachea shows compression and narrowing of its distal end, due to the vascular ring (*arrows*)

Imaging studies are fundamental for diagnosis, and several methods can be used.

Congenital Pulmonary Hyperinflation

Previously called congenital lobar emphysema, this condition is characterized by progressive overdistension of one (or sometimes two) pulmonary lobes without destruction of the alveolar walls. Most often the upper lobes or the right middle lobe are compromised. In the first days of life there is pulmonary fluid trapped in the compromised lobe, so on a chest x-ray this appears opaque and enlarged, with a mass effect on the heart and mediastinum. As vascular and lymphatic reabsorption progresses, the compromised lobe is aerated. It presents a reticular pattern and later a typical pattern of a hyperinflated lobe with reduced density. The pulmonary vessels are markedly attenuated, but there is no alteration in their structure. These alterations are best demonstrated by CT, which can confirm the diagnosis, determine with certainty the compromised lobe or lobes, and differentiate between this lesion and other pathologies such as CPAM (Fig. 11.7). Most patients become symptomatic in the neonatal period.

Bronchial Atresia

Bronchial atresia is characterized by proximal obliteration of a bronchial segment but with preservation of distal structures. The air enters the affected lung through the collateral canals, producing hyperinflation and air trapping. In turn, bronchial mucus secretions accumulate at the site of obstruction, producing mucosal and mucocele impaction. In most cases, only one segment is affected—usually the upper left lobe—and the condition may be associated with other anomalies. Segmental focal air trapping during exhalation can be observed on a chest x-ray, accompanied by a central tubular or rounded appearance of the mucocele. CT shows segmental pulmonary hyperinsufflation and mucosal impaction signs in much more detail (Fig. 11.8).

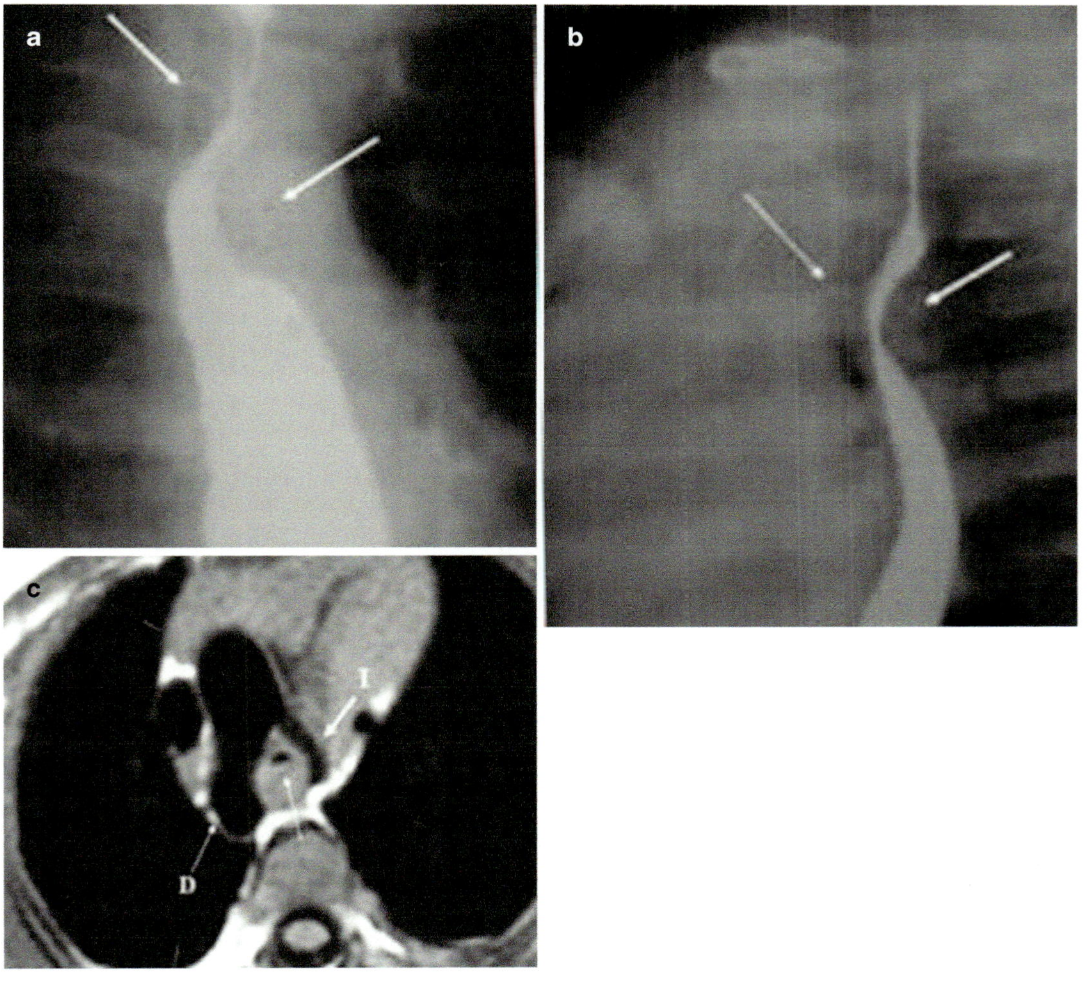

Fig. 11.5 Vascular ring and double aortic arch in a 3-month-old patient with a congenital stridor. An esophagram in the anteroposterior view (**a**) shows posterior compression of the esophagus (*arrows*); the lateral view (**b**) shows posterior compression of the esophagus (*posterior arrow*) and compression of the airway (*thin anterior arrow*). An axial T2-weighted MRI of the chest (**c**) shows the right aortic arch (D) and left aortic arch (I) with airway compression

Isolated or Single Congenital Chest Cysts

This group includes isolated congenital cysts located in the mediastinum or the pulmonary parenchyma (bronchogenic cysts, duplication cysts, or pleuropericardial cysts). Around 85% of such cysts are located in the mediastinum, and the remaining 15% are located within the lung parenchyma. Mediastinal cysts are most often located in the subcarinal region, while pulmonary cysts are most often found in the lower lobes. The cysts contain mucus fluid and may contain air when there is communication with the airway (Figs. 11.9 and 11.10). The cysts sometimes have calcified walls and can also be associated with other anomalies such as pulmonary sequestration or congenital pulmonary hyperinflation.

Congenital Pulmonary Airway Malformation

Previously called a pulmonary cystic adenomatoid malformation, CPAM is a rare anomaly in development of the lower respiratory tract and branching of the tracheobronchial tree, with hamartomatous formations of distal pulmonary

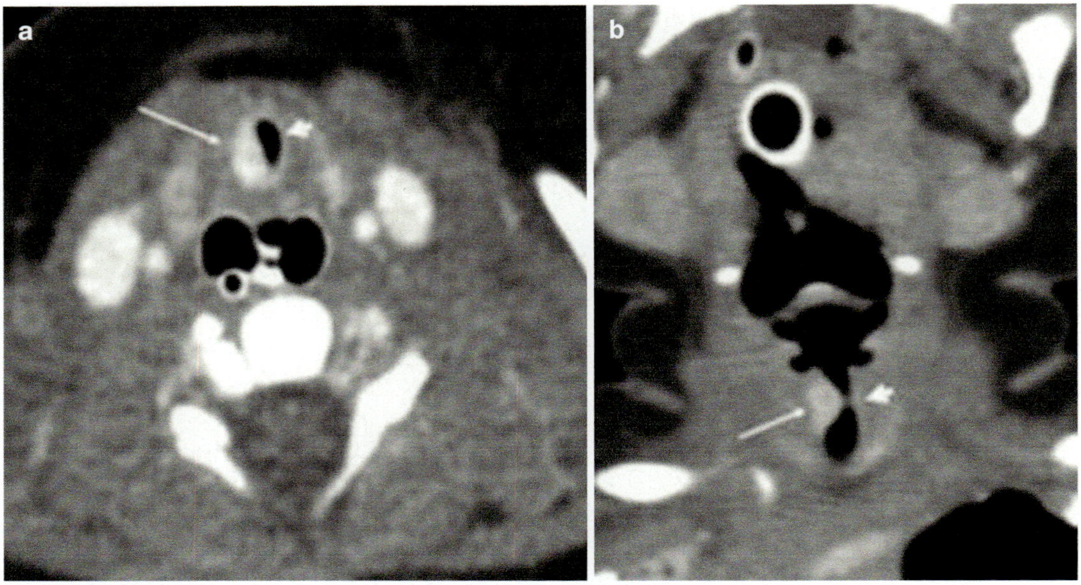

Fig. 11.6 Subglottic hemangioma in a 5-day-old newborn with a progressive stridor. Multidetector helical CT scans obtained after intravenous contrast administration show, in the axial section (**a**) and coronal reconstruction (**b**) of the neck, severe stenosis of the subglottic airway (*arrowhead*) secondary to a lesion intensely impregnated with contrast, compatible with a hemangioma (*thin arrows*)

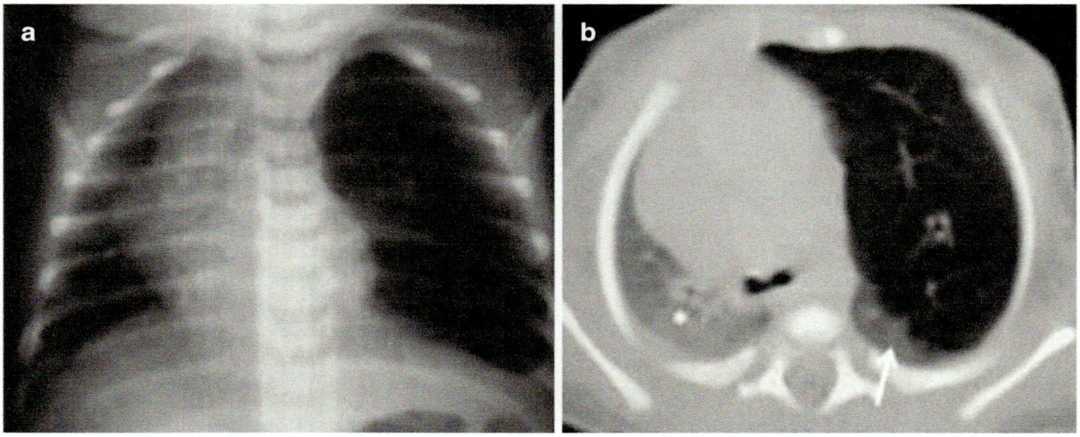

Fig. 11.7 Congenital lobar overinflation in a 3-day-old newborn with progressive difficulty breathing. (**a**) A chest x-ray shows hyperinflation of the left upper lobe with secondary displacement of the heart and mediastinum to the right. (**b**) A CT scan of the chest shows localized hyperinflation of the left upper lobe with displacement of the mediastinal structures and compression of the left lower lobe (*arrow*) and right lung (*asterisk*)

tissue. Histologically, it is characterized by adenomatous proliferation of bronchial-type structures and formation of macro- and microcysts coated with columnar or cuboidal epithelium, with no cartilage or bronchial glands. The different types of CPAM arise from interruption of development at different levels of the tracheobronchial tree and at different stages of pulmonary development. These malformations have been classified into five subtypes according to

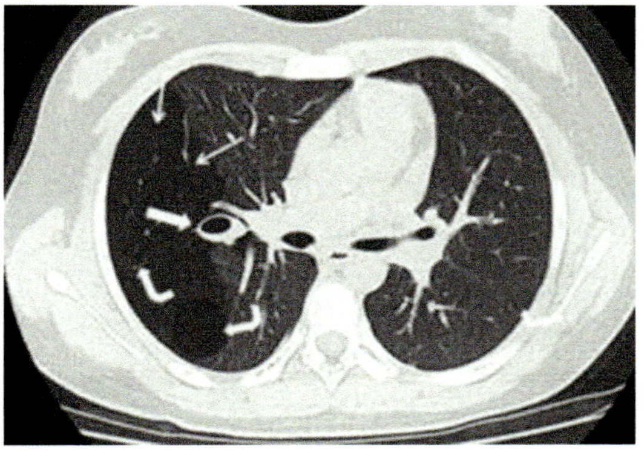

Fig. 11.8 Bronchial atresia in a 12-year-old girl with a history of recent right pneumonia. A CT scan of the chest below the carina shows a zone of greater transparency in the right lung (*thin arrows*), associated with mucosal impaction and a mucocele in the hilar region on the same side (*thick arrow*). There are also two thin-walled cystic masses inside, compatible with a congenital pulmonary airway malformation (formerly known as a congenital cystic adenomatoid malformation) (*curved arrows*)

their clinical, radiological, and histological aspects. The most common (representing 70% of cases) is type I CPAM, which is composed of several cysts of variable size, with at least one being dominant (>2 cm) (Fig. 11.11). Type II is composed of smaller uniform cysts ≤2 cm in diameter and represents 15–20% of cases. Around 10% of cases are type III, which is composed of microcysts, all <0.5 cm in diameter, generally with one lobe completely compromised. Type IV is very rare and consists of one or more very large cysts that are not coated by epithelium and that compromise a pulmonary lobe. Finally, type 0 is an extremely rare and lethal form of CPAM in which lung development fails completely. All types have arterial irrigation and normal venous drainage, and the radiological aspect depends on the type of lesion, the age of the patient, and the presence or absence of complications such as infection.

The clinical picture varies according to the patient's age, the size of the lesion, and whether there are associated anomalies or complications. Patients may present respiratory distress during the neonatal period or remain asymptomatic for variable periods of time. This condition may also appear as recurrent pneumonia; sometimes it appears as an incidental finding or may be detected in routine prenatal ultrasound examinations.

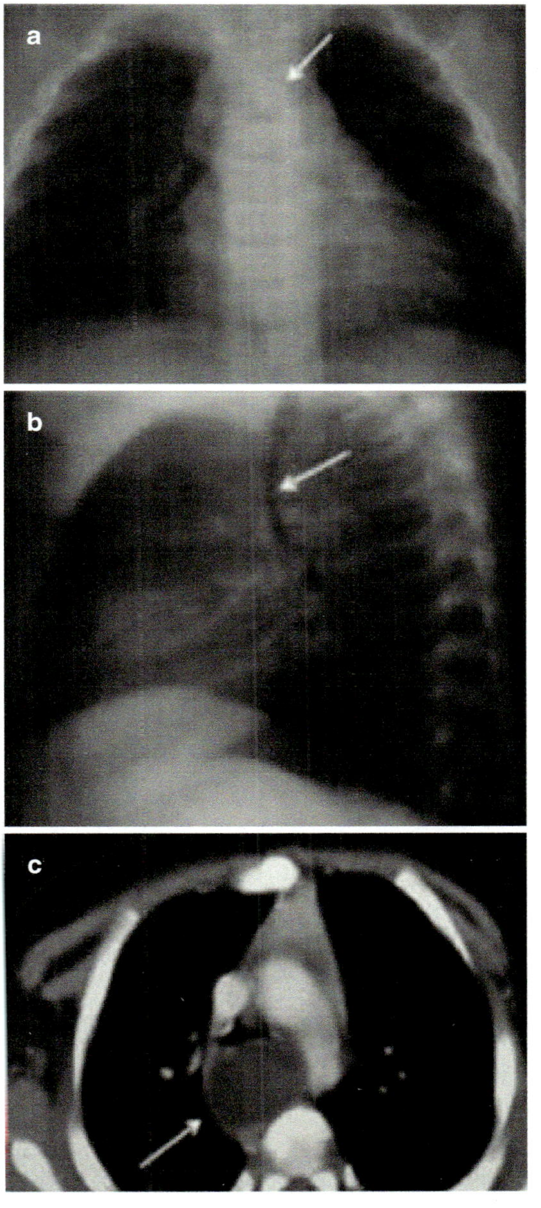

Fig. 11.9 Bronchogenic cysts in a 2-month-old infant with bronchial obstruction syndrome. Chest x-rays in the anteroposterior (**a**) and lateral (**b**) views show a mass in the posterior mediastinum that displaces the trachea to the right and anteriorly (*arrows*). (**c**) An axial CT scan with intravenous enhancement at the carina level confirms a cystic mass that compresses and displaces the trachea anteriorly (*arrow*)

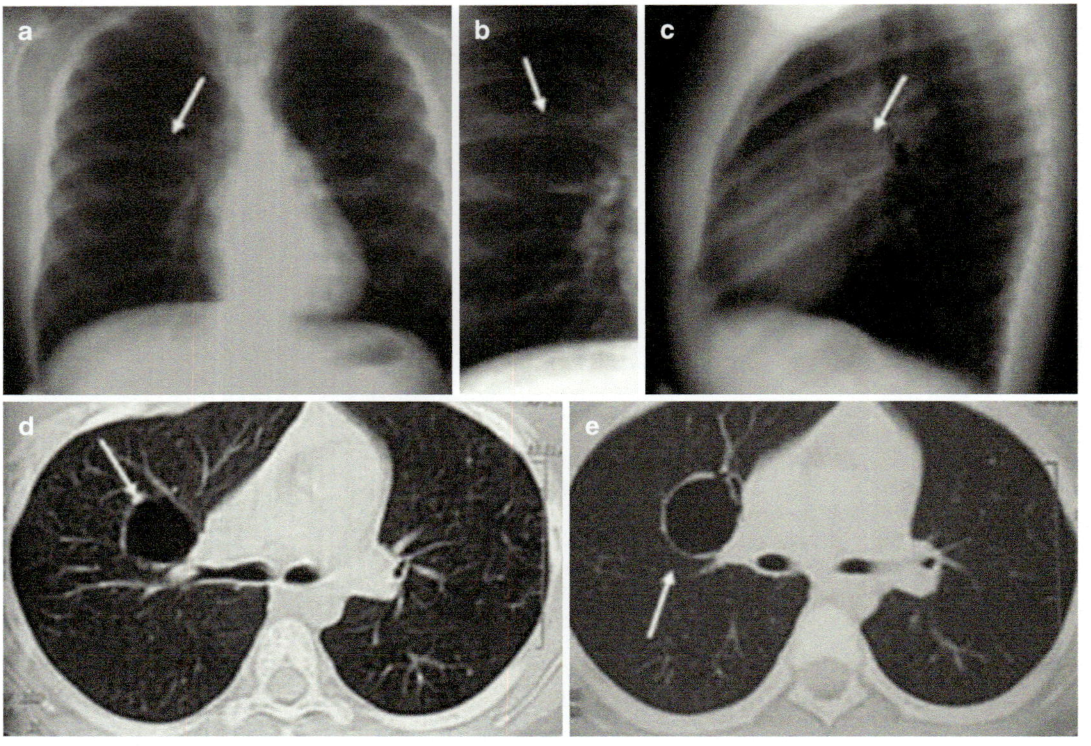

Fig. 11.10 Bronchogenic cysts in an 11-year-old boy with radiographic findings. Chest x-rays in the anteroposterior (**a**), AP localized (**b**), and lateral (**c**) views show a rounded radiolucent image of thin walls with air in the interior of the right upper lobe (*arrows*). Axial CT scanning of the chest (**d**, **e**) below the carina confirms a thin-walled cystic lesion (*arrows*)

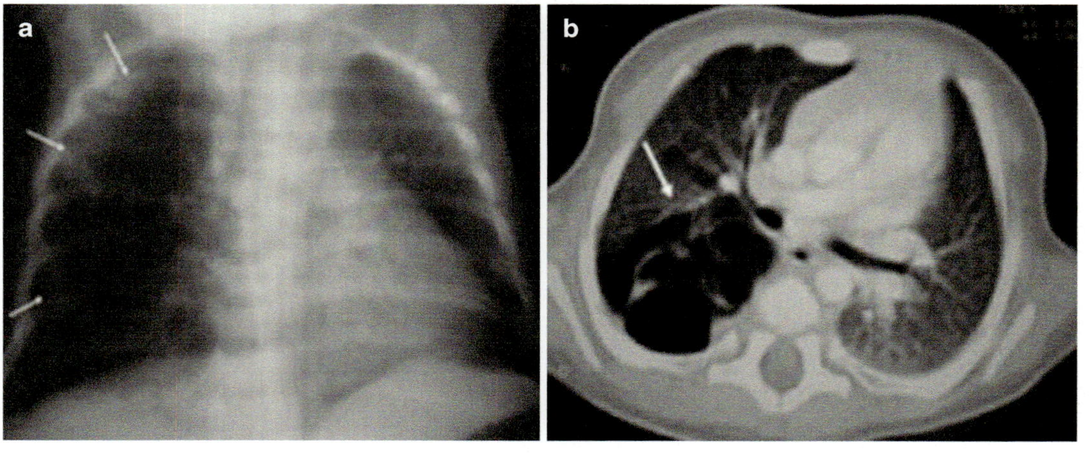

Fig. 11.11 Congenital pulmonary airway malformation in a 2-month-old infant with a cough and breathing difficulty. (**a**) A chest x-ray shows a transparent cystic mass, with thin walls, in the right lung (*arrows*). (**b**) A CT scan of the chest shows that this mass is multicystic in appearance, is in the posterior aspect of the lung on that side (with upper and lower lobe involvement (*arrows*)), and causes a mass effect, with mediastinal displacement toward the left

Types I and II can grow progressively with time, communicate with the airway, and fill with air. According to the type of CPAM, a chest x-ray shows areas of greater or lesser lung transparency, with a mass effect on other chest structures, which can be confused with congenital pulmonary hyperinflation or a diaphragmatic hernia.

Chest CT is fundamental in diagnosis because it not only enables characterization of lesions and shows their location and extension, but also allows them to be differentiated from other diseases. Differential diagnosis for CPAM should include pleuropulmonary blastoma, particularly for type IV.

Pulmonary Sequestration

Pulmonary sequestration is a congenital anomaly characterized by an aberrant pulmonary tissue mass that does not have a normal connection with the tracheobronchial tree or pulmonary arteries. It is usually irrigated by an arterial anomaly that originates directly from the aorta with venous drainage through the azygos system, pulmonary veins, or inferior vena cava. It normally appears as pneumonia, although (depending on its size) it can also appear as a chest mass that causes respiratory distress in newborns.

Pulmonary sequestration is most often found in the basal segments of the lower lobes, particularly in the medial zone of the lower left lobe. It has traditionally been divided into two types: intralobar and extralobar. In the former, sequestration is contained within the adjacent lobe, with which it shares its pleural covering and venous drainage, normally through the pulmonary veins. Extralobar sequestration is most often located between the lower lobe and the diaphragm, and has its own pleural covering. Around 90% of cases are located on the left side, and the venous drainage is commonly via the azygos system.

The clinical picture is diverse. Most cases of intralobar sequestration involve a history of recurrent focal pneumonia, but some of them appear as an incidental finding, particularly in newborns and infants. Extralobar sequestration is most often diagnosed during the first 6 months of life with clinical manifestations such as dyspnea, cyanosis, and difficulty feeding. It can be associated with other anomalies such as pulmonary hypoplasia, a horseshoe lung, CPAM, a bronchogenic cyst, a diaphragmatic hernia, or cardiovascular anomalies such as an arterial trunk and total anomalous pulmonary venous drainage.

The radiological aspect of intralobar sequestration depends on the degree of aeration and on the presence or absence of associated infection. Nonaerated opacity is a common finding on a chest x-ray (Fig. 11.12). Mixed opacity is evident after recurrent or chronic infections, with air and sometime fluid levels in their cavities. Newborns with extralobar sequestration typically show persistently dense images in the posterolateral aspect of the thorax, normally on the left side.

Chest CT is an indispensable tool in the diagnosis of pulmonary sequestration and can confirm the diagnosis through demonstration of aberrant vessels, and also through its extension and venous drainage (Fig. 11.12). If there is a lung infection, the sequestration is commonly multicystic. Fetal MRI can be useful in intrauterine cases when ultrasound findings are inconclusive (Fig. 11.13).

Acute Lower Respiratory Tract Infections

It is generally not possible to determine with certainty the etiology of an acute lower respiratory tract infection with just a radiological study and, because of this, clinical correlation is fundamental. However, there are radiographic characteristics that can orient the clinician and that correlate with anatomopathological manifestations.

Viral infections produce superficial infection of the mucosa, and the bronchial and bronchiolar walls present edema and diffuse infiltration by inflammatory cells. Often there is compromise of the peribronchial tissues and interlobular septa, and this may also extend to the alveolar space. These alterations are manifested in chest x-rays as interstitial compromise, with thickening of the peribronchial and perivascular interstitium, bilateral hyperinflation due to air trapping, and areas of atelectasis (Figs. 11.14 and 11.15). Less often, there can be isolated confluent shadows, usually without pleural effusion. It is important to note

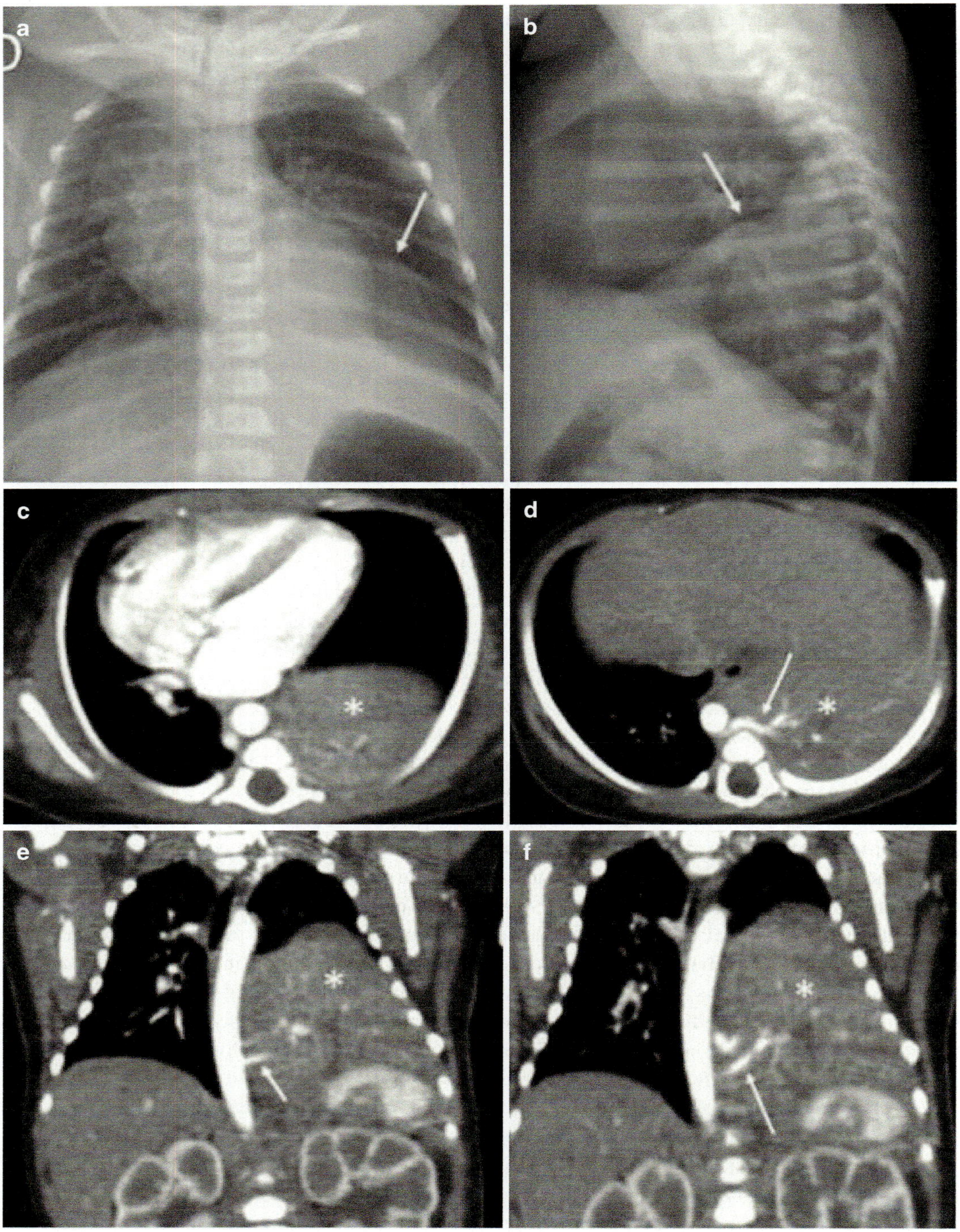

Fig. 11.12 Intralobar pulmonary sequestration of the left lower lobe in a 5-day-old infant who had a prenatal ultrasound suggestive of a congenital pulmonary malformation but was born without respiratory distress. Chest x-rays in the anteroposterior (**a**) and lateral (**b**) views show a mass that occupies much of the left lower lobe (*arrows*). Axial CT scans with intravenous contrast enhancement (**c**, **d**) and coronal reconstruction (**e**, **f**) confirm the presence of the left lung mass (*asterisk*), which receives a systemic arterial supply from at least two aberrant arteries that arise from the thoracic aorta

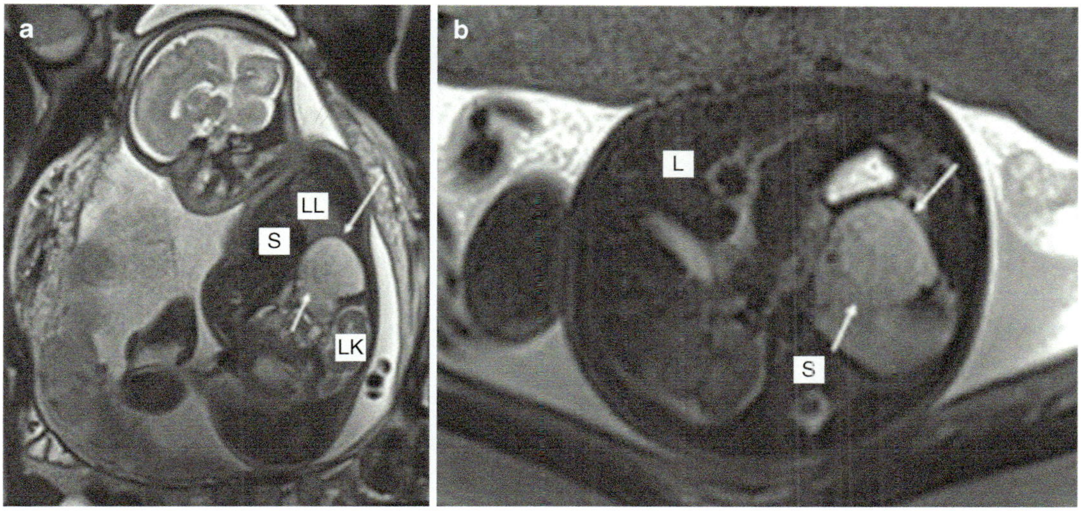

Fig. 11.13 Extralobar pulmonary sequestration in a singleton pregnancy of 34 weeks. Coronal (**a**) and axial (**b**) T2-weighted fetal MRIs show a hypointense mass at the base of the left hemithorax in the posterior situation, adjacent to the diaphragm (*arrows*). *L* liver, *LK* left kidney, *LL* left lung, *S* spine

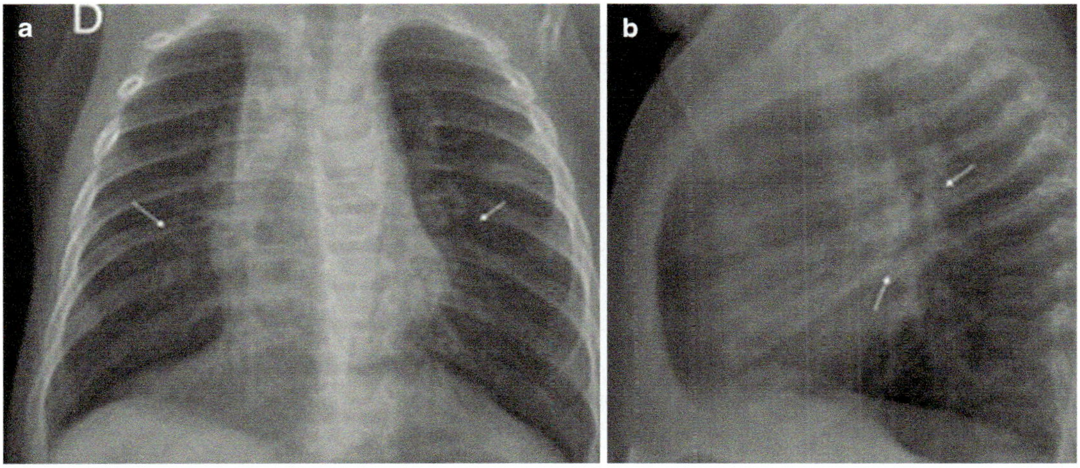

Fig. 11.14 Interstitial lung disease with bronchial obstruction in an 8-month-old infant with a fever, cough, and wheeze. Chest x-rays in the anteroposterior (**a**) and lateral (**b**) views show marked bilateral pulmonary hyperinflation and interstitial shadowing in the central regions of both lungs (*arrows*)

that with viral infections, radiological alterations can take 2–3 weeks to resolve completely, by which time there have been clinical improvements and the child is asymptomatic. Most cases of infection resolve without sequelae. However, some viruses, such as some strains of adenovirus, can leave sequela such as bronchiolitis obliterans and bronchiectasis. When these predominantly affect one lung, this can manifest as a unilateral hyperlucent lung.

Typically, with bacterial infection, there is an exudate that occupies air space and progresses until it compromises a segment or lobe, and it can have multiple foci (Figs. 11.16 and 11.17).

Radiographically, alveolar condensation appears as a confluent opacity with generally lobular or segmentary distribution (Fig. 11.16) and can include an air bronchogram. "Hidden pneumonia" is common in children and may go unnoticed by an inexperienced observer. It is located in

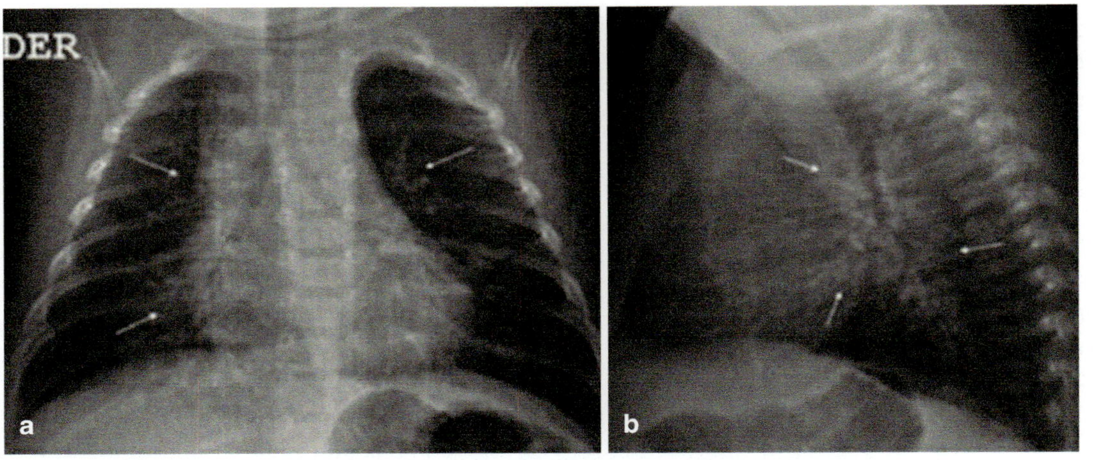

Fig. 11.15 Interstitial pneumonia in a 6-month-old infant with a cough and fever. Chest x-rays in the anteroposterior (**a**) and lateral (**b**) views show interstitial shadowing in the central regions of both lungs (*arrows*)

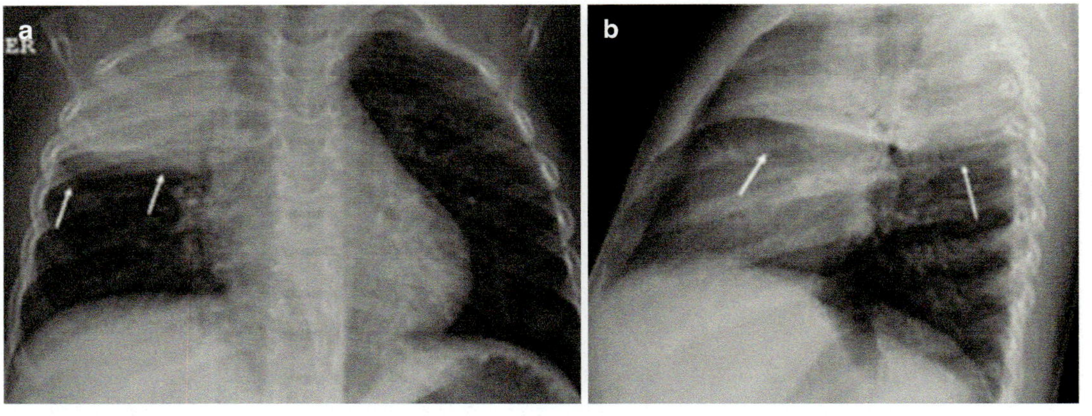

Fig. 11.16 Lobar pneumonia in a 14-month-old infant with a cough and fever. Chest x-rays in the anteroposterior (**a**) and lateral (**b**) views show pneumonic consolidation in the right upper lobe, with signs of volume loss and a shifted minor fissure (*arrows*)

a retrocardiac situation, in the region of the posterior costophrenic sinuses, or in a paramediastinal situation. Because of its morphology, pneumonic condensation is always highly visible in the anteroposterior and lateral planes, in contrast to atelectasis, which, in addition to being associated with volume loss, is generally much more evident in one of the projections. The visualization of a central radiolucid area in the condensation can represent an aerated lung, excavation, or the formation of a pneumatocele. It appears initially as a rounded opaque area (round pneumonia) and is not evident until 12–24 hours after the disease begins (Fig. 11.18). Pleural effusion, a pneumatocele, and a pulmonary abscess can occur as complications (Figs. 11.19 and 11.20). Pneumatoceles are fine-walled air cavities, which commonly appear 10–14 days after the beginning of infection during clinical improvement. A pulmonary abscess is a severe complication of a bacterial infection and tends to occur early in the course of the disease. Radiographically, it appears as a low-density lesion, generally at the center of the condensation of the thick walls, and sometimes with

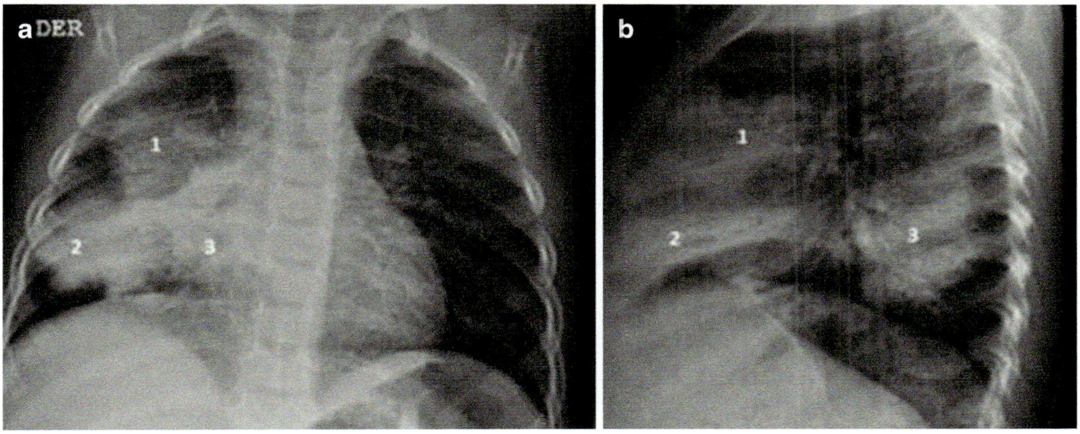

Fig. 11.17 Multifocal pneumonia in a 2-year-old infant with a persistent fever. Chest x-rays in the anteroposterior (**a**) and lateral (**b**) views show three spots of consolidation in the right lung that compromise the upper (1), middle (2), and lower (3) lobes

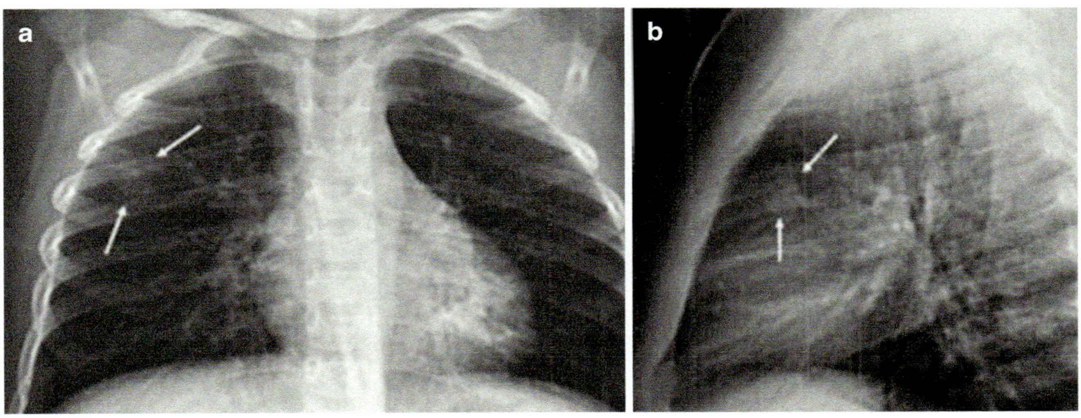

Fig. 11.18 Early pneumonia in a 6-year-old child with an 18-hour fever. Chest x-rays in the anteroposterior (**a**) and lateral (**b**) views show a small nodular mass in the middle third of the left lung (*arrows*), corresponding to early pulmonary consolidation

a fluid level visible on the x-ray, depending on the patient's position during the study (vertical or horizontal).

Infection by *Mycoplasma pneumoniae* can cause more than 30% of pneumonia cases in older children, and radiological alterations can simulate other pulmonary diseases. The most common pattern consists of poorly defined infiltrates (which are predominantly interstitial), with small areas of alveolar compromise, especially in one or both lower lobes, or in one of the upper lobes. This can be accompanied by an atelectatic component with a discrete pleural reaction (usually basal and marginal). A reticulonodular-type pattern can also be present. Presentations of consolidation of the air space or diffuse compromise of both lungs are much less common, are usually associated with greater clinical compromise, and can be associated with immunosuppression.

While chest CT can provide excellent anatomical information in pneumonia, in most cases it does not change therapeutic decisions. We generally do not recommend this technique in the study

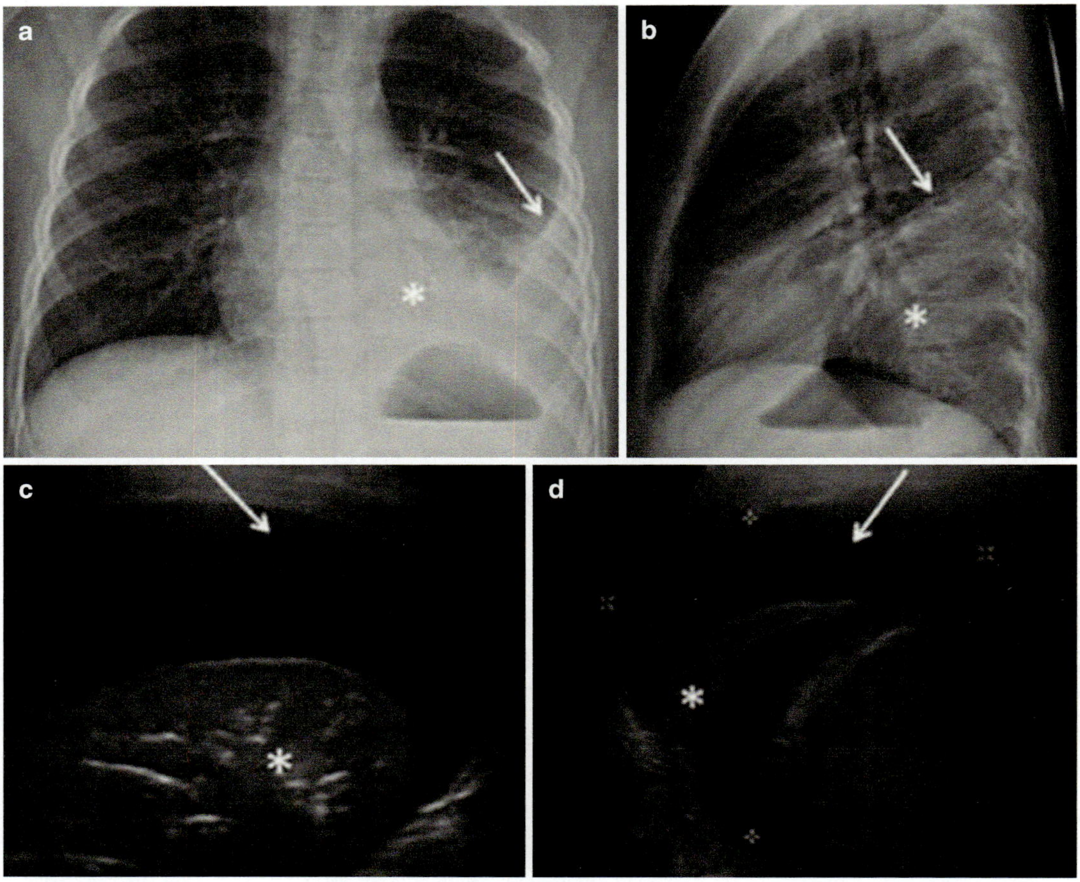

Fig. 11.19 Left basal pneumonia with uncomplicated pleural effusion in a 5-year-old child. Chest x-rays in the anteroposterior (**a**) and lateral (**b**) views show left lower lobe pneumonia (*asterisk*) associated with pleural effusion (*arrows*). Pleural ultrasound shows the consolidated lung (*asterisk*) and the uncomplicated pleural effusion, echo-free and without partitions inside (*arrows*)

of acute lower respiratory infections in children, except in certain specific situations such as complicated pneumonia, a pulmonary abscess, complicated empyema, or a refractory bronchopleural fistula.

Pulmonary tuberculosis (TB) merits a separate mention. The chest x-ray continues to be the fundamental pillar of TB diagnosis in children. In most cases, there is evident localized lung disease, with partially confluent shadows and hilar adenopathies, usually unilaterally (Fig. 11.21). Axial CT is indicated in unusual, complicated, or disseminated cases of the disease. It provides better definition of the extension of lung disease and ganglion compromise. The examination should be done with imaging before and after the use of intravenous contrast, and the finding of adenopathies with central hyperdense areas is highly suggestive of TB. In general, TB should be suspected in all cases of pneumonia with unusual progression, with a poor response to antibiotics, or with hilar and/or unilateral mediastinal adenopathies.

Diffuse or Focal Diseases of the Pulmonary Parenchyma

Simple radiography can be useful in diagnosing diffuse diseases of the pulmonary parenchyma,

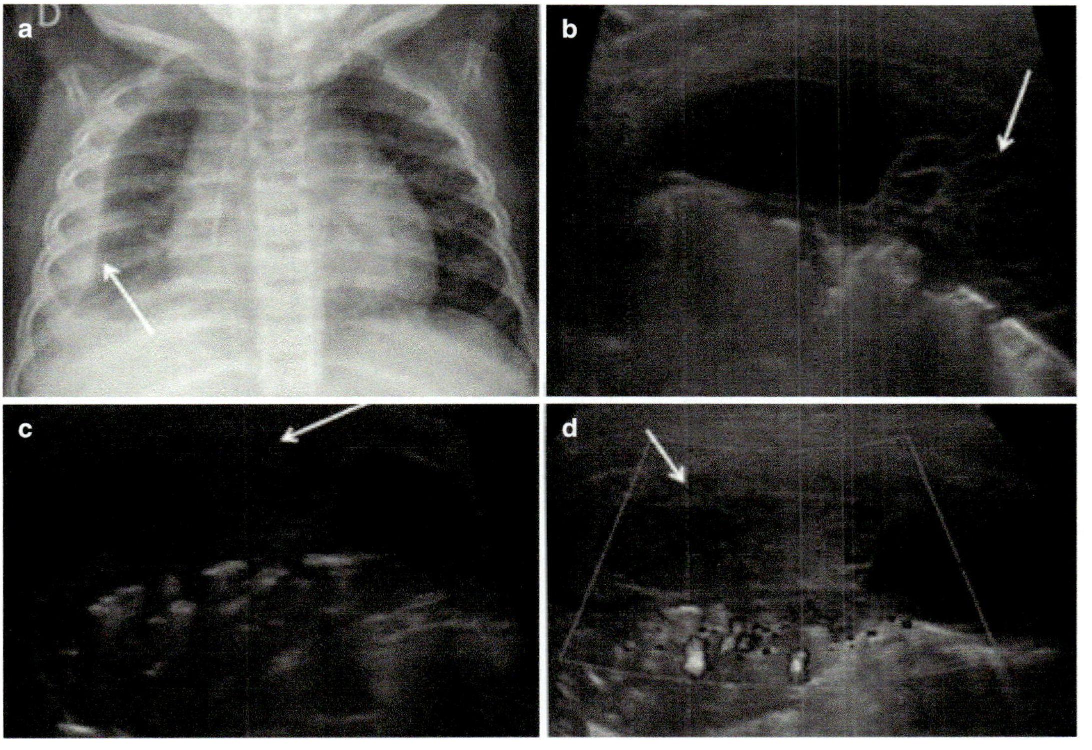

Fig. 11.20 Right-sided pneumonia with parapneumonic pleural effusions and empyema in a 10-month-old infant. A chest x-ray (**a**) shows right pleural effusion (*arrow*). Pleural ultrasounds (**b**–**d**) show echoic, septate pleural effusion with fibrin inside (*arrows*), compatible with empyema. (**d**) The *arrow* shows the Doppler effect

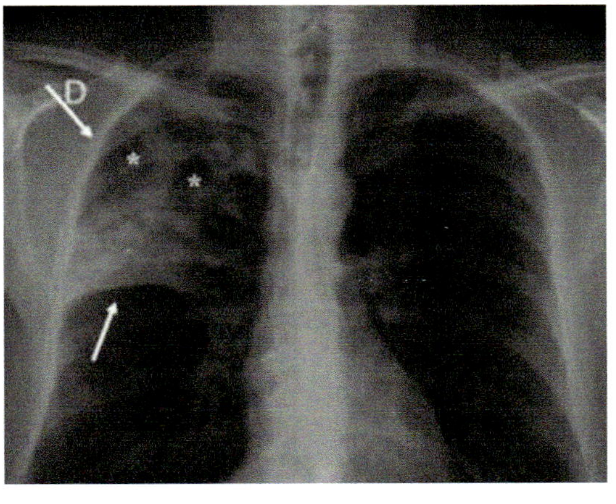

Fig. 11.21 Pulmonary tuberculosis in a 14-year-old adolescent with tuberculosis. An anteroposterior chest x-ray shows an area of consolidation in the right upper lobe (*arrows*), with volume loss and some areas of lower density inside, compatible with excavation zones (*asterisked*)

but high-resolution CT undoubtedly yields the best results, allowing for assessment of the lungs with excellent spatial resolution and providing precise anatomical details of the pulmonary parenchyma. Some of the most common patterns or alterations are:

Ground glass pattern This consists of a slight increase in lung density, with conservation of normal vascular and bronchial margins. This is sometimes associated with an air bronchogram and can be heterogeneous, determining a mosaic pattern. This pattern can be seen in many pediatric diseases, and infectious pneumonia of any etiology is the most common cause. The pattern can also be seen following bronchoalveolar lavage and in pulmonary edema, pulmonary hemorrhage, leukemic infiltrates, pulmonary contusion, respiratory distress syndrome, collagen diseases, extrinsic allergic alveolitis, drug toxicity, interstitial pneumonia, alveolar proteinosis, and idiomatic pulmonary fibrosis.

Consolidation pattern This appears as a homogeneous increase in the density of the parenchyma, which erases the contours of vessels and the walls of the airway, and can include an air bronchogram. By definition, alveolar air is occupied by liquid, cells, tissue, or other matter. The most common causes are pneumonia of any etiology, pulmonary edema, hemorrhage, and pulmonary contusion.

Bronchial disease pattern This is suspected when there is thickening of the bronchial walls or of the peribronchial interstitium, when the bronchial walls in the peripheral third of the lungs are clearly identified, or when the thickness of the wall of the proximal bronchial tree represents more than a third of the bronchial diameter.

Tree-in-bud pattern This pattern represents severe bronchial impaction. The small airway that is dilated and/or filled with mucus, pus, or inflammatory matter appears as small, well-defined nodules associated with structures that branch out. This is commonly seen in infectious bronchiolitis of any etiology, endobronchial dissemination of TB, cystic fibrosis (CF), allergic bronchopulmonary aspergillosis, immobile cilia syndrome, bronchiolitis obliterans, and asthma.

Air trapping This is defined as retention or an excess of air in a lung, which is evident during expiration and is the result of complete or partial obstruction of the airway, or local abnormalities in lung compliance. It is particularly common in bronchiolitis obliterans, CF, bronchiectasis, and asthma. The mosaic pattern consists of the presence of multiple areas of trapped air, generally in both lungs, with segmentary or subsegmentary distribution, appearing as areas with greater transparency and a decrease in the vascular pattern, alternating with normally ventilated areas with normal vascularization.

"Honeycomb" pattern This is indicative of destruction and pulmonary fibrosis involving complete loss of the normal acinus and bronchial architecture in the final stage of chronic lung disease. It takes the form of multiple cyst-like air spaces, with well-defined walls 1–3 mm thick, which are found mainly in peripheral and subpleural areas.

Bronchiectasis This is defined as irreversible dilatation of the bronchial tree. The diagnostic criteria for axial CT are a greater internal diameter of the bronchus in comparison with the diameter of the adjacent pulmonary artery branch, loss of the normal progressive thinning of the bronchus, thickening of the bronchial wall, and identification of bronchus in the periphery of the lung (1 cm apart from the pleural space). According to the morphology, this condition is classified as cylindrical, varicose, or cystic. The cylindrical form is the only form without thinning of the bronchus distally, with smooth or slightly irregular bronchial walls. The varicose form has a pearl-necklace appearance, while the cystic form has a saccular appearance.

Bronchiolitis obliterans This is characterized by thickening of the bronchiolar wall due to submucosal collagenation, with few changes in the distal parenchyma. Progressive narrowing of the bronchioles is associated with lumen distortion, mucus plugs, and chronic inflammation. This condition is usually secondary to viral or bacterial infections, lung or bone marrow transplantation, collagen diseases, or inhalation of toxic substances. A chest x-ray can be normal, while CT shows a mosaic pattern due to air trapping or oligemia, which can be visualized better in exhalation images.

Specific Pathologies of Importance

Cystic fibrosis The role of imaging in CF has changed. Care was historically based on clinical assessment, using chest x-rays to confirm the clinical impression and in the event of suspicion of overinfection. While chest x-rays continue to be the most commonly used images for study of CF patients, CT is becoming increasingly important.

Children with CF are born with normal lungs but rapidly develop a cycle of infection and

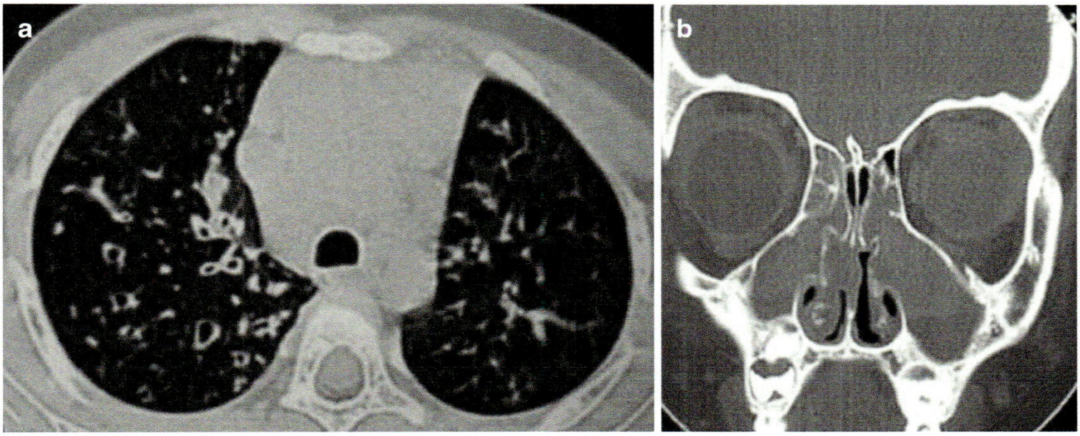

Fig. 11.22 Cystic fibrosis a 5-year-old child. A chest CT scan (**a**) shows multiple cylindrical bronchiectases in the right lung. A coronal CT scan (**b**) shows maxillary sinuses and ethmoidal sinuses filled with fluid and mucosal edema

inflammation that causes airway disease and eventually parenchymal damage. Thus, a chest x-ray will be normal in these infants in their first year of life. Any alterations that do appear can be nonspecific and similar to those observed in viral or atypical infection, with swelling of the bronchial walls. High-resolution CT is the most accurate method for assessment of morphological changes in CF. It can detect bronchiectasis, peribronchial thickening, mucus plugs, air trapping, condensation zones, and lung destruction (Fig. 11.22).

Bronchiectases are usually diffuse, with compromise of the upper lobes occurring in most cases and central and peripheral bronchiectases being present in two thirds of patients. While cystic and varicose bronchiectases are not uncommon, the cylindrical form predominates, particularly in small children. Mucosal impaction and a mosaic perfusion pattern secondary to air trapping are very common findings in CF. Mosaic perfusion can be the only finding in the initial course of the disease, and mucosal impaction can manifest as large nodes or elonelongated central shapes, or as a tree-in-bud pattern in the periphery of the lung. Mucus plugs can, in turn, lead to segmentary or lobar atelectasis. Total or partial resolution of mucus plugs can reflect therapeutic effectiveness and is useful for monitoring the disease. Hilar lymphadenopathy is another relatively common finding. Nuclear medicine has been used to assess the ventilation/perfusion ratio and mucus clearance in patients with CF.

Immotile ciliary syndrome (ciliary dyskinesia) This term includes diseases that occur as a direct result of congenital defects of the airway cilia. The main findings are inflammatory sinus disease (sinusitis), recurring pulmonary infections, situs inversus, and infertility. An association between chronic respiratory disease and immotile ciliary is well known. Kartagener syndrome is characterized by total situs inversus, bronchiectasis, and sinusitis, and it affects 50% of patients with immotile ciliary syndrome. The radiological aspects and clinical manifestations of immotile ciliary syndrome are similar to those of CF but less severe. The most common alterations are hyperinflation, peribronchial thickening, bronchiectasis, mucus plugs, atelectasis, and areas of consolidation.

Sources

Andronikou S, Irving B, Hlabangana LT, Pillay T, et al. Technical developments in postprocessing of paediatric airway imaging. Pediatr Radiol. 2013;43:269–84.

Arce JD. Estudio radiológico de la vía aérea central. Neumol Pediatr. 2012;7:72–83.

Calder A, Owens CM. Imaging of parapneumonic pleural effusions and empyema in children. Pediatr Radiol. 2009;39:527–37.

Carsin A, Mely L, Chrestian MA, Devred P, De Lagausie P, Guys JM, et al. Association of three different congenital malformations in a same pulmonary lobe in a 5-year-old girl. Pediatr Pulmonol. 2010;45:832–5.

Deshmukh S, Rubesova E, Barth R. MR assessment of normal fetal lung volumes: a literature review. AJR Am J Roentgenol. 2010;194:W212–7.

Recio Rodríguez M, Martinez de Vega V, Cano Alonso R, Carrasco Arranz J, Martinez Ten P, Perez Pedregosa J. MR imaging of thoracic abnormalities in the fetus. Radiographics. 2012;32:E305–21.

Dillman JR, Attili AK, Agarwal PP, Dorfman AL, Hernandez RJ, Strouse PJ. Common and uncommon vascular rings and slings: a multi-modality review. Pediatr Radiol. 2011;41:1440–54.

Espinoza A. Ultrasonido del tórax pediatrico. Neumol Pediatr. 2015;10:58–66.

Irodi A, Prabhu SM, John RM, Leena RV. Congenital bronchopulmonary vascular malformations, "sequestration" and beyond. Indian J Radiol Imaging. 2015;25:35–43.

Lee E, Tracy D, Mahmood S, Weldon C, Zurakowski D, Boiselle P. Preoperative MDCT evaluation of congenital lung anomalies in children: comparison of axial, multiplanar, and 3D images. AJR Am J Roentgenol. 2011;196:1040–6.

Lee EY, Boiselle PM, Cleveland RH. Multidetector CT evaluation of congenital lung anomalies. Radiology. 2008;247:632–48.

Lee EY, Dorkin H, Vargas SO. Congenital pulmonary malformations in pediatric patients: review and update on etiology, classification, and imaging findings. Radiol Clin North Am. 2011;49:921–48.

Lee EY, Zucker EJ, Restrepo R, Daltro P, Boiselle PM. Advanced large airway CT imaging in children: evolution from axial to 4-D assessment. Pediatr Radiol. 2013;43:285–97.

Lucaya J, Strife JL. Pediatric chest imaging: chest imaging in infants and children. Berlin: Springer; 2002.

Lyons K, Cassady C, Mehollin-Ray A, Krishnamurthy R. Current role of fetal magnetic resonance imaging in body anomalies. Semin Ultrasound CT MR. 2015;36:310–23.

Mong A, Epelman M, Darge K. Ultrasound of the pediatric chest. Pediatr Radiol. 2012;42:287–97.

Pedata R, Palermo M, Maiello M, Esposito N, Ermito S, Dinatale A, et al. Fetal lung lesions diagnosis: the crucial role of ultrasonography. J Prenat Med. 2009;3:49–52.

Ramos-Duran L, Nance JW Jr, Schoepf UJ, Henzler T, Apfaltrer P, Anthony M, Hlavacek AM. Developmental aortic arch anomalies in infants and children assessed with CT angiography. AJR Am J Roentgenol. 2012;198:W466–74.

Raychaudhuri P, Pasupati A, James A, Whitehead B, Kumar R. Prospective study of antenatally diagnosed congenital cystic adenomatoid malformations. Pediatr Surg Int. 2011;27:1159–64.

Sepulveda W. Perinatal imaging in bronchopulmonary sequestration. J Ultrasound Med. 2009;28:89–94.

Stocker JT. The respiratory tract. In: Stocker JT, Dehner LP, Husain AN, editors. Pediatric pathology. 3rd ed. Filadelfia, PA: Lippincott Williams & Wilkins; 2011. p. 441–515.

Sundarakumar DK, Bhalla AA, Sharma R, Gupta AK, et al. Multidetector computed tomography imaging of congenital anomalies of major airways: a pictorial essay. World J Radiol. 2011;3:289–97.

Zaninovic A, Arce JD, Ferron S. Estudio por imágenes de vía aérea. Utilidad de la tomografía computada multidetector con reconstrucción tridimensional. Neumol Pediatr. 2015;10:72–81.

12 Assessing Arterial Oxygen Saturation

Christian Poets and Pablo Brockmann Veloso

Contents

Oxygen Transport in the Blood

The dissolved oxygen transported in the blood constitutes a small fraction of the total oxygen content, which has a direct relation to the partial oxygen pressure (Henry's law). The solubility coefficient is only 0.003 ml of oxygen for every 100 ml of blood.

Hemoglobin (Hb) is the main oxygen transporter, which bonds with the Fe^{++} of the hemoglobin molecules. Each hemoglobin cell contains four Fe^{++} ions; thus, every Hb molecule transports four oxygen molecules in the form of a compound that easily delivers oxygen to tissue, called oxyhemoglobin (HbO_2). Under normal conditions, every gram of hemoglobin transports 1.34 ml of oxygen. The oxygen content is the sum of dissolved oxygen plus the oxygen that is chemically bonded to the hemoglobin. The oxygen content is determined by both the partial pressure of oxygen (PaO_2) and the quantity of

C. Poets (✉)
Department of Neonatology, University Children's Hospital Tübingen, Alemania, Tübingen, Germany
e-mail: christian-f.poets@med.uni-tuebingen.de

P. Brockmann Veloso
Department of Pediatrics, School of Medicine, Pontificia Universidad Católica de Chile, Santiago, Chile
e-mail: pbrockmann@med.puc.cl

P. Bertrand, I. Sánchez (eds.), *Pediatric Respiratory Diseases*,
https://doi.org/10.1007/978-3-030-26961-6_12

hemoglobin and its degree of arterial saturation (SaO_2), which is represented by the following formula:

$$CaO_2 = Hb \times 1.34 \times SaO_2 + PaO_2 \times 0.003$$

Transcutaneous Measurement of Oxygen Saturation

Pulse oximeters do not measure oxygen concentrations in the plasma; rather, they measure the proportion of hemoglobin that carries oxygen molecules, which is termed oxygen saturation. This technique was first developed in 1975 but not introduced into clinical practice until 10 years later. The terms for the oxygen saturation values are saturated and unsaturated. This technique is based on a simple physiological principle, which determines that oxygenated and unoxygenated hemoglobin absorb light rays differently. The former absorbs more light from the red band (at 600–750 nm), while unoxygenated hemoglobin absorbs more infrared light (at 850–1000 nm). The pulse oximeter emits light at two specific wavelengths (660 and 940 nm), which are transmitted through tissue (a finger, for example) and sensed by a photodetector. The light absorbance radius of the two wavelengths correlates with the saturation of the oxygenated hemoglobin in the tissue blood, in accordance with a pre-established formula (Fig. 12.1). However, of all of the light that is absorbed, only the light absorbed by the pulsatile component of the arterial vasculature correlates with the arterial oxygen saturation. Consequently, the pulse oximeter makes use of the fact that the expansion and contraction of the vasculature causes changes in the distance the light has to travel, which in turn changes the amount that is absorbed. The peaks and nadirs of the amount of light absorbed are determined by measuring the light transmitted several hundred times per second. The peak oximeter divides the absorbance in the peaks by that in the nadirs. This

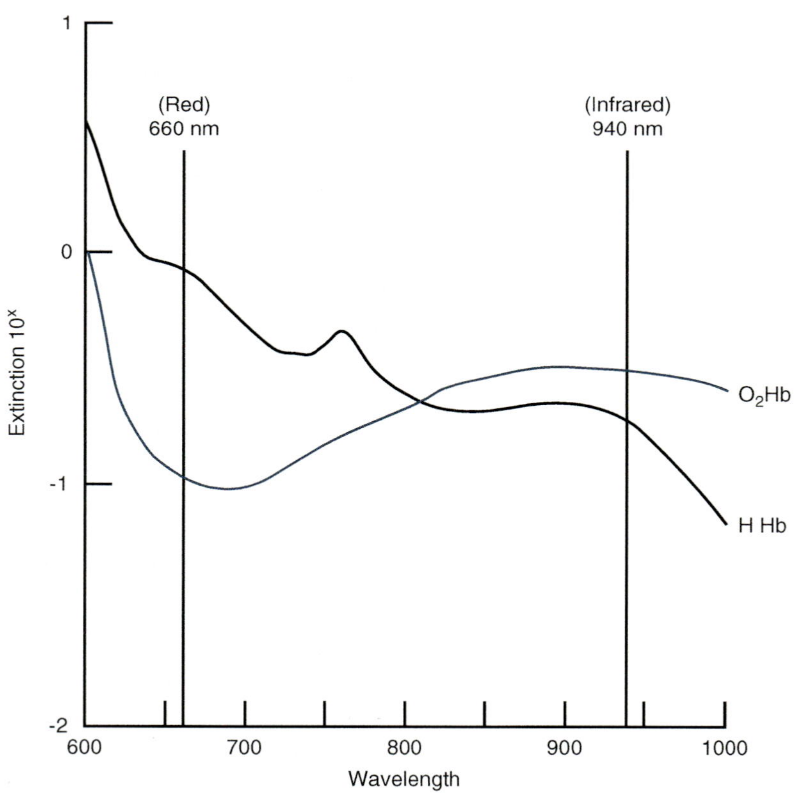

Fig. 12.1 Absorption mechanism used in pulse oximetry

absorbance ratio is different from that in nonpulsatile tissue. The value obtained from the absorbance ratio in pulsatile tissue can be extrapolated to a pre-established scale of oxygen saturation values.

Factors That Affect Oxygen Saturation Measurement

Pulse oximeters are relatively easy to use. They do not require calibration or preheating of the patient's skin, and they can be used immediately with all types of patients of any age. However, there are factors that can affect peripheral oxygen saturation (SpO_2) measurement and interpretation, which are discussed below.

Type of Sensor and Its Placement

The location of the sensor is the most important factor in obtaining a real SpO_2 value. Incorrect placement results in an optical shunt, which happens when the light received by the photodiode does not pass correctly through the tissue to be analyzed. Incorrect placement can also result in exposure to ambient light, which can affect the measurement. In most cases where this occurs, ambient light accounts for 85% of SpO_2 readings, which is approximately the extrapolated value that corresponds to a ratio of 1:0 between red and infrared light. Overestimations occur as a result of exposure to an excess of ambient light, which can lead to a belief that a patient is properly saturated, while in reality the values are low. Actual hypoxemia may pass undetected in these patients.

An optical shunt can also occur in the absence of ambient light. This is because in the majority of oximeter devices, the red light and infrared emission diodes are 2–3 mm apart. If the sensor is detached and one of the diodes is left out, it can produce falsely low (60–70%) or high (95–100%) SpO_2 values, depending whether it is the infrared diode or the red-light diode that is uncoupled, respectively. To avoid this situation, which can result in clinical complications for the patient, proper placement of the sensor should be ensured. The light emitter should be facing the receiver, with both correctly covered to avoid contact with ambient light. The sensors should be fastened to a fabric that does not let light pass through. The sensors should not be fastened to the skin with excessive force (over 50 mm Hg) that could affect the signal-to-noise ratio and severely disturb the operation of the SpO_2 sensor.

Another less common problem with pulse oximeters is skin lesions by burning. This usually occurs when a different type of sensor is used from that determined by the oximetry equipment or when the surface of the sensor has been damaged. The sensor should be checked to ensure it is the correct one, and its position should be changed every 8 hours.

It is worth noting that, to date, little attention has been given to the performance of different types of sensors in newborns and infants. In fact, we know of no study that has systematically assessed the differences among sensors used in this age group. In the experience of the authors, more flexible sensors provide more reliable SpO_2 measurements in young patients, given that these sensors can be applied more easily, without the need for a lot of pressure to fasten them. The problem with flexible sensors is that they tend to be more expensive than more fixed or rigid sensors.

Peripheral Perfusion

Pulse oximeters depend on peripheral perfusion, and most of the equipment currently available requires at least 20 mm Hg of pulse pressure or systolic pressure of over 30 mm Hg to operate adequately and reliably. The efficiency of the pulse oximeter falls significantly if the pressure falls below these thresholds. The most reliable test of correct functioning is the signal-to-noise ratio, which can be appreciated through the pulse curve, built into most new oximeters. There are significant variations among the different pulse meter brands with respect to the SpO_2 reading in situations of hypotension—for example, shock.

Response Time

In theory, the response time of the pulse oximeter depends only on the time it takes the oxygenated blood to reach the point where the sensor is located, which is 4 seconds to the toe of a newborn, 4.5 seconds to that of an infant, and 5.5 seconds to that of a child of around 5 years of age. However, the pulse oximeters available nowadays average the values registered in a range from 2 to 15 seconds (average time) or 4 to 32 beats per minute, to avoid errors and provide a more reliable reading of SpO_2.

This procedure attempts to reduce the number of false alarms. The longer the average time of these values is, the more slowly the equipment reacts to changes. For example, fewer alarms sound with postural changes; however, this extends the time that the physician has to react to real changes in SpO_2 or it can lead to false low SpO_2 values if the patient is constantly moving, and this might falsely suggest the presence of hypoxemia. Erroneous readings can be indistinguishable from real hypoxemia, particularly without pulse plethysmography curves. In addition, the use of the average time can lead to erroneous conclusions in situations in which a very precise measurement of SpO_2 is required. An example is the decision to use supplementary oxygen in newborns and infants with bronchopulmonary dysplasia. The association between oxygen desaturations and cardiorespiratory events such as apnea necessarily require a short average time. Finally, the different average SpO_2 times make it impossible to define normal values in a population and extrapolate them to oximeters with different average times. Therefore, all of the reference values obtained with a specific pulse oximeter can be extrapolated only to subjects in which the same equipment is used.

These problems can be overcome by using the beat-to-beat mode, which provides an SpO_2 value for every heartbeat. However, every clinical unit must decide to what extent it needs SpO_2 measurements and whether oximetry is intended for adequate diagnosis (for example, polysomnography) or for more general monitoring and detection of threatening situations on the basis of determined limits.

Motion Artifacts

The pulsatile (arterial) component contributes only 1–5% of the total absorbance as measured by the pulse oximeter. Consequently, the instrument is very sensitive to signal changes—for example, body movement. It is particularly important to identify the presence of movements in order to discount them. This can be done by analyzing the plethysmograph curve from the SpO_2 reading. Ideally, the plethysmograph curve should be complete. The SpO_2 values are not reliable and must be discarded if the curve is disrupted or incomplete. A less reliable alternative is to compare the pulse rate and the heart rate obtained with the electrocardiograph, because the two rates should be identical. Without a system for validating and excluding artifacts, SpO_2 values should not be interpreted.

Influence of Changes in Hemoglobin and Skin Pigmentation

Pulse oximeters only use two light wavelengths. Consequently, they cannot identify abnormal hemoglobin or pigments that can interfere with the reading. Some of these pigments or distinct forms of hemoglobin—among them fetal hemoglobin—absorb light, which results in false readings. Methemoglobinemia will give values of around 85% of SpO_2, and carbon monoxide intoxication will result in falsely high SpO_2 values. Bilirubin generally does not alter pulse oximeter readings.

Reference studies of skin pigmentation and SpO_2 have yielded variable results. A study involving nine premature African American newborns concluded that a Nellcor N100® overestimated SpO_2 by 5% in two cases, but the others were very precise. Another study showed falsely high SpO_2 levels in black adults but only if the SpO_2 was <90%. At higher levels, there are no discrepancies between SpO_2 and SaO_2. This matter is remains unclear, and more studies are required, especially in relation to children.

Influence of Specific Algorithms

Pulse oximeters extrapolate their measures to a table of predetermined values, which is based on empirical data obtained in adults. Consequently, these instruments should be revalidated to be used in children. Studies that have compared different types of pulse oximeters have found statistically significant differences in their results. Moreover, the same equipment can yield significant differences when applied to different age groups.

These differences among devices can be partly explained by the ways in which the equipment shows or calculates SpO_2. Examples of this are the Nellcor® oximeter, which measures functional SpO ($[HbO_2/(HbO_2 + RHb)] * 100$)—where RHb is reduced hemoglobin—as compared with the Ohmeda® oximeter, which estimates the fractional SpO $[HbO_2/(HbO_2 + RHb + MetHb + CO\ Hb) * 100]$—where MetHb is methemoglobin and COHb is carboxyhemoglobin. The former equipment estimates SaO_2 by simply subtracting 2%, which represents MetHb and COHb concentrations, and displaying an SpO_2 that is 2% less than the fractional SpO_2. However, in the clinical context, functional SpO_2 is preferred, and COHb and MetHb are determined only in patients in whom clinical suspicion requires them.

The differences in the values obtained in studies using the same equipment could be caused by the way in which motion artifacts are discounted. For reasons that are explained below, another important factor is the SpO_2 values that are measured: the lower the SpO_2 range is, the less precise the measurement is. The differences can likewise be explained by different types of software. This can explain why in a 1990 study the same Ohmeda Biox III/3700® underestimated real SaO_2 values by 2.9%, while in 1991 this same equipment overestimated SaO_2 by only 0.4%. Reassessments should be done when every new version of the software is installed.

Precision in Detecting Hyperoxemia and Hypoxemia

Pulse oximeters derive their measurements from algorithms based on empirical in vitro data on oxygen saturation values obtained from healthy adult volunteers, in which SpO_2 generally varies within a normal range around 100%. Most suppliers maintain that their equipment shows SpO_2 values at close to ±4–6% of the real SaO_2 values. Normal SpO_2 levels in infants and preschool children are in the same range as those in adults. However, with SpO_2 below 75–80%, the values are simply extrapolated from the algorithm obtained with higher SpO_2 values. This procedure can result in underestimation of the real oxygen saturation values. Given the above, we do not know the real sensitivity of oximeters to screen for low SaO_2 values in seriously ill children—for example, those in shock or with associated infectious problems.

Given the shape of the hemoglobin dissociation curve, pulse oximeters are not ideal for screening for hyperoxemia. The upper limit above which there is not sufficient sensitivity to screen effectively varies depending on the equipment. There have been few studies involving children that have correlated high SpO levels with SaO_2 and established a threat level (Fig. 12.2).

SpO_2 Reference Values

The correct clinical application of the nocturnal saturometer requires adequate SpO_2 reference values for every age, type of equipment, software, and clinical scenario for the patient. For evident reasons, these are very difficult to obtain, and reference values from healthy populations—mostly, young adult volunteers—have been used to interpret pulse oximeter algorithms.

There have been a series of studies to establish values for pediatric ages, particularly for premature and term newborns and small infants, where the deviation from the reference values for adult populations are the greatest.

Most studies that cite references have provided oxygen saturation averages and means, without

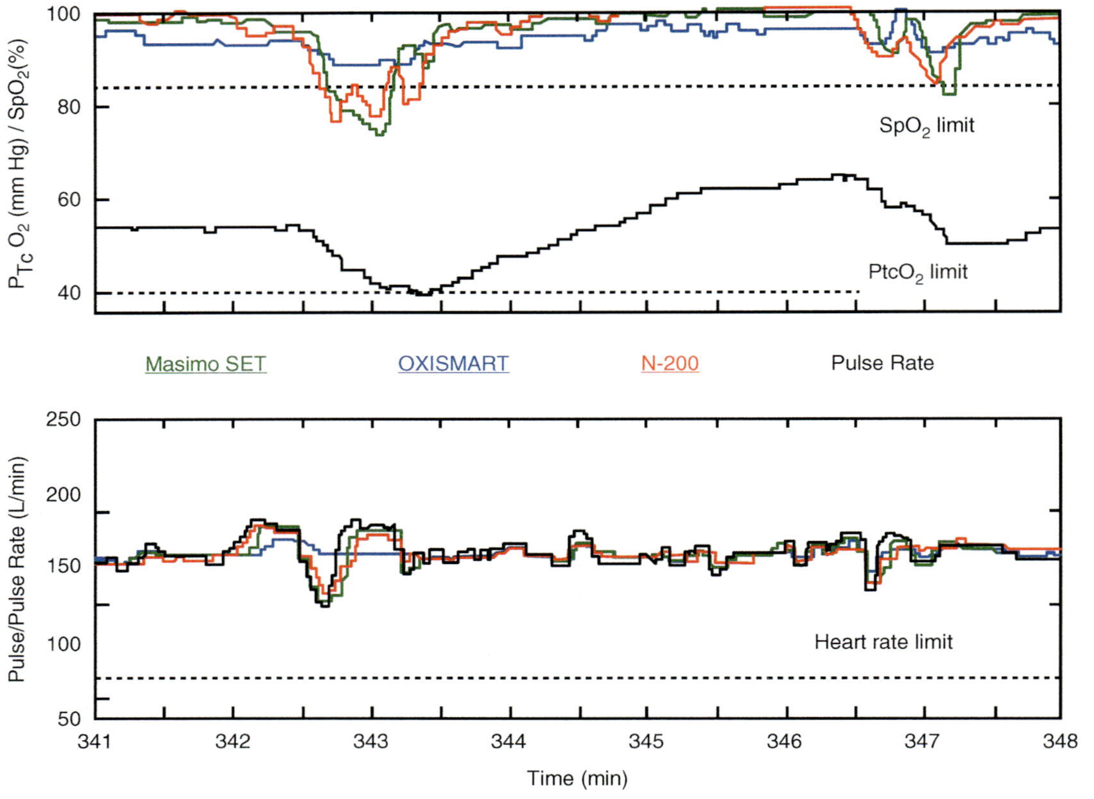

Fig. 12.2 Comparison of different pulse oximetry equipment

fixing on the number and frequency of desaturation events. The desaturation index (DI) is one of the most important elements, especially in newborns and infants, to detect pathological conditions. ID corresponds to the total count of times that SpO_2 values fall 3–4 points during 1 hour. In a study that involved more than 200 child volunteers, our team found a significant presence of desaturation among completely healthy babies less than 3 months of age. This level of desaturation was consistent with those described in other works, emphasizing that desaturation by 3 or 4 points in children in this age range may be physiological. In contrast, in schoolchildren and adolescents, desaturation by 3 or 4 points has a pathological connotation, suggesting obstructive sleep apnea.

Unlike what happens with desaturation events, SpO_2 averages tend to be quite even and are similar at different pediatric ages. SpO_2 is normally expected to be above 95%.

The desaturation index of 4 percent (ID4) of SpO_2 is within normal limits when the index is < 4 points per hour (in children above 1 year of age). We recommend using a saturation index below 80% of SpO_2, which is considered normal if it is less than 1.5 events per hour in infants under 3 months of age.

A consolidated SpO_2 under a specific cutoff is widely used in chronic lung disease, such as bronchopulmonary dysplasia. The cutoff depends on the equipment. For example, when Massimo SET equipment is used, it is considered normal if the patient has an SpO_2 of <90% for <3% of the time.

Transcutaneous Oxygen Measurement

Transcutaneous oxygen ($TCPO_2$) measurement is a noninvasive method to determine the partial oxygen pressure from the surface of the skin, using an electrode that chemically senses the concentration of oxygen molecules circulating in the blood. The oxygen molecules that pass through the skin are illuminated by an optical fiber that emits a specific light. The electrode consists of a platinum cathode and a silver reference anode separated by an electrolyte solution that is permeable to oxygen. The electrode is heated to 42 °C, which diffuses the oxygen molecules from the skin to the electrode. Once they are in the electrode, the oxygen molecules are reduced, generating an electrical current. The red reflection that is produced is interpreted by the probe as the partial oxygen pressure according to an algorithm.

Pulse oximeters and apparatuses that calculate $TCPO_2$ perform measurements in different but related ways. Because the relationship between PaO_2 and SaO_2 is based on the hemoglobin dissociation curve, this is not linear or constant. Thus, the values obtained from measuring the $TCPO_2$ do not necessarily reflect the SpO_2 in the same patient. There are several factors that should be taken into consideration when extrapolating one value to another: the measuring time, the number of measurements, and the peripheral perfusion of the patient. The equipment for measuring $TCPO_2$ also has a series of disadvantages, including the fact that it is difficult to use and the sensors need to be changed often, because of which it is recommended to use the equipment as a complement to the pulse oximeter.

Sources

Bohnhorst B, Geuting T, Peter CS, Dordelmann M, Wilken B, Poets CF. Randomized, controlled trial of oral creatine supplementation (not effective) for apnea of prematurity. Pediatrics. 2004;113:e303–7.

Brockmann PE, Poets A, Urschitz MS, Sokollik C, Poets CF. Reference values for pulse oximetry recordings in healthy term neonates during their first 5 days of life. Arch Dis Child Fetal Neonatal Ed. 2011;96:F335–8.

O'Brien LM, Stebbens VA, Poets CF, Heycock EG, Southall DP. Oxygen saturation during the first 24 hours of life. Arch Dis Child Fetal Neonatal Ed. 2000;83:F35–8.

Poets A, Urschitz MS, Poets CF. Intermittent hypoxia in supine versus side position in term neonates. Pediatr Res. 2009;65:654–6.

Poets CF, Stebbens VA, Alexander JR, Arrowsmith WA, Salfield SA, Southall DP. Oxygen saturation and breathing patterns in infancy. 2: Preterm infants at discharge from special care. Arch Dis Child. 1991;66:574–8.

Poets CF, Stebbens VA, Samuels MP, Southall DP. Oxygen saturation and breathing patterns in children. Pediatrics. 1993;92:686–90.

Poets CF, Urschitz MS, Bohnhorst B. Pulse oximetry in the neonatal intensive care unit (NICU): detection of hyperoxemia and false alarm rates. Anesth Analg. 2002;94:S41–3.

Richard D, Poets CF, Neale S, Stebbens VA, Alexander JR, Southall DP. Arterial oxygen saturation in preterm neonates without respiratory failure. J Pediatr. 1993;123:963–8.

Urschitz MS, Wolff J, Sokollik C, Eggebrecht E, Urschitz-Duprat PM, Schlaud M, et al. Nocturnal arterial oxygen saturation and academic performance in a community sample of children. Pediatrics. 2005;115:e204–9.

Assessment of Sleep in Newborns to Adolescents

13

Óscar Sans Capdevila and David Gozal

Contents

Introduction

Sleep is a physiological state that is reversible, cyclical, and appears in opposition to the state of wakefulness. It presents characteristic behavioral manifestations such as a relative absence of mobility and a higher response threshold for external stimuli. At the organic level, sleep produces a series of modifications of activity in the nervous system, accompanied by variations in intellectual function that constitute dreaming.

Historically, sleep has always been considered a passive state, although today it is seen as a paradoxically active one in which several neural systems intervene that are mutually regulated: the diencephalon, brain trunk, and cerebral cortex. Humans spend approximately a third of their lives sleeping. It has been shown that sleep is absolutely necessary, given that physiological functions occur during sleep that are essential for the physical and psychic balance of individuals, restoration of homeostasis of the central nervous system and of other tissue, reestablishment of cellular energy stores, and consolidation of memory.

The quantitative need for nocturnal sleep varies as a function of age, the state of health, the emotional state, and other factors. The ideal

Ó. Sans Capdevila
Department of Pediatric Neurology,
Hospital Sant Joan de Déu, Barcelona, Spain
e-mail: osans@sjdhospitalbarcelona.org

D. Gozal (✉)
Department of Pediatrics, The University of Chicago,
Chicago, IL, USA
e-mail: gozald@health.missouri.edu

P. Bertrand, I. Sánchez (eds.), *Pediatric Respiratory Diseases*,
https://doi.org/10.1007/978-3-030-26961-6_13

duration is one that allows us to undertake our daily activities with normality. It has always been considered that sleep is related to behavior. However, the specific characteristics of the electrical brain function registered by electroencephalography (EEG) confirm that there is a relationship between base brain activity and the state of sleep. Polysomnography (PSG) was also developed for this purpose and provides standardized and simultaneous reading of several biological signals during the wakeful and sleeping states, allowing for their clear differentiation. These bioelectrical signals are processed digitally.

There are two well differentiated types of sleep: rapid-eye-movement (REM) sleep and non-REM (NREM) sleep. REM sleep is associated with a high level of neuronal activity and dreaming, while NREM sleep is divided into three states according to the new terminology recommended by the American Academy of Sleep Medicine: phase 1 is the shortest phase and represents a superficial level of sleep; phase 2 represents 50% of the total time slept; and phase 3 represents the deepest and most repairing level of sleep.

REM and NREM sleep alternate cyclically (4–6 times) during nocturnal sleep. Deep sleep predominates during the initial phases of the night. The duration of the REM sleep periods increases progressively in successive cycles.

Sleep in Childhood and Adolescence

Sleep behavior varies throughout life in the functioning of intrinsic and extrinsic biological cycles, with changes related to development of the central nervous system and to educational, work-related, and social conditioning factors. These determinants vary depending on the stage of life:

- *At the intrauterine stage*: The human fetus presents wakefulness–sleep cycles (lasting less than 24 hours) at 30–32 weeks of gestation.
- *In newborns and 3-month-old infants*: Active sleep, the precursor to REM sleep, lasts the longest, representing 60% of the total time slept in the first days of life. Newborns sleep for more than 16 hours per day, distributed over several periods. The sleep is characterized by irregular breathing and an irregular heart rate, rapid eye movements, axial muscular atony, and brief muscular contractions accompanied by facial motions such as smiles and sucking.
- *Beginning at 2–3 months of age*: Sleep spindles (characteristic of phase 2) appear. Differentiation of all sleep stages is now possible. The number of hours slept begins to decrease at this age as part of changes relating to cerebral maturation, which is expressed fundamentally by a reduction in REM sleep.
- *At 12 months*: The mean duration of sleep is 12–13 hours per day, 30% of which is in the form of REM sleep.
- *At 2 years*: The child sleeps for an average 13 hours, which falls to 10–12 hours at 3–5 years and 11 hours at 5 years of age.
- *Between 6 and 10 years*: The central nervous system is almost completely mature, and the child sleeps for an average of 10 hours per day.
- *In adolescence*: The number of hours needed for sleep increases, and there is a physiological tendency for individuals to go to sleep at a later hour.
- *In young adults*: Young adults spends some 8 hours per day sleeping, most of which is NREM sleep (phase 1: approximately 5%; phase 2: approximately 50%; phase 3: approximately 20%). At this age, REM sleep does not represent more than 25% of the total time sleeping.

Functions of Sleep

Just as REM and NREM sleep differ physiologically, they also have different functions. NREM sleep has a restorative capacity, favoring energy processes and protein synthesis. It increases the release of growth hormones, decreases the stress response (cortisol synthesis), and favors cellular regeneration. REM sleep plays an important role in attention and memory processes and in consolidation of learning.

Diagnosis

Anamnesis

It is necessary to assess the following aspects:

- *Age at onset*: The presence of processes other than the usual ones for a given age should raise suspicion of a problem; examples include daytime naps beyond the age of 6 years, appearance of parasomnias in adolescence, or persistence of nocturnal enuresis beyond the age of 6 years.
- *Incorrect habits*: Aspects related to healthy sleeping habits should always be valued: the type of response of the parents; bedtime schedules; the types of leisure activities of children/adolescents; and the presence of television, computers, mobile phones, and/or video games in the sleep routines or the room of the patient.
- *Description of sleep over 24 hours*: This refers to how and how much the patient sleeps over the course of a day.
- *Family history of sleep disorders*: There are processes with a hereditary basis that should be considered, such as insomnia, restless leg syndrome (RLS), and phase delay. Sleep apnea has an evident genetic component, because of which we should investigate other cases of this pathology in the family. Likewise, it is advisable to consider unfavorable environmental or socioeconomic situations—for example, smokers in the family.
- *Transitory alterations*: These include the birth of a sibling, a new school, or a change of home.
- *Disorders associated with chronic problems*: These include problems such as asthma, rhinitis, and atopic dermatitis.
- *Effects of other biological functions*: Examples include eating habits, nighttime or daytime behavior, the type of respiration during sleep, the appearance of snoring, the presence of apnea, and leisure habits.
- *Typical sleep-specific sleep disorders*: These include sleep apnea–hypopnea and RLS.

Table 13.1 Indications to perform a polysomnography test

Indications
Excessive daytime sleepiness unrelated to chronic sleep deprivation; for diagnosis of hypersomnia, a multiple sleep latency test (MSLT) may be necessary
Alteration of the respiratory pattern during sleep; suspicion of sleep apnea
Violent motor activity or abnormal behaviors related to sleep; differential diagnosis between parasomnias and nocturnal frontal lobe seizures
Periodic limb movement disorder (PLMD) during sleep

Source: American Academy of Sleep Medicine

- *Use of pharmaceuticals and other drugs that can affect sleep*: These include antihistamines, antidepressants, antismoking drugs, or drugs used in adolescents.
- *The presence of other concomitant pathologies*: These include organic disorders (gastroesophageal reflux, asthma, obesity, atopic dermatitis, blindness, etc.), neurological disorders (headaches, epilepsy, attention deficit disorder, hyperactivity, etc.), psychiatric disorders (depression and anxiety), and social disorders (family problems, mistreatment, abuse, and certain types of parent–child relationship or partner relationship).

In summary, what happens during the night and during the day should be assessed (see the indications suggested in Table 13.1).

Complete Physical Exploration

Mouth breathing does not correlate with the presence of catarrh or adenoid–amygdala hypertrophy, nor does it coincide with aspects of craniofacial anatomy, the upper respiratory tract, retrognathism, the Mallampati score, and midfacial hypoplasia (Fig. 13.1).

The degree of adenoid–amygdala hypertrophy does not correlate linearly with the presence of sleep apnea–hypopnea; small adenoids and a small amygdala do not exclude the condition if other symptoms are present.

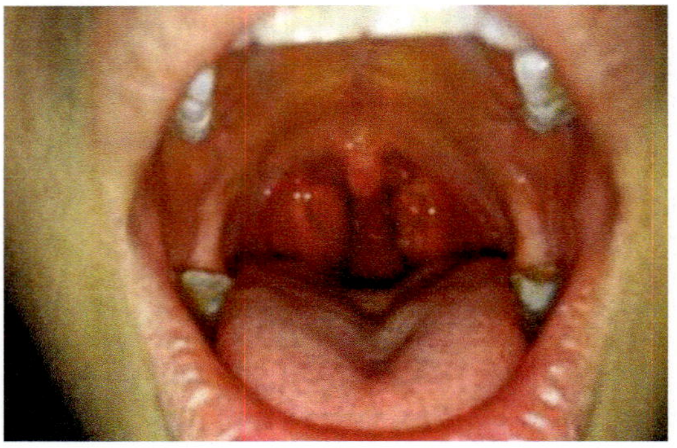

Fig. 13.1 Tonsillar hypertrophy in a 15-year-old patient with obstructive sleep apnea (OSA)

Useful Tools

Some useful tools are available for general assessment of children and adolescents, and these are discussed below.

Sleep Duration Percentiles

Every child has his or her own sleep requirements, and there are no absolute data in this respect. Iglowstein et al. (2003) studied 500 children and adolescents to establish reference values and to establish how naps are distributed according to age. The percentiles help to determine the evolution of sleep, inform doctors if changes have occurred, and allow them to compare a child's habits with those of other children.

Sleep Diary

Knowledge about the number of hours a child spends sleeping and awake over the 24 hours of a day is fundamental and can be obtained and organized with the use of a sleep diary. The health professional can suggest to the patient's parents that they keep a register of when the child goes to bed, the time the child remains awake in bed before going to sleep, the frequency with which the child wakes up at night, the amount of time the child remains awake during the night, what time the child wakes up in the morning, and how the child feels in the morning (quality of sleep). A diary with these characteristics can also be used to assess the appropriateness of daily routines as they relate to sleeping habits. It requires some practice time, because of which it is recommended to have a practice time of about 15 days. Figure 13.2 is an example of a real diary.

This time period provides a baseline that is more reliable and representative of the characteristics of sleep. Likewise, it makes it possible to monitor the progress of the child, facilitating self-assessment of the problem, and at the same time it is reassuring for the parents, who can observe improvements.

A sleep schedule is composed of a table with vertical subdivisions for every day of the month and horizontal subdivisions for every hour of every day. It should indicate times for going to bed and rising, highlighting the hours spent sleeping. In this way, it provides a global view of the subject's sleep: total hours slept, latency, nocturnal awakenings, and bedtime and awakening routines. Using the diary, parents can provide relevant information about the child's sleep and his or her social context.

Actigraphy

An actigraph assesses rest and active phases according to measurement of motor activity, which can be determined in an ambulatory subject with an actigraph/actimeter. The sleep diary and the actigraph provide similar information, but studies have pointed to interesting differences in terms of information on the quality and continuity of sleep. The most notable difference is that the sleep diary fails to register all nocturnal awakenings, given that the parents are often not aware of many aspects of their child's sleep or are confused about times when reporting them.

Actigraph/Actimeter

An actimeter is the size of a watch and detects bodily movements during activities. It provides information about the chronology and duration of sleep phases and events related to them. Periods of inactivity are interpreted as periods of sleep. It constitutes a very useful tool for diagnosing delayed sleep phase syndrome (which is more common in adolescents and young adults). The transition time from wakefulness to sleep in this disorder is generally delayed by more than

	Morning	Afternoon	Evening
Wednesday 10.09.13	10.40-12.20		20.30-23.20 (100ml of milk) / 23:25-3.45 (diaper change) /5.10-7.45 (fell asleep after milk)
Thursday 10.10.13	11.00-14.00	Did not sleep	20.30-23.15 (100ml of milk) / 23.15-1.30 (diaper change) /1.40-7.00 (milk on the recommendation of the kinesiologist)
Friday 10.11.13	Did not sleep	13.30-16.00	21.00-23-15 (milk) / 23.15-00.30 / 00.35-02.00 / 02.05-7.30
Saturday 10.12.13	Did not sleep	12.30-14.00	20.00-22.00 (milk) / 22.00-3.00 / 3.00-4.00 / 4.00-5.00 / 5.00 (milk)-8.00
Sunday 10.13.13	Did not sleep	12.50-14.40	20.10-22.20 (milk) / 22.20-5.30 (woke up but went back to sleep right after) / 5.30-7.40
Monday 10.14.13	Did not sleep	12.55-16.10	20.30-22.20 (leche) / 22.20-1.30 / 1.35-4.00 / 4.45-6.50 (fell asleep only after milk)
Tuesday 10.15.13	Did not sleep	12.00-13.20	20.30-23.00 (milk) / 22.00-1.00 / 2.45-6.50 (restless between 1.30 and 2.45)
Wednesday 10.16.13	9.45-11.50	Did not sleep	20.10-22.35 (milk) / 22.45-1.00 / restless between 1.00 and 3.00 / milk 6.30 / 6.30-7.45
Thursday 10.17.13	10.40-12.50	16.10-17.00	20.30-
Friday 10.18.13			Very bad night (coughing)
Saturday 10.19.13			Bad night
Sunday 10.20.13	11.50-13.15	17.30-18.00	20.30-1.00 (milk) / 1.00-6.00 (milk) 6.00-7.30
Monday 10.21.13	10.40-12.40	Did not sleep	20.00-00.00 (cried, did not drink milk) / 00.00-3.30 (did drink milk) / 3.30-7.30
Tuesday 10.22.13	11.00-12.00	17.30-18.15	20.30-2.00 / 3.00 / 7.30
Wednesday 10.13.13			
Thursday 10.24.13	11.00-12.30	Did not sleep	20.00-00.00 / 00.00-2.45 / 5.15-8.00

Fig. 13.2 Sleep diary of a patient who snores

2 hours in relation to the conventional time needed to fall asleep. Patients have difficulty going to sleep at the start, but once they are asleep, the structure and quality of sleep are completely normal. They also have difficulty waking up in the morning, because the number of hours of sleep is reduced as a result of the delay in beginning sleep.

Domestic Video

This can be a useful tool in diagnosing sleep disorders. It is focused fundamentally on assessing respiratory disorders during sleep (the Sivan video score), parasomnia with rhythmic movements, and periodic movements of the extremities.

With the Sivan video score, the parents are asked to record their child sleeping for 30 minutes. Specifically, the parents should be asked to ensure that the child sleeps with his or her chest and abdomen uncovered. The parents should record any sounds the child makes and not interfere with any position the child assumes while sleeping (hyperextension of the neck is common among these patients to improve the caliber of the upper airway). It is advisable that a recording be obtained during the last hours of the night (between 5:00 a.m. and 5:30 a.m.)—given that obstructive respiratory events are more common during REM sleep—or, failing that, when parents observe that the child's respiratory sounds are more intense. The Sivan score assesses seven parameters. Scores equal to or below 5 indicate normality, scores between 6 and 10 are doubtful for a probable diagnosis of sleep apnea–hypopnea syndrome (SAHS); and scores over 10 are highly suggestive of such a diagnosis (77–89%, respectively).

Sleep Scales/Questionnaires

Studies generally suggest there is not sufficient screening for sleep problems among pediatric populations, which is confirmed by the significant underdiagnosis of sleep disorders.

According to some surveys, more than 20% of pediatricians who are consulted do not screen schoolchildren for sleep problems during routine visits, and up to 40% of them do not ask adolescents directly about their sleeping habits. Taking this into account, the American Association of Sleep Medicine (AASM) recommends regular screening of all children in clinical practice to detect sleep-related problems.

In primary care, structured questionnaires can facilitate screening for sleep disorders among children and adolescents. They are a basic tool to assess healthy children and to diagnose children with behavioral disorders. They can be applied from the neonatal period onward.

There are broader and specific questionnaires that require more time to complete and serve to focus on specific problems such as parasomnias, respiratory disorders during sleep, etc. There are also questionnaires that are simpler and easier to complete for screening for pediatric sleep disorders. Some of these that can be useful in primary health care are described below (for a more complete and in-depth review of sleep questionnaires and methodologies, see Spruyt and Gozal).

- *Brief Infant Sleep Questionnaire* (BISQ): This screening tool is aimed at identifying risk factors for sudden infant death, sleep routines, and sleep problems in infants under 1 year of age, detected by the parents. The questionnaire can be completed in 5–10 minutes. It has been developed on the basis of a series of significant variables through a review of specialized literature: the duration of nocturnal sleep, the duration of daytime sleep, the number of nighttime awakenings, the duration of nocturnal awakenings, the time to go to sleep, the duration of sleep latency, the method used for staying asleep, where the child sleeps, the preferred body position, the age and sex of the child, the child's numeric order among his or her siblings, and the person who completed the questionnaire. A significant correlation has been shown with objective data obtained using an actigraph in children 5–29 months of age in terms of awakenings and the duration of nocturnal sleep. However, this questionnaire has not been validated in a Spanish-speaking context.
- *BEARS Questionnaire* [B = bedtime issues, E = excessive daytime sleepiness, A = night awakenings, R = regularity and duration of sleep, S = snoring]: This questionnaire is aimed at children from 2 to 18 years of age, with questions directed at the children and the parents. It establishes three age groups: 2–5 years old, 6–12 years old, and 13–18 years old. It assesses five aspects of sleep: problems at bedtime, excessive daytime sleepiness, nocturnal awakenings, sleep regularity and duration, and snoring. If there are positive answers to any of the questions, the matter should be

investigated further. However, this questionnaire has not been validated in a Spanish-speaking context.

Once the screening questionnaires described above have been applied, more specific questionnaires can be employed in the search for disorders:

- *Bruni Sleep Disturbance Scale for Children* (SSSC): This scale has 27 items and is designed to detect sleep disorders, including respiratory disorders. It assesses events in the prior 6 months. While its internal consistency is greater in controls (0.79), it maintains a satisfactory level of consistency in children with sleep disorders (0.71). The reliability of the test/retest is satisfactory for the total ($r = 0.71$) and for scoring every individual item. However, this scale has not been validated in a Spanish-speaking context.
- *Chervin Pediatric Sleep Questionnaire* (PSQ): This questionnaire is directed at children from 2 to 18 years of age, and there are two versions of the questionnaire. The reduced version has 22 items, and the original version has been validated. It addresses sleep-related respiratory disorders. Its validity, reliability, and sensitivity are all over 80%. It compares the symptoms of attention deficit and hyperactivity, and correlates them with the polysomnography readings. More than eight positive responses suggest respiratory problems during sleep. The polysomnographic study is necessary to establish the definitive diagnosis of respiratory disorders during sleep. A determination based only on the questionnaire is neither sensitive nor specific. The complete version of the PSQ also explores a wide range of other sleep disorders such as parasomnias and excessive daytime somnolence. This questionnaire has been validated in a Spanish-speaking context, and there is a Chilean version of it.
- *Frontal Lobe Epilepsy And Parasomnias Scale* (FLEP): This scale was developed to differentiate between frontal lobe epilepsy and parasomnias through a series of questions related to the clinical characteristics of the two conditions. It was designed by an expert panel after a literature review. FLEP has sensitivity of 100%, specificity of 90%, a positive predictive value of 91%, and a negative predictive value of 100% in diagnosing frontal lobe epilepsy. Although it is basically used with adults, the questionnaire can also be useful in children and adolescents.
- *Screening Questionnaire for Snoring and SAHS*: This is a very brief and simple questionnaire that serves to identify children at risk and consequently reduces the need for more complicated and onerous tests.

Complementary Tests

Extensive complimentary examinations are usually unnecessary in the study of children with sleep disturbances. However, in some situations, on the basis of the medical history, laboratory studies (such as blood counts and biochemical screening), image studies, psychological studies, and/or laboratory sleep studies (polysomnography, respiratory polygraph, actigraphy, or others), the patient may be referred to a pediatric sleep unit or a sleep center.

Analysis

A basic biochemical examination, which includes cholesterol and high-sensitivity C-reactive protein, is performed.

Respiratory Polygraph

Portable or respiratory polygraph systems (American Sleep Disorders Association (ASDA) levels III and IV) are available for initial use at home. Typically, they include measurement of cardiorespiratory variables but not neurophysiological variables. Polygraphs can register oronasal flow (which is generally measured with a thermocouple/thermistor and/or a nasal cannula), thoracic and/or abdominal respiratory effort, oxygen saturation by pulse oximetry, the body position, snoring, and the heart rate. Another variable that is often incorporated is a tibial electromyogram (two electrodes in the anterior tibial muscle) to evaluate periodic leg movements (PLMs). This technique is not monitored directly and does not allow for intervention while it is being carried out. Like polysomnography, the tibial electromyogram is carried out while the subject is asleep at night. The criteria for analysis of the records should be the same for all polygraphs in terms of the variables they record, in accordance with the AASM criteria.

The respiratory polygraph (PR) presents some limitations that should be noted:

1. It does not detect electroencephalographic arousals, because of which it cannot diagnose upper airway resistance syndrome. In this context, some studies have related arousals to other variables such as a decreased pulse transit time, flattening of the inspiratory flow loop, or reduced amplitude of the bands following hyperventilation.
2. Instead of registering neurophysiological variables to measure the time spent sleeping, it uses the time spent in bed as a denominator of indices such as apnea, hypopnea, and desaturation, which can yield false negatives because more time is spent in bed than is spent sleeping.

There have been few studies of application of a respiratory polygraph in children, and those that exist have been done in populations with high probabilities of sleep apnea–hypopnea, involving small numbers of patients. Moreover, those studies did not involve comparison with polysomnography, and the results were inconsistent.

A recently published study involved 53 children with clinical suspicion of sleep apnea–hypopnea, in which both polysomnography and a respiratory polygraph were applied in the sleep laboratory. Obstructive apnea–hypopnea index (IAH) values of ≥1, ≥3, and ≥5 were considered for the diagnosis, with the receiver operating characteristic (ROC) curve being calculated for each of these and being 4.6 the best respiratory events index for obstructive AHI, with an area under the curve (AUC) of diagnostic efficiency greater than 85% and specificity of up to 91.7%. Consequently, a respiratory polygraph is a valid alternative to diagnose apnea–hypopnea in children, and it is an appropriate screening technique for use in children.

Nocturnal Polysomnography

Nocturnal polysomnography (PSG) is the reference test for diagnosing SAHS or motor or behavioral sleep disorders (for example, the Modified Pediatric Epworth Scale (MPES) score or rhythmic movements during sleep), allowing for registration of physiological variables during sleep, among which are:

- *Neurophysiological variables*: An electroencephalogram, electro-oculogram, and tibial and submental electromyograms to assess sleep states and architecture.
- *Cardiorespiratory variables* with registration of:
  - Oronasal flow to assess respiratory events: apnea, hypopnea, and flow limitations, using thermosensors (a thermocouple/thermistor) and/or a nasal cannula.
  - Respiratory effort: to classify respiratory events as central, obstructive, or mixed, using piezoelectric thoracic and abdominal bands or impedance plethysmography.
  - Gas exchange: oxygen saturation by pulsometry (blood oxygen saturation ($SatO_2$)) and measurement of expired or transcutaneous CO_2.
- *Heartbeat.*
- *Snoring.*
- *Bodily positions*: Analysis of the occurrence of respiratory events in relation to bodily positions.
- *Electromyography of the anterior tibial muscles*: This allows for determination of the presence of myoclonic movement of the legs during wakefulness and/or sleep associated with respiratory events. From a logistical perspective, it is not reasonable to employ nocturnal polysomnography in the context of minimal suspicion of apnea–hypopnea syndrome or other sleep disorders. Consequently, there is growing interest in improving screening techniques or tests for this pediatric syndrome, as well as development of simpler tools that yield reliable diagnostic results, reserving more complex and/or costly tech-

niques (polysomnography, respiratory polygraphs) for cases in which simple tests do not provide certain diagnoses or in which the results of a complex technique can condition therapy (for example, noninvasive ventilation in the context of surgical treatment).

Multiple Latency Sleep Test

The multiple latency sleep test (MLST) is a standardized diagnostic method used to objectively measure daytime drowsiness. After nocturnal polysomnography, the patient has the opportunity to nap during the day (up to five naps between 20–30 minutes long). The naps occur at 2-hour intervals. Sleep latency in these naps is assessed with polysomnography, and it is determined whether the child begins sleep with REM or NREM sleep (two or more initiations of a nap with REM sleep is highly suggestive of narcolepsy).

Conclusion

Approximately 30% of children and adolescents experience some type of sleep disorder, from an isolated difficulty in falling asleep or in remaining asleep to more serious problems such as sleep apnea–hypopnea syndrome.

Sleep disorders present clear clinical manifestations during the night that are easily identifiable: snoring, noisy and difficult breathing, respiratory pauses, mouth breathing, abnormal postures, profuse perspiration, or enuresis. However, given their importance for the quality of life of patients and their families, daytime symptoms such as motor restlessness, somnolence, poor school performance, altered behavior, aggressiveness, and predisposition to accidents should also be considered. Structured questionnaires that facilitate initial screening can be useful for diagnosis, as can complementary tests such as nocturnal polysomnography.

The main cause of sleep disorders at preschool and school ages lies in inappropriate habits—in particular, related to television. Using television as a way to fall asleep and prolonged viewing (for more than 2 hours per day) have been shown to reduce the effective sleeping time, increase nocturnal awakenings, and produce problems at bedtime. Moreover, this type of habit continues into adolescence and adulthood, with consequences for the patient's social and working life. The easy access that children now have to electronic games and the internet should also be considered.

With the beginning of puberty, there is a concurrent physiological shift to a later time to initiate sleep, which does not imply a reduction in the number of hours needed for nocturnal sleep during adolescence. Schools demand specific wake-up times that can result in lack of sleep and affect learning. Healthy sleep habits at this stage of life include avoidance of television, video games, cell phones, and stimulating drinks such as coffee, cola, and alcohol at determined hours of the day. The sleeping schedule for working days should be maintained during the weekend, as should regular physical activities. Exposure to natural morning light favors correct sleep physiology at night. It is also necessary to control other concomitant pathologies that can affect sleep, such as asthma and obesity.

The professionals involved in primary attention play a fundamental role in early detection, diagnosis, treatment, and follow-up of this type of patient, as well as in helping families. Good sleeping habits should be fostered and, when necessary, patients should be referred to sleep specialists. Good communication with experts can provide access to more complex complementary tests such as polysomnography and specific treatment for the disorder.

In conclusion, sleep is a physiological necessity, and an impoverishment in its quality or quantity can have significant repercussions for physical, cognitive, and psychosocial well-being, both for the present and for the future of a child. Likewise, a sleep disorder generates stress and problems in the family environment. Many of these problems can be easily resolved in the first weeks of life with behavioral measures, whereas they could persist for years if not adequately addressed.

Sources

American Academy of Sleep Medicine. International Classification of Sleep Disorders. 3rd ed. Darien, IL: American Academy of Sleep Medicine; 2014.

Arens R, Sin S, McDonough JM, Palmer JM, Dominguez T, Meyer H, et al. Changes in upper airway size during tidal breathing in children with obstructive sleep apnea syndrome. Am J Respir Crit Care Med. 2005;171:1298–304.

Brietzke SE, Katz ES, Roberson DW. Can history and physical examination reliably diagnose pediatric obstructive sleep apnea/hypopnea syndrome? A systematic review of the literature. Otolaryngol Head Neck Surg. 2004;131(6):827–32.

Esteller More E, Pons Calabuig N, Romero Vilarino E, Puigdollers Perez A, Segarra Isern F, Matino Soler E, et al. Alteraciones del desarrollo dentofacial en los trastornos respiratorios del sueño infantil. Acta Otorrinolaringol Esp. 2011;62:132–9.

Friberg D, Sundquist J, Li X, Hemminki K, Sundquist K. Sibling risk of pediatric obstructive sleep apnea syndrome and adenotonsillar hypertrophy. Sleep. 2009;32:1077–83.

Grupo de Trabajo de la Guía de Práctica Clínica Sobre Trastornos del Sueño en la Infancia y Adolescencia en Atención Primaria. Guía de práctica clínica sobre trastornos del sueño en la infancia y adolescencia en atención primaria. Plan de calidad para el Sistema Nacional de Salud del Ministerio de Sanidad, Política Social e Igualdad. Guías de Práctica Clínica en el SNS: UETS no. 2009/8. Madrid: Unidad de Evaluación de Tecnologías Sanitarias de la Agencia Lain Entralgo, 2011.

Hoppenbrouwers T, Hodgman J, Arakawa K, et al. Sleep and waking states in infancy: normative studies. Sleep. 1988;11:387–401.

Howard BJ, Wong J. Sleep disorders. Pediatr Rev. 2001;22:327–42.

Iber C, Ancoli-Israel S, Chesson A, et al. The AASM manual for the scoring of sleep and associated events: rules, terminology and technical specifications. Darien: American Academy of Sleep Medicine; 2007.

Iglowstein I, Jenni OG, Molinari L, et al. Sleep duration from infancy to adolescence: reference values and generational trends. Pediatrics. 2003;111:302–7.

Iwasaki M, Iemura A, Oyama T, et al. A novel subjective sleep assessment tool for healthy elementary school children in Japan. J Epidemiol. 2010;20 Suppl 2:S476–81.

Mindell JA, Owens JA. Symptom-based algorithms. A clinical guide to pediatric sleep: diagnosis and management of sleep problems. Filadelfia, PA: Lippincott Williams & Wilkins; 2003.

Myatt HM, Beckenham EJ. The use of diagnostic sleep nasendoscopy in the management of children with complex upper airway obstruction. Clin Otolaryngol. 2000;25:200–8.

Pijpers M, Poels PJ, Vaandrager JM, De H, Van D, Hoeve HJ, et al. Undiagnosed obstructive sleep apnea syndrome in children with syndromal craniofacial synostosis. J Craniofac Surg. 2004;15:670–4.

Pin Arboledas G, Cubel Alarcon M, Morell Salort M. Del laboratorio del sueño a la práctica clínica: esquemas diagnosticos en medicina del sueño pediátrica. Vigilia Sueño. 2005;17(1):24–8.

Rechtschaffen A, Kales A. A manual of standardized terminology, techniques and scoring system for sleep stages of human subjects. Los Angeles: UCLA Brain Information Service/Brain Research Institute; 1968.

Spruyt K, Gozal D Screening of pediatric sleep-disordered breathing: a proposed unbiased discriminative set of questions using clinical severity scales. Chest. 2012;142(6):1508–15. https://doi:10.1378/chest.11-3164.

Touchette E, Petit D, Seguin JR, et al. Associations between sleep duration patterns and behavioral/cognitive functioning at school entry. Sleep. 2007;30:1213–9.

Velluti RA, Pedemonte M. Fisiologia de la vigilia y el sueño. In: Treguerres JAF, editor. Fisiologia humana. Madrid: McGraw-Hill/Interamericana; 2004.

Wolfson AR, Carskadon MA. Sleep schedules and daytime functioning in adolescents. Child Dev. 1998;69:875–87.

Study of Infectious Agents in Respiratory Diseases

14

Cecilia Perret Pérez

Contents

Virological Diagnosis

A few years ago, it was possible to diagnose a viral infection only on the basis of clinical and epidemiological information about the patient, without going beyond that. Among the large group of viral infections, there are many types of viruses with distinct behavior, and they produce distinct clinical scenarios, affect different age groups in different ways, and require different types of treatment. The capacity to establish a correlation between the different types of viral agents and their clinical manifestations has been possible only through techniques that allow identification of a particular virus.

There have been major advances in the last decade in this respect, and new techniques have emerged that have greater sensitivity to detect a viral causal agent within a wider viral spectrum that we can identify.

Today, the epidemiology of viral respiratory infections is changing with the identification of new agents that help us to better understand this large group of "viral infections."

Viral Cultures

The oldest method used to diagnose respiratory viruses is the viral culture—a cumbersome

C. Perret Pérez (✉)
Department of Pediatrics, School of Medicine, Pontificia Universidad Católica de Chile, Santiago, Chile
e-mail: cperret@med.puc.cl

P. Bertrand, I. Sánchez (eds.), *Pediatric Respiratory Diseases*,
https://doi.org/10.1007/978-3-030-26961-6_14

method that requires laboratories with special characteristics and highly trained staff. Added to this is the cost of identification of each virus, which greatly limits the possibility of more universal diagnosis. The method is used almost exclusively for research.

Accelerated Cultures

An improvement on viral culture is the accelerated culture or viral shell technique appeared, which involves forcing the entry of a sample of a respiratory virus into culture cell lines. However, instead of having to wait for the appearance of cytopathic effects, the presence of the virus can be confirmed by marking of viral replication proteins with fluorescence, which can be seen with immunofluorescence microscopy. This technique allows study of the most common respiratory viruses such as respiratory syncytial virus (RSV), influenza A and B, adenovirus, and parainfluenza 1–3. The method still requires cultures in cell lines and therefore has the same disadvantages as viral culture. Moreover, this method cannot provide results in less than 48 hours.

Immunofluorescence

The technique of using antibodies marked with fluorescence, directed against different antigens of respiratory viruses, is known as direct or indirect immunofluorescence (DIF or IIF) and does not require culturing. It has vastly broadened the possibility of diagnosing viral agents in patients with symptoms that suggest a viral infection (Fig. 14.1). This technique provides a response in less than 24 hours and can simultaneously identify several respiratory viruses. The identification of several respiratory viruses is called a viral panel, which is available in commercial kits that include adenovirus, influenza A and B, parainfluenza 1–3, RSV, and metapneumovirus. The method has good sensitivity and specificity. The sensitivity varies between age groups (being best in subjects under 5 years of age) and between different viruses. The lowest sensitivity is related to adenovirus and is independent of the age of the patient. The sensitivity is higher for the influenza and RSV viruses. In the best scenario, only around 30% of patients who consult a physician because of respiratory symptoms remain without an etiological diagnosis after the application of this method.

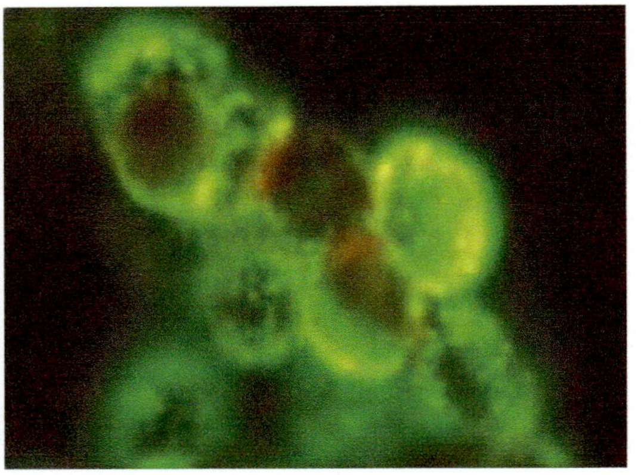

Fig. 14.1 Use of direct immunofluorescence to show a positive result for influenza A virus, observed using immunofluorescence microscopy on a nasopharyngeal swab at 400× magnification

Immunochromatography

Rapid immunochromatographic tests, which can identify the presence of viral antigens directly from patients' samples, also represent an important tool for diagnosing respiratory viruses. They have the advantage of providing results within 2 hours, but their sensitivity to detect viruses is still lower than that of immunofluorescence, and their performance depends on the age of the patient and on the type of respiratory virus. Another disadvantage is that they cover a smaller spectrum of viruses—basically just influenza A and B, RSV, and adenovirus. An immunochromatographic test is a blind test in which the quality of the sample cannot be assessed, because of which it is not possible to determine whether a negative result is valid or due to a scarcity of mucosal epithelial cells in the sample. Another problem with this technique is that it can detect only the specified virus rather than a wide spectrum of respiratory viruses. The ability to identify a spectrum of viruses is particularly important for use in children under 5 years of age, in whom the correlation between the clinical syndrome and the virological diagnosis is inadequate, especially with regard to flu symptoms and the influenza virus status.

Molecular Biology

In recent years, there have been significant advances in the development of molecular biological techniques in the field of virological diagnosis—in particular, the use of polymerase chain reaction (PCR) (Fig. 14.2). This technique amplifies the nucleic acids in respiratory viruses in a sample from a patient with a respiratory infection. Molecular panels have been developed that are comparable to immunofluorescence panels and can identify several respiratory viruses in a single sample. Their advantage over immunofluorescence is that a wider spectrum of respiratory viruses can be identified, including new viruses such as enterovirus, rhinovirus, coronavirus, and bocavirus. This technique is also more sensitive than the others. Distinct sensitivity levels have been described for different respiratory viruses, and the sensitivity for RSV, influenza virus, and metapneumovirus in the pediatric population is over 95%. The sensitivity is somewhat lower for parainfluenza and influenza B, at 90%, while for adenovirus it does not exceed 85% and in the majority of studies is between 75% and 80%. These sensitivity rates are notably better than those achieved by immunofluorescence for viruses such as influenza B and adenovirus.

A study at the Infectology and Molecular Virology Laboratory of the Pontificia Universidad Católica compared the performance of a DIF respiratory virus panel with that of a PCR molecular panel. The viral diagnostic yield of DIF was 35.1%, based on 6743 samples, versus 46.9% for PCR, based on 1792 samples (Table 14.1). As it can be seen in the table, the molecular technique has better performance than DIF, and this is consistent with the results of other laboratory studies. The PCR technique also has higher sensitivity (88%) with 98% specificity, while the sensitivity and specificity of the DIF technique are both around 70%. Another important aspect that can

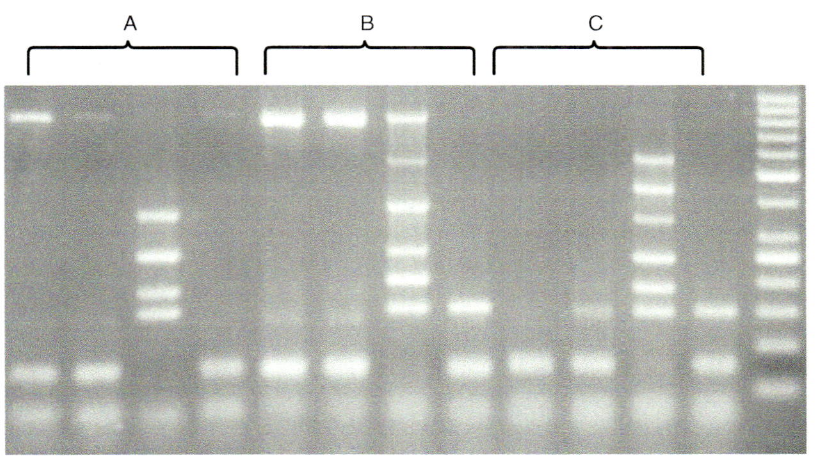

Fig. 14.2 Respiratory virus molecular panel

Table 14.1 Diagnostic performance of direct immunofluorescence (DIF) and polymerase chain reaction (PCR)

	Patients, *n* (%)			
		Age groups		
Technique	Total population	<5 years	5–15 years	>15 years
DIF, *n* = 6743 samples	2368 (35.1)	1874 (46.9)	273 (35.5)	264 (13.3)
PCR, *n* = 1792 samples	841 (46.9)	508 (61.3)	78 (47.8)	255 (31.9)

be appreciated in the table is the performance and sensitivity of the methods in different age groups. The sensitivity of both techniques clearly decreases in persons over 15 years of age and becomes progressively lower with age. This could be due to factors such as later medical consultation and less viral excretion in adults, with consequently lower viral loads in their samples.

Given the wider spectrum of studied viruses, PCR allows identification of respiratory viruses that traditionally have not been diagnosed, such as rhinovirus, coronavirus, bocavirus, and enterovirus. While these viruses are known as causal agents of respiratory infections, it was long thought that their pathogenic role was limited to infections of the upper respiratory tract and other trivial infections. However, the known spectrum of clinical manifestations that these viruses produce has broadened with the appearance of techniques capable of diagnosing them, and it is now possible to understand their frequency, their seasonality, and their pathogenic role in mild or severe infections.

Several clinical studies have shown that rhinovirus is prevalent in all age groups, and it has been identified with greater frequency in some series. The sensitivity and specificity of PCR to identify rhinovirus are 100% and 98%, respectively. This virus has been described as the most prevalent one in pediatric populations and as the second most frequent cause of hospitalization of children under 2 years of age with wheezing.

Another important comparative advantage of PCR over DIF is the possibility of diagnosing viral coinfections in the same patient with greater sensitivity. DIF offers approximately a 2% possibility of diagnosing coinfections, while the possibility can reach 20% with PCR. Coinfections are more common among children under 5 years of age, and bocavirus commonly appears as a copathogen.

Two problems with the molecular technique are its cost and the need for a specialized laboratory. However, given its aforementioned characteristics, PCR should be the technique of choice for use in hospitalized patients, adults, and patients with immunodeficiency. Achievement of a rapid and certain diagnosis with good sensitivity is fundamental in these patients to determine the most appropriate therapeutic strategies, particularly for viruses that require specific therapy, such as influenza.

Bacterial Diagnosis

Traditional Bacteria

Diagnosis of bacterial infections of the respiratory system has also made advances in recent years with the incorporation of techniques to reach rapid and precise diagnoses. Until some years ago, microbiological diagnosis was based mainly on phenotypical characteristics and application of a battery of biochemical tests. Automated methods for applying biochemical tests were then developed, which provided more precision in the identification of bacteria. Now a new method has been introduced that has been used for many years in research laboratories—namely, proteomic or mass spectrometry, in which bacterial protein profiles are identified by their distinct characteristics, on the basis of which the genus and species can be determined rapidly.

This microbiological technique has been developed for a system called MALDI-TOF (matrix-assisted laser desorption/ionization time-of-flight) mass spectrometry, which basically consists of four stages: recovery of a colony under study previously isolated from the culture, running of the mass spectrometry, comparison with databases, and presentation of the results. Once the sample has been prepared, identification takes less than 2 minutes. The results have been very promising for the identification of Gram-negative bacilli such as enterobacteria and nonfermenting Gram-negative bacilli. The incorporation of new protein profiles into the databases has led to more than 94% correct identification of *Stenotrophomonas* and HACEK group bacteria. This technique is also highly sensitive for traditional Gram-positive coccaceae such as *Staphylococcus, Enterococcus,* and *Streptococcus*. The protein profile of *Streptococcus pneumoniae* is very similar to that of streptococci of the viridian group, because of which this method is really only useful for identifying *Streptococcus* species. The percentage of diagnosis of Gram-positive bacilli is only about 85%.

Atypical Bacteria

Diagnosis of atypical bacteria (which are termed "atypical" because of the difficulty in cultivating them in commonly used media) such as *Legionella pneumophila*, *Chlamydia pneumoniae*, and *Mycoplasma pneumoniae* is based on determination of immunoglobulin M antibodies for *Mycoplasma* and *Chlamydia*, and determination of urinary antigens in the case of *Legionella* species. The PCR method is also used to search for these agents and forms part of the expanded panel of many laboratories.

Mycobacteria

Mycobacteria can be identified by different diagnostic methods. Firstly, there is staining applied directly to a respiratory sample, using Ziehl–Neelsen stain, which gives bacilli an intense pink color. Mycobacteria can grow in solid or liquid culture media, and the characteristics of the colonies and the growth velocity indicate whether or not they are tubercular complex bacteria. The culture methods used to identify *Mycobacterium tuberculosis* can take up to 60 days. Molecular methods such as PCR have been of great help for identifying nontubercular mycobacterial species, allowing rapid diagnosis of tubercular complex bacteria with a high degree of sensitivity. The application of mass spectrometry (MALDI-TOF) results in a high percentage of identification, although an additional preparatory step for mycobacteria is to create the necessary conditions for the cellular wall. There is a 97% identification rate when the mycobacteria are grown in a solid medium and a 77% rate when they are grown in a liquid medium.

Diagnosis of Fungi

Yeasts and filamentous fungi should be etiologically suspected in gravely ill patients and patients with immunosuppression. Like bacteria, fungi can be identified by staining samples of respiratory secretions. Gram stain is used for yeasts but not for filamentous fungi. Because of thus, in the case of a suspected fungal infection, the most useful option is calcofluor-white stain, which bonds with the chitin of the fungal walls and can be observed by use of immunofluorescence microscopy (Fig. 14.3). Fungal species grow in special culture media and can be identified by the characteristics of the colony and the types of hypha and conidia. There is no universal PCR that allows diagnosis of all types of fungi with a short diagnostic time and a high level of sensitivity. There are indirect methods, such as identification of antigens in the cell walls of *Aspergillus* (galactomannan) in blood or respiratory samples, or polysaccharides from yeasts and fungi (β-D glucan) in blood. These methods are not widely available, and they have not been well standardized for application in children, as in the case of β-D glucan.

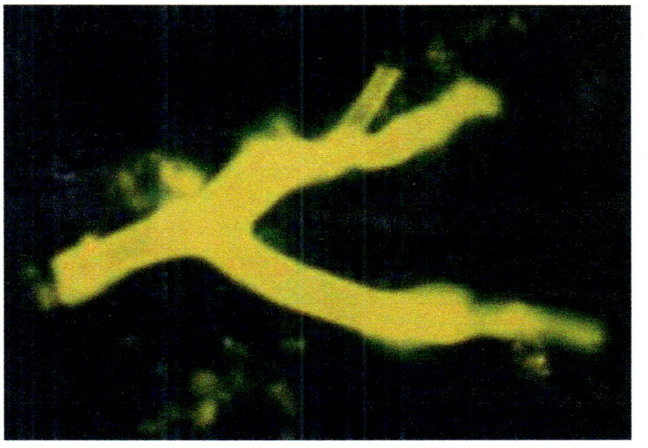

Fig. 14.3 Use of calcofluor-white stain to show fluorescence captured by the wall of *Rhizopus* sp. coenocytic hyphae at 400× magnification

Sources

Bellau-Pujol S, Vabret A, Legrand L, Dina J, Gouarin S, Petitjean-Lecherbonnier J, et al. Development of three multiplex RT-PCR assays for the detection of 12 respiratory RNA viruses. J Virol Methods. 2005;126(1–2):53–63.

Bonzel L, Tenenbaum T, Schroten H, Schildgen O, Schweitzer-Krantz S, Adams O. Frequent detection of viral coinfection in children hospitalized with acute respiratory tract infection using a real-time polymerase chain reaction. Pediatr Infect Dis J. 2008;27(7):589–94.

García P, Allende F, Legarraga P, Huilcaman M, Solari S. Identificación bacteriana basada en el espectro de masas de proteínas: una nueva mirada a la microbiología del siglo XXI. Rev Chil Infectol. 2012;29(3):263–72.

Gharabaghi F, Hawan A, Drews SJ, Richardson SE. Evaluation of multiple commercial molecular and conventional diagnostic assays for the detection of respiratory viruses in children. Clin Microbiol Infect. 2011;17(12):1900–6.

Legarraga P, Moraga M, Lam M, Geoffroy E, Zumarán C, García P. Impacto de la espectrometría de masas por MALDI-TOF MS en la identificación rápida de bacterias aeróbicas y anaeróbicas de importancia clínica. Rev Chil Infectol. 2013;30(2):140–6.

Mahony J, Chong S, Merante F, Yaghoubian S, Sinha T, Lisle C, et al. Development of a respiratory virus panel test for detection of twenty human respiratory viruses by use of multiplex PCR and a fluid microbead-based assay. J Clin Microbiol. 2007;45(9):2965–70.

Mahony JB, Blackhouse G, Babwah J, Smieja M, Buracond S, Chong S, et al. Cost analysis of multiplex PCR testing for diagnosing respiratory virus infections. J Clin Microbiol. 2009;47(9):2812–7.

Olofsson S, Brittain-Long R, Andersson LM, Westin J, Lindh M. PCR for detection of respiratory viruses: seasonal variations of virus infections. Expert Rev Anti-infect Ther. 2011;9(8):615–26.

Tiveljung-Lindell A, Rotzen-Ostlund M, Gupta S, Ullstrand R, Grillner L, Zweygberg-Wirgart B, et al. Development and implementation of a molecular diagnostic platform for daily rapid detection of 15 respiratory viruses. J Med Virol. 2009;81(1):167–75.

Wang W, Ren P, Sheng J, Mardy S, Yan H, Zhang J, et al. Simultaneous detection of respiratory viruses in children with acute respiratory infection using two different multiplex reverse transcription-PCR assays. J Virol Methods. 2009;162(1–2):40–5.

Assessment of the Airway with Flexible Endoscopy

15

Pablo Bertrand, Nils Linus Holmgren Palmen, and Francisco Prado Atlagic

Contents

P. Bertrand (✉)
Department of Pediatrics, School of Medicine, Pontificia Universidad Católica de Chile, Santiago, Chile
e-mail: pbertrand@med.puc.cl

N. L. Holmgren Palmen
Department of Pediatrics, Clínica Alemana and Universidad del Desarrollo, Santiago, Chile

F. Prado Atlagic
Department of Pediatrics, Hospital Clínico San Borja Arriarán, Santiago, Chile

P. Bertrand, I. Sánchez (eds.), *Pediatric Respiratory Diseases*,
https://doi.org/10.1007/978-3-030-26961-6_15

Indications

The indications to employ flexible bronchoscopy can be diagnostic or therapeutic. The most common diagnostic indications include the assessment of persistent stridor and wheezing, atelectasis, recurrent pneumonia, and suspicion of malformation of the upper or lower airway (Table 15.1). The most common therapeutic indications are bronchoalveolar lavage (BAL) for expansion of atelectasis and as a complement to extraction of a foreign body (Table 15.2).

Contraindications

The contraindications for flexible bronchoscopy are generally relative, because these situations will be transitory; therefore, they do not involve major risk. The only real contraindications are scenarios in which the procedure will not be useful diagnostically or the patient's guardians do not give consent for its use.

A relative contraindication is performance of a procedure without the necessary rigid bronchoscopy support or in an unstable airway condition in which predictable failure of the procedure forces the physician to take invasive measures to recover the airway. The following conditions are relative contraindications that should be corrected before the procedure is undertaken:

1. Hemodynamic instability
2. Intracranial hypertension
3. Hemorrhagic diathesis
4. Pulmonary hypertension
5. Massive hemoptysis
6. Respiratory insufficiency

Table 15.1 Diagnostic indications for flexible bronchoscopy

Indication
Assessment of the airway
Suspicion of a foreign body
Malformation of the upper airway
Obstructive sleep apnea syndrome
Persistent/recurrent symptom (cough, stridor, wheezing)
Persistent/recurrent disease (atelectasis, pneumonia, etc.)
Follow-up of some conditions (tracheostomy, transplantation, surgery)
Bronchoalveolar lavage
Pulmonary hemorrhage
Interstitial lung disease
Pneumonia in immunosuppressed patients
Severe pneumonia in immunocompetent patients
Suspicion of endobronchial tuberculosis
Suspicion of pulmonary aspiration

Table 15.2 Therapeutic indications for flexible bronchoscopy

Indication
Aspiration of a foreign body
Assessment before and after extraction of a foreign body
Extraction of a distal foreign body
Bronchoalveolar lavage
Expansion of persistent or massive atelectasis
Inhalation of highly irritating matter (barium, soot, blood, etc.)
Selective/massive cleaning of alveolar proteinosis
Application of medication (DNase, surfactant, cold serum, etc.)
Difficult intubation
Monointubation for thoracic surgery
Seldinger endoscopic intubation technique
Additional procedures (unusual indications)
Airway biopsy
Distal airway laser surgery
Dilatation of the airway with an inflatable balloon
Sealing of a persistent tracheoesophageal fistula

Technical Aspects

Equipment

There are two types of instruments currently available: the fiber bronchoscope, which has an optical fiber that sends images to a simple viewer or an external camera and then to an image processor; and the more recently introduced video endoscope, featuring a camera at one end of the instrument that sends images directly to a processor. The latter instrument has better optical resolution, being termed "high definition", when the image is translated into a determined number of

Table 15.3 Types and sizes of instruments, their applicability in different age groups, and their compatibility with other equipment

Patient age	Instrument type	External diameter (mm)	Working Channel (mm)	BAL	Biopsy	Laryngeal mask (minimum size (mm))	Endotracheal tube (minimum size (mm))
Premature/ newborn	Fiberscope	2.2	No	No	No	1	≥3
0–2 years	Fiberscope/video endoscope	2.7–2.8	1.2	Yes	Yes[a]	1.5	≥3.5
0–5 years	Fiberscope/video endoscope	3.4–3.6	1.2	Yes	Yes[a]	2	≥4.5
2–5 years	Fiberscope	4	2	Yes	Yes	2.5	≥5.5
>5 years	Fiberscope/video endoscope	4.9–5.1	2–2.2	Yes	Yes	3	≥6
>15 years	Fiberscope/video endoscope	5.9–6	2.2–2.8	Yes	Yes	4	≥7.5

BAL bronchoalveolar lavage
[a]Only with difficulty

pixels on a screen. Both types of equipment should include a working channel for aspiration of secretions, instrumentalization, and drug instillation.

The equipment necessary to adequately view the airway depends on the fundamental characteristics of the patient, such as his or her age and the estimated diameter of the airway, but it also depends on the characteristics of the disease or the proposed objectives of the procedure: biopsy, BAL, etc. (Table 15.3). Equipment with an external diameter of 3.6 mm is most often used, given that it can have a broad reach and is useful for access via the nasal passage of patients ranging from newborns to children 10 years of age. An instrument with an external diameter of around 2 mm is needed for small children (weighing <3 kg) and children with airway stenosis or an artificial airway (an endotracheal tube or tracheostomy cannula), in order to obtain a peripheral view of the airway. In contrast, in children over 6 years of age, it is essential that the instruments have an external diameter of approximately 5 mm for improved illumination, particularly for management of excessive secretions and for BAL. The equipment should ideally have an image processor for real-time viewing, as well as partial or complete documentation of the procedure with photography or videography.

Procedure

Flexible bronchoscopy is a clean procedure, but it is not sterile, because the route of entry—nasal, tracheostomy, laryngeal mask, etc.—is always contaminated. The risk of intrahospital infection by flexible bronchoscopy is low if protocols for disinfection, storage, and handling of equipment are adequately followed. Sterilization can be done with ethylene oxide, ortho-phthalaldehyde, or glutaraldehyde for high-level disinfection. In this scenario, disinfection with glutaraldehyde is very practical, given that it takes only 60 minutes to have the equipment available for reuse, but it does require a central unit with staff trained to ensure adherence to standards of efficacy, as well as the safety of the personnel who handle the disinfectant. There is now equipment that includes a disposable outer jacket with a suction channel. The external jacket is sterile and is discarded after the procedure; thus, multiple procedures can be conducted without the need for disinfection intervals.

First, the procedure is explained in detail to the parents before it begins, and informed consent is obtained in accordance with the protocols of the specific center, with the objective of clarifying the procedure, its usefulness, and potential complications. The procedure room should be equipped with oxygen, central aspiration, a resuscitation cart, a manual ventilator, a laryngoscope, tracheal tubes, masks, aspiration cannulas, monitors, drugs for sedation, and inputs. Other situations in which flexible bronchoscopy is applied are the critical care unit and the operating room, which allows us to carry out the procedure without any additional risk. The procedure is carried out with noninvasive cardiovascular monitoring (heartbeat and blood pressure) and continuous registering of peripheral oxygen saturation (SpO_2) until the patient recovers completely. The procedure should be carried out by a doctor trained in endoscopy, accompanied by another doctor trained in deep sedation and monitoring. It is also necessary to have the help of a nurse and a high-level technician trained in the procedure, administration of drugs, and high-level disinfection. The members of the team have specific responsibilities during the procedure, which are coordinated prior to the procedure, such as drug labeling, registration of vital signs, and positioning of the patient, nasal or oral aspiration of secretions, and assisting the operator in other tasks.

Sedation

The patient should have a clinical assessment for potential problems associated with the procedure, including a consultation between an anesthesiologist and the doctor in charge of sedation for the procedure. The patient should have a permeable venous access inserted before the procedure begins. The sedation depends on the access and the characteristics of the patient, and can range from deep sedation with access through the nose (with spontaneous ventilation) to profound anesthesia and a muscular block (with assisted manual ventilation with the airway maintained). For patients at risk of respiratory insufficiency or a minimal ventilatory reserve, the use of a laryngeal mask, an endotracheal tube, or manual ventilation should be considered before the procedure is conducted. A laryngeal mask can be used in procedures in which the objective is not to view the airway dynamics but, rather, to perform more invasive exploration, whether it is to search for a foreign body or to perform BAL for culturing, bronchial brushing, or bronchial biopsy. The idea is to anticipate hypoxemia to avoid systemic consequences. The most useful medications for this sedation are those that, in combination, offer sedation and analgesia for short periods, with minimal effects on spontaneous respiration. The most widely used medications are midazolam with morphine, midazolam with ketamine, and propofol. To some degree, and depending on their doses, all of the medications that are used can have a depressive effect on the respiratory system and increase secretions in the airway; thus, there are adverse effects that must be monitored throughout the procedure. Topical sedation is necessary from the nasal passage to the main carina to avoid pain, reflexive spasms, and coughing. Lidocaine in either a liquid or gel form is used to an obtain an adequate level of sedation. Lidocaine is preferably administered at 2% in the upper airway and 1% in the lower airway, and not exceeding a total dose of 7 mg/kg. The administration of lidocaine in the upper airway should be preceded by adequate visualization of the epiglottis and of the movement of the vocal cords, so as to not attribute exaggerated collapse of these structures to a pathological condition rather than to the effect of anesthesia, especially in patients in whom paralysis of the vocal cords is suspected.

Administration of atropine, which was a common practice in instrumentation of the airway in the past, is now reserved for patients who present an excessive vagal response or for infant under 6 months of age. Administration of oxygen is considered in all procedures from the beginning because of the high risk of hypoxemia when the instrument is inserted into the airway, to which is added an exaggerated spasm reflex, coughing, and the excess of secretions produced by the introduction of the instruments. Oxygen is provided by means of a nasal cannula with a flow of $\geq$2 l/min, so as to obtain a reservoir of the inhaled fraction of oxygen in the rhinopharyngeal space of a patient breathing spontaneously.

Another way to administer oxygen is by manual ventilation with an inflatable bag, whether through an endotracheal tube or a laryngeal mask. Finally, oxygen can be administered for bronchoscopy. However, this should be done only in the central airway and intermittently, because of the high risk of increasing pressure in the airway and an associated pneumothorax. Ideally, an SpO_2 of >93% is maintained continuously and the procedure is temporarily interrupted if this level is not maintained. In this context, hypoxemia is always considered a late indicator of hypoventilation because oxygen is administered concomitantly throughout the procedure.

Bronchoalveolar Lavage

Bronchoalveolar lavage consists of administration of a physiological serum in a specific area for diagnostic or therapeutic purposes. The procedure involves positioning the point of the instrument in a bronchus with a caliber similar to that of the device, such that it allows for a certain degree of bronchial sealing when the physiological serum is transferred, which is termed "interlocking." The procedure is done in the selected area either because it is a collapsed pulmonary area (in the case of lobar atelectasis) or because it presents infectious compromise, in which case the procedure is expected to determine the etiological agent (pneumonia in the case of immunocompromised patients). Upon reaching the desired location, 1–2 ml/kg of physiological serum is instilled in the working channel on at least three occasions (with a volume not greater than 25% of the functional residual capacity), to be subsequently aspirated through the same channel, with recovery of approximately 30–50% of the instilled volume. If a good seal is achieved during the maneuver, the liquid that is obtained contains cells from the respiratory bronchiole and the alveolar territory.

The risk of contamination of equipment that enters the upper airway can be reduced with the use of a laryngeal mask and with bronchial brushing, using brushes with protected ends that are only exposed when they reach the area to obtain a culture sample.

Recovery

The patient recovers from flexible bronchoscopy in the procedure room, the critical care unit, or the anesthetic recovery room, under the same noninvasive monitoring that is described above, and under the responsibility of the physician in charge of sedation. Once the patient awakens from sedation and his or her respiratory and cardiovascular condition is stable, he or she is taken to the unit of origin. Depending on the sedation that is used, and once the patient is fully awake, he or she can be fed within 2 hours after the procedure. This safety interval also allows for full recovery of the protective reflexes of the airway following the use of local lidocaine. A routine chest x-ray is not necessary unless there is respiratory deterioration with increased oxygen requirements and breathing difficulty. Following the application of flexible bronchoscopy with BAL, the patient can present a fever, which is usually limited and is not associated with any intercurrent infection. This can be prevented with administration of paracetamol (15 mg/kg every 6–8 hours, orally) within hours after the procedure or dexamethasone (0.3 mg/kg) during the procedure.

Complications of Flexible Bronchoscopy

Complications of flexible bronchoscopy are common; most of them are transitory. The complications are directly related to the duration of the procedure, because of which it is vital to reduce the procedural time as much as possible. The most common complications are the result of the partial occlusion of the airway and the effects of sedation. The most frequent complication is transitory hypoxemia, which occurs as a result of hypoventilation while the equipment is in the airway, and it is resolved by temporarily removing the equipment. An excessive cough reflex is also common, which is generally controlled with the application of local lidocaine. The use of topical anesthesia in patients with excessive secretions (e.g., due to cystic fibrosis) is decisive to prevent this complication. Less common, but no less important, are complications arising from the sedation, such as hypoventilation secondary to the use of depressor drugs and accumulation of secretions due to the lack of a cough reflex. Rapid diagnosis allows for immediate resolution with regard to the positioning of the upper airway, manual ventilation with a mask, and sometimes intubation of the airway. In patients with respiratory difficulty prior to the procedure, endotracheal intubation and mechanical ventilation should be considered. Epistaxis during or after the application of flexible bronchoscopy is common in infants, where the narrow nasal passage is similar in size to the equipment. This condition often resolves spontaneously or after application of cold serum at the end of the procedure. Other complications are also common, such as postprocedural hemorrhaging of the distal airway, pneumothorax, laryngospasms, and pneumonia.

Performance of Flexible Bronchoscopy

Congenital Stridor

Most patients who consult physicians because of a congenital stridor have laryngomalacia, a condition that is suspected on the basis of a characteristic medical history, which can be confirmed by nasal fibroscopy conducted with topical anesthesia. However, flexible bronchoscopy is necessary to confirm the causes of the condition in patients with a severe stridor, episodes of cyanosis or apnea, or with eating difficulties. Likewise, flexible bronchoscopy should be applied when the stridor has an uncommon temporal profile, when a condition other than laryngomalacia is suspected, and, above all, when there is a therapeutic possibility. The procedure is sometimes justified by parental anxiety caused by the stridor. Common causes are vocal cord paralysis and subglottic stenosis, both of which are generally related to a previous treatment: surgery for patent ductus arteriosus in the former case, and prolonged intubation in the latter case. More uncommon conditions that are nevertheless important to rule out are a tracheal cleft, laryngeal membrane, tracheal stenosis, and tracheal hemangioma.

Acute Stridor

In patients suffering from an episode of acute obstructive laryngitis, flexible bronchoscopy is justified only when the patient has not improved despite treatment or when intubation is needed because of deterioration of the condition. The findings can be compatible with bacterial tracheitis, a foreign body, or unexpected congenital malformations, which is particularly relevant information for treating the patient.

Recurrent Laryngitis

If there are more than three recurrent episodes of acute obstructive laryngitis, especially when they occur within a year, a flexible bronchoscopy study is mandatory. There is evidence from such cases in children under 3 years of age that a third of them present some degree of alteration of the airway that explains the recurrence of this condition.

Upper Airway Obstruction

Assessment of the upper airway of patients with upper airway obstruction (UAO) is facilitated by directed viewing through a flexible bronchoscopy, where the potential therapeutic value of medical or surgical solutions in specific situations can be evaluated. In patients with craniofacial malformations or neuromuscular disease, repositioning of the tongue or collapse of the tonsils can be very evident with the patient under sedation but not when the patient is awake. The procedure in this scenario tends to be highly risky because of the possibility of destabilizing the airway.

Atelectasis

In the context of lobar or massive atelectasis, flexible bronchoscopy has a mainly diagnostic objective, whether this situation is the result of a bronchial malformation, vascular compression, a foreign body, a mucosal plug, or an endobronchial lesion. In conditions in which bronchial cleaning with physiological serum facilitates the expansion of the tributary area, bronchial lavage, which expands the area in 70% of cases, can be attempted. It is useful to apply diluted adrenaline (epinephrine) and/or DNase in this procedure to facilitate the removal of mucus plugs. In other situations, the treatment is done according to the endoscopic findings.

Pneumonia in Immunocompetent Patients

The performance of BAL through a flexible bronchoscope in patients with an acute lower respiratory infection is variable but does not achieve etiological identification in more than 50% of cases. The performance is affected by prior use of antibiotics, the timing of the disease, and the quality of the samples obtained. New techniques such as polymerase chain reaction and quantitative bacterial culturing have improved etiological identification. The procedure is thus justified in patients who have a severe condition without a known agent and who do not respond to treatment.

Pneumonia in Immunocompromised Patients

In immunocompromised patients, pulmonary infections by the usual and opportunistic agents are a common cause of complications, and their identification is usually difficult. The agents involved vary according to when the disease appears and its treatment: neutropenia, chemotherapy, antibiotics, etc. BAL is effective in more than 50% of cases under these conditions, and it is even more justified in immunocompromised patients because noninvasive tests have poorer results. Bronchial lavage has a high negative predictive value for some infectious agents, so therapeutic decisions can be facilitated by reducing antibiotic coverage. However, the time available to perform the procedure may be limited by the presence of hypoxemic respiratory failure because of the high risk, under these conditions, of the patient's condition worsening and the need to resort to ventilatory support. Other complications are more common in immunocompromised patients; thus, the potential benefits must always be weighed against the risks.

Recurrent Wheezing and Pneumonia

In patients with episodes of bronchial obstruction or recurrent pneumonia that do not respond well to treatment, it may be necessary to perform flexible bronchoscopy to rule out conditions that can imitate this clinical presentation (tracheomalacia (Fig. 15.1), a foreign body, etc.). A cellular study of BAL fluid and a tissue study by means of a carinal biopsy (Fig. 15.2) can help in the diagnosis of other conditions.

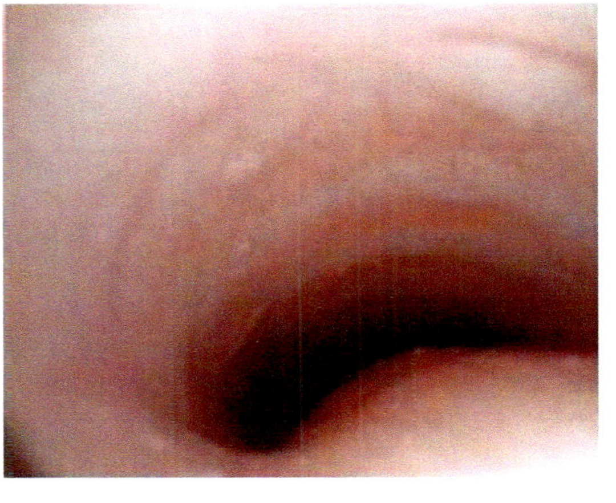

Fig. 15.1 Tracheomalacia. Endoscopic visualization of significant collapse of the posterior wall of the middle third of the trachea in a 15-month-old infant with persistent wheezing

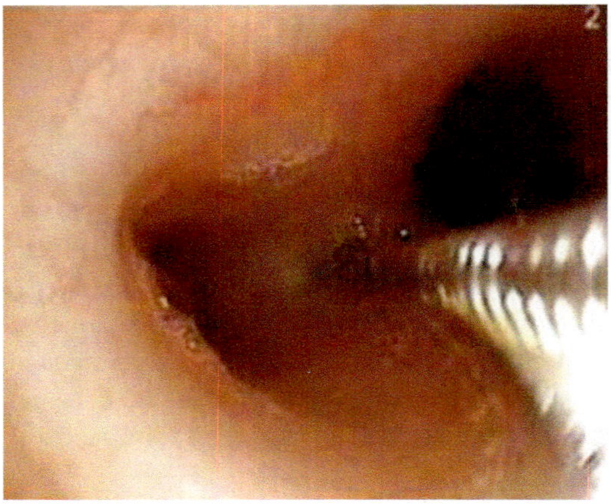

Fig. 15.2 Biopsy of the main carina. Endoscopic visualization of biopsy forceps in the carina of a 6-year-old child with suspected ciliary dyskinesia

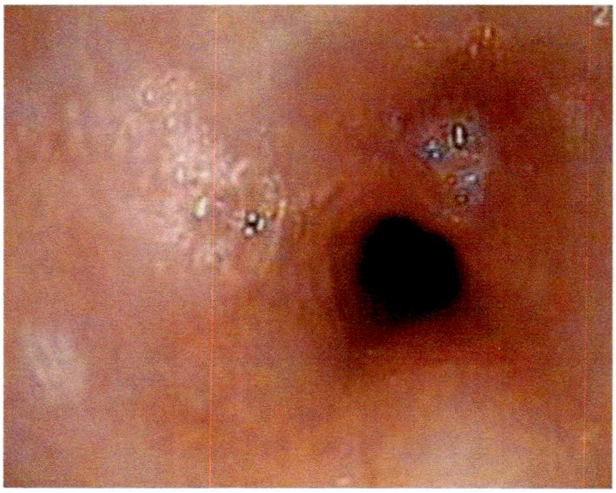

Fig. 15.3 Subglottic stenosis. Endoscopic visualization showing 60% lumen tightness in the subglottic region, due to the presence of an eccentric membrane in a 15-month-old infant after mechanical ventilation for 30 days during recovery from a Glenn procedure

Hemoptysis

Hemoptysis is an uncommon situation in pediatrics in which fiberoptic bronchoscopy can identify a source of bleeding, rule out the presence of a foreign body in the airway, and perform a bronchoalveolar lavage to rule out bacterial, fungi, and tuberculosis infections. Fiberoptic bronchoscopy should be considered for all patients with repeated mild or moderate hemoptysis in whom medical evaluation and noninvasive tests have not clarified the diagnosis. If the patient's age allows it, it is necessary to consider proceeding with equipment that has a suction channel measuring $\geq$2 mm for adequate aspiration in the event of active bleeding. In cases of massive hemoptysis, flexible bronchoscopy is indicated.

Extubation Failure

It is often necessary to assess the airway of an infant after a severe and acute illness or when the infant exhibits an abrupt deterioration after a long period of connection to ventilatory support. Once correctable conditions have been ruled out, it is essential to assess the airway to rule out the presence of vocal cord paralysis, subglottic stenosis (Fig. 15.3), or other acquired or congenital lesions.

Difficult Intubation

Flexible bronchoscopy is used as an alternative in patients who need an artificial airway, especially in children with craniofacial anomalies or genetic syndromes. In these cases, the instrument is used as a guide for an endotracheal tube. The airway is first accessed in a controlled manner, then the tube is advanced for its final positioning or to position semiflexible guides to help in the intuba-

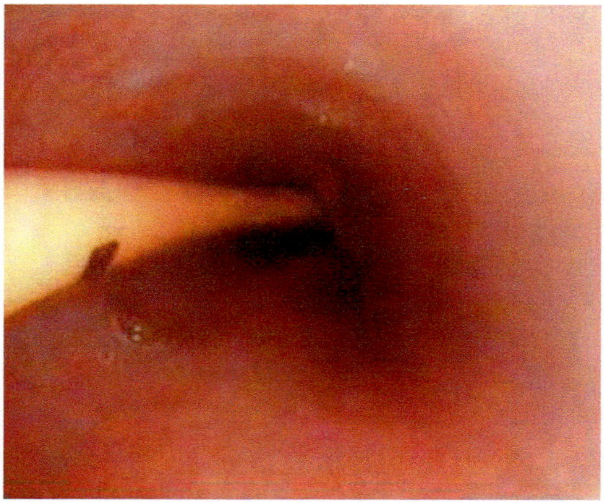

Fig. 15.4 Difficult intubation. Airway scoring with a semiflexible guide lead by means of bronchial video endoscopy in a 20-day-old patient with Pierre Robin syndrome

tion (Fig. 15.4). The flexible bronchoscope is also useful for selective bronchial intubation, either to perform asymmetrical ventilation or to facilitate selective thoracic surgery.

Foreign Bodies

Extraction of a foreign body by means of a flexible bronchoscope has become a routine procedure. The advantages of the bronchoscope are that it provides diagnostic certainty and certainty about the location of the foreign body, especially in the case of objects that are radiolucent or that can fragment after extraction. In older children in whom it is possible to use bronchoscopes with working channels 2 mm in diameter, some low-risk foreign bodies can be extracted with tweezers or cryoprobes. The tip of the latter is frozen to catch foreign bodies with a liquid content, although this alternative should be considered only at centers where flexible bronchoscopy and emergency airway surgery can be performed in case the procedure fails.

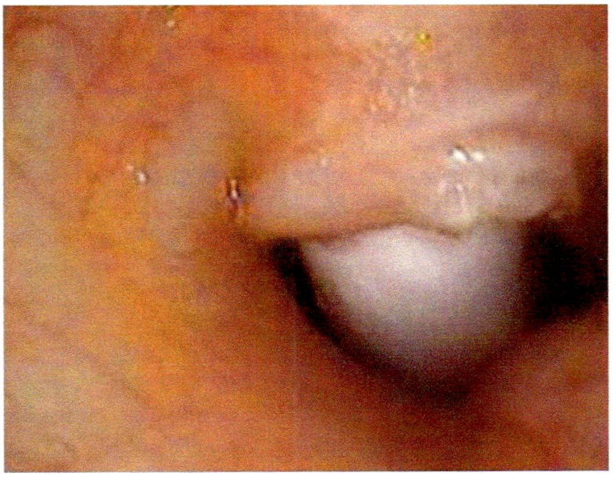

Fig. 15.5 Tracheostomy. Endoscopic view of a tracheostomy cannula in its correct position in a 5-year-old patient with nemaline myopathy who is dependent on long-term mechanical ventilation

Miscellaneous Applications

Fiberoptic bronchoscopy has advanced rapidly as new devices have become available that facilitate the procedure and allow for assistance with other diseases. It is used routinely in children with a tracheostomy (Fig. 15.5) to determine the size of the trachea, the position of the cannula, and the presence of complications before decannulation is performed. At our center, we have performed permeabilization of a congenital tracheoesophageal fistula (Fig. 15.6) as a way to ease the surgery process during the fistula identification. This technique for tracheal intubation has also been used as part of the EXIT (Ex Utero Intrapartum Treatment) technique. The objective of this is to

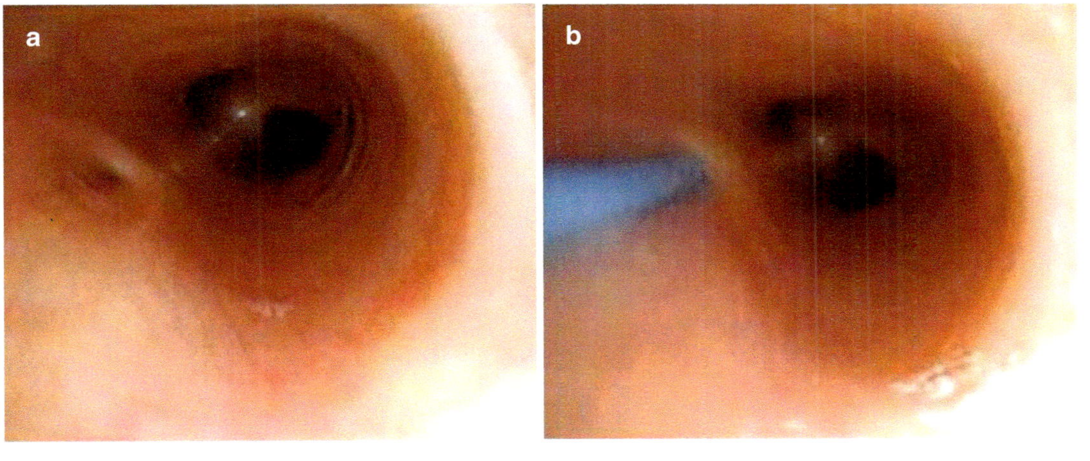

Fig. 15.6 Tracheoesophageal fistula. Endoscopic visualization of a congenital tracheoesophageal fistula (**a**) and scoring with a semiflexible guide lead by means of bronchial video endoscopy (**b**) to facilitate surgical closure

safeguard the airway of the newborn during a partial cesarean section, and it is also used as a rescue hygiene measure for the bronchi in patients connected to extracorporeal membrane oxygenation for long periods.

Sources

Álvarez C, Rodríguez J, Ronco R, Castillo A, et al. Uso de mascarilla laríngea para fibrobroncoscopia durante ventilación mecánica. Rev Chil Enf Respir. 2002;18:103–11.

Barch B, Rastatter J, Jagannathan N. Difficult pediatric airway management using the intubating laryngeal airway. Int J Pediatr Otorhinolaryngol. 2012;76:1579–82.

Bar-Zohar D, Suan Y. The yield of flexible fiberoptic bronchoscopy in pediatric intensive care patients. Chest. 2004;126:1353–9.

Cakir E, Hamutcu Ersu R, Seda Uyan Z, et al. Flexible bronchoscopy as a valuable tool in the evaluation of persistent wheezing in children. Int J Pediatr Otorhinolaryngol. 2009;73:1666–8.

Cutrone C, Pedruzzi B, Tava G, et al. The complimentary role of diagnostic and therapeutic endoscopy in foreign body aspiration in children. Int J Pediatr Otorhinolaryngol. 2011;75:1481–5.

Davies J, Payne D. Research applications of bronchoscopy. Paediatr Respir Rev. 2003;4:230–6.

De Blic J, Midulla F, Barbato A, Clement A, Dab I, Eber E, Green C, Grigg J, Kotecha S, Kurland G, Pohunek P, Ratjen F, Rossi G. Bronchoalveolar lavage in children. ERS Task Force on Bronchoalveolar Lavage in Children. European Respiratory Society. Eur Respir J. 2000;15:217–31.

Fidkowski C, Zheng H, Firth P. The anesthetic considerations of tracheobronchial foreign bodies in children: a literature review of 12,979 cases. Anesth Analg. 2010;111:1016–25.

Hertzog H, Campbell J, Dalton H, Hauser G. Propofol anesthesia for invasive procedures in ambulatory and hospitalised children: experience in the pediatric intensive care unit. Pediatrics. 1999;104:e30.

Holmgren NL, Cordova M, Ortuzar P, Sanchez I. Rol of flexible bronchoscopy in the re-expansion of persistent atelectasis in children. Arch Bronchoneumol. 2002;38:367–71.

Kamat P, Popler J, Davis J, et al. Use of flexible bronchoscopy in pediatric patients receiving extracorporeal membrane oxygenation (ECMO) support. Pediatr Pulmonol. 2011;46:1108–13.

Labbé A, Meyer F, Albertini M. Bronchoscopy in intensive care units. Paediatr Respir Rev. 2004;5 Suppl A:S15–9.

Medulla F, de Blic J, Bush A, Eber E, et al. Flexible endoscopy of paediatric airways. ERS Task Force. Eur Respir J. 2003;22:698–708.

Midyat L, Cakır E, Kut A. Upper airway abnormalities detected in children using flexible bronchoscopy. Int J Pediatr Otorhinolaryngol. 2012;76:560–3.

Naguib ML, Streetman DS, Clifton S, Nasr SZ. Use of laryngeal mask airway in flexible bronchoscopy in infants and children. Pediatr Pulmonol. 2005;39:56–63.

Nicolai T. The role of rigid and flexible bronchoscopy in children. Paediatr Respir Rev. 2011;12:190–5.

Ondik M, Kimatian S, Carr M. Management of the difficult airway in the pediatric patient. Oper Techn Otolaryngol. 2007;18:121–6.

Pérez-Frías J, Moreno Galdó A, Pérez Ruiz E, Barrio Gómez De Agüero MI, Escribano Montaner A, Caro Aguilera P, Sociedad Española de Neumología y Cirugía Torácica. Normativa de broncoscopia pediátrica. Arch Bronconeumol. 2011;47:350–60.

Prado F, Boza ML, Isamitt D. Bronchopleural fistula in children: treatment with endoscopic sealing. Eur Resp J. 2002;20(Suppl):s149.

Sánchez I, Pesce C, Navarro H, Holmgren L, Bertrand P, Álvarez C. 10-Year experience in flexible bronchoscopy in pediatric patients. Rev Méd Chil. 2003;131:1266–72.

Vega-Briceño LE. Utility of bronchoalveolar lavage in immunocompromised children: diagnosis yield and complications. Arch Bronconeumol. 2004;40(12):570–4.

Assessment of the Airway with Rigid Endoscopy

16

Harlan Muntz and Constanza Beltrán Morales

Contents

History

Historically, many attempts were made to examine the human airway, and it was not until 1854 that Manuel García was able to do so with the use of a mirror. Before that, in 1828, Babington used what he called a glotoscope—a mirror attached to a tongue depressor. In 1837, Liston tried to obtain

H. Muntz
Health Sciences Center, Universidad de Utah, Salt Lake City, UT, USA
e-mail: harlan.muntz@intermountainmail.org

C. Beltrán Morales (✉)
Department of Otorhinolaryngology, School of Medicine, Universidad de los Andes, Santiago, Chile
e-mail: cbeltran@clinicauandes.cl

P. Bertrand, I. Sánchez (eds.), *Pediatric Respiratory Diseases*,
https://doi.org/10.1007/978-3-030-26961-6_16

a better view of the airway with a dental mirror. García reported his advance to the Royal Society in London in 1855, but it was not until 1858 that Czemark (in Budapest, Hungary) popularized the clinical use of García's laryngeal mirror.

Direct examination of the larynx became possible near the end of the nineteenth century (1888) with the use of cocaine as a local anesthetic. Killian developed suspension laryngoscopy in 1912. Thanks to Kleinsasser, the surgical microscope was later developed, which allowed for laryngeal microsurgery. Killian introduced the bronchoscope in 1897, but it was Chevalier Jackson (who is now considered the inventor of the rigid bronchoscope) who introduced instruments with distal light. Jackson dedicated his life to clinical and technological developments for direct assessment of the human upper airway. Together with Pilling, in the first two decades of the twentieth century, Jackson developed the angulated telescope and a bronchoscope with the capacity for ventilation, which has made rigid endoscopy a safe procedure in most cases. Toward the end of his life in 1937, Jackson stated, "A new era has dawned. The day of inferential diagnosis of the airway has ended. The larynx of any human being, from newborn to century old can be examined in the entirety." This is true today and indicates the need to endoscopically and thoroughly assess any patient with upper airway pathologies.

Assessment of the Patient

Rigid endoscopy of the airway can be used diagnostically, therapeutically, or both. The diagnosis is sometimes known, as in the case of laryngeal papillomatosis, while in other cases there may not be a clear diagnosis or any diagnosis at all, but all of these cases can require assessment of the airway.

The patient's medical history is very important, and particular attention should be given to the beginning of symptoms:

1. *Rapid beginning*: A rapid beginning of the symptoms suggests the cause is infection (croup) or inhalation of a foreign body. If the latter is suspected, rigid endoscopy should be applied urgently for both diagnosis and treatment. It should be noted that the presence of a foreign body in the airway cannot be ruled out with an x-ray, which is useful only if the object is radiopaque. Thus, the need for airway endoscopy is determined clinically and by the need for an adequately ventilated airway.
2. *Chronic airway symptoms*: In children with chronic airway symptoms where the pathology is well known, periodic airway assessment may be required—for example, to rule out stenosis or for therapeutic purposes, such as bronchoalveolar lavage or resection of tracheal granulomas. In these cases, endoscopy is generally an elective procedure, where the child is assessed in good conditions if it is possible.
3. *Severity of symptoms*: The severity of the child's symptoms can determine the need for airway endoscopy and its urgency. This is a rather dynamic determination, as it depends on the severity of the symptoms, and that in turn depends on the degree of obstruction in the child. This can be resolved only through frequent observation and measurement of parameters such as the pulse rate, respiratory rates, and saturation. Timely intervention is important because there is a direct relationship between the magnitude and the severity of the obstruction.

Symptoms and Signs of Airway Obstruction

It is important to determine the degree of airway obstruction, for which there are signs and symptoms such as:

1. Oxygen saturation
2. Respiratory frequency
3. Use of accessory musculature
4. Costal retraction
5. Level of awareness

This clinical observation has been formalized in the croup score, which assigns points to the parameters (Table 16.1). This helps in determining

Table 16.1 Severity score for obstructive laryngitis

	Score		
Parameter	0	1	2
Respiratory sounds	None	Rough	Delayed
Stridor	None	Inspiratory	Biphasic
Cough/voice	None	Dysphonic cry	Canine cough
Retraction	None	Suprasternal	1 + intercostal
Cyanosis	None	With air	With 40% O_2
Level of consciousness	Normal	Lethargic	Obtunded

A score of ≥30 minutes requires more airway support

when intervention should occur, which generally consists of controlling the airway with endotracheal intubation or a tracheotomy.

Indications for Airway Endoscopy

A severe stridor generally goes hand in hand with significant airway obstruction. It is important to know how much air the patient is moving. If there is no movement of air through the airway, because of a severe obstruction, the symptom of a stridor will not be noticeable. Whenever possible, flexible endoscopy should be considered as a first step in assessing the larynx in any patient with a moderate to severe stridor. This test can provide the diagnosis, and a rigid endoscope can be used if necessary.

The best way to make a good assessment is with laryngoscopy or with flexible or rigid bronchoscopy prior to endotracheal intubation, because afterward the opportunity for a good diagnosis decreases.

If the stridor and airway obstruction are progressive—and to this can be added a weight increase and difficulty in feeding—rigid endoscopy is generally indicated not only for diagnosing the pathology but also with the aim of applying immediate treatment. For example, this can occur with laryngomalacia.

Endoscopy is often complemented with x-rays, while computerized axial tomography can also be useful when the endoscopic study suggests the presence of an abnormality, such as a vascular ring. In children with symptoms of severe obstruction, radiographic or magnetic resonance tests that require sedation should not be done before the diagnosis has been established by means of rigid endoscopy. As with the diagnosis of a foreign object, upper airway lateral and anteroposterior plaques do not provide sufficient resolution to rule out a large number of common pathologies. Consequently, direct visual observation by flexible or rigid endoscopy is more useful than imagery for assessing the airway in pediatrics.

When Is Rigid Endoscopy, Rather than Flexible Endoscopy, Appropriate?

Rigid and flexible endoscopy are complementary. Flexible endoscopy is used to examine the larynx of a child who is awake, and it allows useful information to be obtained about cordal mobility and laryngeal dynamics.

Lesions in the pharynx and lower airway can be viewed only with rigid endoscopy. If necessary, with general anesthesia after suspension of the larynx, the vocal cords can be viewed with a binocular microscope, providing a stereoscopic view. Rigid endoscopy allows for a good and detailed view, while control of the airway is maintained. Flexible bronchoscopy does not allow for absolute control of the airway and can obstruct it entirely in small children. The quality of the image with a rigid Hopkins rod-type telescope is superior to that obtained with a flexible bronchoscope, and its documentation is undoubtedly much clearer.

Rigid Instruments

Instruments can be considered under two headings:

1. Laryngoscopy and bronchoscopy
2. Documentation and teaching

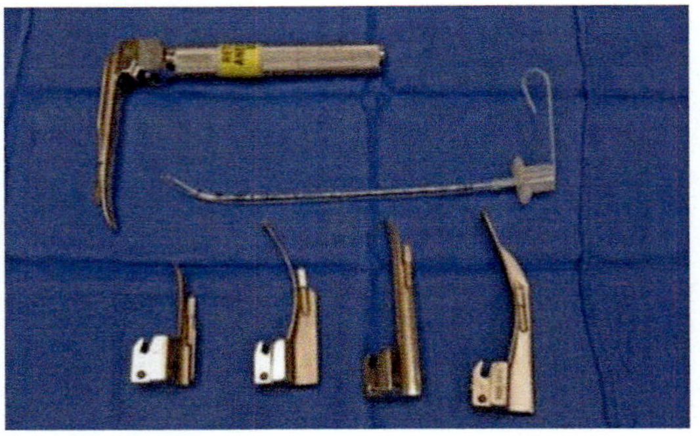

Fig. 16.1 Laryngoscopes for intubation

Laryngoscopy and Bronchoscopy

Laryngoscopes

There are a wide variety of laryngoscopy approaches and devices, and they can be divided into those that are designed for suspension and those that are not. It is important to know how to employ the different types, including those for intubation. There are two types of nonsuspension laryngoscope: straight bladed and curved bladed (Fig. 16.1). The straight blades are more compatible with rigid endoscopy. Among the straight blades are the Miller, Wis-Hipple (or Wisconsin), and Philips; the Philips provides the most space in the oropharynx to pass the endoscope and facilitate intubation. An important feature of suspension laryngoscopes is that they have a xenon light source and consequently provide more illumination than intubation laryngoscopes do. Suspension is also necessary for endolaryngeal surgery with a microscope. The most commonly used suspension laryngoscope in pediatrics is the Parsons type (Karl Storz), of which there are several sizes for all ages, and it is partially open, allowing for its use in suspension or intubation. It is also useful to have small closed laryngoscopes to view the anterior of the larynx, such as the Hollinger anterior commissure laryngoscope. Finally, the closed Benjamin–Lindholm laryngoscope, which is available in many sizes for all ages, offers the possibility of a broad posterior view.

Bronchoscopes

Telescopes

In 1966, Hopkins introduced the long telescope with different lenses, which improved the resolution and the angle of viewing, and revolutionized pediatric bronchoscopy, providing the potential to see into very small spaces. For example, a 4.0 mm by 20 cm zero-degree telescope is ideal for passing through a laryngoscope in the subglottis or trachea.

A Hopkins rod telescope alone (bare) or with a ventilating bronchoscope can be used for rigid assessment of the upper airway. Both visualize the larynx, trachea, and bronchi with magnification. The advantage of using the telescope alone is that it minimizes the trauma to the airway walls, given that the diameter of the endoscope is less than that of the ventilating bronchoscope. The diameters of Hopkins rod telescopes (the most widely used) are 1.9, 2.7, and 4 mm, while the lengths vary. There are also lenses with 30- and 70-degree angles. When a bare telescope is used, the patient cannot be actively ventilated, and so the endoscopy is usually conducted under spontaneous ventilation (see below for more information on this).

A ventilating bronchoscope is much wider and thicker than a bare telescope, given that the Hopkins rod is inserted inside the bronchoscope light. The size of the telescope that is inserted depends on the size of the bronchoscope. Sometimes it is useful that the telescope is longer than the bronchoscope, because more peripheral areas can be examined. Ventilating bronchoscopes allow for ventilation of the patient while therapeutic maneuvers are being conducted in the trachea. These bronchoscopes are characterized in the following manner:

1. Connection of a closed gas system to the anesthesia circuit so that the bronchoscope also acts as an endotracheal tube, which can serve to provide spontaneous ventilation and positive ventilation
2. A rigid optical Hopkins rod inside its light, to provide distal illumination

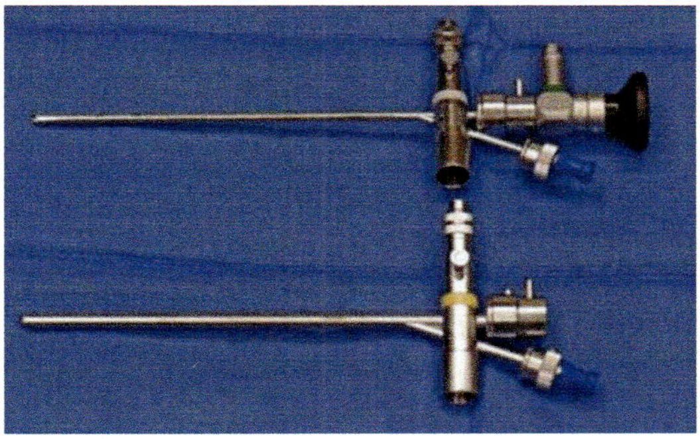

Fig. 16.2 Storz bronchoscopy with zero-degree optics

Table 16.2 Bronchoscope size

Nominal size of bronchoscope (mm)	Internal optical telescope size (mm)	External diameter (mm)	Age range
2.5	1.9; 2.7	4.0	Preterm, newborn
3.0	1.9; 2.7	5.0	Newborn to 6 months
3.5	2.7; 4.0	5.7	6–18 months
3.7	2.7; 4.0	6.0	6–24 months; a peanut clamp can be inserted
4.0	4.0; 5.0	7.0	18–36 months
5.0	4.0; 5.0	7.8	3–8 years
6.0	4.0; 5.0	8.2	>8 years

3. A lateral channel for passing a suction catheter or flexible forceps

Ventilating bronchoscopes in different sizes are fabricated by Karl Storz (Fig. 16.2). Table 16.2 shows bronchoscope sizes for use in children of different ages. It should be kept in mind that the size of the optics depends on the size of the bronchoscope. Small bronchoscopes cannot accommodate a suction catheter. Optical forceps or a clamp are highly useful for removing foreign bodies and granulomas. Optical forceps, which are available in a variety of sizes and shapes, can be introduced into the airway by use of a rubber cap.

Documentation and Teaching

Cameras have, without doubt, been of great help to endoscopy. The camera is connected to the telescope in bronchoscopy or microscopy—the latter in the case of suspension laryngoscopy—and projects images to monitors; the images can also be digitally recorded.

Anesthesia

It is important to maintain the patient's spontaneous ventilation during the induction of anesthesia and during laryngoscopy or bronchoscopy. If there is significant stenosis in the airway, it causes major resistance to ventilation with positive pressure. However, it can be difficult to maintain spontaneous ventilation in newborns or very sick infants under deep anesthesia. In most cases the patient can be anesthetized under spontaneous ventilation with a combination of inhaled and intravenous agents (propofol, dexmedetomidine, ketamine).

The following considerations are also critical:

1. Work as a team with the anesthesiologist and have a good working relationship with him/her.
2. Never start an endoscopy procedure without a safe venous line, even if it means waiting.
3. Apply local anesthesia in the larynx and trachea, using 4 mg/kg of lidocaine at 2–4% to minimize the risk of laryngospasm.
4. Conduct the laryngoscopy without the endotracheal tube getting in the way.
5. If the larynx cannot be visualized directly with the laryngoscope, because of a very anterior position, it can often be accessible to the rigid bronchoscope.
6. If the upper airway is obstructed, it is better to conduct a tracheotomy, even as an emergency (for which you should be prepared).
7. There should be mutual confidence between the anesthesiologist and the endoscopist to maintain control of the process.

Operative Techniques

Laryngoscopy

In most cases the larynx can be visualized by telescope or microscope. The patient lies face up in hyperextension, with his or her shoulders raised. The laryngoscope is inserted on the right side of the mouth while the jaw is held in the physician's left hand. Care must be taken not to harm the lips or teeth. The laryngoscope is inserted to the vallecula, following the tongue and moving the tongue to the left. Then the tip of the laryngoscope should be hooked to the epiglottis, to observe the vocal cords, arytenoid folds, arytenoid cartilage, and subglottis. The telescope is then passed into the trachea and advanced to the main bronchi. If a ventilating bronchoscope is used, the laryngoscope must be removed because of its size. The physician should withdraw it with his or her left hand to advance the bronchoscope in the trachea.

If it is planned to use suspension laryngoscopy, the laryngoscope is placed in position and suspended from an arm that is inserted into the handle of the laryngoscope. Once in position, a telescope or microscope is put in place with a 400 mm lens.

Bronchoscopy

Before the procedure, the instruments should be completely assembled, and their sizes should be appropriate for the patient. As noted above, after exposure of the larynx, a bare telescope or a ventilating telescope is inserted into the airway. When a bare telescope is used, it is important that the patient ventilates spontaneously with the help of oxygen insufflation administered via the nose or into the hypopharynx by a tube during the bronchoscopy. If a ventilating bronchoscope is used, it is necessary to remove the laryngoscope as the bronchoscope advances. Once the bronchoscope is inserted, it reaches to the carina to recognize structures and possible pathologies in the trachea. To get the bronchoscope to enter the main bronchi, it is often useful to move the patient's head from side to side, allowing access to the bronchi from right to left. Viewing should continue until removal of the bronchoscope.

Complications of Airway Endoscopy

Loss of Control of the Airway

Loss of control of the airway can result in the patient suffering hypoxia or respiratory/cardiac arrest. To avoid these complications, the attending physician must be familiar with the procedure, the instruments, and the problems that can lead to loss of control. The factors that can precipitate this are:

1. An airway that is already compromised
2. Occurrence of laryngospasm when insertion of the bronchoscope is attempted, especially when this occurs early in the procedure
3. An undiscovered cardiovascular abnormality in which the positive ventilation pressure impedes venous return
4. Unfamiliarity with the instruments
5. Inexperience

Excessive Injury to the Subglottis and Edema During Recovery from Anesthesia

The use of a very large bronchoscope can result in injury to the subglottic mucosa, provoke postoperative edema and major obstruction of the airway, and even precipitate the need for tracheal intubation or a tracheotomy. When the rigid endoscope does not enter easily, it should be exchanged for a smaller gage or a bare telescope.

Injury to the Teeth or Gums

Dental injury is more common with the laryngoscope than with the bronchoscope. Children's jaws, which are relatively small and mobile, can also suffer injury and can be displaced when the laryngoscope is inserted.

Hemorrhaging

Hemorrhaging of the airway can become severe. The predisposing factors are:

1. Vascular lesions, such as laryngeal papillomas
2. Hemangiomas
3. Removal of a foreign body, particularly when it has been there for a long time and is surrounded by granulating tissue

Pneumothorax

This occurs when there is a major respiratory obstruction or unnecessary positive pressure to ventilate. In such cases, pleural drainage should be put in place.

Failure to Recognize Abnormalities

Strictly speaking, this is not a complication, but it can require other interventions, which is why it is best to seek assistance from someone with more experience if one is not familiar with the methods.

Sources

Cotton RT, O'Connor DM. Evaluation of the airway for laryngotracheal reconstruction. Int Anesthesiol Clin. 1992;30(4):93–8.

Doherty JS, Froom SR, Gildersleve CD. Pediatric laryngoscopes and intubation aids old and new. Paediatr Anaesth. 2009;19 Suppl 1:30–7.

Fidkowski CW, Zheng H, Firth PG. The anesthetic considerations of tracheobronchial foreign bodies in children: a literature review of 12,979 cases. Anesth Analg. 2010;111(4):1016–25. https://doi.org/10.1213/ANE.0b013e3181ef3e9c.

Muntz HR. Therapeutic rigid bronchoscopy in the neonatal intensive care unit. Ann Otol Rhinol Laryngol. 1985;94(5 Pt 1):462–5.

Nicolai T. The role of rigid and flexible bronchoscopy in children. Paediatr Respir Rev. 2011;12(3):190–5.

Niggemann B, Haack M, Machotta A. How to enter the pediatric airway for bronchoscopy. Pediatr Int. 2004;46(2):117–21.

Reilly J, Thompson J, MacArthur C, Pransky S, Beste D, Smith M, Gray S, Manning S, Walter M, Derkay C, Muntz H, Friedman E, Myer CM, Seibert R, Riding K, Cuyler J, Todd W, Smith R. Pediatric aerodigestive foreign body injuries are complications related to timeliness of diagnosis. Laryngoscope. 1997;107(1):17–20.

Reilly BK, Holliday MA, Rock AN, Kang X, Shekhar R, Preciado DA. Three-dimensional direct laryngoscopy and bronchoscopy: enhanced visualization of the airway. JAMA Otolaryngol Head Neck Surg. 2013;139(4):367–70.

Tucker JA, Reilly BK, Tucker ST, Reilly JS. Pediatric otolaryngology in the United States: Chevalier Jackson's legacy for the 21st century. Otolaryngol Head Neck Surg. 2012;146(1):5–7.

Children with Respiratory Failure

17

Juan Andrés Carrasco Orellana
and Andrés Castillo Moya

Contents

Definition

Respiration is the exchange of gases between the organism and the external environment, providing the body with the oxygen (O_2) necessary for aerobic metabolism and removing carbon dioxide (CO_2). This is done through three processes: (1) ventilation, which allows air to reach the alveoli in the areas where there is blood exposed; (2) diffusion, which is the movement of gases (O_2 and CO_2) between the alveolar and capillary walls; and (3) circulation, through which O_2 is distributed to the tissues and the CO_2 resulting from metabolism is removed.

According to this concept, respiratory insufficiency is defined as an alteration in the capacity of the respiratory system to maintain an adequate exchange of oxygen and carbon dioxide, expressed as hypoxemia, with or without hypercapnia. This causes serious dysfunction of other organs, with a consequent risk to life.

Classification

While the respiratory system can be divided into two major functional components (pump and gas exchange components), anatomically it can be divided into at least seven components: (1) the central nervous system, (2) the spinal medulla;

J. A. Carrasco Orellana
Department of Pediatrics, School of Medicine, Universidad del Desarrollo, Santiago, Chile

A. Castillo Moya (✉)
Department of Pediatrics, School of Medicine, Pontificia Universidad Católica de Chile, Santiago, Chile
e-mail: acastill@med.puc.cl

P. Bertrand, I. Sánchez (eds.), *Pediatric Respiratory Diseases*,
https://doi.org/10.1007/978-3-030-26961-6_17

(3) the neuromuscular system; (4) the rib cage and pleura; (5) the upper airway; (6) the cardiovascular system (including hemoglobin); and (7) the lower airway until the alveoli. Normal respiration depends on proper interaction of all of these components, because an alteration in any of them (see Table 17.1) can lead to respiratory insufficiency.

Physiopathology

There are five physiopathological mechanisms that can alter the homeostasis of gases and lead to respiratory insufficiency: (1) an alteration in the alveolar ventilation and pulmonary perfusion ratio (V/Q ratio); (2) a shunt (short circuit); (3) hypoventilation; (4) an alteration in the diffusion of gases in the alveolocapillary membrane; and (5) a decrease in the concentration of inhaled oxygen. The three most important are the V/Q ratio, hypoventilation, and a shunt, with a decrease in inhaled O_2 being considered a minor clinical implication of acute respiratory insufficiency.

Table 17.1 Anatomical classification of types and causes of respiratory insufficiency

Type	Cause
Respiratory drive	
Pharmacological	Drug overdose, anesthesia
Congenital	Central hypoventilation syndrome
Acquired	Cerebrovascular accident
Neuromuscular	
Cervical spinal cord injury	Trauma
Chronic inflammatory demyelinating polyneuropathy	Guillain–Barré syndrome
Anterior horn disease	Poliomyelitis
Phrenic nerve injury	Trauma, cardiac surgery
Muscles of respiration	
Pharmacological	Neuromuscular blocks
Congenital	Hypophosphatemia
Acquired	Kyphoscoliosis, trauma
Rib cage	
Decreased mobility	
Alt. Pleura	
Extrapulmonary restriction	Pneumothorax, pleural effusion
Airway	
Upper airway obstruction	Epiglottitis, foreign body
Lower airway obstruction	Asthma
Increase in dead space	
Increased ventilation/perfusion ratio	Emphysema
Decreased ventilation/perfusion ratio	Acute respiratory distress syndrome
General pulmonary hypoperfusion	Hypovolemia, cardiogenic shock
Localized hypoperfusion	Thromboembolism

Ventilation/Perfusion Alterations

An alteration in the V/Q ratio is the most common cause of arterial hypoxemia. The concentration of O_2 in the alveoli and capillary blood depends on the relative concentrations of inhaled O_2 and unsaturated blood in the pulmonary artery, which is termed the ventilation/perfusion ratio. The same applies to CO_2. While it could be expected that there is an adequate ratio for every alveolar unit, the lung does not act as a multitude of identical gas exchange units; rather, it acts as a multitude of parallel and serial perfusion and ventilation units, which vary, even in healthy individuals, because of age, physical activity, bodily posture, and other factors, with some poorly ventilated but well perfused areas, and other areas that are well ventilated but poorly perfused (Fig. 17.1).

Alveolar oxygen pressure (P_aO_2) is determined by the pressure of inhaled oxygen, the pressure of alveolar carbon dioxide (P_aCO_2), and the respiratory quotient, while P_aCO_2 is determined by alveolar ventilation (V_A) and the range of corporeal CO_2 production. When the pulmonary blood flow of the unit decreases (i.e., the V/Q ratio increases), P_aO_2 and the capillary oxygen pressure approach the partial inhaled oxygen pressure. When the ventilation of the unit decreases (i.e., the V/Q ratio decreases), P_aO_2 and PcO_2 approximate the P_aO_2 of mixed venous blood. In the normal lung, the V/Q ratio ranges between 0/6 and 3.0, concentrated mostly at 1.0. Hypoxemia occurs when perfusion exceeds ventilation—that is, when the V/Q ratio is <1 (Fig. 17.2).

In a person who is breathing spontaneously, there are compensatory mechanisms to correct

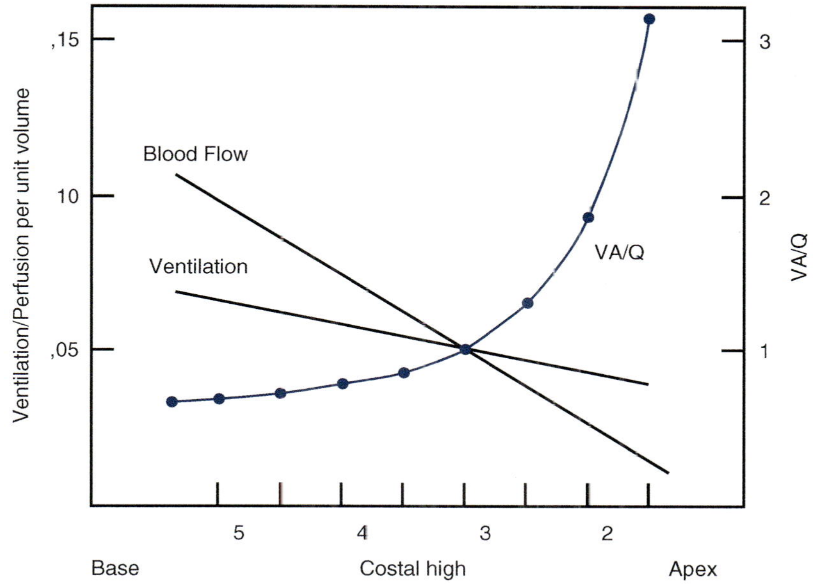

Fig. 17.1 Ventilation distribution, blood flow, and ventilation/perfusion (V/Q) ratio

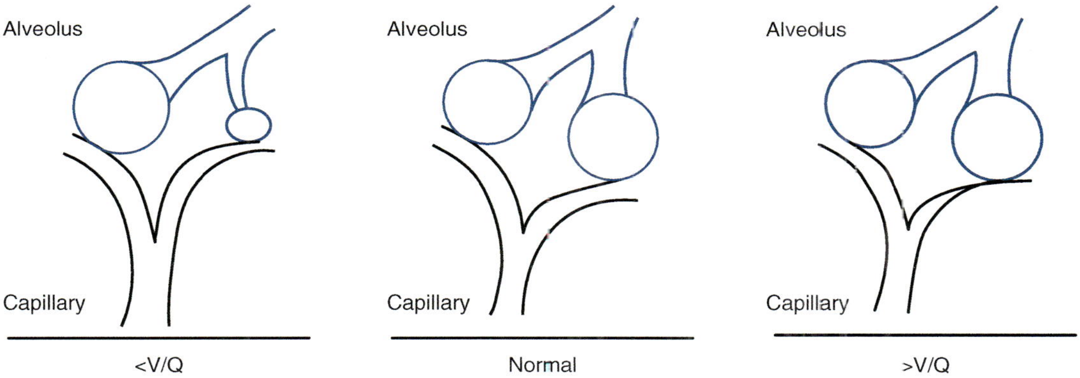

Fig. 17.2 Ventilation/perfusion alteration

hypoxia and/or hypercarbia. In the context of hypoxemia, pulmonary vascular vasoconstriction consists of the alveolar units with better V/Q ratios an excluding those that are poorly ventilated, while the increase in V_A as a response to hypoxia prevents an increase in PcO_2, including lowering it to below normal levels.

Hypoventilation

P_aO_2 is determined by the balance between oxygen provided by V_A (which provides oxygen from inhaled air) and the extraction of oxygen by capillary blood. Consequently, when V_A decreases significantly, P_aO_2 decreases and PcO_2 increases, which are the fundamental characteristics of hypoventilation.

PcO_2 is determined by V_A and the production of CO_2 (VCO_2), multiplied by the K constant, as is seen in the formula $P_aCO_2 = (VCO_2/V_A) \times K$, from which it can be deduced that increased CO_2 production or a decrease in V_A increases P_aCO_2. As the compensatory renal response to hypercarbia is slow (bicarbonate retention), there is an acute fall in arterial pH.

Given that minute ventilation includes both V_A and dead space, its reduction or increase implies an increase or decrease in V_A. The ratio between the decrease in P_aO_2 and the increase in PcO_2 that

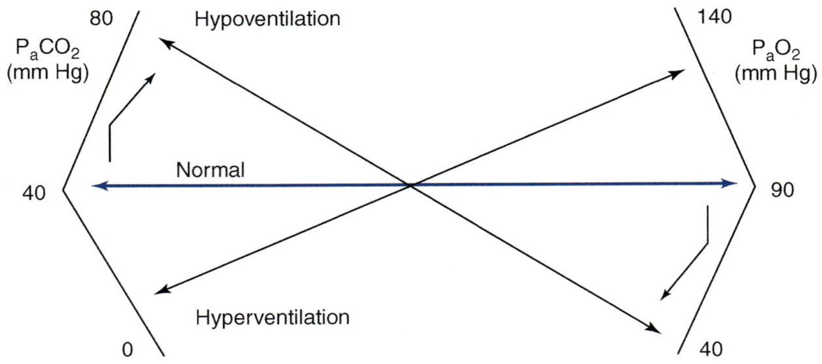

Fig. 17.3 Relationship between arterial P_aO_2 (P_aO_2) and arterial PcO2 (P_aCO_2) with changes in ventilation. An alveolar–arterial difference of stable P_aO_2 and a respiratory change ratio of 0.8 are assumed

occurs in hypoventilation can be calculated by the alveolar gas equation, (P_aO_2 = PIo_2 − (P_aCO_2/R) + F, where PIo_2 is the inhaled oxygen fraction multiplied by barometric pressure, minus water vapor; R is the gas exchange ratio (CO_2 production/oxygen consumption), which is determined by the metabolic state of the tissue; and F is a minimal correction. This formula makes it clear that hypoventilation responds to the contribution of oxygen without necessarily decreasing PcO_2. The effects of the equation at the arterial level can be seen in Fig. 17.3.

Shunting

This is the extreme case in which the V/Q ratio is zero; that is, there are unventilated but perfused alveolar units, so the blood that drains them does not participate in gas exchange, or the blood circulates in an arteriovenous short circuit and does not participate in gas exchange (a cardiac shunt). This can be calculated by comparing the oxygen content in arterial, mixed venous, and pulmonary capillary blood, according to the formula:

$$Qs / Qt = CcO_2 - CaO_2 / CcO_2 - Cvo_2$$

Where Qs is blood flow through the shunt per minute, Qt is total cardiac output per minute, CcO_2 is pulmonary end-capillary O_2 content, CaO_2 is arterial O_2 content and Cvo_2 venous O_2 content.

The percentage of a shunt in a healthy individual is <10%. When it exceeds 30%, it produces hypoxia refractory to the administration of O_2, given that it no longer is in contact with the blood. In contrast, PcO_2 remains constant because of the compensatory increase in minute ventilation caused by hypoxemia.

Clinical Effects

There is a series of anatomical and functional considerations that explain why the incidence of respiratory insufficiency is higher in the pediatric age group, particularly among infants. The difference is found in the extrathoracic airway and the respiratory pump (Table 17.2).

Mild hypoxemia produces few symptoms, although it can be clinically perceptible in the presence of compensatory symptoms. In this way, the patient will initially present tachypnea, tachycardia, arterial hypertension, and sensory restlessness, which can progress from nasal fluttering to use of accessory musculature and active respiration in exhaling, associated with wheezing. Only when the level falls below 40–50 mmHg are any effects on different organs observed, with headaches, sleepiness, compromised awareness, convulsions, and subsequent permanent brain damage. The cardiovascular system, which initially reacts with tachycardia and arterial hypertension, progresses to bradycardia and hypotension, with pulmonary hypertension.

At the tissue level, anaerobic glycolysis begins, with formation of lactic acid and consequent metabolic acidosis. The effects of hypercapnia overlap with those of hypoxia. Cerebral vasodilation produces headaches, increased cerebrospinal fluid

Table 17.2 Anatomical and functional considerations in children

A. Extrathoracic airway	
	Neonates are absolute nasal respirators, so nasal congestion can precipitate significant respiratory distress
	The airway is smaller in infants and young children than in patients ≥ 8 years old
	Infants and young children have larger tonsils in a smaller oropharynx
	The larynx of the infant is more anterior and more cephalic (being positioned at the C3–C4 level) than that of adults (which is positioned at the C6–C7 level)
	The epiglottis is longer and horizontal to the pharyngeal wall
	The subglottic area is smaller and cone shaped, with the narrowest area being the cricoid cartilage
	Adenoid and tonsil tissue can grow considerably in preschool children and schoolchildren, contributing to high airway obstruction
B. Intrathoracic airway	
	Infants and young children have fewer alveoli and thus a smaller gas exchange area
	The alveoli are smaller
	Collateral ventilation is not very developed, facilitating the formation of atelectasis (few pores of Kohn and canals of Lambert)
	Smaller intrathoracic airway
	Less cartilaginous support
C. Respiratory muscle pump	
	Immature respiratory center, with irregular breathing and risk of apnea
	More horizontal ribs with a smaller displaced volume
	Smaller area of interaction between the diaphragm and the thorax
	Less developed musculature
	More compliant thorax, with a greater tendency for deflation, with a decrease in residual capacity in comparison with adults

pressure, and qualitative compromise of consciousness, ranging from restlessness to obtundation.

Diagnosis

Suspicion and early diagnosis are critical, given that lack of treatment can result in respiratory failure, irreversible brain damage, and ultimately cardiorespiratory failure, with all of the associated risks and prognoses. It is also important to have blood gas measurements to determine the level of compromise and the evolution time (the presence or absence of renal compensation, based on bicarbonate levels). The diagnostic criteria for respiratory insufficiency are arbitrary. The most widely accepted one is a partial arterial CO_2 pressure (P_aCO_2) of >50 mmHg or a partial arterial oxygen pressure (P_aO_2) of <60 mmHg in a person breathing ambient air at sea level, which can vary according to the fraction of inspired oxygen (FiO_2), barometric pressure, and the patient's age and prior gasometric condition.

In accordance with the recommendations of the American Heart Association (AHA) for dealing with respiratory insufficiency (Fig. 17.4), rapid assessment of the patient includes a general cardiopulmonary assessment, characterized by an initial impression prior to physical contact with the patient. This general assessment includes three elements: the aspect ("looks well/poorly", muscle tone, and interaction with the environment); respiration (respiratory work, effort, signs of respiratory difficulty); and skin color and temperature (which indicate oxygenation; thus, pallid cyanotic or cold skin indicates inadequate oxygenation). If there are no signs of a life-threatening risk, the team in direct contact with the patient should then carry out a primary ABCDE (airway, breathing, circulation, disability (neurological state), and exposure) assessment and a secondary SAMPLE (signs and symptoms, allergies, medications, past medical history, last oral intake, and events) assessment, which includes the history of the patient.

Treatment Management of respiratory insufficiency begins with the early recognition proposed by this guideline, followed by application of the measures proposed. This chapter discusses the first two steps.

Airway

The airway of the pediatric patient poses inherent anatomical difficulties. In comparison with

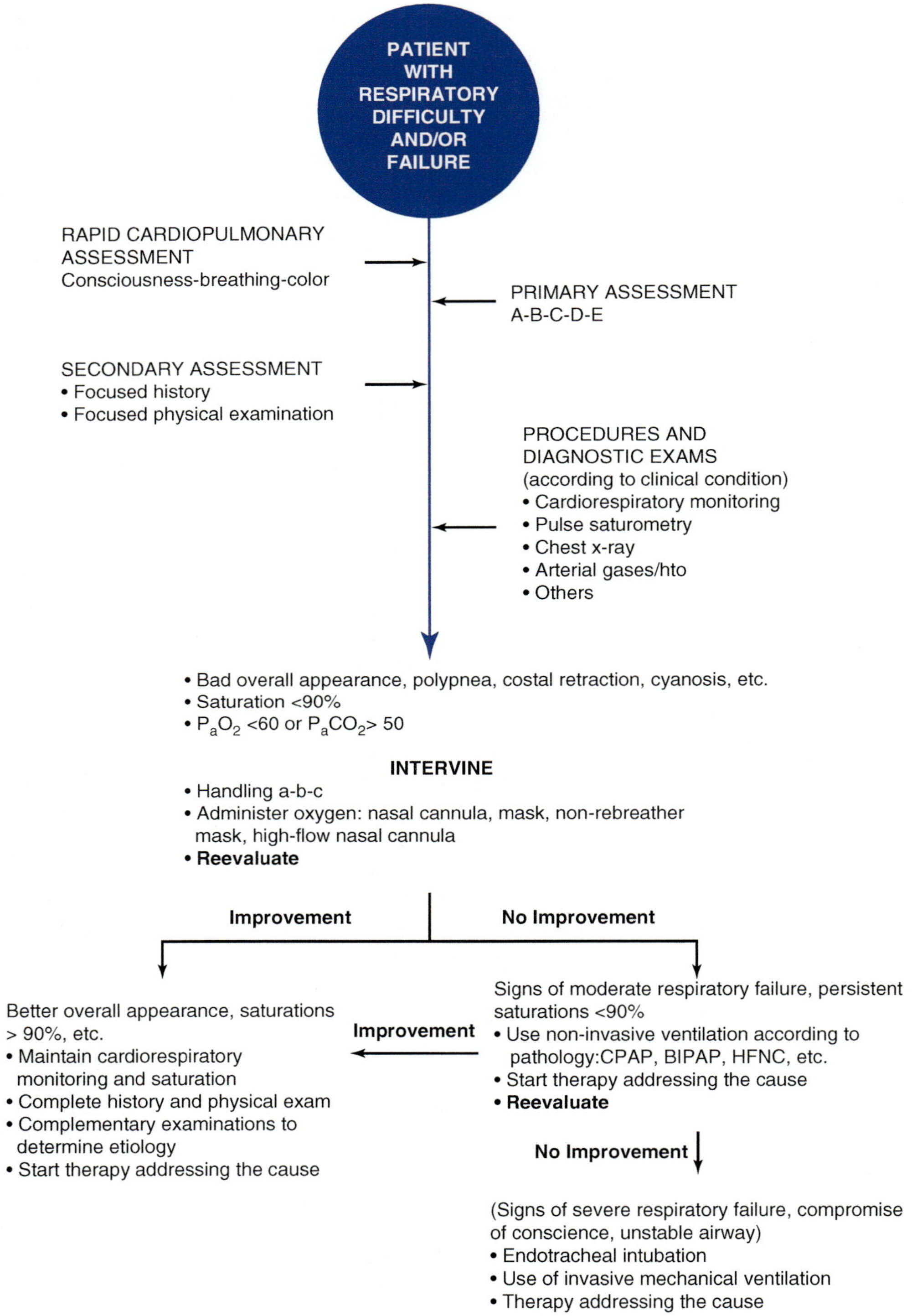

Fig. 17.4 Algorithm for management of respiratory failure

adults, the infant tongue is larger in relation to the mouth, and the larynx is higher, more posterior, and smaller, which means it fills with secretions, blood, or other elements more easily. All of this implies the need for greater care in aligning the airway, without hyperextending it. This involves the technique of elevating the head and chin, leaving the head in a sniffing position. One hand holds the child's head, while the other hand holds his or her chin. The chin is raised, while the head is turned downward and back. This raises the tongue and aligns the pharynx with the larynx, allowing for the entrance of air. Once the airway is open, it is reviewed visually for secretions and other elements. The airway can be categorized as permeable, sustainable, or unsustainable, provided that the necessary elements are available. An endotracheal tube is the element of choice for airway intervention, using the orotracheal route when the patient is unconscious. The correct tube diameter is of utmost importance to avoid damaging the airway. The airway into which the endotracheal tube is inserted should be examined clinically, with observation of chest movements (which should be symmetrical), bilateral auscultation over the armpits (which should also be symmetrical), and auscultation over the epigastrium (which can indicate whether or not the tube is in the trachea). Clinical examination is still the method used for confirmation, but this can also be done with devices such as a colorimetric CO_2 detector, a capnographic exhaled CO_2 detector, and a self-inflating esophageal bulb, which is used in children who weigh ≥20 kg.

Respiration

In relation to respiration, it is important to assess how the patient ventilates and oxygenates; thus, determination of the respiration rate is essential in the assessment. It is important to know the ranges of normal respiratory rates at different ages (Table 17.3). Very high or low and/or irregular rates constitute ominous signs. The state of respiratory mechanics and effort also need to be assessed, including the presence of costal retraction or use of accessory musculature, besides grunting and nasal flaring.

Table 17.3 Respiratory frequency at different ages

Age group	Frequency (breaths per minute)
Infants <1 year	30–60
1–2 years	25–35
Preschool children (2–5 years)	25–30
Schoolchildren	18–30
>12 years	15–20
Adolescents and adults	12–15

With this information, we can determine how air enters, whether there is good thoracic expansion, and whether there are respiratory noises such as a stridor or wheezing. Categorization of the respiratory status and support with oxygen and ventilation equipment have now been implemented. Respiratory compromise can be categorized by the degree of severity in respiratory difficulty and respiratory failure, which are part of a single progression. Respiratory difficulty is characterized by an increased respiratory rate, with signs of respiratory distress: nasal flaring, increased effort, intercostal retraction, etc. Respiratory failure is characterized by an inappropriate rate and effort for the condition of the patient, with poor ventilatory mechanisms and signs of hypoxia: hypoventilation, cyanosis, and gasping. At this level, the state of consciousness is compromised. Oxygen support should be provided once it is available. There have been no comparative studies of different oxygen concentrations, because of which oxygen support is maintained at 100% during resuscitation and is adjusted afterward as necessary. If the patient has a pulse with adequate perfusion, an oximeter can be excellent for monitoring. Ventilatory support is indicated for patients with poor ventilatory mechanics or if there is no spontaneous respiration. Among the ventilation methods, use of a mask and bag is the method of choice. To achieve adequate ventilation, it is important to choose the right mask and bag for the child. The mask should cover the patient's face. If the right mask is not used, it will not be possible to have a good seal that would provide good ventilation. The bags differ in size according to the volume that can be infused with each breath: a bag that is too large puts the safety of the lung at risk, while one that is too small can result in part of the lung collapsing, resulting in hypoventilation and thus not meeting the primary objective. Good ventilation with a bag and a mask is as effective as ventilation with a bag and an endotracheal tube; thus, if experience in intubation is lacking and the objective is achieved with a mask, the process should continue with it. It is common that in stressful situations such as resuscitation, there is a tendency to hyperventilate the patient. Observational studies show that even personnel who are experienced in resuscitation tend to do this.

Hyperventilation leads to an increase in transthoracic pressure with a decrease in venous return, which implies a decrease in cardiac output and, consequently, decreases in coronary and cerebral blood flow, compromising the survival rate. In the absence of cardiac arrest, or in its presence (but with an isolated airway), the objective must be to maintain ventilation of 8–10 breaths per minute in children and adolescents and 12–20 breaths per minute in infants. During ventilation with a bag and mask, it should be remembered that the airway is not isolated; thus, air can pass into the esophagus, with the risk of gastric distension and possible regurgitation. Finally, it should be remembered that the first action when evaluating respiration is to determine if the patient is breathing. This is done by observing if the chest rises and falls, and if breathing sounds can be heard. If the patient is not breathing, the physician should begin basic and then advanced resuscitation.

Once the patient is stabilized, the process to determine the cause of the patient's condition continues and specific treatment begins, concomitantly with the introduction of therapies to improve oxygenation, correction of secondary alterations (metabolic, hemodynamic, etc.), and, depending on the severity, different degrees of ventilatory support to reduce respiratory work, such as a high-flow nasal cannula, noninvasive mechanical ventilation, and, if necessary, invasive ventilation modalities.

Treatments are as varied as the causal pathologies: bronchodilators, steroids, antibiotics, respiratory kinesiology, and others, alone or in different combinations, depending on the triggering pathology. Oxygen therapy is a fundamental therapeutic pillar and, depending on the seriousness of the clinical picture, there are different methods for aiding patients without external ventilatory support, ranging from a nasal cannula to a nonrebreather mask with a reservoir bag. Therapy for support and correction of secondary alterations depends on the degree of compromise associated with the respiratory insufficiency. There are common base acid, electrolyte, and hemodynamic alterations, each of which has specific therapeutic requirements. Finally, another pillar in managing severe respiratory insufficiency is ventilatory support, the purpose of which is to reduce or support the ventilatory function of the patient. As noted, this ranges from noninvasive mechanical support to invasive mechanical ventilation—therapies that are analyzed in other chapters of this book.

Sources

Bateman S, Arnold J. Acute respiratory failure in children. Curr Opin Pediatr. 2000;12:233–7.

Mason RJ, Broaddus VC, Murray JF, Nadel JA. In: 4th, editor. Murray and Nadel's textbook of respiratory medicine. Philadelphia: Saunders; 2005.

Chameides L, Ralston R; American Academy of Pediatrics, American Heart Association. Pediatric advanced life support: provider manual. Dallas: American Heart Association, 2011.

Prodhan P, Noviski N. Pediatric acute hypoxemic respiratory failure: management of oxygenation. J Intensive Care Med. 2004;19:140–53.

Rubenfeld GD. Epidemiology of acute lung injury. Crit Care Med. 2003;31(4 Suppl):S276–84.

Taussig LM, Landau LI. Pediatric respiratory medicine. St. Louis: Mosby; 1999.

Children with Persistent Cough

18

Katalina Bertrán Salinas, Ricardo Saranz, Alejandro Lozano, and José Antonio Castro-Rodríguez

Contents

Definition and General Concepts

Cough is a complex physiological reflex that protects the airway from chemical, mechanical, and thermal injury. It consists of violent expiration with the objective of freeing the airway of secretions and foreign material. Nevertheless, as a result of its chronic evolution or intensity, it can become an annoying symptom that seriously affects the quality of life of the child, interrupting sleep, studies, and sports, and creating anxiety in the family. It is of great clinical use to define cough according to its duration, its association with specific causes, and its response to rationally indicated therapy.

Cough is defined as acute when it lasts for at least 3 weeks and is defined as subacute when it continues for 3–8 weeks. Cough is recurrent when there are more than two episodes per year that are not associated with the common cold and that last for more than 1–2 weeks. Cough is defined as chronic in pediatric patients when it persists for more than 8 weeks. It is not a disease

K. Bertrán Salinas
Department of Pediatrics, Hospital Clínico Universidad Católica de Chile, Santiago, Chile

R. Saranz · A. Lozano
Department of Allergy and Immunology, Faculty of Medicine, Universidad Católica de Córdoba, Córdoba, Argentina
e-mail: aloza@vccor.edu.ar

J. A. Castro-Rodríguez (✉)
Department of Pediatrics, School of Medicine, Pontificia Universidad Católica de Chile, Santiago, Chile

P. Bertrand, I. Sánchez (eds.), *Pediatric Respiratory Diseases*,
https://doi.org/10.1007/978-3-030-26961-6_18

per se; rather, it is a cardinal symptom of numerous respiratory and nonrespiratory pathologies, and it is responsible for a large number of medical consultations. Cough is the reason for 10% of primary health care consultations for schoolchildren and 20% of consultations for preschool children.

Assessment and diagnosis of chronic cough in pediatrics require adequate knowledge of the possible causes. Consequently, correct identification of the cause is a priority for etiological treatment in order to avoid a symptomatic approach with antitussives or expectorants, which most often have disappointing results and pose risks of addiction and negative side effects.

Cough Reflex Anatomy

Key Concepts

1. Cough is an integral part of the defensive system of the respiratory tree, together with mucociliary clearance, alveolar macrophages, and the immune system.
2. The reflexive mechanism of cough is very complex and consists of five components (Fig. 18.1):
   (a) Cough receptors: These are distributed throughout the respiratory tract and extrarespiratory locations: the outer ear, stomach, pericardium, and diaphragm. There are rapid-adaptation irritant receptors (mainly concentrated in the higher-caliber airways on the luminal side of the basal membrane, close to the cilia of the pseudostratified epithelium), mechanical receptors (which are sensitive to changes in the caliber of the airway), and chemical receptors (which are sensitive to gases and smoke).
   (b) Afferent nerves: The afferent tracts reflect their origin in the different locations of the aforementioned receptors. Laryngeal impulses go through the homonymous nerve, while tracheobronchial impulses go through the vagus nerve—the high-velocity myelinated fibers being the most important in mediating centripetal stimulus. The phrenic nerve is responsible for passing a stimulus from the diaphragm and pericardium, and the trigeminal nerve passes a stimulus from the nose and paranasal sinuses to the cough center.
   (c) Medullary center: The integrating center is at the level of the medulla, although its existence is controversial.
   (d) Efferent nerves: The efferent–effector response is transmitted to the expiratory and diaphragmatic muscles by the spinal and phrenic motor nerves and to the larynx by the recurring branches of the vagus nerve. The ends of the parasympathetic nerve system supply the trachea and bronchi, and through their effect of contracting the smooth muscle, they contribute to the effort of cough by narrowing the airway and consequently increasing the velocity of airflow.
   (e) Effector muscles.

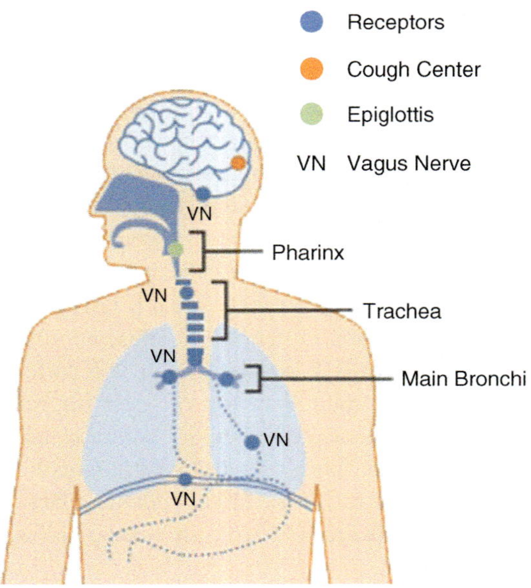

Fig. 18.1 Anatomy of cough

Etiology

Key Concepts

1. The causes of chronic cough in children and adults are different, and within pediatrics they can differ among infants, preschool children, and schoolchildren and adolescents.

2. The etiological spectrum can include one or more coexisting causes.

There are numerous causes of chronic cough as a consequence of the interaction of the mechanisms summarized in Fig. 18.2.

The cause of cough can vary according to age. In infants, cough in early life suggests the presence of congenital anomalies such as a tracheoesophageal fistula, vascular ring, innominate artery, neuromuscular disorders, or other abnormalities or malformations of the airways. Viral infections such as *Chlamydia*, *Bordetella pertussis*, mycobacteria (tuberculosis), and others should not be ignored, nor should the possibility of gastroesophageal reflux (GER), cough-equivalent asthma, or cystic fibrosis.

In preschool children, upper airway cough syndrome (UACS)—including rhinosinusitis, adenoiditis, infection, and inflammation of Waldeyer's lymphatic ring—and the effects of cigarette smoke (passive smoking) are added to the aforementioned range of causes. This is one of the periods of life when the possibility of asthma (cough-variant asthma) is particularly important. Cough caused by inhalation of a foreign body is typically paroxysmal but can be delayed and become chronic. Prolonged bacterial bronchitis, described above, is characterized by chronic productive cough caused by *Moraxella catarrhalis*, *Haemophilus influenzae*, or *Streptococcus pneumoniae*. It produces intense neutrophilic inflammation in the airways and characteristically resolves within 2 weeks of administration of amoxicillin and clavulanic acid or clarithromycin acid.

In schoolchildren and adolescents, postnasal discharge rhinosinusitis (UACS) is the main cause. Cough-equivalent asthma, exacerbated by smoking, and eventually a psychogenic cough, which characteristically calms during sleep, also acquire relevance and should be considered in the differential etiological diagnosis of this frequent symptom. The diagnosis of bronchiectasis should not be overlooked, especially in patients who have suffered severe pneumonia during childhood. Table 18.1 shows the main causes of chronic cough according to pediatric age.

Diagnosis

Key Concepts

1. The clinical history (interview and physical examination) is the fundamental diagnostic pillar.
2. Confirmation of a cause does not necessarily mean that it is responsible for the cough.

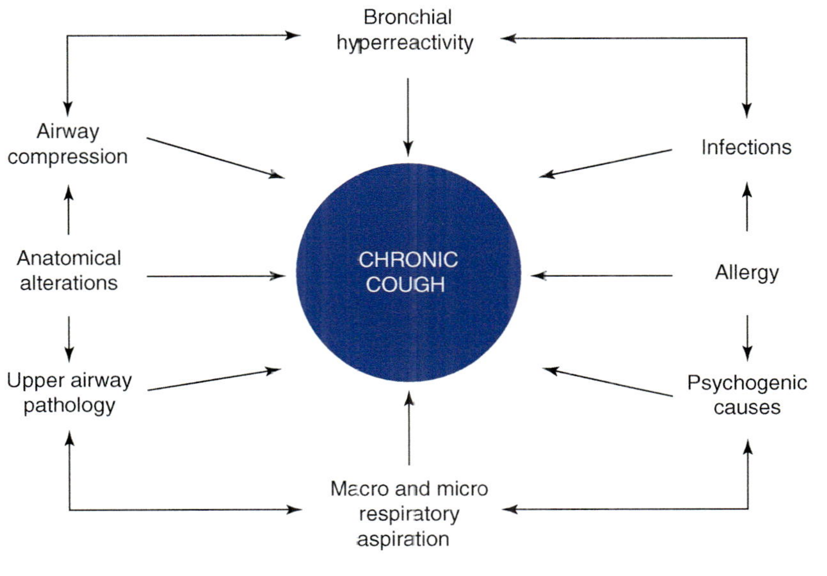

Fig. 18.2 Interaction of etiological factors in chronic cough

Table 18.1 Causes of chronic cough by age

Infant	Preschool	School and adolescence
Congenital anomalies	Infections	Asthma
Tracheoesophageal fistula	Bacterial	Rhinosinusitis
Vascular ring	Viral	Psychogenic
Airway malformation	*Mycoplasma*	Gastroesophageal reflux
Neuromuscular disorders	Tuberculosis	Infections
Infections	Rhinosinusitis	Tuberculosis
Viral	Asthma	*Mycoplasma*
Bacterial	Gastroesophageal reflux	Bronchiectasis
Tuberculosis	Foreign body	Irritative
Chlamydia	Irritative	Environmental pollution
Asthma	Passive smoking	Smoking
Gastroesophageal reflux	Cystic fibrosis	
Cystic fibrosis	Bronchiectasis	

3. The sensitivity, specificity, positive predictive value, and negative predictive value of the different diagnostic methods should be adequately considered.
4. A diagnostic test is accurate only if the cough is resolved with the specific therapy for that diagnosis.
5. Complementary studies should always be supported by the clinical history.

The anamnesis should detect and characterize the time of onset and evolution, type of cough, hourly rhythm, aggravating and triggering factors, production and quality of sputum, and presence of associated symptoms. Orienting signs and the growth and development of the child should be assessed in a detailed physical examination (Table 18.2).

In particular, consideration should be given to infants' neonatal and feeding history, any habits relating to putting foreign objects in the mouth, and the personal and family background in relation to allergies. The pediatrician should review the history of vaccinations, irritants, and allergies at home and the prescribed medications: the dosages, durations of treatment, adherence, and responses to medication. The use of angiotensin-converting enzyme (ACE) inhibitors should be investigated.

Asthma-associated cough is typically nocturnal and exacerbated by cold air, irritants, allergens, and exercise. Cough can be the only manifestation for a long period and can delay a definitive diagnosis. Knowledge of the personal and family history of atopy can be orienting.

Table 18.2 Symptoms and signs associated with specific causes of chronic cough in childhood

Symptom/sign	Possible etiology
Pulmonary auscultatory findings	Asthma, bronchitis, foreign body, aspiration, congenital anomalies, cystic fibrosis
Heart murmur	Heart disease
Chest pain	Asthma, pleurisy
Thoracic deformity	Severe chronic obstructive pulmonary disease
Productive cough	Chronic bronchitis, suppurative lung disease, cystic fibrosis
Nail clubbing	Suppurative lung disease, cystic fibrosis
Dyspnea on exertion/ at rest	Airway or lung parenchymal disease, heart disease
Growth retardation	Severe lung or heart disease, cystic fibrosis
Deglutition disorders	Gastroesophageal reflux, primary aspiration
Immunodeficiency	Suppurative lung disease, atypical infections
Recurrent pneumonia	Immunodeficiency, congenital anomalies of the lung, tracheoesophageal fistula
Fever	Tuberculosis, suppurative lung disease, bacterial bronchitis, other infections
Hemoptysis	Suppurative lung disease, vascular anomalies, bronchitis

This is only a partial list of associated symptoms and signs

A chronic cough associated with purulent expectoration indicates bronchiectasis, suppurative pulmonary, or cystic fibrosis. An association with chronic diarrhea, slow growth, nasal polyposis, and/or nail clubbing provides strong evidence of cystic fibrosis.

Postnasal discharge in children often indicates nasal obstruction and mucopurulent rhinorrhea. Persistent headaches and eventually facial pain and pain around the eyes are symptoms suggestive of sinusitis, while a history of recurrent febrile syndrome, with general malaise and generally productive cough, indicates the need to inquire about contacts and raises suspicion of tuberculosis.

Cough can be linked in aspiration syndromes to regurgitation and choking, and can be exacerbated during or after eating. Occasionally, wheezing and basal crackling can be heard. Finally, psychogenic cough is unproductive, relaxes while the subject is sleeping, and does not improve with antitussive drugs. It is usually diagnosed by a process of elimination.

The pediatrician should carefully consider complementary studies, which will depend on the initial clinical assessment. A chest x-ray is the first indicated study and should be done in almost all cases. It can confirm the existence of an organic pulmonary cause of cough, and it is the guide for an algorithm of subsequent complementary studies. If the chest x-ray is abnormal—for example, if it shows the presence of localized shadows or diffuse infiltrates—more complex imaging techniques, cultures, sputum cytology, and/or diagnostic bronchoscopy should be employed.

In children under 3 years of age, spirometry can contribute to detection of reversible bronchial obstruction, which is compatible with a diagnosis of asthma. If the results are normal, with a strong suspicion of asthma, a bronchial provocation test with either exercise or methacholine, and an airway inflammation study measuring exhaled nitric oxide or induced sputum, are indicated if they are available. The sensitivity and specificity of the method that is employed should be considered in order to optimize the diagnostic utility.

X-rays of the paranasal sinuses offer low diagnostic specificity, but it improves significantly when combined with clinical findings for etiological determination of cough syndromes associated with upper airway pathologies (UACS). Computerized tomography is not generally recommended to assess sinusitis, although it can provide more diagnostic precision.

Rhinopharyngeal assessment can contribute to detection of organic pathologies of the upper airway and provide indirect signs of a laryngopharyngeal reflux that is responsible for cough. An esophagogastroduodenal transit study allows us to study GER, foreign bodies in the esophagus, tracheoesophageal fistulas, and exogenous compressions of the esophagus. GER and/or laryngopharyngeal reflux should be suspected in all cases of cough with an undetermined cause. In this respect, 24-hour esophageal pH monitoring may be useful, although a normal study does not rule out nonacid reflux as a cause of associated cough, which can be detected by impedance measurement.

Allergological assessment (skin tests for immediate detection of allergens, immunoglobulin dosages, etc.) should be reserved for specialist use for proper interpretation.

A study of tuberculin sensitivity is absolutely necessary if epidemiological evidence of tubercular contacts is found, including the entire family if necessary.

Figure 18.3 shows a diagnostic algorithm for chronic cough in pediatrics.

Treatment

Key Concepts

1. The treatment of chronic cough has a greater possibility of success when the precise cause has been identified and is specifically addressed.
2. Before prescribing any symptomatic medication, the pediatrician should perform an exhaustive causal investigation of the symptoms.
3. Analysis of the evidence according to the Grading of Recommendations, Assessment, Development, and Evaluations (GRADE) system supports more precise therapeutic recommendations.

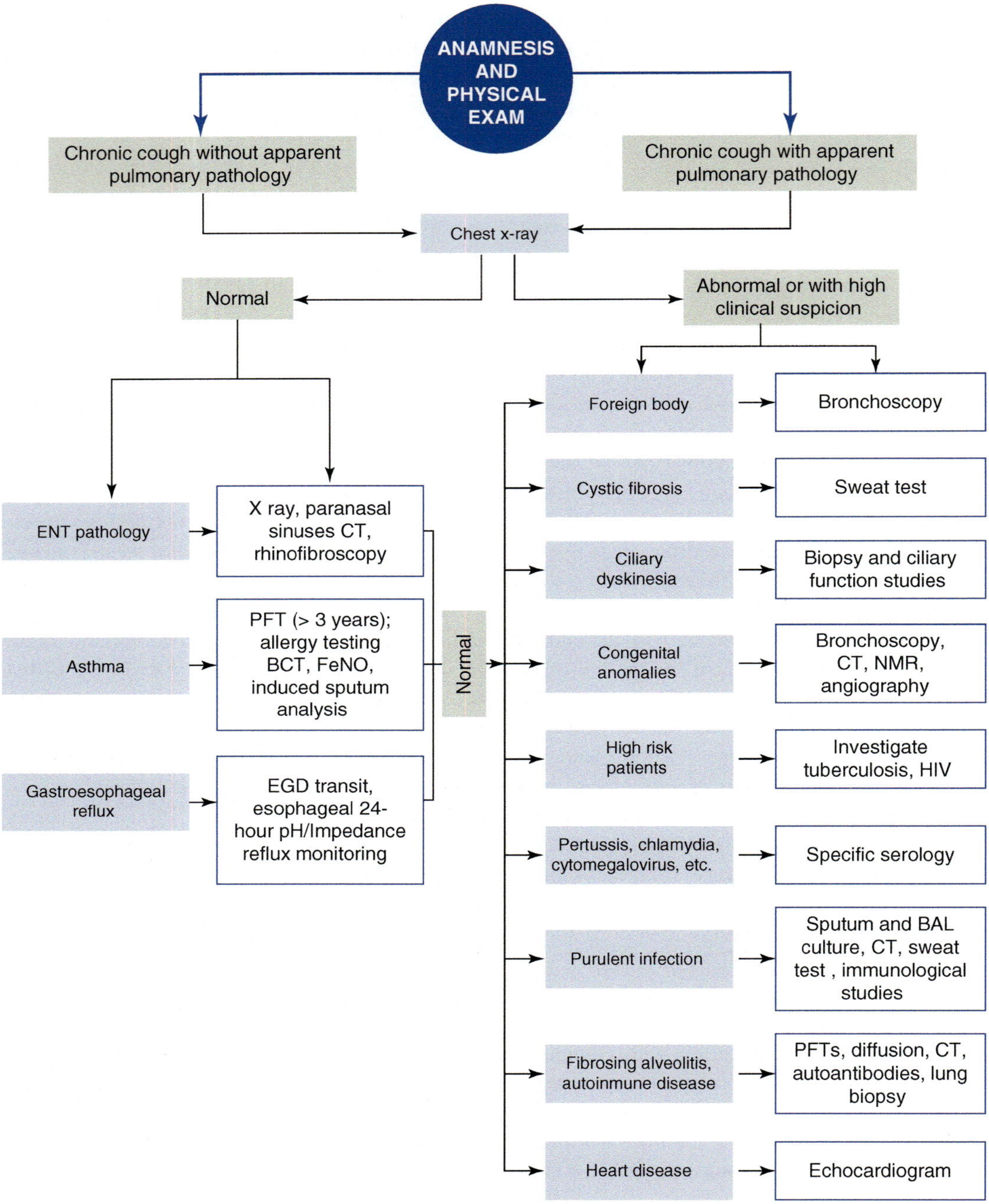

Fig. 18.3 Algorithm suggested for diagnosis of chronic cough in pediatrics. *BAL* bronchoalveolar lavage, *BCT* bronchial challenge test, *CT* computerized tomography, *EGD* esophagogastroduodenal transit, *ENT* ear, nose, and throat, *FeNO* fraction of exhaled nitic oxide, *PFT* pulmonary function test

At the beginning of the twentieth century, Chevalier Jackson said, "The cough is the guard dog of the lungs that protects them from external damage and internal enemies. However, doctors often give us drugs that put the guard dog to sleep just when we need it most." This author considered that cough was a physiological defense mechanism and that doctors of that time were, wrongly, more concerned with treating symptoms than identifying the origins of them; the same occurs today.

The objectives of treating chronic cough can be summarized as follows:

1. Remove the causal agent or irritant.
2. Mobilize and facilitate expectoration.
3. Suppress stimulation of peripheral receptors.
4. Depress the cough center.

Treatment of Chronic Cough with an Identified Cause

1. Chronic cough due to asthma requires treatment with a bronchodilator, antileukotrienes, and/or steroids via inhalers. These treatments should be accompanied by measures to avoid allergens and irritants, such as avoiding cigarette smoke (GRADE recommendation strength: strong).
2. For cough associated with allergic rhinitis, allergens should be avoided, and nasal antihistamines and steroids should be applied (GRADE recommendation strength: weak). If there is bacterial sinusitis, antibiotic therapy is imperative.
3. There is no specific GRADE recommendation for use of a proton pump inhibitor assay in children for 8–12 weeks. Laparoscopic fundoplication is not advised for relief from cough caused by GER.
4. For cough produced by prolonged bacterial bronchitis, antibiotic therapy with amoxicillin and clavulanic acid or clarithromycin is useful for 2–6 weeks (GRADE recommendation strength: strong). Antituberculosis therapy should be given in response to a confirmed diagnosis of tuberculosis. The most common viral causes of respiratory infection are generally not self-limited.
5. Psychogenic cough requires detailed exploration of the family situation and dynamics, and of stressful aspects of the family and school environments. This can require the involvement of a psychologist.
6. For any type of cough, smoking cessation by the parents (where applicable) carries the strongest GRADE recommendation.

Chronic Cough Without an Identified Cause: Is Symptomatic Treatment Useful?

Key Concepts

1. The cause of cough can sometimes not be determined, or it can present prejudicial effects such as chest pains, fatigue, vomiting, headaches, or disturbed sleep, making symptomatic treatment necessary.
2. Nonspecific therapy tends to provide relief from symptoms when the cough does not serve any physiological reason (such as irritative, dry, and prolonged postviral cough) or to avoid these complications or pernicious effects.
3. Productive cough should not be suppressed, given that retention of secretions can prolong the base disease and the consequent symptoms.
4. Many therapeutic combinations used in symptomatic treatment of cough (antitussives and mucolytics) do not make sense, given that their components have contradictory effects, as well as toxic and addictive side effects.

The practice of "observe, wait, and review" is strongly recommended to avoid unnecessary medication, given that the benefit of such medication generally does not exceed that of a placebo, and because in a high percentage of cases, nonspecific cough resolves spontaneously.

1. Antitussive drugs: There is a wide variety of commercial antitussive drugs, which are classified according to their site of action. Narcotic and non-narcotic centrally acting agents depress the integrating medullar reflex center, while peripherally acting agents depress or anesthetize the receptors where the cough reflex originates.

2. Centrally acting antitussives are most widely used. Codeine, a narcotic antitussive par excellence, is one of the most potent cough suppressants and has addictive effects. It is usually well tolerated but can provoke drowsiness, dizziness, symptoms of digestive intolerance, and a dry mouth. It is contraindicated in all guidelines.
3. Synthetic derivatives of codeine and morphine, such as oxycodone and hydrocodone, can be found in many preparations. They are highly effective but can have the same side effects as their parent drugs. There are strong GRADE recommendations against their use in all cases.
4. Dextromethorphan is one of the most important non-narcotic antitussive agents. Acting at the central level, it appears to be as potent as codeine. It is better tolerated but can sometimes have unwanted gastrointestinal effects, although the recommended dose does not produce the types of sedative and respiratory depressant effects that often accompany codeine. Dextromethorphan is rarely addictive. Noscapine, chlophedianol (clofedanol), clofedianol, clobutinol, oxeladin, and butamirate complete the list of non-narcotic antitussives recommended for children over 6 years of age.
5. Mucolytic and expectorant drugs: These liquefy mucus, reduce retention of secretions, and increase mucociliary clearance, because of which they are used in patients who have difficulties in expectorating abnormally viscous secretions.

Guaifenesin and iodine compounds are present in several commercial preparations, but as iodine-containing drugs they carry the risk of causing hypothyroidism, skin rashes, and mouth infections. More modern drugs such as bromhexine and ambroxol are available in our pharmacopoeia, but their effectiveness does not exceed the mean range of the other drugs mentioned above. As a mucolytic agent, N-acetylcysteine interferes with disulfide bonds in the mucus, reducing its viscosity. However, these drugs can increase bronchial hyperresponsiveness. GRADE strongly recommends minimizing the use of mucolytics and demulcents.

Despite these warnings—and although symptomatic cough medicines are not recommended by the American Academy of Pediatrics and the US Food and Drug Administration (FDA) did not approve their use in children under 4 years of age in 2008—they continue to be the drugs most commonly prescribed by doctors and consumed by patients.

Advantages of Managing Chronic Cough with Diagnostic–Therapeutic Algorithms

The clinical performance of chronic cough management is improved by incorporation of a standardized diagnostic–therapeutic sequence. The more rapidly an algorithm is applied, the sooner the problem is resolved and the sooner the quality of life of the patient is improved. Chang et al. (2013) conducted a multicenter study to test the hypothesis that management of chronic cough in children according to an evidence-based algorithm is feasible and improves clinical outcomes (Fig. 18.4). Two groups, with early use and late use, were compared with the aid of the algorithm shown in the figure. The percentage of cough-free children at 6 weeks (the primary outcome) was significantly higher ($p < 0.0001$) in the early use group (54.3%) than in the late use group (29.5%). The absolute reduction in risk among the intention-to-treat groups was 24.7% (95% confidence interval (CI) 13–35), with an NNT of 4 during a 6 week period (95% CI 3–8). In effect, 85% of the diagnoses were made following this protocol, without the need for specialized investigation, showing that standardized management of chronic cough leads to improved results in practice.

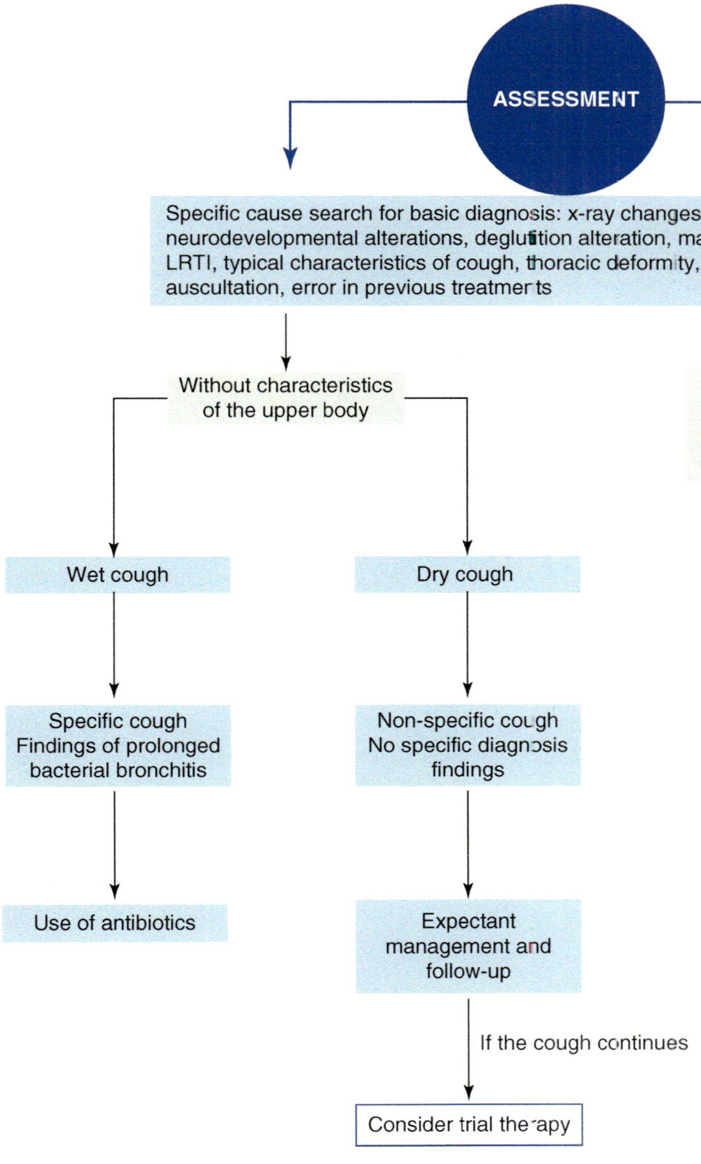

Fig. 18.4 Algorithm for diagnostic and therapeutic management of chronic cough. *CSLD* chronic suppurative lung disease. (Adapted from Chang et al. 2013)

Conclusion

1. Cough is a cardinal symptom of numerous respiratory and nonrespiratory diseases. In pediatrics, cough is defined as chronic when it persists for more than 8 weeks, and chronic cough requires an ordered and precise diagnosis.
2. A careful and exhaustive anamnesis and physical examination are fundamental pillars of the diagnosis.
3. The etiological spectrum is different in children and adults, with consequent therapeutic implications.
4. The causes of chronic cough in childhood vary with age. The most common causes are cough syndrome related to upper airway

pathologies, cough-variant asthma, and prolonged bacterial bronchitis.

5. The exact etiological identification should be followed by specific treatment. If this does not prove effective, the following should be considered:
   (a) The cause is partially identified and undertreated.
   (b) The diagnosis is incorrect.
   (c) The treatment is not appropriate.
   (d) The patient is not compliant with the treatment.
6. Symptomatic therapy is necessary in rare instances if the cause is properly determined. Treatment with antitussives, mucolytics, and expectorants is often disappointing. It has undesirable side effects and should be considered for use only as an adjuvant in the case of an "irritating" cough that does not respond to a demonstrable cause, or used as a complement to a specific therapy.
7. New symptomatic therapies are being developed with specific effects on peripheral receptors and channels involved in the cough reflex and in the modulation of the sensorial peptides of the respiratory tract. These therapies are opening promising new fields of treatment for cough.

Sources

Asiloy S, Bayram E, Agin H, Apa H, Can D, et al. Evaluation of chronic cough in children. Chest. 2008;134:1122–8.

Chang AB, Glomb WB. Guidelines for evaluating chronic cough in pediatrics: ACCP evidence-based clinical practice guidelines. Chest. 2006;129:260–83.

Chang AB, Lasserson TJ, Kiljander TO, Connor FL, Gaffney JT, Garske LA. Systematic review and meta-analysis of randomized controlled trials of gastro-oesophageal reflux interventions for chronic cough associated with gastro-oesophageal reflux. BMJ. 2006;332:11–7.

Chang AB, Redding GJ, Everard ML. Chronic wet cough: protracted bronchitis, chronic suppurative lung disease and bronchiectasis. Pediatr Pulmonol. 2008;43:519–31.

Chang AB, Robertson CF, van Asperen PP, Glasgow NJ, Masters IB, Teoh L, Mellis CM, Landau LI, Marchant JM, Morris PS. A cough algorithm for chronic cough in children: a multicenter, randomized controlled study. Pediatrics. 2013;131:e1576–83.

Chow PY. Chronic cough in children. Singap Med J. 2004;45(10):462–8.

de Jongste JC, Shields MD. Cough 2: chronic cough in children. Thorax. 2003;58:998–1003.

Ali M. Laryngopharyngeal reflux: diagnosis and treatment of a controversial disease. Curr Opin Allergy Clin Immunol. 2008;8:28–33.

Gibson PG, Chang AB, Glasgow NJ, Holmes PW, Katelaris P, Kemp AS, et al. CICADA: cough in children and adults: diagnosis and assessment. Australian cough guidelines summary statement. Med J Aust. 2010;192:265–71.

Goldsobel AB, Chipps BE. Cough in the pediatric population. J Pediatr. 2010;156:352–8.

Irwin RS. Chronic cough due to gastroesophageal reflux disease: ACCP evidence-based clinical practice guidelines. Chest. 2006;129:80S–94S.

Marchant JM, Masters IB, Taylor SM, Chang AB. Utility of signs and symptoms of chronic cough in predicting specific cause in children. Thorax. 2006;61:694–8.

Marchant JM, Newcombe PA, Juniper EF, Sheffield JK, Stathis SL, Chang AB. What is the burden of chronic cough for families? Chest. 2008;134:303–9.

Pratter MR. Chronic upper airway cough syndrome secondary to rhinosinus diseases (previously referred to as postnasal drip syndrome). ACCP evidence-based clinical practice guidelines. Chest. 2006;129:63S–71S.

Ramanuja S, Kelkar P. Habit cough. Ann Allergy Asthma Immunol. 2009;102:91–5.

Rank MA, Kelkar P, Oppenheimer JJ. Taming chronic cough. Ann Allergy Asthma Immunol. 2007;98:305–13.

Saranz RJ, Lozano A, Lozano N, Castro Rodríguez JA. Diagnóstico y tratamiento de la tos crónica en pediatría. Arch Arg Pediatr. 2013;111(2):140–7.

Schaefer MK, Shehab N, Cohen AL, Budnitz DS. Adverse events from cough and cold medications in children. Pediatrics. 2008;121:783–7.

Schroeder K, Fahey T. Over-the-counter medications for acute cough in children and adults in ambulatory settings. Cochrane Database Syst Rev. 2008;1:CD001831.

Shields MD, Bush A, Everard ML, McKenzie S, Primhak R, et al. Recommendations for the assessment and management of cough in children. Thorax. 2008;63(Suppl III):iii1–iii15.

Infants with Persistent Tachypnea

19

Pablo Bertrand and Ana Moya Olivares

Contents

Definition

Tachypnea is an increased respiratory rate above the reference value for the patient's age. This clinical sign is extremely useful and forms part of the basic vital signs necessary for good clinical assessment of a child. The respiratory rate changes over the course of childhood and, on the basis of curves by age, it is possible to characterize a physiological decrease and narrowing of the dispersion range as the child grows toward adolescence (O'Leary et al.).

In newly emerging conditions, tachypnea is a symptom in the course of a clinical picture with or without respiratory symptoms. It can result from physiological phenomena such as fear, anxiety, crying, and exercise, as well as being influenced by organic causes such as pain, fever, neurological alterations, or metabolic alterations. Above all, it is a good indicator of respiratory illness. Tachypnea is defined as persistent when it continues for more than a month as the main symptom in an infant who has overcome the original cause of the condition. The respiratory rate that qualifies as tachypnea depends on the age of the patient, as defined by the World Health Organization (Table 19.1).

Table 19.1 Tachypnea according to the World Health Organization

Patient age	Respiratory rate (respirations per minute)
Newborn	>60
2–12 months	>50
1–5 years	>40

P. Bertrand (✉) · A. Moya Olivares
Department of Pediatrics, School of Medicine, Pontificia Universidad Católica de Chile, Santiago, Chile
e-mail: pbertrand@med.puc.cl

P. Bertrand, I. Sánchez (eds.), *Pediatric Respiratory Diseases*,
https://doi.org/10.1007/978-3-030-26961-6_19

Respiration Control Mechanisms

Respiration begins in the nervous system by means of centers located in the brain stem (which automatically command every inhalation–exhalation cycle) but is influenced by voluntary cortical control.

Most of the time, respiration is under the control of the automatic respiratory center, which can alter respiration to meet the metabolic demand, activating the respiratory system in a highly sensitive manner by a system of negative feedback in response to the partial pressures of oxygen and carbon dioxide (PaO_2 and $PaCO_2$) and the pH. The ventilatory response to hypoxemia emerges when PaO_2 values reach 50–60 mmHg, when the afferent influence of peripheral chemoreceptors (especially carotid bodies) on the regulatory center increases. The ventilatory response increases significantly when there is a slight concomitant increase in $PaCO_2$ values (42–48 mmHg) and follows a logarithmic curve as PaO_2 decreases. The ventilatory response to hypercapnia is determined by a rapid response at the central level, where the $PaCO_2$ of the cerebrospinal liquid, which is in balance with the blood because of its capacity to easily diffuse through the blood–brain barrier, stimulates the central chemoreceptors linearly (Fig. 19.1). Parallel to this, ventilation increases along with a rise in the concentration of hydrogen ions of between 20 and 60 nEq/L, whether they are of respiratory or metabolic origin. If the respiratory system is in a condition to respond to the stimuli of hypoxemia and hypercarbia, the increase in alveolar ventilation improves $PaCO_2$ levels, which significantly decreases the afferent influence of carotid chemoreceptors in the respiration process (Fig. 19.2).

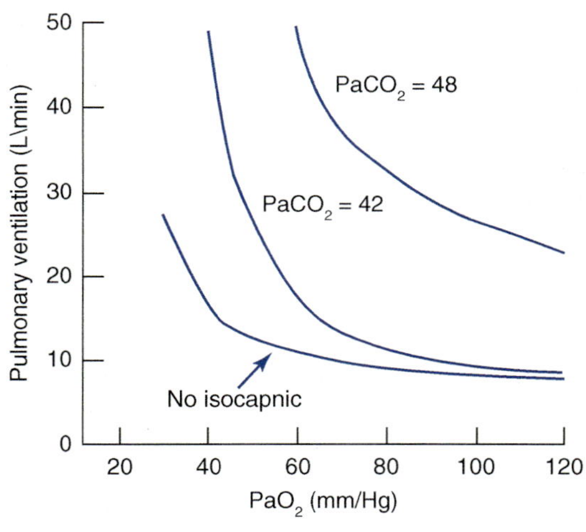

Fig. 19.1 Respiratory response to partial pressure of O_2 (PaO_2)

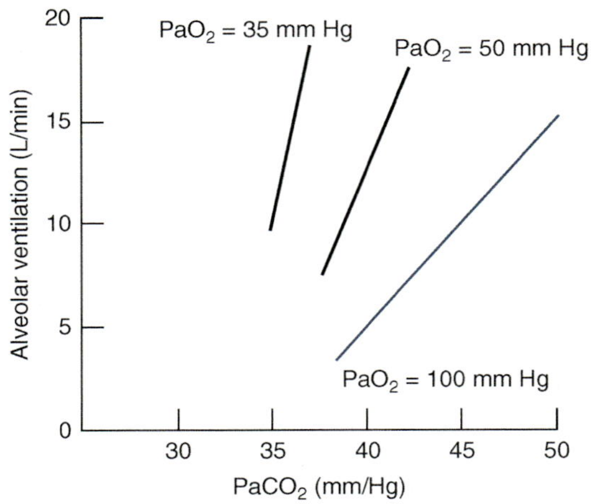

Fig. 19.2 Respiratory response to partial pressure of CO_2 ($PaCO_2$)

The respiratory cycle is influenced by afferent receptors of diverse voluntary and involuntary respiratory control mechanisms, such as the reflexes of the lungs and respiratory tract, the cardiovascular system, and the reflexes of stretched muscles and articulations. Moreover, the respiratory cycle is influenced by higher centers such as the hypothalamus and areas of the cerebral cortex that take control over the automatic system when we speak, cry, or laugh.

Etiology

Assessment of persistent tachypnea requires adequate knowledge of the possible causes. Identification of the probable etiology is necessary to appropriately deal with and manage the condition. Once the influences of fever, crying, and pain on the respiratory rate have been assessed, it is important to determine the respiratory and nonrespiratory causes of tachypnea in infants (Table 19.2).

Table 19.2 Organic causes of tachypnea

Respiratory causes	Nonrespiratory causes
Hypoxemia (persistent pneumonia, bronchopulmonary dysplasia, pulmonary aspiration, hemorrhage, alveolar proteinosis, interstitial pneumonitis) Trauma (pneumothorax, rib cage fracture, interstitial emphysema) Pulmonary edema Pulmonary hypertension Pulmonary embolism Pleural effusion	Psychogenic (anxiety, irritability) Metabolic (acidosis, liver failure) Poisoning (salicylates, methylxanthines) Central nervous system (tumors, infections) Cardiovascular (cardiac insufficiency) Miscellaneous (fever, pain, sepsis)

Diagnosis

The history of the course of tachypnea is essential for a diagnostic approximation. It is necessary to characterize the initial symptoms and the evolution over time, the type of respiration, aggravating and triggering factors, and associated symptoms. A rapid general assessment is recommended prior to a physical examination, observing the appearance, respiratory work, and circulation to determine whether the phenomenon is potentially serious or not. In the physical examination, it is imperative to observe respiratory patterns: the rate, rhythm, efforts, and associated respiratory sounds. The respiratory rate should be determined over a minute, ideally with the subject at rest and in the most comfortable position for him or her.

The breathing rate increases with fever by 5–7 rpm (respirations per minute) for every degree over 37 °C, with metabolic acidosis. In the assessment of small children, consideration should be given to the significant changes that occur in the respiratory rhythm, including periodic respiration, which can reach up to 20% of the time in newborns, but in infants over 3 months old, this is clearly abnormal and suggests neurological disease. Cheyne–Stokes breathing is not a common finding in children, but it can appear with congestive cardiac insufficiency or intracranial hypertension. Most often, tachypnea is related to hypoxemia, because of which the examining physician should look for signs of increased respiratory effort, which may be indicative of the physiopathological situation. In this scenario, in which a small child is not able to communicate his or her respiratory difficulty or dyspnea, the examining physician should look for nasal flaring, retraction of the thoracic wall, use of accessory musculature, and/or paradoxical movement, as well as determining if there is asymmetry in the rib cage. Tachypnea is sometimes not associated with significant respiratory symptoms or signs, and it constitutes a clinical challenge.

Requests for tests depend on the initial diagnostic suspicion. When a disease of respiratory origin is suspected, a chest x-ray is the first-line examination to determine whether there is an organic cause of the tachypnea, as occurs with atypical pneumonia, pneumothorax, and x-ray patterns for interstitial diseases. A chest x-ray is also indicated to search for heart disease when there is cardiomegaly or pulmonary congestion that suggests heart insufficiency. In this scenario, it is recommended to perform an echocardiogram for a more complete assessment of the cardiological situation. Immunofluorescence and polymerase chain reaction tests are very useful in identifying viral or bacterial etiology. An abnormal chest x-ray indicates that the study must be complemented by axial computerized tomography (CT) of the helical thorax to better classify images suggesting chronic lung damage, interstitial disease, malformations, or a pulmonary embolism. When tachypnea appears to be attributable to nonrespiratory causes, the x-ray investigations are directed according to the suspicion. Respiratory patterns such as acidotic or Kussmaul respiration provoke significant metabolic acidosis, making it necessary to conduct arterial gas analysis and a biochemical profile that includes glycemia, creatinine, and hepatic tests. When tachypnea of a central origin is suspected, the investigations should be complemented with axial CT scanning of the brain to rule out brain or cerebellar tumors and malformations of the central nervous system. In the case of suspicion of infection, it is important to perform a lumbar puncture.

Figure 19.3 shows a proposed algorithm for diagnostic study.

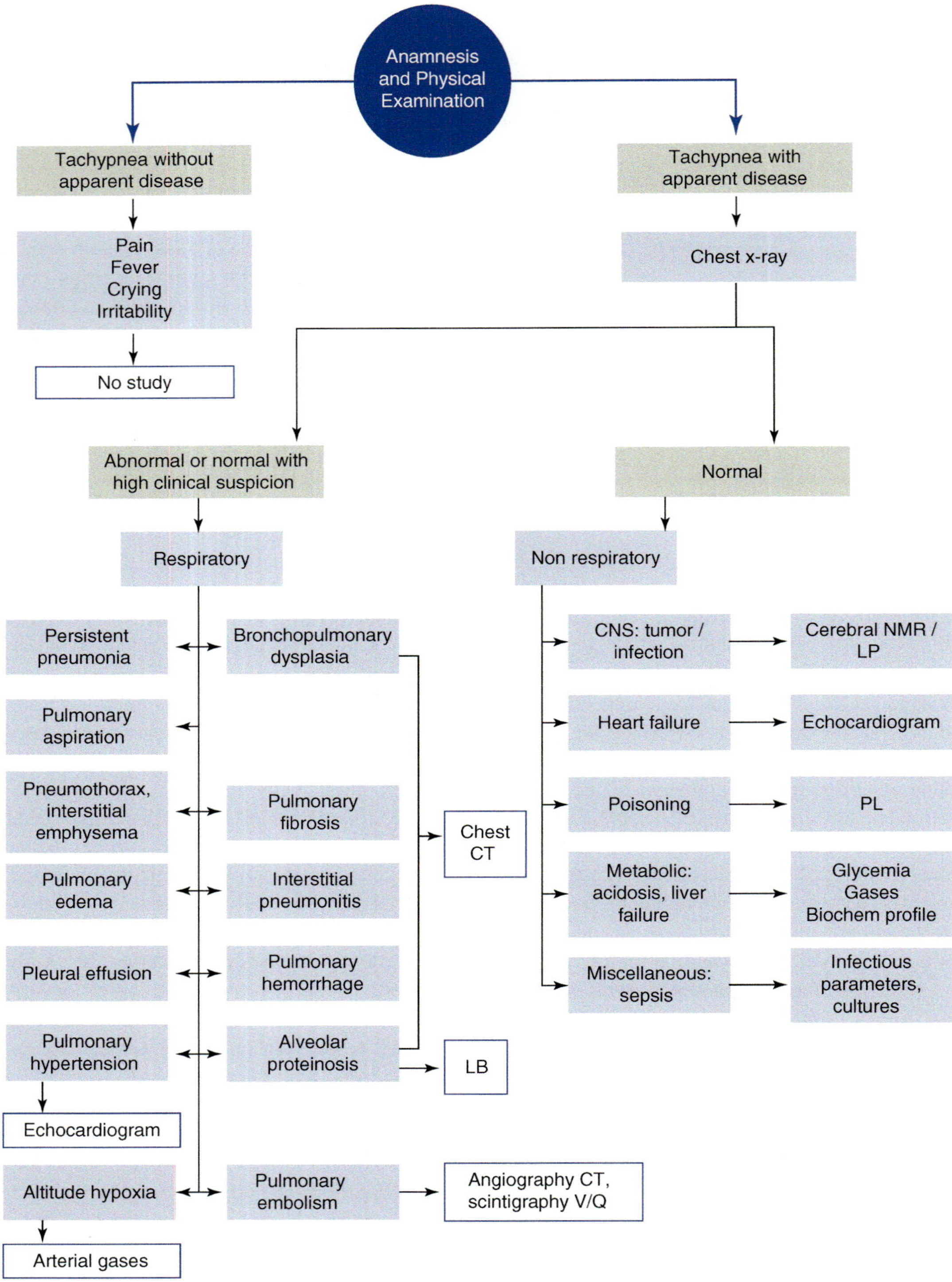

Fig. 19.3 Algorithm for study of persistent tachypnea. *Biochem* biochemical, *CT* computerized tomography, *LB* lung biopsy, *LP* lumbar puncture, *NMR* nuclear magnetic resonance, *PL* plasma levels

Sources

Bloomfield D. Tachypnea. Ped Rev. 2002;23:294–5.

Chernick V, Boat T, Wilmott R, Bush A, Deterding R, Ratjen F. Kendig and Chernick's disorders of the respiratory tract in children. 8th ed. Filadelfia, PA: Elsevier; 2012.

De Groot EP. Review breathing abnormalities in children with breathlessness. Paediatr Respir Rev. 2011;12:83–7.

Dijk F, Curtin J, Lord D, Fitzgerald DA. Pulmonary embolism in children. Paediatr Resp Rev. 2012;13:112–22.

Kossowsky J, Wilhelm F, Schneider S. Responses to voluntary hyperventilation in children with separation anxiety disorder: implications for the link to panic disorder. J Anxiety Disord. 2013;27:627–34.

Levitzky M. Pulmonary physiology. 8th ed. New York: McGraw-Hill; 2013.

O'Leary F, Hayen A, Lockie F, Peat J. Arch Dis Child. 2015;100:733.

Palafox M, Guiscafré H, Reyes H, Muñoz O, Martínez H. Diagnostic value of tachypnoea in pneumonia defined radiologically. Arch Dis Child. 2000;82:41–5.

Perpiñá M. Síndrome de hiperventilación y asma. Arch Bronconeumol. 2004;40 Suppl 3:6–10.

Rothrock G, Green S, Fanelli JM, et al. Do published guidelines predict pneumonia in children presenting to an urban ED? Pediatr Emerg Care. 2001;17:240–3.

Taylor J. Beccaro M, Dune S, et al. Establishing clinically relevant standards for tachypnea in febrile children younger than two years. Arch Pediatr Adolesc Med. 1995;149:283–7.

Children with Persistent Stridor

20

Solange Caussade Larraín
and Carlos Flores Berríos

Contents

Definition

Stridor is the main symptom or sign of obstruction of the upper airway. It can be congenital or acquired, and acute or chronic. The latter is a form that persists for more than 4 weeks. It is defined as a high-pitched (>500 Hz) musical respiratory sound and is predominantly inspiratory. Stridor that is solely inspiratory suggests obstruction of the extrathoracic airway. Fixed lesions of the extrathoracic airway are manifested by a biphasic stridor. When airflow decreases because of a severe obstruction of the airway, stridor can disappear.

Epidemiology

Obstruction of the upper airway is more common in children than in adults because children have a greater risk of infections and their anatomical features differ from those of adults.

The incidence of stridor in the general pediatric population is unknown. Acute conditions are usually the result of inflammation or infection, and chronic conditions are due to anatomical or pathological alterations. The most common cause of acute stridor in preschool children is viral laryngotracheobronchitis (LTB), which has been identified

S. Caussade Larraín (✉)
Department of Pediatrics, School of Medicine, Pontificia Universidad Católica de Chile, Santiago, Chile

C. Flores Berríos
Department of Pediatrics, Hospital de Ovalle, Ovalle, Chile

P. Bertrand, I. Sánchez (eds.), *Pediatric Respiratory Diseases*,
https://doi.org/10.1007/978-3-030-26961-6_20

Table 20.1 Causes of chronic stridor

Cause
Laryngomalacia
Vocal cord paralysis
Congenital or acquired congenital stenosis
Laryngeal cleft
Laryngeal membrane
Subglottic hemangioma
Laryngeal papillomatosis
Cysts and laryngoceles
Laryngeal condylomatosis
Proximal tracheomalacia
Foreign body

in Chilean and international endoscopic studies as the cause of 40–70% of stridors. With endoscopic studies, it has been possible to determine the association of two or more airway anomalies in 10–50% of patients with congenital stridor.

Table 20.1 lists the causes of chronic stridor.

Applied Physiopathology

Stridor is related to the anatomy of the central airway and airflow dynamics. There is a natural anatomical division of the airway at the level of the glottis or vocal cords. However, from the physiological point of view, the central airway is composed of an extrathoracic part (the nose, nasopharynx, larynx, and upper part of the trachea) and an intrathoracic part (the rest of the trachea and the bronchi). The thorax meets the neck at the level of the first dorsal vertebra, the first ribs, and the sternal manubrium.

The upper airway in children, and especially in infants, is funnel shaped and has a smaller diameter than that in adults; the tongue is proportionally larger, the location of the larynx is closer to the brain and to the anterior section, the tissues are more lax, and there is greater cartilaginous flexibility of the support structures. The cricoid cartilage is the narrowest airway segment in infants and preschool children, while the narrowest segment in newborns is the nose. In schoolchildren, the narrowest airway segment is the vocal cords.

There are two physical principles that play a role in generating stridor. The first is Poiseuille's law of fluid dynamics, which shows a direct proportional relationship between resistance (R), fluid viscosity (η), and the length of the tube (L), and a proportional inverse relationship to the fourth power of the radius (r^4) of the tube:

$$R = 8\eta L / \pi r^4$$

According to this formula, a 50% decrease in the radius increases airflow resistance by 16 times and consequently produces a notable decrease in airflow. When the lumen of the airway is reduced, the velocity of the flow increases and induces the Bernoulli effect, which establishes that when the air velocity increases, the pressure exerted by the airflow in the lumen decreases and, in this case, facilitates the collapse of the airway. Finally, stridor is produced by distortions of the laminar flow and turbulence, with a vibratory effect on the adjacent tissue.

The diaphragm descends during inspiration; the ribs ascend and are in a horizontal position, generating negative pressure within the chest cavity and the airway. The structures that surround the extrathoracic airway are at atmospheric pressure, and so a pressure gradient is created that compresses this segment of the airway during inspiration. Stridor is produced when the airway is collapsible or is partially obstructed (for example, in patients with laryngomalacia or laryngitis, respectively).

The most common cause of chronic stridor in infants is laryngomalacia, located anatomically in the extrathoracic and supraglottic region. This can include a tubular and collapsible epiglottis, with redundant supra-arytenoid and/or short arytenoepiglottic folds, which anatomically and/or dynamically impede the passage of air (as a result of collapse of the supraglottic structures during inspiration) (Fig. 20.1). Viral laryngotracheal bronchitis fundamentally affects the subglottic space, and stridor can be solely inspiratory or biphasic, according to the severity of the obstruction (Fig. 20.2). The subglottic region is formed by cricoid cartilage, which is the only complete cartilage in the airway and is the narrowest part of the larynx in infants and preschoolers. Because it is a rigid area, it facilitates significant obstruction of the airway.

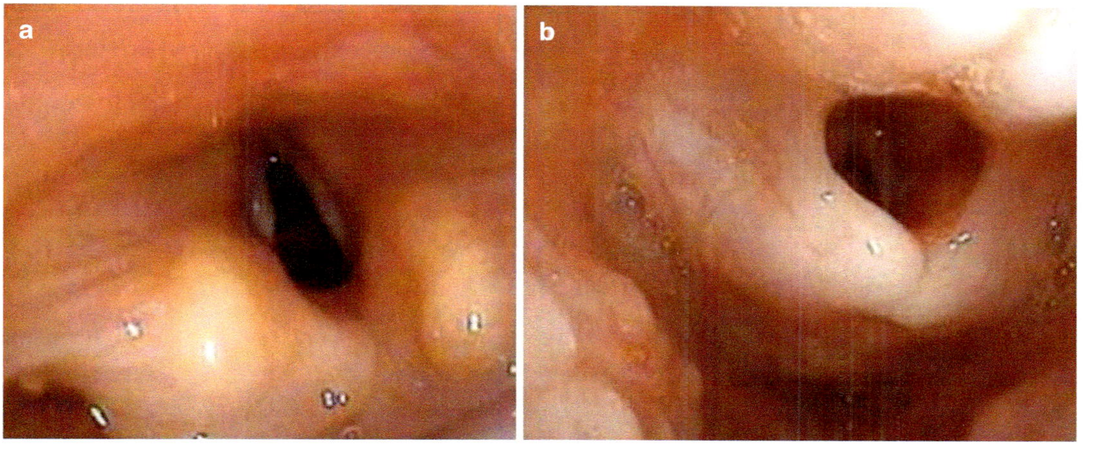

Fig. 20.1 Laryngomalacia. On expiration (**a**), redundant mucosa is visible. On inspiration (**b**), the arytenoids partially obstruct the lumen and the epiglottis collapses in a cross direction

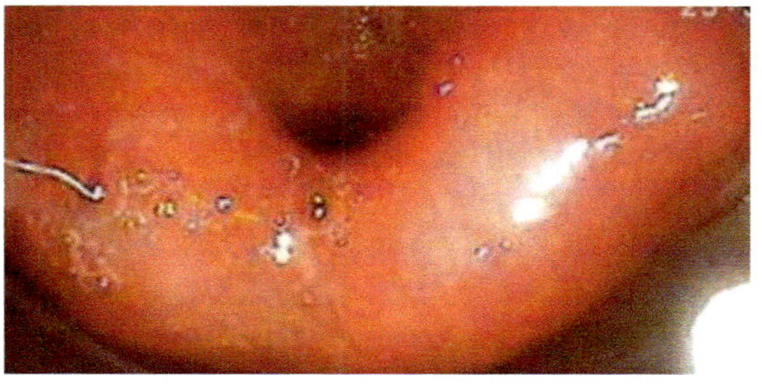

Fig. 20.2 Viral laryngotracheobronchitis. The larynx shows erythema and edema in the entire glottis, including the cord and arytenoids

Clinical History

The clinical history is very helpful for diagnosing stridor, assessing its severity, and deciding on the therapeutic approach, including referral to a specialist.

The data to consider in the anamnesis are:

- *Age at initiation*: Congenital causes are most common in newborns, and the most common of these is laryngomalacia. The most common cause among preschool children is LTB, although the possibility of foreign body aspiration should always be considered. Croup usually presents in patients between 6 months and 6 years of age. An infant under 6 months of age with repeated LTB could have a subglottic anatomical anomaly.
- *Form of initiation*: If stridor is acute and is associated with a fever, the etiology probably involves viral or bacterial infection. Abrupt initiation with respiratory difficulty or asphyxia suggests aspiration of a foreign body or an inflammatory cause (an allergic reaction).
- *Evolution timeline*: A patient with stridor for more than a week after viral laryngitis could be suffering a complication such as bacterial tracheitis.
- *Chronology*: Stridor caused by laryngomalacia becomes notable at 1–2 weeks after birth and can increase until 3 months of age, after which it decreases progressively, generally disappearing by 1 year of age. A subglottic hemangioma often appears at 2 months of age and is progressive, following the same course as hemangiomas of the skin.
- *Conditions that modify stridor*: In children with laryngomalacia, stridor increases when they eat, cry, or lie on their back; it decreases when they lie face down or are asleep.
- *History of cervical or thoracic trauma or surgery*: Lesions of the vagus nerve or its upper laryngeal or recurrent laryngeal branches can decrease the mobility of the vocal cords, including paralysis.
- *Association with apnea and cyanosis*: This can occur in cases of laryngomalacia, but it can also appear in the presence of vascular

rings and external causes not related to the airway.
- *History of intubation*: This indicates the presence of acquired subglottic stenosis.
- *Association with feeding difficulty*: This can indicate the presence of acid reflux or an anatomical anomaly, such as a laryngeal cleft or a tracheoesophageal fistula. It also constitutes a symptom of the seriousness of the airway obstruction.
- *Physical growth*: Alterations can be due to greater respiratory work that indicates the seriousness of the obstruction.

The general aspects that should be taken into consideration in the physical examination are:

- *Signs of respiratory failure*: Intercostal and subcostal retraction, use of accessory musculature, state of awareness, cyanosis, decreased arterial oxygen saturation.
- *Associated cough*: A barking cough associated with stridor suggests LTB.
- *Presence of craniofacial malformations*, especially those that compromise the middle third of the face and the base of the tongue. Stridor and snoring can coexist because of their association with diseases such as adenotonsillar hypertrophy and laryngomalacia.
- *Presence of cutaneous hemangiomas*: In 50% of subglottic hemangioma cases, there are similar lesions on the skin. Subglottic hemangiomas are observed in 1% of children who present cutaneous hemangiomas.
- *Presence of cervical malformations or a mass*, which can compress the airway.

The characterization of the stridor should take into account the following:

- *Phase of the respiratory cycle of stridor*: The stridor is generally inspiratory if the compromise is extrathoracic. If the compromise is glottic, the stridor can be inspiratory or biphasic. If the subglottic space is affected, the stridor is usually biphasic.
- *Accompanying signs*: Chronic dysphony can suggest the presence of a glottic mass (papilloma) or a lesion of the vagus nerve or of its branches, with a compromise of the vocal cords. A "potato voice" suggests abscessed tonsils.

Figure 20.3 shows the clinical approach to differential diagnosis of acute-onset stridor.

Assessment

Images

Radiology has been somewhat useful as a diagnostic tool. Traditionally, soft tissue cervical radiography has been used to look for reductions of the airway lumen in cases of LTB and congenital subglottic and tracheal lesions. When a patient has aspirated a radiopaque foreign body, a radiological study is genuinely useful. Uroscopy is a complementary method, which provides dynamic information on the airway from the nasopharynx to the main bronchi, taking pictures in different phases of breathing. A contrast study of the esophagus is useful for diagnosing vascular rings.

Computerized tomography (CT) with three-dimensional reconstruction helps to delimit and characterize lesions, particularly when they are complex and poorly defined anatomically, or when there is a severe stenosis of the airway that does not allow for an endoscope entering the airway. In this way, CT can contribute to planning for surgery, when it is appropriate. Nuclear magnetic resonance imaging is useful for assessing aberrant cervical and vasculature masses (vascular rings).

Respiratory Function

In cooperative patients, the spirometric flow–volume curve can be useful to distinguish between a fixed obstruction of the central airway (in which both the inspiratory and expiratory segments are affected) and a variable obstruction (in which only the inspiratory phase is compromised) (Figs. 20.4 and 20.5). The inspiratory and expiratory phases of the flow/volume are affected (with flattening). It is not possible to determine if the obstruction is intra- or extrathoracic.

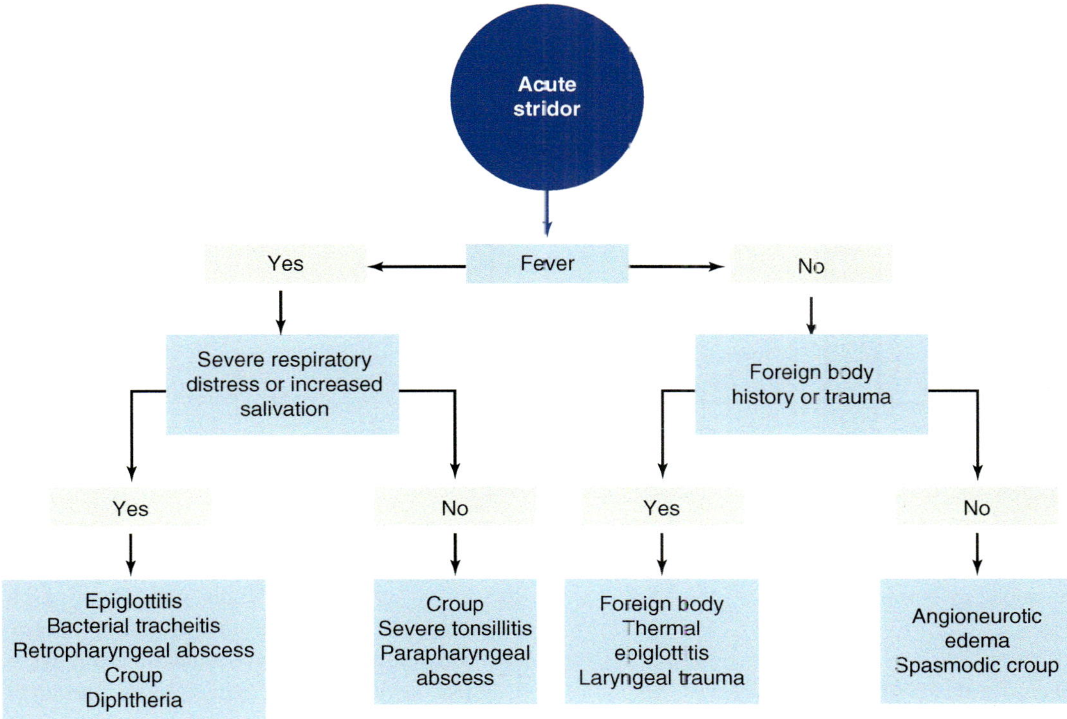

Fig. 20.3 Diagnostic approach to an acute-onset stridor

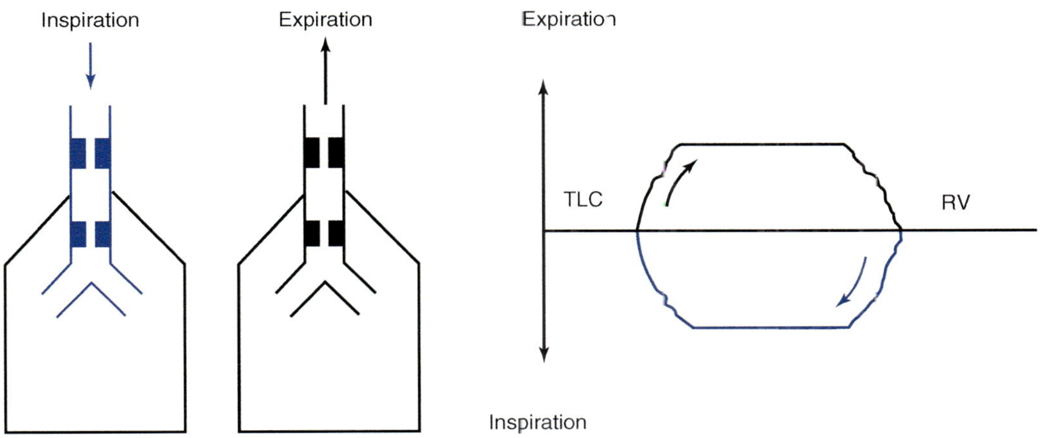

Fig. 20.4 Fixed obstruction of the intra- or extrathoracic central airway

The pressure of the airway is lower than the atmospheric pressure during inspiration, and if this is unstable, its cross-sectional area decreases, decreasing the flow, which is manifested as a flattening of the inspiratory phase of the flow/volume curve.

In more severe cases, gas exchange is assessed by measurement of arterial or venous gases, and measurement of arterial oxygen saturation.

If there is suspicion of obstructive apnea during sleep in patients with persistent stridor,

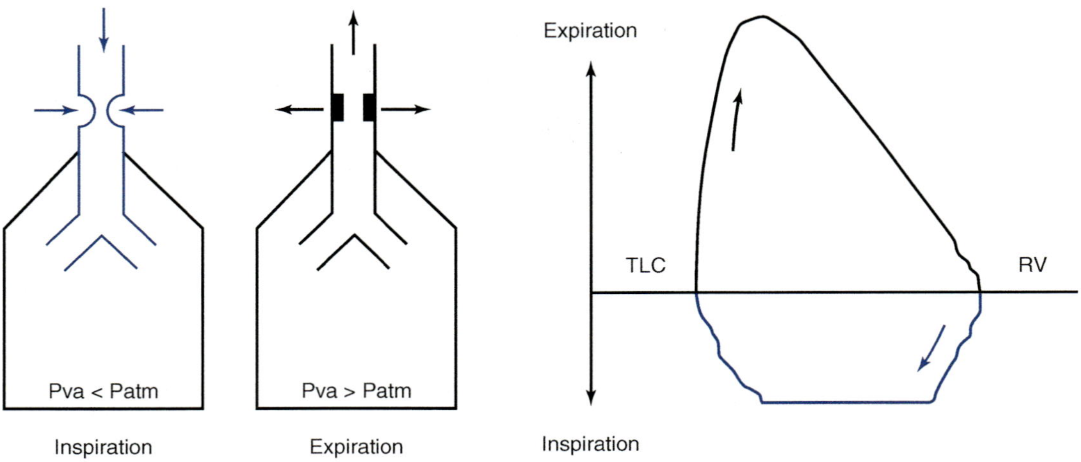

Fig. 20.5 Variable obstruction of the extrathoracic central airway

polygraph monitoring of ventilatory parameters during sleep is indicated.

Visualization of the Airway

Direct laryngoscopy and bronchoscopy currently constitute the gold-standard treatments for etiological diagnosis of chronic stridor.

In diagnosing laryngomalacia, flexible bronchoscopy has 93% sensitivity and 92% specificity, while laryngoscopy scores 100% for both parameters. However, laryngoscopy is not optimal for searching for associated lesions in the airway, as it does not allow for viewing below the vocal cords. According to some authors, these lesions associated with the cause of stridor are not clinically significant and only rarely require specific treatment. If they implied any serious condition, there would be clinical manifestations. The indications for comprehensive viewing of the airway are shown in Table 20.2. Figure 20.6 shows a proposed algorithm for endoscopic study of stridor. The treating physician should make a decision on referral to a specialist for partial or complete visualization of the airway.

If the stridor suggests laryngomalacia, there is no need for invasive studies (Table 20.2), and if regression is observed, flexible bronchoscopy is not absolutely indicated.

Table 20.2 Indications for bronchoscopy

Indication
Signs of respiratory distress
Two-phase stridor
Laryngomalacia with an unusual course
Stridor starting on the first day of life
Apnea and/or cyanosis
Feeding difficulty
Failure to grow
Normal or inconclusive nasal fibroscopy

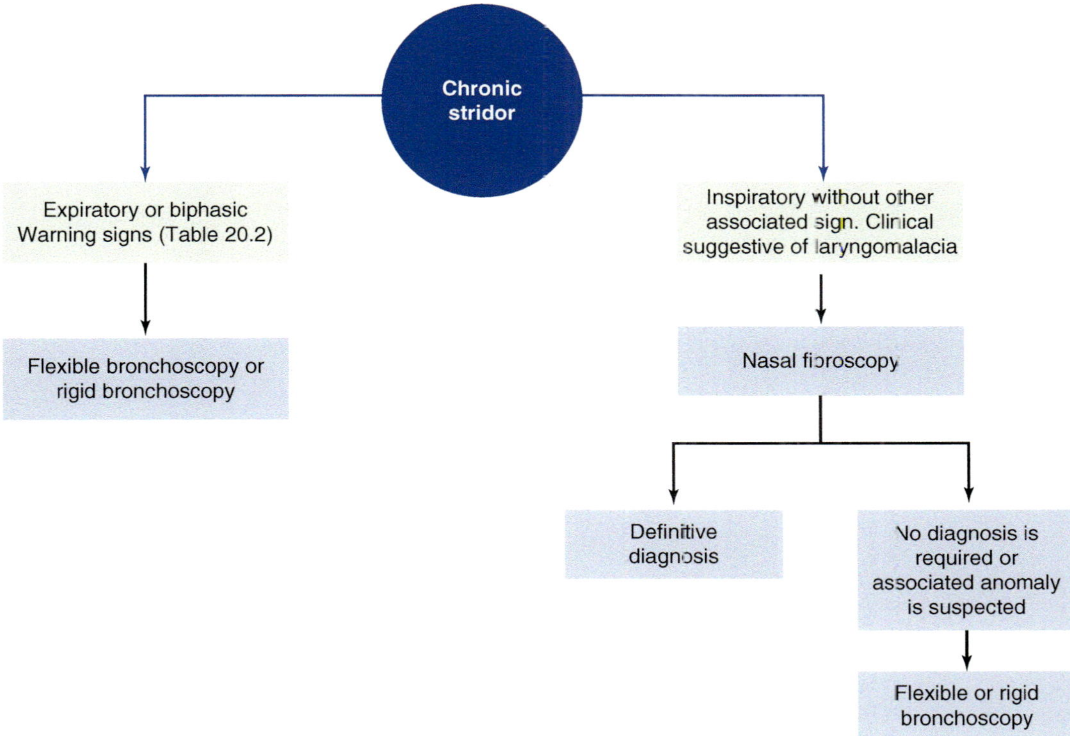

Fig. 20.6 Algorithm for endoscopic study of chronic stridor

Sources

Bodahana A, Izbicki G, Kraman S. Fundamentals of lung auscultation. N Engl J Med. 2014;370:744–51.

Boudewyns A, Claes J, Van de Heyning P. An approach to stridor in infants and children. Eur J Pediatr. 2010;169:135–41.

Carter E. Evaluating noisy breathing in children: how far down the airway should one look? Chest. 2004;125:1185–6.

Contreras I, Rosa G, Navarro H, Bertrand P, Cuevas M, Sánchez I, Caussade S. Estridor en el paciente pediátrico: estudio descriptivo. Rev Chil Pediatr. 2004;75:247–53.

Doherty G. Acute and chronic airway obstruction in children. Anaesth Int Care Med. 2012;13:220–5.

Ida J, Thompson D. Pediatric stridor. Otolaryngol Clin N Am. 2014.47:795–819.

Kubba H. An infant with stridor. Clin Otolaryngol. 2007;32:283–4.

Laya B. Lee E. Congenital causes of upper airway obstruction in pediatric patients: updated imaging techniques and review of imaging findings. Semin Roentgenol. 2012;47:147–58.

Petrocheilou A, Tanou K, Kalampouka E, Malakasioti G, Giannios C, Katidis A. Viral croup: diagnosis and a treatment algorithm. Pediatr Pulmonol. 2014;49:421–9.

Pfleger A, Eber E. Management of acute severe upper airway obstruction in children. Paediatr Respir Rev. 2013;14:70–7.

Children with Snoring

21

Daniel Zenteno Araos, José Luis Pérez Sánchez, and Pablo Brockmann Veloso

Contents

Introduction

Habitual snoring is the cardinal symptom of respiratory sleep disorders (RSDs) and arises from a series of causes that are classified into three large groups: adenotonsillar hypertrophy without obesity, adenotonsillar hypertrophy with obesity, and a group that includes neuromuscular diseases, Down syndrome, cerebral paralysis, and craniofacial syndromes (Table 21.1).

D. Zenteno Araos (✉)
Department of Pediatrics, Universidad de Concepción, Concepción, Chile

J. L. Pérez Sánchez
Department of Pediatrics, Universidad Austral de Chile, Osorno, Chile

P. Brockmann Veloso
Department of Pediatrics, School of Medicine, Pontificia Universidad Católica de Chile, Santiago, Chile
e-mail: pbrockmann@med.puc.cl

The prevalence of snoring in the general pediatric population is 3–12%. Among individuals with obstructive sleep apnea (OSA) it is 0.7–2%, mainly associated with adenotonsillar hypertrophy.

The notable increase in the prevalence of child obesity has changed the demographic and anthropometric characteristics of children who

Table 21.1 Classification of causes of sleep breathing disorders (SBDs)

Type I SBD	Type II SBD	Type III SBD
Adenotonsillar hypertrophy without obesity	Obesity with mild-to-moderate adenotonsillar hypertrophy	Neuromuscular diseases Down syndrome Arnold–Chiari malformation Cerebral palsy Craniofacial syndromes: Pierre Robin syndrome, Apert syndrome, Goldenhar syndrome, Crouzon syndrome, achondroplasia

P. Bertrand, I. Sánchez (eds.), *Pediatric Respiratory Diseases*,
https://doi.org/10.1007/978-3-030-26961-6_21

Table 21.2 Differences between type I and type II sleep breathing disorders (SBDs)

Symptoms	Type I SBDs*	Type II SBDs*
Somnolence	+	++++
Weight gain	–	++
Hyperactivity	++++	–/+
Attention deficit disorder	++++	+++
Truncal/visceral obesity	–/+	+++
Increased cervical girth	–/+	+++
Increased adenotonsillar size	++++	++
Acute otitis media/tympanostomy	+++	+
Depression and low self-esteem	+	+++
Shyness and social isolation	+	+++
Left ventricular hypertrophy	++	++++
Hypertension	+	++++
Insulin resistance	–	++++
Dyslipidemia	+	++++
Elevated C-reactive protein	++	++++
Elevated liver enzymes	–	++

*+ to ++++ infrequent to very frequent, – absent

are referred to sleep units. In the USA, fewer than 15% of children were obese in the 1990s, but in the last decade more than 50% were.

Several authors have argued that type I and II SBDs should be considered specific phenotypes with different characteristics and forms of presentation (Table 21.2).

In children and adolescents with neuromuscular diseases, obesity, or craniofacial malformations, the prevalence of SBDs with clinical significance can be as high as 50%.

While there are symptoms associated with SBDs, the clinical history and directed anamnesis have low sensitivity and/or specificity, because of which complementary examinations are necessary to obtain an early examination and timely interventions, thus reducing the possibility of neurocognitive alterations and deleterious biological effects on the child's metabolic, cardiovascular, and other systems, with the possibility of affecting the quality of life throughout his or her lifetime.

Associated Risk Factors

There are factors that we can consider to be associated with snoring, which have not been well studied despite their high prevalence and potential influence on the therapeutic focus. Some authors have even proposed these as specific phenotypes.

Asthma

A recent meta-analysis, which included 17 studies, found that asthmatic children have SBDs more often than nonasthmatic children (24% versus 17%), which implies that just being asthmatic increases the risk of having this disorder by almost.

Rhinitis

The coexistence between rhinitis and SBDs has been reported and discretely studied, although the focus remains on treatment to control rhinitis. A recent study confirmed this coexistence (in 43% of study participants with rhinitis) but without considering the severity of sleep disorders in the pediatric population.

Poor Dental Occlusion

Different anatomical alterations can affect respiratory flows and resistance in the upper airway, and thus facilitate the appearance of SBD. These alterations sometimes coexist with other possible causes. Therapeutic treatment of these children should be considered.

Diagnosis

Habitual snoring is defined as the presence of snoring on three or more nights per week. The anamnesis should serve to determine if the snoring is independent from colds or respiratory infections, the position the child is in when snoring occurs, and whether the snoring is associated with buccal breathing or apnea that is evident to the observer.

The precise diagnosis to rule out OSA is based on nocturnal polysomnography in a sleep laboratory. This examination is the only one currently considered a gold standard. However, there are

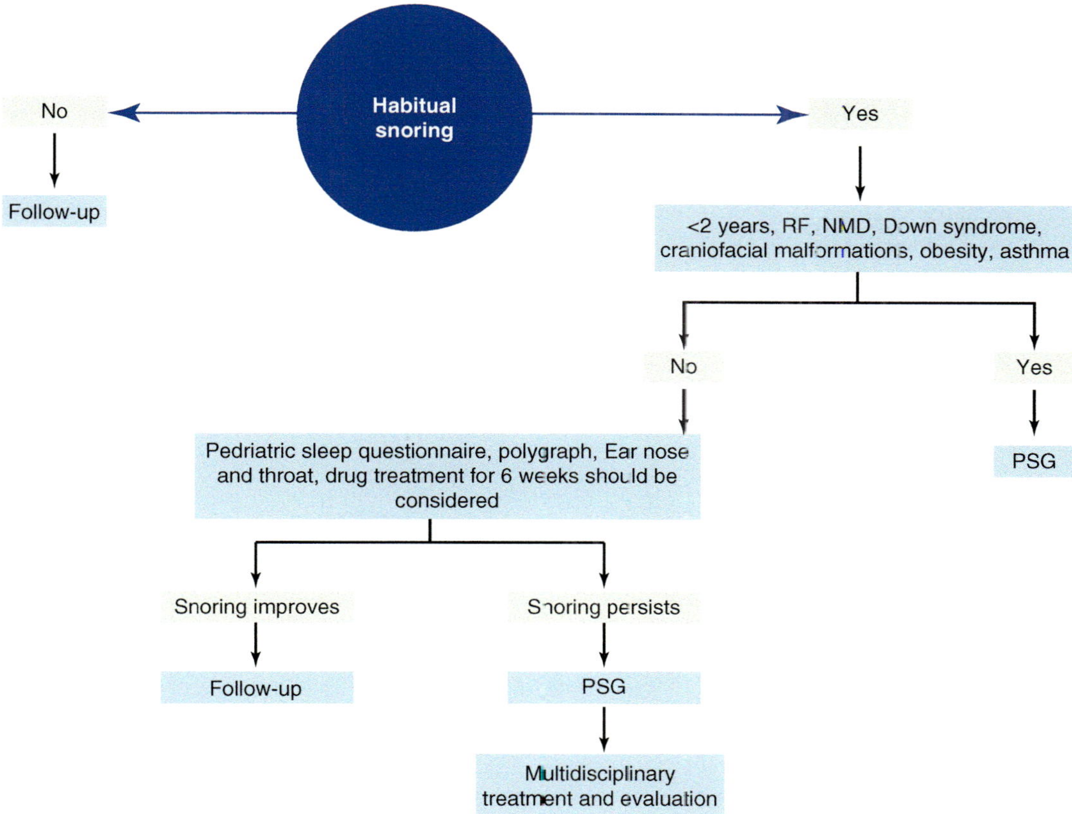

Fig. 21.1 Diagnostic and therapeutic approaches

abbreviated studies that play a role in screening for patients who snore.

It is important to incorporate screening for habitual snoring into all care for children and adolescents, given its association with risk factors (type II SBDs, obesity, craniofacial malformations, Down syndrome, etc.). Sleep studies should be conducted as early as possible and ideally should involve polysomnography (Fig. 21.1).

In children between 2 and 8 years of age, when the main cause of OSA is adenotonsillar hypertrophy, an abbreviated diagnosis and empirical treatment can be introduced, such as nasal corticoids for 6 weeks. The persistence of nocturnal and diurnal symptoms at the end of this period should be assessed, and it should be decided if polysomnography and a multidisciplinary study are necessary.

Clinical and physical examinations do not have sufficient sensitivity and specificity to rule out OSA, because of which a combination of different tools such as questionnaires, polygraph tests, and an established system of referrals is proposed as an option for screening of the general population.

Sources

Brockmann PE, Schaefer C, Poets A, Poets CF, Urschitz MS. Diagnosis of obstructive sleep apnea in children: a systematic review. Sleep Med Rev. 2013;17:331–40.

Brockmann P, Bertrand P, Castro-Rodríguez JA. Influence of asthma on sleep disordered breathing in children: a systematic review. Sleep Med Rev. 2014;18:393–7.

Elso MJ, Brockmann P, Zenteno D. Consecuencias del síndrome de apnea obstructiva del sueño. Rev Chil Pediatr. 2013;84(2):128–37.

Gozal D, Simakajornboon N, Holbrook CR. Secular tends in obesity and parentally reported daytime sleepiness among referred to a pediatrics center for snoring and suspected sleep-disorders breathing. Sleep. 2006;29:A74.

Huseni S, Gutierrez MJ, Rodriguez CE, Nino CL, Perez GF, Pancham K, Nino G. The link between rhinitis and rapid-eye-movement sleep breathing disturbances in children with obstructive sleep apnea. Am J Rhinol Allergy. 2014;28:56–61.

Kaditis A, Kheirandish-Gozal L, Gozal D. Algorithm for the diagnosis and treatment of pediatric OSA: a proposal of two pediatric sleep centers. Sleep Med. 2012;13:217–27.

Mellies U, Dohna-Schwake C, Voit T. Respiratory function assessment and intervention in neuromuscular disorders. Curr Opin Neurol. 2005;18:543–7.

Sans-Capdevila O, Gozal D. Neurobiological consequences of sleep apnea syndrome in children. Rev Neurol. 2008;47:659–64.

Urschitz MS, et al. Snoring in children: algorithm for diagnostic approach. Monatsch Kinder. 2013;161:347–50.

Zenteno D, Salinas P, Vera R, Brockmann P, Prado F. Enfoque pediátrico para el estudio de los trastornos respiratorios del sueño. Rev Chil Pediatr. 2010;81(5):445–55.

Children with Recurrent Wheezing 22

Luis Enrique Vega-Briceño, Ilse Contreras Estay, and Ignacio Sánchez

Contents

Epidemiology

Close to 50% of children experience wheezing during the first 6 months of life, but not all of them experience bronchial asthma. Long-term follow-up studies have shown that in approximately 30% of cases, wheezing begins before the children are 1 year old, with significantly poorer pulmonary function test results (before the first infection) than those of children who never experience wheezing. Many researchers agree that many early-age episodes of wheezing are associated with infections of viral origin. Several studies have shown that these infections are associated with abnormal pulmonary functioning during adolescence, even in the absence of respiratory symptoms.

The observational Avon Longitudinal Study of Parents and Children (ALSPAC) identified that 26% of a cohort of 6265 children experienced at least one episode of wheezing by the age of 18 months.

L. E. Vega-Briceño (✉)
Faculty of Medicine, Universidad del Desarrollo, Santiago, Chile
e-mail: levega@udd.cl

I. Contreras Estay
Department of Pediatrics, Hospital Padre Hurtado, Santiago, Chile

I. Sánchez
Department of Pediatrics, School of Medicine, Pontificia Universidad Católica de Chile, Santiago, Chile

P. Bertrand, I. Sánchez (eds.), *Pediatric Respiratory Diseases*, https://doi.org/10.1007/978-3-030-26961-6_22

Etiology

Recurrent wheezing in infants raises serious problems with regard to determining its etiology or nature, owing to the clinical similarities of different conditions (Table 22.1). While viral respiratory infections represent the main causal factor in many obstructive episodes, it is recognized that there are environmental factors that can result in wheezing episodes. There are important anatomical differences between the airway of an infant or a preschool child and the airway of an adult—differences that can favor the development of obstructive conditions in small children. It is also recognized that a state of bronchial hyperresponsiveness (BHR) is normal in the first years of life, but it decreases progressively with age, although it increases significantly after certain viral infections (respiratory syncytial virus (RSV), influenza, parainfluenza). This indicates that the causes of many obstructive episodes in children are multifactorial. It is estimated that in almost 80% of children with wheezing, the condition is associated with a viral infection.

Physiopathology

The term "wheezing" is often used imprecisely. It has been assessed in diverse epidemiological studies that have employed video questionnaires and works that have quantified wheezing. In some European languages, there is no appropriate translation for the English word "wheezing." Wheezing is the audible clinical manifestation of the small airway obstruction. It consists of high-pitched musical sounds generated by the flow of air through the narrow intrathoracic airway. It usually is perceived during expiration, and it is associated with increased work of breathing, although it can also occur during inspiration. Studies of pulmonary sounds have quantified wheezing directly through the use of microphones on the chest surface, which is ideal, but it is not very useful in clinical situations. This method has shown that doctors do clearly identify this symptom, although parents and nurses often do not, as it is not easily reproducible. As noted earlier, wheezing is common among infants.

It is possible that more than one physiopathological mechanism is involved in generating

Table 22.1 Differential diagnosis of infants with recurrent wheezing

Etiology	Clinical characteristics	Tests and investigations
Bronchopulmonary dysplasia	Prematurity, respiratory distress of the newborn, mechanical ventilation in the neonatal period, O_2 needed for >28 days	Chest x-ray, nocturnal SpO_2
Cystic fibrosis	Malnutrition, malabsorption syndrome, pneumopathy, or recurrent sinusitis	Sweat electrolyte test, genetic testing
Congenital heart disease	Heart murmur, heart failure	X-ray, ECG, Doppler echocardiogram
Foreign body aspiration	Acute episode of asphyxia, asymmetrical lung signs	X-ray, flexible or rigid bronchoscopy
Gastroesophageal reflux	Recurrent vomiting	X-ray, pH measurement
Dysphagia due to neurological damage	Recurrent or persistent pneumopathy	Pulmonary aspiration scintigraphy
Lung malformations	Radiological finding	Prenatal ultrasound, chest x-ray, CT scan, angiography, MRI
Vascular malformations	Stridor	X-ray, esophagogram, endoscopy, Doppler echocardiogram, angiography, MRI
Primary ciliary dyskinesia	Sinus pathology, recurrent acute otitis media, bronchiectasis, situs inversus	X-ray, saccharin test, respiratory epithelium biopsy

CT computerized tomography scan, *ECG* electrocardiogram, *MRI* magnetic resonance imagining, *SpO_2* peripheral capillary oxygen saturation recurrent wheezing: intraluminal obstruction due to inflammation, edema, contraction of the smooth muscle, or BHR; extraluminal obstruction due to compression by vascular rings, adenopathy, or congenital pulmonary malformations; and structural defects that condition dynamic obstruction of the airway: hemangiomas, polyps, bronchomalacia, and tracheomalacia, among others.

Airway inflammation: While bronchial asthma has been considered an inflammatory disease of the airway induced by eosinophils and mediated by type 2 helper T (T_h2) lymphocytes, studies of bronchial lavage fluid, bronchial biopsies, and induced sputum have identified noneosinophilic forms of recurrent wheezing in preschool children that may be a form of nonallergic child asthma. Other inflammatory diseases (such as cystic fibrosis) present a neutrophilic cell preference, with an increase in interleukin-8 (IL-8), including before the presence of a bacterial colony. The participation of inflammation in the pathogeny of other respiratory diseases, such as bronchopulmonary dysplasia in premature infants, is well recognized.

Limitation of airflow: Limitation of airflow can be secondary to pre- or postnatal anatomical reduction of the airway caliber. Different alternations of the distensibility of the airway wall can occur (a primary defect in the structure of the wall, or loss of the alveolar framework). Prenatal factors include a mother who smokes, hypertension during the pregnancy, and atopy. While changes in the distensibility of the airway wall have been suggested as being important, this is difficult to establish without histological studies. The most common causes at the postnatal stage are bronchopulmonary dysplasia, postinfectious bronchiolitis obliterans (generally caused by an adenovirus), gastroesophageal reflux, and aspiration syndromes. There are also flow limitations secondary to aspiration of a foreign body, congenital and acquired stenosis of the airway, cicatricial polyps in patients with bronchopulmonary dysplasia, hemangiomas, vascular rings, compression by vascular structures (the ligamentum arteriosum or the pulmonary artery trunk), lymph nodes, bronchogenic cysts, and pulmonary sequestration, among others.

Bronchial hyperresponsiveness: This is one of the components of bronchial asthma. The traditional model maintains that inflammation produces hyperresponsiveness and is responsible for the symptoms. While there is a good correlation between BHR and the severity of asthma in preschool children, this is not certain when the response to medication is being assessed at an individual level. BHR is a nonspecific condition of asthma, often secondary to other causes such as viral infections, *Mycoplasma Pneumoniae*, exposure to cigarette smoke or other types of smoke, environmental contamination, and allergies, among others. For clinical effects, BHR and inflammation should be considered as independent and overlapping conditions. Children are born with a predisposition to develop BHR, which disappears with age. However, viral infections can aggravate the condition and even make it permanent. Figure 22.1 summarizes the possible mechanisms involved in the development of recurrent wheezing in preschool children.

Clinical Characteristics

Once it has been determined that a child is suffering an acute episode of wheezing, an adequate clinical history and a complete physical examination are required to place the child in one of the three categories mentioned in Table 22.2. The medical history and the physical examination are essential to categorize a child and to decide if further investigation is needed. The reasons for referring a child to a specialist in respiratory diseases are if there is doubt about the diagnosis, if the treatment that is applied does not work, or if the parents are not satisfied with the results. Most preschool children with recurrent wheezing do not require any further laboratory study. Diagnostic confusion increases with the use of terms such as "bronchiolitis," "obstructive bronchitis," and "asthmatic bronchitis," which refer

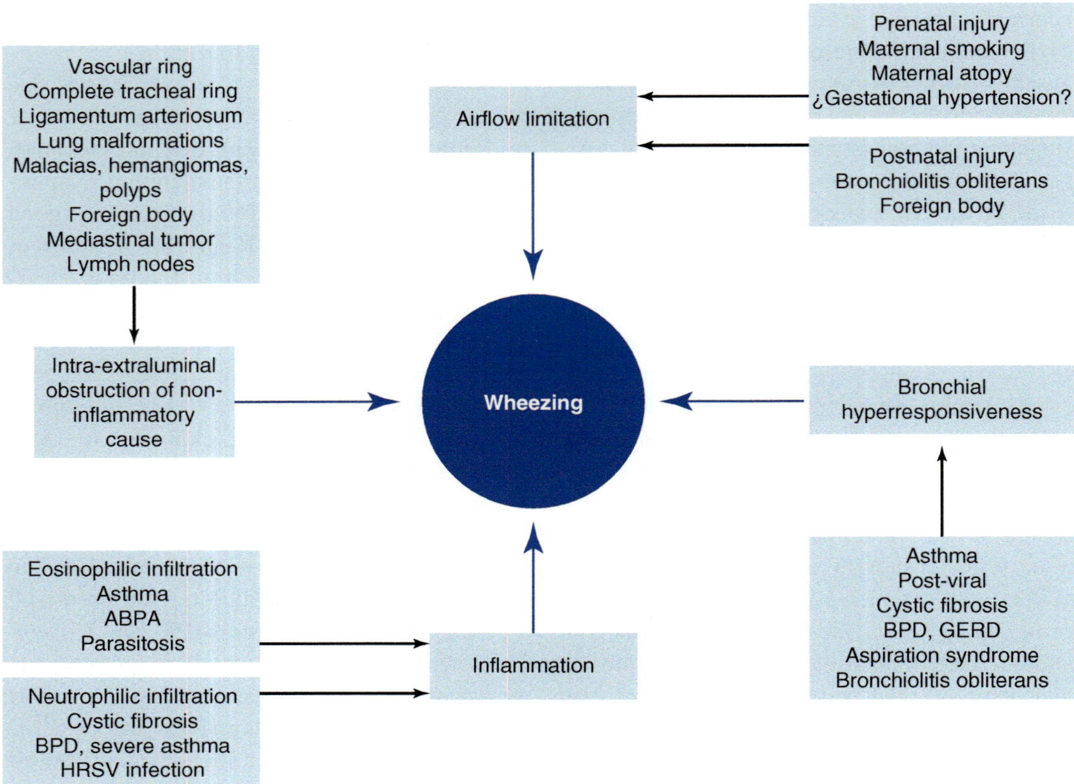

Fig. 22.1 Etiopathogenesis of recurrent wheezing. *ABPA* allergic bronchopulmonary aspergillosis, *BPD* bronchopulmonary dysplasia, *GERD* gastroesophageal reflux disease, *HRSV* human respiratory syncytial virus

Table 22.2 Causes of recurrent wheezing

Frequent causes	Infrequent causes	Rare causes
Viral infections	Cystic fibrosis	Mediastinal masses (tumors, tuberculosis)
Asthma	Bronchopulmonary dysplasia	Immunodeficiencies
	Congenital heart disease	Primary ciliary dyskinesia
	Foreign bodies	Bronchiolitis obliterans
		Bronchiectasis
		Aspiration syndromes
		Vascular and pulmonary malformations

to different clinical conditions. In UK, the first term refers to a condition characterized by respiratory difficulty, with the presence of fine crepitant crackles (alveolar noises) in children under 1 year of age. While wheezing can be present, UK authors consider that crepitant crackles define the illness. No rigid definition based on age should prevail, given that any generalization is artificial. In the USA and elsewhere, for example, bronchiolitis is synonymous with wheezing diseases.

Many classifications that use different categories for children with recurrent wheezing have been published, and these are outlined below.

(a) *Epidemiological phenotype*: In this context, the wheezing phenotypes are “transitory or early” (occurring only during the first 3 years after birth) and persistent wheezing (continuing until the age of 6 years). This study from Tucson (AZ, USA) was focused on the evolution of symptoms (wheezing) and long-term pulmonary function, but its categories can be determined only retrospectively and are not clinically useful.

(b) *Phenotype based on the presence/absence of atopy*: Early sensitization to aeroallergens is the best predictor of development of symptoms and loss of pulmonary function by school age, such that assignment to an atopic category or a nonatopic category can be useful as a guide for treatment.

(c) *Phenotype based on triggers for wheezing*: The Task Force of the European Respiratory Society recommends that preschool children with a recurrent sibilant wheeze should be put into one of two categories—episodic wheezing or multitriggered wheezing—which is also what we propose.

- *Wheezing episodes*: These children present wheezing solely in the context of upper respiratory tract infection of viral etiology but are free of symptoms between such episodes.
- *Multitriggered wheezing*: These children have wheezing in the context of upper respiratory infections of viral etiology and also in the context of other triggers such as exercise, exposure to cigarette smoke, exposure to allergens, and others.

The ERS-recommended classification is now used in many publications to guide treatment. Since its publication, it has been criticized for the fact that children can change between categories over time; consequently, the drug treatment can also change. This is analogous to what occurs in schoolchildren with asthma, in which the treatment does not remain fixed over time; rather, dose increases or reductions are introduced (and are eventually suspended), depending on the presence of symptoms and their severity. Unfortunately, few studies have adopted this classification, because many epidemiological studies and clinical assays have combined the two phenotypes as being more relevant.

Obstructive conditions in infants are manifested by the presence of coughing, wheezing, audible or prolonged expiration, costal retraction, an increased anteroposterior diameter, and dullness to percussion. While these findings are nonspecific and do not point to a determined etiology, their absence does not rule out the possibility that a process is under way. The presence of nail clubbing, a heart murmur, postbronchodilator clinical deterioration, a stridor, lack of growth, craniofacial malformation, compromise of the branchial arches (CHARGE and velocardiofacial syndromes), recurrent pneumonia, or other parenchymal infections are indications for ruling out conditions associated with a secondary cause.

Infants with more intense respiratory symptoms or with a chronic base condition (neurological, comorbid, digestive, cardiological, genetic, dysmorphic, or growth related) require further study to determine bronchial, inflammatory, or infectious compromise. Any atypical clinical or radiological presentation—such as the onset of symptoms during the neonatal period, asymmetrical wheezing, localized hyperinflation, bronchiectasis, diaphragmatic asymmetry, radiological patterns, or persistent or recurrent atelectasis—indicates the need to consider another disease.

Diagnosis

The assessment of a child with recurrent wheezing begins with a good anamnesis and a complete physical examination. To establish the diagnosis of asthma in children under 2–3 years of age, certain chronic diseases need to be ruled out (particularly in children who do not present the aforementioned risk factors). A family history of asthma or a personal or parental history of allergies can be very important. The diagnosis of asthma should always include anatomical or structural considerations. While asthma is a chronic inflammatory disease of the small airway and preferentially eosinophilic, with changes in expiratory flows, these characteristics are not usually assessed in clinical practice, particularly in infants and preschool children. Flow reversibility with pulmonary studies and exhaled nitric oxide measurements do not yet have practical application in differentiating the aforementioned clinical patterns. A chest x-ray can confirm the elements of air trapping and rule out associated anatomical conditions. The most common radiological findings in relation to an obstructive bronchial crisis are hyperinsufflation, diaphragmatic flattening, increased retrosternal space, increased interstitial and peribronchovascular trauma, segmental atelectasis, and subsegmentation. When there is clinical evidence suggesting a determined etiology, complementary examinations can be useful, such as esophagography, bronchoscopy, chest echography, and echocardiography. Axial computerized tomography (CT) and nuclear magnetic resonance imaging allow diagnosis of vascular malformations such as rings and vascular compressions of the airway, as well as confirming pulmonary, airway, or digestive tract malformations (tracheoesophageal fistulas or recurrence of tracheoesophageal fistulas in patients with a history of esophageal atresia), aspiration of a foreign body, tracheomalacia, or bronchomalacia. Video deglutition is useful to establish the diagnosis of aspiration syndromes and pharyngeal incoordination, particularly in children with cerebral paralysis or psychomotor retardation. During an acute episode, some laboratory examinations should be considered that can point toward or confirm the responsible etiological agent in some uncommon conditions. In such conditions, it can be necessary to determine the esophageal pH, total immunoglobulin, and immunoglobulin subclasses, and to perform fiber bronchoscopy (with a mucosal biopsy, alveolar lavage, and eventually electron microscopy) or an echocardiogram. A sweat test should be always be requested for children with recurrent wheezing, given that this is a way to diagnose cystic fibrosis, particularly if there is nutritional compromise and suspicion of digestive compromise.

Management

Before any medication is prescribed to a child with episodic or multitriggered wheezing, it is essential to ensure that the environment in which the child lives is controlled, particularly with regard to exposure to smoking: smoking outside the house (not in front of the child) does not protect the child from harm. A follow-up study cohort from birth found that environmental contamination increases the probability of developing wheezing in the preschool period, but currently there is no clear recommendation based on individual exposures—only recommendations at the population level.

Medication should be considered in order to avoid complications such as remodeling of the airway and persistent obstruction of airflow, as well as for treatment of symptoms. In practice, we do not have a clear strategy to reduce the risk of developing asthma, even through continuous or intermittent use of inhaled corticosteroids. When prescribing an inhaled medication, it is essential to be prepared to stop the inhalation technique and use of the spacer at any time if the prescribed aerosol does not appear to be working. Proper administration should be determined, rather than escalating the treatment.

Episodic Wheezing

Children with episodic wheezing are not at greater risk of atopy or respiratory symptoms, according to follow-up series that have studied children up to 14 years old. The evidence is clear and comes from clinical studies showing that early treatment, whether intermittent or continuous, does not affect the progress of the disease. This means that we do not have treatments that modify the disease, and that treatment should be focused on controlling symptoms.

Intermittent symptoms should be treated with intermittent drug strategies, which in practice is what parents do. It is important to determine which patients require ongoing treatment. The use of inhaled medication to treat mild respiratory sounds with minimal respiratory pressure can be more problematic than the disease itself. The treatment should start with intermittent use of bronchodilators (either short-acting agonists or anticholinergics). If the treatment needs to be staggered from bronchodilators because of lack of symptom control, the next option is intermittent use of antileukotrienes, corticosteroids, or both. There have been recent and important randomized, controlled clinical studies assessing intermittent therapy. One study compared intermittent use of antileukotrienes with a placebo in children who received the treatment from the time of onset for a minimum of 7 days or until the symptoms of respiratory tract infection disappeared. The study found that the children who received the treatment required fewer unscheduled medical consultations because of asthma exacerbations (odds ratio 0.65; 95% confidence interval 0.47–0.89) and had fewer days away from school or kindergarten, with fewer days being lost from work by the parents (37% versus 33%, $p < 0.001$). In a pre-established analysis of a subgroup of patients, the benefits were greater among children 2–5 years of age (close to 80%). However, these findings have not been confirmed by subsequent studies. A comparative study of standard treatment for children versus intermittent antileukotriene and intermittent budesonide, showed that the active treatment and standard strategy provided similar benefits. On the basis of such studies, we recommend a trial of antileukotrienes for preschool children with virus-induced symptoms. We recommend beginning the treatment when the first sign of a cold appears and stopping it when the child is well, rather than continuing it for a fixed number of days.

A Cochrane review identified that intermittent use of inhaled corticoids is a partially effective strategy in response to episodic wheezing in preschool children. A study in children between the ages of 1 and 6 years showed that use of fluticasone for 10 days at the beginning of cold symptoms was responsible for reducing the use of rescue prednisone in comparison with a placebo. However, this use of inhaled corticoids is associated with adverse effects, because of which it is not recommended. Another study that compared continuous versus intermittent use of budesonide from the onset of a cold did not show differences in any parameter, but the absence of a placebo group meant that it could not be determined which of the two strategies was more beneficial. What this study did show is that daily doses of inhaled budesonide do not prevent the development or onset of viral exacerbations with wheezing. Older small-scale studies that used beclomethasone also failed to demonstrate this preventive effect. There is currently no evidence to support the use of inhaled corticosteroids at the usual doses in children with episodic wheezing. There are studies that have recommended more research into intermittent use of inhaled corticoids in response to virus-triggered wheezing to clarify the doses, the timing, and the benefits of this intervention in this context. It appears inappropriate and unsafe to use fluticasone twice a day in doses above 150 μg in healthy preschool children (without base conditions) with viral colds, given the risk of adverse effects such as axis suppression and adrenal failure with high doses. To date, no studies have combined intermittent doses of inhaled corticoids with montelukast to treat episodic wheezing.

There is no evidence supporting regular use of inhaled corticoids in preschool children who wheeze between colds. However, if children experience severe episodic exacerbations that require frequent hospitalization, or if they have prolonged symptoms, with interruptions in the quality of their home life, prophylactic doses of inhaled corticosteroids can be tested. In some cases, it may seem that fluctuations in symptom control are not fully perceived by the parents. A trial of an inhaled corticoid should always be avoided in milder cases of episodic wheezing. The treatment should be reviewed and discontinued if there is no benefit. There is no evidence establishing the optimal duration of the treatment, but 6–8 weeks appears to be a reasonable period. If the episodic wheezing improves with treatment, a brief interruption and reduced doses should be considered according to the clinical evolution of the condition. If it is suspected that the child has symptoms between colds that are not perceived by the parents, a trial of inhaled corticosteroids can reveal whether the child was really more symptomatic than previously believed. Whatever the context of a therapeutic trial in preschool children is, the treatment period must be predetermined and the treatment must be suspended at the end of the trial to determine if the symptoms reappear and if the treatment is indeed necessary.

Recent evidence has called into question the use of oral prednisone in acute episodes of viral wheezing in preschool children. There have been at least two well-designed studies in children with recurrent wheezing and at least one hospitalization, where the use of prednisone was compared with use of a placebo. No differences were found between the two groups in either study. This indicates that preschool children who have virus-triggered episodic wheezing and who are well enough to not be hospitalized do not receive any benefit from oral steroids. Moreover, many children who are hospitalized should not receive oral steroids either. These studies considered children with mild cases, since many were discharged in the first 24 hours, so this experience cannot be extrapolated to children with severe exacerbations triggered by viruses. In the absence of evidence, it is probable that prednisone continues to be prescribed for a small subgroup of hospitalized children.

Multitriggered Wheezing

In preschool children with wheezing or coughing who respond to bronchodilators with reduced breathing difficulty even in the absence of viral infections, prophylactic treatment should be considered, whether it is inhaled corticoids or antileukotrienes. As inflammation of the airway cannot be ruled out in this age group, and many children are asymptomatic until school age, it is wrong to assume that the physiopathology of this disease is the same as that of asthma. Furthermore, eosinophilic inflammation is less likely in small children, because of which the use of inhaled corticoids is more problematic. The final objective is to avoid incorrectly diagnosing children as having asthma and, as a consequence, prescribing inappropriate treatment, given that most children begin treatment when there is a strong probability that they will improve spontaneously. Long-acting β-adrenoceptor antagonist (LABA) treatment is not approved for this age group.

In a small, double-blind study, 451 children between 1 and 6 years of age were randomly assigned to receive hypertonic saline at 7% or normal saline at 0.9%, both combined with salbutamol. The treatments were administered twice, 20 minutes apart, in the emergency ward, and four times, separated by 20-minute intervals, if the child was hospitalized. The hospital admission rate and the duration of hospitalization were measured, and were lower in the hypertonic saline group, but there were no significant differences in the severity score, probably because the study included only a small number of patients. Since hypertonic saline can produce bronchospasm, it should be used only in the hospital. Palivizumab has been used to prevent RSV infections in high-risk children, such as extreme premature survivors. However, because of cost and inconvenience, it is not the treatment of choice for all children. In a recent study, 429 children born at gestational ages from 33 to 35 weeks were randomly given palivizumab or a placebo. Palivizumab reduced the number of days with wheezing in the first year of life by 61% and reduced the percentage of children with recurrent wheezing from 21% to 10%. The most interesting question this study could resolve—provided that the children are followed up from infancy to school age—is the controversy as to whether early RSV infection causes asthma or is simply a sign that a child has a predisposition to develop asthma. The current position is that this is a work in progress, rather than an indication of a change in public policy.

Treatment plans highlight the importance of self-management, depending on the severity of symptoms and the measurement of peak flow at school age. A controlled trial involved 200 children between 18 months and 5 years of age with a history of unscheduled visits to a hospital or emergency room because of wheezing. The children were divided into two groups; one group received standard treatment, while the parents of the other group received two education sessions and an instruction booklet with a plan of guided action to manage the symptoms. No differences were found in any of the outcomes. Although there is no evidence of their effectiveness, education sessions and action plans are widely employed.

Assessment of Severity

In determining the seriousness of recurrent obstructive symptoms, consideration should be given to the number of hospitalizations or emergency visits, the presence of nocturnal respiratory symptoms or associated conditions (for example, gastroesophageal reflux), tolerance of exercise and eating, frequency of oral steroid use, and other factors. Several clinical scores have been developed to determine the severity of acute episodes and to provide an objective assessment of the degree of obstruction and the most appropriate treatment. While all of these scoring systems are assessment tools and they are used widely, the quality of the evaluators varies greatly, and so the sensitivity of scoring systems depends on the operators. We consider that the scoring system developed by Tal et al. is useful, reproducible, objective, and easy to use. The clinical score should be determined under basal conditions and also after every medical intervention, complemented with determination of arterial oxygen saturation, at least.

Evolution and Prognosis

There is a particular association between wheezing during the first year of life and subsequent development of asthma. More than 60% of infants with recurrent postbronchiolitis wheezing do not present obstructive symptoms beyond the age of 3 years, and fewer than 15% present persistent wheezing afterward. This symptom disappears in most children by the time they are 6 years old. The influence of viral infections declines dramatically during school age. While it is recognized that the small size of the airway is conditioned by intrauterine exposure to smoking and arterial hypertension, many of these factors are corrected with the growth and development of the child, because of which the prognosis is generally good.

Sources

Andersen ZJ, Loft S, Ketzel M, Stage M, Scheike T, Hermansen MN, et al. Ambient air pollution triggers wheezing symptoms in infants. Thorax. 2008;63:710–6.

Bisgaard H, Hermansen MN, Loland L, Halkjaer LB, Buchvald F. Intermittent inhaled corticosteroids in infants with episodic wheezing. N Engl J Med. 2006;354:1998–2005.

Blanken MO, Rovers MM, Molenaar JM, Winkler-Seinstra PL, Meijer A, Kimpen JL, Dutch RSV Neonatal Network, et al. Respiratory syncytial virus and recurrent wheeze in healthy preterm infants. N Engl J Med. 2013;368:1791–9.

Brand PL, Baraldi E, Bisgaard H, Boner AL, Castro-Rodriguez JA, Custovic A, et al. Definition, assessment and treatment of wheezing disorders in preschool children: an evidence-based approach. Eur Respir J. 2008;32:1096–110.

British Thoracic Society. British guideline on the management of asthma. 2012 update. www.brit-thoracic.org.uk/guidelines/asthmaguidelines.aspx.

Bush A. Practice imperfect—treatment for wheezing in preschoolers. N Engl J Med. 2009;360:409–10.

Devulapalli CS, Carlsen KC, Håland G, Munthe-Kaas MC, Pettersen M, Mowinckel P, et al. Severity of obstructive airways disease by age 2 years predicts asthma at 10 years of age. Thorax. 2008;63:8–13.

Ducharme FM, Lemire C, Noya FJ, Davis GM, Alos N, Leblond H, et al. Preemptive use of high-dose fluticasone for virus-induced wheezing in young children. N Engl J Med. 2009;360:339–53.

Guilbert TW, Morgan WJ, Zeiger RS, Mauger DT, Boehmer SJ, Szefler SJ, et al. Long-term inhaled corticosteroids in preschool children at high risk for asthma. N Engl J Med. 2006;354:1985–97.

Henderson J, Granell R, Heron J, Sherriff A, Simpson A, Woodcock A, et al. Associations of wheezing phenotypes in the first 6 years of life with atopy, lung function and airway responsiveness in mid-childhood. Thorax. 2008;63:974–80.

Illi S, von Mutius E, Lau S, Niggemann B, Grüber C, Wahn U, Multicentre Allergy Study (MAS) Group. Perennial allergen sensitisation early in life and chronic asthma in children: a birth cohort study. Lancet. 2006;368:763–70.

McKean M, Ducharme F. Inhaled steroids for episodic viral wheeze of childhood. Cochrane Database Syst Rev. 2000;(2):CD001107.

Murray CS, Woodcock A, Langley SJ, Morris J, Custovic A, IFWIN Study Team. Secondary prevention of asthma by the use of inhaled fluticasone dipropionate in wheezy infants (IWWIN): double-blind, randomized controlled study. Lancet. 2006;368:754–62.

Oommen A, Lambert PC, Grigg J. Efficacy of a short course of parent-initiated oral prednisolone for viral wheeze in children aged 1–5 years: randomized controlled trial. Lancet. 2003;362:1433–8.

Panickar J, Lakhanpaul M, Lambert PC, Kenia P, Stephenson T, Smyth A, et al. Oral prednisolone for preschool children with acute virus-induced wheezing. N Engl J Med. 2009;360:329–38.

Pool J, Petrova N, Russell RR. Exposing children to secondhand smoke. Thorax. 2012;67:926.

Robertson CF, Price D, Henry R, Mellis C, Glasgow N, Fitzgerald D, et al. Short-course montelukast for intermittent asthma in children: a randomized controlled trial. Am J Respir Crit Care Med. 2007;175:323–9.

Saglani S, Malmstrom K, Pelkonen AS, Malmberg LP, Lindahl H, Kajosaari M, et al. Airway remodeling and inflammation in symptomatic infants with reversible airflow obstruction. Am J Respir Crit Care Med. 2005;171:722–7.

Saglani S, Payne DN, Zhu J, Wang Z, Nicholson AG, Bush A, et al. Early detection of airway wall remodelling and eosinophilic inflammation in preschool wheezers. Am J Respir Crit Care Med. 2007;176:858–64.

Savenije OE, Kerkhof M, Koppelman GH, Postma DS. Predicting who will have asthma at school age among preschool children. J Allergy Clin Immunol. 2012;130:325–31.

Schultz A, Devadason SG, Savenije OE, Sly PD, Le Souef PN, Brand PL. The transient value of classifying preschool wheeze into episodic viral wheeze and multiple trigger wheeze. Acta Paediatr. 2010;99:56–60.

Sonnappa S, Bastardo CM, Wade A, Saglani S, McKenzie SA, Bush A, et al. Symptom-pattern and pulmonary function in preschool wheezers. J Allergy Clin Immunol. 2010;126:519–26.

Sonnappa S, Bastardo CM, Saglani S, Bush A, Aurora P. Relationship between past airway pathology and current lung function in preschool wheezers. Eur Respir J. 2011;38:1431–6.

Stevens CA, Wesseldine LJ, Couriel JM, Dyer AJ, Osman LM, Silverman M. Parental education and guided self-management of asthma and wheezing in the preschool child: a randomized controlled trial. Thorax. 2002;57:39–44.

Tal A, Bavilski C, Yohai D, Bearman JE, Gorodischer R, Moses SW. Dexamethasone and salbutamol in the treatment of acutewheezing in infants. Pediatrics. 1983;71:13–18.

Valovirta E, Boza ML, Robertson CF, Verbruggen N, Smugar SS, Nelsen LM, et al. Intermittent or daily montelukast versus placebo for episodic asthma in children. Ann Allergy Asthma Inmunol. 2011;106:518–26.

Warner JO, ETAC Study Group. Early Treatment of the Atopic Child. A double-blinded, randomized, placebo-controlled trial of cetirizine in preventing the onset of asthma in children with atopic dermatitis: 18 months' treatment and 18 months' posttreatment follow-up. J Allergy Clin Immunol. 2001;108:929–37.

Zeiger RS, Mauger D, Bacharier LB, Giobert TW, Martinez FD, Lemanske RF Jr, CARE Network of the National Heart, Lung, and Blood Institute, et al. Daily or intermittent budesonide in preschool children with recurrent wheezing. N Engl J Med. 2011;365:1990–2001.

Hemoptysis in Children

23

Julio Maggiolo Massone, Carlos Mendoza Fox, and Ricardo Kogan Alterman

Contents

J. Maggiolo Massone (✉)
Department of Pediatrics, Hospital Exequiel González Cortés, San Miguel, Chile

C. Mendoza Fox
Department of Pediatrics, Hospital Nacional Hipólito Unanue, Lima, Peru
e-mail: ginp@upch.edu.pe

R. Kogan Alterman
Department of Pediatrics, Faculty of Medicine, Universidad de Chile, Santiago, Chile
e-mail: ricardokogan@med.uchile.cl

P. Bertrand, I. Sánchez (eds.), *Pediatric Respiratory Diseases*,
https://doi.org/10.1007/978-3-030-26961-6_23

Epidemiology and Etiology

Hemoptysis is an infrequent condition in children although some of the diseases that can cause it are not uncommon—such as bronchiectasis in patients with cystic fibrosis (CF) or chronic lung disease postadenovirus—or it may be caused by other conditions such as aspiration of a foreign body or a respiratory infection. It can also occur in much less frequent conditions such as diffuse alveolar hemorrhage syndrome (DAHS), the most important causes of which are pulmonary–renal syndrome (PRS) and idiopathic pulmonary hemosiderosis (IPH).

The frequency varies between different centers. Coss-Bu and collaborators published a study of 228 children and young adults over a period of 10 years, and they found that in 65% of cases, it was caused by CF. Among the remainder of the cases, the main causes were congenital cardiopathies (16%), infections (16%), tumors (2.6%), and miscellaneous (14%).

Godfrey and collaborators evaluated indications for fibrobronchoscopy over a period of 6 years, during which 2148 procedures were performed in children younger than 18 years of age. Hemoptysis was the indication in just 0.8% of cases and, of this group, 29.4% of cases were indicated for lower airway disease, 17.6% for tracheostomy bleeding, 17.6% for an unidentified reason, and the rest for miscellaneous reasons.

Table 23.1 lists conditions associated with hemoptysis in children, differentiated by their frequency.

Physiopathology

The lung receives blood from two systems: the arterial lung circulation (an extensive vascular, complacent, low-pressure bed, which irrigates up to the alveoli) and the bronchial circulation (a minor system, which perfuses up to the terminal bronchioles). Although bleeding can originate from any of these systems, massive hemoptysis usually originates from the bronchial circulation because its pressure is systemic.

Infections in the respiratory tract produce minor bleeds in the lower airway, which are of little clinical importance. Foreign bodies can cause hemoptysis in the bronchial circulation by damaging the airway wall. Hyperplasia, tortuosity, and dilation of bronchial arteries exist in bronchiectasis, provoking anastomosis between both systems. As a result of chronic inflammation, recurrent infections may cause erosion and tearing of abnormal bronchial arteries, which explains the hemorrhage. In DAHS, bleeding is produced by an injury in the lung microcirculation, which later extends to the alveoli.

Etiology

Aspiration of a Foreign Body

Aspiration of a foreign body is relatively common, especially in children younger than 3 years. Hemorrhage is more frequent during extraction

Table 23.1 Conditions associated with hemoptysis

Frequent conditions	Infrequent conditions
Aspiration of a foreign body	Lung malformations
Infection	Pulmonary sequestration
Tracheobronchitis	Tumor
Pneumonia	Adenoma
Influenza (e.g., H1N1)	Carcinoid
Lung abscess	Diffuse alveolar hemorrhage syndrome
Bronchiectasis (cystic fibrosis and noncystic fibrosis)	Pulmonary–renal syndrome
Echinococcosis	Goodpasture syndrome
Tuberculosis	Wegener granulomatosis
Aspergillosis (e.g., aspergilloma)	Microscopic polyangiitis
Trauma	Systemic lupus erythematosus
Accidental	Henoch–Schonlein purpura
Lung puncture	Idiopathic pulmonary hemosiderosis
Bronchoscopy	Factitious hemoptysis
Tracheostomy-related	
Intentional (suffocation)	
Cardiovascular	
Congenital cardiopathies	
Lung hypertension	
Arteriovenous fistula	
Lung thromboembolism	

of the foreign body if enough time has elapsed for it to cause infection.

Infections

Hemoptysis caused by an acute infection of the lower airway, as in tracheobronchitis, is of little clinical significance, although this is the most common cause, accounting for around 40% of cases.

In Chile, cavitary lung tuberculosis is an infrequent cause, but in endemic zones it is not rare for it to cause hemoptysis, which may become massive. Another cause is bronchiectasis after pneumonia due to an adenovirus. These two causes can result in hemoptysis in older children.

Cystic Fibrosis

Patients with advanced disease present extensive bronchiectasis, which can cause massive hemoptysis.

Trauma: Accidents, Surgery, and Other Causes

Direct trauma to the thorax in a motor vehicle accident or other causes of lung contusion can cause hemorrhage. Children with tracheostomies can also bleed, especially during aspiration. A significant number of children with suspected sudden death present with bleeding in the mouth, nose, or lungs at autopsy, suggesting accidental or intentional suffocation.

Cardiovascular Causes

Arterial or venous lung hypertension due to congenital or acquired diseases was an important cause of hemoptysis in children without CF in the series described by Coss-Bu and collaborators. Other relevant diseases are pulmonary veno-occlusive disease and congestive heart failure, among others. Nowadays, congenital cardiopathies are a less relevant cause because of the availability of early correctional surgery.

Tumors and Vascular Malformations

Adenoma and carcinoid tumors are the types of tumor that present hemoptysis more frequently, and they are more important in older patients. Hemoptysis with a tumor-related etiology is not very prevalent, although it can result in a massive hemorrhage. The most common type of vascular malformation is multiple arteriovenous fistulas, related to hereditary hemorrhagic telangiectasia (Osler–Weber–Rendu syndrome).

Hemorrhagic Diathesis

Occasionally, hemoptysis has been reported in patients with von Willebrand disease and hemophilia.

Diffuse Alveolar Hemorrhage Syndrome

This occurs as a result of an injury in small vessels, mainly capillaries, as well as arterioles and venules from the lung microcirculation. The current classification of DAHS subclassifies the diseases according to whether or not they present capillaritis on histopathological study.

Capillaritis can appear in isolation or as part of a systemic compromise, as happens in PRS. Other cases occur in the absence of capillaritis, not associated with vascular or systemic inflammatory disease (as in IPH), and are subclassified according to whether or not they are associated with cardiopathies.

Clinically, DAHS can appear in a spectrum that ranges from life-threatening acute respiratory failure to a more insidious appearance with few symptoms. During the hemorrhage, hemoptysis, coughing, paleness, dyspnea, respiratory difficulties, crackles, and hypoxemia can be observed; meanwhile, characteristic chest x-rays show cottony, shifting, and usually bilateral interstitial alveolar infiltrates.

In entities that present capillaritis, alongside lung compromise, some signs of an associated systemic disease can appear as a result of an immune-mediated condition.

Patients with nonimmune lung hemorrhage cannot be clinically differentiated. When there is suspicion of vasculitis, a lung biopsy must be done.

Diffuse Alveolar Hemorrhage Syndrome Associated with Capillaritis: Pulmonary–Renal Syndrome

In Wegener granulomatosis or microscopic polyangiitis, ANCAc and ANCAp (antineutrophil cytoplasmatic antibodies), which directly damage the lung microvasculature, are usually present. In Goodpasture syndrome or systemic lupus erythematosus, lung hemorrhage is produced by vasculitis, while in Wegener granulomatosis and microscopic polyangiitis it results from the presence of cavitary injuries.

Similar findings have been reported in children with Henoch–Schonlein purpura and other infrequent conditions such as antiphospholipid antibody syndrome or immunoglobulin A nephropathy.

Other Causes of Diffuse Alveolar Hemorrhage Syndrome with Lung Capillaritis

Idiopathic lung capillaritis, polyarteritis nodosa, cryoglobulinemia, and, lastly, medicines such as propylthiouracil, amiodarone, or penicillamine can provoke hemoptysis, even in therapeutic doses.

Diffuse Alveolar Hemorrhage Syndrome Not Related to Idiopathic Pulmonary Hemosiderosis Capillaritis

Idiopathic pulmonary hemosiderosis is a rare disease, limited to the lungs; there is no kidney or systemic compromise. The prognosis of this disease has improved because of early diagnosis and more effective treatments, with use of systemic steroids and immunosuppressive drugs, besides inhaled steroids in high doses.

Eighty percent of cases appear in the first decade of life. Clinical cases are characterized by recurrent hemoptysis (although this is not present in up to 33% of cases) and anemia, which is usually important. Severe episodes can put the patient's life at risk because of respiratory insufficiency and hemodynamic instability.

During an acute episode, shifting interstitial alveolar forms, usually symmetrical, are apparent on chest x-rays, which predominate in the perihilar regions and the bases of the lungs, without compromise of the apical zones and costophrenic angles (Fig. 23.1). Computerized tomography (CT) scans of the chest show cottony forms and a frosted glass effect (Fig. 23.2). The x-rays studies in both figures are from patients in our series. From the hematological standpoint, anemia with reticulocytosis exists depending on the availability of spinal deposits of iron and can subsequently turn into microcytic, hypochronic anemia if recurrences of the lung hemorrhage occur.

Lung function can be normal or show a restrictive ventilatory pattern. The CO diffusion capacity can be diminished, although it increases during

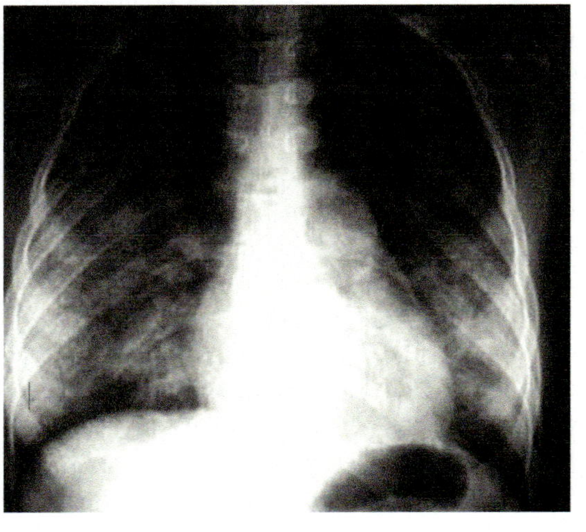

Fig. 23.1 Chest x-rays showing idiopathic pulmonary hemosiderosis (IPH) in a 13-year-old girl with an active hemorrhage, showing cottony, bibasilar, symmetrical forms without compromise of the lung apexes and costophrenic angles

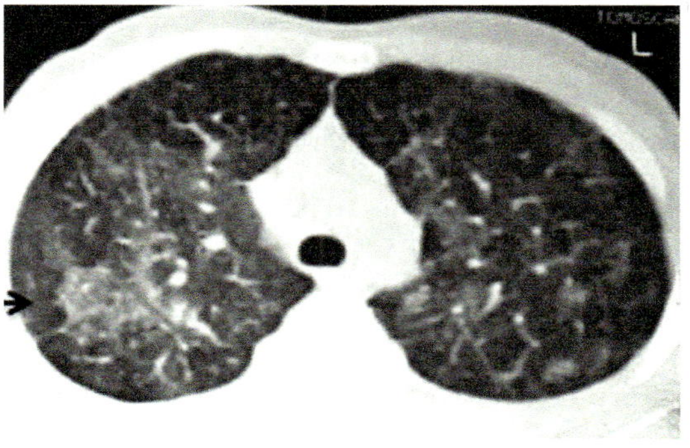

Fig. 23.2 CT scanning of idiopathic pulmonary hemosiderosis (IPH) in a 7-year-old boy with an active hemorrhage, showing cottony, bilateral shapes and a frosted glass effect in the right lung area (*arrow*)

active bleeding, which indicates intra-alveolar hemoglobin, representing a useful and sensitive indicator of hemorrhage during treatment.

Tests to exclude other causes of lung hemorrhage, such as PRS or disease of a cardiac origin, give negative results.

Acute Idiopathic Pulmonary Hemorrhage in Infancy: Epidemic in Cleveland

Dearborn and collaborators described a pulmonary hemorrhage epidemic that affected 30 infants. All of them presented severe DAHS. In some of them, the bleeding stopped spontaneously; in others, steroids had to be applied. The researchers found an association with environmental exposure to fungi, especially *Stachybotrys chartarum*, which was present in the damp houses of these patients, and the damaging mechanism acted through a mycotic angiotoxin. These children showed stunting and hemoglobinuria—characteristics suggesting that this entity should be differentiated from classical idiopathic pulmonary hemorrhage.

Other Causes of Diffuse Alveolar Hemorrhage Syndrome Without Lung Capillaritis

Other causes of idiopathic pulmonary hemorrhage include Heiner syndrome or allergy to cow's milk protein, von Willebrand disease, celiac disease, infanticide (suffocation), medications in therapeutic doses or overdoses (such as acetylsalicylic acid), cocaine abuse, inhalation of trimethyl anhydride, or exposure to pesticides.

Factitious Hemoptysis

Within this group is Munchausen syndrome, which presents especially in emotionally unstable adolescents, who self-provoke injuries that simulate hemoptysis.

Diagnostic Approach to Hemoptysis in Children

It is necessary to establish whether the presenting problem is hemoptysis or a hemorrhage in the upper airway (pseudohemoptysis) or in the upper digestive tract (hematemesis).

An upper airway hemorrhage—such as epistaxis or bleeding due to gingivitis, a pharyngeal ulcer, or tonsillar or adenoidal bleeding—can simulate hemoptysis. Hematemesis, which is infrequent in children, can occasionally be hard to differentiate from hemoptysis (Table 23.2).

Table 23.2 Differential diagnosis of hemoptysis and hematemesis

	Hemoptysis	Hematemesis
Color	Bright, foaming red	Dark red or brown
pH	Alkaline	Acidic
Consistency	May be mixed with sputum	May contain food particles
Background	Lung disease	Gastroesophageal or hepatic disease
Symptoms	Coughing may be preceded by a gurgling noise	May be preceded by nausea and vomiting
Confirmation	Bronchoscopy	Endoscopy

On the other hand, the fact that young children swallow blood that originates in the lung should be kept in mind; this can rarely cause hemoptysis (except when the hemorrhage is significant), hindering the diagnosis. Furthermore, children can vomit blood without coughing, which forces us to consider a diagnosis of hemoptysis in children with presumed hematemesis of unclear etiology in the presence of abnormalities on chest x-rays.

In many cases, the clinical history and physical tests do not considerably help to define the cause. Occasionally, the etiology is relatively obvious, such as in the case of patients with CF, chronic lung disease, or systemic diseases associated with lung hemorrhage, such as PRS. Other scenarios require more investigation.

Chest x-rays are mandatory, specifying whether the hemorrhage is unilateral or bilateral, and additionally showing the extension. The most common findings are atelectasis, and alveolar and interstitial cottony infiltrates; nevertheless, up to a third of children with hemoptysis have normal chest x-rays.

CT scanning of the chest with contrast dye is necessary to define bronchiectasis, cavitary injuries, malformations, arteriovenous fistulas, or tumors.

Computerized angiotomography and angiography—the latter being less used nowadays—help to evaluate pulmonary sequestration, which denotes the presence of an aberrant vessel, arteriovenous malformation, and other vasculature anomalies or a pulmonary thromboembolism.

Despite scintigraphy ventilation/perfusion being progressively less used, it is useful if a pulmonary thromboembolism is suspected. Magnetic resonance imaging has better resolution in soft tissues such as the mediastinum, hilum, and blood vessels, but it is less useful for the lung parenchyma. Finally, ultrasound scanning contributes only limited information.

Administration of red blood cells marked with technetium 99 is useful for identifying an active hemorrhage with a flow rate as low as 0.1 ml/min. The source of the hemorrhage is identified in 50% of patients.

Fibrobronchoscopy is prescribed if the hemorrhage is persistent, significant, or recurrent, or if its origin is not identified through imaging procedures, since it allows visualization of both the upper and lower airways, being able to determine the place of bleeding. However, when the hemorrhage is profuse, it is very hard to pinpoint; on the other hand, if bronchoscopy is done when the hemorrhage has stopped, the origin may not be located. Likewise, through fibrobronchoscopy, the esophagus can be observed in order to dismiss a high digestive hemorrhage.

Use of a flexible bronchoscope allows us to obtain samples for microbiological, cytological, and histopathological studies, and it can be used to perform bronchoalveolar lavage (BAL). A rigid bronchoscope is useful for extracting foreign bodies and in cases of a massive hemorrhage, for keeping the airway permeable while appropriate aspiration is conducted.

When there is not an obvious cause, BAL must be performed to search for hemosiderophages, which can also be found in induced sputum and gastric contents, with Prussian blue dye (Perl's reaction). In this regard, an experimental study in a murine model by Epstein and collaborators demonstrated that hemosiderophages start appearing within 3 days (2.8% cellularity) after the appearance of blood in the lungs. The numbers peak between the sixth and tenth day (60%) and drop to 10% in the following 1–2 months. A hemosiderophage count higher than 20% starting from the third to the fourth day of hemorrhage indicates IPH.

Once the bleeding has stopped and the results of imaging studies, bronchoscopy, and BAL are normal, it is reasonable to wait for another episode of hemorrhage before inquiring in further investigation.

If there is evidence of hemorrhage not due to airway injury, a foreign body, or CF, and there is no bronchiectasis due to other disease, a cardiological evaluation must be performed (including an electrocardiogram, an echocardiogram with color Doppler), with studies for PRS and hemorrhagic diathesis. If these diseases are dismissed, the lung hemorrhage may be due to IPH, the diagnosis of which is exclusionary.

Figure 23.3 shows a diagnostic algorithm for hemoptysis/lung hemorrhage.

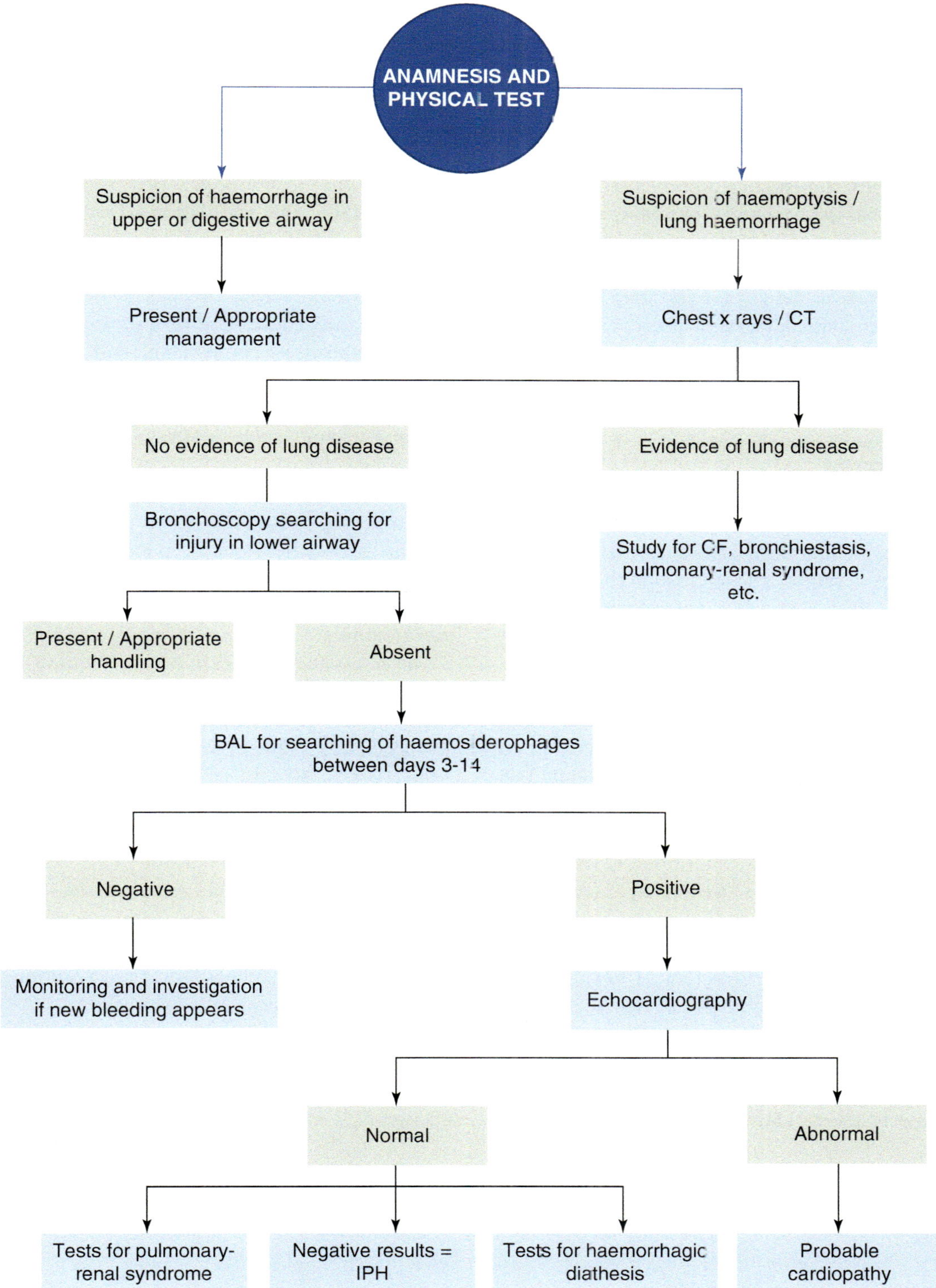

Fig. 23.3 Algorithm for diagnosis of hemoptysis/lung hemorrhage in children. *BAL* bronchioalveolar lavage, *CF* cystic fibrosis, *IPH* idiopathic pulmonary hemosiderosis

A lung biopsy is needed to dismiss systemic diseases associated with vasculitis, veno-occlusive disease, or pulmonary capillary hemangiomatosis. It is rarely performed in IPH; its diagnosis is based on the clinical and radiological findings, besides the finding of hemosiderophages, although it has been observed that this entity can evolve into a systemic autoimmune disease. Histopathology in IPH during active bleeding shows a large number of intact red blood cells in the alveoli and lung interstitium, and after some days, hemosiderophages appear; there is no evidence of vasculitis, granulomas, or immune complexes.

Treatment

Hemoptysis can be slight and transient, depending on its etiology and magnitude, or, conversely, it can be a severe and even fatal event. In this last case, the management approach must be proactive in order to establish appropriate treatment.

In patients with hemoptysis with an acute onset, the therapeutic objectives are, firstly, stabilization (which includes a permeable airway), oxygen administration, and eventual use of noninvasive or invasive mechanical ventilation. Positive pressure at the end of expiration can produce compression of vessels, thereby limiting the hemorrhage, and this is the reason why the patient must be kept in a lateral decubitus position, with the bleeding site downward. Furthermore, if hemodynamic instability exists, appropriate management for hypovolemic shock must be instituted through administration of a crystalloid bolus and/or a blood transfusion. If respiratory insufficiency persists, the patient must be connected to high-frequency mechanical ventilation. If this therapy is not effective, extracorporeal ventilatory support must be considered. Death in patients with a massive hemorrhage results more from acute respiratory insufficiency than from the extent of blood loss.

During the hemorrhage, BAL with cold saline solution and instillation of adrenaline (epinephrine) 1:10,000 must be performed for vasoconstriction, using a rigid bronchoscope; furthermore, extraction of clots is performed during this procedure. Use of tranexamic acid must be considered in patients with CF, on top of providing vitamin K, with avoidance of physical therapy, medicines that alter coagulation, and irritants such as DNase or nebulized antibiotics.

Some alternative treatments in the case of persistence of the hemorrhage are plugging with an inflatable Fogarty balloon catheter installed for 24 hours a day, application of fibrinogen and thrombin, carbon dioxide, or laser treatment.

The next step is selective embolization of the lung or bronchial vessels—a procedure that is relatively frequent in patients with advanced CF—and a satisfactory response is observed in 80% of cases. At our hospital, we have used it successfully in two instances (Fig. 23.4). If the objective is not accomplished, re-embolization must be done, associated with use of tranexamic acid. Lastly, if the hemorrhage still persists, surgical resection of the bleeding zone must be performed, such as a segmentectomy, lobectomy, or, exceptionally, pneumonectomy.

In cases of lung hemorrhage due to DAHS, systemic steroids are accepted as first-line medicines. Aggressive therapy has been used successfully, such as intravenous pulses of

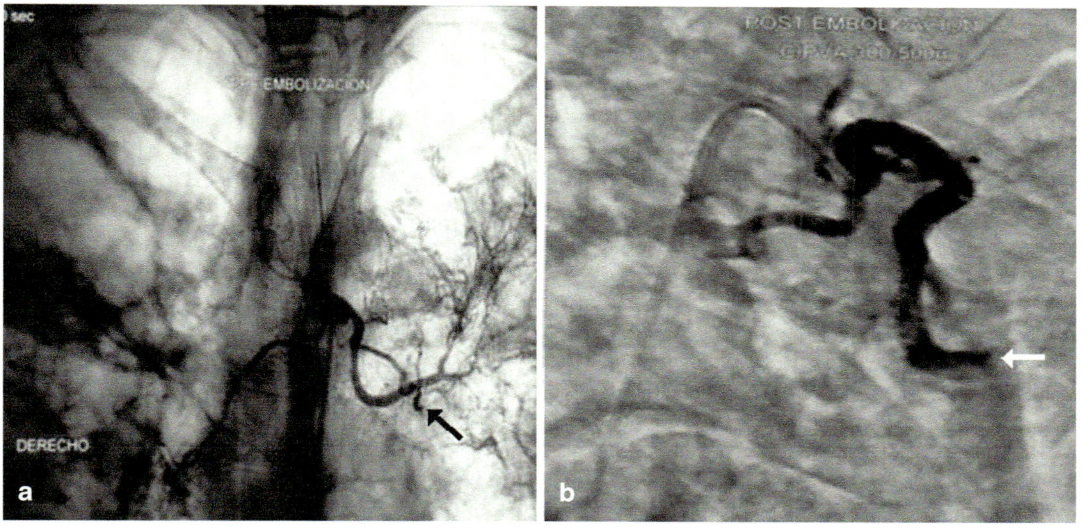

Fig. 23.4 Angiography and embolization of the left bronchial artery in an 18-year-old patient with advanced cystic fibrosis and a recurrent hemorrhage. (**a**) Pre-embolization, the left bronchial artery shows hyperplasia, tortuosity, and dilation (*arrow*). (**b**) Post-embolization with polyvinyl alcohol (*arrow*)

methylprednisolone 10–30 mg/kg (1 g maximum) per day for three consecutive days. Then, daily administration of oral prednisone (2 mg/kg/day) should be started, associated with an immunosuppressant such as azathioprine, hydroxychloroquine, mycophenolate, cyclophosphamide, or methotrexate, followed by an inhaled steroid in long-term high doses, to induce remission and improve the prognosis. Recently, monthly intravenous immunoglobulin has been used in immunomodulating doses (2 mg/day). Although there have been few publications describing such an approach, the results have been successful.

Finally, plasmapheresis is employed in Goodpasture syndrome. Lately, there have been reports of its utility for refractory hemorrhage in isolated lung vasculitis and for cases associated with connective tissue disease.

Figure 23.5 shows an algorithm for management of hemoptysis.

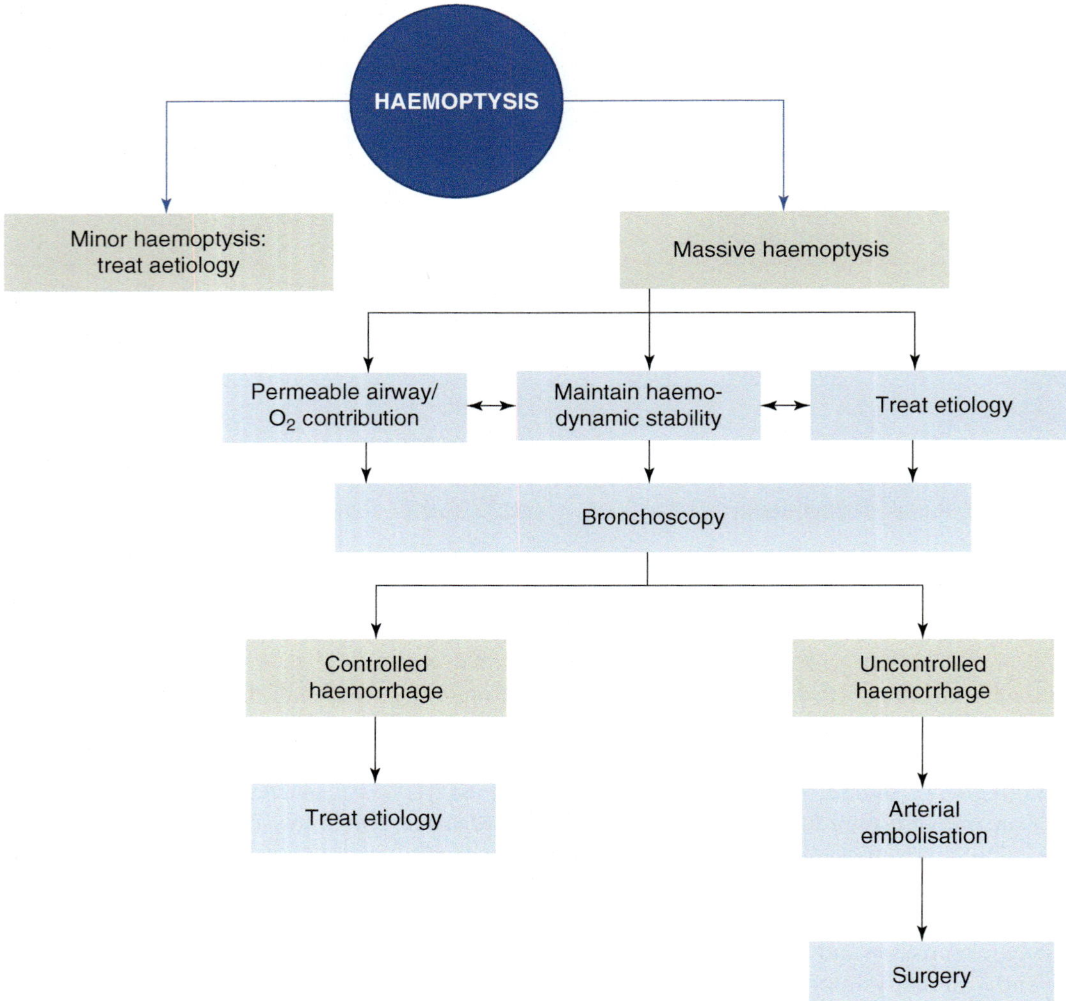

Fig. 23.5 Algorithm for management of hemoptysis in children

Conclusion

Hemoptysis in children is infrequent but can be caused by common diseases; generally, it is of minor magnitude but occasionally can manifest because of a severe case of hemorrhage that could be fatal if not appropriately managed.

The most likely causes are bronchiectasis associated with CF, chronic lung disease, injuries located in the airway, foreign bodies, coagulopathies, or cardiopathies. Other less frequent causes include serious pathologies that are a part of DAHS, such as PRS or IPH.

Sources

Batra PS, Holinger LD. Etiología y manejo de la hemoptisis pediátrica. Arch Otolaryngol Head Neck Surg. 2001;127:137.

Boat TF. Pulmonary hemorrhage and hemoptysis. In: Chernick V, Boat TF, Wilmatt RW, Bush A, editors. Kendig's disorders of the respiratory tract in children. 7th ed. Philadelphia: Saunders; 2006. p. 676–85.

Coss-Bu JA, Sachdeva RC, Bricker JT, Harrison GM, Jefferson LS. Hemoptysis: a 10-yr retrospective study. Pediatrics. 1997;100:E7.

Dearborn DG, Smith PG, Dahms BB, Allan TM, et al. Clinical profile of 30 infants with acute pulmonary hemorrhage in Cleveland. Pediatrics. 2002;110:627–37.

Epstein CE, Elidemir O, Colasurdo GN, Fan LL. Time course of hemosiderin production by alveolar macrophages in a murine model. Chest. 2001;120: 2013–20.

Fontenot AP, Schwarz MI. Hemorragia alveolar difusa. In: King Jr TE, Schwarz MI, editors. Enfermedad pulmonar intersticial. 4th ed. Hamilton: Decker; 2003. p. 632.

Gaude GS. Hemoptysis in children. Indian Pediatr. 2010;47:245–54.

Godfrey S. Pulmonary hemorrhage/hemoptysis in children. Pediatr Pulmonol. 2004;37:476–84.

Ioachimescu OC, Sieber S, Kotch A. Idiopathic pulmonary haemosiderosis revisited. Eur Respir J. 2004;24:162–70.

Khalil A, Soussan M, et al. Utility of high-resolution chest CT scan in the emergency management of hemoptysis in the intensive care unit: severity, localization and etiology. Br J Radiol. 2007;80(949):21–5.

Lara AR, Schwarz MI. Hemorragia alveolar difusa. Chest. 2010;137:1164.

Le Clainche L, Le Bourgeois M, Fauroux B, Forenza N, et al. Long-term outcome of idiopathic pulmonary hemosiderosis in children. Medicine (Baltimore). 2000;79:318–26.

Maggiolo J, Farbinger F, Rubilar L. Hemoptisis/hemorragia pulmonar en pediatría. Neumol Pediatr. 2009;4(2):65–72.

Pianosi P, Al-Sadoowh. Hemoptisis en niños. Pediatr Rev. 1997;18:16–9.

Rubilar L, Maggiolo J, Girardi G, González R. Hemosiderosis pulmonar idiopática: evolución de 5 niños. Neumol Pediatr. 2006;1:30–3.

Shah MK, Hugghins SY. Characteristics and outcomes of patients with Goopasture's syndrome. South Med J. 2002;95:1411–8.

Susarla SC, Fan LL. Diffuse alveolar hemorrhage syndromes in children. Curr Opin Pediatr. 2007;19:314–20.

Von Vigier RO, Trummler SA, Laux-End R, et al. Pulmonary renal syndrome in childhood: a report of twenty-one cases and a review of the literature. Pediatr Pulmonol. 2000;29:3.

Infants with an Apparent Life-Threatening Event

24

Pablo Brockmann Veloso, Daniel Zenteno Araos, and José Luis Pérez Sánchez

Contents

Diagnosis

Apparent life-threatening events (ALTEs) tend to be difficult to assess, given that, by definition, they present a subjective element based on the view of the observer. In this sense, it is expressly recommended to avoid terms such as "apnea crisis" and "aborted sudden death," which suggest a physiopathological process not necessarily related to ALTE. The risk factors for ALTE are exposure to cigarette smoke—in particular, intrauterine exposure—and premature birth. The risk factors for severe ALTE are prematurity, gestational age, symptoms of respiratory infection, and a history of sudden death of a sibling. The cause is found, in most cases, after an exhaustive review of the medical history (which is repeated in many cases), an extensive physical examination, and basic laboratory examinations (with sampling for viral agents, glycemia, and blood gases). ALTE cases generally have the following causes: a poor feeding technique associated with regurgitation, respiratory infections, gastroesophageal reflux, or convulsions. The causes in a minority of cases are metabolic diseases, poisoning, arrhythmia, Munchhausen syndrome, or others in a long list of associated diseases and syndromes.

P. Brockmann Veloso
Department of Pediatrics, School of Medicine, Pontificia Universidad Católica de Chile, Santiago, Chile
e-mail: pbrockmann@med.puc.cl

D. Zenteno Araos (✉)
Department of Pediatrics, Universidad de Concepción, Concepción, Chile

J. L. Pérez Sánchez
Department of Pediatrics, Universidad Austral de Chile, Osorno, Chile

Management Algorithm

ALTE patients should be assessed comprehensively with all clinical examinations that appear necessary. However, the decision as to which steps to follow and when to undertake a particular

P. Bertrand, I. Sánchez (eds.), *Pediatric Respiratory Diseases*,
https://doi.org/10.1007/978-3-030-26961-6_24

examination is difficult and costly. As a general recommendation, most ALTE cases should be hospitalized in a facility where monitoring is provided for at least 24–48 hours, because of which the following factors should be considered as risk factors in making such a decision: premature birth, age <2 months, vigorous resuscitation, recurrent condition, background disease, history of sudden death of a sibling, and social background.

The diagnosis should be made in stages, always considering details of the medical history and of physical examinations that may prove to be key in the final diagnosis: the family history, previous events, respiratory symptoms, sickness in a family member, history of epilepsy, the time of day when the event occurred, and other factors. Specific examinations are recommended in the context of symptoms indicating a particular disease (Table 24.1). It is critically important to determine whether the event occurred while the child was awake or asleep, as that information is helpful for determining the cause. In most series in Chile and other countries, even after an exhaustive evaluation, up to 30% of ALTE cases end up being diagnosed as "idiopathic." A sleep study (polysomnography) is particularly important in these patients to determine the presence of any sleep pathology. The algorithm shown in Fig. 24.1 (adapted from the Chilean consensus statement) orients the stages of the study of an infant with ALTE.

Table 24.1 Possible causes, symptoms and findings, and suggested studies in infants with an apparent life-threatening event

Possible causes	Symptoms and findings	Suggested studies
Gastrointestinal causes GERD Aspiration	Vomiting Blockage or coughing with food	pH metry Video swallow study Speech therapy assessment
Respiratory causes Viral infection/pertussis Aspiration/foreign body Anatomical airway alteration	Cor yza, cough, wheezing, fever, hypothermia History of foreign body ingestion Stridor, feeding difficulties, dysmorphisms (especially craniofacial dysmorphisms)	Viral panel, viral DIF PCR testing for *Bordetella* Endoscopic airway evaluation
Trauma Munchhausen syndrome by proxy	History of trauma, blood in the mouth or nose Previous ALTE, SIDS in a sibling, discordant history	Radiological clinical evaluation Rule out abuse Clinical suspicion
Neurological/convulsive causes	Loss of consciousness Eye deviation Seizure, hypotonia/hypertonia Microcephaly/macrocephaly Dysmorphia	EEG Brain echocardiogram CT scan/brain MRI Glycemia; Ca, P, Mg, PLD levels Metabolic study
Emotional apnea	Suggestive clinical history without other findings (while awake)	Rule out associated anemia
Metabolic causes	Family history Seizures Feeding difficulties Consciousness compromise Dysmorphia	Glycemia Lactate, ammonium, pyruvate Aminoacidemia, aminoaciduria, etc.
Cardiovascular causes Congenital heart disease Arrhythmia	Feeding difficulties Diaphoresis Central cyanosis, syncope	ECG (QTc) 24-hour Holter monitoring Doppler echocardiography
Infectious causes Meningitis Septicemia UTI	Fever, hypothermia, lethargy, and/or shock	Hemogram, blood culture PCR, complete urine, urine culture Lumbar puncture
Medications or toxicity	Consciousness compromise Lethargy, previous history	Toxicology screening of blood and/ or urine

CT computerized tomography, *DIF* direct immunofluorescence, *ECG* electrocardiogram, *EEG* electroencephalogram, *GERD* gastroesophageal reflux disease, *MRI* magnetic resonance imaging, *PCR* polymerase chain reaction, *PLD* phospholipase D, *QTc* corrected QT interval, *SIDS* sudden infant death syndrome, *UTI* urinary tract infection

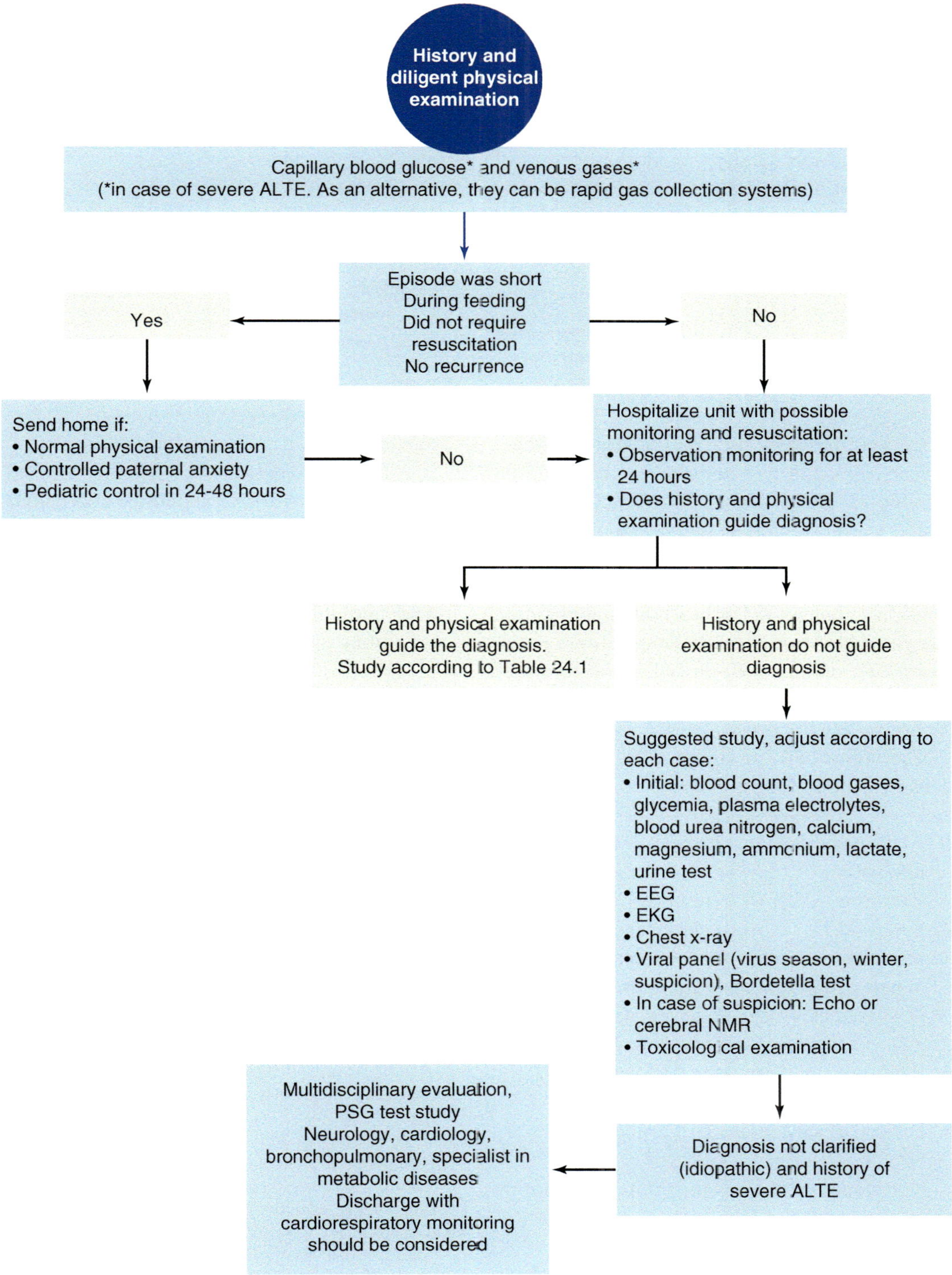

Fig. 24.1 Algorithm for study of an infant with an apparent life-threatening event (ALTE)

The objectives of hospitalization are clinical observation and treatment of a recurrent event, general and specific studies according to indicative symptoms, and education of the parents in cardiopulmonary resuscitation and safe sleeping conditions. If the standard monitoring period of 24–48 hours ends without occurrence of any events of concern and the study results are in the expected ranges, the treating physician can plan to release the patient to go home.

Indications for Cardiorespiratory Monitoring

Monitoring has been used for 40 years in ALTE patients, although, as noted above, it has not been possible to prevent incidents of sudden infant death. Cardiorespiratory monitoring does not detect obstructive apnea nor episodes of oxygen saturation decline. It detects only central-type apnea and changes in the heart rate (tachycardia, bradycardia). Apart from cardiorespiratory monitoring, we do not recommend other forms of monitoring that measure infant movements on the bed or that are superimposed.

The indications for comprehensive investigations in a child who has suffered ALTE are:

1. ALTE without a specific diagnosis (i.e., idiopathic)
2. Recurrent ALTE (≥2 episodes)
3. Severe ALTE without a clear cause, with formal resuscitation, or with persistent cyanosis; history of base disease (prematurity, bronchopulmonary dysplasia, Down syndrome, neuromuscular disease, craniofacial malformations, etc.)
4. Requirement for domestic ventilation or oxygen
5. History of sudden death of a sibling

Our recommendations regarding the duration of monitoring are as follows:

1. In cases where real alarms or events have occurred, but without apnea or bradycardia, monitoring should continue for a minimum of 6 weeks. The minimum age to suspend monitoring is 3 months in patients without risk factors or 6 months in those with risk factors.
2. In patients who depend on oxygen or assisted ventilation, monitoring should be continuous for as long as this type of support is required.
3. In the case of a patient with a history of sudden death of a sibling, monitoring should continue until the patient reaches the age at which the sibling died.

Table 24.2 Recommended variables for cardiorespiratory monitoring in preterm and term infants with an apparent life-threatening event

Infant age	Bradycardia (beats/minute)	Apnea duration (seconds)
Preterm infants[a]		
<40 weeks	100	15
40–44 weeks	80	15
>44 weeks	70	15–20
Term infants		
<1 months	80	20
1–3 months	70	20
3–12 months	60	20

[a]Corrected gestational age

The variables for cardiorespiratory monitoring are flexible and can be adjusted for each patient. Monitoring of the variables listed in Table 24.2 is recommended in patients with idiopathic ALTE.

Sources

Brockmann P, González X, Bertrand P, Sánchez I, Holmgren NI. Perfil clínico de lactantes hospitalizados por un episodio de ALTE (apparent life-threatening event). Rev Chil Pediatr. 2006;77(3):267–73.

Brockmann PE, et al. Consenso sobre el manejo de eventos de aparente amenaza a la vida del lactante (ALTE) Comisión de Sueño, Sociedad Chilena de Neumología Pediátrica 2013. Rev Chil Pediatr. 2014;85(3):378–87.

Esani N, Hodhman JE, Ehsani N, Hoppenbrouwers T. Apparent life-threatening events and sudden infant death syndrome: comparison of risk factors. J Pediatr. 2008;152(3):365–70.

Fu LY, Moon RY. Apparent life-threatening events: an update. Pediatr Rev. 2012;33(8):361–8.

Kaji AH, Claudius I, Santillanes G, Mittal MK, Hayes K, Lee J, Gausche-Hill M. Apparent life-threatening event: multicenter prospective cohort study to develop a clinical decision rule for admission to the hospital. Ann Emerg Med. 2013;61(4):379–87.

Khushi A, Côté A. Apparent life-threatening events: assessment, risks, reality. Paediatr Respir Rev. 2011;12(2):124–32.

McGovern MC, Smith MB. Causes of apparent life-threatening events in infants: a systematic review. Arch Dis Child. 2004;89(11):1043–8.

National Institutes of Health Consensus Development Conference on Infantile Apnea and Home Monitoring, Sept 29 to Oct 1, 1986. Pediatrics. 1987;79(2):292–9.

Ross-Russell R, Ravikumar K. Apparent life-threatening episodes in children. Paediatr Child Health. 2007;17(5):188–92.

Zenteno D, Quiroz G, Celis M, Tapia J. Causas atribuidas a eventos de aparente amenaza a la vida del lactante. Rev Chil Pediatr. 2008;79(2):163–71.

25 Immunosuppressed Children with Lung Infection

Alejandra Zamorano Wittwer and Marcela Ferrés Garrido

Contents

Epidemiology

Respiratory infections are the most common cause of morbidity in children. The World Health Organization (WHO) calculates that there are 1.9 million cases of pneumonia that result in death each year. In Chile, half of all hospital admissions in the early years of life are due to this cause, and it is the cause of death in 1.38 of every 1000 live births. Development of serious illnesses is more concerning in high-risk populations such as immunosuppressed patients.

Infectious agents that cause respiratory problems in immunocompetent and immunosuppressed patients are also opportunistic, remaining latent in the body and being reactivated in the situation of immunosuppression. The immune deficiencies in this patient group are diverse, and the orientation of the etiological diagnosis will depend on knowledge of the specific condition in every case.

With the optimization of treatments for oncological diseases (which have resulted in greater

A. Zamorano Wittwer · M. Ferrés Garrido (✉)
Department of Pediatrics, School of Medicine, Pontificia Universidad Católica de Chile, Santiago, Chile
e-mail: mferres@med.puc.cl

P. Bertrand, I. Sánchez (eds.), *Pediatric Respiratory Diseases*,
https://doi.org/10.1007/978-3-030-26961-6_25

numbers of survivors) and increases in the numbers of solid organ transplant and hematopoietic precursor recipients, patients with human immunodeficiency virus (HIV) infection, and patients with primary immunodeficiency, well-informed management of respiratory infections—which are the main causes of morbidity and mortality in these groups—is becoming increasingly important.

Physiopathology

Lung infection occurs generally through contact with droplets from people who are infected with, or who are carriers of, an infectious agent, or through exposure in a contaminated environment; for example, filamentous fungal infections occur this way. The infection is disseminated from the higher airway through the descending bronchogenic airway, finding a host with altered natural barriers, a deficient systemic or local immune response, alteration of the ciliary response, or decreased phagocytosis, among other factors, which in turn depend on the basic pathology of the patient. This group of weakened elements creates an environment for the settling of a bacterial, viral, fungal, or parasitic infection. All of the infectious processes that are a result of reactivation of latent infections acquired previously are added to the acute episode—for example, *Mycobacterium tuberculosis*, *Pneumocystis jirovecii*, *Toxoplasma gondii*, or *Cytomegalovirus* (CMV).

The clinical approach to a process that raises suspicion of pneumonia in these patients is not easy, since the symptomatology is not always typical and depends on the type of immunodeficiency and the etiological agent involved. Thus, there are cases of febrile pneumonia with lung condensation, pneumonia with torpid evolution despite broad-spectrum antimicrobial treatment, recurrent pneumonia, lung suppuration, or respiratory symptoms with or without fever. In many cases, radiological images are not typical, because it is impossible to focus on an infection. Some patients will develop respiratory insufficiency, which is often fatal. Added to this difficulty are the noninfectious processes that simulate or complicate pneumonia. Some of these noninfectious causes with early or late and diffuse or local infiltrates are listed in Table 25.1. An example of this is diffuse alveolar bleeding, which may compromise or even endanger life and manifests as anemia, hemoptysis, diffuse respiratory infiltrates, and development of acute lung insufficiency. In immunocompromised patients, drugs are the main cause of infections.

Table 25.1 Etiology of infection according to the radiological pattern

Pattern	Incidence	Causal agent
Diffuse	Common	*Pneumocystis* *Cytomegalovirus* *Mycobacterium*
	Rare	*Cryptococcus* *Aspergillus* *Candida*
Nodular or cavitary	Common	*Cryptococcus* Bacteria *Nocardia* *Aspergillus* *Mycobacterium*
	Rare	*Legionella* Septic embolism
Focal	Common	Bacteria *Cryptococcus* *Aspergillus* *Mucor*
	Rare	Tuberculosis Viruses *Legionella*
Local infiltrates	Bronchiolitis obliterans with organizing pneumonia Diffuse alveolar bleeding Metastasis Pharmacological toxicity Graft-versus-host disease Post-transplantation lymphoproliferative disease Radiotherapy toxicity Pulmonary alveolar proteinosis	
Diffuse infiltrates	Metastasis Pharmacological toxicity engraftment syndrome	
Early infiltrates	Pulmonary edema Pulmonary embolism Atelectasis Bleeding Aspiration, acute respiratory distress syndrome Chemotherapy	
Late infiltrates	Radiation Tumors Chemotherapy	

In patients with hematopoietic precursor transplants, the associated mortality exceeds 50% within 3 weeks after diagnosis.

Etiology

The spectrum of microorganisms is very wide, so it is very important to identify the causal agent. For this, we must take the following parameters into account:

1. The type of immunosuppression that the patient has.
2. The medical history, physical examination, epidemic status, clinical presentation, and speed at which the respiratory disorder has developed: acute, subacute, or chronic.
3. The timing of the appearance of the respiratory disorder relative to that of the base illness, transplantation, or immunosuppressive drug administration.
4. The preliminary results of general and specific examinations to establish the etiology.
5. The type of radiological infiltrate (diffuse, focal, nodular, cavitated) and the images obtained from computerized tomography (CT scanning), ultrasound scanning, or nuclear magnetic resonance imaging.
6. The drugs and treatments the patient has received, considering that some of them might favor immunosuppression and/or lung damage. The use of immunosuppressive treatments needs to be noted in patients with transplants, such as cyclosporin, steroids, mycophenolate, monoclonal antibodies, or antithymocyte globulins.
7. Chemotherapy drugs such as bleomycin, cyclophosphamide, and methotrexate can cause lung damage, while radiotherapy can cause myelosuppression and lung fibrosis.

Because of their base condition and chemotherapy/radiotherapy, oncological patients have periods of neutropenia and secondary cell immunodeficiency, with a higher risk of developing viral pneumonia due to respiratory syncytial virus (RSV), adenovirus, enterovirus, or varicella zoster; or mycotic pneumonia due to *Aspergillus*, *P. jirovecii*, *Mucor*, *Rhizopus*, or occasionally *Candida*. The possibility of pneumonia associated with *M. tuberculosis*—or, less often, *Toxoplasma* or *Cryptococcus neoformans*—must also be taken into account.

In patients who have undergone bone marrow or solid organ transplantation, lung complications will depend on the period of immunosuppression associated with the transplantation.

In general terms, lung infections occurring early after solid organ transplantation are linked to the surgery and invasive procedures performed in hospitalized patients. After the first month and up to 6 months afterward, the level of immunosuppression that is achieved favors infection by organisms that are dormant in the donor or the recipient, opportunistic infections, and infections acquired in the community. After 6 months the predominant infections are those contracted from both viral and bacterial communities (Fig. 25.1). It is important to bear in mind that the risks are higher in lung transplantation when acquired agents have tropisms for the respiratory tract.

During the first 15 days after hemopoietic precursor transplantation, neutropenia and severe damage of the mucosa, due to chemotherapy, favor bacterial infections that can focus on the lung. At the following stage, after bone marrow grafting, CMV is one of the most common problems that can affect the lung, together with opportunistic filamentous fungal infections. At the third stage, 3 months after the transplantation, the cell response and humoral response remain weak, and infections due to encapsulated bacteria, filamentous bacteria, and opportunistic bacteria are frequent (Fig. 25.2).

Patients with common variable immune deficiency and agammaglobulinemia present recurrent bacterial pneumonia, normally produced by encapsulated germs; they are rarely present in pneumonia caused by *P. jirovecii*. Children with T cell immunodeficiency, serious combined immunodeficiencies, etc., have a higher risk of contracting the same type of opportunistic diseases as patients with acquired immunodeficiency syndrome (AIDS), as well as recurrent and persistent infections caused by *Candida albicans*

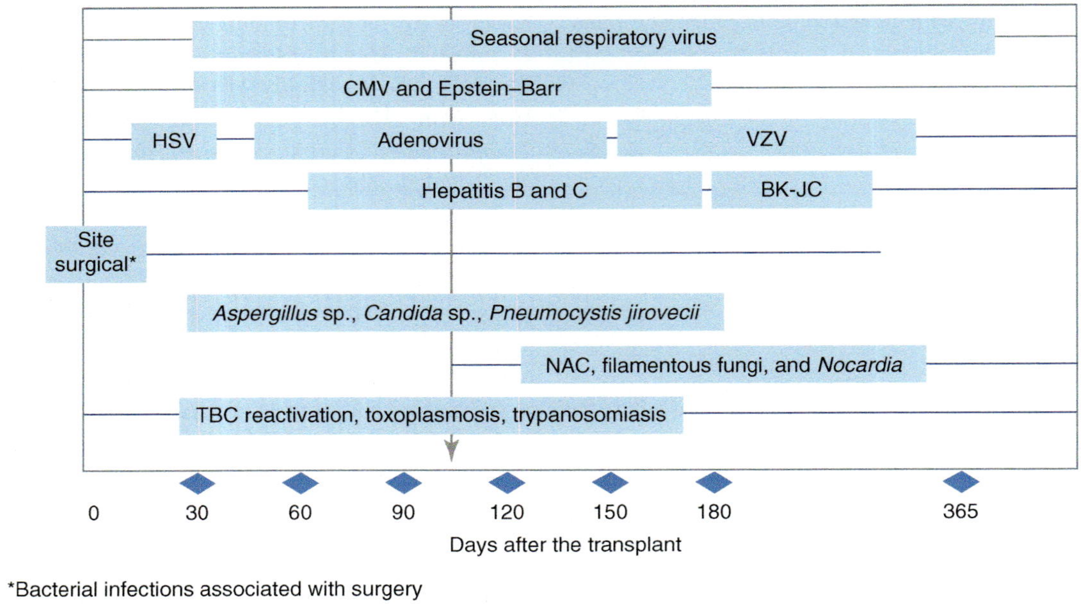

Fig. 25.1 Timing of infections in solid organ transplant recipients

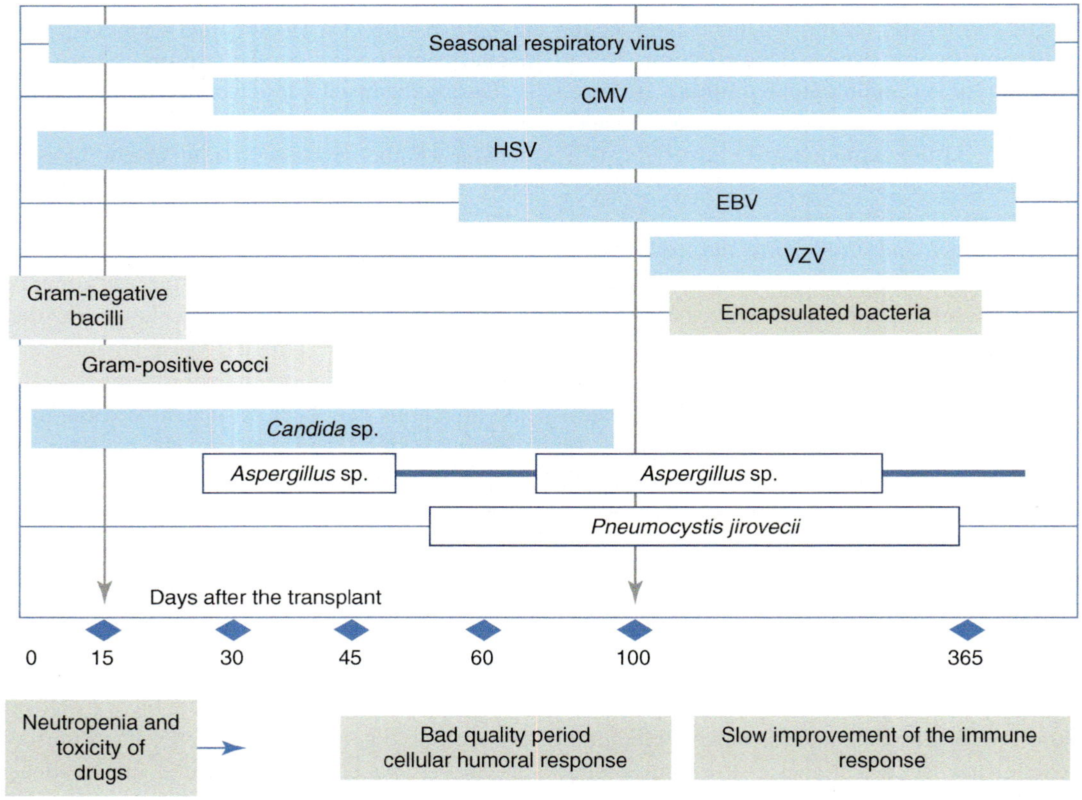

Fig. 25.2 Timing of infections in hematopoietic precursor transplant recipients

Table 25.2 Immunosuppression and infectious etiology

Type of immunosuppression	Mechanisms compromised	Favored organisms	Common causes
Phagocytosis	Engulfment of bacteria and fungi by mononuclear cells (monocytes and macrophages) and polymorphonuclear cells (neutrophils) Antigen presentation	*Staphylococcus aureus*, bacilli, Gram-negative aerobes (*Pseudomonas aeruginosa*, *Klebsiella pneumoniae*, *Escherichia coli*), *Candida* spp., *Aspergillus* spp.	Neutropenia (leukemia, bone marrow suppression due to chemotherapy) Chronic granulomatous diseases Corticotherapy Hyper-IgE (Job syndrome)
Humoral immunity	B lymphocytes Neutralization Opsonization Complement activation	Extracellular encapsulated bacteria: *Streptococcus pneumoniae, Haemophilus influenzae, Staphylococcus aureus*	Primary: agammaglobulinemia, IgA deficiency, IgM deficiency Secondary: myeloma, Waldenström macroglobulinemia, lymphocyte leukemia
Complement	Mediation of opsonization Attraction of inflammatory cells Elimination of microorganisms through damage to their membranes	C3-C5: encapsulated bacteria C5–C9: *Neisseria gonorrhoeae*, *Neisseria meningitidis*	C3–C5: encapsulated bacteria C5–C9: *Neisseria gonorrhoeae*, *Neisseria meningitidis*
Cellular immunity	T lymphocytes Killing of pathogen-infected cells by cytotoxic T (CD8) cells Macrophage activation by T_h1 (CD4) cells B lymphocytes activation by T_h2 (CD4) cells to produce antibodies	*Mycobacterium tuberculosis*, *Mycobacterium avium*-c, *Nocardia asteroides*, *Legionella* spp., *Cryptococcus neoformans*, *Histoplasma capsulatum*, *Coccidioides immitis*, varicella zoster, herpes simplex, *Cytomegalovirus*, Epstein–Barr virus, *Pneumocystis jirovecii*, *Toxoplasma gondii*	Primary Secondary: malnutrition, lymphoma, leukemia, old age, drugs, AIDS Corticosteroids
Hyposplenia/ asplenia	Blood filtration Production of bacteria-specific antibodies Removal of bacteria covered in antibodies	Encapsulated bacteria	Thrombotic thrombocytopenic purpura, Hodgkin lymphoma

AIDS acquired immunodeficiency syndrome, *IgA* immunoglobulin A, *IgE* immunoglobulin E, *IgM* immunoglobulin M, T_h1 type 1 helper T cell, T_h2 type 2 helper T cell

in the mucosa or the skin. Patients with chronic granulomatous disease suffer lung infections caused by *Aspergillus* or *Staphylococcus aureus*—agents that require effective phagocytosis for their destruction. Children with primary immunodeficiency always present severe lung complications: bronchiectasis, empyema, lung abscesses, etc.

In patients with AIDS, there is a long list of associated lung infections, including those caused by *P. jirovecii*, CMV, Epstein–Barr virus, and mycobacteria, both typical and atypical. These are detailed in the corresponding chapter.

The most frequent etiologies for severe pneumonia according to the type of immunosuppression are listed in Table 25.2.

Bacteria

In addition to bacterial infection caused by common pathogens such as *Streptococcus pneumoniae* or *Haemophilus* spp., we find agents selected by broad-spectrum antimicrobial therapies or long stays in the hospital, such as *S. aureus*,

Pseudomonas aeruginosa, and resistant Gram-negative bacilli such as *Stenotrophomonas maltophilia* and *Burkholderia cepacia* complex.

Viruses

Viral infections are the most frequent cause of respiratory infection in immunosuppressed patients with pneumonia. The diseases have an atypical course, which can be severe, and they can lead to respiratory failure with a high death rate. This is especially serious in patients with bone marrow transplants, in whom RSV, adenovirus, and parainfluenza 3 result in death rates of 60–70%. A favorable prognosis in these patients is determined by early suspicion, diagnosis, and therapy, if available.

Infections can be due to seasonal viruses present in the community, such as influenza A and B viruses, parainfluenza (1–4), RSV, adenovirus, metapneumovirus, or rhinovirus. With advances in molecular diagnostic techniques, it is increasingly common to find coinfections by both respiratory viruses and latent bacteria or viruses that have reactivated, such as viruses in the Herpesviridae family, among which CMV can be highlighted.

Unfortunately, there are few antiviral drugs available as a therapeutic resource. Influenza vaccination must be targeted toward close contacts of the patients, especially within the first 3 months after transplantation. Beyond this period, it can be used in transplant recipients themselves, who can progressively mount an immune response.

Cytomegalovirus

Cytomegalovirus is a herpes virus and infects 40–100% of the general population in adulthood. After the primary infection, it persists as a latent infection for long periods and can reactivate in states of cellular immunosuppression, as in the case of patients treated with a lymphocyte immunosuppressant (OKT3).

The infection and disease caused by CMV are the main complications in patients who undergo bone marrow transplantation and in patients with AIDS; the latter have a high risk of reaching CD4 counts as low as <50 cells/mm^3.

The clinical picture is acute or subacute with fever, tachypnea, a dry cough, and, in serious cases, respiratory failure. The radiological pattern is very varied, ranging from presentation of slight interstitial infiltration to a diffuse alveolar filling pattern.

An accurate disease diagnosis for CMV requires demonstration of tissue damage with the characteristic cytopathic effect caused by the virus, with intranuclear or intracytoplasmic inclusion bodies, or positive immunohistochemistry. However, collection of tissue samples is an invasive procedure, and so it is generally avoided in these patients. Nowadays, other methods for diagnosis are used, such as detection by quantification of viral genomes in the blood (using quantitative polymerase chain reaction (PCR) for CMV or the CMV viral load), which provides the etiological diagnosis and confirms pulmonary involvement. A finding of inclusion bodies on cytological analysis of bronchoalveolar lavage (BAL) fluid or PCR for CMV in BAL fluid is helpful. However, these findings must be interpreted cautiously because such detection may signify contamination of the higher respiratory tract, where CMV can exist without causing disease.

It is important to regularly monitor the primary infectious condition or reactivation in patients who have undergone solid organ or bone marrow transplantation, at least during the higher-immunosuppression phase (corresponding roughly to the 3-month period after the transplantation). Appropriate prophylaxis and early treatment can prevent severe infection.

Fungi

Fungal infections in immunosuppressed patients can be divided into opportunist infections caused by organisms that invade the lung primarily (*Aspergillus* or *C. neoformans*), opportunistic infections that reach the lung through hematogenous dissemination from another site, fungal overinfection of lung tissue previously damaged by a viral or bacterial infection (*Candida* or *Aspergillus*), and reactivated secondary systemic mycosis (in the context of immunosuppression) from previously acquired infections, as occurs in cases of blastomycosis, coccidioidomycosis, and histoplasmosis.

Aspergillosis

The genus *Aspergillus* (especially the species *A. fumigatus* and *A. flavum*) is the most frequent cause of fungal pneumonia in neutropenic patients and in bone marrow transplant recipients (it can affect up to 20% of recipients). There is a lower incidence (between 1% and 8%) in solid organ transplant recipients. This invasive pulmonary infection is associated with prolonged neutropenia, graft-versus-host disease, and use of steroids. The incidence depends on antifungal prophylaxis and the kind of immunosuppression.

The infection is acquired by inhalation, and the clinical picture consists of a high fever, cough, dyspnea and hemoptysis, with pleuritic chest pain. It usually occurs after a previous bacterial infection.

From a radiological point of view, many alveolar infiltrates, which can coalesce, may be observed. A thoracic CT scan presents typical findings of nodules with central density and a peripheral halo with intermediate density, and sometimes these lesions can cavitate (Fig. 25.3). CT scanning is the preferred imaging test for diagnosis. Aspergilloma does not usually occur in immunosuppressed patients, although it can happen in patients with an alteration of the underlying lung architecture.

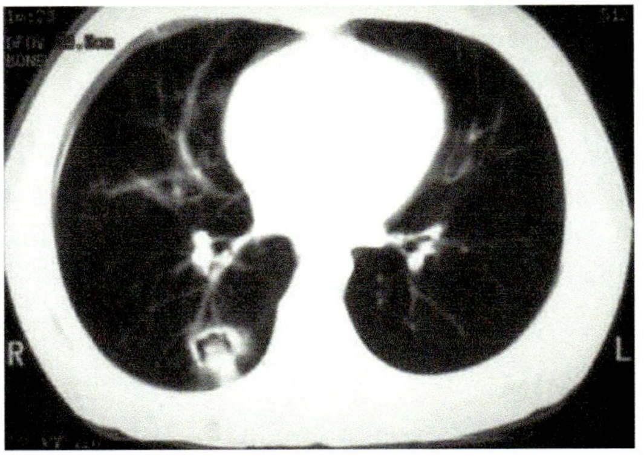

Fig. 25.3 Aspergillosis. "Half-moon" shaped, cavitated nodular opacity in an axial section of a CT scan, due to *Aspergillus* infection in a child with acute lymphoblastic leukemia

Measurement of galactomannan antigen in BAL fluid has 90% sensitivity and 94% specificity for invasive lung aspergillosis. Detection of the fungus in significant amounts in BAL fluid or in three repeat samples of sputum can be enough to establish the diagnosis.

Molecular diagnosis of fungal infections is not as advanced as molecular diagnosis of viral or bacterial infections. Biopsy with histopathological analysis of the lung tissue is still the gold standard but is rarely done, because of the risks associated with collection of samples.

Lung angiography can be useful in the search for an angioinvasive disease. Untreated infections can have a mortality rate as high as 90%.

Voriconazole is the first-line treatment for invasive lung aspergillosis, and the duration of the treatment depends on clinical improvement, resolution of galactomannan antigenemia, and radiological confirmation of lesion improvement.

Lobectomy has a limited role in neutropenic patients and is reserved for patients with potentially lethal massive hemoptysis.

Mucormycosis

Mucormycosis is the second most common type of invasive lung infection and is caused by *Rhizopus*, *Mucor*, or *Rhizomucor*. It manifests as lung nodules in patients with bone marrow transplants. It evolves faster than aspergillosis in causing angioinvasion. A definitive diagnosis requires histological evidence. The first-line treatment for this etiology is liposomal amphotericin B.

Candida

Neutropenia, cell immunity alterations, diabetes mellitus, and the use of immunosuppressants and broad-spectrum antibiotics are predisposing factors for infection with *Candida albicans*, which usually manifests as widespread pneumonia with focal or diffuse alveolar infiltrates. Isolated lung infections are uncommon.

In HIV-positive patients, *C. neoformans* is the fungus that most frequently causes lung infiltrates. It usually produces a disseminated infection that affects the central nervous system, causing meningitis, which is the most common manifestation; this can conceal the respiratory clinical condition, but in up to a 40% of cases, pulmonary impairment can also be present, with interstitial reticulonodular opacities or well-delimited nodules.

Pneumocystis jirovecii

Despite prophylaxis with sulfamethoxazole trimethoprim, *P. jirovecii* is a common infection in immunocompromised patients. Risk factors include immunosuppressant therapies, both in transplant patients and in oncological patients, and systemic steroid use for long periods of time.

Patients can have the following clinical manifestations: a cough, progressive shortness of breath (especially during exercise), and hypoxia. Chest x-rays can be normal or can present diffuse interstitial infiltrates, which can evolve to become alveolar, bilateral, or perihilar (Fig. 25.4). The changes are more evident on CT scans, and *P. jirovecii* cysts can be identified in sputum or BAL fluid. In patients with a compatible clinical picture, a serum β-D-glucan test can be used to confirm the diagnosis in immunocompromised patients with 94.8% sensitivity and 86.3% specificity.

A death rate of up to 34% has been reported for this etiology in patients with oncological pathologies that require mechanical ventilation.

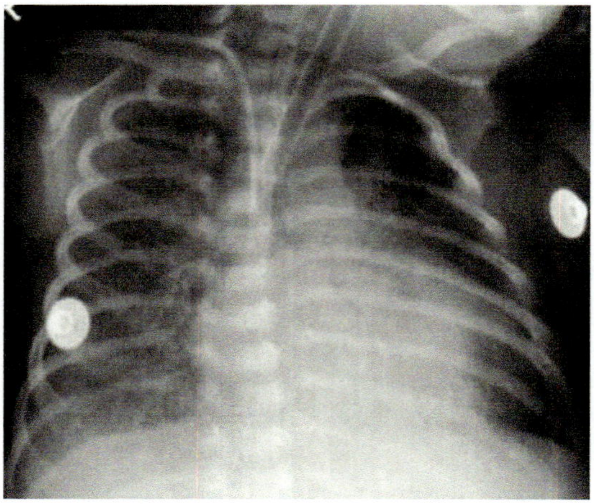

Fig. 25.4 *Pneumocystis jirovecii*. Anteroposterior chest x-ray showing bilateral pneumonia caused by *P. jirovecii* in an infant with cellular immunodeficiency

The treatment of choice is sulfamethoxazole/trimethoprim with added corticosteroids in hypoxemic patients.

Prophylaxis for *P. jirovecii* is recommended for at least 6 months after transplantation, or for longer if immunosuppression persists. A specific length of time has not been defined for oncological patients.

Mycobacteria

Reactivation of latent tuberculosis is the most common form of disease in patients from countries with a high tuberculosis prevalence. Chemoprophylaxis before immunosuppression reduces but does not eliminate the risk of reactivation.

The clinical picture is usually insidious, with general discomfort, a low-grade fever, a wet cough, and dyspnea. The most common clinical presentation is that 1 year after transplantation the patient develops fever without respiratory symptoms but with nonspecific radiological changes, including lymphadenopathy with pleural effusion and patchy pulmonary infiltrates.

Nontubercular Mycobacteria

In patients with significant immunosuppression, such as AIDS patients and recipients of solid organ or bone marrow transplants, *Mycobacterium* can cause pulmonary bacterial infections and disseminated disease, with *M. avium* and *M. kansasii* being the most frequently causal species.

In patients with cystic fibrosis, colonization by *M. avium* and *M. abscessus* complex are common, becoming worse in the state of post-transplantation immunosuppression.

Automatized culture methods such as molecular techniques allow for quick diagnosis.

Treatment is maintained for 12–18 months with three or more drugs.

Parasites

The most common parasite is *Toxoplasma*, which usually causes fever, a dry cough, and dyspnea. Its radiological presentation usually shows a diffuse interstitial pattern.

Diagnostic Studies

Early commencement of adequate therapy is crucial; thus, empirical therapy is initiated and then adjusted according to the evolution of the disease and the results of investigations.

Clinical Presentation

It is important to know what the cause of the immunosuppression is, whether it is primary or secondary, and what the relationship is between the start of the symptoms or pulmonary infiltrates and the immunosuppression.

Radiology

Radiological findings are very useful, and even though no radiological pattern is pathognomonic of an etiology, differentiation of diffuse, nodular, and focal patterns can provide an initial orientation (Table 25.1).

Early axial CT scanning is important for diagnosis, because in neutropenic patients with fever, up to 50% of pulmonary lesions diagnosed with CT may not be observable with simple radiography.

Microbiological Diagnosis

Sampling

Sampling of spontaneous sputum or sputum induced by nebulization of hypertonic serum can be performed before collection of BAL fluid by bronchoscopy, which can be useful if germs that do not belong to the oropharyngeal cavity grow in the culture.

Blood cultures are useful mainly in neutropenic patients and for germs that invade the bloodstream, such as *S. pneumoniae*. Special culture media are required if *Nocardia* or atypical *Mycobacterium* are present.

BAL with bronchoscopy is the main diagnostic procedure performed in an immunosuppressed patient with pulmonary infiltrates. It enables identification of the causal agents, adjustment of treatment according to the etiology, and exclusion of infections that are not present, allowing suspension of any empirically initiated therapies that are inappropriate and could be harmful to the patient.

While a surgical pulmonary biopsy allows us to obtain an adequate amount of lung tissue for complete microbiological and pathological diagnosis, in these patients it presents a high risk of complications, and often the diagnostic capability is low, so the decision to perform such a biopsy must be made on a case-by-case basis. The possibility of reaching a correct diagnosis that might change the treatment must be evaluated, along with the likelihood of tolerance and surgical complications.

Figure 25.5 shows an algorithm for microbiological diagnosis on the basis of pulmonary infiltrates in immunosuppressed patients with fever.

Treatment

Given the severity of the clinical picture and the importance of early commencement of treatment, the normal way of managing an immunosuppressed patient with a respiratory infection is to start empirical therapy while waiting for test results.

The initial empirical therapies that may be instituted according to the clinical picture are listed in Table 25.3.

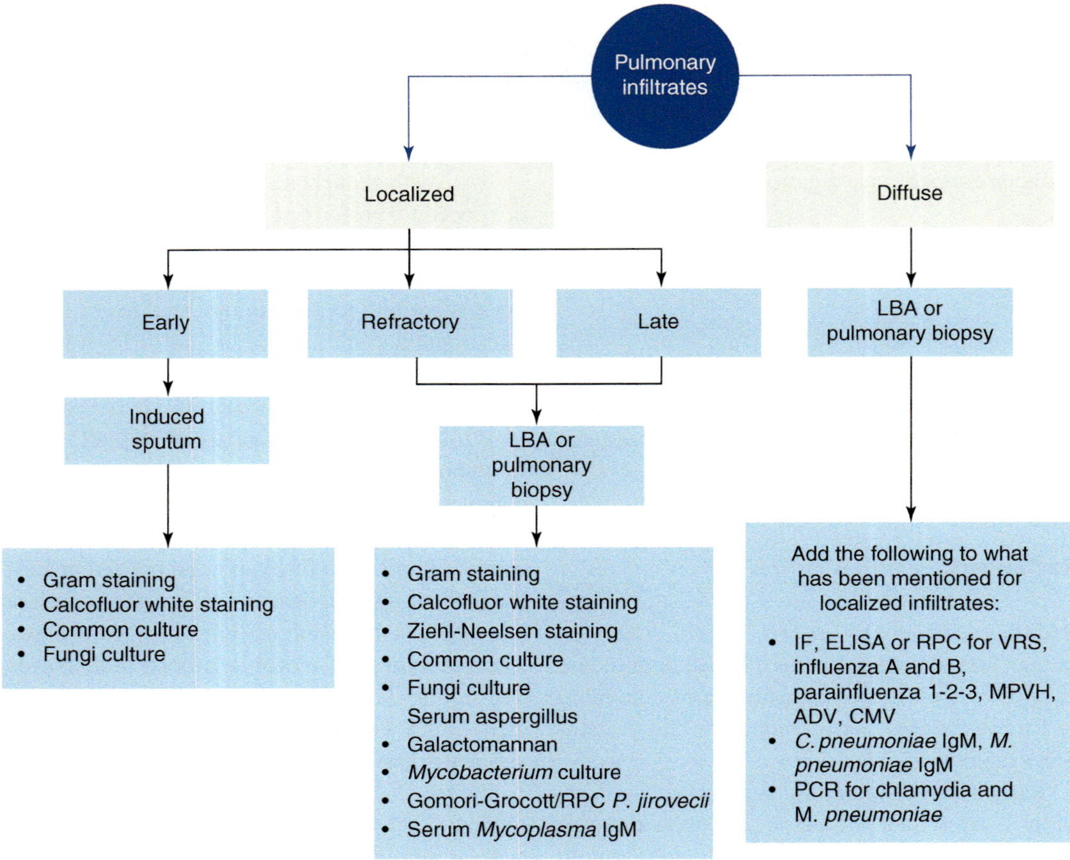

Fig. 25.5 Microbiological diagnosis in immunosuppressed patients with fever

Table 25.3 Initial empirical therapeutic management

Indication	Therapy
Febrile neutropenia (Gram-negative bacteria, *Staphylococcus*, fungi)	Broad-spectrum β-lactam with antipseudomonal activity + quinolone or aminoglycoside
No response	Addition of glycopeptide
Patchy/diffuse infiltrates	
If neutropenia is prolonged	Addition of amphotericin B or voriconazole
Solid organ transplantation	Cotrimoxazole + ganciclovir
Interstitial pattern (pneumonia due to *Pneumocystis* or *Cytomegalovirus*)	
Lobar infiltrates (pneumococcus, *Haemophilus influenzae, Staphylococcus*)	Broad-spectrum β-lactam with antipseudomonal activity + aminoglycoside
Diffuse process (*Pneumocystis*, viruses, fungi)	Cotrimoxazole + ganciclovir + amphotericin B
Atypical agents	Macrolide or quinolone
Hypogammaglobulinemia (bacterial process)	Intravenous immunoglobulin + β-lactam with antipseudomonal activity ± macrolide
HIV infection	Cotrimoxazole
Interstitial process (*Pneumocystis*, viruses)	Cotrimoxazole
Lobar infiltrates (bacteria)	Third-generation cephalosporin + macrolide
Nosocomial pneumonia (Gram-negative resistant *Staphylococcus*)	Broad-spectrum β-lactam with antipseudomonal activity + aminoglycoside

(continued)

Table 25.3 (continued)

Indication	Therapy
Bone marrow transplantation	Ganciclovir + immunoglobulin
Allogenic	Ganciclovir + immunoglobulin
Interstitial process	
Patchy/diffuse	Ganciclovir + immunoglobulin + amphotericin B + β-lactam + aminoglycoside

HIV human immunodeficiency virus

Sources

Bosque M, Larramona H, Asensio O, Tardío E. Pulmón en el paciente inmunodeprimido. In: Protocolos diagnóstico terapéuticos de la AEP: neumología. Madrid: Asociación Española de Pediatría; 2008. p. 133–43.

Canals M, Sabbagh E, Chernilo S. Neumonías en el inmunocomprometido: perspectiva desde el diagnóstico por imágenes, e inferencia Bayesiana. Rev Chil Infectol. 2014;31(2):139–52.

Doan TT, Phung TT, Pham HV, Pham SH, Nguyen LT. Effect of ganciclovir for the treatment of severe *Cytomegalovirus*-associated pneumonia in children without a specific immunocompromised state. BMC Infect Dis. 2013;13:424.

Eslamy H, Newman B. Pneumonia in normal and immunocompromised children: an overview and update. Radiol Clin N Am. 2011;49:895–920.

Gambra MP, Bidart T. Profilaxis de neumonía por *Pneumocystis jirovecii* en niños y adultos sometidos a trasplante de órganos sólidos y de precursores hematopoyéticos. Rev Chil Infectol. 2012;29(Suppl 1):19–22.

Gilberta C, Lernerb A, Baramc M, Bharat K. Utilidad de la broncoscopía flexible en la evaluación de infiltrados pulmonares en la población con trasplante de células madre hemopoyéticas: experiencia de 14 años en un solo centro. Arch Bronconeumol. 2013;49(5):189–95.

Godbole G, Gant V. Respiratory tract infections in the immunocompromised. Curr Opin Pulm Med. 2013;19:244–50.

Letourneaua A, Issaa N, Baden L. Pneumonia in the immunocompromised host. Curr Opin Pulm Med. 2014;20:272–9.

Paganini H, Santolaya ME. Diagnóstico y tratamiento de la neutropenia febril en niños con cáncer. Consenso de la Sociedad Latinoamericana de Infectología. Rev Chil Infectol. 2011;28(Suppl 1):10–38.

Santolaya ME. Rabagliati R. Bidart T, Payá E, Guzmán AM, et al. Consenso manejo racional del paciente con cáncer, neutropenia y fiebre. Rev Chil Infectol. 2005;22(Suppl 2):S80.

Silva RF. Fungal infections in immunocompromised patients. J Bras Pneumol. 2010;36(1):142–7.

Steen B. La neumonía en el paciente inmunodeprimido: un problema en aumento. Rev Patol Respir. 2005a;8(2):157–8.

Steen B. Neumonía en el inmunodeprimido. In: García Satué JL, Aspa Marco J, editors. Monografías Neumomadrid, vol. IX. Madrid: Neumomadrid; 2005b. p. 159–78.

Stocchi R, Ward K, Fanin R, Baccarani M, Apperley J. Management of human *Cytomegalovirus* infection and disease after allogeneic bone marrow transplantation. Haematologica. 1998;84:791–7.

Vega-Briceño LE, Holmgren NL, Bertrand P, Rodríguez JI, Barriga F, Contreras I, Sánchez I. Utilidad del lavado broncoalveolar en niños inmunodeprimidos: rendimiento y complicaciones. Arch Bronconeumol. 2004;40(12):570–4.

Respiratory Complications in Children with Neurological Diseases

26

Raúl Escobar Henríquez
and Bernardita Chateau Infante

Contents

R. Escobar Henríquez
Department of Pediatrics, School of Medicine, Pontificia Universidad Católica de Chile, Santiago, Chile
e-mail: rescobar@med.puc.cl

B. Chateau Infante (✉)
Department of Pediatrics, Clínica Los Andes, Santiago, Chile
e-mail: bchateau@clinicauandes.cl

Epidemiology

Respiratory disorders are one of the main causes of morbidity and mortality among patients with neurological diseases. They have multifactorial causes, their prevalence is variable, and they depend on the type of neurological disease.

P. Bertrand, I. Sánchez (eds.), *Pediatric Respiratory Diseases*,
https://doi.org/10.1007/978-3-030-26961-6_26

The most common condition that affects the central nervous system is cerebral palsy, with an estimated incidence of 1.5–2.5 cases per 1000 live births. The prevalence and intensity of respiratory alterations within this disease depend on the type of motor compromise. The worst prognosis is quadriplegic cerebral palsy. In highly disabling neurological diseases, of which spastic quadriplegic cerebral palsy is the most common, factors such as immobility, feeding via a nasogastric tube and not by gastrostomy, and epilepsy have significant effects in increasing mortality. Recurrent pneumonia appears in almost 70% of this patient population, and there is a 77% mortality rate among those who contract pneumonia.

Diseases that compromise the peripheral nervous system, known as neuromuscular diseases (NMDs), have an estimated prevalence of 63 cases per 100,000 people under the age of 16 years. The most common conditions are spinal muscular atrophy (SMA), with an incidence of 1 in every 6000 live births, and Duchenne muscular dystrophy (DMD), with an incidence of 1 in every 3500 live male births. We do not have specific information about the prevalence rates of SMA and DMD in Chile.

In NMDs, respiratory compromise can be very rare, as happens in Charcot–Marie–Tooth neuropathy, or it can affect 100% of patients, as in the case of children over 10 years of age with DMD. By the time these children are 10 years old, they show a progressive decrease in respiratory force, which is accentuated by loss of the ability to walk. All of them require assisted ventilation before they reach the age of 20 years. In patients with SMA, the level of respiratory compromise can vary depending on the type. In the case of SMA type 1, 100% of patients will die from respiratory insufficiency within a year if they do not receive ventilatory support. In patients with SMA types 2 or 3 (as in those with DMD), a progressive decline in respiratory force begins around 8 years of age, which leads to respiratory insufficiency that requires assisted ventilation.

Etiology and Physiopathology

Respiratory disorders in patients with neurological diseases have multifactorial causes, the importance of which depends fundamentally on the base neurological disease.

Diseases of the central nervous system can present alteration of respiratory control and muscular weakness of the upper airway. Alteration of respiratory control is manifested by progressive hypoventilation. The process can be slow and overlapping, with subtle clinical signs, at first during sleep with hypopneas and/or hypercapnia, and finally with evident central apnea. Muscular weakness of the upper airway determines a higher risk of obstructive apnea and alters the protection of the airway, with a greater risk of aspiration and consequent damage. Repeated and persistent aspiration causes repeated pneumonia, besides progressive damage to the pulmonary parenchyma, with ventilation/perfusion (V/Q) mismatch in which dead space and hypoxemia increase, leading to a restrictive respiratory pattern and increasing the load on the system.

The problem with NMDs is essentially the failure of the pump: there is an imbalance between the muscular force and the load on the respiratory system, and this finally causes hypoventilation and hypercapnia, which is characteristic.

Respiratory muscular weakness translates into incapacity to generate pressure and normal flows during inhalation and exhalation, increasing the mechanical load, thus altering the mechanics and gaseous exchange. Inspiratory muscular compromise decreases the corresponding reserve volume and total lung capacity, causing a characteristically restrictive respiratory pattern. There is also a decrease in the vital capacity (VC), which is not linearly proportional to the reduction in the expiratory force, because of the mechanical effect of the elastic retraction of the system, which maintains a higher VC than might be expected. However, expiratory muscular compromise reduces the expiratory reserve volume, increasing the residual volume and maintaining an almost constant functional reserve capacity. Alterations in inspiratory and expiratory muscles are manifested in weak coughing and inadequate maneuvers in both phases, increasing the risks of aspiration, atelectasis, and pneumonia.

Associated Conditions

Sleep disorders are common in patients with neurological diseases, although they tend to be underdiagnosed. The factors that determine these alterations are respiratory muscular weakness of the upper airway, deformities of the rib cage and spine, obesity, craniofacial alterations, and alterations in respiratory control. It is important to suspect and search for these conditions in a directed manner. Weakness of the respiratory pump—in particular, during rapid-eye-movement (REM) sleep, or the active sleep stage—accentuates the normal situation of muscular atony, resulting in hypoventilation and apnea.

Orthopedic alterations are common and should be diagnosed early so that appropriate interventions can be instituted. They are caused by damage to the spinal extensor muscles, the effect of gravity, nonharmonic movements, and axial rotation. Kyphoscoliosis, which is progressive and difficult to control, contributes to the alteration of respiratory mechanics. It has been shown that there is a directly proportional relationship between the degree of kyphoscoliosis, as defined by the Cobb angle, and respiratory insufficiency.

Clinical Manifestations

There is a wide variety of neurological diseases and consequently a wide variety of clinical manifestations, which are summarized in Table 26.1.

Muscular weakness is a cardinal sign of neurological diseases with respiratory compromise. Depending on which respiratory muscle group is compromised, a clinical examination may reveal the condition. Preferential involvement of the inspiratory muscles is related to nocturnal hypoventilation syndrome as an initial clinical presentation, which often goes unnoticed if it is not looked for directly. If there is preferential involvement of the expiratory muscles, the symptoms include a weak cough and more frequent atelectasis. If there is compromise of the musculature of the upper airway, the mechanisms of swallowing and aspiration are affected. The physiopathological relationships are multiple and complex, as shown in Fig. 26.1.

Table 26.1 Forms of clinical presentation of neurological diseases

Presentation
Hypotonic infant
Delayed psychomotor development
Swallowing disorder
Gait alteration, frequent falls
Central neurological symptoms: epileptic seizures
Lack of strength, fatigability
Muscular pain, cramps
Orthopedic alterations: clubfoot, equinus foot, pes cavus, scoliosis
Recurrent pneumonia, recurrent or persistent atelectasis with no clear respiratory cause
Sleep disturbances, snoring, obstructive and central apneas

The respiratory clinical picture depends on the severity and timing of respiratory muscular compromise. For example, in patients with SMA type 1, who have an early and severe presentation, the infant's chest is bell shaped, with tachypnea and paradoxical breathing, in a context of generalized hypotonia. With diseases that progress more slowly, such as DMD, the respiratory symptoms are insidious and often go unnoticed, such as sleep alterations due to nocturnal hypoventilation, resulting in hypoxia and sleep fragmentation, in turn leading to neurocognitive and behavioral problems, hyperactivity or lethargy, morning headaches, and anorexia.

There are various signs and symptoms caused by compromise of the respiratory system in neurological diseases. It is important for physicians to know of these and seek them in a directed manner in an anamnesis and a thorough physical examination (Table 26.2).

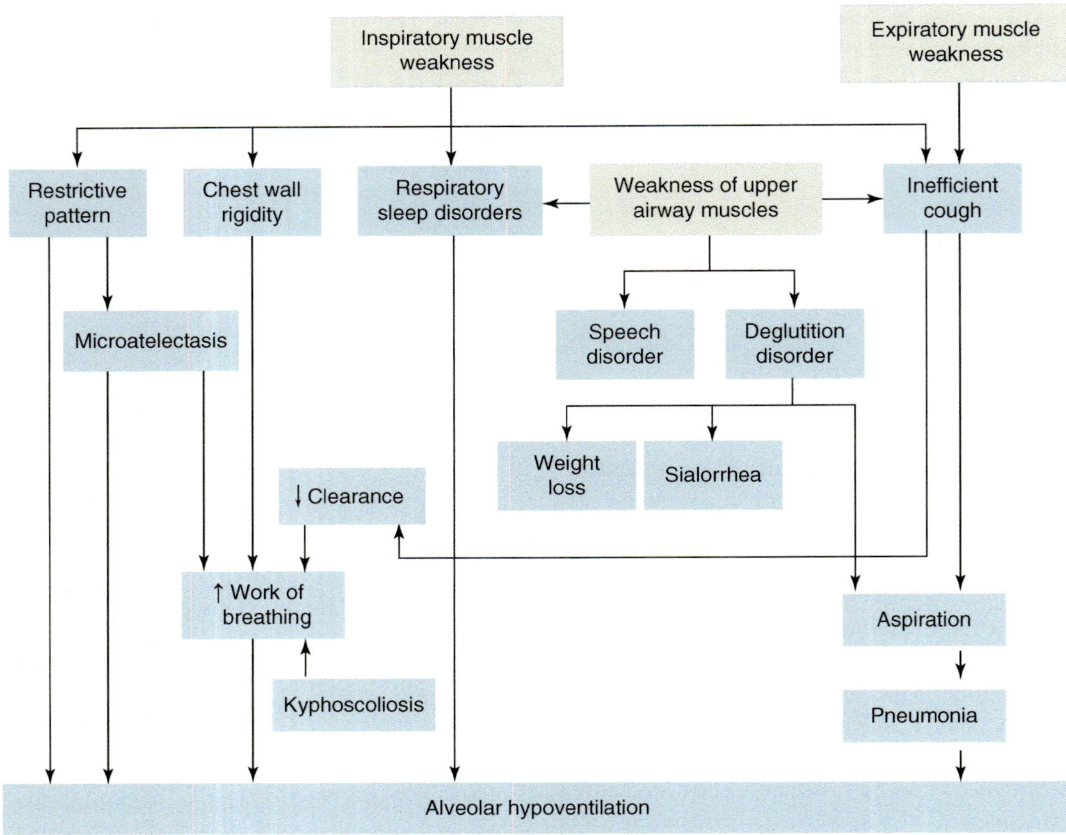

Fig. 26.1 Pathophysiology and clinical signs in neurological disease

Diagnostic Foci

A complete initial assessment that includes the medical history is needed, besides a complete physical examination that seeks the signs and symptoms described above, with evaluation by specialists in the relevant fields.

Neurological Focus

To determine the prognosis, it is necessary to have a topographical neurological diagnosis that identifies the level of compromise of the nervous system. A complete neurological examination is essential, which includes nuclear magnetic resonance (NMR) imaging of the brain and/or bone marrow; neurophysiological studies such electroencephalography, evoked potentials, muscle enzyme levels, electromyography, and peripheral nerve conduction velocity; muscular imaging studies; muscle and/or nerve biopsies; and specific molecular and genetic studies.

Respiratory Focus

Evaluation of Sleep Alterations

Peripheral oxygen saturation: The peripheral oxygen saturation (SpO_2) can be assessed continuously during sleep to determine the base and average levels, besides the levels during desaturation events or clusters in relation to snoring or sleep stages in particular. More sophisticated and sensitive equipment has been developed in recent years, using signal purification techniques that better show periods of desaturation, although this test does not adequately identify

Table 26.2 Symptoms and signs of alterations of the respiratory system in neurological disease

System	Symptoms and signs
Constitutional	Fatigue Weakness Retarded growth
Cardiopulmonary	Cyanosis Tachycardia Dyspnea Tachypnea Diaphragmatic paradox Use of accessory muscles Decreased diaphragmatic excursion Bell-shaped thorax Weak cough Recurrent or persistent atelectasis Recurrent pneumonia
Central nervous	Morning headache Hypersomnolence Neurocognitive alterations Hyperactivity Speech disorder
Sleep	Restless sleep Nightmares Nocturnal enuresis Frequent awakenings Snoring Apneas
Others	Blockages Sialorrhea Speech disorder

respiratory sleep disorders (RSDs) in this type of patient.

Capnography: Expirated or transcutaneous carbon dioxide levels can be measured. This parameter indicates alveolar ventilation. This measurement is more useful as a complement to sleep study than in isolation.

Gases in arterial blood: The partial pressure of carbon dioxide ($PaCO_2$) shows the severity of hypoventilation, while the pH, bicarbonate, and base excess indicate the repercussions in terms of the acid–base balance and the degree of metabolic correction, adding specificity to the diagnosis. Studies by Hukins (2000) and Mellies (2003) showed that $PaCO_2$ values above 40 mmHg and 45 mmHg, respectively, correlated with nocturnal hypoventilation, with sensitivity of more than 90% and specificity of around 75%.

Polysomnography: Polysomnography studies play an important role in early detection of RSDs among patients with neurological diseases, including in the absence of significant clinical manifestations and in the absence of examinations of pulmonary function in normal wakefulness. Active (REM) sleep inhibits muscular activity, and slow-wave non-REM (NREM) sleep impedes nonchemical afferences to the respiratory center, increasing the risk of nocturnal hypoventilation, obstruction of the upper airway, and apnea. Polygraph testing, which is derived from polysomnography, uses other criteria besides electroencephalographic waves to determine sleep stages. The polygraph has the advantage of being portable, and this type of test is relatively inexpensive. Respiratory alterations during sleep should be assessed at least once a year in patients presenting any of the following criteria: VC <60% of the predicted value, loss of mobility, symptoms or signs of obstructive apnea–hypoventilation, and diaphragmatic weakness (level of recommendation: D). If rapid worsening, repeated infections, or sleep alteration symptoms occur, the studies should be repeated with the necessary frequency for early diagnosis and intervention.

Assessment of Pulmonary Force and Function

Spirometry: There is a characteristically restrictive pattern (reduced forced vital capacity (FVC) and reduced forced expiratory volume in 1 second (FEV_1)). The flow curve is useful to show a reduction in force-dependent respiratory flows: the maximum inspiratory flow (MIF) and maximum expiratory flow (MEF). VC should be measured as part of lung function studies in all patients diagnosed with NMDs who can perform this maneuver (level of recommendation: C).

Muscular strength assessment: Decreases in muscular strength and resistance in the context of fatigue are the first clinical elements that present in NMDs. The assessment includes measurement of the maximum voluntary ventilation (MVV), maximum inspiratory pressure (MaxIP), and maximum expiratory pressure (MaxEP), and it is more sensitive than VC measurement at the initial stages of the disease. MaxIP is the maximum pressure generated during inspiration with the airway occluded and is based on the residual volume or the functional reserve capacity. MaxEP is the maximum pressure generated during expiration with the airway occluded and is based on the total lung capacity. The effort should be maintained for 1 second, and at least five maneuvers of each type should be done until at least two reproducible results are obtained. A MaxIP value of >80 cm H_2O is of great value in excluding muscular compromise of clinical importance. A 75% decrease in the MaxIP value or a predicted value close to 30% is needed to observe a significant decrease in FVC. Thus, spirometry and the volume/time relationship are not very sensitive tests to evaluate muscular failure at the initial stages.

Maximum flow with cough: This is a tool to assess the effectiveness of coughing and can be measured using a mask or mouthpiece. There is evidence in adults that a minimum of 160 l/min is necessary to adequately mobilize secretions, and that values above 270 l/min represent respiratory indemnity (level of evidence: 3). Although no specific values have been established in children, this test is recommended for respiratory evaluation in subjects over 12 years of age.

Evaluation of Complications

Imaging studies: A chest x-ray determines the presence of associated pneumonia or atelectasis. Radioscopy and echoscopy assess diaphragmatic mobility.

The chest of a patient with NMDs is bell shaped when there is thoracic muscle involvement. The esophagus–stomach–duodenum (ESD) transit, assessed with a specific videodilution study, evaluates the presence of gastroesophageal reflux (GER) and deglutition disorders as causes of pulmonary aspiration, recurrent pneumonia, or chronic interstitial lung compromise.

Assessment of the airway: Suspicion of bulbar or pharyngeal and suprahyoid musculature compromise makes it necessary to evaluate the airway. Fiber bronchoscopy is useful to diagnose hypotonic or pharyngeal incoordination and vocal cord paralysis or paresis, which is related to a potentially unstable airway. In patients with a tracheostomy, it is useful to anatomically evaluate the intervened airway. In the case of persistent atelectasis, fiber bronchoscopy can indicate appropriate therapy.

Cardiological Focus

Patients with neurological disease can have primary or secondary compromise of the cardiovascular system. Primary myocardial involvement must be ruled out in myopathies such as DMD or Becker disease, some congenital myopathies, mitochondrial diseases, and other conditions, as determined by a specialist in NMDs. Cardiovascular compromise is secondary to muscle-based diseases or to the development of pulmonary hypertension due to chronic hypoxemia, which at the advanced stage constitutes pulmonary heart disease. Hyperpulmonary flow, due to increased transpulmonary pressures, is also a cause of pulmonary hypertension, as occurs in patients with obstructive sleep apnea. Other alterations of the airway, such as heart rhythm disorders, should be evaluated in patients with central hypoventilation syndromes and patients with specific NMDs, such as Emery–Dreyfus syndrome or certain congenital myopathies.

Treatment

In neurological diseases, respiratory failure accounts for most acute and chronic morbidity, as well as mortality. Until curative therapies are available for the underlying neurological disease, efforts must be made to slow the progressive deterioration of musculoskeletal and respiratory function, thus improving the quality of life. The treatment is multidisciplinary, including respiratory medicine, neurology, nutrition, kinesiology, gastroenterology, orthopedics, and other specialties.

Nutrition

Patients with neurological diseases often suffer from malnutrition, due to both deficiency and excess. Situations of malnutrition occur more in a context of low nutritional intake (due to difficulty in swallowing) or greater energy expenditure (due to excessive respiratory work). Excesses occur in a context of assured nutrition, without consideration of the fact that the patients have lower basal energy expenditure, so their requirements are also lower.

Malnutrition affects the functioning of the respiratory musculature, and at the same time it facilitates recurrent infections. Thus, when diagnosed, the patient must be supported until an acceptable nutritional status is reached, which varies from one person to another. Slow growth is common, so it is advisable to adapt the height/weight ratio to limit the diet in order to avoid overfeeding. Enteral feeding via a nasogastric tube or gastrostomy is usually necessary. It is also useful to consider specific nutritional gaps—in particular, those related to bone metabolism—because of a higher risk of multicausal osteopenia and related fractures.

Respiratory Kinesiotherapy

The main objectives of respiratory kinesiotherapy are to prevent and treat atelectasis, permeabilize the airway, and assist respiratory rehabilitation. Multiple maneuvers of successive inspirations and forced expirations with assisted coughing add to the workload and to respiratory muscle fatigue in children with ventilatory insufficiency, so this therapy should be conducted with caution.

There are now cough assist devices that can be used in patients with neurological disease. These devices are applied through interfaces such as masks, mouthpieces, and tracheostomies as part of the management of respiratory exacerbations, minimizing the risk of intubation and providing mechanical cough assistance for stable patients who are too weak to cough.

Respiratory muscle training with adjustable valves has allowed the development of training plans for adult patients with chronic obstructive pulmonary disease. These have begun to be applied to children, with positive results, although long-term research will be needed, especially considering that the muscles of patients with NMDs are diseased and their training capacity does not necessarily follow the same principles that apply to healthy muscles.

Scoliosis

The rapid progression of scoliosis in patients with neurological diseases is directly related to the progression of the disease and to the sitting postures that patients maintain, which do not always preserve correct alignment, making the gravitational effect on the curvature of their spine accelerate the progression of the kyphoscoliosis. Respiratory complications are an indication for treatment with arthrodesis, because systems for support and maintenance with corsets in these cases have not been shown to be useful, while hindering respiratory mechanics. Surgery should be deferred for as long as possible; however, the presence of a Cobb angle of >40° correlates with respiratory failure.

Neurorehabilitation

Neurorehabilitation aims to improve the general functioning of the patient in relation to the activities that correspond to their age. Two types of interventions are generally carried out: one involves techniques to stimulate the generation or restoration of central or peripheral motor circuits to improve motor functionality, while the other employs external support for neuromuscular functioning—for example, padding to keep the head erect, chairs adapted for sitting requirements, a tilting table to put patients without control over head movement in a standing position, or a prone-position table for patients with partial control over their heads.

Standing systems are based on the extensive published evidence of the benefits of patients being in a standing position in several respects: it improves gastric and urinary emptying, and it strengthens ossification, according to studies in quadriplegic patients, who stand for an hour five times a week. This evidence can be extrapolated to patients with more serious NMDs, who commonly experience fractures of long bones as a result of low-impact trauma associated with movement and postural changes.

Evaluation and management of swallowing are essential to avoid pulmonary complications. Although oral feeding is not an objective, techniques of desensitization and intra- and perioral management are essential for development of reflexes. Establishment of motor sequences and muscle strengthening through speech therapy intervention techniques must also be considered early on. Swallowing rehabilitation is aimed at maintaining and/or recovering suction–swallowing mechanisms.

Pharmacological Treatment

The use of steroids is indicated in patients with DMD; prednisone and deflazacort have been shown to be effective in increasing force and delaying loss of force, prolonging autonomy for around 2 years. The increase in strength, and especially the increase in the time spent walking, has a direct effect on the ventilatory capacity of affected children, although side effects must be monitored. Recent studies have shown that treatment with lower doses of corticosteroids in nondaily regimens has the same beneficial effects as daily use of prednisone, but without the traditional side effects. However, once the ability to walk is lost, this therapy merely increases potential adverse effects such as osteoporosis.

Creatine is a dietary supplement that has been shown to improve strength in both healthy individuals and carriers of disabling diseases. The beneficial effect is due to increased muscle protein synthesis—in particular, heavy chain myosin—and to increased intramuscular glycogen. However, it should be kept in mind that this effect is beneficial only when it supplements creatine associated with strength training and antiresistance techniques. Carnitine may be useful in patients with myopathies secondary to metabolic syndromes with carnitine deficiency.

Assisted Ventilation

Publications on the impact of noninvasive assisted ventilation—especially in relation to NMDs and thoracic deformities such as kyphoscoliosis—recommend its use in investigation of nocturnal hypoventilation, a condition associated with disorders of pulmonary function and blood gases during wakefulness.

Thus, investigation of nocturnal hypoventilation and RSDs, involving sleep and pulmonary function studies, makes it possible to decide whether or not to employ noninvasive ventilatory assistance.

Long-term follow-up of this type of assistance has shown improvements in the quality of life, RSDs, nocturnal hypoventilation, and daytime hypercapnia, with decreased health care costs. It has also been recently verified that the frequency and severity of respiratory infections are reduced, with a decreased incidence of hospitalizations for complications of infections.

Oxygen Therapy

The cardinal disorder in NMDs is hypoventilation. Treatment should aim to correct this situation; thus, ventilation support is fundamental. In the case of chronic hypercapnic respiratory insufficiency, oxygen therapy can accentuate hypoventilation by inhibiting the only other stimulus for ventilation that remains: hypoxemia. Therefore, special care should be taken when considering indications for oxygen therapy in these patients.

Prognosis

On the basis of their clinical progression, NMDs can be classified as shown in Table 26.3.

Ethical Dilemmas

The survival of children with neurological diseases and dependence on medical technologies has improved because of specialized respiratory

Table 26.3 Prognostic features of neuromuscular diseases

Feature	Disease
Early appearance of acute respiratory failure	Spinal muscular atrophy type 1 Congenital myotonic dystrophy Some congenital myopathies
Continuous slow progression	Duchenne muscular dystrophy Some congenital myopathies Myotonic dystrophy Spinal muscular atrophy types 2 and 3 Some polyneuropathies
Stable slow progression	Some congenital muscular dystrophies Some polyneuropathies Some congenital myopathies
Improvement with development	Congenital myotonic dystrophy Some congenital myopathies

care, such as prolonged mechanical ventilation, among other factors.

This has been related to improvements in the quality of patients' lives and their family environment. However, the desired results are not always obtained, and the psychological, social, and financial burdens need to be evaluated in the framework of bioethics. The challenges and clinical dilemmas involved in establishment of noninvasive ventilatory assistance differ according to the pathologies and their prognoses. An evident reduction in respiratory effort is achieved in some patients, improving the growth and development of the pulmonary system, and allowing suspension of ventilatory assistance for a time or maintaining it in a stable long-term manner.

However, in other situations where there is progressive functional deterioration, the indications for starting or continuing mechanical ventilation or making a transition to another more complex strategy may be controversial. The therapeutic challenges include bioethical considerations that rationally guide human actions to do good and prevent evil. Participation in the decision-making process for patients and their families must honor the principle of autonomy.

Sources

Allen J. Pulmonary complications of neuromuscular disease: a respiratory mechanics perspective. Paediatr Respir Rev. 2010;11:18–23.

Arens R, Muzumdar H. Sleep, sleep disordered breathing, and nocturnal hypoventilation in children with neuromuscular diseases. Paediatr Respir Rev. 2010;11:24–30.

Bach JR, Saltstein K, Sinquee D, Weaver B, Komaroff E. Long term survival in Werdnig–Hoffmann disease. Am J Phys Med Rehabil. 2007;86:339–45.

Benditt JO, Boitano LJ. Pulmonary issues in patients with chronic neuromuscular disease. Am J Respir Crit Care Med. 2013:187(10):1046–55.

Hukins CA, Hillman DR. Daytime predictors of sleep hypoventilation in Duchenne muscular dystrophy. Am J Respir Crit Care Med. 2000;161(1):166–70.

Hull J, Aniapravan R, Chan E. British Thoracic Society guideline for respiratory management of children with neuromuscular weakness. Thorax. 2012;67:i1–i40.

Katz SL. Assessment of sleep-disordered breathing in pediatric neuromuscular diseases. Pediatrics. 2009;123:S222–5.

Kennedy JD, Martin AJ. Chronic respiratory failure and neuromuscular disease. Pediatr Clin N Am. 2009;56:261–73.

Khirani S, Colella M, Caldarelli V, Aubertin G, Boulé M, Forin V, Ramirez A, Fauroux B. Longitudinal course of lung function and respiratory muscle strength in spinal muscular atrophy type 2 and 3. Eur J Paediatr Neurol. 2013;17:552–60.

Khirani S, Ramirez A, Aubertin G, Boulé M, Chemouny C, Forin V, Fauroux B. Respiratory muscle decline in Duchenne muscular dystrophy. Pediatr Pulmonol. 2014;49:473–81.

Kwon YH, Lee HY. Differences of respiratory function in children with spastic diplegic and hemiplegic cerebral palsy, compared with normally developed children. J Pediatr Rehabil Med. 2013;6:113–7.

Mellies U, Ragette R, Schwake C, et al. Long-term noninvasive ventilation in children and adolescents with neuromuscular disorders. Eur Respir J. 2003;22:631–6.

Panitch HB. The pathophysiology of respiratory impairment in pediatric neuromuscular diseases. Pediatrics. 2009;123:S215–8.

Rajatonirina S, Razanajatovo NH, Ratsima EH, et al. Outcome risk factors during respiratory infections in a paediatric ward in Antananarivo, Madagascar 2010–2012. PLoS One. 2013;8:1–9.

Sharma GD. Pulmonary function testing in neuromuscular disorders. Pediatrics. 2009;123:S219–21.

Vega-Briceño LE, Contreras I, Prado F. Evaluación respiratoria de la enfermedad neuromuscular en niños. Rev Neumol Pediatr. 2007a;2(1):6–10.

Vega-Briceño LE, Prado F, Bertrand P, Sánchez I. Soporte ventilatorio no invasivo en enfermedades neuromusculares. Rev Neumol Pediatr. 2007b;2:15–20.

Wallgren-Pettersson C, Bushbyb K, Melliesc U, Simonds A. Ventilatory support in congenital neuromuscular disorders—congenital myopathies, congenital muscular dystrophies, congenital myotonic dystrophy and SMA (II). Neuromuscul Disord. 2004;14:56–69.

Yang ML, Finkel RS. Overview of paediatric neuromuscular disorders and related pulmonary issues: diagnostic and therapeutic considerations. Paediatr Respir Rev. 2010;11:9–17.

A Children with an Airway Foreign Body

27

Jacques de Blic and Agustín León Cortés

Contents

Epidemiology

Inhalation of a foreign body is a common cause of morbidity and mortality among children. In 2001, there were more 17,000 pediatric consultations in emergency rooms because of airway obstruction by a foreign body, representing a rate of 140 per 100,000 infants. A foreign body in the airway is the most common cause of accidental death among children under 1 year of age. Although mortality has decreased with the development of bronchoscopy, it remains at 5–7% according to a meta-analysis by Foltran et al. involving 174 multinational publications describing almost 40,000 cases.

While inhalation of a foreign body can occur at any age, the majority of cases (80%) occur between the ages of 9 months and 3 years, and they are more common among males. At a younger age, children are at greater risk because they explore their surroundings with their mouths,

J. de Blic (✉)
Université Paris Descartes, Hôpital Necker Enfants Malades, Paris, France
e-mail: j.deblic@aphp.fr

A. León Cortés
Pediatrics, Respiratory Diseases, Clínica Santa María, Providencia, Chile

P. Bertrand, I. Sánchez (eds.), *Pediatric Respiratory Diseases*,
https://doi.org/10.1007/978-3-030-26961-6_27

they lack molars to chew properly, their swallowing–glottic function is still immature, and they often play, run, laugh, or cry with food in their mouths.

The diagnosis is delayed by more than 24 hours in 50–60% of cases, typically in the <3-year age group, because the penetration is not reported by the child and is not witnessed by an adult, and any accompanying respiratory sounds are attributed mainly to an infection. Thus, the reason for consultation is coughing or wheezing rather than a suffocation crisis.

The nature of the foreign body varies according to age and cultural habits. Organic foreign bodies—usually dried fruit, but also nuts, beans, rice, and popcorn—are most common in subjects at a younger age, representing up to 80% of cases. Inorganic foreign bodies as varied as parts of toys, pen nibs, pins, stones, pearls, and others are more common in children >3 years of age. The high rate of inhalation of food as a foreign body among infants and preschool children makes evident the responsibility of adults in charge of children in relation to permitting access to potentially inspirable foods.

Foreign bodies reach the bronchi in more than 80% of cases, according to the different published series, with a slightly higher preponderance of the right bronchus after 2 years of age. While the less common larynx–trachea location can produce potentially fatal asphyxia or severe respiratory distress, bronchial foreign bodies can remain asymptomatic for a variable duration, although if the foreign body is vegetal, the symptomatology usually does not last long, given the significant inflammatory reaction that is triggered.

Clinical Presentation

Penetration Syndrome

Penetration syndrome refers to a coughing attack with dyspnea, an inspiratory stridor, and cyanosis in situations in which a child has put a solid object in its mouth. When penetration syndrome occurs, it does not always prompt immediate consultation with an emergency service, because its importance may be minimized when an asymptomatic period ensues following the accident. The most common reason for consultation is coughing and, although the triad of a persistent cough, abolition of a lung murmur, and localized wheezing has a good positive predictive value, the absence of symptoms of penetration syndrome does not rule out the presence of a bronchial foreign body.

The Acute Clinical Situation

The clinical situation depends on the level of obstruction. Muscular retraction and/or cyanosis indicate obstruction of the proximal airway. Laryngeal obstruction is manifested by a hoarse cough, a muffled voice or dysphonia, hypersalivation, and a stridor with dyspnea. Tracheal obstruction produces a stridor or wheezing on both inspiration and expiration, sometimes with a thrill and bilateral diminution of a lung murmur. The most distal obstruction causes auscultatory asymmetry, with a unilateral manifestation of hypersonority and wheezing, and a localized decrease in the lung murmur.

Chronic Complications

Chronic complications occur if the foreign body is not suspected and not removed, and remains at the bronchial level, which occurs especially when the penetration syndrome has gone unnoticed or its importance has been minimized. The manifestations are diverse, such as persistent wheezing, asthma that does not respond to treatment, chronic coughing (Fig. 27.1), atelectasis or persistent or recurrent pneumonia (particularly in the same area), a lung abscess, and hemoptysis.

Radiological Study

In the case of a radiolucent foreign body, which is the most common type, localized hyperinflation is the most evocative radiological sign (occurring in 30–60% of cases). This results from air trap-

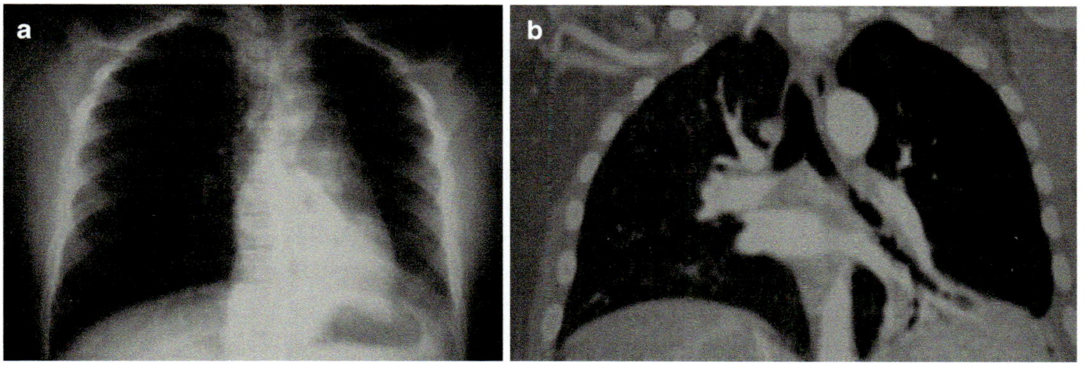

Fig. 27.1 Bronchial sequelae of a foreign body. Anteroposterior chest x-ray of a 5-year-old child presenting with chronic atelectasis in the left inferior lobe (**a**). Axial CT scan of the chest, showing bronchiectasis in the left lung (**b**)

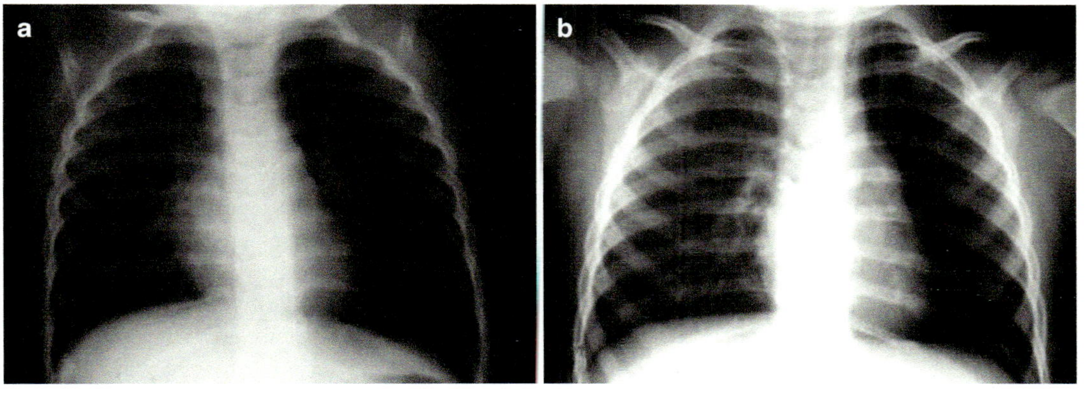

Fig. 27.2 Lung hyperinflation. Anteroposterior chest x-rays of a 4-year-old child during inhalation (**a**) and during exhalation, showing hyperinflation of the left hemithorax (**b**)

ping secondary to partial obstruction of the airway, where the foreign body represents a valve that allows greater air passage on inspiration than on expiration (Fig. 27.2). This sign is more evident on forced expiratory or lateral decubitus radiography, which should be done systematically when there is suspicion of a foreign body. Atelectasis is a product of complete bronchial obstruction, particularly in the case of infants, in whom reabsorption of distal air causes alveolar collapse because of the absence of well-developed collateral ventilation. Other suggestive radiological findings are mediastinal deviation, interruption of an air bronchogram, and radiopaque foreign bodies, such as metal, bone, a tooth, or a stone (Figs. 27.3 and 27.4). A normal chest x-ray (which is present in up to 30% of cases) does not rule out the presence of a foreign body, which is why the clinical picture is the most important factor in deciding whether or not to perform bronchoscopy.

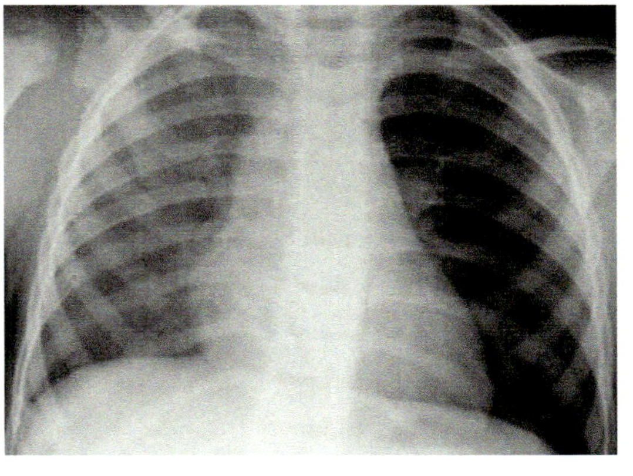

Fig. 27.3 Radiotranslucent foreign body in the left source bronchi, with secondary left lung hyperinflation

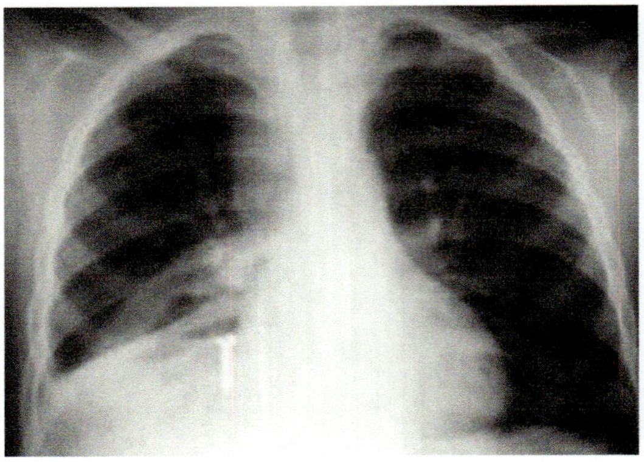

Fig. 27.4 Radiopaque foreign body (a screw) in the right posterior basal bronchi

If the foreign body remains in the bronchi for an extended period, radiography may show atelectasis or bronchiectasis, the extent of which depends on the level of interlocking.

The usefulness of computerized tomography (CT) and virtual endoscopy is debatable. It has been suggested that these are indicated in cases of penetration syndrome with normal radiography, to avoid the anesthesia required for rigid bronchoscopy. However, in these cases, fiber bronchoscopy evaluation under sedation is more advantageous than CT, which, in addition to involving a radiation dose and being less readily available, also does not show the nature of the foreign body or the presence of granulation tissue, and thus has no therapeutic value.

Treatment

Immediate action in response to penetration syndrome can result in dislodgement of the foreign body. In an infant, this involves slapping the child's back while he or she is being held with his or her head downward, with or without chest compression. In an older child, the classic Heimlich maneuver can be performed.

Treatment in response to inhalation of a foreign body is based on endoscopic extraction. There is no consensus as to the best anesthetic protocol, but there is more support for having the patient pharmacologically paralyzed than for maintaining spontaneous ventilation.

The most universal therapeutic approach is based on the degree of certainty about the presence of the foreign body.

Absolute certainty: There is absolute certainty in the case of dyspnea or persistent coughing after penetration syndrome, with asymmetry on pulmonary auscultation, localized hyperinsufflation, or a radiopaque foreign body. In these cases, the use of therapeutic bronchoscopy is indicated. Most often, the clinical situation is stable because the foreign body is located in the bronchi; thus, removal can wait for the recommended fasting time and to ensure the availability of the ideal equipment for extraction. On the other hand, extraction is urgently required if there is severe respiratory distress, mediastinal diversion, massive atelectasis, a pneumothorax, or, in the case of a particularly harmful foreign body such as a battery, because it can cause tissue necrosis, or spikes, that rapidly migrate distally.

Suspicion of a foreign body: In cases where there are few specific symptoms following penetration syndrome (especially if the child was symptomatic before the syndrome), or when the chest x-ray is normal or there are chronic or recurring radiological abnormalities, diagnostic exploration by flexible bronchoscopy is performed, which requires simple sedation (Fig. 27.5).

Most foreign bodies are extracted with use of a rigid bronchoscope. This is the mandatory method in an asphyxia crisis, where the foreign body is in the larynx, subglottis, or trachea, and where it is probably large or has an irregular surface that anchors it to the walls. In this scenario, rigid bronchoscopy offers high-caliber instruments for dealing with different types of foreign bodies, together with good control of the airway during the extraction.

Extraction with flexible bronchoscopy is also possible according to the experience of different centers. In the largest series (described by Tang et al.) involving 1027 cases between 2000 and 2008, which included children between the ages of 5 months and 14 years (average age 17 months), 938 foreign bodies (91.3%) were extracted by flexible bronchoscopy, and only 34 (3.5%) required use of a rigid bronchoscope after an

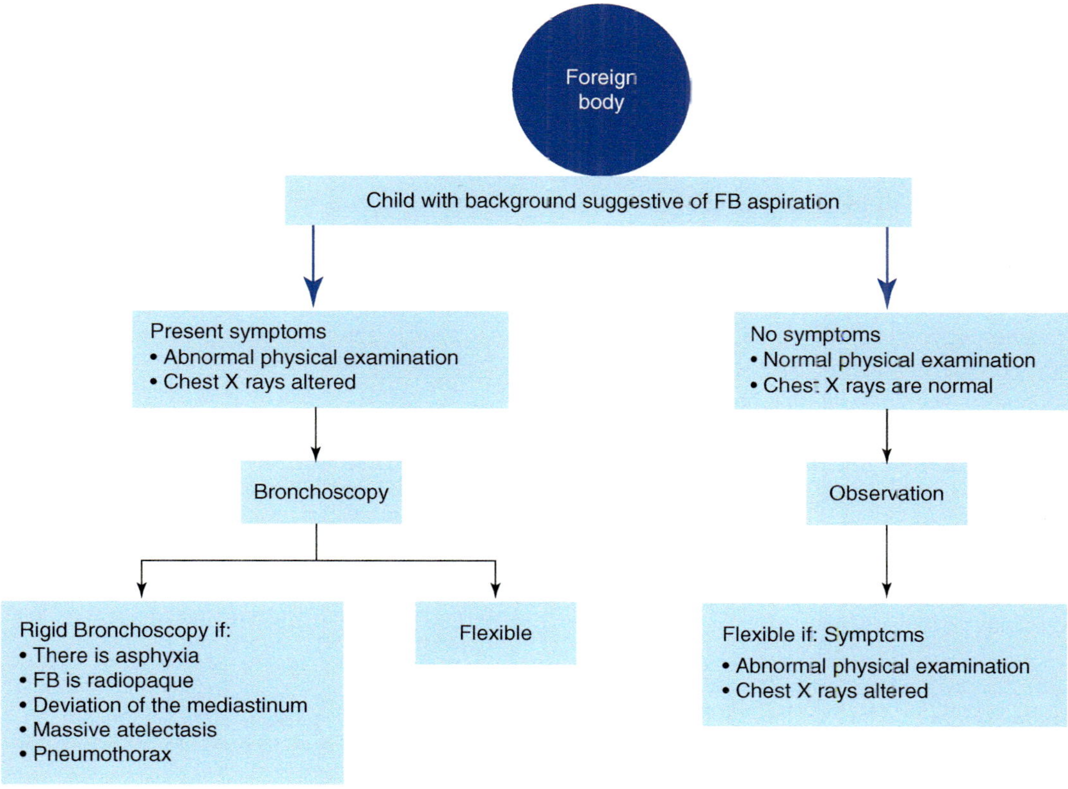

Fig. 27.5 Algorithm for studying foreign bodies

attempt with a flexible one. The flexible bronchoscopes that were used had external diameters of 2.8–3.9 mm, with a 1.2 mm working channel. The most commonly used extraction tools are basket forceps with three or four spiral strands, and biopsy and mouse-toothed forceps, the most popular being the basket forceps. A laryngeal mask is currently considered to provide the best control of the airway when a flexible endoscope is used, although it can also be introduced through an endotracheal tube or a rigid bronchoscope.

Flexible endoscopy may be preferable when dealing with a distal foreign body and particularly in the upper lobules, which are difficult to access with a rigid endoscope. The consistency, size, and shape of the foreign body should always be considered in order to assess the risk of fragmentation or laryngeal interlocking during its extraction, which should be done in a way that keeps it intact during its removal by the endoscope. The option of converting to extraction by rigid bronchoscopy should be available in case of failure with a flexible bronchoscope, because of which it is necessary to have an operator familiar with both techniques or to have two operators, usually a pulmonologist and an otolaryngologist.

Periendoscopic morbidity is higher if the foreign body remains in the airway for more than 7 days (in particular, in the case of dried fruit), a period during which more severe edema and inflammation develop and the consistency of the foreign body diminishes, making treatment more difficult. In this respect, it can be very difficult to dislodge a vegetal foreign body trapped in the granulated tissue that it triggers, to which must be added possible loss of visibility in the area of work because the inflamed mucosa can easily bleed. Systematic application of steroids for several days is recommended, followed by antibiotics, before another attempt at extraction is made. Another consideration is that if pressure is lost during the extraction and the foreign body falls into the trachea, it should be pushed until it reaches the bronchi again. If the foreign body begins to move and it lodges in the bronchi, it is preferable to invest 20 seconds in optimizing the permeability of the inflamed bronchus where the foreign body is located (using adrenaline, lavage, aspiration) before attempting another extraction.

The complementarity of rigid and flexible bronchoscopy should be emphasized. Together, they provide maximum yield and safety in the extraction, where the flexible bronchoscope contributes the diagnostic certainty of a minimally invasive procedure, the ability to remove a distal foreign body, and an easier and better view of the airway following extraction. The need for a thoracotomy is becoming rare, but this procedure is done in cases with very distal migration of a foreign body in the airway.

Prevention

Minimization of risks associated with children aspirating a foreign body is a responsibility shared by society, parents, and all adults with responsibility for children. Some important considerations are:

- Educating the general population to avoid children under the age of 3 years having access to objects or foods that can be inhaled because of their shape and size.
- Expressly warning about the danger of asphyxia through inhalation on the packaging of risky foods (e.g., peanuts, popcorn, hard candies, and beans).
- Complying with recommendations regarding age limits on toy packaging and not allowing children under these age limits to have access to toys with small parts.
- Not trying to abruptly remove an object from a child's mouth, as this can provoke crying, which in turn can result in the child aspirating the object.
- Not feeding children while they are playing, laughing, crying, or frightened.
- Training the general population in the classic Heimlich maneuver and the modified maneuver for infants.

Sources

AAP policy statement: prevention of choking among children. Pediatrics. 2010;125:601–7.

Adaletli I, Kurugoglu S, Ulus S, et al. Utilization of low-dose multidetector CT and virtual bronchoscopy in children with suspected foreign body aspiration. Pediatr Radiol. 2007;37:33–40.

Bhat KV, Hegde JS, Nagalotimath US, Patil GC. Evaluation of computed tomography virtual bronchoscopy in paediatric tracheobronchial foreign body aspiration. J Laryngol Otol. 2010;124:875–9.

Boufersaoui A, Smati L, Benhalla KN, et al. Foreign body aspiration in children: experience from 2624 patients. Int J Pediatr Otorhinolaryngol. 2013;77:1683–8.

Centers for Disease Control and Prevention (CDC). Nonfatal choking-related episodes among children: United States, 2001. MMWR Morb Mortal Wkly Rep. 2002;51:945–8.

Cohen S, Avital A, Godfrey S, et al. Suspected foreign body inhalation in children: what are the indications for bronchoscopy? J Pediatr. 2009;155:276–80.

Fidkowski CW, Zheng H, Firth PG. The anesthetic considerations of tracheobronchial foreign bodies in children: a literature review of 12,979 cases. Anesth Analg. 2010;111:1016–25.

Foltran F, Ballali S, Passali FM, et al. Foreign bodies in the airways: a meta-analysis of published papers. Int J Pediatr Otorhinolaryngol. 2012;76(Suppl 1):S12–9.

Foltran F, Ballali S, Rodríguez H, et al. Inhaled foreign bodies in children: a global perspective on their epidemiological, clinical, and preventive aspects. Pediatr Pulmonol. 2013;48:344–51.

Heyer CM, Bollmeier ME, Rossler L, et al. Evaluation of clinical, radiologic, and laboratory prebronchoscopy findings in children with suspected foreign body aspiration. J Pediatr Surg. 2006;41:1882–8.

Karakoc F, Karadag B, Akbenlioglu C, et al. Foreign body aspiration: what is the outcome? Pediatr Pulmonol. 2002;34:30–6.

Karakoc F, Cakir E, Ersu R, et al. Late diagnosis of foreign body aspiration in children with chronic respiratory symptoms. Int J Pediatr Otorhinolaryngol. 2007;71:241–6.

Kiyan G, Gocmen B, Tugtepe H, et al. Foreign body aspiration in children: the value of diagnostic criteria. Int J Pediatr Otorhinolaryngol. 2009;73:963–7.

Midulla F, Guidi R, Barbato A, et al. Foreign body aspiration in children. Pediatr Int. 2005;47:663–8.

Ramirez-Figueroa JL, et al. Foreign body removal by flexible fiberoptic bronchoscopy in infants and children. Pediatr Pulmonol. 2005;40:392–7.

Righini CA, Morel N, Karkas A, et al. What is the diagnostic value of flexible bronchoscopy in the initial investigation of children with suspected foreign body aspiration? Int J Pediatr Otorhinolaryngol. 2007;71:1383–90.

Rodrigues AJ, et al. Bronchoscopic techniques for removal of foreign bodies in children's airways. Pediatr Pulmonol. 2012;47(1):59–62.

Tang LF. Airway foreign body removal by flexible bronchoscopy: experience with 1027 children during 2000–2008. World J Pediatr. 2009;5(3):191–5.

WISQARS [Web-Based Injury Statistics Query and Reporting System]. Leading causes of death reports, 1999–2001. National Center for Injury Prevention and Control. https://webappa.cdc.gov/sasweb/ncipc/leadcaus10_us.html.

Epidemiology of Respiratory Infections

28

Luis Avendaño Carvajal and Cecilia Perret Pérez

Contents

The relationship between living disease agents—viruses, bacteria, fungi, and parasites—and their human or animal hosts can be studied at different levels. Biologists and biochemists analyze this relationship at the molecular and cellular levels, and are constantly making advances in knowledge about the pathogenesis of infections, as well as diagnosis and control through use of vaccines and medicines. Clinicians play the leading roles in the study and application of advances in individual curative medicine.

Epidemiology is the study of health at a human population scale, including transmissible and nontransmissible diseases. It also considers diseases that affect animals. It analyses factors depending on the agent, host, and environment that come into play in the population's health. Its contribution to the health field can be summarized as the following goals:

1. *Collaboration with clinical and laboratory diagnosis*: Epidemiology functionally defines suspicious and confirmed cases, using specific laboratories with validated techniques.
2. *Prediction of the appearance tendencies of infectious and noninfectious diseases*: Epidemiology provides a record of information and an appropriate collection of samples.

L. Avendaño Carvajal
Faculty of Medicine, Universidad de Chile, Santiago, Chile
e-mail: lavendan@med.uchile.cl

C. Perret Pérez (✉)
Department of Pediatrics, School of Medicine, Pontificia Universidad Católica de Chile, Santiago, Chile
e-mail: cperret@med.puc.cl

P. Bertrand, I. Sánchez (eds.), *Pediatric Respiratory Diseases*,
https://doi.org/10.1007/978-3-030-26961-6_28

(a) *Impact*: Epidemiology describes mortality, morbidity, life-years lost through death or disability, and other parameters to measure the impact of different agents; it also predicts the appearance tendencies of infectious and noninfectious diseases.
(b) *Pathogeny*: Epidemiology analyses the successive stages of disease, considering the source, transmission mechanism, portal of entry, human dissemination, defense mechanisms, and elimination from the community.

3. *Proposition and evaluation of measures of control*, including resource planning.
   (a) *Prevention*: These measures include (i) vaccines, (ii) education, (iii) the environment, (iv) biosecurity, (v) chemoprophylaxis, and (vi) passive immunization.
   (b) *Treatment*: This involves application of antibacterials, antivirals, antifungals, and other support measures such as oxygen treatment or mechanical ventilation.

Viral Respiratory Infections

Several indicators illustrate the big global impact that acute respiratory infections (ARIs) have on public health, through morbidity and mortality. According to the World Health Organization (WHO), respiratory infectious diseases take first place in the ranking of the burden of disease measured by years lost through death or disability (disability-adjusted life-years (DALYs)). Lower respiratory tract infections represent the third leading cause of death in the world, after cardiac and encephalic vascular illnesses; however, in countries of low economic status, they take first place.

Many regional or global estimates have identified acute respiratory infections as a primary cause of ambulatory consultations, hospitalizations, and deaths. In Chile, they take second place and third place in the leading causes of death in children and adults, respectively. Furthermore, several studies point toward them as the main causes of ambulatory consultations and absenteeism from both school and work. Their seasonal form of appearance and high infectivity place viruses as being responsible for the majority of acute respiratory infections. According to post-neonatal mortality estimates, lower respiratory tract infections cause 20% of deaths, with respiratory syncytial virus (RSV) and influenza virus being most common (9.5%). Advances in viral diagnosis have confirmed the participation of viruses in respiratory pediatric pathology, with frequencies that go from more than 50% (if they compromise the lower respiratory tract) to 90% (if they affect the upper respiratory tract). In adults, the scenario of upper respiratory tract infections is similar, but in lower respiratory tract infections a predominance of bacterial etiologies has been described. However, application of molecular viral diagnosis shows significant participation of respiratory viruses in lower respiratory tract infections. This fact acquires more relevance when considering the aging of a population.

Several viruses are included in the group of "respiratory viruses" because they have the respiratory system as a target organ. Nevertheless, other viruses can also compromise the respiratory system while a systemic infection takes place (measles, chickenpox, enterovirus, hantavirus), especially in immunocompromised individuals (cytomegalovirus, herpesvirus, shingles). Furthermore, studies always show an important group of cases without a proven etiology, although the number of such cases has diminished with the application of molecular diagnosis techniques because many potentially pathogenic agents are now being detected or discovered (Table 28.1).

The clinical manifestations of viral respiratory diseases vary from asymptomatic cases to fatal infections, with several intermediate scenarios. Some viruses tend to produce infections mainly in the upper respiratory tract (rhinovirus, coronavirus, adenovirus), while others can similarly compromise the lower respiratory airways, with variable severity (adenovirus, RSV, metapneumovirus, influenza, and parainfluenza). In general, it is an accepted fact that any respiratory virus can compromise one or several levels of the

Table 28.1 Main causes of disease worldwide (World Health Organization 2004)

	Disease or injury	DALYs (millions)	Total burden (%)
1	Lower respiratory tract infection	94.5	6.2
2	Diarrhea	72.8	4.8
3	Unipolar depression	65.5	4.3
4	Cardiac ischemia	62.6	4.1
5	HIV/AIDS	58.5	3.8
6	Encephalic vascular disease	46.6	3.1
7	Prematurity	44.3	2.9
8	Asphyxia and neonatal trauma	41.7	2.7
9	Traffic accidents	41.2	2.7
10	Neonatal infections	40.4	2.7

AIDS acquired immunodeficiency syndrome, *DALYs* disability-adjusted life years, *HIV* human immunodeficiency virus

Table 28.2 Predominant viruses in the respiratory system

Virus	Varieties: types, serotypes, genotypes, and other
Rhinovirus	Species A, B, and C: >101 serotypes
Coronavirus	Alpha: 229E, NL63; beta: OC43, HKU1, SARS, MERS
Respiratory syncytial virus	A and B groups; genotypes and lineage
Metapneumovirus	A and B groups; genotypes
Adenovirus	55 serotypes
Influenza	Types A, B, and C; subtypes A H1–3, N1–2; several strains
Parainfluenza	4 serotypes
Bocavirus	? 1 serotype
Others	Hantavirus, enterovirus, measles, chickenpox, cytomegalovirus

MERS Middle East respiratory syndrome, *SARS* severe acute respiratory syndrome

respiratory system and cause clinical and subclinical infections, but there is a certain preference of viruses for compromising specific levels of the respiratory system (Table 28.2). In this way, during an epidemic of a virus such as RSV or influenza, the major proportion of upper and lower respiratory tract infections will be caused by the prevalent virus. In addition, there will be an important incidence of subclinical infections, which act as efficient sources of transmission. As a result of herd immunity, important epidemics of multiple different viruses do not usually coexist in a community; instead, they alternate in terms of their presence in the community. For example, in Chile, the most commonly observed pattern involves parainfluenza outbreaks, followed by influenza outbreaks, and then RSV outbreaks; later, during winter–spring, metapneumovirus appears. Thus, the apexes of the epidemics follow one another and rarely overlap unless they affect populations of different ages. This phenomenon of viral interference may be explained by generation of interferon in infected patients, which "interferes" with the development of an infection of other viruses circulating at the same time.

These characteristics allow us to suspect specific causes of outbreaks or epidemics with reasonable certainty, considering associated clinical cases and detection of viruses at sentinel sites. Thus, a winter outbreak that involves infants under 1 year old and causes cases of obstructive bronchial illness will be due to RSV. A characteristic trait of influenza is an epidemic of disease that is marked by fever, cough, headache, and musculoskeletal aches, and that compromises preschool children, schoolchildren, and young adults. Parainfluenza virus outbreaks are associated with symptoms of hoarseness, gruffness, and cough, besides lower respiratory tract infections, in infants. Adenoviruses are feared because they sometimes cause intense feverish conditions and severe nosocomial infections.

Epidemiology contributes a lot to clarifying these situations, because alongside defining "suspicious cases" it implements diagnostic systems for circulating viruses (Fig. 28.1). The high infectivity of viruses makes epidemiological information vitally important in etiological clinical diagnosis, especially in terms of contact between sick patients and their relatives or close people in the community. The two kinds of respiratory virus that have the greatest impact on global health are RSV, which affects infants and elderly patients, and influenzas A and B, which compromise all of the population. Vaccines and

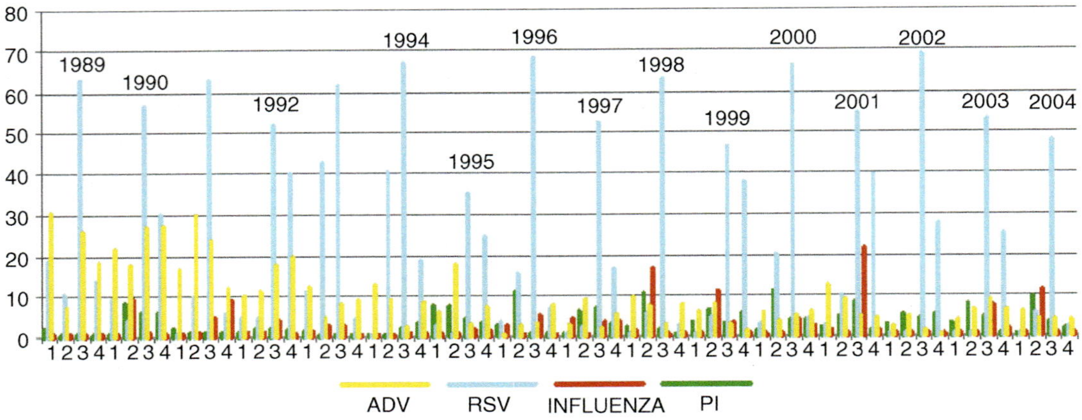

Fig. 28.1 Viral monitoring at Hospital Roberto del Río (Santiago, Chile). Detection of respiratory viruses (adenovirus, RSV, influenza, and parainfluenza) by immunofluorescence in infants hospitalized for acute lower respiratory tract infection in 1989–2004

antivirals have been developed just for influenza virus.

Viral respiratory infections are a very good example of a model of acute viral infection, in which viruses affect the individual, with or without symptoms, and then they leave him or her within a period of days or weeks. The course of infection depends on the interaction of various factors depending on: (1) the human host: age, immune status (based on previous infections and vaccinations), activity, tobacco use, etc.; (2) the virus: infecting dose, type, serotype, and viral strain; and (3) the environment: season, weather, humidity, contamination, geographical location, rural/urban setting, hospital/community, etc. From the host standpoint, acute respiratory infections are more frequent in childhood, particularly in infants and children under 2 years old, who represent the group with the biggest serious risk.

Diagnosis

Specific diagnosis of respiratory viruses is quite attainable nowadays because there are several immunodiagnostic techniques (immunofluorescence, enzyme-linked immunosorbent assay (ELISA), immunochromatography) available at public and private centers. They are easy to implement, with reasonably acceptable sensitivity and specificity, allowing appropriate study of cases that need it. Nowadays, molecular techniques (polymerase chain reaction (PCR) and reverse transcription PCR) are also available in many laboratories; they have high sensitivity and specificity, and provide results in less than 24 hours. The great sensitivity of these techniques enables detection of many agents, even in the same sample, raising questions about their interpretation. In severe cases or in deceased patients, they should always be implemented to establish the causes.

Emergent Infections

Among respiratory viruses, very good examples of "viral emergencies" are found, the most classic being the occurrence of global epidemics of influenza A virus derived from birds or pigs in 1918, 1957, 1968, and 2009; on these occasions, the virus broke through the species barrier and, thanks to multiple mutations, was able to transmit itself efficiently and establish itself as a "human virus." A pandemic of severe acute respiratory syndrome (SARS) due to a coronavirus is another example of a phenomenon that has threatened the world and was able to be controlled. During August 2014, an outbreak of lower respiratory tract infections in children, associated with enterovirus D68, started in the USA, and its evolution is ongoing. Likewise, an emergency involving the Middle East respiratory syndrome (MERS) coronavirus (MERS-CoV) started in Saudi Arabia in 2012. Probably of animal origin (camels and bats) and transmissible through air, it has caused over 900 cases (30% lethal); luckily, it has not expanded efficiently in other territories.

Pathogeny of Viral Infections

Some viruses have certain particularities that require special consideration (Table 28.3). This process is described considering a population as a host. There are over 200 respiratory viruses capable of infecting humans, with diverse structures—RNA or DNA, naked or enveloped—and although they can be grouped into a few families, the great variety of serotypes, genotypes, and strains that can be identified entails the existence of many different potential pathogens.

The source of infection is usually another human carrier of the virus with or without an evident clinical infection. Even though viral shedding is greater in symptomatic cases, the relative isolation that viruses suffer when the host is resting in bed makes viral dissemination less efficient; in contrast, in slight or subclinical cases, despite eliminating smaller amounts of the virus in secretions, patients continue doing their normal activities, actively contributing to viral diffusion. In many respiratory infections, preschool children and schoolchildren are the main disseminators of the virus because they satisfy the following two conditions: shedding of high virus concentrations through secretions, and regular and close contact with their schoolmates and relatives.

Likewise, the chance of infection from animals exists, as in hantavirus cardiopulmonary syndrome, in which the source of the virus is a rodent. Emergence of influenza pandemics always represents a latent threat because they have origins in avian or swine viruses. These new strains have been able to adapt to the human host, converting him or her into a viral reservoir. Also, coronaviruses, which usually cause upper respiratory tract infections, have represented global threats because of the emergence of animal strains that have acquired the character of pandemics (e.g., SARS).

Table 28.3 Respiratory syndromes

Syndrome	Responsible virus[a]
Common cold	Rhinovirus ++++ Coronavirus ++
Pharyngitis	Adenovirus +++ Influenza virus ++ Parainfluenza virus ++
Laryngitis	Parainfluenza virus ++++ Influenza virus ++
Influenza	Influenza viruses A and B ++++ Parainfluenza viruses 1–3 ++ Hantavirus
Bronchiolitis	Respiratory syncytial virus ++++ Metapneumovirus +++ Parainfluenza virus ++
Pneumonia	Respiratory syncytial virus +++ Influenza virus ++ Metapneumovirus ++ Parainfluenza virus 3 ++ Adenovirus + SARS virus Hantavirus
Subclinical infection	Any of the viruses listed above

SARS severe acute respiratory syndrome

[a]The number of plus symbols listed for each virus denotes its relative degree of responsibility for the relevant syndrome

The infection mechanism works through respiratory secretions that are eliminated as big particles (>5 μm in size), which remain both on the hands and in the environment (on aprons, toys, medical instruments, and furniture), or small particles (<5 μm in size: Flügge droplets), which can form aerosols and stay suspended in the environment. A sneeze or a cough can expel secretions at 65 km/h over a distance of 9 meters. For some viruses, such as rhinovirus or RSV, contact with contaminated hands represents the main form of transmission.

The upper respiratory mucosa is the portal of entry (including the ocular conjunctiva for some viruses) and also represents the target organ of these viral infections. Dissemination within the organism happens because of the contiguity of the mucosa, contaminated secretions, or virus diffusion due to the proximity of infected cells and healthy cells. Even though the virus can escape into the blood and other territories, this phase of viremia is not essential to the pathogeny of the infection, and this is why respiratory virus are considered localized infections.

The following pathogenic facts explain five basic clinical and epidemiological concepts shared by respiratory viruses:

1. The incubation time is very short, from hours to 5 days.
2. There is abundant production of the virus at the portal of entry, which facilitates viral shedding and high infectivity.
3. Viral diffusion via mucosal proximity causes simultaneous and bilateral compromise of more than one segment of the respiratory airways and their annexes—for example, the paranasal sinuses and the middle ear.
4. The defense mechanisms in play—both innate and specifically acquired (immunoglobulin A)—are mainly of a local character.
5. Specific immunity is temporary and lasts only for some months (Table 28.4).

Table 28.4 Clinical and epidemiological consequences of the pathogeny of respiratory viral infections

Consequences
Transmission
Directly from person to person
Through big droplets (>5 μm in size) deposited in the environment (secretions on hands, clothes, furniture, toys) and small droplets (<5 μm in size) that form aerosols
Potential animal sources of influenza virus (birds, pigs, and others) and hantavirus
Portal of entry = target organ
Short incubation time, from hours to a few days
High infection rate in the community
Localized infection = local defense mechanisms prevail
Innate immunity: epithelial barrier (cilia, coughing, associated lymphatic tissue) and inflammatory response (leukocytes, macrophages, fever, cytokines)
Acquired immunity: local (immunoglobulin A) and general (immunoglobulin G), T lymphocytes CD8–CD4 (type 1 and type 2 helper T cells); short-duration immunity with frequent reinfections
Propagation by proximity
In individuals, it simultaneously compromises many levels of the respiratory system in a bilateral way
In the community, it affects various members with close contact within the family, at school, or at work; it is hard to contain with isolation measures or physical barriers

Prevention of viral respiratory infections is difficult because high infectivity is favored by the presence of subclinical infections, human sociability, and unavailability of vaccines, except for influenza virus vaccines. Treatment is fundamentally symptomatic and essentially consists of maintenance of the permeable airway, oxygen administration, and assisted mechanical ventilation in extreme cases. Use of antiallergics, anti-inflammatories, steroids, bronchodilators, and prophylactic antibiotics is very controversial, and this is discussed in other chapters in this book. Antivirals are available just for influenza viruses and, if they are administrated early, they shorten the symptomatic period but seemingly do not prevent development of serious illness in high-risk patients.

Epidemiological Management: The Winter Plan

In countries with temperate weather, the incidence of acute respiratory infections increases in cold seasons because of the appearance of viral epidemics. RSV is the virus most responsible for this and usually coincides with influenza outbreaks. In addition, respiratory adenoviruses appear endemically, with unpredictable increases that can acquire relevance because of their clinical seriousness and propensity to cause inpatient infections at times of overload in hospitals. Despite prevention not being efficient and the fact that there is no specific treatment for respiratory viruses, health care (both public and private) can be organized for prevention of severe cases and deaths.

RSV appears "all winter" and its outbreak lasts for 3–5 months. It has been estimated that 60% of children who are born are infected during the first year of life, and all children have had contact with it by their second year; 25–40% of primary infections evolve as acute lower respiratory tract infections, and 2% of them require hospitalization. Influenza viruses usually appear in autumn in epidemics that last for 6–8 weeks. Accordingly, the demand for pediatric care increases during every winter; the emergence of RSV dominates bed availability for infants in hospitals and increases the need for ambulatory care, while influenza viruses dominate consultations for preschool children, schoolchildren, and adults.

This increase in the demand for pediatric ambulatory and hospital care forces us to adopt special measures for management of acute lower respiratory tract infections—the most serious pathology. They have to be implemented at both the ambulatory and hospital levels. The objective of this "winter campaign" is to prevent deaths from acute lower respiratory tract infections, and it should be directed preferentially toward those children and adults who are at greater risk of developing severe illness.

At the ambulatory level, the campaign should be focused on two aspects:

- Education of the population for recognition of serious symptoms (long-lasting fever, respiratory distress, wheezes, apnea, etc.) to encourage early medical consultation, particularly in higher-risk populations such as preterm infants, chronic disease patients, immunosuppressed patients, and, in general, patients under 3 months of age.
- Increased pediatric ambulatory care, including prolongation of clinic hours (afternoons, nights) for pediatric and kinesiotherapy care, increased availability of bronchodilators (salbutamol) and antimicrobial medication (amoxicillin), and implementation of ambulatory oximetry and oxygen therapy.

At the hospital level, the following measures are recommended:

- Anti-influenza and antipneumococcal vaccination.
- Local implementation of rapid diagnosis of RSV, influenza, and adenovirus (using immunofluorescence or ELISA).
- Reinforcement of medical and paramedical at emergency medical clinics and in hospital emergency rooms and intensive care units. For this purpose, operating rooms are "repurposed" and realigned for attention to respiratory cases, with equipment for administration of oxygen. Institutional conventions are also established for facilitating transfer of severely ill patients.
- Ensuring the availability of cubicles for isolation of individual patients (for admissions and for cases of suspected or confirmed adenovirus).

In Chile, these measures have been applied every year since 1990, with great success in reducing deaths, though morbidity has not decreased, because that depends on the development of vaccines of high effectiveness (Fig. 28.2).

Epidemiology of the Most Frequent Bacterial Infections

Unlike respiratory infections with a viral cause, infections of bacterial origin, while frequent, affect a smaller group of the population, given their characteristics in terms of pathogenicity, transmissibility, and preventive measures such as use of specific vaccines.

In the following sections, we discuss the epidemiology of respiratory infections caused by *Streptococcus pneumoniae* and *Bordetella pertussis*.

Streptococcus pneumoniae

Pneumococcus is the main cause of bacterial pneumonia in all age groups across the globe. Its incidence varies according to the age group, the development status of the country, and employment of specific vaccines. It is now by far the most frequent causal agent of pneumonia since the incidence of pneumonia caused by *Haemophilus influenza* type B was reduced by introduction of a specific vaccine, which practically made infections with that causal agent disappear. The most relevant risk groups are infants <2 years old, adults over 60 years old, and immunosuppressed patients. The WHO estimates that this agent causes the deaths of 700,000 to one million people every year.

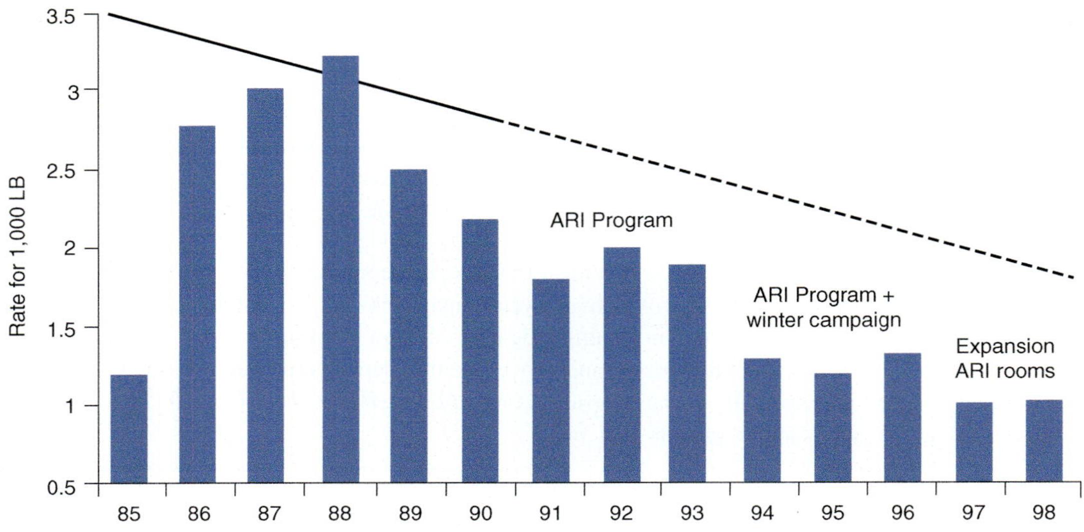

Fig. 28.2 Infant mortality due to pneumonia in Chile, 1985–1998 (Rev Chil Pediatr (2001))

In Chile, we know, with reasonable accuracy, the epidemiology of invasive pneumococcal infections (meningitis, septicemia, bacteremia), since they are under laboratory monitoring. Nevertheless, the great majority of pneumococcal pneumonias are not bacteremic, which is why the incidence of pneumococcal pneumonia is unknown; there are just data extrapolated from monitoring of pneumonia in hospitalized patients, assuming that pneumococcus is the primary cause of bacterial pneumonia at any age.

Before universal vaccination with a pneumococcal conjugate vaccine was introduced, the incidence of this disease in Latin America was between 61/100,000 in patients under 2 years old and 32/100,000 in patients under 5 years old, subsequently decreasing with age.

In Chile, vaccination with a 10-valent pneumococcal conjugate vaccine was introduced in 2011 for children born since November 2010. Between 2011 and 2014 the rate of invasive infections in patients under 2 years old decreased from approximately 39/100,000 to 8.7/100,000, although there has been no impact of vaccination in other age groups; on the contrary, an increase in cases has been seen among patients over 65 years old (Fig. 28.3).

The most prevalent serotypes prior to the use of vaccines were 5, 14, and 1. In the last postvaccination period they were serotypes 15, 1, and 7F, followed by serotypes 3, 19A, 6A, and 6B, although there were reductions in serotypes 15, 1, 5, and 6B. Since the introduction of vaccines, the proportions of serotypes 3, 19A, and 6A have increased in all age groups; those serotypes are not contained in the 10-valent vaccine but are included in the 13-valent one.

Susceptibility to penicillin in pneumococcal infection is an emergent topic that greatly worries clinicians, although management of pneumonias is not as important as management of pneumococcal meningitis. Since changes in the cut-off points in the definition of resistance to infections outside the central nervous system, susceptibility to penicillin has remained low. Resistance to penicillin is greater in patients under 5 years old than in other age groups, which is why this topic is more relevant to pediatric populations.

The most recent report of the Chilean Public Health Institute showed that the rates of intermediate sensitivity to penicillin and cefotaxime were 1–3% in the preceding 2 years, and the rate of resistance was 0%. When analyzed by age group, it was observed that for patients under 5 years old, the rate of intermediate sensitivity was 4% for penicillin and 5% for cefotaxime between 2007 and 2014, with a 0% rate of resis-

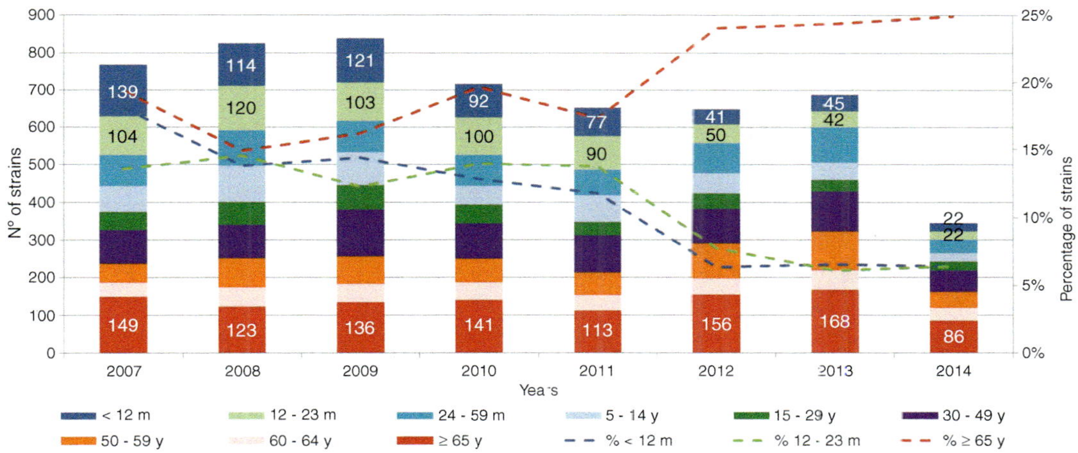

Fig. 28.3 Confirmed cases of invasive pneumococcal disease in Chile

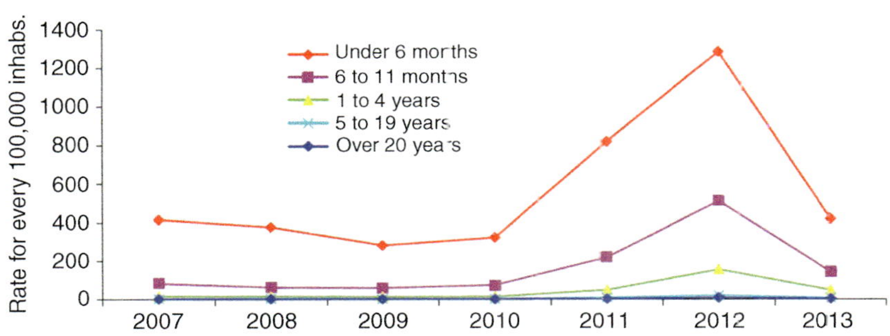

Fig. 28.4 Incidence of whooping cough in Chile

tance to these antibiotics. The rate of resistance to macrolides in the same age group reached 47%, while the rate of susceptibility to levofloxacin and vancomycin remained at 100%.

Bordetella pertussis

B. pertussis is a causal agent of respiratory infections that pose a serious risk of mortality in young infants, especially those under 6 months old. Thanks to the introduction of vaccines in the 1950s and 1960s, the incidence and mortality rates have decreased significantly. However, despite the high coverage rates for the vaccine, and although humans are the only reservoir for *B. pertussis*, control and elimination of its circulation have not yet been accomplished.

Its distribution is ubiquitous, with over 50 million cases and 300,000 deaths annually. The majority of the mortality is concentrated in patients under 1 year old, particularly in those under 6 months old.

In Chile, during the early 1990s, a sustained increase in the incidence started to be registered, starting from less than 4/100,000 and reaching 25/100,000 between 1996 and 2000. After 2010 and 2012, a new increase in cases, with incidence rates of up to 35/100,000, was observed.

Incidence rates vary according to the age group, reaching the highest rate (136/100,000) in infants under 12 months old and then dropping to 19/100,000 in children between 1 and 4 years old (Fig. 28.4). Cases in patients under 1 year old represent 42% of all notified cases and, of those, 82% are under 6 months old.

A feature shared by all of these epidemic outbreaks is that mortality is concentrated in young infants, who are not protected by the primary scheme of three vaccine doses, which is not completed until the child is 6 months of age.

Several studies on the source of infection of *B. pertussis* in young infants have shown that the main sources are intrafamily contacts. The vaccine loses its effectiveness 5 to 7 years after the vaccination is completed, which is why adolescents and adults can be infected.

Since whooping cough does not always manifest as classic clinical cases in adolescents and adults but, rather, is characterized by a persistent cough, suspicion levels are low and appropriate diagnosis is often not made; thus, there is no timely treatment. This situation facilitates infection of infants within a family group.

On the basis of this epidemiology, between 2011 and 2012 the Capullo control program took place in Chile, in which the entire family groups of newborns and vaccination of adolescents in the eighth grade was performed. In 2013 the incidence dropped to less than 12/100,000, and in 2014 the aggregated incidence reached 4.6/100,000.

These numbers show us that whooping cough is a disease that affects all age groups, but its biggest impact in terms of both morbidity and mortality is in patients under 6 months old.

Multiple strategies have been tested internationally, but none of them have been very effective. A combination of different strategies seems to be the key, such as systematic and permanent vaccination in pregnant women, adolescents, and family groups. Creation of a vaccine with proven high efficacy in controlling this disease in the short term has not yet been accomplished.

Clinical suspicion is very important for appropriate treatment of cases, in both adults and infants, to reduce the risk of transmission in the former and to reduce mortality in the latter.

Sources

Avendaño LF, Palomino MA, Larrañaga C. Surveillance for respiratory syncytial virus in infants hospitalized for acute lower respiratory infection in Chile (1989 to 2000). J Clin Microbiol. 2003;41:4879–82.

Bill & Melinda Gates Foundation Group. Global and regional mortality from 235 causes of death for 20 age groups in 1990 and 2010: a systematic analysis for the Global Burden of Disease Study 2010. Lancet. 2012;380:2095–128.

Departamento de Epidemiologia, Ministerio de Salud. Buscar influenza o infecciones respiratorias agudas, por años de informes. http://epi.minsal.cl. Accessed March 2019.

Girardi G, Astudillo P, Zúñiga F. El programa IRA en Chile: hitos e historia. Rev. chil. pediatr. 2001; 72(4):292–300. ISSN 0370–4106.

Luchsinger V, Ruiz M, Zunino E, Martínez MA, Machado C, Piedra PA, Fasce R, Ulloa MT, Fink MC, Lara P, Gebauer M, Chávez F, Avendaño LF. Community-acquired pneumonia in Chile: the clinical relevance in the detection of viruses and atypical bacteria. Thorax. 2013;68:100–6.

Mahony JB. Detection of respiratory viruses by molecular methods. Clin Microbiol Rev. 2008;21(4):716–47.

Perret C, Viviani T, Peña A, Abarca K, Ferrés M. Fuente de infección de *Bordetella pertussis* en lactantes hospitalizados por coqueluche. Rev Méd Chile. 2011;139:448–54.

Unidad de Epidemiología, Ministerio de Salud. Tos ferina o coqueluche. Boletín Epidemiológico Trimestral 2014; 110(3).

Valenzuela MT, O'Loughlin R, De La Hoz F, Gomez E, Constenla D, Sinha A, et al. The burden of pneumococcal disease among Latin American and Caribbean children: review of the evidence. Rev Panam Salud Publica/Pan Am J Public Health. 2009;25(3): 270–9.

Vigilancia de enfermedad invasora *Streptococcus pneumoniae*. Chile, 2007–2014. Boletín de Instituto de Salud Pública de Chile 2014;4(11).

World Health Organization. The global burden of disease. 2004. https://www.who.int/healthinfo/global_burden_disease/GBD_report_2004update_full.pdf. Accessed 15 October 2019.

Laryngitis (Croup) 29

Ida Concha Murray and Cecilia Perret Pérez

Contents

Epidemiology

Acute laryngitis (croup) is more common in the cold months of autumn and winter, but it can occur throughout the year. It affects 2% of preschool children, with a 3:2 male-to-female ratio.

The causal agent is spread by direct person-to-person contact through sneezing, coughing, and droplets of contaminated nasopharyngeal secretions on the hands. The most common etiological agent identified in monitoring studies of respiratory viruses is the parainfluenza virus, which is active throughout the year but usually has a higher incidence during winter (Fig. 29.1). Serological studies have shown that 50% of

I. Concha Murray · C. Perret Pérez (✉)
Department of Pediatrics, School of Medicine, Pontificia Universidad Católica de Chile, Santiago, Chile
e-mail: iconcha@med.puc.cl; cperret@med.puc.cl

P. Bertrand, I. Sánchez (eds.), *Pediatric Respiratory Diseases*,
https://doi.org/10.1007/978-3-030-26961-6_29

children have acquired the parainfluenza virus by the time they are 1 year old. In terms of its incidence, it is generally the third most common virus after influenza and the respiratory syncytial virus (RSV), depending on the season. In infants under 1 year of age, it occupies second place for incidence (Fig. 29.2). Acute obstructive laryngitis accounts for 7% of fever- and respiratory-related hospitalizations of children under 5 years old. Half of these situations are due to parainfluenza 3.

Etiology and Physiopathology

The most common etiological agents are parainfluenza viruses 1 and 3. Less common agents are parainfluenza 2, influenza viruses A and B, RSV, adenovirus, measles, and *Mycoplasma pneumoniae*.

Parainfluenza is a single-strand, enveloped RNA virus that belongs to the Paramyxoviridae family. It is pleomorphic, measures between 100 and 200 nm, and has six proteins. There are four types of parainfluenza virus, the most common of which are types 1–3. Types 1 and 2 generally produce acute or obstructive laryngitis, while type 3 produces infections of the lower respiratory tract, such as bronchitis and pneumonia. Type 4 is less often detected and can cause upper and lower respiratory infections.

The HN glycoprotein adheres to the host cell and facilitates F protein initiation of virus–cell

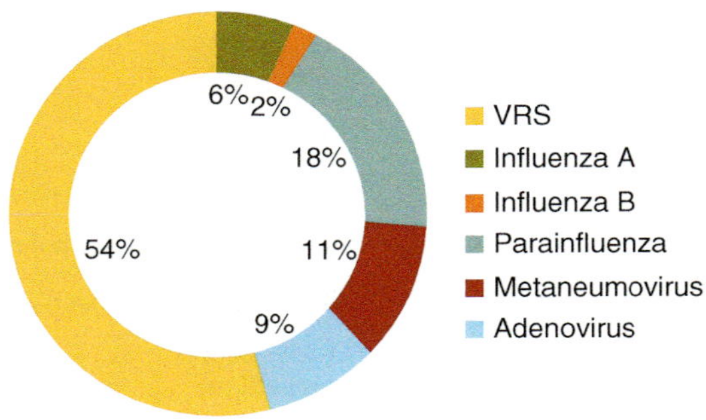

Fig. 29.2 Respiratory virus

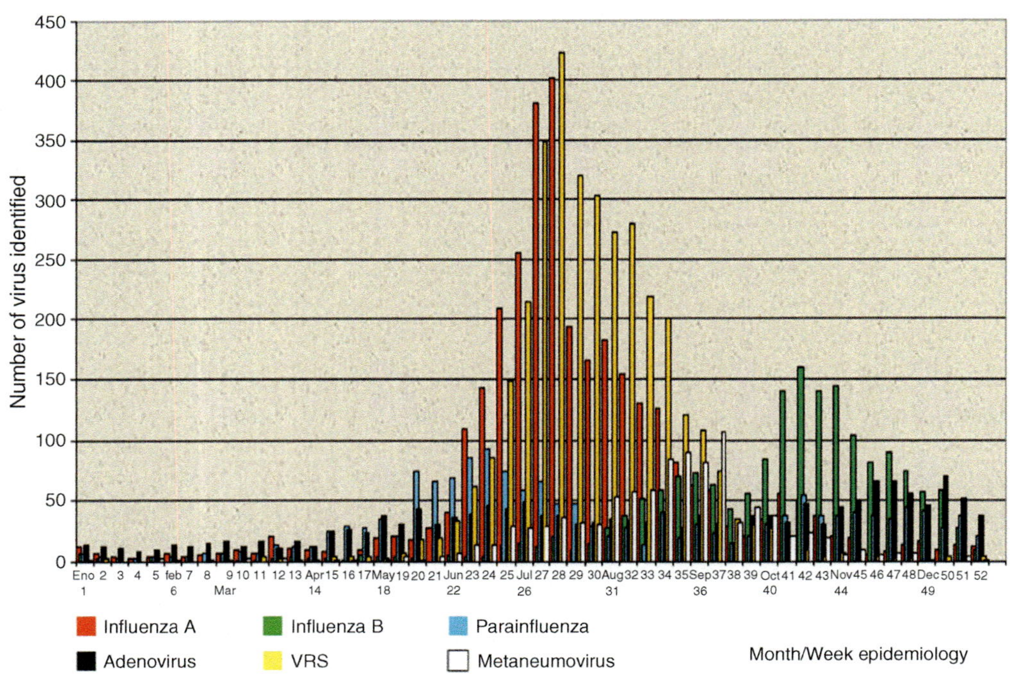

Fig. 29.1 Vigilance against respiratory virus infections

membrane fusion. It also facilitates the binding of the nucleocapsid (formed by NP, P, and L proteins linked to the viral genome) to the genome of the host cell, thus initiating viral replication. In addition to its basic proteins, the parainfluenza virus expresses other proteins such as C, V and D. V and C neutralize innate immunity through suppression of activity by interferon 1.

Initially, the virus infects epithelial cells of the nose and oropharynx, and then it extends to the cell cilia and bronchial epithelial alveoli, as well as to the large and small airways. Viral replication peaks at 2–5 days and begins to decline by the seventh day.

Cellular or tissue damage is fundamentally caused by the host response, with minimal direct cytopathic effects of the virus itself. It induces an innate immune response with production of CD4 and CD8, interferon, and local and systemic immunoglobulin A and immunoglobulin G, all of which contribute to elimination of the virus. The hyperresponsiveness that is often seen in patients may be due to immunoglobulin E production and histamine release.

The result of this process is diffuse inflammation of the airway, with a greater intensity at the levels of the larynx and trachea, particularly in the subglottic space. This causes a reduction of the lumen and increased resistance to the entry of air in the lungs, resulting in greater work of breathing and appearance of the cardinal sign, a stridor.

Clinical Manifestations

After an incubation period of 2–7 days in the case of parainfluenza virus, the patient presents coryza and a fever, which can be high or low, and in 24–48 hours the characteristic signs appear: a barking cough and a stridor. If the edema and narrowing of the airway increase, the breathing rate rises, the patient becomes increasingly more agitated (to the extent that respiration is more difficult), and the use of accessory musculature appears, with suprasternal drainage, intercostal and subcostal retraction, and even cyanosis. Changes in the mental state occur in this phase, with agitation or lethargy. The patient is unable to cry or speak, and there is no stridor and no air entering the lungs, but there is a paradoxical movement of the chest, with signs of hypoxemia and respiratory failure.

Fortunately, the majority of cases of acute obstructive laryngitis are mild and resolve within 7 days, although coughing can continue for weeks.

Severity Scores

There are different severity scores to assess the seriousness of the clinical picture, such as the Downes score and the Wesley score, the latter being the most often used for studies.

Downes Score

- *Grade I—mild*: stridor during crying or activity, absence of retraction
- *Grade II—moderate*: inspiratory stridor at rest, suprasternal and intercostal retraction at rest, but without agitation
- *Grade III—severe*: major inspiratory or biphasic stridor, with marked suprasternal and intercostal retraction, and with agitation; signs of respiratory difficulty
- *Grade IV—imminent respiratory failure*: weak cough, altered level of consciousness, signs of hypoxemia

Westley Score

- *Stridor*:
  - 0: absent
  - 1: during crying
  - 2: at rest
- *Retraction*:
  - 0: absent
  - 1: slight
  - 2: moderate
  - 3: severe

- *Entry of air*:
  - 0: normal
  - 1: reduced but audible
  - 2: very reduced, hardly audible
- *Cyanosis* (O_2 saturation <92%; fraction of inspired oxygen (FiO_2) 0.21):
  - 0: absent
  - 4: with agitation
  - 5: at rest
- *Level of awareness*:
  - 0: normal
  - 5: diminished
- *Total score*: 0–1 = mild; 2–7 = moderate; ≥8 = severe

Diagnostic Focus

The diagnosis is clinical. A virus identification study is sometimes requested in severe cases, which can include a viral etiological study of a respiratory sample (either a nasopharyngeal swab, nasopharyngeal aspirate, bronchoalveolar lavage fluid, or tracheal aspirate). The parainfluenza virus can be identified by direct immunofluorescence or polymerase chain reaction (PCR). There are rapid immunochromatographic tests for RSV, influenza, and adenoviruses.

X-ray examinations are done only when there is suspicion of a differential diagnosis.

The airway is assessed endoscopically only in severe cases in which an adequate response to the established therapy is not observed and significant obstructive symptoms persist after 48 hours of treatment.

Differential diagnosis: In general, the other diagnostic alternatives are much less common but, because they require other assessments and/or treatments, the clinician should always keep them in mind, especially if the patient does not evolve as expected.

The most common infectious causes are:

- Bacterial tracheitis
- Epiglottis
- Retro- or parapharyngeal abscess

Possible noninfectious causes are:

- Foreign body in the airway
- Airway trauma
- Congenital caustic injuries and/or scarring (stenosis)
- Spasmodic croup
- Angioneurotic edema

Treatment

First, a rapid primary evaluation should be performed to assess the patient's awareness, stridor intensity, and respiratory distress, using the Downes score or Westley score and the patient's hemodynamic parameters (distal perfusion, heart rate, and blood pressure, among others). With this, it is possible to determine if the patient requires immediate therapy. The intensity of the stridor can be used to classify the patient's status as mild, moderate, or severe, in order to then adopt an appropriate clinical management algorithm for acute obstructive laryngitis (Fig. 29.3).

If the patient's state of awareness is compromised, there is severe retraction with no air entry or with poor air entry at the pulmonary level, or the oxygen saturation is <92%, the patient has severe laryngitis (grade III–IV) according to the Downes score or a Westley score of ≥8, and rapid intervention is required to avoid further deterioration such as respiratory or cardiorespiratory arrest. As a first measure, to reduce respiratory difficulty, nebulized adrenaline (epinephrine) should be administered in either a general form or a racemic form diluted in physiological serum, with an air or oxygen flow of at least 6–8 l/min.

Epinephrine reduces edema in the airway by producing vasoconstriction, given its α-adrenergic effect. It has become the standard therapy for treatment of moderate and severe laryngitis. Traditionally, racemic adrenaline (composed of the same proportions of L and D isomers) was used for treatment of acute laryngitis on the basis that its cardiovascular effects would be less than those of common adrenaline (L-adrenaline). Three studies have confirmed a moderate to

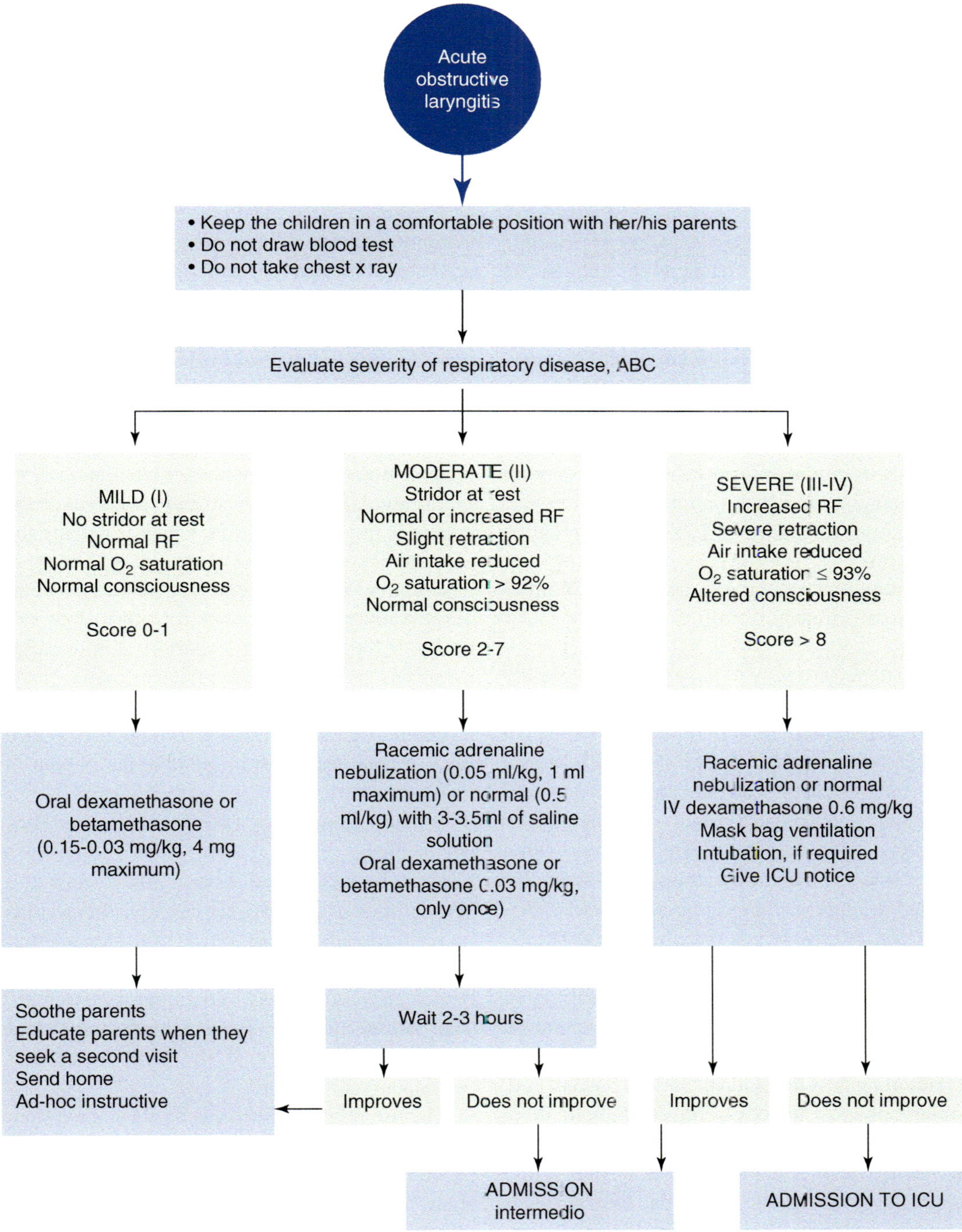

Fig. 29.3 Algorithm for clinical management of acute obstructive laryngitis

major reduction in the severity score at 30 minutes after nebulization. This effect lasts for 2 hours (level of recommendation: A).

A small-scale study showed that common adrenaline is as effective as the racemic form if it is used in an equimolar dose. The frequency of adverse effects is similar with use of either of the two forms. Neither should be used according to a schedule; rather, they should be used according to need. There is a report in the literature of a previously healthy patient who had an acute myocardial infarction after three nebulizations within 1 hour. Vital signs should be monitored, and the nebulization should consist of a 0.05 ml/kg/dose with a maximum of 1 ml of racemic adrenaline, with the medication diluted in 3–3.5 cc of physiological serum for a maximum of 10 minutes with an air or oxygen flow of 6–8 l/min. The equivalency of racemic and common adrenaline is described below:

- 2.25% racemic adrenaline = (L + D) adrenaline 22.5 mg/ml = L-adrenaline 11.25 mg/ml + D-adrenaline 11.25 mg/ml
- Common adrenaline 1/1000 = L-adrenaline 1 mg/ml
- Consequently, racemic adrenaline 0.5 ml = common adrenaline 5 ml

Secondly, 0.6 mg/kg of dexamethasone should be administered venously. If there are hemodynamic alterations, 20 cc/kg of physiological serum is recommended. Patients should be monitored and watched, with adequate oxygenation maintained above 94% through a reliable oxygen delivery system such as a Campbell mask with a venturi system. A nonrebreathing mask is recommended in more serious cases. If an intense stridor at rest returns or persists, the patient should be nebulized with adrenaline again. If this does not work, there have been reports that delivery of a mixture of helium with oxygen through a mask has decreased respiratory difficulty.

Helium is less dense than air and oxygen, and, with use of a mixture of oxygen and helium, there is less resistance to gas flow in narrow airways and hence less respiratory work. This option should be used only in units that have this gas available and have experience in critical airway treatment. Routine use of it is not recommended (level of recommendation: C).

Along with clinical evaluation of critically ill patients, it is recommended to determine the degree of compromise by, at least, venous blood gas monitoring to show the severity of the obstruction. If respiratory acidosis persists and the partial pressure of carbon dioxide (pCO_2) remains elevated, intubation is recommended. This is a dangerous procedure in inexperienced hands, so it should be done by the most expert member of the team—ideally, an anesthesiologist.

Fortunately, moderately severe laryngeal symptoms (grade II or a Westley score of 2–7) are more common, with a normal oxygen saturation of >92%, a stridor at rest, and a normal or slightly elevated respiratory rate, which on auscultation is accompanied by decreased air intake. In this case, there is an indication to nebulize the patient with adrenaline and give a dose of oral dexamethasone (0.3 mg/kg) if the patient can tolerate it. If not, it is administered intravenously or intramuscularly. If the stridor stops and the patient is in good condition, which is usually the case, he or she should be observed for 2 hours to ensure that greater respiratory distress (previously known as respiratory rebound) does not return. If the patient has no stridor 2 hours after nebulization, he or she can be sent home. If the stridor returns, nebulization with adrenaline can be applied again, but if the stridor appears a third time, it is advisable to hospitalize the patient in an intermediate unit.

When patients have a stridor only when they cry or during physical effort, or if they have a history of a stridor (mild laryngitis grade I or a Westley score of 0–1), only one dose of steroids is recommended, preferably oral dexamethasone (0.15–0.3 mg/kg) or its equivalent (betamethasone) in an anti-inflammatory strength. The patient can then be sent home with clear instructions to return if the stridor becomes permanent.

The use of glucocorticoids has become a standard treatment for croup and has been supported by numerous works: 30 randomized studies and controlled studies, and three meta-analyses (level of recommendation: A). Steroids improve the symptoms of obstructive laryngitis as fast as within 6 hours and for up to 12 hours after treatment. They lower the Westley score at 6 hours and 12 hours after being administered and reduce the number of consultations with emergency services, the need for hospitalization, the use of adrenaline, the number and duration of intubations, and the need for reintubation in an intensive care unit.

In a Canadian study that included administration of dexamethasone versus placebo in response to mild croup, dexamethasone reduced the number of patients requiring further consultations (7% versus 15%) and notably decreased the stridor score at 48 hours. Consequently, dexamethasone is recommended for even mild croup.

The standard dose of dexamethasone is 0.6 mg/kg, but studies have shown the value of lower doses (0.15–0.3 mg/kg), because of which we recommend lower doses in mild to moderate cases.

These medications are equally effective when administered parenterally or orally; thus, oral administration is recommended except when the patient is intolerant of it.

There have been no studies that support the use of repeated doses versus a single dose. Some authors recommend a repeat dose 24 hours later if there have been no clinical improvements.

Nebulized budesonide at 2 mg is equally effective and is recommended in several English-speaking countries for moderate croup, but it is not available in Chile. Budesonide can be mixed with adrenaline and administered together with it in serious cases.

Because an oral formulation of dexamethasone is not available, a vial for injection can be administered orally and has proven efficacy.

Betamethasone has the same potency and duration of action as dexamethasone, so it is a suitable replacement at equimolar doses. Oral betamethasone comes in a 0.5 mg/ml presentation (Cidoten or Coritex), giving a dose of 0.15–0.3 mg/kg. Prednisone 1 mg/kg/day for 2–3 days can be used to give a comparative dosage in terms of potency and duration.

In effect, the degree of benefit provided by steroids in response to acute obstructive laryngitis is so remarkable that if five patients are treated, an improvement in the symptoms of one of them will be obtained (number needed to treat (NNT) = 5).

Other therapies—such as cold vapor, nonsteroidal anti-inflammatories, antitussives, and decongestants—have been widely used, but they have not been shown to be useful in clinical studies.

There have been no controlled studies of use of antibiotics that have shown their utility.

Etiological Treatment

Treatment is generally symptom driven. There are no specific treatments for infections by parainfluenza virus, RSV, or adenovirus. The presence of laryngitis as the only manifestation of infection by influenza virus or *M. pneumoniae* is very uncommon, and the impact of specific treatments in these cases has not been assessed.

Hospitalization

It is recommended that the patient remains in an intermediate unit during the first 24 hours to monitor airway stability and provide any necessary treatment in a rapid and timely manner. The patient's condition can worsen to a point where emergency intubation is required, so the patient must be monitored. Given the degree of inflammation of the airway that is characteristic of acute obstructive laryngitis, this is a more difficult procedure that should be performed by the most expert professional available—ideally, an anesthesiologist.

The patient should continue to be nebulized with adrenaline as needed and monitored in the intermediate unit.

There is no evidence recommending new doses of steroids, although some experts recommend repeat doses of dexamethasone after 24 hours if the stridor has not improved.

Indications for Hospitalization

A patient should be hospitalized if respiratory symptoms such as retraction and a stridor persist or recur within 2 hours of therapy (two nebulizations with adrenaline and a steroid). When a patient arrives at an emergency service in a serious condition (with compromised awareness, cyanosis, or with a toxic appearance) or if evaluation of the patient raises suspicion of bacterial tracheitis or another serious differential diagnosis, he or she should be hospitalized. Infants and children who have acute obstructive laryngitis and require oxygen, have poor ingestion of liquids, or are dehydrated should also be hospitalized.

The indications for hospitalization are relative. How far away the patient is from a health care center and how easy it is to get there should be taken into account when hospitalization of the patient is being considered. It is also recommended to hospitalize patients if the parents are experiencing severe anxiety and have made repeated visits to emergency services within the last 24 hours.

Criteria for Patient Release from an Emergency Service

If the patient has minimal symptoms and does not have a stridor at rest, or after a period of observation of 2–3 hours after one or two nebulizations, he or she can be sent safely home. This must be carefully evaluated beforehand; the patient must have normal oxygen saturation, show a normal level of awareness, have good intake of air into the lungs, and be able to drink fluids.

The parents should be instructed as to what clinical conditions they should describe in any subsequent consultation with an emergency service. It is expected that around 5% of patients will present for another consultation because their symptoms have worsened.

Complications

It is necessary to intubate fewer than 1% of hospitalized patients with acute obstructive laryngitis, since there are now equally effective therapies such as nebulized adrenaline and steroids.

The appearance of bacterial tracheitis can complicate and aggravate an initial condition of viral laryngotracheobronchitis and should be treated vigorously with intravenous antibiotics that cover *Staphylococcus aureus*, the most common causative organism.

Another feared complication is complete obstruction of the airway, which can lead to respiratory or cardiorespiratory arrest and eventual death or neurological sequelae. Therefore, it is essential that the patient's first hours of hospitalization are monitored adequately. Finally, pneumonia is an uncommon complication and is usually a result of the same virus that causes laryngitis.

Specialist Follow-Up

Patients with a number of conditions should be seen by an otolaryngologist and a bronchopulmonary specialist to evaluate possible differential diagnoses that can be confirmed or discarded by fiber bronchoscopy, laryngoscopy, or other examinations. The conditions include a long-term stridor (lasting >1 week), severe acute obstructive laryngitis, obstructive laryngitis with atypical evolution, acute obstructive laryngitis in a child under 3 months of age, or craniofacial dysmorphism.

Summary

The prognosis of acute obstructive laryngitis is generally benign without sequelae when treatment is timely.

If the patient has moderate to severe obstructive laryngitis, he or she should receive racemic adrenaline or an equimolar dose of common adrenaline to relieve the obstructive symptoms rapidly.

A single dose of a steroid is the standard therapy for all degrees of laryngitis. If the patient has good tolerance, the oral route should always be chosen.

If the patient is hospitalized, he or she should be monitored for at least the first 24 hours in an intermediate unit.

Sources

Beckmann KR, Brueggemann WM. Heliox treatment of severe croup. Am J Emerg Med. 2000;18:753–6.

Bjornson C, Russell K, Vandermeer B, Klassen TP, Johnson DW. Nebulized epinephrine for croup in children. Cochrane Database Syst Rev. 2013;10:CD006619.

Bjornson C, Klassen TP, Williamson RN, et al. Randomized trial of a single dose of oral dexamethasone for mild croup. N Engl J Med. 2004;351(13):1307–13.

Fitzgerald DA. The assessment and management of croup. Paediatr Respir Rev. 2006;7:73–81.

Holmgren N, Concha I. El niño hospitalizado. Laringitis. http://escuela.med.puc.cl/publ/pediatriaHosp/Laringitis.html. Accessed August 2016.

Luria JW, et al. Efectiveness of oral or nebulized dexamethasone for children with mild croup. Arch Pediatr Adolesc Med. 2001;155(12):1340–5.

Russell KF, Liang Y, O'Gorman K, Johnson DW, Klassen TP. Glucocorticoids for croup. Cochrane Database Syst Rev. 2011;1:CD001955.

Terregino CA, Nairn SJ, Chansky ME. The effect of heliox on croup: a pilot study. Acad Emerg Med. 1998;5:1130–3.

Waissman Y, et al. Prospective randomized double-blind study comparing L-epinephrine and racemic epinephrine aerosols in the treatment of laryngotracheitis (croup). Pediatrics. 1992;89:302–6.

Bronchiolitis

30

Miriam Pérez and Giovanni Piedimonte

Contents

Historical Perspective

Bronchiolitis is the most frequent disease of the lower respiratory tract in infants and small children. Its most common cause is respiratory syncytial virus (RSV). In 1850, John Eberle published the first medical description of acute bronchiolitis. He described a "catarrhal effect" in children under 1 year old, which was accompanied by breathing difficulty, coughing, and wheezing, similar to an "asthma crisis." By the end of 1930, the United States had witnessed several serious outbreaks of respiratory diseases in infants, which led John Adams to publish several reports related to these epidemics, wherein he described the seasonal variety as well as the physical and pathological manifestations of the disease, relating it to a viral infection.

In 1955, some scientists from the Walter Reed Army Institute of Research isolated a virus from the nasal secretions of young chimpanzees who had sneezing and mucopurulent rhinorrhea. Having identified this new virus, which they called "chimpanzee coryza agent," they could reproduce the same viral syndrome after having exposed other chimpanzees to the same agent. Robert J. Chanock isolated the same virus in two children: one child had bronchiolitis and the other child had pneumonia that replicated in cellular cultures and had the ability to produce

M. Pérez
Cleveland Clinic Children's Hospital,
Cleveland, OH, USA

G. Piedimonte (✉)
The Cleveland Clinic at Cleveland,
Cleveland, OH, USA
e-mail: piedimg@ccf.org

P. Bertrand, I. Sánchez (eds.), *Pediatric Respiratory Diseases*,
https://doi.org/10.1007/978-3-030-26961-6_30

giant multinuclear cells, which are characteristic of a massive syncytium, and therefore he called it RSV.

Chanock continued studying this disease, and during the 1960s he published a more detailed description of the epidemiology, recurrent infections, and clinical manifestations of RSV. During this period, with collaboration with Robert Parrott, he started to develop a vaccine against this virus. The first tests using a formol-inactivated virus began in 1966. The vaccine was at first administered to the children of military personnel in Washington, DC, Colorado, and California. During the outbreaks of that year, infants who were vaccinated developed infections at the same rate as those who had received a placebo, but a greater cause for concern was that 80% of the children who received the vaccine had to be hospitalized because of bronchiolitis or serious pneumonia, in comparison with only 5% of children in the placebo group.

In this study, two children who were vaccinated died, which caused serious concern relative to the safety of the following implemented clinical trials that aimed to develop a new vaccine against RSV, and to date there is no available vaccine. Nevertheless, it is important to highlight that today there are several trials assessing the administration to healthy children of intranasal vaccines with attenuated live virus. These studies seek to prevent the onset of lower respiratory tract infections caused by RSV, and some of the vaccines are in preclinical and early clinical testing phases (including Phase I/II).

Up to today, investigation of RSV is still being developed, but a great obstacle has been the lack of an adequate animal model to faithfully reproduce the clinical and pathological characteristics of the infection in human beings. The virus only produces a clinically identical syndrome in chimpanzees, which is a very costly animal model, and therefore it is a great limitation for research. The animal model has had a very important role in understanding the clinical progression of the infection caused by this virus, as well as the safe development of experimental vaccines against it.

Epidemiology

The World Health Organization (WHO) estimates that RSV causes more than 60% of acute viral infections in children around the globe, and more than 80% of these infections appear in children who are under 1 year old: this places it as the most common cause of bronchiolitis and pneumonia in pediatric populations.

Seasonal outbreaks during winter months happen each year around the world, but the beginning, peak, and duration period of the season changes from one year to the next, and the outbreaks are very difficult to predict. In the United States of America (USA) and in the Northern Hemisphere, the outbreak generally starts in November, reaching a maximum peak between January and February and ending in May. Regional variability is significant, and subtropical zones such as Florida show a stable pattern during the year, with no seasonal predisposition and epidemic peaks that are difficult to predict. Throughout the Southern Hemisphere, outbreaks are similarly present during the winter months.

At 2 years of age, all children have been infected with RSV at least once, and half the children will have had two or more infections. In total, approximately 40% will develop an acute infection of the lower respiratory tract. It is estimated that each year in the USA about 126,000 children (24.3 per 1,000) are hospitalized because of bronchiolitis, and approximately 2% to 5% of them require mechanical ventilation. Even though this is a burden for the country, the numbers in other parts of the world are also impressive. At the worldwide level, it is considered that yearly 1 of every 200 children is hospitalized for treating bronchiolitis caused by RSV, with a worldwide mortality rate that ranges from 5% to 25%. The infection has a great morbidity rate, especially in preterm newborns (<35 weeks of gestation), children with pulmonary chronic disease (for example, pulmonary dysplasia or cystic fibrosis), and in children with significant congenital heart disease.

The maximum incidence of serious disease appears between 2 and 3 months of age when the infant reaches the lowest point of postnatal maternal immunoglobulin, which passes through the placenta during the last trimester of pregnancy. Because premature newborns miss this window for IgG transplacental transfer, they are born with minimum humoral protection against infections, if they have any at all, and this causes increased risk of serious disease and hospitalization in this age group. This risk is even greater when a chronic pulmonary disease has progressed, as well as any other illness that may impair pulmonary functional reserve.

Other risk factors for serious disease include male gender, overcrowding, lack of maternal breastfeeding, and any other type of immunodeficiency. Besides numerous publications that have explored the role of environmental exposure to tobacco smoke, there is still no definitive recommendation. RSV mortality in the world is greater than 1 million children per year. In infants under 1 year old, this rate is 10 times higher than the mortality rate related to influenza. Although there has been an important reduction in the mortality rate (from 4500 deaths in 1985 to 390 deaths in 1999), the economic burden is still very high, and the yearly hospitalization cost from bronchiolitis is more than 700 million dollars. Infection caused by RSV does not grant persistent immunity, even when there are significant antibody titers against the virus. Nevertheless, it has been proven that a high presence of antibody titers may alleviate the course of the disease. Reinfection is very common, and the disease can repeat itself in all age groups during the same epidemic. The first and second infection episodes usually appear during the first 2 years of life, and they tend to be more serious. Most subsequent infections affect the upper respiratory tract and have a much more benign progression, although the disease may progress with more serious symptoms and respiratory difficulty along with lower respiratory tract compromise.

Pathogenesis and Physiopathology

Transmission Respiratory syncytial virus (RSV) transmission is mainly caused through direct contact with infected respiratory secretions and their subsequent inoculation via large respiratory droplets in the nose or eyes. Small aerosolized particles seem less likely to propagate the infection. The virus can persist intact on hard surfaces (for example, counters) up to 6 h, on rubber gloves up to 90 min, and in the skin as long as 20 min. Because of this prolonged survival rate, measures such as handwashing and contact precautions are important to limit the propagation of the infection. The incubation period can vary from 2 to 8 days, and immunocompetent subjects may excrete the virus up to 3 weeks, although on average this is limited to 8 days. Excretion in immunocompromised subjects may continue for several months.

During the past decades we have achieved a better understanding of the physiopathological effects caused by RSV infection, which has made possible the developing and testing of new therapies for the treatment of this disease. Particularly, the purine ribosine rivabirin analogue was developed for the treatment of active infection caused by RSV, as well as IV immunoglobulin. Both approaches were very promising in the beginning, but they turned out to be very disappointing. Palivizumab, a humanized monoclonal antibody, has proven to be an effective and safe method to prevent the serious presentation of the disease caused by this virus in high-risk infants. Currently, it is the only approved strategy for protection against the infection caused by RSV in this population. In developed countries, a remarkable reduction in the mortality caused by this virus has been achieved, and this is in part thanks to palivizumab use, in addition to the advances achieved relative to the supportive care for children infected by this virus.

Microbiology

Respiratory syncytial virus (RSV) is a single-stranded RNA virus that belongs to the Paramyxoviridae, genus *Pneumovirus* (Fig. 30.1). The virion is composed of a nucleocapsid contained within a lipid double layer, created from the plasma membrane of the cell of the host. The

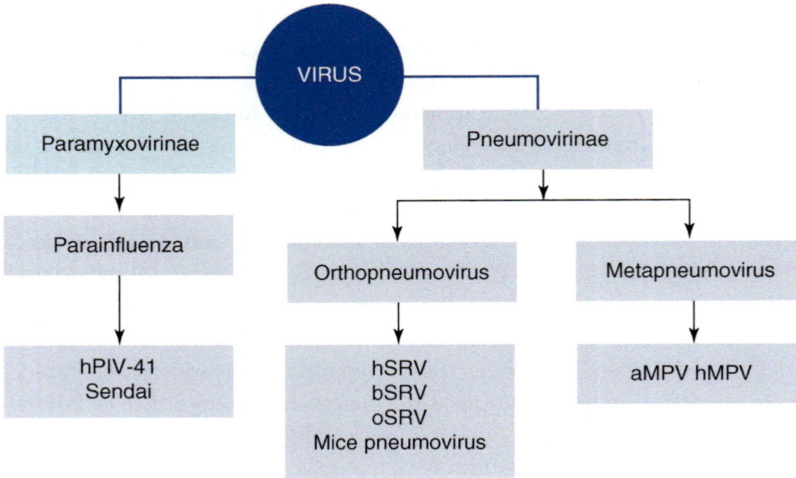

Fig. 30.1 Taxonomy of Paramyxoviridae virus

nucleocapsid contains the viral genome, which consists of a single strand of nonsegmented RNA and negative polarity, including 10 genes, which code a total of 11 proteins. Eight of these function as structural proteins and superficial glycoproteins, and the rest directly handle viral replication.

RSV, particularly, expresses two superficial glycoproteins: fusion (F) protein and binding proteins (G). These glycoproteins are very important in the virus lack of effectiveness and viral pathogenesis, and they are the main objectives of the host's protective antibody production. G protein regulates the binding to the cell of the host. Then, F protein allows the binding of the plasma membranes of the virus and the host, which allows the virus to move into the cell. F protein also promotes the fusion of its plasma membranes, through which the virus can be transmitted from one cell to another. An interesting note is that these "syncytia" are rarely seen in vivo, but they are commonly observed by in vitro viral detection.

There are two generic subgroups of the RSV: A and B. Within these subgroups there is great variability and a general antigenic reaction of approximately 25%, mostly caused by G protein, which shows only 1% to 7% of antigenic activity. F protein is much less variable, with approximately 50% of antigenic reaction. During outbreaks, both subtypes are generally present; however, it is still debatable if the subtype A is related to more serious disease, and therefore it may be the cause of an increasing number of cases admitted into the intensive care unit.

Replication Viral replication takes place at the beginning of the nasopharyngeal epithelium, and it then propagates toward the bronchiolar epithelium, where replication is much more efficient (Fig. 30.2). This progression can be caused by the cell itself, through direct transmission from one cell to another, or through direct aspiration of upper respiratory tract secretions. Additionally, the virus can be propagated through blood flow, or through the infection of inflammatory cells (monocytes, for example), which can also cause the dissemination of the disease in immunocompromised patients. Nevertheless, in most cases the infection is limited to the respiratory tract. Viral replication is followed by necrosis of the bronchiolar epithelium, which is accompanied by peribronchiolar lymphocytic infiltration and submucosal edema. Mucus secretions increase in quantity and viscosity, and also mix with cellular detritus, which causes the blockage of small airways and also increases expiratory resistance, causing partial air trapping. With the combination of these factors, the classic triad of wheezing, atelectasis, and hyperinflation is formed.

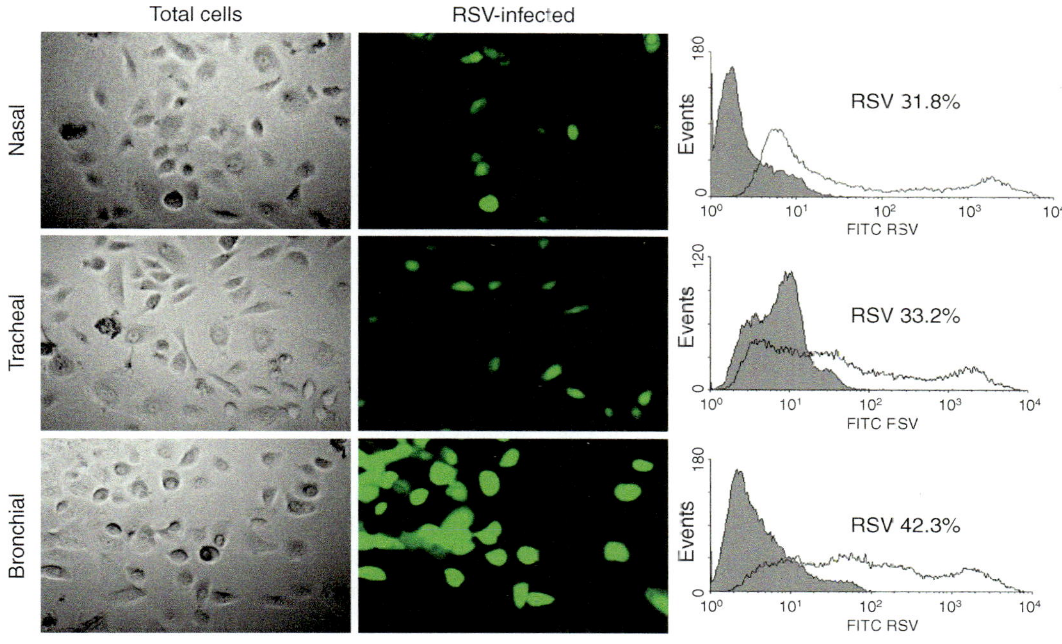

Fig. 30.2 Epithelial cell infection in the respiratory tract. (**a**) Cells from human nose, trachea, and bronchial epithelial cells after being infected with RSV GFP expressing (rgRSV) to 1 MOI (multiplicity of infection) for 48 h. The clear field panels (*left*) show the total number of cells. The green fluorescence color (*center*) represents those actively infected with RSV. (**b**) Bronchial epithelial cells are more susceptible to RSV infection. Flux cytometry data show the percentage of fluorescent cells (infected) on each panel in comparison to control cells (not infected) (*shaded* histogram). Data are expressed as median ± SEM ($n = 4$ experiments). $***P < 0.001$ when compared to nasal or tracheal cells

Immune Response Historically, it has been considered that the seriousness of the disease caused by RSV is related to the intensity of the host immune response. This perception comes from the postmortem examination of two children who died because of a pneumonia caused by this virus during the study of the formol-inactivated vaccine. These findings suggest that immunopathological mechanisms have an important role in the serious presentation of the disease caused by RSV. Also, studies done in animal models have indicated an amplified immunity for Th2 and activated cytotoxic cells, which would be responsible for this response, although several aspects of the physiopathology are still very controversial. Formol inactivation has been involved in what seems to be the cause of the immunogenicity amplification of the specific viral antigen, especially for the G protein of RSV. Nevertheless, the inactivation also caused an alteration in the capacity to induce a protective response of the neutralizing antibodies.

The infection caused by the RSV induces both humoral and cellular immune activity, and although this response does not achieve a complete response in relation to reinfection, it does seem to reduce the seriousness of subsequent infections. In infants, high titers of neutralizing antibodies against RSV, which come from the mother and are located in the umbilical cord serum, are related to much less risk of hospitalization because of bronchiolitis caused by this virus. This protection can also be obtained by the exogenous administration of specific immunoglobulin. Also, reduction of titers against RSV in the serum has been linked to a significant increase in the risk of developing a symptomatic infection. Cellular immunity probably has a function in the control of the active infection and the elimination of the virus. This idea is highlighted by the observation that immunocompromised subjects, whose cell-mediated immunity is reduced, tend to suffer a much more serious and extended RSV infection; also, they eliminate the virus for longer periods of time.

A recent study offers an alternate explanation of the physiopathology of serious diseases caused by this virus. This study examined the autopsy samples of 20 Chilean children who died of pneumonia with no intervention with mechanical respiration assistance. The authors compared the results with those of other infants who died of an infection caused by influenza, and there was no evidence of an inflammatory response in the most serious stage of the disease. There was no activation of cytotoxic T cells, but there was significant apoptosis induced by epithelial detachment. The authors interpret that the serious infection caused by RSV is the result of an insufficient adaptive immunity, and the elimination of the virus still depends greatly on a less efficient innate immunity.

Neuroimmune Interactions Some recent studies have shown that RSV infection during the early stages of life promotes a great increase in nerve growth factor (NGF) and its receptors during the development of the respiratory tract, proteins that control the structural development of peripheral neurons, both afferent and efferent, and these cause changes in their functional activity in several ways that collectively define their "neural plasticity." NGF overexpression induced by RSV may cause changes in both the short and long term related to the distribution and reactivity of sensorial and motor nerves through the respiratory tract. This change causes the unspecific hyperreactivity of the airway before and after the infection, which can be increased by chronic exposure to environmental pollution.

Studies in animal models indicate that overexpression in the NGF is crucial for the production of mucosal edema, mediated by neurogenic response, as well as innate lymphocytic and monocytic responses in the respiratory tract, when they have been infected by the RSV. This finding suggests that neuroimmune interactions created by neurotrophic pathways are very important in the systemic and local inflammation against viral pathogens. This important inflammatory mechanism is to a great extent resistant to steroids, which would give a plausible explanation for the poor therapeutic activity of these drugs in children with wheezing induced by this virus.

Mastocytes and Leukotrienes Some studies in animal models indicate that RSV has a dramatic impact on the number, distribution, and function of mastocytes in the mucosal respiratory tract (Fig. 30.3). Histopathological examination with an antibody against tryptase has identified numerous mastocytes in the secretions originated in rat lungs infected by RSV. The data show an increase of approximately sevenfold in comparison to noninfected control lungs. Further, most of these mast cells were spatially closely related to nerve fibers, which suggests that there may be a functional interaction in nerve cells that could be similar to what has previously been observed in other organs and systems, specially the central nervous system, gastrointestinal tract, and the skin.

Among the inflammatory mediators released by the mastocytes, the cysteinyl leukotrienes (CysLT) have been proven to cause inflammation of the respiratory tract, besides the contraction of smooth muscle, during RSV infection, which causes the wheezing observed in bronchiolitis. Greater levels of LTC4 have been detected in the nasopharyngeal secretions of children who are undergoing the acute phase of RSV infection, and its concentration is related to the clinical seriousness of the disease, which is more severe when the lower respiratory tract has been affected, in comparison to children who only manifest the disease in the upper respiratory tract. Another clinical study showed that urinary LTE4 (the terminal product of the CysLT metabolism) is considerable higher during bronchiolitis caused by

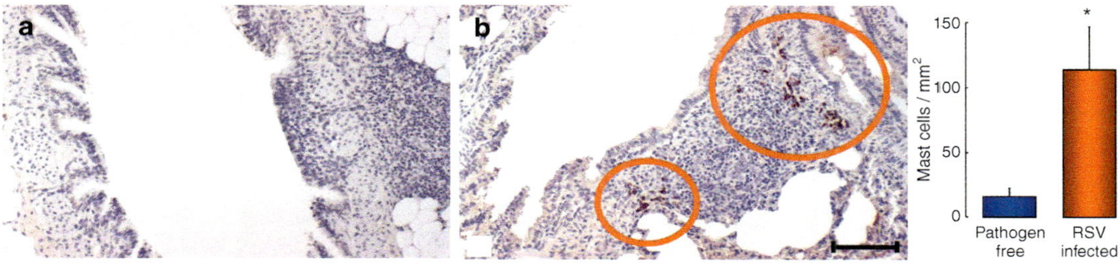

Fig. 30.3 Mastocytes in pulmonary tissue. Lung sections of weanling rats, killed 5 days after being intranasally inoculated with virus-free environment (**a**) or suspension (**b**). Mastocytes have been identified through immunohistochemistry, using a tryptase-specific monoclonal antibody. A sevenfold average increase in mastocyte density was found in the lung sections of rats infected with respiratory syncytial virus (RSV), in comparison to those who were free of the pathogen (*right*). Inner scale = 40 m. $*P < 0.05$ significantly different to the rats who were free of the pathogen

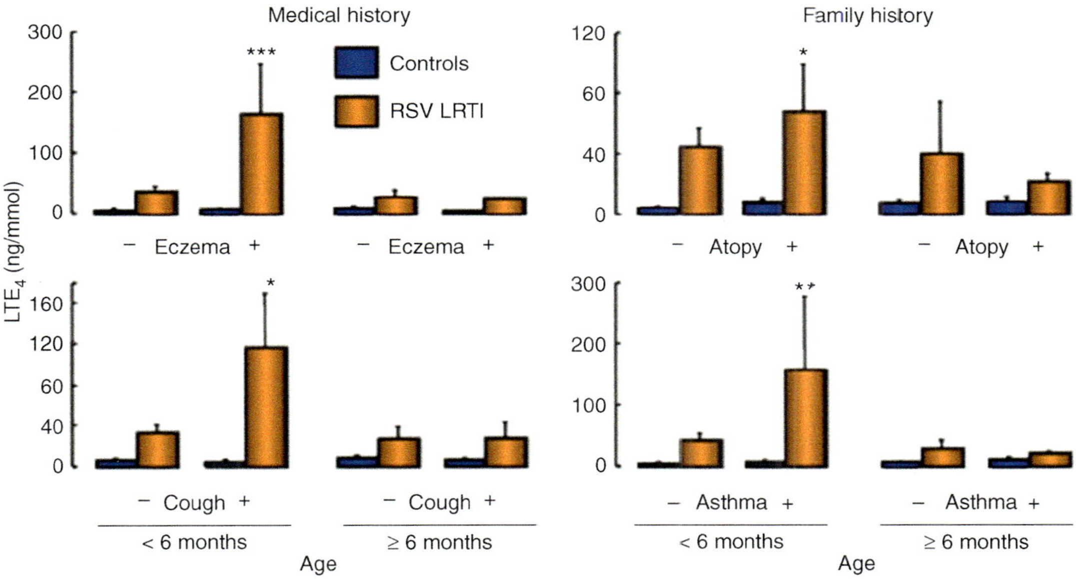

Fig. 30.4 Leukotrienes synthesis. Urinary excretion of LTE4 (terminal product of CysLT metabolism) is increased in children with bronchiolitis caused by RSV when compared to control samples with no respiratory infection. Overproduction of CysLT shown by this marker is accentuated in younger patients (<6 months old) infected with this virus. Further, the effect of the virus seems to be amplified in infants with a higher concentration of LTE4, clinical history of eczema or dry coughing, and/or a familial history of asthma, an intrinsic predisposition to develop atopy, or hyperreactivity of the respiratory tract. Age or atopy alone does not seem to affect leukotriene synthesis when there is no infection. $*P < 0.05$, $**P < 0.01$, $***P < 0.001$ significantly different from the control group of the same age free from respiratory infection

RSV in younger children (<6 months old) who have an atopic/asthmatic background (Fig. 30.4). As is already known, CysLT not only seems to develop a crucial role in asthma physiopathology but could also be an important factor in the link between RSV and asthma.

Analysis of infected pulmonary tissue has shown that the RSV effect in the leukotriene synthesis is temporary. The maximum levels are present during days 3 to 5 after the beginning of the infection and then return to baseline state after 30 days. These findings collectively suggest that the acute inflammatory response of the respiratory airways infected by RSV during the first years of life involves releasing CysLT, as well as the activation of the CysLT receptor. This effect can be observed in the antiinflammatory effect found in animal and human models in relationship to the leukotriene receptor antagonists, such as Montelukast. After the early phase of viral respiratory infection, leukotriene production and release quickly return to basal levels, but they can be reactivated when there are irritants present in the air (such as tobacco smoke), which can once again stimulate the nerve nociceptive fibers connected to the numerous mastocytes, which are still present in the pulmonary tissue.

Clinical Manifestations

The RSV infection in children almost always causes clinical manifestations, although it may vary greatly in its seriousness, depending on the age of the patient, present comorbidities, environmental exposure, and history of previous infections. Infants generally present with symptoms related to the upper respiratory airway, such as congestion and rhinorrhea. These symptoms can progress in 2 to 4 days and involve the lower respiratory tract, accompanied by cough, wheezing, increase of respiratory effort, and cyanosis. During auscultation, diffuse polyphonic wheezing and gross crackles can be heard. Chest X-rays usually show bilateral hyperinflation, irregular atelectasis, and peribronchial enlargement (Fig. 30.5).

Patients undergoing serious involvement of the lower respiratory tract can also show changes on chest X-ray images that are more consistent with pneumonia, presenting areas of interstitial infiltration. The resulting respiratory difficulty may differ greatly in seriousness, ranging from minimum to extensive, and it can even be fatal. Infants tend to be lethargic, lack appetite, and present with otitis media. Elderly patients, as well as patients with cardiorespiratory disease or immunodeficiency, are also at risk to suffer a serious infection of the lower respiratory tract. Older children and healthy adults usually manifest symptoms compromising the upper respiratory airway, but they may as well present with a tracheobronchitis.

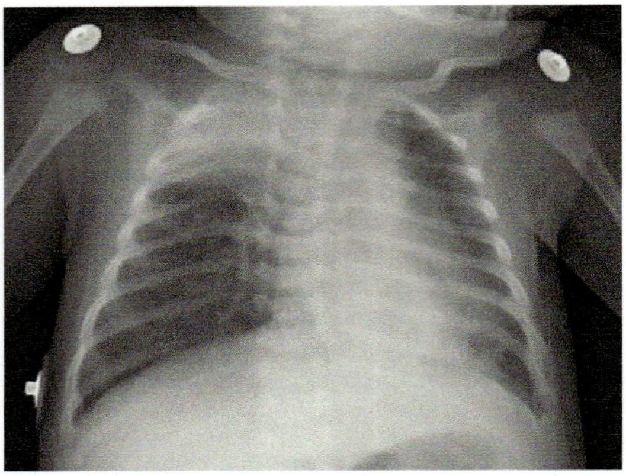

Fig. 30.5 Acute bronchiolitis. Chest X-ray obtained from a child with bronchiolitis caused by RSV shows bilateral hyperinflation, irregular atelectasis, and peribronchial enlargement. Seriously ill patients may also present symptoms consistent with pneumonia, with interstitial infiltration areas

Apnea is a well-known complication of RSV in small infants and can be sufficiently serious to cause death. It affects about 20% of babies younger than 6 months of age who have undergone hospitalization. It is frequently the first clinical manifestation of virus infection, and its presence is not related to the seriousness of the disease or other related symptoms. Because of this, it is believed that the virus may be involved in at least some cases of infant sudden death, which also shares several epidemiological similarities with RSV infection, such as seasonal impact and risk factors.

Some studies suggest that infection by RSV significantly prolongs the duration of central apnea caused by a peripheral sensorineural stimulation reflex. The specific blockage of the central GABA-A receptors or the P (NK1) substance, as well as their high-affinity receptors, suppresses the influence originated by the RSV infection in relation to the apnea caused by sensorineural stimulation. This finding suggests that the P substance, released by the primary sensorineural neurons in the nodose ganglion, activates second-order GABAergic interneurons in the dorsal horn at the medulla. This process inhibits the function of the medullary inspiratory neurons, which causes the apnea.

Treatment

Support Measures Most children infected by RSV have a mild disease, which is self-limited, and may only require symptomatic treatment that consists of a close follow-up, especially related to the progression of respiratory difficulty, oxygen need, and hydration. Children who refuse to be fed, who present with respiratory distress or need of supplemental oxygen, must be admitted into the hospital for closer observation and more aggressive management. Independently of where the patient is being treated, the base of the treatment is always to provide support care: this includes respiratory assistance and an adequate management of liquids and nutrition.

Children whose oxygen saturation levels are 92% or less must receive oxygen through a thermal humidification system. Nasal obstruction is a very frequent problem, and considering that small children are compulsory nasal breathers, this can cause a significant worsening of the respiratory difficulty. Simple nasal cleaning using saline solution drops as well as a suction bulb may improve respiratory function. Chest physiotherapy is usually administered in an effort to mobilize secretions and rescue the lung segments with atelectasis; nevertheless, the evidence shown by a Cochrane systematic review does not recommend its use. Children with supplemental oxygen refractory hypoxemia, with persistent respiratory difficulty, or who present with increasing respiratory insufficiency may require noninvasive support, continuous positive nasal pressure, or endotracheal intubation. Mechanical ventilation with positive pressure has been an important type of treatment for children with bronchiolitis and significantly reduces the mortality rate.

Hospitalized infants reduce their nutrient intake because of respiratory difficulty and the increase of insensible losses, and therefore they may require volume and nutritional support. When there is significant respiratory difficulty in these patients, continuous oral feeding may increase the risk of aspiration. If the patient cannot tolerate oral feeding and enteral nutrition is considered unsafe, a feeding tube, nasogastric or orogastric, must be used to ensure that an adequate amount of fluids and nutrition is being delivered.

Pharmacological Interventions Although many efforts have been made to identify pharmacological therapies that may improve the clinical progression of this infection, the most effective treatment is still limited to the support measures already mentioned.

Bronchodilators Bronchodilators are frequently used in infants with wheezing secondary to lower respiratory tract infections caused by RSV. Nevertheless, their routine use is still controversial, and most randomized controlled assays have failed to find objective evidence of clinical benefit. In a recent Cochrane review comprising 22 studies, which combined in total 1428 infants with bronchiolitis, the efficiency of salbutamol in acute treatment was evaluated. The measured results included improvement in the clinical score, oxygenation, hospital admittance, and the duration of time in the hospital. The authors found that there was a minimally significant improvement in the clinical scores of the children who received a bronchodilator treatment in comparison to those who received a placebo, but this improvement was not clinically relevant. In the same way, there was no statistically significant improvement in oxygenation, hospital admission rate, and length of stay in the hospital. The authors concluded that bronchodilators are not recommended for routine use in infants with bronchiolitis and a first wheezing episode. An attempt to use bronchodilators while monitoring the patient may be justified, but the treatment must be suspended if there is no objective improvement. A Cochrane review that intended to evaluate the efficacy of epinephrine, through the comparison of albuterol and epinephrine versus placebo, including hospitalized and ambulatory patients, concluded that the available information does not support using epinephrine in hospitalized patients. However, its use in ambulatory patients may offer a modest short-term improvement, and therefore it would be preferable to use in comparison to albuterol or nebulized saline solution for bronchiolitis treatment. Anticholinergics have not proven to be effective for treating bronchiolitis caused by RSV.

Systemic Steroids A systematic review of 13 trials including 1198 children under 30 months old with wheezing showed a reduction in the hospital stay of 0.38 days per patient; however, it was not statistically significant. There were no differences in the clinical scores of severity, respiratory frequency, and oxygen saturation. Related to patients treated in the emergency department, there was no difference in the rates of hospital admissions. The authors warn about the significant heterogeneity of the studies included, as well as their results, which makes it difficult to have a final analysis to interpret with confidence. However, the authors concluded that this therapy offers no significant clinical benefit when compared to a placebo, and therefore it is not indicated for this group of patients.

Inhaled Steroids Several studies have evaluated the use of inhaled steroids in patients with bronchiolitis and have showed no significant benefit. Bloom et al. carried out a Cochrane review of five studies, totaling 374 newborns, in whom they evaluated the use of inhaled steroids to prevent post-bronchiolitis wheezing. This analysis showed no reduction in the rates of wheezing or admission when systemic steroids were used, and the same result was seen with the use of bronchodilators.

Combination Therapy Several studies have evaluated the usefulness of the combined administration of steroids and nebulized racemic epinephrine. The results have been very promising. A recent randomized clinical trial compared 61 children randomly assigned to receive nebulized dexamethasone or saline solution. Both groups also received nebulized epinephrine. This study did not show any statistically significant differences in the clinical scores or in oxygen saturation. Nevertheless, there was significant reduction in the length of stay in the hospital for the dexamethasone group, especially in the subgroup of premature newborns. Another study carried out by Plint et al., which was conducted as a large multi-centric study, attempted to evaluate the hospital admittance rates after the administration of treatment with oral dexamethasone and nebulized racemic epinephrine. This study showed that the combination therapy was efficient in the reduction of hospital admittance rates. Some specific patient populations may benefit from a steroid therapy attempt, depending on the personal medical history (eczema, atopy), family history of atopy (parental asthma or atopy), and according to the atopic predisposition.

Antivirals The only licensed antiviral drug that can be used in the therapy of serious infections caused by RSV is ribavirin, a synthetic nucleoside analogue with a broad-spectrum virustatic activity in vitro. The first studies were promising, but a recent review conducted by Ventre, which included 12 studies published between 1983 and 1999, showed only small improvements with no statistical significance related to mortality, length of time for mechanical ventilation, clinical condition, or length of stay in the hospital. Although ribavirin efficiently inhibits RSV replication in vitro, its failure to do so in vivo is not surprising, because the first clinical symptoms begin to appear (acute rhinitis) toward the end of the virus exponential replication in the lungs, and after this, a fast reduction of the virus titers can be observed. For now, when the classical signs of bronchiolitis are diagnosed, few virus remain in the lungs, while the immune response of the host is the predominant trait in the physiopathology. Today, ribavirin is used to treat infections caused by RSV by itself or combined with anti RSV antibodies, but only for some selected immunocompromised hosts.

Antibiotics It is not unusual for children with bronchiolitis to receive antibiotic therapy. It is estimated that antibiotics are used in 34% to 99% of the cases of non-complicated bronchiolitis. This therapy is administered early during the treatment because the patient is febrile, but considering the fever itself, viral infections cannot be accurately differentiated from bacterial ones. As a matter of fact, the risk of bacterial superinfection in febrile infants with bronchiolitis is quite low (0.2%), even when the body temperature is greater than 39 °C. Nevertheless, in the case of intubated infants with acute bronchiolitis, the rate of secondary bacterial infection is much higher, reaching 26%.

When a secondary bacterial infection is diagnosed, the most common affected structures are the urinary tract and the middle ear. In particular, children with secondary infections tend to have infections in the urinary tract, rather than a bacteremia or meningitis (12% versus 0.43%). Acute otitis media can also be seen as a complication of the infection caused by the RSV (57–67%), but its presence does not seem to impact the seriousness of the fever, respiratory difficulty, or the global clinical progression of the disease.

A study that included 24 children with bronchiolitis examined middle-ear aspirations and confirmed the presence of RSV in the middle ear of 17 patients. Bacterial pathogens were also isolated in all the patients who suffered from acute otitis media. The most common were *Streptococcus pneumoniae*, *Haemophilus influenzae*, and *Moraxella catarrhalis*. Otitis media should be treated according to the current recommendations of the American Academy of Pediatrics (AAP).

Antibiotics should be used in patients with bronchiolitis only when there is specific evidence of a coexistent bacterial infection.

Recombinant Human Deoxyribonuclease (rhDNase) Because neutrophils are important for the early immune response against RSV infection and the DNA released from its lysis is often found in the thick secretions present when there is bronchiolitis, it seems reasonable to think that the treatment with rhDNase as a mucolytic should yield some benefit. Nevertheless, a recent multicentric, randomized, placebo-controlled study assessed the efficacy of rhDNase in 225 hospitalized children, who were oxygen dependent, and no actual benefit was found.

Hypertonic Solution Hypertonic saline solution has been previously used to improve mucociliary clearance in patients with asthma and cystic fibrosis, and it has drawn interest as a potential therapy for infants with bronchiolitis. A Cochrane review conducted in 2008 by Zhang et al. discussed four trials totaling 254 infants with acute bronchiolitis (189 hospitalized patients and 65 ambulatory patients) who received nebulized saline solution at 3% versus 0.9%, with or without a bronchodilator. The primary results were related to the length of stay in the hospital for the admitted patients and admittance rates for ambulatory patients. This review concluded that nebulized saline solution may reduce by nearly 1 day (25.9% reduction) the length of stay in the hospital for infants who were already hospitalized in comparison to infants who received placebo. Considering the enormous financial burden that signifies the hospitalization of infants with bronchiolitis, for their parents and also for healthcare systems all over the world, its small cost makes it seem even more attractive.

Surfactant Beyond its function in reducing the superficial tension in alveoli and bronchioles, with subsequent improvement of alveolar permeability and the small airways, surfactant has protein components (A and D) that bond to superficial markers, both viral and bacterial, facilitating the immune-mediated elimination. It has also been proven that surfactant protein D promotes the production of free radicals in alveolar macrophages. In the presence of acute bronchiolitis, the production of these proteins is reduced; these return to their normal levels after disease resolution.

The administration of exogenous surfactant to newborns with severe respiratory failure caused by bronchiolitis seems promising, and the several meta-analyses that have been conducted to assess this therapy have yielded encouraging results. A recent meta-analysis by Ventre et al. included three studies, totaling 79 patients. The authors reported a decrease in the length of mechanical ventilation use and length of stay in the intensive care unit. Besides this, it seems to show some improvement in pulmonary mechanics and gas exchange. It is important to note that available studies are scanty and have small statistical power, so larger additional studies are needed. Nevertheless, the treatment with exogenous surfactant does seem promising for patients who have severe respiratory failure secondary to bronchiolitis.

Heliox Barach described for the first time the use of helium for treating asthma and the obstruction of upper respiratory airways during the 1930s. Heliox is a mixture of helium and oxygen in a proportion of 70:30 or 80:20. Its theoretical advantage lies in the fact that it sustains the laminar flow, and therefore there is less turbulence in the airways, in comparison to air. In patients with a disease of the lower tract airways, this translates into ventilation improvement with reduced work of breathing. Several investigators have studied heliox for the treatment of bronchiolitis. Some of the authors have obtained small improvements in clinical scores, as well as a reduction in both tachypnea and the effort of breathing. The equipment needed to administer heliox is large and cumbersome, which can make its use problematic. Also, as the therapy is more effective when it uses high helium concentrations in relation to oxygen, it would be minimally efficient for patients who have significant oxygen needs. The current evidence for heliox use in the treatment of bronchiolitis is scarce, conflictive, and has small statistical power.

Antileukotriene Drugs As was previously discussed, strong experimental evidence in animal models and several clinical studies indicates that CysLT are released during the infection caused by RSV, which contributes to hyperreactivity and the inflammation of respiratory airways. Therefore, it could be thought that leukotriene antagonists may have a therapeutic use in the configuration of acute bronchiolitis, and they could possibly avoid or reduce the recurrence of wheezing episodes post bronchiolitis. A small pilot study involving hospitalized children with acute bronchiolitis drew great interest and hope, but another recently finished study, which was larger, multi-centric, and double blind, found no significant differences between montelukast and placebo in relationship to the symptom-free days. It would be interesting to compare the effect of the antileukotriene therapy during the infection along with its prophylactic use before the RSV season, as well as its posterior effect on subsequent asthma incidence.

Prevention

In the nonclinical setting, several interventions have proven to be effective in limiting the probability of acquiring an infection caused by RSV. Handwashing is probably the most effective way to prevent its propagation. Specific recommendations for those who take care of high-risk babies are advisable, as well as avoiding the exposure to tobacco smoke and restricting the use of nurseries during the yearly seasonal activity. Besides this, considering the available evidence relative to the transmission of immunoglobulin from mother to child during breastfeeding, it is important to support the recommendation for breastfeeding, especially for high-risk infants.

Immunoprophylaxis To this day, only two products have been developed for clinical use: IGIV-RSV, which is a polyclonal hyperimmune immunoglobulin, and palivizumab, which is a humanized monoclonal antibody. Motivzumab is a second-generation humanized monoclonal antibody that is still not available for commercial use.

Immunoglobulin Against the SRV (IGIV-RSV) IGIV-RSV is a purified polyclonal human immunoglobulin, elaborated from donors with high titers of neutralizing antibodies against RSV. In high-risk infants who are premature or who have a chronic pulmonary disease, a significant reduction in hospitalizations was shown, as well as a reduction in the duration of the hospitalization period. Nevertheless, its use was also related to an increase in surgical morbidity and in the mortality rate of children with congenital heart disease. As IGIV-RSV may interfere with the immune response to vaccines with attenuated live virus, it is necessary to delay the administration of the vaccine against measles, mumps, and rubeola (MMR). The MMR vaccine can be administered 9 months after the last dose of IGIV-RSV vaccine. The main disadvantages of using IGIV-RSV involved the need of a repeated IV access, as well as a long IV infusion period (4–6 h), and therefore it requires medical supervision in the hospital. The administered volume was also quite considerable: The recommended dose was 15 ml/kg, which importantly increases the risk of fluid overcharge in babies, who are naturally sensitive to fluids, and therefore treatment with diuretics was frequently needed. It also had the potential to transfer pathogens through blood flow, and the supply of eligible donors was not trustworthy. Another practical disadvantage was the high combined costs, resulting from the acquisition and supervised administration of this immunoglobulin.

Palivizumab The use of monoclonal antibodies has several advantages. These drugs tend to have no immunosuppressive effect in children, and essentially they have no contagion risk for diseases transmitted by blood or other adverse effects involved in the use of plasma. Besides this, these drugs tend to have greater titers of neutralizing antibodies, and therefore they can be prepared in smaller volumes, which makes them appropriate for intramuscular administration in ambulatory patients, or even at home, which eliminates the risk of fluid overcharge and the subsequent need of diuretic rescue.

Palivizumab is an IgG_1-humanized monoclonal antibody developed using recombining DNA technology. It has been considered as a very successful treatment, which has placed it as one of the pioneers in the worldwide expansion and successful use of biological products. With this technology, specific complementary sequences of the A antigenic site in the F protein of the mouse RSV are inserted within a human frame (Fig. 30.6). The effectiveness of pavilizumab lies in limiting the spread toward the lower respira-

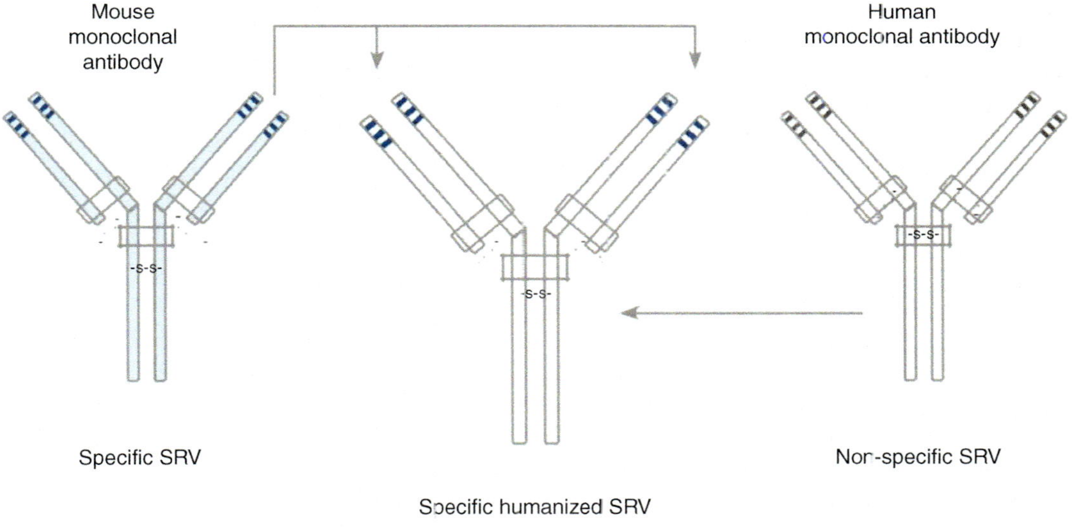

Fig. 30.6 Humanized monoclonal antibodies. This schematic representation shows mouse-originated free sequences for the A antigenic site of F protein corresponding to RSV inserted on a human IgG frame. The result is palivizumab, an antibody that is considered to be human in 95% or more; it is not immunogenic, and has a wide reactive activity to both RSV subtypes. The substitution of 13 amino acid residues in the definition complementarity regions of palivizumab originates motavizumab, a second-generation antibody, which has an affinity 70 times greater relative to the F protein present in RSV

tory tract. The Impact-RSV assay included 1502 preterm infants, who had been born before 35 weeks of gestation and/or who had pulmonary chronic disease. The children were randomized to receive either placebo or palivizumab as monthly doses of 15 mg/kg IM, during the RSV seasonal activity time. The children who received palivizumab showed a reduction of 55% in hospitalization rate, and the hospitalization periods were reduced from 62.6 days per 100 children to 36.4 days. A dramatic reduction in the clinical score used to evaluate the seriousness of the disease was observed. Other reductions observed were related to the use of the intensive care unit and supplemental oxygen. In spite of this, no difference was observed for the use of mechanical ventilation. Another multicenter clinical trial evaluated the effectiveness of prophylaxis using pavalizumab. Included were 1287 children with significant congenital heart disease, for whom a 45% relative reduction rate in hospitalizations was observed in comparison to the placebo group. For acyanotic patients, a 58% reduction in the hospitalization rates was observed, and for cyanotic patients this reduction was 29%. Therefore, combining the data of the aforementioned pivotal studies, we can conclude that pavilizumab is an effective protection for preterm newborns without bronchopulmonary dysplasia. This conclusion also applies for children with significant acyanotic congenital heart disease. The protective effect of pavilizumab in infants with bronchopulmonary dysplasia or cyanotic congenital heart disease is less dramatic (Fig. 30.7).

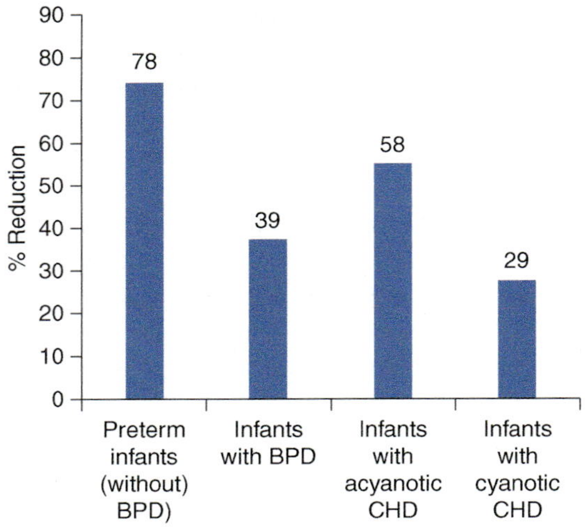

Fig. 30.7 Palivizumab protection effects. Combined data from the fundamental randomized clinical trials show that palivizumab is a good protective agent for newborns without borderline personality disorder (BPD), as well as children with acyanotic congenital heart disease. In contrast, this protection is less dramatic in infants with bronchopulmonary dysplasia or cyanotic congenital heart disease. It is also worth noting that most of the post-commercialization information suggests that the protection granted by palivizumab may be substantially greater than the protection estimated using the randomized clinical trials, but because there is no control information, these data can be difficult to interpret

Palivizumab is usually well tolerated and is administered monthly as a 15 mg/kg intramuscular dose during the RSV active season (Table 30.1). Adverse events most commonly reported are upper respiratory tract infections, otitis media, fever, rhinitis, skin rash, diarrhea, cough, vomiting, gastroenteritis, and wheezing. An acute hypersensitivity may appear, but its incidence is rare, with fewer than 1 anaphylaxis case per 100,000 patients.

A recent study sponsored by the industry proposed the hypothesis that palivizumab, through the improvement or early prevention of bronchiolitis caused by the RSV in preterm newborns, could later reduce recurrent wheezing. A cohort of 191 preterm newborns who received palivizumab and who were not hospitalized because of RSV was compared to 230 preterm newborns who never received palivizumab (76 of those were hospitalized because of RSV and 154 were not hospitalized). The follow-up of these children lasted 24 months, and their average age of the beginning of the follow-up was 19 months. The incidence of recurring wheezing diagnosed by a physician was approximately 50% lower in those subjects treated with pavilizumab when compared to all the subjects who did not receive this treatment, as well as the 154 patients in the subgroup who were not hospitalized because of bronchiolitis caused by the RSV. This finding suggests that using pavilizumab to prevent bronchiolitis caused by RSV may reduce the subsequent recurrent wheezing in preterm babies. This study needs to be repeated and confirmed in

Table 30.1 Prophylaxis recommendations for respiratory syncytial virus (RSV) (Academy of Pediatrics, AAP)

1.	Infants with chronic pulmonary disease under 24 months old who have received medical treatment within the 6 months after the beginning of the RSV season may benefit from a monthly dose beginning the first month of the RSV season, totaling 5 doses.
2.	Infants born before the 28th week of gestation can benefit from monthly doses, starting the first month of the RSV season, totaling 5 doses.
3.	Infants born between the 29th and 32th weeks of gestation, and who are under 6 months old at the beginning of the RSV season, may benefit from a monthly dose beginning the first month of the RSV season, totaling 5 doses
4.	Infants born between the 32th and 35th weeks of gestation, who are under 3 months old at the beginning of the RSV season, and who attend daycare, or have a sibling who is under 5 years old, can benefit from monthly doses until they reach 3 months of age. In this category, the maximum number of doses that may be administered for this category is 3, and in many cases only 1 or 2 doses will be administered.
5.	Infants with respiratory tract congenital anomalies and who are under 1 year old can benefit from a monthly dose beginning the first month of the RSV season, totaling 5 doses.
6.	Infants with neuromuscular disease who are under 1 year old can benefit from a monthly dose beginning the first month of the RSV season, totaling 5 doses.
7.	Infants with hemodynamically significant congenital heart disease and who are under 2 years old can benefit from a monthly dose beginning the first month of the RSV season, totaling 5 doses.
8.	Infants with serious immunodeficiency can benefit from a monthly dose beginning the first month of the RSV season, totaling 5 doses.

larger samples, including term infants in double-blind protocols. Once this is done, a formal and widespread recommendation could be done relative to RSV prophylaxis to independently reduce the incidence of postviral wheezing in infants.

Sources

Bruhn FW, Mokrohisky ST, McIntosh K. Apnea associated with respiratory syncytial virus infection in young infants. J Pediatr. 1977;90:382–6.

Chanock R, Roizman B, Myers R. Recovery from infants with respiratory illness of a virus related to chimpanzee coryza agent (CCA). I. Isolation, properties and characterization. Am J Hyg. 1957;66:281–90.

Gadomski AM, Bhasale AL. Bronchodilators for bronchiolitis. Cochrane Database Syst Rev. 2006;3:CD001266.

Hall CB, McBride JT, Walsh EE, Bell DM, Gala CL, Hildreth S, Ten Eyck LG, Hall WJ. Aerosolized ribavirin treatment of infants with respiratory syncytial viral infection. A randomized double-blind study. N Engl J Med. 1983;308:1443–7.

Hartling L, Wiebe N, Russell K, Patel H, Klassen TP. Epinephrine for bronchiolitis. Cochrane Database Syst Rev. 2004(1):CD003123.

Hu C, Wedde-Beer K, Auais A, Rodriguez MM, Piedimonte G. Nerve growth factor and nerve growth factor receptors in respiratory syncytial virus-infected lungs. Am J Physiol Lung Cell Mol Physiol. 2002;283:L494–502.

IMPACT-SRV. Palivizumab, a humanized respiratory syncytial virus monoclonal antibody, reduces hospitalization from respiratory syncytial virus infection in high-risk infants. The IMpact-SRV Study Group. Pediatrics. 1998;102:531–7.

Johnson S, Oliver C, Prince GA, Hemming VG, Pfarr DS, Wang SC, Dormitzer M, O'Grady J, Koenig S, Tamura JK, Woods R, Bansal G, Couchenour D, Tsao E, Hall WC, Young JF. Development of a humanized monoclonal antibody (MEDI-493) with potent in vitro and in vivo activity against respiratory syncytial virus. J Infect Dis. 1997;176:1215–24.

Kapikian AZ, Mitchell RH, Chanock RM, Shvedoff RA, Stewart CE. An epidemiologic study of altered clinical reactivity to respiratory syncytial (RS) virus infection in children previously vaccinated with an inactivated RS virus vaccine. Am J Epidemiol. 1969;89:405–21.

Legg JP, Hussain IR, Warner JA, Johnston SL, Warner JO. Type 1 and type 2 cytokine imbalance in acute respiratory syncytial virus bronchiolitis. Am J Respir Crit Care Med. 2003;168:633–9.

Piedimonte G. Neural mechanisms of respiratory syncytial virus-induced inflammation and prevention of respiratory syncytial virus sequelae. Am J Respir Crit Care Med. 2001;163:S18–21.

Piedimonte G, Renzetti G, Di Marco A, Auais A, Tripodi S, Colistro F, Villani A, Di Ciommo A, Cutrera R. Leukotriene synthesis during respiratory syncytial vi-rus bronchiolitis: influence of age and atopy. Pediatr Pulmonol. 2005;40:285–91.

Sabogal C, Auais A, Napchan G, Saguihara C, Bancalari E, Piedimonte G. Effect of respiratory syncytial virus on apnea in weanling rats. Pediatr Res. 2005;57:819–25.

Shay DK, Holman RC, Newman RD, Liu LL, Stout JW, Anderson LJ. Bronchiolitis-associated hospitalizations among US children, 1980–1996. JAMA. 1999;282:1440–6.

Sigurs N, Bjarnason R, Sigurbergsson F, Kjellman B. Respiratory syncytial virus bronchiolitis in infancy is an important risk factor for asthma and allergy at age 7. Am J Respir Crit Care Med. 2000;161:1501–7.

Simões EA, Carbonell-Estrany X, Rieger CH, Mitchell I, Fredrick L, Groothuis JR. The effect of respiratory syncytial virus on subsequent recurrent wheezing in atopic and nonatopic children. J Allergy Clin Immunol. 2010;126:256–62.

Tortorolo L, Langer A, Polidori G, Vento G, Stampachiacchere B, Aloe L, Piedimonte G. Neurotrophins overexpression in lower airways of infants with respiratory syncytial virus infection. Am J Respir Crit Care Med. 2005;172:233–7.

Ventre K, Randolph A. Ribavirin for respiratory syncytial virus infection of the lower respiratory tract in infants and young children. Cochrane Database Syst Rev. 2007(1):CD000181.

Walsh EE, Falsey AR, Hennessey PA. Respiratory syncytial and other virus infections in persons with chronic cardiopulmonary disease. Am J Respir Crit Care Med. 1999;160:791–5.

Welliver TP, Garofalo RP, Hosakote Y, Hintz KH, Avendano L, Sanchez K, Velozo L, Jafri H, Chavez-Bueno S, Ogra PL, McKinney L, Reed JL, Welliver RC Sr. Severe human lower respiratory tract illness caused by respiratory syncytial virus and influenza virus is characterized by the absence of pulmonary cytotoxic lymphocyte responses. J Infect Dis. 2007;195:1126–36.

Zhang L, Mendoza-Sassi RA, Wainwright C, Klassen TP. Nebulized hypertonic saline solution for acute bronchiolitis in infants. Cochrane Database Syst Rev. 2008(4):CD006458.

Community-Acquired Pneumonia

31

María Lina Boza Costagliola

Contents

Definition

Community-acquired pneumonia (CAP) is an infection of the distal part of the breathing airway and the pulmonary parenchyma in the extra-hospital environment.

M. L. Boza Costagliola (✉)
Pediatrics, Respiratory diseases, University of Chile, Santiago, Chile

Epidemiology

In spite of the development of new antibiotics and vaccines, community-acquired pneumonia is still a frequently occurring disease, which usually presents in children under 5 years of age. It is one of the main causes of mortality annually worldwide, especially in developing countries: 2 million deaths, of which 20% correspond to children. In Chile, it is the main cause of pediatric hospital-

P. Bertrand, I. Sánchez (eds.), *Pediatric Respiratory Diseases*,
https://doi.org/10.1007/978-3-030-26961-6_31

ization during winter and spring, corresponding to 52% of hospital admissions to the hospital in the first 2 years of life. It is the first cause of late infant mortality, with a 0.18/1000 ratio in children under 1 year old (2010), although it has experimented a dramatic decrease since 1990, when the mortality rate of community-acquired pneumonia was 60% (see Minsal 2013). Currently, the infection caused by the human immunodeficiency virus (HIV) has increased the number of deaths caused by pneumonia (with a risk six times higher in comparison to those not infected), particularly in underdeveloped countries.

Etiology

The biggest challenge in pneumonia is to determine the causative agent. The identification depends on such factors as age, disease severity, immunological condition, geographic location, year season, epidemiological situation, and immunizations. Therefore, identification of the causative agent varies between 10% and 85%, depending on the method used.

Etiology differs according to the patient's age. In newborns, group B *Streptococcus* and gram-negative bacteria are the most common agents; in infants, the most common agent is usually a virus, corresponding to 50% to 60% in Chile, for example, whereas in developed countries this percentage increases to 80%. Among the viral agents, respiratory syncytial virus (RSV) is the most frequent agent, and adenovirus causes the most serious disease (B7h serotype). Among common etiological agents, we can mention influenza, parainfluenza, and metapneumovirus: human metapneumovirus (hMPV) causes about 7% to 20% of lower respiratory infections in this age group. In past years, rhinovirus and coronavirus have also been described as causing community-acquired pneumonia.

Bacterial etiology increases with age: as many as 50% of hospitalized children are older than 5 years. *Streptococcus pneumoniae* causes the most common bacterial infection at any age, about 20–30%. It is predominant during winter and spring times. Other bacteria include *Haemophilus influenzae*, which is a rare causative agent because of mandatory vaccination, although nontypified serotypes can cause serious presentations: *Staphylococcus aureus*, which has a quick and serious progression, but currently is exceptional; and *Streptococcus pyogenes*, which has a variable clinical course, but may cause serious disease with shock and pulmonary suppuration.

Other less frequent agents include *Chlamydia trachomatis*, which is an infection acquired through the birth canal, with a clinical onset between 2 to 12 weeks of life. It does not include fever, but it does involve tachypnea, rhinitis, conjunctivitis, and coughing fits. A hemogram shows eosinophilia, and the chest X-ray is unspecific, but shows interstitial pattern predominance. *Bordetella pertussis* causes a whooping cough clinical syndrome and mainly interstitial pulmonary compromise. Atypical agents such as *Mycoplasma pneumoniae* and *Chlamydia pneumoniae* are common causes agents in children between the ages of 5 and 10 years, respectively (Table 31.1).

Coinfection with different pathogens is possible. The most frequent combinations are RSV or influenza virus with *Streptococcus pneumoniae*, in 30% of the cases, and *Mycoplasma pneumoniae* with *Streptococcus pneumoniae* or *Chlamydia pneumoniae* in 15% of cases (Table 31.2).

Table 31.1 Etiological orientation for pneumonia

Etiology	Bacterial	Viral	Mycoplasma
Age	Any	<2 years	5–15 years
Season	All year	Winter	All year
Presentation	Sudden	Variable	Insidious
Fever	High	Variable	Low
Tachypnea	Common	Common	Infrequent
Coughing	+	++	+++
Related symptoms	Chest pain	Acute rhinitis, conjunctivitis	Pharyngitis

Table 31.2 Etiological agents according to age

	RN	1–3 months	4–24 months	Preschool	School
Virus					
RSV	+	+++	++++	++	–
ADV	–	+	++	+	–
Influenza	–	–	+	++	+++
Parainfluenza	–	+	+	+	–
Metapneumovirus	–	+	+	+	–
Bacteria					
Streptococcus pneumoniae	+	+	++	++++	++++
Mycoplasma pneumoniae	–	–	+	++	++++
Haemophilus influenzae	–	+	+	–	–
Staphylococcus aureus	+	+	+	+	+
Streptococcus agalactiae	+++	+	–	–	–
Escherichia coli and other gram-negative bacilli	++	+	–	–	–
Chlamydia trachomatis	–	–	–	+	+
Chlamydia pneumoniae	–	–	+	+	++
Streptococcus pyogenes	–	–	–	+	+

Physiopathology

The following factors protect the respiratory system from infections:

1. *Mechanics*: nasal filter of inhaled air, gag reflex, cough reflex, and mucociliary clearance
2. *Immunological*, involving: alveolar macrophages, immunoglobulins, local inflammatory response, complement, cytokines, antiproteases, lysozyme, fibronectins
3. *Immune cellular response*.

Under normal circumstances, mucociliary clearance removes efficiently inhaled agents; however, if the inoculum is big, the agent is especially aggressive, or the defense mechanisms are altered, the pulmonary parenchyma will develop an infection. The inhalation of infectious agents (virus or bacteria), or the aspiration of germs through the mouth and upper airway (bacteria), is common. Contiguous hematogenous spread or endogenous reactivation, as in tuberculosis, is rare.

Bacteria cause alveolar damage accompanied by inflammatory exudate, edema, fibrin, and afterward, invasion of polymorphonuclear leukocytes. General resolution is complete almost always, with no functional compromise. Virus cause epithelial damage which may progress to necrosis and diffuse alveolar damage in varying degrees. There is evidence suggesting that the virus could be a factor for the increase of bacterial infections, because it may take advantage of the alterations of the mechanical or immunological barrier of the host.

Clinical Manifestations

The clinical picture fluctuates in seriousness and depends on age, etiological agent, and extension. The classic triad is fever, cough, and respiratory distress Nevertheless, cough may appear later, because there are a few receptors in the lower airways that are only irritated when cellular lysis and inflammatory exudate appear.

In the newborn, when there is a history of premature membrane rupture related to respiratory distress during the first hours of life, along with cardiovascular collapse, group B *Streptococcus* must be suspected. Infants under 3 months old frequently present with tachypnea, usually above 60 breaths per minute, along with a retraction of the soft chest structures. This is frequently associated to unspecific symptoms such as hypothermia, hyperthermia, fatigue food intolerance, somnolence, diarrhea, or apnea. High fever must alert the clinician to rule out septic shock secondary to a respiratory infection.

In older infants, there is usually a history of upper airway symptoms with coughing and rhinorrhea. Soon after, fever, tachypnea (>50/min), general status deterioration, and grunting and nasal flaring appear. High fever, especially in those under 2 years old, can be related to the seriousness of the disease, although it is not a sign that can be used to determine a specific etiology. Preschool and school-age children present with high fever, accompanied by shivers, coughing, and chest pain (pain resembling a side stitch). Abdominal pain may be present when there is compromise of the inferior lobules, and often acute appendicitis must be ruled out, particularly in school-age children. Pain in the shoulder area suggests pleural compromise. Dry or productive cough, rhinorrhea, general discomfort, headache, myalgia, and abdominal pain are nonspecific signs that may or may not accompany bacterial and viral infections. Physical examination results vary and fluctuate depending on the age of the patient. Tachypnea is a very sensitive sign in patients under 5 years old. Younger infants and newborns present with reduced breath sounds but only a few crackles. Condensation syndrome—bronchophony, dullness when percussing, bronchial murmur, and fine crackles—is frequently present in children over 2 years of age. Crackles have a sensitivity of 75% and specificity less than 60%. Wheezing may be present in infants with viral pneumonia or, in children over 5 years old with atypical pneumonia agents such as *Mycoplasma pneumoniae*. A normal respiratory examination does not rule out pneumonia, especially during the first 48 h, named the "silent period."

Diagnostic Approach

Diagnosis suspicion is mainly clinical.

Chest X-ray

No routine chest X-rays are needed for the diagnosis in the ambulatory setting, and administration of treatment must not be delayed. However, the chest X-ray is considered the gold standard to confirm the diagnosis of community-acquired pneumonia, except when acquired very early (24 h) in the clinical progression when sensibility is low.

Chest X-rays do not differentiate among bacterial, viral, or atypical agents, but a lobar condensation pattern suggests bacterial infection and an interstitial pattern suggests viral or atypical agent infection (Figs. 31.1 and 31.2). Chest X-rays are best when used to rule out pneumonial complications such as empyema or abscess. When the clinical picture shows a persistent fever after starting antibiotic treatment and/or dullness

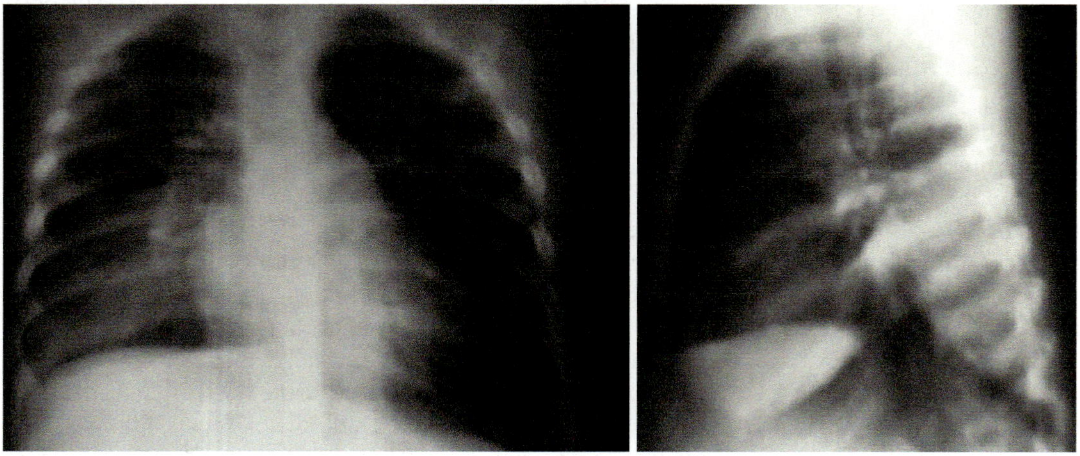

Fig. 31.1 Consolidated pneumonia

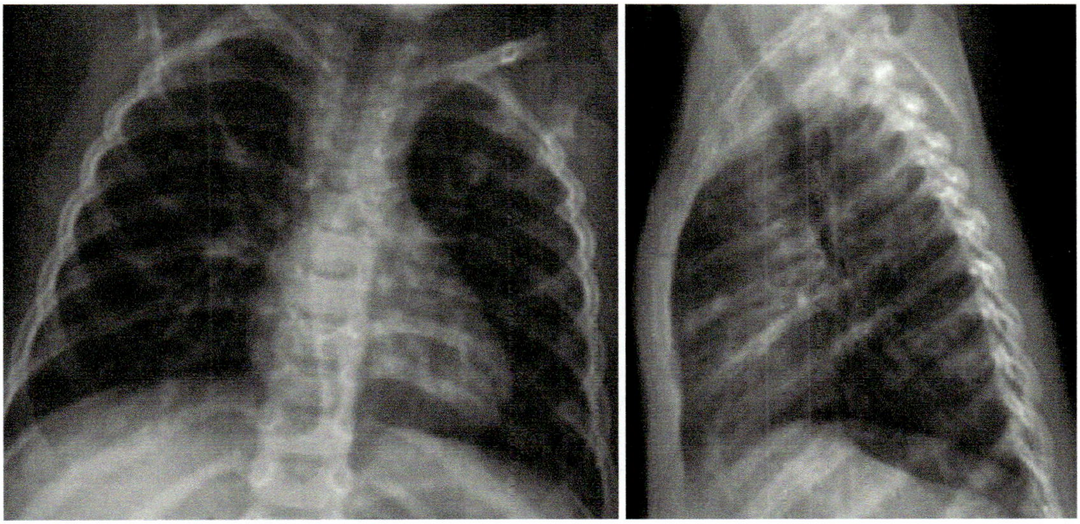

Fig. 31.2 Interstitial pneumonia

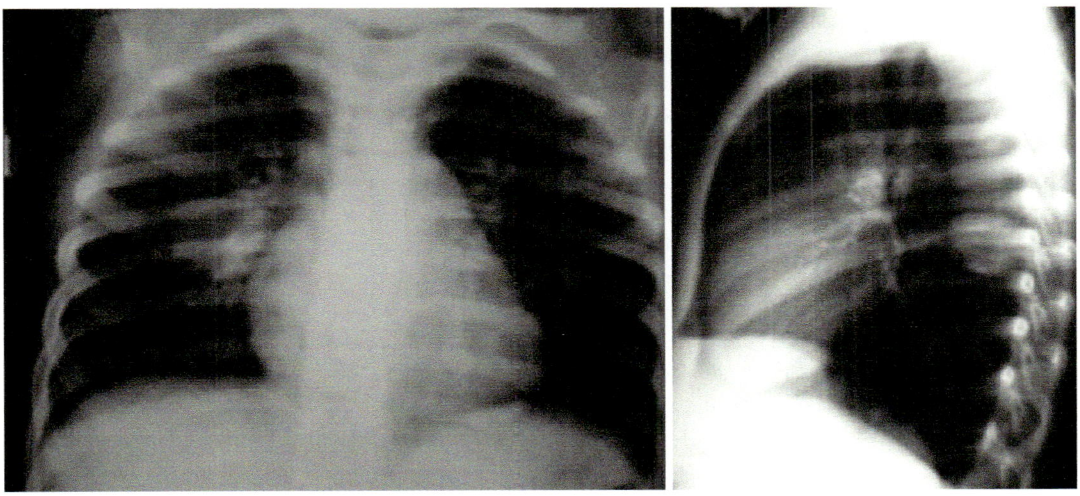

Fig. 31.3 Rounded pneumonia

when percussing the chest, which can be presented as an acute respiratory difficulty syndrome, accompanied by hypoxemia, and/or hemodynamic instability, a chest X-ray is mandatory. This test also must be considered in patients with no response to treatment, lobar atelectasis, round-shaped consolidation, persistent symptoms, and complicated pneumonia.

A chest X-ray follow-up at 4 weeks must be done in cases of recurrent pneumonia, lobar atelectasis, suspicion of malformation, or slow-resolution pneumonia (Fig. 31.3). Chest echography is useful when there is a suspicion of effusion to evaluate the amount and presence of septa or recollection areas.

Basic Laboratory Analysis

White cell blood count, neutrophil count, C-reactive protein, sedimentation rate, and procalcitonin are not useful to identify the etiology. Several prospective studies have proven that acute-phase reactants have a low sensitivity and specificity when it comes to distinguishing between a viral or bacterial infection.

Microbiology

Microbiological identification does not have any clinical impact for most children with community-acquired pneumonia. Nevertheless, for patients undergoing the most serious course and/or hospitalized, etiological investigation is important. When facing the possibility of a viral etiology, direct immunofluorescence (DIF) or ELISA tests are useful, although it must be considered that for adenovirus the sensitivity is not greater than 50% in most cases. DIF on incubated cells (shell-vial technique) yields better results. It is advisable to request this technique in cases having negative results with a high clinical suspicion. Currently, the amplification of specific viral genome fragments has a high sensitivity and specificity. It uses minimum quantities of DNA, with the simultaneous detection of multiple virus; it is easy to standardize, with quick results (8 h), and therefore it is very useful in hospitalized patients. When facing the possibility of a bacterial infection, hematic cultures have a low positive rate, so they are considered only for patients who show poor clinical response. In infants, hematic culture yields poorly (around 2%) but it is similar in older children (about 10%). In patients with pleural effusion, direct pleural space, Gram stain, and culture are less than 30% positive. Nevertheless, cytochemical analysis can help to precisely locate an empyema. In older children, Gram stain and expectoration culture may be useful when there are agents that differ from those that usually colonize the upper airway, particularly when its intracellular location corresponds to macrophages or polymorphonuclear leukocytes. To validate the sample, it is necessary to have at least 25 white blood cells and fewer than 25 epithelial cells per field. Serum antigen detection for *Streptococcus pneumoniae* and *Haemophilus influenzae* in blood, urine, or pleural effusion liquid has a low specificity and sensitivity, yielding false-positives in nasopharyngeal colonization or in patients who have recently received immunization, and therefore they are not recommended. The combination of urine antigen with acute-phase reactants may be a good predictor for bacterial pneumonia. The effectiveness of the immune complex for *Streptococcus pneumoniae* has shown better specificity and sensitivity to diagnose *Mycoplasma pneumoniae*, and for *Chlamydia pneumoniae* serum tests such as IgM are used. They have the limitation of allowing the diagnosis only after the first week, and therefore they are not useful for early diagnosis.

Protein chain reaction (PCR) technique has a 73% sensitivity and a specificity of 94%, so the diagnosis can be done early and rapidly within the progression of the disease. Invasive methods such as bronchoalveolar lavage (BAL) may have better results, but their indication for community-acquired pneumonia is restricted to patients with a complicated course, generally with a poor response to empirical treatments, and when serological or fast microbiological methods (PCR, ELISA, DIF) have failed to yield a diagnosis. These observations are especially true for immunocompromised patients presenting with feverish neutropenia, lymphopenia, AIDS, or bone marrow or another organ transplant. When treating these patients, especially those in whom *Pneumocystis jirovecii* is suspected, it is suggested to obtain an induced sputum sample, which can be a noninvasive method that may be effective and secure in relationship to bronchoalveolar lavage.

Differential Diagnosis

It is difficult to make an etiological differential diagnosis in pneumonia. For some recurrent events, other diseases may explain its origin (Table 31.3).

Table 31.3 Pneumonia differential diagnosis

Recurrent pneumonia: same location	Foreign body aspiration
	Pulmonary malformation
Recurrent pneumonia: different location	Cystic fibrosis
	Chronic aspiration Immunosuppression
Noninfectious pneumonia	Gastric content aspiration
	Hydrocarbon aspiration
	Lipid aspiration
Pneumonia in immunodeficient patients	Noncommon agents

Treatment

Outpatient

General Measures

Most patients will respond to outpatient treatment. For infants, medical monitoring is recommended at 24 h, and for preschoolers this can be up to 48 h. Monitoring must be foreseen for worsening of the condition caused by food rejection, medication intolerance, increase in respiratory difficulty, irritability (persistent crying), or compromised consciousness. The use of antipyretics and analgesics is indicated to keep the child in better condition and to reduce the metabolic and oxygen requirements. The physician must insist that the caregivers look for medical advice in case of symptom worsening, axillar fever greater than 38.5°C for longer than 3 days, respiratory difficulty (tachypnea, cyanosis, rib retraction), food rejection, or notable weakness.

Kinetic Therapy

Kinesiotherapy is not indicated for pneumonia management. It does not accelerate the recovery process and may delay symptom progression. Cough assistance techniques, postural drainage, diaphragmatic reeducation, and early mobilization may help to expand poorly ventilated areas and improve symptoms of respiratory distress to achieve these objectives.

Antibiotics

Antibiotic treatment is empirical, and given the difficulty in isolating the etiological agent, it should be based on the best possible etiology, depending on the patient's age and the epidemiological timing. In children under 5 years old, antibiotics should not be routinely indicated, because in most cases the disease will be caused by a virus. If bacterial etiology is suspected, amoxicillin should be prescribed at 80–100 mg/kg/day, fractioned every 12 h during 5 to 7 days (using a maximum of 2 g/day). In children who are over 5 years old, amoxicillin can be prescribed at 50–80 mg/kg/day. If there is poor oral tolerance, sodium penicillin should be used as follows: 200,000 U/kg/day IV every 12 h (maximum of 4 million U/day) until tolerance is recovered, and continue with oral amoxicillin. The use of macrolides is considered for older children who are suspected of having *Mycoplasma pneumoniae,* or *Chlamydia pneumoniae*, or penicillin allergy: azitromicin 10 mg/kg/day on a daily dosage, without food, for 5 days (maximum 500 mg/day); claritromicin 15 mg/kg/day every 12 h for 10 days (maximum 1 g/day); or erythromycin 50 mg/kg/day divided into four doses, for 10 days (maximum 2 g/day). As an alternative to macrolides use, quinolones can be indicated: daily levofloxacin in 10 mg/kg doses for 10 days. In epidemic episodes, influenza A virus must be ruled out, and early treatment with antivirals (oseltamivir) must be started.

In Hospital

Hospitalization Criteria

- No clinical response to outpatient therapy
- Vomiting and dehydration, which may make oral treatment difficult
- Total or partial respiratory insufficiency: transcutaneous saturation <93%
- Under 3 months of age, because of apnea and risk of cardiorespiratory arrest
- Relevant comorbidity: cardiac, pulmonary, neuromuscular, immunological
- Complicated pneumonia: effusion, excavated lesions
- Serious disease: Hemodynamic instability, alteration of consciousness, seizures, toxic presentation

General Measures

Oxygen for patients whose saturation is less than 93 mmHg in environment air.

Avoid prolonged fasting, especially in infants who are under 1 year old. Because of this, it is recommended to administer fractionated feeding, feeding in small volumes, or through a small nasogastric tube, to avoid worsening the respiratory difficulty.

Antibiotics

Newborns and infants who are under 6 weeks old: ampicillin 100 mg/kg/day every 8 h, IV, plus amikacin 15 mg/kg each 24 h, IV, during 7–10 days to ensure a good coverage for enteric gram-negative bacteria: group B *Streptococcus*, type D *Enterococcus*, and *Listeria monocytogenes*. After the first week of life, as an alternative to amikacin, cefotaxime can be indicated (150 mg/kg/day), given a lower risk of *Listeria monocytogenes*, which may require adding ampicillin to the synergic effect of an aminoglycoside. In patients with progressive worsening, or for whom a resistant *Streptococcus pneumoniae* is suspected, high doses of amoxicillin, of third- or second-generation cephalosporins, or IV ampicillin, should be used. Ampicillin, which is a derivative from penicillin, is a very good choice for patients who are under 24 months of age, and it has a similar efficiency to oral amoxicillin or parenteral cephalosporins, with a significantly lesser cost. The association of macrolides with a beta lactam antibiotic is indicated in hospitalized children when there is a strong suspicion of atypical agents. In the infections caused by *Staphylococcus aureus*, depending on the sensitivity, cloxacillin, clindamycin, or vancomycin is indicated.

Antibiotic Resistance of *Streptococcus*

The appearance of resistant *Streptococcus* is a worldwide concern, and its degree of resistance degree is variable, depending on geographic distribution. The risk of having an invasive disease caused by a resistant *Streptococcus pneumoniae* is related to being 5 years old or younger (specially under 2 years old), use of antibiotics within the precedent month, middle-ear infection, and daycare attendance. Resistance is caused by mutations of penicillin protein-binding (PPB) sites, with a reduction in the protein affinity that binds to the antibiotic. This genetic change is caused by the DNA acquisition from resistant species such as *Streptococcus viridans*. The reduction of the affinity could be countered by increasing the penicillin dosage or with the use of third-generation cephalosporins. Observations made in patients with community-acquired pneumonia caused by resistant *Streptococcus pneumoniae* who still have a good response to treatment have increased the chosen cutoff points to determine penicillin and cefotaxime resistance (CIM > 8 ug/ml).

Complications

Whenever a patient persists with fever after 48–72 h, the presence of some complication such as effusion, pleural empyema, abscess, pneumatocele, bacterial resistance, or choice of an inadequate antibiotic must be suspected. The presence of some extrapulmonary focus (pericardium, joints, meninges) must be ruled out. Pleural effusion or empyema is a possible complication in up to 40% of hospitalized children.

Prevention

The use of vaccines for *Bordetella pertussis*, measles, *Haemophilus influenzae*, and influenza have reduced the occurrence of community-acquired pneumonia. Important effects have been registered in relation to its prevention and suppurative complications after the incorporation of vaccines for type B *Haemophilus influenzae*. The national rate of invasive disease reported for 2003 was of 2.5/100,000 inhabitants, and the effectivity prevention for the bacterial community-acquired pneumonia and empyema was 80%. It must be considered that 6% to 16% of infections caused by *Haemophilus influenzae* are caused by noncapsulated agents against which the vaccine offers no protection. Influenza vaccine has a double effect: it reduces virus infection rate in high-risk populations, and, as a parallel effect, it decreases bacterial community-acquired pneumonia caused by *Streptococcus pneumoniae* and *Staphylococcus aureus*, related to post-influenza virus infection. In Chile, when mandatory vaccination was introduced in 2000 for risk groups, pneumonia incidence was clearly reduced. For those children under 2 years old, 10- and 13-valent pneumococcal conjugate vaccines are less effective for preventing pneumonia (30%) than other invasive diseases such as sepsis and meningitis (97%). Both vaccines have a good immunogenicity and herd immunity. The 13-valent vaccine includes 1, 3, 4, 5, 6A, 6B, 7F, 9 V, 14, 18C, 19A, 19F, and 23F serotypes. Premature newborns, with chronic lung damage and other risk factors, must receive monoclonal antibody prophylaxis for syncytial respiratory virus.

Conclusion

Community-acquired pneumonia is still a prevalent disease in children. The etiological diagnosis cannot be done by X-ray studies, hemograms, or acute-phase reactants, so the development of materials for rapid diagnosis is an unmet need required to avoid the indiscriminant use of antibiotics, which is an important factor in the appearance of bacterial resistance. Penicillin derivatives, especially oral amoxicillin, continue to be the treatment of choice when *Streptococcus pneumoniae* is suspected; macrolides are used when a pneumonia caused by atypical agents is suspected, especially in schoolchildren more than 5 years old. Coverage with effective vaccines is important, according to the regional needs, which may contribute to the prevention of the disease. National programs, when systematically applied to have primary care coverage, have contributed to the significant decrease of morbidity and mortality.

Sources

Bradley JS, Byington CL, Shah SS, Alverson B, Carter ER, Harrison C, Kaplan SI, Mace SE, MacCracken GH Jr, St Peter SD, Stockwell JA, Swanson JT. Executive summary: the management of community-acquired pneumonia in infants and children older than 3 months of age: clinical practice guidelines by the Pediatric Infectious Diseases Society and the Infectious Diseases Society of America. Clin Infect Dis. 2011;53(7):617–30.

Coria de la HP. Recomendaciones para el manejo en niños de las neumonías adquiridas en la comunidad. Rev Chil Infect. 2004;21(S1):S7–S12.

Galetto-Lacour A, Alcoba G, Posfay-Barbe KM, Cevey-Macherel M, Gehri M, Ochs MM, Brookes RH, Siegrist CA, Gervaix A. Elevated inflammatory markers combined with positive pneumococcal urinary antigen are a good predictor of pneumococcal community-acquired pneumonia in children. Pediatr Infect Dis J. 2013;32(11):1175–9.

Harris M, Clark J, Coote N, Fletcher P, Harmen A, McKean M, Thompson J. British Thoracic Society guidelines for the management of community-acquired pneumonia in children. Thorax. 2011;66:1–23.

Heffelfinger J, Dowell S, Jorgensen J, Klugman K, Mabry L, Musher D, et al. Management of community-acquired pneumonia in the era of pneumococcal resistance: a report from the drug-resistant *Streptococcus pneumoniae* therapeutic Working Group. Arch Intern Med. 2000;160:1399–408.

Kronman MP, Hersh AL, Feng R, Huang YS, Lee GE. Ambulatory visit rates and antibiotic prescribing for children with pneumonia, 1994–2007. Pediatrics. 2011;127:411.

Lee GE, Lorch SA, Sheffler-Collins S, Kronman MP, Shah SS. National hospitalization trends for pediatric pneumonia and associated complications. Pediatrics. 2010;126(2):204–13.

Lynch JP III, Zhanel G. *Streptococcus pneumoniae*: epidemiology and risk factors, evolution of antimicrobial resistance, and impact of vaccines. Curr Opin Pulmon Med. 2010;16:217–25.

Minsal. Guía Clínica Auge Infecciones respiratorias agudas en menores de 5 años. 2013. https://www.minsal.cl/portal/url/item/7220fdc4341244a9e04001011f0113b9.pdf.

Plosker GL. 13-Valent pneumococcal conjugate vaccine: a review of its use in infants, children, and adolescents. Paediatr Drugs. 2013;15(5):403–23.

Swingler GH, Zwarenstein M. Chest radiograph in acute respiratory infections in children. Cochrane Database Syst Rev. 2000;2:CD001268.

Williams JV, Harris PA, Tollefson SJ. Human metapneumovirus and lower respiratory tract disease in otherwise healthy infants and children. N Engl J Med. 2004;350:443–50.

Atypical Pneumonia

32

Ricardo Kogan Alterman
and Julio Maggiolo Massone

Contents

Definition

Atypical pneumonia is known as a pneumonia that differs in the clinical picture and chest reticulonodular images from the usual presentation of classic bacteria or virus infections. Cough appears as the main characteristic symptom, and there is a dissociation between the severity of the

R. Kogan Alterman (✉)
Department of Pediatrics, Faculty of Medicine, Universidad de Chile, Santiago, Chile
e-mail: ricardokogan@med.uchile.cl

J. Maggiolo Massone
Department of Pediatrics, Hospital Exequiel González Cortés, San Miguel, Chile

P. Bertrand, I. Sánchez (eds.), *Pediatric Respiratory Diseases*,
https://doi.org/10.1007/978-3-030-26961-6_32

symptoms and the findings of the respiratory physical examination, which tend to be inconstant and slow or late on onset. The main etiological agents that cause atypical pneumonia in the pediatric population are *Mycoplasma pneumoniae* and *Chlamydophila pneumoniae*. Sometimes this terminology is used for *Legionella pneumophila* and *Chlamydia psittaci*, which are very infrequent in pediatrics. These pathogens are not considered in this chapter, because in our opinion they deviate from the characteristic atypical profile.

Pneumonia Caused by *Mycoplasma pneumoniae*

Microbiology

Thirteen species of *Mycoplasma pneumoniae* (*MP*) can infect humans; however, only 4 have been identified as pathogens. It is the smallest known bacterium in relation to cellular dimensions: 1–2 nm in length and 0.1–0.2 nm wide, as in the size of the genome. The bacteria have an autonomous life; they are prokaryotes with no cell wall, pleomorphic, and surrounded by a triple cellular membrane containing sterols, which determines their antigenicity and allows their adherence to the respiratory epithelium. They grow in environments where there are no cells, contain DNA and RNA, and require a great amount of nutrients for their growth. *Mycoplasma* are facultative anaerobes and their way of life is strictly parasitic. They are demanding and grow slowly; they develop well in anaerobic environments and ferment glucose. When placed on agar, they create colonies with a dense central zone and a peripheral region with lower density in the shape of blackberries.

Mycoplasmas produce enzymes such as nucleases and proteases, and they find nutrients in eukaryotic cells, using their ability to lyse red blood cells through the production of hydrogen peroxide.

Mycoplasmas are short bacilli, rod shaped, with an organelle on one end. The main protein, called adhesin (P1), is responsible for its attachment to the membrane cells of the respiratory epithelium. *Mycoplasma pneumoniae* reproduces through binary fission, which takes 6 h to accomplish, and therefore its culture process is slow (5–20 days). Because it lacks a cell wall, these pathogens are not affected by beta-lactam antibiotics and cannot be visualized by Gram stain.

MP has a great affinity with the respiratory epithelium: it adheres to the ciliary cells, causes tissue destruction, and produces cytotoxic products, such as hydrogen peroxide and superoxide anion. Ciliary paralysis explains the irritating cough that accompanies the disease during days or weeks. Other biological properties that determine its virulence are the competition for nutrition consumption, antigenic variation which avoids the host defenses, and the secretion of enzymes such as phospholipases, ATPases, hemolysin, proteases, and nucleases, which cause localized tissue alteration and intracellular hosting. This effect creates chronic latent states, and the immune mechanisms are avoided through its identification in cerebrospinal fluid and serum, which supports its dissemination.

MP has been considered an extracellular organism, although its genomic structure suggests that it is the product of a genetic reduction process, which is characteristic of intracellular bacteria, inducing oxidative stress, damage to the host membrane, and nutrients obtained from the inside of the cell. This mechanism would be an adaptive process, which would explain the observation of *MP* in respiratory secretions for a prolonged period of time, even after successful therapy, and this contributes to the presence of the pathogen agent in nonrespiratory tissues.

Pathogenesis

MP enters the body through a canicular line, descendant, and bronchogenic. After this, it binds to the cells of the respiratory tract through adhesin P1, which allows it to bind to the cells of the host, with other adherence proteins also. Thus, the pathogen can colonize mucous membranes and their cell surface. This cytoadherence is the first step in the pathogen virulent process, which is accompanied by ciliostasis and exfoliation of the infected cells. Cytotoxicity is caused by hydrogen peroxide, which causes oxidative stress. After opsonization of the *MP*, whether it is by complement or by antibodies, macrophagic activation takes place as well as proinflammatory cytokine releases that infiltrate the lung with a mononuclear response, CD4, T and B cells, plasma cells with lymphocyte proliferation, antibody production, and tumor necrosis factor-alpha (TNF-α) release, as well as interferon, interleukin (IL)-1, IL-5, and IL-6, and chemokine IL-8 (which is a powerful neutrophil activator). These immunological processes may stop the disease, reinforcing the defensive mechanisms, or exacerbate the clinical condition through lesions secondary to the immunological damage. The autoimmune reaction occurs as a consequence of the homology between the adhesin sequence of the *MP* and a variety of human tissues, red blood cell antigen I, CD4, and immune complexes, and because of the polyclonal activation of B and T cells.

During the progression of the infection, neutralizing antibodies and autoantibodies are produced. Among these, agglutinins against the lung, brain, and smooth muscle can be included, which explains the systemic compromise. The immunopathological process, which involves epithelial damage ciliary dysfunction, is stimulated through the generation of specific IgE or inflammatory cytokines, especially type 2 interleukins (IL-6). The dimension of the cytokine- and cell-mediated immune response corresponds to the extent of tissue damage. The host immunity does not efficiently block the cell adherence of the *MP*, which would explain the high reinfection rates. Adhesins have sequence homology with the host structural proteins, and this mimicry explains the appearance of autoimmune events, which are mainly expressed as extrapulmonary manifestations. Direct invasion and dissemination have been verified as damage mechanisms in different parts of the body. It is likely that the intracellular localization is mediated by the fusion of the pathogen with the host cells through the membranes that contain cholesterol and protect the *MP* against antibiotics and antibodies. The antigenic variation of the surface adhesins may explain the ability of the MP to cause a chronic infection and transform healthy hosts into carriers. The immunopathological processes triggered by the infection are responsible for the appearance of the clinical conditions, which are generally moderate in 5-year-old or younger children (pharyngitis, tracheobronchitis) and more severe (pneumonia) in older children, because of the immune hyperresponse.

Epidemiology

MP causes between 20% and 40% of pneumonia cases in the pediatric population, and its incidence is greater among schoolchildren who are 5 years old or younger, with the incidence decreasing during adolescence. It is necessary to highlight the pneumonia caused by *MP* in children under 5 years of age, and even in infants (10%). In our experience, *MP* is responsible for 28% of outpatient pneumonia, usually in springtime. The infection is endemic, with epidemic outbreaks every 4 or 5 years. *MP* infection is 10 to 20 times higher as the cause for tracheitis, bronchitis, and other diseases than pneumonia. The distribution of the infection is worldwide, and children represent an asymptomatic reservoir for family outbreaks. Transmission takes place from person to person, through infected droplets. Possible transplacental transmission has been described, which causes a congenital pneumonia. Reinfections can be observed throughout the lifetime because of the lack of protection after the first infections. Mortality is low, although the infection can progress to a serious pneumonia, with serious extrapulmonary manifestations, which has become more frequent as resistance to macrolides has emerged in some countries. Family outbreaks appear slowly, given the long incubation period (2–3 weeks), and this can also be observed among children in kindergartens, schools, and other closed environments where an easier dissemination of the microorganism can occur. Pharyngeal carriers can be observed in 2% to 15% of the cases, depending if they are related to intrafamilial contacts with index patients infected by *MP* during epidemic outbreaks or children with no contact with infected patients during usual periods.

Clinical Presentation

Pneumonia caused by *MP* has some special characteristics. After a long period of incubation, it gradually begins with malaise, headache, myalgia, fever that can vary in its magnitude, cough, which starts as dry cough, and then progresses to productive cough, with some mucous expectoration, of paroxysmal frequency, which seriously bothers the patient and can be accompanied by odynophagia, acute rhinitis, and, in some patients, otalgia. Cough, which gradually becomes more cumbersome, is the central sign in the clinical progression (Tables 32.1 and 32.2). Physical examination usually reveals a patient who does not seem to be in a serious condition; there is no dyspnea, and during auscultation in the pulmonary examination fine crackles can be heard in compromised areas, usually at the lobar bases. Sometimes there is wheezing, pulmonary sounds are reduced, and in cases where there is a related atelectasis, a condensation syndrome can be auscultated. It is possible, in some cases, to identify a painful enlargement of the cervical ganglia, pharyngeal erythema with no exudate, bullous myringitis, dysphonia, conjunctivitis, or skin rash. It is important to highlight the frequent clinical dissonance with the radiological findings: there are few findings related to the physical examination, whereas the chest X-ray is quite expressive. The progression of the disease includes moderate fever that does not persist during more than 5 to 7 days, but the cough persists for a long period of time (2–3 weeks). Timely treatment reduces the persistence of the symptoms. The clinical and radiological profile, which is usually composed by a typical condensing syndrome (10–20%), can be similar to pneumonia caused by *Chlamydia pneumoniae* (*CP*), and sometimes it can also be similar to the infection caused by *Streptococcus pneumoniae* (*SP*). *MP* has an unfavorable progression in patients who present with an extensive bilateral compromise, pleural effusion, or respiratory failure, which may even require hospitalization in the intensive care unit. The disease can progress to a serious pneumonia in patients with sickle cell disease, Down syndrome, or immunosuppression. When there is coinfection (*CP* and *SP* are most frequent), the clinical condition tends to be severe, with prolonged hospitalization and greater risks of complications. *MP* is occasionally responsible for pulmonary sequelae, such as bronchiectasis and bronchiolitis obliterans.

Table 32.1 Etiological and clinical orientation for pneumonia

	Bacterial	Viral	Mycoplasma
Age	Any	Mainly less than 2 years old	3–15 years old
Season	Year-round	Winter	Spring
Presentation	Sudden	Variable	Insidious
Fever	High	Variable	Variable
Tachypnea	Common	Common	Infrequent
Cough	Scarce	Frequent	Frequent and intense
Related symptoms	Chest pain	Acute rhinorrhea Conjunctivitis	Exanthema
			Arthralgias
			Otalgia
Pulmonary examination	Condensation syndrome	Wheezing is frequently present	
		Condensation is sometimes present	Wheezing or condensation syndrome
	Bronchial sounds, fine crackles		
	Bronchophony		Localized fine crackles

Table 32.2 Clinical manifestations of pneumonia caused by *Mycoplasma*

Very frequent	Frequent	Regular frequency	Infrequent
Cough	Headache	Myalgias	Conjunctivitis
			Odynophagia
Fever	Lack of energy	Wheezing	Skin rush
			Otalgia
	Expectoration		Vomiting
			Acute rhinitis
	Crackles		Adenopathy
			Pharyngitis

Extrapulmonary Manifestations

According to the subsets of patients studied, a variable percentage (10–20%) may have extrapulmonary compromise, which happens before, during, or after the pulmonary infection caused by *MP*, even when no symptoms are present. The most common ones are these:

Cutaneous Present in 15–20% of the patients and are self-limited. Among them we have the following skin conditions: maculous eruptions, morbilliform rashes, papulovesicular rash, urticaria, erythema nodosum, erythema multiforme major (Steven–Johnson), and bullous.

Neurological The first cause of extrapulmonary pathology. There have been cases of encephalitis, meningitis, aseptic meningoencephalitis, transverse myelitis, Guillain–Barré syndrome, peripheral neuropathy, cerebellar syndrome, and mental confusion. There is evidence that direct invasion and autoimmunity are the pathogenesis of neurological compromise.

1. *Hematological*: Hemolytic anemia caused by cold agglutinins, autoimmune hemolysis, disseminated intravascular coagulation, thrombocytopenic purpura, and aplastic anemia.
2. *Articular*: Mono- or polyarthritis (most frequent cause according to our experience in Chile).
3. *Cardiac*: Myocarditis, pericarditis, arrhythmia, and heart failure.
4. *Renal*: Acute nephritis, IgA nephropathy.
5. *Oculars*: Conjunctivitis, anterior uveitis, iritis, hemorrhagic retinitis (very rare).

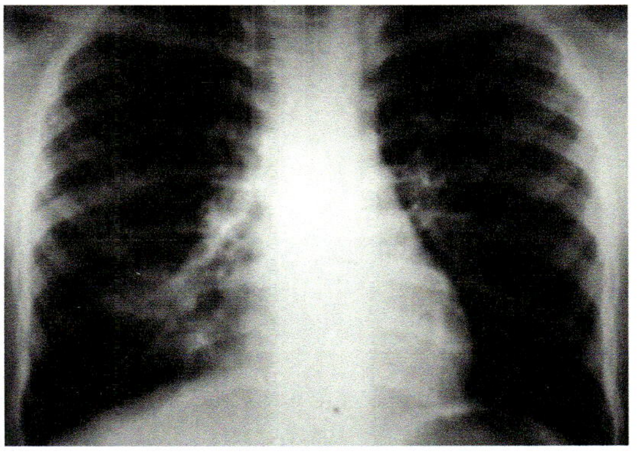

Fig. 32.1 Interstitial-alveolar pneumonia. Chest X-ray of 9-year-old schoolchild shows a right lower lobe interstitial-alveolar image

Radiology
The chest X-ray usually shows a segmented condensation that compromises the inferior lobes, in one or both sides, or the central perihilar regions. The usual image is nonhomogeneous, irregular, with interstitial or alveolar shadows, and sometimes atelectasis may be present. Sometimes the following can be observed: a lobar or multilobar condensation of a greater extension, small pleural effusions, diffuse or nodular interstitial infiltrations, hilar adenopathy, abscess, or peribronchovascular enlargements, which are rare (Figs. 32.1, 32.2, and 32.3). Our studies show interstitial images in 22.6% of patients, mixed in 28%, and alveolar in 48%; 10% presented with pleural compromise, and no chest tubes were needed for the pleura. Local experience suggests that 20% of the pulmonary images caused by *MP* are indistinguishable from those of classic pneumococcal pneumonia or of the *CP* chest X-ray pattern. X-ray findings may persist

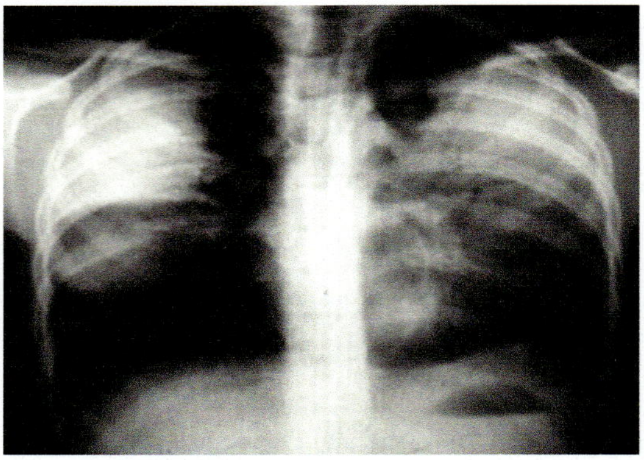

Fig. 32.2 Alveolar pneumonia. Chest X-ray of 6-year-old schoolchild presenting with an extensive bilateral lobar consolidation (similar to that caused by *Streptococcus pneumoniae*)

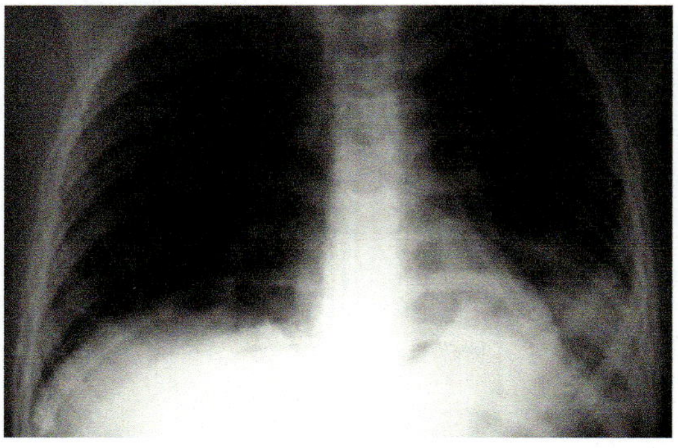

Fig. 32.3 Alveolar pneumonia and pleural effusion. Chest X-ray of 7-year-old schoolchild presenting with nasal bilateral condensation and left pleural effusion

during 2 to 6 weeks, depending on how early the antibiotic treatment is prescribed.

Laboratory Diagnosis

Classic Diagnosis Techniques

Culture and serology using the complement fixation (FC) test have their limitations in clinical practice. Complex nutritional sources are required for isolation, and although the specificity of the procedure is total (100%), its sensitivity varies between 60% and 70%. *MP* grows slowly in culture media; it is a cumbersome microorganism, and visible colonies take from 2 to 6 weeks to appear. Consequently, most laboratories do not conduct this test. FC is a technique that measures a mixture of IgM and IgG. The antigens used are related to several microorganisms and tissues, which causes unspecific reactions and yields false-positives. Because there usually is a high IgG level in the population, caused by previous infections, this technique requires serum-matched samples to prove seroconversion.

Serological Diagnosis

IgM detection is the most common test ordered in general pediatrics to diagnose pneumonia caused by *MP*. Although its sensitivity depends on the humoral immune response and the time at which the test was taken, generally IgM appears somewhere between 7 to 10 days after the onset of the clinical condition, and it rapidly increases, which makes it a fundamental pillar in the diagnosis of the infection caused by this microorganism, with a sensitivity of 80% or more. Nevertheless, in some patients, especially those under 2 years old, the IgM does not develop until 2 weeks after the beginning of the disease, which limits the sensitivity of this diagnostic procedure. IFI to determine IgM considers as a positive a number of 1/32 titers, and it is a classic technique for the diagnosis, but its reading requires trained personnel. Enzyme immune assays (EIA) are techniques that are easy to implement in clinical laboratories and can detect IgM and IgG separately, which eases the differentiation between an active infection and a previous one. It has been proven that IgM in children can have sensitivity levels as high as 89% to 92%. Also, the specificity of IgM detection done through enzyme-linked immunosorbent assay (ELISA) can vary in about 25% to 90%, depending on the commercial kit being used.

DNA Amplification Polymerase Chain Reaction (PCR)

Nucleic acid amplification techniques have a great potential for *MP* diagnosis, because of their specificity and because they quickly deliver results. Also, they are the best diagnostic tool when treating immunocompromised children and infants who have not reached the first year of life. These patients have a lower humoral immune response when facing this agent. Nevertheless, the presence of *MP* in the upper respiratory tract may be an obstacle, particularly during epidemics. In Chile, it has been detected in 2% of healthy children. In children between 1 to 4 years of life, it was detected in 1.9%, and in children between the ages of 4 to 15 it appeared in 5% of cases. During the periods in which the incidence of *MP* is greater, the presence of *MP* also increases. A 15% increase in relationship to the *MP* presence has been observed in children who are in contact with family members who are undergoing respiratory infections caused by these bacteria. The new nucleic acid amplification techniques, such as the nucleic acid sequence-based amplification (NASBA) and conventional, nested, or real-time PCR (Fig. 32.4), are attractive alternatives when determining the diagnosis. For ARN, NASBA is intrinsically more sensitive than conventional amplification techniques, and further, NASBA can also measure the microbial load in the sample. PCR in real time can identify an active infection through the detection and quantification of the accumulation of amplified DNA as the reaction develops.

Pathology

There are not many pathological findings about community-acquired pneumonia caused by *MP* because of its low severity and mortality rates. In deadly cases where the patient was previously healthy, diffuse alveolar pneumonia can develop, with infant respiratory distress syndrome, besides involving the liver, spleen, and brain. Other evidence shows myocarditis and interstitial lung disease. Lung biopsies show that tracheal, bronchiolar, and peribranchial tissues are affected, with purulent exudate. There are metaplastic cells in both bronchi and bronchoalveolar linings, besides monocytes (plasma cells), enlargement of the peribranchial septa, and type II monocyte hyperplasia. There is also scalping in the ciliary epithelium, which explains the intense cough that is the main symptom of pneumonia.

Treatment

Antimicrobial therapy significantly reduces the progression of the pneumonia caused by *MP*, reducing the intensity and frequency of the cough, lowering the fever, and improving the

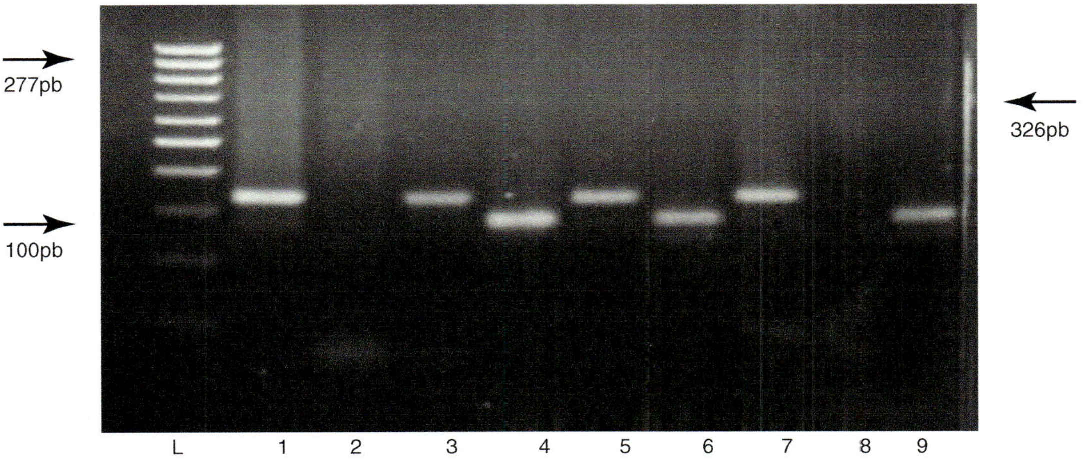

Fig. 32.4 Electrophoresis for *Mycoplasma pneumoniae* in agarose gel for the amplification products using simple polymerase chain reaction (PCR) for *M. pneumoniae* (gene 16S rRNA) and human β-globulin gene. Channels 1, 3, 5, and 7 present positive beta-globulin; Channel 2 is negative for *M. pneumoniae*; Channels 4 and 6 are positive for *M. pneumoniae*; Channels 8 and 9 are negative control and positive for *M. pneumoniae*, respectively. *L*, marker of molecular weight of 100 pb

general condition of the patient. In the same way, it partially avoids the dissemination of the agents among the contacts of the patients through the reduction in the number of microorganisms per sputum volume unit. Because the microorganism does not have a cell wall, it is refractory to beta-lactam antibiotics, but it responds adequately to the use of macrolides. *MP* can live intracellularly, which explains the difficulty for eradicating it, as it survives in bronchial secretions during a long time after the end of treatment. The effect of antibiotic therapy in relation to the extrapulmonary manifestations is unknown; nevertheless, it is always used even when there is no extrapulmonary compromise. In our environment, resistance to macrolides is a rare exception because of the reduction of antibiotic affinity in relation to ribosomes. However, during the past 10 years we have observed an alarming resistance increase, which has been reported in several studies, especially in Asia. This new reality has caused, in some situations, the combination of a refractory disease evolution and a longer disease progression. Also, during epidemic outbreaks, we have observed a more severe presentation of the disease with a greater number of complications. Mutations A20636, A20646, and A20676 constitute 98% of the resistance cases. Involved factors are progressive increase of macrolides usage, which triggers a selective pressure phenomenon; a greater demographic density in some geographic areas, and the increase of travel between neighboring countries with large populations. The appearance of this resistance creates a challenge in the management of the refractory patient or the patient who progresses to a serious condition, which requires administration of medications that are not free of controversy, such as quinolones, doxycycline, and even steroids. In Chile vigilance is scarce, as well as the information available about the issue, although clinical published experience shows a good response to macrolides in the pediatric population. Sensitivity tests are not performed in the management of individual cases. See Table 32.3 for the treatment scheme in case of *MP*; Table 32.4 specifies the hospitalization criteria.

Table 32.3 Treatment for infection caused by *Mycoplasma pneumoniae*

Medications
Antibiotics:
Oral erythromycin at 50 mg/kg/day in 4 doses, 10–14 days
Oral clarithromycin at 15 mg/kg/day in 2 doses, 10–14 days
Oral azithromycin at 10 mg/kg/day in 1 dose, without food, during 5 days if there is resistance or clinical refractory disease
Oral ciprofloxacin at 20 mg/kg/day in 2 daily doses during 10 days
Doxycyclines for children over 8 years old at 100 mg in 1 dose or 50 mg every 12 h during 10–14 days
Bronchodilators
Beta-adrenergic dilators are used if there is airway obstruction (7–10 days)
Kinesiotherapy
Kinesiotherapy treatment for bronchial hypersecretion or atelectasis
Hospitalized patients
Medications
Antibiotics: As indicated for ambulatory patients. In patients with a serious disease, use IV ciprofloxacin at 10 mg/k/day during 10–14 days
Bronchodilators for airway obstruction
Systemic steroids in usual dosage for serious cases with severe obstruction and neurological manifestations (methylprednisolone)
Kinesiotherapy: Bronchial hypersecretion or atelectasis
Chest drainage: Only if significant effusion is present

Table 32.4 Hospitalization because of infection caused by *Mycoplasma pneumoniae*

Patient in serious condition with toxic appearance since admittance
Poor response to initial ambulatory treatment (fever persistence, dyspnea, or significant cough increase)
Extensive bilateral compromise
Clinical and radiological progression
Respiratory failure
Important pleural effusion, abscesses, necrosis
Extrapulmonary manifestations

Prevention

The use of prophylactic antibiotics in a member of a family who has been exposed to *MP* shows a reduction in the clinical disease appearance, although seroconversion is not avoided. Some authors believe that antibiotics should be used in the case of intrafamilial index only when symptoms start. We agree with this opinion, and we recommend it to our patients. There has been no success in the use of protective vaccines against *MP*, and during past years the interest in these has decreased.

Prognosis

In most cases, pneumonia caused by *MP* progresses positively with adequate treatment, although there may be some severe cases that may involve hospitalization, with oxygen or ventilation support. Depending on the affected system or organ, extrapulmonary manifestations may also need to be treated with a more strict and specific treatment, especially in neurological or cardiac cases. In asthma patients, this pneumonia can trigger the acute obstruction of the airways or worsening of the chronic asthma symptoms. There are reports of lung sequelae after suffering from an infection caused by *Mycoplasma pneumoniae*. Computed tomography scans of the chest show mosaic attenuation, peribronchovascular enlargement, bronchiectasis, bronchiolitis obliterans, and even pulmonary fibrosis.

Pneumonia Caused by *Chlamydophila pneumoniae*

Microbiology

Chlamydophila pneumoniae (*CP*) is an intracellular bacterium that grows through binary division and uses the energetic system of the cells. The TWAR serovariety for *CP* has been established using DNA homology studies and the unique morphology of its elementary body (EB), which is pear shaped and is functionally important, contrasting with the round body of the other species. *CP* is more homogeneous than the other two species (*Chlamydophila trachomatis* and *C. psittaci*) and the main protein (adhesin) of its external membrane is less complex. The small distal end is the location site of adherence to the cell, which causes a cell invasion (endocytosis) adhering to the base of the microvilli and several entrance mechanisms that depend on the cell and the infection route (Fig. 32.5).

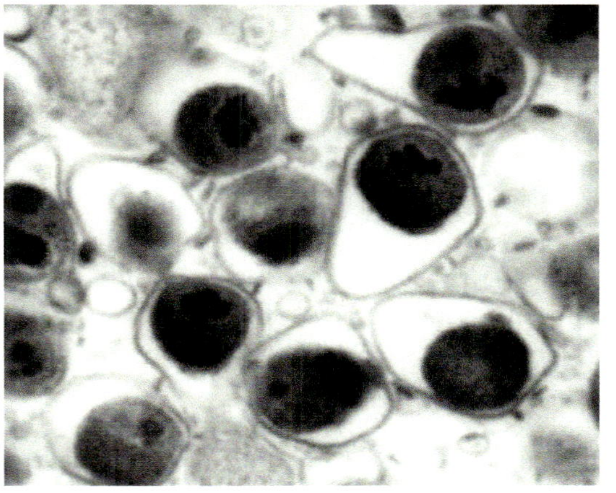

Fig. 32.5 *Chlamydophila pneumoniae*

Etiopathogenesis

CP is characterized by a unique development cycle, which has a different morphology depending on whether it is in its infectious or reproductive form, EB or reticulate body (RB), and also has a gram-negative coating. Some recent studies have revealed that EB and RB code proteins creating a complete pathway for the synthesis of peptidoglycan, including proteins that bind to penicillin, which would make them relatively sensitive to beta-lactam antibiotics. After the infection, EB (which has a 0.3 μm diameter) binds to the host cell through electrostatic union and enters the cell by endocytosis. In this way, the EB remains in the phagosome membrane, which does not fuse together with the lysosome. EB differentiates from RB, which divides by binary fission after 36 h. Then, 48 h later, all the RB is expelled by cytolysis or exocytosis, leaving the cells intact. CP can progress to a persistent state after the effect of cytokines, such as interferon-gamma (IFN-γ), antibiotic treatments, or restriction of certain nutrients. In that state, metabolic activity is reduced, which explains its ability to cause a subclinical infection. CP enters through the airway and infects the leukocytes and pulmonary macrophages, which enter the blood flow once they are infected (marker of chronic infection). Infection of endothelial cells in smooth muscle takes place, as well as microvascular activation in the NF-KB pathway, expressing adherence molecules and proinflammatory cytokines (IL-1, IL-6, TNF-α, IFN-γ) and procoagulant proteins. The *CP* life cycle during the intracellular period favors the development of chronic infections, which also happens because of its ability to survive in monocytes and macrophages, allowing the bacteria to disseminate to different organs of the host. On the one hand, the presence of *CP* stimulates the inflammatory reaction and the tissue damage that is secondary to infection; on the other hand, it produces pathogenic activity against the host, and it also affects the immunological response against foreign antigens. This action creates chronic inflammation, which is usually accompanied by a very broad noninfectious pathology.

Epidemiology

CP is a common human pathogen, with a wide geographic distribution, and it affects patients of all ages. Evidence indicates that even though the microorganism was recently discovered, its capacity to cause disease in humans is not new. Current published information suggest that pneumonia caused by this pathogen is infrequent in preschool-age children and more common in school-age children and during adolescence. The greatest incidence is observed in older adults and in patients with comorbidity (asthma and chronic pulmonary obstructive disease). Virtually all people are infected at some point in their lives, and reinfection is common. Also, the infection would be more common in tropical weather countries, and, for reasons unknown, in males. Chile has a high seroprevalence, which is low in those under 5 years old, but it gradually increases until it reaches 32% in children who are between 10 and 14 years old (Table 32.5).

We have published our results about pneumonia etiology in children 1–14 years of age, in whom we found 2.3% of *CP* (3 cases of 108 pneumonias). Other studies around the world suggest a frequency of about 5% to 20% of pneumonia is caused by *CP* in school-age children and adolescents. *CP* transmission is probably person to person through respiratory secretions, although there is no direct evidence. Dissemination of the disease is very slow, and the interval between each case can span up to 30 days, which explains the slow spreading of epidemic outbreaks. In some people, asymptomatic infections are crucial in the dissemination of the disease, whereas others are ineffective transmitters. Infections caused by *CP* are endemic and epidemic, with an increase in the incidence during 2 to 3 years, or with short 4-month outbreaks. The periods of low incidence can last up to 3 years. Around 2–5% of adults and children are asymptomatic carriers, and only a small percentage of those infected progress to pneumonia.

Table 32.5 Presence of IgG antibodies for *Chlamydia pneumoniae* sorted by age (Santiago, Chile)

Age (years)	Samples	Number of seropositive serum samples (IgG > 1:32), *n* (%)
6 months–4 years	22	1 (4.5)
5–9 years	28	4 (14.3)
10–14	41	10 (31.7)
15–19	27	15 (37.0)
20–29	62	31 (50.0)
30–39	61	34 (55.7)
40–49	65	40 (61.5)
50–59	43	28 (65.2)
60–89	54	39 (72.2)

Clinical Presentation

The clinical characteristics of *CP* can be similar to those presented by *MP*, and in some cases it may be similar to a pneumococcal pneumonia. Nevertheless, it frequently presents a symptomatology with some features that differentiate it from other respiratory pathogens. It has a gradual onset, starting with odynophagia, hoarseness, dysphonia, and moderate fever. It improves after days or even weeks, when persistent dry cough appears, which progresses to productive cough, and, sometimes, to paroxysmal cough. In this way, the progression profile of the disease turns biphasic. Sometimes it is accompanied by headache and rhinorrhea (rhinosinusal compromise); pulmonary auscultation is variable, sometimes with isolated fine crackles, or wheezing and rhonchus. Pneumonia caused by *CP* resolves adequately with standard therapy, but cough and lack of energy can persist for weeks. Hospitalized patients are few, usually older adults or, at any age, patients who are chronic carriers of the disease.

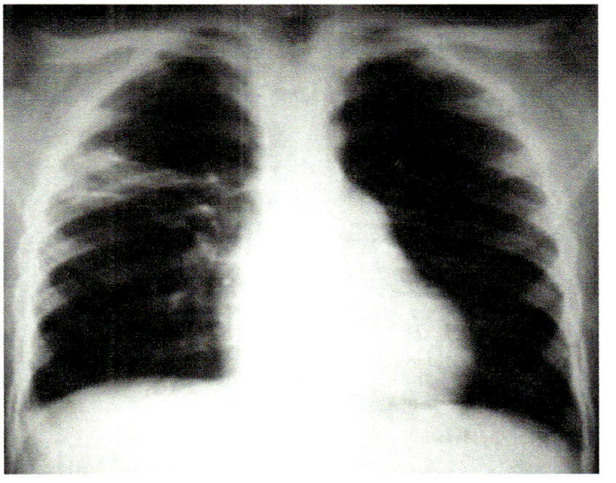

Fig. 32.7 Interstitial-alveolar pneumonia. Chest X-ray of 11-year-old schoolchild presenting with interstitial-alveolar compromise in the right superior lobe, caused by *Chlamydophila pneumoniae*

Radiology

Chest X-ray presents isolated subsegmented images, with alveolar-interstitial shadows, non-homogeneous, and with irregular borders. In some cases, there is lobar or multi-lobar compromise of a greater extension, which usually has a more serious progression, especially for *MP* coinfection (Figs. 32.6 and 32.7). Pleural effusion is exceptional and scarce.

Specific Diagnosis

Indirect immunofluorescence is used in the serological diagnosis of *Chlamydophila pneumoniae*, although its real usefulness is debatable. Some commercial kits use antigens from which the lipopolysaccharide (LPS) (which is a common antigen among the *Chlamydia* species) has been removed to reduce cross reactions between species. The cutoff points for acute infection caused by *CP* are the presence of IgM titers ≥1:16, or at least a fourfold increase in the IgG titers for matched serum samples (acute and convalescent). IgG titers ≥1:512, whether they are unique or sustained, should be considered as previous infections. For now, no serological procedure can overcome two important problems in the serological study of *CP*: the slow appearance of antibodies for this species and its high seroprevalence in the adult population, caused by past infections or even current asymptomatic infections. There are two serological patterns: primo-infection, which is usually present in children, and the reinfection pattern, caused by this agent and seen in adults. During primo-infection, IgM appears after the third week, and IgG appears between 7 and 8 weeks after the infection has taken place. During the reinfection, generally there is no IgM response, and IgG appears between 3 and 5 weeks after the infection has occurred. The serology study provides retrospective results, which have little clinical application as a diagnostic technique. The technique of nucleic acid amplification (PCR) is a quick and sensitive alternative for the diagnosis of *CP*. Nasopharyngeal aspiration samples are the most used samples for the diagnosis. Nested PCR has proven to be more sensitive relative to conventional PCR for the *CP*

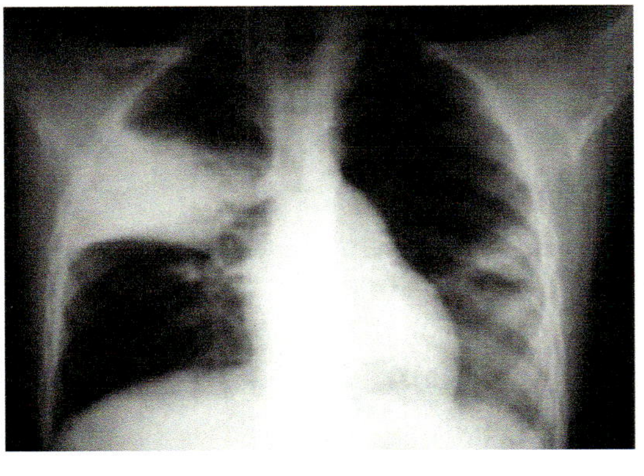

Fig. 32.6 Condensing pneumonia. Chest X-ray of 10-year-old schoolchild presenting with bilateral alveolar compromise caused by *Chlamydophila pneumoniae* and *Mycoplasma pneumoniae*

diagnosis in respiratory samples. Besides this, about 2% to 5% of children and adults have been identified as asymptomatic respiratory carriers, which emphasizes the need to critically analyze the microbiological results for each patient. As happens with *MP*, the molecular techniques that can be used to quantify the microbial load in clinical samples have great potential for future differentiation between carriers and infected patients. Currently, cell culture is used with a variable correlation along with PCR.

Relationship of *CP* with Other Diseases

For some time, asthma and lower tract respiratory infection caused by *CP* have been known to be related, and it has been proven that acute infection may trigger an asthma crisis in the same way as other pathogens, such as viruses and *MP*. Reinfections or persistence can be the cause of exacerbations of asthma episodes. In these cases, treatment with macrolides improves the clinical evolution and the functional parameters. The hypothesis is that chronic infection causes hyperreactivity and inflammation in susceptible children. There are numerous studies relating *CP* with ischemic disease (atherosclerosis), acute infarction, chronic obstructive pulmonary disease, arthritis, pericarditis, thyroiditis, multiple sclerosis, Alzheimer's, erythema nodosum, Guillain-Barré, or lung cancer. An increase in the antibodies, as well as the evidence of the agent presence in atheromatous plaques obtained through PCR and electronic microscopy, have been proven, although the role of *Chlamydophila pneumoniae* in these pathologies is still not sufficiently clear.

Treatment

The main drugs used are macrolides or doxycyclines (patients >8 years old) and cephalosporins, in prolonged therapies to avoid relapses. Most cases respond favorably. Our suggestion for children who are 5 years or older is to use 50 mg/kg/day of oral erythromycin every 6 h during 2 to 3 weeks; or 15 mg/kg/day of oral clarithromycin every 12 h during 2 to 3 weeks, or 10 mg/kg/day of oral azithromycin as a daily dose for 5 days, combined with oral cefuroxime in doses of 20 to 30 mg/kg/day every 12 h during 2 to 3 weeks. For children younger than 5 years old, use only oral cefuroxime in doses of 20 to 30 mg/kg/day every 12 h during 2 to 3 weeks. If the patient has been hospitalized and is in serious condition, cefuroxime should be used in doses of 100 mg/kg/day combined with an oral macrolide.

Summary

Atypical pneumonia is a disease caused by *MP* and *CP*. *MP* is a small bacillus, with autonomous life, pleomorphic, with no cell wall, which produces enzymes and has an organelle that attaches to the respiratory epithelium. *CP* has a DNA homology that differs from other *Chlamydia*: its body has a characteristic pear-shaped form. These pathogens share their clinical presentation of frequent and tormenting cough, moderate fever, and a progression profile that is insidious, gradual, and usually not serious. *MP* and *CP* are community acquired, and the contagion is produced by droplets.

The typical chest X-ray shows interstitial infiltrations, although there is a minor percentage where a great variety of mixed images can be observed: reticulonodular infiltrations, atelectasis, and even lobar shadows (*MP* and *CP*). The diagnosis is made through laboratory exams, particularly PCR and serology (ELISA and IFI) for *MP*, and only PCR for *CP*. Pulmonary examination usually reveals crackles and/or wheezing. Both *MP* and *CP* can cause extrapulmonary complications or serious progression of the disease, related to complex immunological events. *MP* is accompanied by the presence of cytokines, CD4, T and B cells, and interferon; *CP* is accompanied by cytokines, TNF-α, IFN-γ, and HSP60.

Treatment for complicated atypical pneumonia caused by *MP* involves macrolides, and if the response is not favorable, or there is resistance, or if the progress of the disease is serious, ciprofloxacin or doxycycline can be used (>8 years old), with or without steroids. For *CP*, in children who are 5 years old or older, macrolides combined with cefuroxime are used, and for those under 5 years old, only cefuroxime.

Sources

Abramo C, Leinonen M, McCracken GH. *Mycoplasma pneumoniae* treatment of community-acquired pneumonia in ambulatory disease: clinical spectrum, pathophysiology, epidemiology, and children. Pediatr Infect Dis J. 1999;18:98–104.

Aizen L, Wang L. Combined treatment for child refractory *Mycoplasma pneumoniae* pneumonia with ciprofloxacin and glucocorticoid. Pediatr Pulmonol. 2011;46:1093–7.

Averibrich D, Hidalgo-Grauss C. Macrolide resistance in *Mycoplasma pneumoniae*, Israel, 2010. Emerg Infect Dis. 2011;17(6):1079–82.

De Barbeyrac B, Bébéar C. Histoire naturelle des infections à *Chlamydia* physiopathologie des infections à *Chlamydia*: conséquences diagnostiques et thérapeutiques. Arch Pèdiatr. 2005;12:526–31.

Dowel SF, Peeling RW, Boman J. Standardizing *Chlamydia pneumoniae* assays: recommendations from the Centers for Disease Control and Prevention (USA) and the Laboratory Centre for Disease Control (Canada). Clin Infect Dis. 2001;33:492–503.

Hammerschlag MR. Pneumonia due to *Chlamydia pneumoniae* in children: epidemiology, diagnosis, and treatment. Pediatr Pulmonol. 2003;36:384–90.

Hong BK, Choi EH. Macrolide resistance of *Mycoplasma pneumoniae*, South Korea, 2000–2011. Emerg Infect Dis. 2013;19:19.

Kim CK, Chung CY, Kim JS, Kim WS. Late abnormal findings on high-resolution computed tomography after *Mycoplasma* pneumonia. Pediatrics. 2000;105:372–8.

Kogan R, Astudillo P, Maluenda J, Cortés C. Clinical and epidemiologic characteristics of *Mycoplasma pneumoniae* infections in Santiago, Chile. Eur Respir J. 2002;20:S337.

Kogan R, Martínez MA, Rubilar L, Puppo H, Girardi G, Castro-Rodriguez JA. Comparative randomized trial of azithromycin versus erythromycin and amoxicillin for treatment of community acquired pneumonia in children. Pediatr Pulmonol. 2003;35:91–8.

Kicinski P, Wisniewska-Ligier M. Pneumonia caused by *Mycoplasma pneumoniae* and *Chlamydophila pneumoniae* in children: comparative analysis of clinical picture. Adv Med Sci. 2011;56(1):56–63.

Kurz H, Gopfrich H. Role of *Chlamydophila pneumoniae* in children hospitalized for community-acquired pneumonia in Vienna, Austria. Pediatr Pulmonol. 2009;44:873–6.

Martínez MA, Diomedi A, Kogan R, Borie C. Taxonomía e importancia clínica de las nuevas familias del orden Chlamydiales. Rev Chil Infect 2001;18:203–11.

Michelow IC, Katz K. Systemic cytokine profile in children with community-acquired pneumonia. Pediatr Pulmonol. 2007;42:640–5.

Mulholland S, Gavranich JB. Antibiotic for community-acquired lower respiratory tract infections secondary to *Mycoplasma pneumoniae* in children (Review). Cochrane Library 2010 issue 7

Lung DC, Lam Shu Yan D. Rapid defervescence after doxycycline treatment of macrolide-resistant *Mycoplasma pneumoniae*-associated community-acquired pneumonia in children. Pediatr Infect Dis J. 2013;32:1396.

de los Ángeles Paúl DM, Vega-Briceño L, Sánchez I. Características clínicas de la enfermedad respiratoria causada por *Mycoplasma pneumoniae* en niños hospitalizados. Rev Chil Infect 2009;26(4):343–349.

Shen Y, Zhang J. Combination therapy with immune modulators and moxifloxacin on fulminant macrolide-resistant *Mycoplasma pneumoniae* infection: a case report. Pediatr Pulmonol. 2013;48:519–22.

Complicated Pneumonia

33

Francisco Prado Atlagic,
Rodrigo Vásquez-De Kartzow,
Pamela Salinas Flores,
and Pamela Navarrete Contreras

Contents

F. Prado Atlagic (✉)
Department of Pediatrics, Hospital Clínico San Borja Arriarán, Santiago, Chile

R. Vásquez-De Kartzow
Department of Pediatrics, Faculty of Medicine, Universidad de Chile, Santiago, Chile

P. Salinas Flores
Pediatric Service, Clínica Las Lilas, Providencia, Chile

P. Navarrete Contreras
Department of Pediatrics, Hospital de Los Ángeles, Los Ángeles, Chile

Definition

Complicated pneumonia includes all clinical situations in which the deterioration caused by the disease jeopardizes complete recovery. These are classified as suppurated or nonsuppurated complications (Table 33.1). Suppurated complications are related to the extension of the inflammatory component, mainly considering the pleura, with an increase of pleural fluid, which in

P. Bertrand, I. Sánchez (eds.), *Pediatric Respiratory Diseases*,
https://doi.org/10.1007/978-3-030-26961-6_33

Table 33.1 Complications in community-acquired pneumonia

Pulmonary complications	Extrapulmonary complications
Suppurated pleuropulmonary complications	Immunological/ infectious complications
Necrotizing pneumonia Pneumatocele, pyopneumatocele Pulmonary abscess Parapneumonic pleural effusion Pleural empyema Mechanical complications of suppurated pneumonias: Air escaping (pneumothorax and bronchopleural fistula)	Sepsis Toxic shock syndrome Hemolytic-uremic syndrome Distant focus: septic arthritis, meningitis, myocarditis, pericarditis, endocarditis
Nonsuppurated complications	
Acute respiratory failure	
Atelectasis	

the beginning is sterile (parapneumonic effusion), but afterward becomes infected and is named an empyema.

Among other complications we can consider pulmonary abscess, as cavitated pulmonary parenchyma with pus-filled material. In contrast to pyo-pneumatocele, which presents with a thin wall and with an appearance secondary to abscesses in the terminal bronchiole, pulmonary abscess is less frequent in patients with community-acquired pneumonia. Pulmonary abscess presents with thick and irregular walls and usually requires prolonged antibiotic treatment. Surgery may be an option of treatment for some patients when there is a bronchopleural fistula with no response to medical therapy, the presence of persistent hemoptysis, or if the airway is compressed. Pulmonary abscess is observed in patients with massive aspiration pneumonia, chronic lung damage with bronchiectasis, pulmonary malformations, or in patients with complicated pulmonary hydatidosis. Infection by *Streptococcus pneumoniae* and *Staphylococcus aureus*, which have become agents seen as suppurating more often than previously, produces necrotizing pneumonia, which presents as pneumonia with multiple confluent microabscesses, usually septic, that follow quickly to multiple cavitations within the consolidated parenchyma, associated with ipsilateral empyema. This suppurated complication is different from the appearance of a thin-walled air-filled image, named a pneumatocele, within the resolution of a pneumonia. In necrotizing pneumonia, it is possible to observe a bronchopleural fistula, corresponding to the communication between the pleural space and the peripheral airway, which is caused by the infected and necrotized parenchyma. A pneumatocele may cause mechanical complications because of the hyperinsufflation and parenchyma or airway compression, or because of a pleural tear, if its location is subpleural, with the formation of a secondary pneumothorax.

Epidemiology

Pneumonia is one of the most common infections in children around the world, with associated morbidity and mortality, but it is especially severe in children under 1 year old in developing countries.

WHO has estimated that every year about 156 million cases of pneumonia affect children under 5 years old, of which about 12.5 million children are hospitalized (8%) because of serious and/or complicated pneumonias. Pneumonia is the main cause of death in children under 5 years old, reaching 1.4 million deaths/year over all the world.

In Latin America, pneumonia is one of the most frequent causes of hospital admission for children under 5 years of age. Mortality varies from 4 to 300 deaths/1000 live births. Considering the Latin American countries, Chile and Uruguay have the lowest mortality rate related to *Streptococcus pneumoniae*, whereas Bolivia, Peru, and Guyana have the highest mortality rate.

In Chile, pneumonia is an important public health issue, with a rate per year of 2000 to 3000 cases per 100,000 children less than 2 years of age. Half of those who seek attention in the emergency room require admission to the hospital, most because of acute respiratory failure and suppurative complications. Estimation of the frequency in which bacterial pneumonias progress to parapneumonic effusion, or noncomplicated exudate, is about 0.6–5%. Empyema has been estimated at about 3.3 per 100,000 children with community-acquired pneumonia.

Pleural empyema is the main suppurated complication. Around 40% of children with pneumonia who require hospitalization present with pleural effusion, and up to 2% of these present with empyema. Its incidence is greater during winter and spring. Epidemiological reports from Europe and the United States have confirmed an increase of this complication over recent years.

Etiology

The agents most commonly involved in empyema are *Streptococcus pneumoniae*, *Streptococcus aureus*, *Haemophilus influenzae*, and *Streptococcus pyogenes*.

Currently, *S. pneumoniae* is the bacterial agent that causes most complicated pneumonias. The use of systematic conjugated vaccines against *S. pneumoniae* has modified their behavior, which may have been related to the recent appearance of serotypes related to a greater frequency of pulmonary suppuration (19A, 7F, 1, and 5). In spite of this, etiological identification by hemocultures and pleural fluid culture is low. It is possible to isolate this bacterium using hemoculture in up to 10% of children hospitalized with pneumonia. Nasopharyngeal culture does not yield further information about the etiology, because generally the isolated agents are commensal flora of the upper respiratory system. Determining the urinary antigen as a pneumococcus has a limited sensitivity and specificity. There is no solid basis to recommend the routine use of fiberoptic bronchoscopy with a protective catheter or bronchoalveolar lavage for children.

The use of polymerase chain reaction (PCR) for *S. pneumoniae* in pleural fluid samples has increased isolation in more than 75% of the cases. Pneumonia caused by *Staphylococcus aureus* and *Streptococcus pyogenes*, as happens with anaerobic microorganisms, often tends to present complications with empyema, and to have a higher rate of positive cultures.

A study conducted in the United States between 1993 and 2001 showed an increase of 24% of cases of pneumonia with pulmonary empyema. After 2000, the cases reduced in rate because of the introduction of the anti-pneumococcal conjugate vaccine. Since 2002, and mainly among children under 1 year old, an increase of pneumonia resulting in pleural effusion caused by *Staphylococcus aureus* has been observed.

Among other microorganisms that may cause pleural effusion less frequently, such as virus (adenovirus, influenza, parainfluenza), we can mention *Mycoplasma pneumoniae*, which may present pleural effusion in 5–20% of the cases, but which rarely requires a pleurocentesis. *Mycobacterium tuberculosis*, gram-negative, and anaerobic bacilli are much less common than in the adult population, in which they must only be suspected in the presence of aspiration pneumonia, pulmonary abscesses, and subdiaphragmatic abscesses. *Haemophilus influenzae* is an infrequent etiological agent in empyemas, but it must be considered as a potential infectious agent.

Community-acquired strains of *S. aureus* resistant to methicillin that have emerged over recent years are responsible for serious suppurated pneumonias.

Empyema Physiopathology

Pleural space is virtual and is limited by the visceral and parietal pleura. There is a continuous fluid filtration process from the capillary space to the subpleural one, and to the pleural cavity, which depends on the balance between the hydrostatic and oncotic pressures of both spaces, in accordance with the Starling law.

The presence of bacteria activates the inflammatory cascade in mesothelial cells, which release cytokines that cause the appearance of neutrophils, lymphocytes, and eosinophils in the pleural space, which breaks the balance between filtration and reabsorption of the pleural liquid. At the same time, the coagulation cascade activates, reducing fibrinolysis and fibrin deposit in the pleural space, which causes loculations or segmentations. This process causes an increase in the metabolic activity of inflammatory cells and bacteria, which initiates a decrease in pH and glucose levels of the pleural fluid, as well as an increase in the LDH concentration.

Pleural Effusion, Classification, and Progression Phases

Pleural empyema has different progression phases that are well defined and impact treatment success. This process is dynamic and can be approached through escalated treatments. The *exudative phase* is the starting phase, usually within the first 48 h of febrile progression; free and sterile fluid is present. In the *fibrinopurulent phase*, segmentations appear and loculations are formed in the pleural space. In the *organization or late phase*, fibroblasts and pleural enlargement appear. Nevertheless, children achieve a complete recovery and rarely present restrictive adherences that may compromise respiratory mechanics.

Pleural effusions related to pneumonia can be classified as follows:

1. *Parapneumonic effusion*: Accumulation of pleural fluid related to a pneumonia or pulmonary abscess. At first the exudate is sterile, with a pH > 7.2 and glucose >40 mg/dl. In adults it is related to an LDH < 1000 UI/l.
2. *Empyema*: Pus presence in pleural fluid, bacteria in the direct study (Gram or acridine orange stain) or culture or pleural fluid pH < 7.20. The presence of one or more of these criteria sets the diagnosis of pleural empyema. Other biochemical characteristics may suggest empyema, but they do not determine it.
3. *Segmented empyema*: Occupation of the pleural space without displacement in the chest X-ray in lateral recumbent position with horizontal ray, or the presence of loculations with segmentations in the chest echography.

Clinical Manifestations

Complications of pneumonia must be suspected in every patient with probable bacterial community-acquired pneumonia who persist febrile after 48 h of adequate antibiotic treatment or who seek attention after 72 h of disease deterioration. The first possibility to rule out is pulmonary empyema.

The classic clinical picture includes lethargy, anorexia, persistent fever, usually above 39 °C with chills, cough (it is not the main symptom), and tachypnea. Chest pain and grunting may be present. Abdominal pain is a frequent symptom of pneumonia located in the lower lobes. In the most serious cases, the child may adopt an antalgic position (scoliosis toward the affected side).

The physical examination of the affected side will reveal a diminished chest excursion, dullness at percussion, and abolished normal breath sounds. In the upper limit of the effusion a pleural murmur may be heard, besides egophony and aphonic pectoriloquy. In infants and preschoolers, these signs are partially present and often absent. Dullness is the most important clinical sign. Large effusions may produce contralateral mediastinum deviation.

Diagnosis

Chest X-ray (anteroposterior and lateral) is the first image to acquire when a complicated pneumonia is suspected. There is controversy about the real utility of a projection of the affected side in lateral recumbent position with horizontal ray to evaluate fluid displacement as an indicator of free effusion. The earliest sign is the obliteration of the costophrenic angle and the meniscus sign, in which the rim of the effusion ascends toward the lateral chest wall (Figs. 33.1 and 33.2).

If there are greater amounts of fluid, enlargement of the intercostal spaces can be seen, as well as mediastinal displacement. When there is a "white lung" image, it may not be possible to differentiate pleural effusion from a consolidated pneumonia pulmonary mass or pulmonary filled cyst.

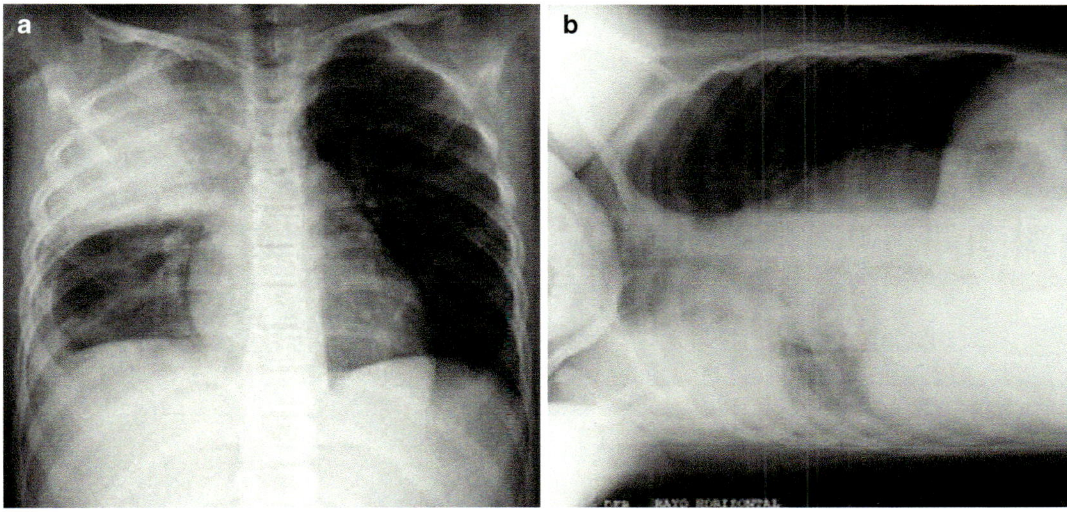

Fig. 33.1 (**a**) Pleural effusion. Chest X-ray of 8-year-old schoolchild presenting with high fever for 48 h showing a consolidated pneumonia in right upper lobe, costophrenic recess obliteration, and pleural meniscus sign. (**b**) Chest X-ray of the same patient in lateral recumbent position with horizontal ray showing displacement of pleural effusion <10 mm on the left side

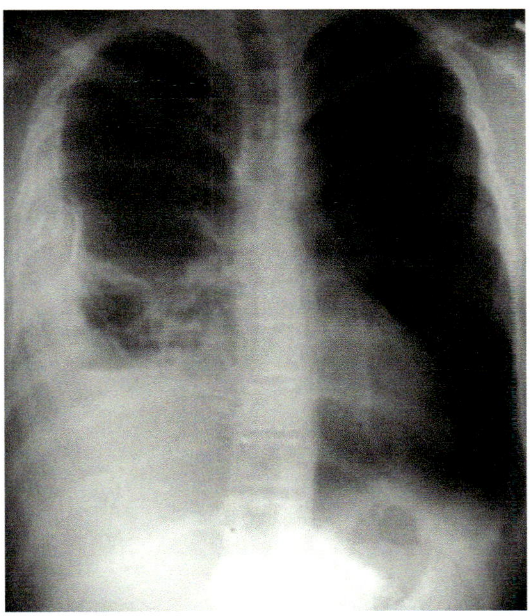

Fig. 33.2 Empyema. Chest X-ray in 10-year-old schoolchild shows necrotizing pneumonia in the right lower lobe and right medial lobe, besides ipsilateral empyema

Chest echography may detect fluid in the pleural cavity, and therefore it is useful for "white lung" evaluation. Although the stage of the effusion cannot be determined, the amount of fluid present can be estimated, as well as differentiating if it is free or loculated and determining its echogenicity (Figs. 33.3 and 33.4).

At the same time, chest echography is useful for therapeutic procedures, as a guide of puncture site and for the insertion of a pleural chest tube. It has the disadvantage of depending on availability and the operator's experience.

Chest computerized axial tomography is not considered a routine examination because it does not differentiate a parapneumonic effusion from an empyema. Also, it does not provide information about the stage of the condition. It is indicated for special cases, such as suspicion of pulmonary abscesses, bronchopleural fistulas, immunodepressed patients, or in empyemas that do not respond to the usual medical management. In those cases, it is necessary to define anatomical details before a surgical intervention (Figs. 33.5 and 33.6).

Basic Laboratory Tests

C-reactive protein is useful for follow-up. A study conducted in Chile showed that when a final control after 48–72 h showed reduction up

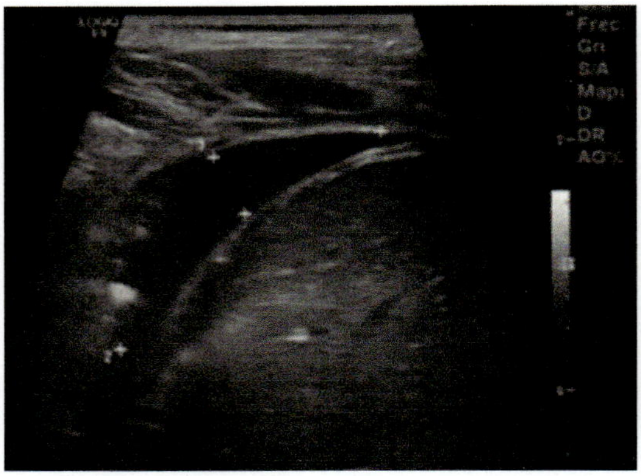

Fig. 33.3 Chest echography of 10-year-old schoolchild with evolving pneumonia shows free anechoic fluid with no septum

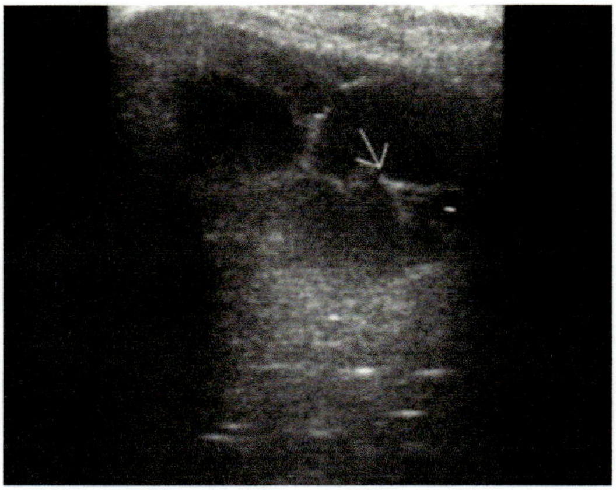

Fig. 33.4 Chest echography of 6-year-old child evolving with empyema shows septum (*arrows*) and anechoic fluid collected

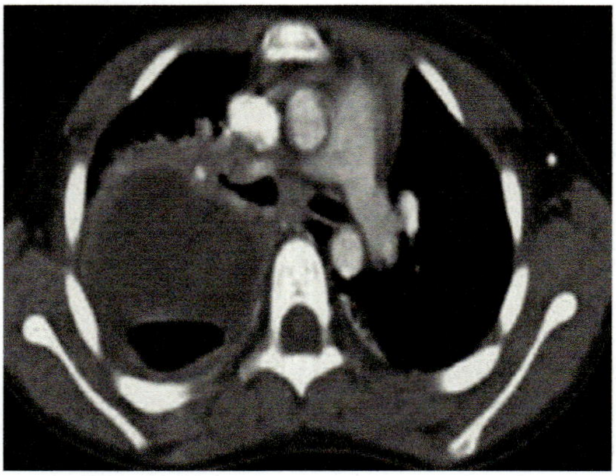

Fig. 33.5 Computerized axial tomography of the chest shows right upper lobe pulmonary abscess: thick wall, filled cavity, and air level

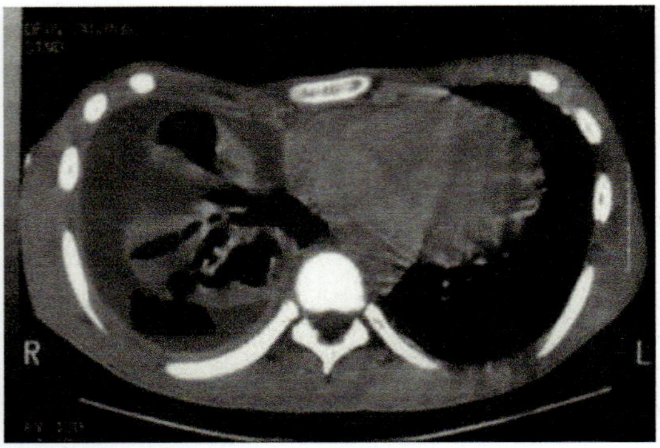

Fig. 33.6 Computerized axial tomography of the chest shows right lower lobe with empyema, necrotizing pneumonia, and bronchopleural fistula

to 50% relative to the initial value of the CRP, it could be used to predict a shorter hospitalization stay (<10 days). The use of procalcitonin may have prognostic importance when assessing the suppuration risk.

Microbiological Study

If there is a suspicion of pneumonia that has been complicated by pleural effusion, or if there are risk factors related to the patient of severe deterioration, two hemocultures must always be taken. For complicated pneumonia, positive results increase up to 10% to 22%, and it gives information about etiology in accordance to the antibiogram and minimum inhibitory concentration (MIC), especially for pneumococcal suppurated pneumonias.

Sputum study is not recommended in children, with the exception of special cases, such as if there is suspicion of tuberculosis.

Thoracentesis

This procedure must be performed when the pleural space is filled and larger than 10 mm, more than a fourth of the hemithorax is compromised, and also when a differential diagnosis is needed. Before the procedure, certain possible situations that would increase the complication risks must be assessed: hemorrhagic diathesis, thrombocytopenia <50,000, dermic compromise in the puncture site, and mechanical ventilation using high pressures. The pleural fluid sample must be taken under anaerobic conditions and its pH must be tested immediately. The amount of pleural fluid to be obtained must be sufficient for microbiology and cytochemistry analysis.

A pleural sample can be analyzed by different studies:

- Microbiology: Gram staining, aerobic culture, anaerobic culture (infrequent), latex agglutination test or PCR for pneumococcus, microbacteria, or other agents, staining for acid/alcohol-resistant bacillus, culture for microbacteria
- Cytology: Differential cell count, analysis of malignant cells
- Biochemistry: pH, glucose, LDH, proteins, adenosine deaminase (ADA), amylase, cholesterol, and triglycerides

Treatment

The objectives of treatment are to stop the infection, restore the normal physiology of the pleural fluid, and restore the normal function of the lung. To achieve this, the pleural cavity has to be sterilized and the lung expanded as early as possible.

Nevertheless, treatment of septic compromise must be a priority. Patients must be admitted to intensive medical care units according to the seriousness of their condition.

Available treatment alternatives include these:

- Intravenous antibiotics.
- Therapeutic thoracentesis.
- Chest pleural tube.
- Intrapleural fibrinolytics (IPF).
- Surgery: Minimally invasive thoracotomy, video-assisted thoracoscopic surgery (VATS), and, rarely, open decortication. In these cases, it is necessary to create a tiered work algorithm to minimize hospitalization days while at the same time ensuring the best efficacy and efficiency (Fig. 33.7).

Antibiotics

Antibiotics use is guided by local epidemiology (most frequent bacteria, antibiotic resistance) and how serious is the clinical condition of the child.

Antibiotics must cover *Streptococcus pneumoniae*. In our environment in Chile, ampicillin and penicillin are the first choice for antibiotics, and they reach adequate concentrations in the pleural fluid. *Staphylococcus aureus* coverage must be considered, especially when managing a pneumatocele (Fig. 33.8) or when there is a previous history of transient immune suppression of viral infections such as smallpox, influenza, and measles. The addition of antibiotic coverage for anaerobic and gram-negative microorganisms must be considered in children with aspiration risk and with secondary pulmonary abscess (Fig. 33.9), surgery, or trauma. When the culture results are ready, the antibiotic therapy is adjusted according to the microorganism and its sensitivity.

Intravenous antibiotic therapy is always recommended, for no less than 7 days, and it should be maintained during 3 days after the fever has resolved and after the chest tube has been removed, to complete 2–3 weeks of full treatment. The initial schedule is ampicillin (200 mg/kg/day) for children who are under 2 years old, and penicillin G sodium (200,000 U/kg/day) for patients over 2 years old. When a resistant strain is suspected, cefotaxime (150 mg/kg/day) or ceftriaxone (75–100 mg/kg/day) may be used. For patients whose condition is serious, other treatment is used in combination ($FiO_2 > 40\%$, ICU admittance, related shock, abscess present), such as cloxacillin (150–200 mg/kg/day) or clindamycin (30 mg/kg/day), plus a third-generation cephalosporin (ceftriaxone or cefotaxime). Rarely, vancomicine is used at 40–60 mg/kg/day.

Repeated Thoracentesis

Thoracentesis is a procedure that requires sedation and technical ability. As part of the diagnosis process, its usefulness is clear to define what

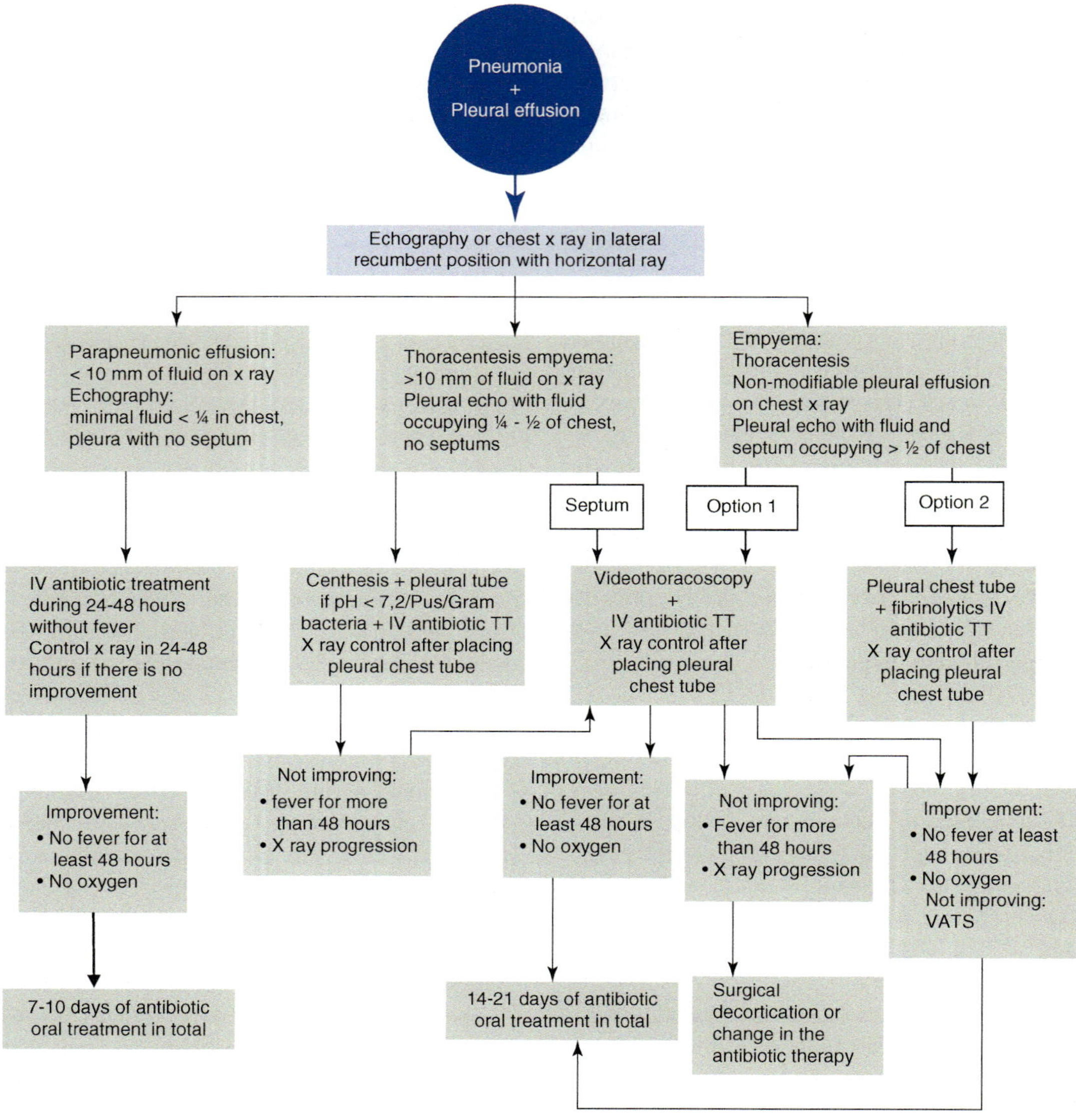

Fig. 33.7 Treatment algorithm for pleural empyema

approach to follow, although as a therapeutic measure in children it has not been validated, and even though it is less invasive, it represents a repeated trauma, and therefore early insertion of a chest tube is preferable.

Pleural Chest Tube

In the same way as happens with thoracentesis, this insertion must be done in the medial axillary line, over the superior rim of the rib, in the point where an imaginary line goes from the nipple to the tip of the scapula.

The placement of a chest tube is indicated for every complicated pleural effusion or empyema occupying more than half the thorax, or more than a fourth of the thorax, which does not respond to antibiotics or diagnostic and evacuation thoracentesis, or if there is related respiratory difficulty.

It is recommended to perform this as early as possible, because as time passes fluid aspiration

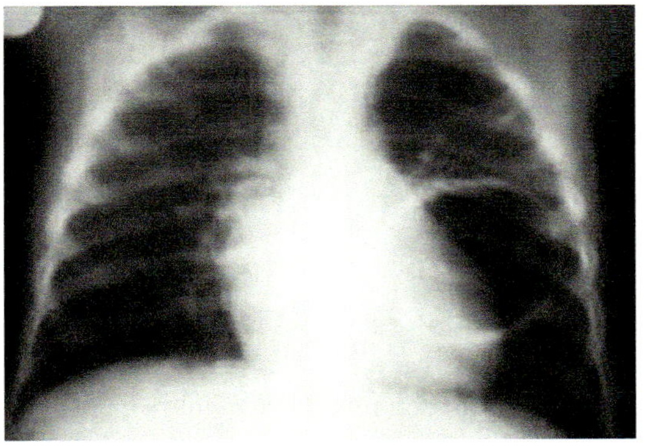

Fig. 33.8 Pneumatocele. Chest X-ray in 10-month-old infant shows left upper lobe pneumatocele

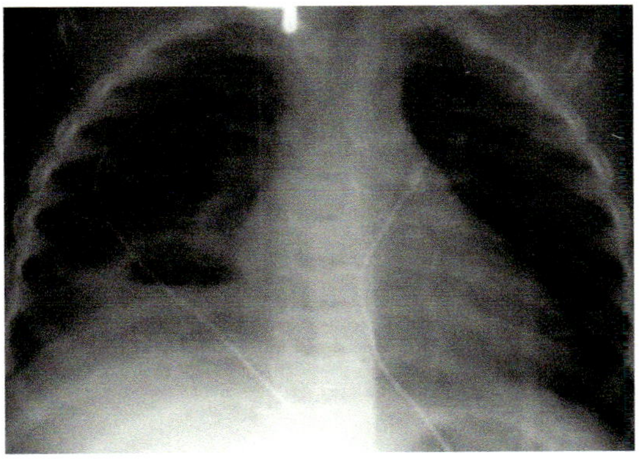

Fig. 33.9 Pulmonary abscess. Chest X-ray in 14-month-old infant evolving with sepsis and pulmonary abscess in the right middle lobe

becomes more complicated, because of the quick appearance of septa.

This procedure must be performed by trained medical personnel, under adequate sedation and anesthesia, using sterile technique, and ideally using chest echography visualization.

The patient must be connected to a drainage system with unidirectional flow, which must be positioned lower in relation to the patient and must have a water seal. Every pleural chest tube must be controlled with X-rays and the output and permeability must be regularly checked. The use of pigtail chest tubes placed using the Seldinger technique has advantages when placing the optimum drainage of the pleural cavity, and even more so when used in combination with fibrinolytics.

If after 48 h there is still high fever, the output is scarce or nonexistent, or there is no improvement in the chest X-ray, the recommendation is to conduct an echography to rule out the presence of liquid in cysts, or extensive or necrotizing underlying pneumonia.

The chest tube must stay in place until the output is less than 25–50 ml/day, or 1–1.5 ml/ kg/ day for infants, with improvement in the X-ray and clinical conditions.

Pleural Drainage Tube with Associated Fibrinolytics

The pleural drainage tube is the recommended nonsurgical option in septated empyemas. The use of intrapleural fibrinolytics (IPF) is based on the idea of smoothing the fibers and cleaning the lymphatic pores, thus improving the drainage of the accumulated fluid. The most frequent adverse effects described are fever, sometimes pain, hypersensitivity reactions, and, rarely, pleural hemorrhage. Nevertheless, urokinase has been studied only in randomized and controlled studies in children, showing effectivity and safety, and reducing the days of use of the pleural tube and hospitalization.

The recommended dose of urokinase for those patients over 10 kg is 40,000 U in 40 ml intravenous saline at 0.9%, twice per day for 3 days. If the patient's weight is less than 10 kg, the dose must be reduced to 10,000 U diluted in 10 ml intravenous saline. The results reported are similar for children with septated empyemas in comparison to children who underwent primary video-assisted thoracoscopic surgery.

Surgery

Surgery is indicated in situations of complicated empyema, with multiple segmentations, or when conservative treatment with antibiotics and drainage using pleural tubes has failed.

Among the surgical possibilities we have minimum thoracotomy or video-assisted thoracoscopic surgery. In both procedures the purulent material, with nonrecoverable tissue and detritus, is removed, and then the area is profusely irrigated to clean the cavity. It is important to conduct these procedures when the patient is hemodynamically stable and with a postsurgical phase in a critical care unit.

Video-assisted thoracoscopic surgery is done using two or three small chest incisions through which the instruments and the camera are inserted. It allows conducting an early cleaning of the pleural space in those empyemas that have progressed to phase II or are fibrinopurulent, with inefficiently drained loculations. During the past years its superiority over the minimum thoracotomy has been proven, because it is less invasive, compromises fewer structures, and reduces pain, infection, movement limitation, and allows healing. In the beginning it was used as rescue therapy when the initial treatment of the empyema failed. The average of hospitalization days for a child with pleural empyema treated with the classic treatment is between 15 and 21 days, which is significantly superior to the average number of hospitalization days for other acute pediatric pathologies. Hospitalization extension is a factor that increases the costs of any pathology, and in this way the impacts of these prolonged hospitalizations are translated into a high economic and social cost, besides school and work absenteeism, along with a greater risk of nosocomial infections.

There is recent evidence suggesting that the use of video-assisted thoracoscopic surgery reduces hospitalization days, as well as fever and needed pleural drainage, in hospitalized pediatric patients because of a septated empyema, with a minimal post-procedure morbidity if the procedure is done by experienced surgery groups. Nevertheless, all the published studies are retrospective, and therefore the results do not provide concluding evidence that may allow us to recommend video-assisted thoracoscopic surgery as the primary choice treatment when facing a septated empyema. For complicated empyema in children, the use of intrapleural fibrinolytics is one option whose results are comparable to those obtained when primary video-assisted thoracoscopic surgery is used. So, the controversy about the optimal management of this pathology persists, and the therapeutic choice is still dependent on the experience of the facility where treatment takes place.

Follow-Up

A chest X-ray must be done as a control test 4 to 6 weeks after hospital discharge. In this control, the pulmonary examination still may be altered, with reduced pulmonary murmur and some degree of dullness in the affected area, which can be explained by the residual pleural enlargement.

Immunity studies are recommended in patients with recurrent infections or an infection caused by atypical agents. It is recommended to conduct a sweat test in patients who have complicated pneumonias caused by *Staphylococcus aureus* or *Pseudomonas aeruginosa*.

Prognosis

The prognosis of pleural empyema in children is excellent. Follow-up studies have shown that no matter what treatment was administered, most of the children fully recover and pulmonary function returns to normal levels. Chest radiography is normal in 60% to 80% of the cases after 3 months, 90% at 6 months, and all cases after 18 months.

Summary

Suppurated complications of pneumonia during pediatric age are more frequent in infants, especially in the population with little to no coverage of conjugate vaccines for *Haemophilus influenzae* and *Streptococcus pneumoniae*. Special populations such as immunosuppressed or immunodeficient patients, and patients with nosocomial pneumonia, particularly those using invasive mechanical ventilation, require a special approach, wherein a different microbiology as well as the risk factors must be considered.

Empyema is the most common suppurated complication. It causes prolonged hospitalizations, although when compared to the adult population, there is a lower death rate. During the past years, this pathology has increased even in developed countries or slightly underdeveloped, as Chile is within Latin America. This epidemiological fact is related to pneumococcus strains, which are more suppurated, even when they are at MIC less than 2 μg/ml, and it is also related in some countries to methicillin-resistant community *Staphylococcus aureus*.

Management should be gradual in accordance with the amount and presence of suppuration in the pleural space. An important support element in the diagnosis is chest echography with Doppler, which shows the extension of the effusion and the presence of loculations. Computerized axial tomography must be reserved for studying complications that may potentially require a surgical solution, such as bronchopleural fistulas or pulmonary abscesses that do not respond to medical treatment.

In fibrinopurulent states, where more than 25% of the pleural space is occupied and the patients have a septic appearance, besides respiratory failure, chest tubes should be placed early in the therapy. The use of pigtail chest tubes inserted using the Seldinger technique, in association with IV beta-lactam antibiotics, yields an adequate disease resolution in most cases. When there are partitioned empyemas, usually at more than 72 h of evolution when the diagnosis is done (late diagnosis), or in patients who do not respond to early chest tube insertion, a video-assisted thoracoscopic surgery (VATS) can be used, as well as intrapleural fibrinolytics. In relation to antibiotic treatment, beta-lactam antibiotics, especially ampicillin for patients less than 2 years old, is still the treatment of choice because of its favorable MIC. The exception are those countries that have high rates of resistant pneumococcus (MIC >2 μg/ml), community-resistant *Staphylococcus aureus*, or low adherence to conjugated immunization against *Streptomyces aureus*.

Sources

Arancibia F, Vega-Briceño L, Pizarro ME, Pulgar D, Holmgren P, Bertrand P, Rodríguez JI, Sánchez I. Empiema y efusión pleural en niños. Rev Chil Infect. 2007;24(6):454–61.

Avansino JR, Goldman B, et al. Primary operative versus nonoperative therapy for pediatric empyema: a meta-analysis. Pediatrics. 2005;115:1652–9.

Balfour-Lynn IM, Abrahamson E, Cohen G, Hartley J, King S, Parikh D, Spencer D, Thomson AH, Urquhart D, Paediatric Pleural Diseases Subcommittee of the BTS Standards of Care Committee. BTS guidelines for the management of pleural infection in children. Thorax. 2005;60:i1–i21.

Bradley J, Byington CL, Shah S, et al. The management of community-acquired pneumonia in infants and children older than 3 months of age: clinical practice guidelines by the Pediatric Infectious Diseases Society and the Infectious Diseases Society of America. Clin Infect Dis. 2011;53:e25–76.

Fuchs S, Fischer GB, Black RE, Lanata C. The burden of pneumonia in children in Latin America. Pediatr Respir Rev. 2005;6:83–7.

Holmgren L, Chateau B. Pleuroneumonía. In: Sánchez I, Prado F, editors. En: Enfoque clínico de las enfermedades respiratorias del niño. Santiago: Ediciones Universidad Católica de Chile; 2007.

Liu YH, Lin YC, Liang SJ, et al. Ultrasound-guided pigtail catheters for drainage of various pleural diseases. Am J Emerg Med. 2010;28:915–21.

Paz F, Céspedes P. Derrame pleural y empiema complicado en niños. Evolución y factores pronósticos. Rev Méd Chile. 2001;129:1289–96.

Rudan I, Boschi-Pinto C, Biloglav Z, et al. Epidemiology and etiology of childhood pneumonia. Bull WHO. 2008;86:408.

Schultz KD, Fan LL, Pinsky J, Ochoa L, Smith EO, Kaplan SL, Brandt ML. The changing face of pleural empyemas in children: epidemiology and management. Pediatrics. 2004;113(6):1735–40.

Pneumonia Caused by Emerging Viral Agents

34

Cecilia Perret Pérez and Marcela Ferrés Garrido

Contents

Emerging viruses that cause pneumonia in humans have a common trait: they are all zoonoses. Normally, these agents circulate in the animal population, often without causing morbidity, but under certain circumstances they can move to human hosts, which determines the occurrence of a new type of disease. Nature holds many examples of such diseases, including avian influenza, Ebola, and severe acute respiratory syndrome (SARS). In this chapter we review agents that have provoked major concern outside their country of origin, but also Hanta virus, because of the endemic nature it has acquired in Chile.

Middle East Respiratory Syndrome

The Middle East respiratory syndrome (MERS) is caused by MERS-CoV, a recently identified coronavirus. Several coronaviruses can cause upper respiratory tract infections, but in some cases they can also produce lower respiratory tract infections and flu-like states. The SARS coronavirus and MERS-CoV are two pathogens from the coronavirus family that predominantly cause serious lower tract respiratory infections with a high mortality rate, but they are genetically different viruses.

C. Perret Pérez · M. Ferrés Garrido (✉)
Department of Pediatrics, School of Medicine, Pontificia Universidad Católica de Chile, Santiago, Chile
e-mail: cperret@med.puc.cl; mferres@med.puc.cl

P. Bertrand, I. Sánchez (eds.), *Pediatric Respiratory Diseases*,
https://doi.org/10.1007/978-3-030-26961-6_34

MERS-CoV was first identified in 2012 following the death of a patient in Saudi Arabia with a serious respiratory infection. This finding led to the retrospective diagnosis of the first cases of an in-hospital outbreak during 2012 in Jordan. Most cases have been recorded in the Middle East, with more than 75% of the cases in Saudi Arabia and some cases outside this region affecting travelers. The mortality rate of MERS is approximately 30%.

Information about the MERS mechanism of transmission is still limited, but it is likely to occur through droplets and by direct and indirect contact with infected respiratory secretions. Aerosol transmission has not been ruled out. Currently, transmission between humans is limited and occasional, with a low secondary attack rate. Isolated cases have been recorded, consisting of nosocomial and household outbreaks, but transmission is not sustained over time. This was the situation in the major South Korean outbreak, which originated through a case in Saudi Arabia and affected more than 180 people. Adequate infection control measures in healthcare rapidly limit in-hospital transmission.

Genetic analysis shows that the human MERS-CoV is quite similar to the virus found in bats and essentially identical to that observed in camels. The virus appears to have originated in bats, transitioning through camels, probably in Africa, and afterward being transmitted to humans. Serological studies do not show its presence in humans before 2012, but it has been observed in camels since the 1990s. This observation suggests that camels are the reservoirs of the virus, which can be transmitted to humans through direct contact with these animals or through consumption of their milk: 1599 cases had been diagnosed by July 2015, with 574 deaths [World Health Organization (WHO)]. Of these patients, 63% are male, with an average age of 48 years (Fig. 34.1). In children, the disease tends to be milder or asymptomatic, with severe cases resulting from a comorbidity. Incubation, defined as the period between the primary and the secondary case, is estimated to last an average of 5 days (2–14 days).

Clinical presentation is characterized by fever, cough, myalgia, and diarrhea. The disease has a wide symptomatic spectrum, which can range

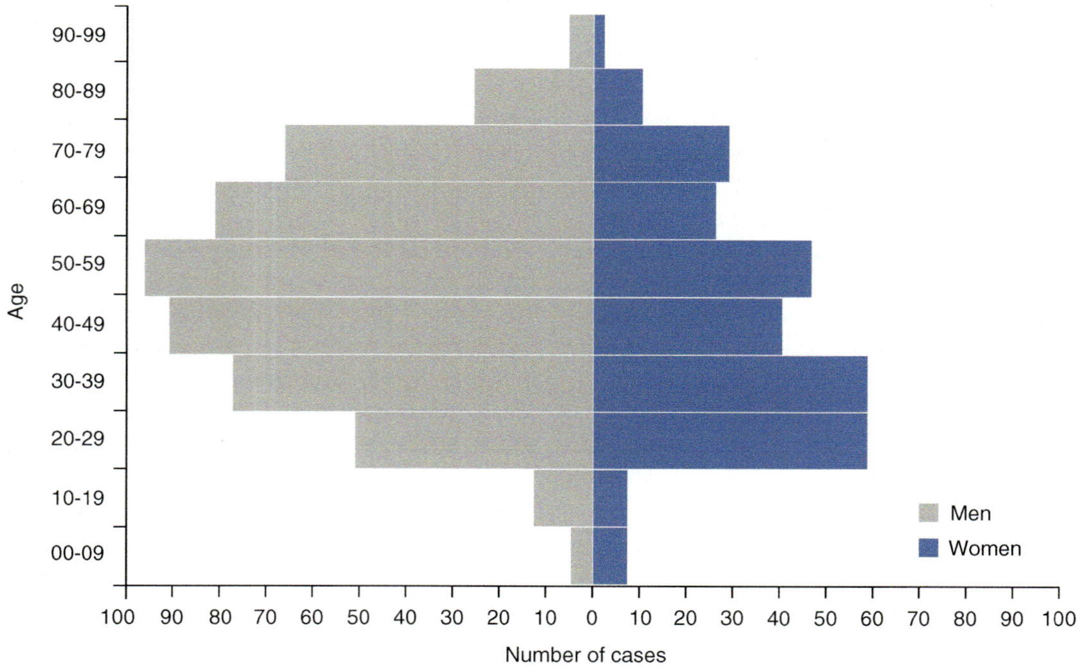

Fig. 34.1 Age distribution for MERS. (Source: http://ecdc.europa.eu/en/publications/Publications/RRA-MERS-CoV-thirteenth-update.pdf)

from asymptomatic infections to fulminant respiratory failure, which is related to high mortality. Patients evolve rapidly (5-day period on average) to respiratory and kidney failure, requiring ventilation support and intensive care management in more than 60% of cases. Diagnostic confirmation is achieved through viral isolation in laboratories with biosecurity clearance level 3; alternatively, the virus is detected in respiratory samples through molecular biology techniques (polymerase chain reaction, PCR), which are only available in reference laboratories. In patients who have displayed symptoms for more than 14 days, the determination of specific antibodies is recommended.

There is no specific treatment, because no antiviral therapy is available, only support measures in intensive care for the most serious cases. There is no specific preventive vaccine. This infection should be suspected in every traveler who reports having traveled to the Arabian Peninsula during the past 14 days and who also presents with respiratory symptoms and fever.

Severe Acute Respiratory Syndrome/Asian Pneumonia

SARS is the first identified coronavirus capable of producing a serious pulmonary disease, unlike those previously known (HCoV-229E and HCoV-OC 43), which cause the common cold. SARS emerged in late 2002 in China and quickly disseminated through Southeast Asia, Europe, Africa, and America. Bats were its presumed reservoir, and it was transferred to humans through civets. This virus caused great international alarm because of its rapid progression and its seriousness, resulting from extensive and rapidly progressing pneumonia with a mortality rate around 50%. Health workers were particularly affected. The most constant symptoms during admissions were high fever, malaise, cough, and headache, followed by diarrhea and prolonged fever.

More than 8000 cases were noted, causing more than 700 deaths. Thanks to international coordination under WHO leadership, the epidemic was controlled in July 2003. There were five clear objectives, which were achieved in record time: identification of the etiological agent, development of diagnostic tests for virus detection, creation and evaluation of epidemiological treatment protocols to reduce morbidity and mortality, definition of key epidemiological parameters to control transmission, and formulation of appropriate public health measures.

SARS demonstrated that coronaviruses can cause serious lower respiratory infections, which would later be observed for HCoV-NL63 and HCoV-HKU 1. To date, no new circulation of this agent has been proven.

HCoV-NL 63 and HCoV-HKU1

Coronavirus NL 63, which belongs to coronavirus group I, was discovered for the first time in a child with bronchiolitis in the Netherlands in 2004, and then ratified in small children hospitalized for serious respiratory infections. HKU1, which belongs to the coronavirus group II identified in 2005, was also shown to be capable of causing a lower respiratory tract infection. Both have been described throughout the world, proving their ubiquity. This virus is detected in up to 10% of acute respiratory disease cases, and its symptoms range from upper respiratory disease, including flu-like disease, fever, rhinitis, odynophagia, and cough, to serious conditions with a rapidly progressing respiratory disease. Infection by HCoV-N63 in children manifests as an obstructive laryngotracheitis in up to 45% of cases in comparison with children not infected by this virus.

The first HCoV-HKU1 viruses were described in elderly patients with preexisting conditions that caused their death. Some later studies, which considered children as well as adults, have confirmed that infection caused by this coronavirus may worsen the health status of individuals with underlying diseases, so that they need to be hospitalized more often. As with HcoV-N63, infection causes upper respiratory tract symptoms, such as fever, coryza, odynophagia, and coughing. Wheezing, pneumonia, and bronchiolitis may also be present. In children a greater frequency of feverish convulsions has been observed in comparison with children who were not infected by HCoV-HKU1.

HCoV-NL63 and HCoV-HKU1 are viruses that tend to manifest as a common cold, just as the usual coronaviruses HCoV-229E and HCoV-OC43; nevertheless, in small children, elderly patients, and immunosuppressed patients, they can cause serious respiratory disease with a high mortality rate.

Avian Influenza

The influenza A virus is widespread in nature: its main reservoir is domestic and feral birds. Several types exist, according to their hemagglutinin (H) and neuraminidase (N) makeup, only two of which have recently circulated among humans and are causing seasonal outbreaks: H1N1 and H3N2.

The animal reservoir of the virus is large and varied. Several subtypes have been described, which include 17 hemagglutinin and 9 neuraminidase types. These zoonotic viruses may cause diseases and infections in several animals, generally pigs and poultry. These zoonotic viruses in particular adapt very poorly to humans, so they seldom cause human diseases, which are limited to outbreaks circumscribed in terms of time and population. Nevertheless, human cases of A H5N1 were observed in Hong Kong for the first time in 1997 and have continued being reported to date. More than 700 cases have been notified, all in Asia and Northern Africa, with 413 deaths. Most cases are isolated, with some intrafamilial clusters being described. Human-to-human transmission is rare, which reflects the poor ability of the virus to adapt to human respiratory mucosa. The persistence of the circulation of these viruses and the great genetic variability of the influenza A virus make us fear that the avian virus may adapt to humans, which would ease its transmission among the human population, potentially causing a pandemic: this is what happened with the H1N1 influenza A, which had a porcine origin and adapted to humans, creating a pandemic in 2009.

The first cases of human infection caused by H7N9 influenza A were reported in China during 2013, and most of these were related in one way or another to contact with poultry, whether direct or environmental in markets where live birds are commercialized. By 2015 there had been 488 confirmed H7N9 influenza cases in China since the beginning of the outbreak, with 185 deaths. This virus does not seem to spread easily among humans, and there has been no proof of sustained human transmission, although its transmission potential seems to be more effective than that of the H5N1 influenza A virus. A couple of cases have been reported outside China: a traveler in Malaysia who stayed in China and a man and his wife who were diagnosed in Canada in January 2015 after traveling to China (WHO). There are no recorded secondary cases in these countries, which confirms its low probability of human-to-human transmission.

Cases have been observed during the coldest seasons in China. From December 2014 to February 2015, 83 new cases were diagnosed, with an average age of 56 years and 19 deaths. Of these newly diagnosed patients, 72% are male, and 93% of patients have had direct contact with poultry markets. The incubation period is 4 days (2–8 days). Even though mild cases have been described, most diagnoses have been serious, with a mortality rate close to 35%. Hospitalized patients have a febrile disease, with temperatures above 102.2 °F and cough. The disease progresses swiftly from moderate to severe. In contrast to human seasonal influenza, most patients do not report rhinorrhea or odynophagia.

In a set of hospitalized patients, the disease progressed swiftly for an average of 3 days after its onset, counting from the beginning of the symptoms until hospitalization. Almost 70% required invasive mechanical ventilation, with a death rate of 30%. Deaths from respiratory failure reached 38%, and 62% were caused by septic shock. Most deaths corresponded to elderly patients and with a underlying disease, as well as to the use of systemic steroids. Diagnosis is performed by identifying viral RNA through RT-PCR in respiratory tract samples, obtained through swabbing or nasal suctioning.

As well as other avian influenza A virus, this virus is sensitive to oseltamivir and is resistant to adamantines. Oseltamivir is indicated for hospitalized or ambulatory patients, whether they have been confirmed or are under suspicion of being infected by H7N9 influenza, even if more than 48 h have passed since the onset of symptoms. The dosage and timeframe of therapy are not clearly established for serious patients, but a longer timeframe is suggested, around 10 days and in higher doses. In patients with mild and noncomplicated infections, therapy must continue for 5 days. Patients with mild infection, who require ambulatory treatment and whose only exposure factor is travel to an area where there are recorded cases, in humans or birds, have no empirical indication for oseltamivir.

Isolated cases of avian origin in humans caused by the influenza H10N8 virus and H6N1 have been observed in China. These facts prove that in these zoonotic influenza cases vigilance is extremely important, given its pandemic potential, so it is crucial to pay close attention to travelers and enforce local vigilance.

Hantavirus

In 1993, a new virus from the the Bunyaviridae family was identified in the United States of America. It was named "virus with no name" and was deemed responsible for what is now known as cardiopulmonary hantavirus syndrome (síndrome cardiopulmonar por hantavirus, SCPH), a feverish disease characterized by respiratory insufficiency and shock. This discovery, which was a new zoonosis, in practice extended over the next years across the whole American continent. In this process, new clinical manifestations were recognized and new agents identified, including the Andes, Laguna Negra, Araquara, and Choclo viruses, which are prevalent in Chile, Argentina, Paraguay, Brazil, and Panama, respectively.

Their natural reservoir are Sigmondontinae rodents, which belong to the Muridae family. These animals develop a chronic infection with an intermittent viral and asymptomatic excretion. Stress situations, such as lack of food during birthing periods, cold, or habitat interventions such as logging, have been associated with greater virus excretion in these rodents. Mice excrete the virus through their feces, urine, and saliva, contaminating the environment. The most representative virus-carrying rodents are *Peromyscus maniculatus* or "deer mouse" (which carries the no-name virus), *Oligoryzomys longicaudatus* or "long-tailed mouse," and *Calomys laucha*, among others. Humans acquire the infection through the inhalation of secretions (stools, urine, saliva) of infected rodents. The Andes virus, predominant in Southern Argentina and the single causal agent in Chile, is only transmitted through close human-to-human contact.

Hantaviruses are spherical viruses with a trisegmented RNA genome with a lipid envelope through which two glycoproteins (Gn and Gc) protrude. These three segments code through proteins such as RNA polymerase (L segment); glycoproteins Gn and Gc (M segment), which are important in the recognition of β3 integrins that the virus use as receptors; and nucleoprotein (S segment), a highly conserved protein used for the laboratory diagnosis of these agents. The lipid envelope is sensitive and is destroyed by detergents, chloride, desiccation, and sun exposure. All these actions form the basis of the prevention and control recommendations for hantavirus infections.

The agent enters the respiratory tract through inhalation of the aerosolized virus in the environment or through contaminated human secretions. After an incubation period that ranges from 1 to 6 weeks (18 days on average), nonspecific symptoms begin, including fever, myalgias, and headache, plus digestive symptoms (more common in children). This stage is followed by progressive respiratory disease and finally by respiratory failure, which is the most serious manifestation of this infection. In 100% of the cases of acute infection, the virus is present in all the white cells and, in variable proportions, in plasma, respiratory secretions, saliva, and urine. Also, viral RNA has been detected in white cells up to 15 days before and 90 days after the first symptoms.

Interaction with β3 integrins and the replication of viral endothelial cells of various tissues appear to alter the modulation functions of permeability in these cells, especially increasing the permeability in small lung vessels, which favors arterial hypotension, thrombocytopenia, and hypoxia from plasma flooding into alveolar spaces. Protein N and superficial glycoproteins stimulate the production of specific and neutralizing antibodies, which have been associated with better survival outcomes when they increase prematurely.

Patients who progress to the cardiopulmonary phase, where respiratory failure sets in, require supplementary oxygen; in addition, more than two thirds need mechanical ventilation, and 50% of patients develop cardiogenic shock, which constitutes a poor prognosis factor. The increased vascularity rate explains the pulmonary edema observed during this stage. This functional alteration is transitory, lasting from 48 to 72 h; afterward, pulmonary function is quickly recovered following a brief period of noticeable diuresis. Cardiogenic shock is difficult to manage and is the main cause of death. The lethality of hanta cardiopulmonary syndrome is about 35%, and most deaths occur during the first 48 h of evolution.

The hemogram is the most useful general laboratory test for hypothesizing a diagnosis, because it can, from an early stage, reveal manifest reductions in the number of platelets as well as the presence of lymphocytes, which take the shape of immunoblasts. A late onset of hematocrit increase has been observed, which is concomitant with the beginning of the cardiopulmonary phase of the disease.

It is also helpful to test for LDH and transaminases, which increase nonspecifically. A chest X-ray may change in a matter of hours from a nonspecific interstitial pattern to diffuse pulmonary edema. The virological diagnosis is confirmed through RT-PCR in white cells or through the ELISA detection of specific IgM/IgG for each regional virus.

Currently, there is no specific treatment for hantavirus infection other than cardiopulmonary support. Patient should be monitored closely, preferably in an intensive care unit, to provide measures such as mechanical ventilation for breathing support, restriction of liquids, and vasoactive drugs. The use of an antiviral such as ribavirin has not been shown to be an effective treatment. Extracorporeal membrane oxygenation (ECMO) has been used as a rescue therapy in some cases of serious cardiopulmonary failure that do not respond to conventional ventilation and vasoactive drugs.

In Chile, two therapeutic options have been investigated for hantavirus: methylprednisolone in high doses and immune plasma with high neutralizing antibody titers. Only the latter strategy has shown promising results relative to mortality rate reduction when used immediately after symptom onset.

As a control measure in hospitalized patient management, and considering that hantavirus has been described as capable of causing nosocomial transmission, standard precautions must be taken: ideally, interning the patient in an individual room and wearing protection equipment [apron, gloves, face mask (no. 95) with a high efficiency filter, and security glasses], especially in procedures during which there is close contact with the patient's fluids, such as intubation, secretion suctioning, and retrieval of samples for laboratory tests.

Enterovirus D68

This viral agent, enterovirus D68, has been known since 1962, when it was isolated in children suffering from bronchiolitis and pneumonia. Because no widely available trials have been conducted, not much is known about its epidemiology and clinical manifestations. During the fall of 2014, Missouri and Illinois hospitals reported an unusual rise in the number of serious cases of children, with or without a background of obstructive disease, who presented with acute respiratory infection. Enterovirus D65 was detected in these patients by applying molecular biology techniques to respiratory samples.

The infection is more frequent in school-age children, whose most relevant clinical antecedent was the presence of previous persistent coughing, asthma, or wheezing episodes that may have required intensive care unit (ICU) management. The virulence of this agent is more impressive than that of other enteroviruses, considering that it was also identified as a causal agent of obstructive episodes in previously healthy children who, when treated with antiasthma therapy, did not respond adequately and had to be hospitalized in intensive care because of hypoxemia and, with some exceptions, had to receive mechanical ventilation.

The most common laboratory findings were high total neutrophils and chest X-ray showing peribronchial interstitial infiltrations, hyperinsufflation, and atelectasis.

As diagnostic tests improve in sensitivity and specificity, and their use becomes more widespread in pediatric centers, our understanding of the epidemiology and pathogeny of this viral agent will increase.

Polyomavirus

Two polyomaviruses with respiratory tropism were discovered in 2007 through deep sequencing of samples taken from respiratory secretions of symptomatic patients: polyomaviruses KI (KIPyV) and WU (WUPyV). These viruses can be found in the lower and upper respiratory tract of immunocompetent as well as immunocompromised patients. Their pathogenic role is not completely clear, because they usually occur at low frequency, have a low viral load, and are related to pathogens whose morbidity is better characterized. Diagnosis requires molecular techniques (real-time PCR), whose inclusion in future research will allow us to better characterize the epidemiology and clinical spectrum of the infections caused by these agents.

Sources

Arabi YM, Arifi AA, Balkhy HH, Najm Hani, Aldawood AS, Ghabashi A et al. Clinical course and outcomes of critically ill patients with Middle East respiratory syndrome coronavirus infection. Ann Intern Med 2014;160:389–397.

Confirmed human cases of avian influenza A (H7N9) reported to WHO. Report 18: data in WHO/HQ as of 14 July 2001. Disponible en: http://www.who.int/influenza/human_animal_interface/influenza_h7n9/18_report-webh7n9number_20140714.pdf?ua=1.

Ferres M, Vial P, Marco C, Yanez L, Godoy P, Castillo C, et al. Prospective evaluation of household contacts of persons with hantavirus cardiopulmonary syndrome in Chile. J Infect Dis. 2007;195(11):1563–71.

Figueiredo LT, Souza WM, Ferres M, Enria DA. Hantaviruses and cardiopulmonary syndrome in South America. Virus Res. 2014;187:43–54.

Forster J, Ihorst G, Rieger CH, Stephan V, Frank HD, Gurthet H, et al. Prospective population-based study of viral lower respiratory tract infections in children under 3 years of age (the PRIDE study). Eur J Pediatr. 2014;163:709–16.

Gao R, Cao B, Hu Y, Feng Z, Wang D, Hu W, et al. Human infection with a novel Avian-origin influenza A (H7N9) virus. N Engl J Med. 2013;368:1888–97.

Manigold T, Vial P. Human hantavirus infections: epidemiology, clinical features, pathogenesis and immunology. Swiss Med Wkly. 2014;144:w13937.

Martinez-Valdebenito C, Calvo M, Vial C, Mansilla R, Marco C, Palma RE, et al. Person-to-person household and nosocomial transmission of Andes hantavirus, Southern Chile, 2011. Emerg Infect Dis. 2014;20(10):1629–36.

Memish ZA, Al-Tawfiq JA, Assiri A, Al Rabiah FA, Al Hajjar S, Albarrak A, et al. Middle East respiratory syndrome coronavirus disease in children. Pediatr Infect Dis J. 2014;33:904–6.

MINSAL. Guía Clínica de Prevención, Diagnóstico y Trata-miento del Sindrome Cardiopulmonar por Hantavirus web site MINSAL. 2013.

Pyrc K, Berkhout B, van der Hoek L. The novel human coronaviruses NL63 and HKU1. J Virol. 2007;81(7):3051–7.

Rha B, Rudd J, Feikin D, Watson J, Curns AT, Swerdlow DL, et al. Update on the epidemiology of Middle East Respiratory Syndrome Coronavirus (MERS-CoV) infection, and guidance for the public, clinicians, and public health authorities: January 2015. MMWR. 2015;64(3):61–2.

Schountz T, Prescott J. Hantavirus immunology of rodent reservoirs: current status and future directions. Viruses. 2014;6(3):1317–35. https://doi.org/10.3390/v6031317.

WHO. Middle East respiratory syndrome coronavirus (MERS-CoV). Summary of Current Situation, Literature Update and Risk Assessment. 7 July 2015 WHO/MERS/RA/15.1.

Yang Y, Guo F, Zhao W, Gu Q, Huang M, Cao Q, et al. Novel Avian-Origin Influenza A (H7N9) in critically ill patients in China. Crit Care Med. 2015;43:339–45.

Pulmonary Tuberculosis

35

Carlos Casar Collazo, María Elena Guarda Barros, and Carolina Gvirtzman

Contents

Introduction

Tuberculosis has been present throughout the history of mankind since ancient times and has been variously described as "consumption," "White Plague," "lung weakness,", or "phthisis." Only in the 1890s was Robert Koch able to demonstrate that the disease was caused by *Mycobacterium tuberculosis*.

Currently, tuberculosis is still the most common disease in the world, causing the death of almost 2 million people per year and infecting almost a third of the world's population. Tuberculosis is an infectious disease caused by *Mycobacterium tuberculosis*, known as Koch's bacillus. This bacterium grows slowly, has a low primary toxicity, and is light sensitive.

C. Casar Collazo (✉) · M. E. Guarda Barros
Department of Pediatrics, Hospital Roberto del Río, Santiago, Chile

C. Gvirtzman
Department of Pediatrics, Hospital Garrahan, Buenos Aires, Argentina

P. Bertrand, I. Sánchez (eds.), *Pediatric Respiratory Diseases*,
https://doi.org/10.1007/978-3-030-26961-6_35

Epidemiology

Tuberculosis distribution is universal, although there are great differences in the incidence of different countries, with very high rates in Africa and Northern Asia and very low rates in North America and Western Europe. In America there are also notable differences between countries, with rates ranging from 12 per 100,000 inhabitants, as in Chile, Uruguay, Costa Rica, and Cuba, up to rates of 200 per 100,000 inhabitants in countries such as Haiti. Large differences can be observed in each country. In Chile, for instance, there are regions with a rate of 40 per 100,000 inhabitants and other areas with a rate of 9 per 100,000 inhabitants, which yields an average of 13 per 100,000 inhabitants for the total population and an average of 1.4 per 100,000 inhabitants under 15 years old.

The fact that a country or region may have a low tuberculosis rate does not mean that the disease has been eradicated from that area, because we know that tuberculosis infections acquired during childhood or youth can be reactivated during adulthood or old age. This realization forces us to sustain elimination and disease control programs for many years before eradication can be declared.

Factors such as overcrowding and poor-quality housing permit the transmission of the disease. Koch's bacillus is very light sensitive: just 5 min of light exposure are enough to inactivate this organism. Another important factor to consider is the reappearance of tuberculosis toward the end of the 1980s in developed countries, caused by the human immunodeficiency virus (HIV) epidemic, which in itself constituted a determinant factor for the death of these patients.

Vaccination programs using the Calmette and Guérin Bacillus, or BCG, vaccine have not changed the general tuberculosis prevalence for some of the countries in the region, but they have made a difference for the most serious presentations, miliary tuberculosis and tuberculous meningitis, especially in countries where coverage is very high (98%), as in Chile.

Etiology and Pathophysiology

The tuberculosis bacillus has multiple defensive mechanisms to protect itself against the immune system and to avoid being promptly recognized, which allows the affected individual to remain asymptomatic until the invasion has reached an advanced level. The main mechanism of immunological defense for Koch's bacillus is cellular immunity, which manages to isolate and eliminate the bacillus, although this often causes tissue damage.

Tuberculosis transmission is mostly transmitted through the airway, with the exception of gastrointestinal infection acquisition through contaminated milk, which has been solved by controlling bovine tuberculosis and industrializing milk production.

Pediatric tuberculosis is closely related to adult tuberculosis. When a child has tuberculosis, an adult gave that child the disease. If tuberculosis increases in a population under 15 years old, it must be assumed that the tuberculosis program is not functioning well.

In children, bacteriology has a low yield for bacilloscopy and positive culture, because these patients tend to have a low bacillus count and the bacteria are often absent from the airway, which serves as a communication path for the environment. So, providing accurate diagnoses in this population is difficult. Most of the tuberculosis cases in children are related to a primary infection caused by Koch's bacillus.

Most children who are exposed for the first time to *Mycobacterium tuberculosis* do not develop the disease, but only a latent infection, so they do not present with clinical or radiological evidence of the disease. Only children under 5 years old (and particularly those under 2 years old) and those who have some kind of immunosuppression develop tuberculosis. Pulmonary and extrapulmonary compromise commonly appears between 2 and 12 months after the primary infection.

Bacilli that manage to enter the bronchial airways reach the alveoli and produce a localized inflammatory process in the pulmonary parenchyma. From there, the bacilli will pass through

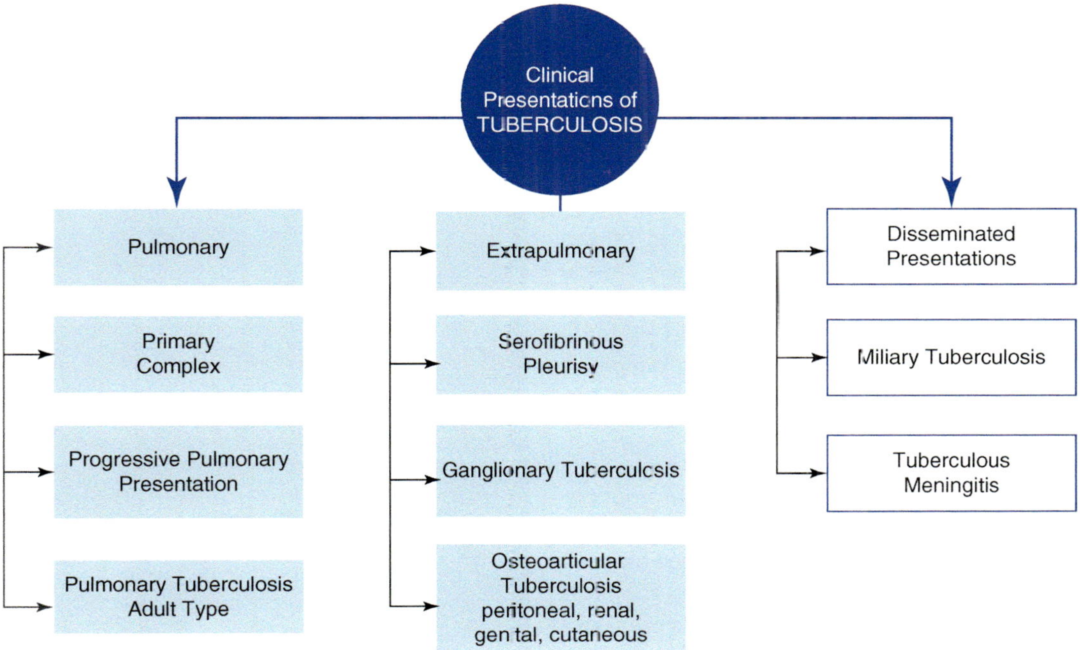

Fig. 35.1 Tberculosis clinical manifestations

the regional lymph nodes and, therefore, to the lymphatic system. The triad of pulmonary focus, local lymphangitis, and lymph nodes compromise is called the primary complex or "Ghon complex." Bacilli enter the systemic circulation through either the bloodstream or the lymph nodes. So, a hidden bacteremia is caused before the body can develop an adequate immune response to control the infection. Once Koch's bacillus reaches the target organs, it can survive as a latent infection during a long period and will cause extrapulmonary tuberculosis. Patients in whom the bacteremia is not controlled through their immune response will present with dissemination (miliary tuberculosis). During adolescence, reactivation of Koch's bacillus can produce tuberculosis with pulmonary or extrapulmonary presentations (Fig. 35.1).

Pulmonary Presentations

Pulmonary Infection or Classic Primary Complex

This presentation is the most common one (90%) and appears in a self-limited form. By having nonspecific respiratory symptoms such as cough and secretions, often it goes unnoticed and is confused with a banal viral infection. Phlyctenular keratoconjunctivitis and nodular erythema are infrequent signs. Small children and adolescents tend to be more symptomatic. Chest X-ray may show the classic radiological image of hilar adenopathy and, less frequently, a figure resembling a loaded barbell, which denotes Ghon's primary complex. Radiological signs tend to take 6–12 months to disappear, although calcifications may develop in the future.

Patients are diagnosed through a positive PPD test or a boosted PPD test, in the context of a contact study of a bacilliferous case. In these cases, it is important to implement a treatment, because the probability of developing the disease with pulmonary or extrapulmonary presentations increases during the first 2 years after the primary infection.

Pulmonary Disease: Progressive Pulmonary Presentations

Nowadays, this presentation is highly exceptional. The development of this clinical manifestation is basically determined by the immunity of the host, so it increases in children younger than 2 years old, children with a poor nutritional state, those who did not receive the BCG vaccine, or are HIV positive, as well as those who are exposed to close contact with bacilliferous sick patients. The pulmonary manifestation is very similar to the clinical presentation of any pneumonia: coughing, fever, expectoration, and dyspnea, and the differential diagnosis includes the suspicion of this possibility when there is no adequate clinical response. When there is a parenchymal progression to cavitary presentations, caseous pneumonia, or primary phthisis, the following symptoms can also be observed: asthenia, adynamia, night sweats, weight loss, and hemoptysis.

Chest X-ray shows condensations that become cysts from necrosis, which happens in necrotizing pneumonia in connection with the presence of large adenopathies. These adenopathies are rarely symptomatic, except when they compress a main bronchus or erode and drain the brionchus (bronchogenic dissemination). A positive culture result for Koch's bacillus is observed in more than 80% of the cases (Fig. 35.2). At times, bronchial compromise may progress to a complete expansion of the lung. In such situations, distal lesions disappear with radiological resolution.

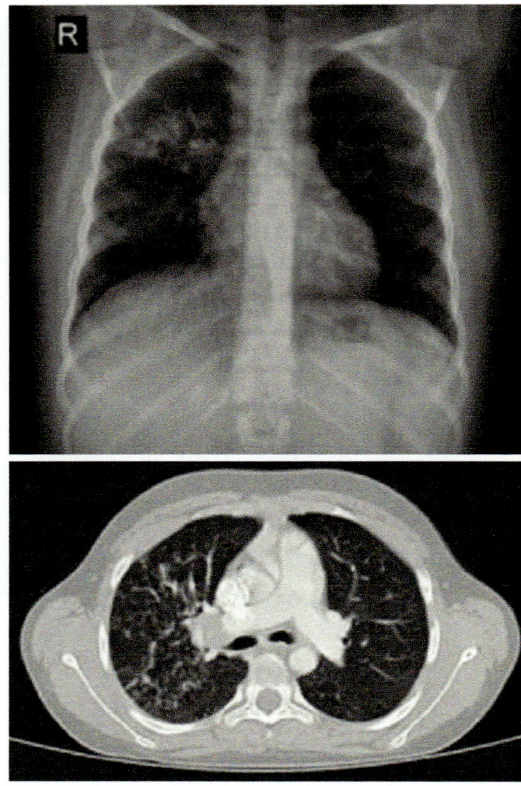

Fig. 35.2 Tuberculosis with bronchogenic dissemination in 10-year-old patient with an HIV infection responding poorly to antiretroviral therapy. Anteroposterior (AP) chest X-ray shows primary alveoli compromise in right upper lobe (RUL) (**a**) and during computed tomorgraphy (CT) (**b**), where bronchial invasion is observed in RUL bronchus and subsequent lumen obstruction

Adult-Type Tuberculosis

In high school seniors or adolescents, primary infection progresses to adult-type manifestations. In these patients there is a general health state compromise, fever, coughing, expectoration, hemoptoic or hemoptysis tear, and weight loss. Radiological images show infiltration, predominantly apical, in addition to excavations or caverns. Lesions in these patients are highly bacilliferous and connected to the external environment, so bacteriological tests are usually positive (Fig. 35.3).

Tuberculous Adenitis

Tuberculous adenitis is the most frequent extrapulmonary presentation. It usually presents as a localized adenopathy on a lymph node or lymph pack. It can involve any lymph group, but it usually appears on the head and neck.

Adenopathy can cause a subacute presentation with mild general symptomatology or none. During the examination, the adenopathy is mobile, painless, and without erythema. If it is not treated, it increases in size and a caseous necrosis appears. In this stage, the adenopathy acquires a typical erythema tone, with a fluid texture in the centre. If this adenopathy breaks, it may cause a skin fistula or scrofula, which chronically leaks. Pulmonary compromise must be ruled out for these patients. Differential diagnoses include lymphoma and certain infectious causes, so a biopsy is fundamental for making a definitive diagnosis.

Others

Patients can present with osteoarticular, renal, genitourinary, abdominal, adrenal, parotid,

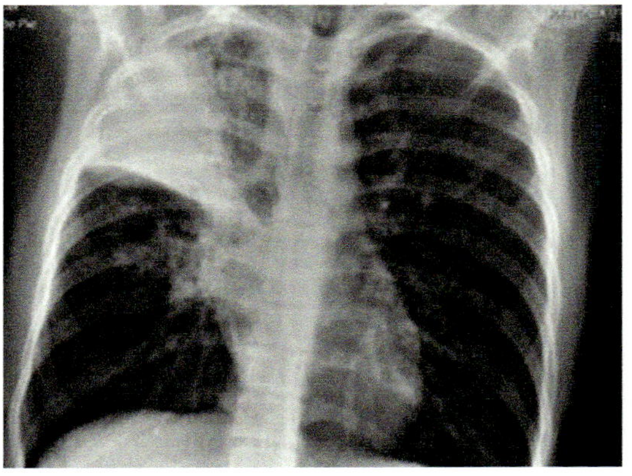

Fig. 35.3 Adult-type tuberculosis. AP radiography of 14-year-old adolescent who presented clinically with a prolonged fever and coughing with bacilliferous expectoration. Condensation in RUL is observed, secondary to alveolar compromise and atelectasis of the same zone, probably caused by lymph node compression of the corresponding bronchus

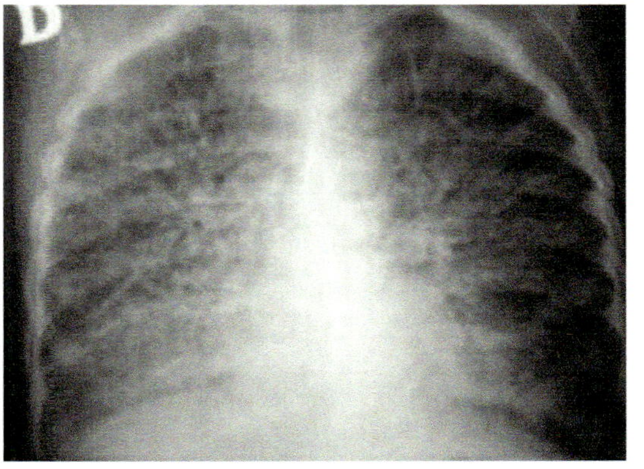

Fig. 35.4 Miliary tuberculosis. AP chest X-ray of an infant with no BCG vaccine and intrafamilial contact with an adult with bacilliferous tuberculosis. Diffuse bilateral granular compromise can be observed, consistent with miliary tuberculosis

ocular, and skin compromise. However, these extrathoracic presentations of tuberculosis are infrequent.

Disseminated Presentations

Disseminated presentations are serious and are characterized by a high mortality rate. They can be clinically present in three ways, depending on the immunological state of the patient and the number of bacilli that enter the bloodstream.

Miliary Tuberculosis

This presentation is more common in children who are younger than 5 years old, have with a poor nutritional state, and are immunosuppressed. The onset is 2–6 months after the first infection. Clinical manifestations are mixed and may depend on the number of bacilli that enter the bloodstream and the patient's immune response. Miliary tuberculosis can present itself as an unspecific infection, with an insidious onset, and without apparent seriousness or acute symptoms. As the infection progresses, fever, coughing, weight loss, anorexia, and night sweats start to appear. Three weeks after the onset of the symptoms, chest X-ray shows diffuse micronodular images (<2 mm) in both lung areas. Lesions can be detected early in the retrocardiac space of a lateral radiography. PPD tends to be negative in these patients, and diagnosis is made through physical examination, thoracic radiography, thoracic computed axial tomography scan, and eye examination (choroidal tuberculous can be seen). Confirmation can be obtained through bacteriological tests of expectorations, gastric content, pulmonary puncture, or mieloculture. Given the high meningitis risk, lumbar puncture is always recommended. Early clinical suspicion of meningitis is very important given its high morbidity and mortality rate as well as its neurological sequelae (Fig. 35.4).

Tuberculous Meningitis

This presentation is a meningoencephalitis that mostly compromises the base of the brain and the circle of Willis. Three developmental stages can be identified, which progress during 1 to 2 weeks. In infants and small children, progression can be faster, lasting only a few days. During stage 1, nonspecific signs are predominant, including fever, lack of energy, irritability, vomiting, constipation, and delays in psychomotor development. During stage 2, an intense headache appears, as well as explosive vomiting, disorientation, and seizures. In this stage, physical examination shows meningeal signs, compromise of the cranial pairs, focal neurological signs, or hemiparesis and endocranial hypertension. Stage 3 is the most serious one, as patients display severe consciousness impairment, which ranges from stupor to coma, hemiplegia, or tetraplegia. Severe endocranial hypertension, besides decerebrate or decorticate posture, can also be observed. These patients tend to have a negative PPD test, with thorax chest X-ray revealing parenchymal compromise. Computerized tomography (CT) shows several brain areas affected by strokes and infarctions, although in some cases tuberculomas may also be observed in the cerebral parenchyma. Diagnosis is based on alterations of the cerebrospinal fluid (CSF), which is characteristically clear and low in glucose. Cytochemical analysis also shows a minor presence of chloride, a high protein level, and a slight increase in predominantly mononuclear cells. Koch's culture, amplification methods, and adenosine deaminase (ADA) in the CSF are useful.

Connatal Tuberculosis

Connatal tuberculosis is fortunately a rare disease. It has a very high mortality rate, even when treated. It is sanguineously transmitted through the umbilical cord or through amniotic fluid aspiration during childbirth. Symptoms include respiratory failure, hepatosplenomegaly, lymphadenopathies, fever, abdominal distension, lethargy, and irritability. Skin lesions, jaundice, seizures, otorrhea, and diarrhea are seen less frequently. Some newborns present with severe septic shock.

Diagnostic Approach

Tuberculosis diagnosis in children is still a major challenge. In spite of numerous studies aimed at developing new techniques or improving on traditional ones, especially those associated with HIV infection, these techniques are not within the reach of the general population; therefore, treatment onset is frequently delayed.

In children, the diagnostic process starts when the clinician suspects the following situations:

1. Children exposed to a bacilliferous patient.
2. Children with an unresolved pneumonia, which does not respond to normal antimicrobial treatment, or with persistent signs in images.
3. Children with an adult-type presentation and compatible clinical findings.

The process begins with chest X-ray, both projections (anteroposterior and lateral), PPD testing, and expectoration bacilloscopy. Thorax radiography will show different images depending on the tuberculosis presentation affecting the patient. Complementary imaging with a computerized axial tomography scan is recommended when diagnosis is uncertain.

There are tests showing immune response to Koch's bacillus:

PPD Testing

The PPD test (*protein purified derivative*) is a protein concentrate of Koch's bacillus, Calmette–Guérin (BCG), and nontuberculous mycobacteria. The PPD test is highly sensitive but nonspecific for *Mycobacterium tuberculosis* infection. The test consists of 2–10 U of this concentrate delivered intradermally in the external radial side of the left forearm. Subsequently, the cellular immunity response to PPD inoculation is measured. The test uses a hypersensitive delayed response, the value of which peaks at 72 h. At this point, the extent of the transverse induration is measured (pencil test). Internationally, a PPD test is considered positive when it has an induration area equivalent to or greater than 10 mm. In children younger than 4 years old, with malnutrition, immunosuppression (HIV infection), or without BCG vaccine, a test is considered positive if induration reaches or surpasses 5 mm. A tuberculous boost is defined as an induration increase greater or equal to 10 mm with a difference greater than 6 mm, which happens in 3-month intervals (up to 2 years). This reaction is compatible with a recent infection. The PPD test can yield a "false negative" after a viral infection, live virus vaccination, immunosuppression, and in severe tuberculosis presentations, especially for the most widespread forms: 5% to 10% of tuberculous diseases yield a negative PPD test.

PPD test interpretation is difficult and may lead to confusion, particularly in countries with high BCG vaccine coverage. The PPD test is useful for diagnosing double tuberculous infections in countries with a low endemic rate of *Mycobacterium tuberculosis*, low infection incidence for nontuberculous mycobacteria, and high BCG vaccine coverage.

IGRAS

IGRAS assays (*interferon-gamma release assays*) measure lymphocytic response to interferon-γ when lymphocytes have been exposed to the Koch's bacillus antigen. Assays are more specific than PPD tests when diagnosing an infection, but their sensitivity varies. Because of this, they do not discriminate between latent and active infection. The current techniques are Quantiferon-TB GIT and Elispot-TB. IGRAS assays are mainly recommended for patients under high clinical suspicion in whom PPD or culture have produced negative results. The widespread use of IGRAS assays is limited by their high cost.

- *Bacteriological study. Mycobacterium tuberculosis* must be identified, which is especially difficult in children, because their lesions have a low bacillus count and they are usually poorly connected to the central airway.

Bacilloscopy requires at least 5000 BK/ml (two samples) to yield a positive result. A Ziehl–Neelsen stain is used, which requires a microscope with 1000× or greater magnification, and 10–15 min of exposure; alternatively, it is possible to use a fluorophore stain, which requires a 400× reduction in the magnification, and takes 2–3 min of exposure. WHO recommends the latter technique.

Culture requires 10 BK/ml to get a positive result and is the gold standard for diagnosis. In children it is rarely positive, except for the cases in which there are excavated lesions communicating with the central airway. Löwenstein–Jensen culture requires from 3 to 6 weeks, plus 3 additional weeks when resistance is suspected. This is a slow process, but it provides a better identification of Koch's bacillus and drug resistance. This medium is available in regional laboratories throughout our country. The liquid medium technique takes from 1 to 3 weeks and relies on a continuous automated reading of bacterial growth, which affords greater sensitivity. It has a higher contamination rate, although it is difficult to identify the morphology of the colonies. There are also nonradiometric cultures, such as MGIT (Mycobacteria Growth Indicator Tube), the BACTEC9000MB system, and ESP Culture System II Myco, available in central laboratories.

Samples for bacteriological studies rarely come from the expectorations of sick children. In these cases, it is recommended to obtain samples by sputum induction, using a nebulized hypertonic saline solution, or aspiration of gastric content (three samples). The output of this sample is up to 30% in children, even for immunosuppressed patients with extrapulmonary tuberculosis. If the sample cannot be obtained with the aforementioned techniques, a bronchoalveolar lavage can be performed through bronchoscopy.

Samples from other parts of the body, such as pleural effusion, cerebrospinal fluid, pericardial fluid, peritoneal fluid, synovial fluid, and urine, are useful when extrapulmonary presentations are suspected.

- *Amplification technique for nucleic acids.* These techniques can be considered in patients under suspicion of resistance to anti-tuberculosis drugs. They have a high sensitivity (96%) and specificity (85–95%) for positive bacilloscopy samples, so they can rapidly detect a few copies of nucleic acid. They do not need to be performed in a high security laboratory (level 3), and the newest techniques also detect drug resistance and identify specific microbacteria. Nevertheless, they are not too sensitive (66%) for negative bacilloscopy samples, which is the most common situation in children, and they are not available in higher prevalence areas, where they are most needed.

At present, the most frequently used tests are these:

a. Line probe assays (LPA) (2–7 days). Recommended by WHO for BK+ and cultures. These assays detect infections and genetic resistance to RIF: rpoB (INNO-Lippa Mycobacteria, Genotype Mycobacterium Assay).
b. Xpert MTB/RIF Assay. Fully automated, very fast: 100 min. It can be used to detect MTB + gen for R to RIF at S = 98%. In 2010, WHO recommended this test to be used in countries prone to epidemic or HIV-related TB, also declaring it to be a diagnostic cornerstone.

Treatment

Tuberculosis control is only possible with a national or regional program suited to the population's epidemiological and clinical characteristics.

BCG Vaccination

BCG vaccination (Calmette–Guérin bacillus) consists of the application of a measured dose of attenuated *Mycobacterium bovis* in noninfected children under risk of exposure to create a primary and nonpathogenic infection. When exposed to Koch's bacillus, it protects against tuberculous meningitis and miliary forms of TB, although it does not grant immunity against the primary infection or late reactivation.

In Chile, this vaccine is part of the Expanded Immunization Programme (Programa Ampliado de Inmunizaciones, PAI) and is mandatory from the moment of birth.

Contraindications:

- Newborns who weigh less than 2000 g
- Newborns whose mothers have active tuberculosis
- Newborns whose mothers are HIV positive, until reaching a normal CD4 lymphocyte count
- Children with disseminated and infected skin conditions, which may compromise the injection site

The vaccine is intradermally delivered in the left shoulder, although in some countries, such as Peru, the right shoulder is used. It produces a subcutaneous reaction and an adenopathy (primary complex) around the fourth week which progresses for 2–4 months and even longer periods.

Complications associated to the vaccine are very rare, consisting mostly of local lesions in the injection site and axillary adenopathy. The skin in these areas can sometimes become enlarged, turn soft, and even fistulize. Progression is generally benign, but on occasion treatment is required. In patients with some kind of immunodeficiency, BCG spreading may be developed. This situation has a high rate of morbidity and mortality. BCG modifies the PPD reaction, so in countries with a broad vaccination coverage it is difficult to interpret this test.

Chemoprophylaxis

The rationale for treating pediatric patients is that children younger than 5 years old with a recent infection may develop the disease, with dissemination risk being proportionally inverse to the patient's age. In addition, children with a latent infection are at risk of developing an active disease during adulthood and then transmitting it. Isoniazid yields good results and has a very low probability of developing resistance as the bacillus population is small.

Two types of chemoprophylaxis can be identified: chemoprophylaxis, which is indicated in patients with a particular susceptibility for contagion (negative PPD test) to protect them from tuberculous infection; and secondary chemoprophylaxis, which is used in patients who are already infected with *Mycobacterium tuberculosis* (positive PPD test) to prevent them from developing the disease.

Chemoprophylaxis is contraindicated for patients with active tuberculosis, liver damage secondary to isoniazid, adverse reactions to this drug, or decompensated liver failure. The recommended approach for individuals in contact with tuberculous patients and newborns whose mother has tuberculosis is summarized in Tables 35.1 and 35.2.

Table 35.1 Management of tuberculosis exposure

Health state of mother	Management	Follow-up
PPD (+) with or without BCG Normal radiography	Chemoprophylaxis during 6 months HIV chemoprophylaxis during 9 months	
PPD (−) without BCG Normal radiography	Chemoprophylaxis during 3 months Repeat PPD and thorax radiography	PPD (−) and normal Rx: vaccinate PPD (+) (boosted) and normal Rx: HIN 6 months in total
PPD (−) with BCG Normal radiography	Chemoprophylaxis during 3 months Evolution follow-up	PPD (−): suspend HIN PPD (+) (boosted) and normal Rx: HIN 6 months in total

The child must not be separated from the mother unless he/she is seriously ill. Suspend maternal breast feeding

Table 35.2 Management for newborns born to mothers with tuberculosis

Health state of mother	Child management	Follow-up
Bacilloscopy (−)	BCG vaccination	
Bacilloscopy (+) during pregnancy or childbirth	Clinically ill children or under suspicion of congenital TB: obtain samples and provide full treatment for TB	
	Normal radiography and clinical condition: chemoprophylaxis during 3 months and PPD and Rx	PPD (−) Normal Rx: suspend HIN and introduce BCG vaccination PPD (+) (boosted): complete 6 months for HIN; strict follow-up

Treatment

The treatment for all types of tuberculosis is based on the use of bactericidal and bacteriostatic drugs. As a general principle, this treatment must be associated, extended, and supervised. Empirically, three or more drugs are used, which are then adjusted in accordance to bacillary sensitivity. Monotherapy should be avoided, as it entails the risk of producing resistant strains. The treatment must be long enough to eliminate or reduce bacillary population to a minimum. It must be a Directly Observed Treatment, Short Course (DOTS), because this is the only way to ensure that the foregoing conditions are met. The scheme to be used depends on the estimation of bacillary load as per the extension of lesions and bacillus elimination rate. It comprises a daily initial phase and a triweekly continuation phase (Table 35.3).

Simple Primary Complex

Simple primary complex is the most benign form of pulmonary tuberculosis in children. Because of the low estimation of bacillary load, a simplified primary scheme is indicated, consisting of 50 daily doses of isoniazid and rifampicin followed by 48 triweekly doses of isoniazid and rifampicin (Table 35.4).

Table 35.3 Tuberculosis treatment scheme

Drug	Daily phase	Triweekly phase
	50 doses (10 weeks)	48 doses (16 weeks)
Isoniazid	10 mg/kg (max. 400 mg)	15 mg/kg (max. 600 mg)
Rifampicine	15 mg/kg (max. 500 mg)	20 mg/kg (max. 600 mg)
Pirazinamide	35 mg/kg	
Ethambutol	20 mg/kg	

Table 35.4 Treatment for the simple primary complex

Drug	Daily phase	Triweekly phase
	50 doses (10 weeks)	48 doses (16 weeks)
Isoniazid	10 mg/kg (max. 400 mg)	15 mg/kg (max. 600 mg)
Rifampicine	15 mg/kg (max. 600 mg)	20 mg/kg (max. 600 mg)

Pulmonary Tuberculosis with Negative Bacteriology

Treat as primary complex, adding pirazinamide during the first phase (Table 35.5).

Pulmonary Tuberculosis with Positive Bacteriology

First phase with four treatment drugs, consisting of isoniazid, rifampicin, pirazinamide, and ethambutol, followed by 48 doses of isoniazid and rifampicin triweekly (Table 35.6).

Extrapulmonary Tuberculosis

Extrapulmonary tuberculosis requires the same treatment as pulmonary tuberculosis with positive bacteriology, unless there is tuberculous meningitis or miliary meningitis.

Tuberculous Meningitis and Miliary Tuberculosis

Treatment is the same as for pulmonary tuberculosis, extending the triweekly phase to 7 months (Table 35.7).

Table 35.5 Pulmonary tuberculosis with negative bacteriology

Drug	Daily phase	Triweekly phase
	50 doses (10 weeks)	48 doses (16 weeks)
Isoniacid	10 mg/kg (max. 400 mg)	15 mg/kg (max. 600 mg)
Rifampicine	15 mg/kg (max. 600 mg)	20 mg/kg (max. 600 mg)
Pirazinamide	35 mg/kg	

Table 35.6 Pulmonary tuberculosis with positive bacteriology

Drug	Daily phase	Triweekly phase
	50 doses (10 weeks)	48 doses (16 weeks)
Isoniazid	10 mg/kg (max. 400 mg)	15 mg/kg (max. 600 mg)
Rifampicine	15 mg/kg (max. 600 mg)	20 mg/kg (max. 600 mg)
Pirazinamide	35 mg/kg	
Ethambutol	20 mg/kg	

Table 35.7 Disseminated tuberculosis

Drug	Daily phase	Triweekly phase
	50 doses (10 weeks)	84 doses (28 weeks)
Isoniazid	10 mg/kg (max. 400 mg)	15 mg/kg (max. 600 mg)
Rifampicine	15 mg/kg (max. 600 mg)	20 mg/kg (max. 600 mg)
Pirazinamide	35 mg/kg	
Ethambutol	20 mg/kg	

Adjunct Drugs

For tuberculous meningitis, corticoid use reduces morbidity and mortality through reduction of vasculitis, inflammation, and intracranial hypertension.

Adjunct drugs are indicated when there is compression of the bronchial tree caused by pericarditis-related adenopathies. Prednisone is the most widely used steroid, with a dose of 1–2 mg/kg/daily during 4–6 weeks.

HIV Coinfection

Coinfections of HIV with tuberculosis are possible, and in small children dissemination caused by BCG must be ruled out. The treatment must be discussed with infectious disease specialists, given the interaction between antiretroviral and anti-tuberculosis drugs. It is advisable to start the anti-tuberculosis treatment first and add the antiretroviral treatment afterward (because of the risk of causing an immune recovery syndrome). The triweekly treatment phase should be extended for 7 months at least, depending on the immunological condition of the patient.

Follow-Up and Control

Bacilliferous patients require monthly bacilloscopy and bacterial susceptibility tests.

Adverse Reaction to Anti-tuberculosis Drugs

If an adverse reaction to anti-tuberculosis drugs is suspected, therapy must be suspended and

Table 35.8 Adverse reactions to anti-TB drugs

Drug	Adverse reaction
Isoniazid	Jaundice and increase in transaminases (infrequent)
	Peripheral neuritis that can be treated with pyridoxine (infrequent)
	Dermatitis and lupus-like reactions (rare)
Rifampicin	Skin rash, jaundice, and transaminases increase (infrequent in children, information to consider in patients with liver damage)
	Flu-like reactions followed by renal impairment
	Thrombocytopenia
Pirazinamide	Liver damage
	Hyperuricemia, arthralgia, vomiting, dysuria, and fever (rare)
Streptomycin	Skin rash
	VIII pair injury, vertigo and/or hearing loss
	Kidney damage
Ethambutol	Optical neuritis

complications must be ruled out. After this has been resolved, the treatment may be reintroduced with a programmed and independent desensitization scheme. These adverse reactions are extremely infrequent (Table 35.8).

Sources

Center for Disease Control and Prevention. Essential components of a tuberculosis prevention and control program: recommendations of the Advisory Council for the Elimination of TB. MMWR. 1995;44:1–15.

Crofton J, Horne N, Millar F. Tuberculosis Clínica. MacMillan Education Ltd. 1992 (Unión Internacional contra la Tuberculosis y Enfermedades Respiratorias).

Farga V. Tuberculosis. Santiago: Mediterráneo, 2011. 3rd edn. Auspiciado por la Unión Internacional Contra la Tuberculosis y Enfermedades Respiratorias.

Garcia-Peña P, Guillerman RP, editors. Pediatric chest imaging, medical radiology Diagnostic imaging. Berlín-Heidelberg: Springer; 2013.

Hamzaoui A, Yaalaoui S, Tritar F, Slim L, Berraies A. European Respiratory Update Tuberculosis. Childhood tuberculosis: a concern of the modern world. Eur Respir Rev. 2014;23:278–91.

Marais BJ, Rabie H, Cotton MF. TB and HIV in children advances in prevention and management. Paediatr Respir Rev. 2010;12:39–45.

Miller FJW. Tuberculosis in children evolution, epidemiology, treatment, prevention. Edinburgh: Churchill Livingstone; 1982.

Ministerio de Salud, Subsecretaría de Salud Pública, División de Prevención y Control de Enfermedades. Programa.

Nacional de Control de la Tuberculosis. Actualización de Normas Técnicas. 2014.

Pediatrics. Vol 134, Number 6, December 2014. Technical Report Interferon-γ Release Assays for Diagnosis of Tuberculosis Infection and Disease in Children. Jeffrey R. Starke, MD, FAAP and Committee on Infectious Diseases.

World Health Organization. Global tuberculosis report. The burden of disease caused by TB. Geneva: World Health Organization; 2012. WHO/HTM/TB/2012.6

World Health Organization, Global Tuberculosis Report. Drug resistant TB. Geneva: World Health Organization.; 2012. WHO/HTM/TB/2012.6

Respiratory Diseases in the Newborn

36

José Luis Tapia Illanes, Paulina Toso Milos, and Javier Kattan Said

Contents

Respiratory Physiology

To understand respiratory diseases during this period, knowledge of normal respiratory physiology is helpful. During intrauterine life, the lungs produce liquid and are filled with it. During the last trimester of pregnancy, this lung fluid goes through the trachea and provide all the substances to the amniotic fluid, even surfactant. Lung maturity can be measured using this information in the amniocentesis, as well as the analysis of the lecithin–sphingomyelin ratio (L/E) and phosphatidylglycerol (PG).

The fetus has intermittent respiratory movements, which may work to move this lung fluid out, with the objective to train its postnatal function. During childbirth, lymphatic reabsorption of the lung fluid takes place, probably through cortisol, thyroid hormones, and catecholamines, which are boosted with the air pulmonary expansion when the child has been born. Once the newborn starts to breathe, the first efforts must be very vigorous (around 40 cm H_2O of pressure) to expel lung fluid and establish a residual lung volume. The beginning of breathing facilitates an important reduction in lung vascular resistance caused by the mechanical expansion of the lung as well as the increase in PaO_2 and pH, and

J. L. Tapia Illanes · P. Toso Milos · J. Kattan Said (✉)
Department of Pediatrics, School of Medicine, Pontificia Universidad Católica de Chile, Santiago, Chile
e-mail: jlta@med.puc.cl; kattan@med.puc.cl

P. Bertrand, I. Sánchez (eds.), *Pediatric Respiratory Diseases*,
https://doi.org/10.1007/978-3-030-26961-6_36

release of humoral vasodilators. Increase in PaO_2 is also responsible for constraining and functionally closing the patent ductus arteriosus (preterm infants are more resistant to this closure). Besides this, systemic pressure rises when circulation to the placenta is stopped. These changes allow the transition of the blood flow from fetal to neonatal. Pulmonary arterial smooth muscle is proportionately greater in the newborn; therefore, when hypoxemia arises, pulmonary hypertension may easily develop, and thus the lung would go back to a "fetal circulation."

Breathing control is more vulnerable during the neonatal period. Although there is a ventilation response to CO_2 level increase, it is less powerful in the preterm newborn and is further reduced by hypoxemia. Newborns present a paradox response to hypoxemia. For a few seconds, a transient hyperventilation occurs (caused by stimulation of chemoreceptors), which then progresses to a central respiratory depression. In the preterm newborn, the hyperventilation phase is reduced, and it can even be absent in those who are very immature. Respiratory reflexes such as the Hering-Breuer (vagal inhibition) and Head (inspiratory response to lung inflation) are fully functional (Table 36.1).

Distensibility of the rib cage is greater in the newborn, especially in the preterm infant, which makes it difficult to maintain an adequate lung residual capacity, and can also ease alveolar collapse when there is a low lung distension.

Of the resistance forces, 20% correspond to the friction of the lung against the rib cage and 80% correspond to airway resistance. In the newborn, the nostrils are the point of greatest airflow resistance in the airway. This is important, considering that during this period, breathing is done mostly through the nose. Lung airway resistance is greater in the newborn than in the adult. In addition, because of the small size of the airway in the newborn, any obstructive process will noticeably increase lung resistance.

In absolute terms, lung distensibility is less in the newborn than in the adult, but when correction per weight is done the values are similar. Respiratory rate in the newborn is greater than at other ages, and this higher rate may be useful to maintain keep lung volume through the reduction in expiratory time (Table 36.2).

Table 36.1 Respiratory physiology of the newborn

High pressures in the first breaths
Expulsion of lung fluid
Decrease in lung vascular resistance
Constriction and functional closure of the arteriosus ductus
High distensibility of the rib cage
Low functional residual capacity
Increased pulmonary resistance
Low lung distension
High respiratory rate
Nasal breathing
Lower CO_2 ventilatory response in preterm infants
Paradoxical hypoxemia response
High minute ventilation
Increase of dead space in preterm infant
High oxygen consumption
Active Hering-Breuer's and Head's reflexes
Pulmonary arteries with larger muscles

Approaching the Newborn with Respiratory Disease

The respiratory distress syndrome (RDS) symptoms are tachypnea, retraction, grunting, cyanosis, and apnea. Nevertheless, these can present from pulmonary and extrapulmonary causes (Fig. 36.1). A detailed perinatal anamnesis based on risk factor determination and an exhaustive physical examination are essential for determining a precise diagnosis and adequate management.

Excluding hyaline membrane disease, the risk factors related to respiratory diseases are as follows:

- *Conatal pneumonia*: Masculine sex, feverish mother, chorioamnionitis, premature labor, prolonged membrane rupture, prolonged labor, streptococcal maternal colonization, Guillain–Barré syndrome, tracheoesophageal fistula.
- *Meconium aspiration syndrome*: (TTN) Amniotic fluid stained by meconium, fetal distress, post maturity, small for gestational age.

Table 36.2 Comparison of respiratory variables per age

		Newborn	Adult	
Respiratory frequency	(f)	34–45	13	rpm
Tidal volume	(Vt or Vc)	6–8	7	ml/kg
Alveolar volume	(Va)	3.8–5.8	4.8	ml/kg
Anatomical dead space	(VD)	2–2.2	2.2	ml/kg
Minute ventilation	(Ve)	200–260	90	ml/kg/min
Alveolar ventilation	(Va)	100–150	60	ml/kg/min
Functional dead space	(VD)	77–99	30	ml/kg/min
Dead space/tidal volume	(VD/Vt)	0.27–0.37	0.3	
Oxygen consumption	(VO_2)	6–8	3.2	ml/kg/min
Lung resistance	(R)	20–30	3–4	cm H_2O/l/s
Dynamic lung distensibility	(Cd)	4–6	100–150	ml/cm H_2O
Functional residual capacity	(FRC)	20–30	34	ml/kg

BPM breaths per minute

Note: Preterm newborns have a higher dead space/tidal volume ratio (0.5) and greater pulmonary resistance

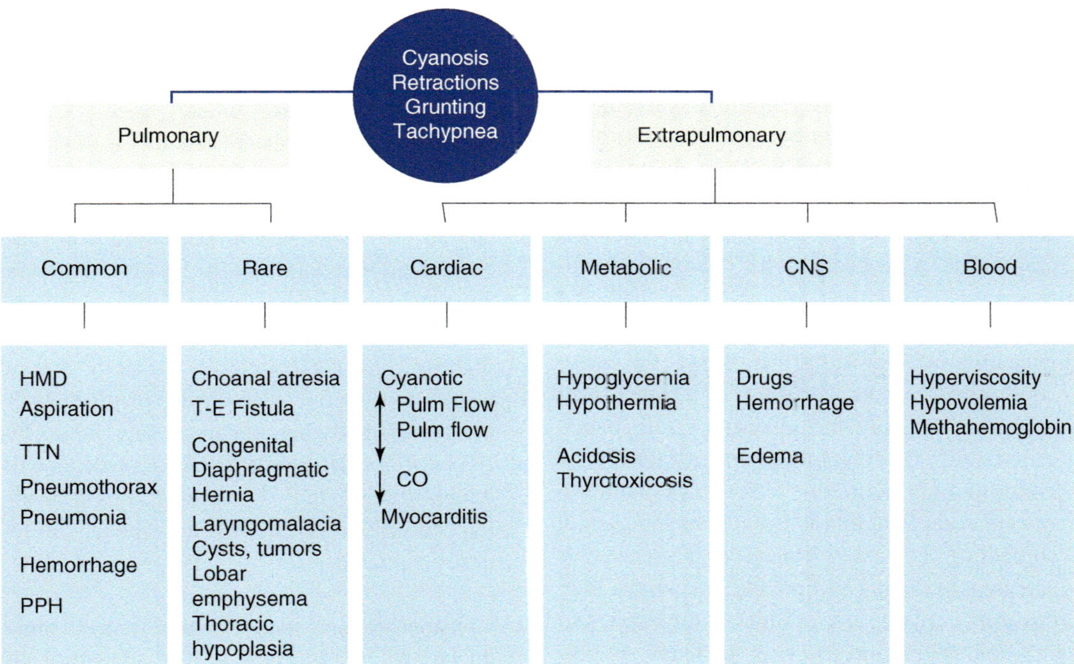

Fig. 36.1 Differential diagnosis for RDS

- *Transient tachypnea of the newborn*: Cesarean section, fast labor, neonatal depression, maternal sedation.
- *Pneumothorax*: History of resuscitation through manual ventilation.
- *Persistent pulmonary hypertension*: (PPH) Meconium aspiration syndrome, neonatal depression, pneumonia, polycythemia, congenital diaphragmatic hernia, ingestion of aspirin or antiinflammatories, hyaline membrane disease, cold stress.

A history of polyhydramnios is related to diaphragmatic hernia and tracheoesophageal fistula. A history of oligohydramnios is related to pulmonary hypoplasia, prolonged membrane rupture, and renal agenesis. In relation to the anamnesis, it is important to consider the following issues:

- *Maternal history*: Health state before pregnancy and during previous pregnancies, prenatal care, prenatal ultrasound, family diseases, pregnancy diseases, drugs and medications, cause of hospital admittance, labor time, fetal state, amount of amniotic fluid (maturity, infection signs, meconium), bleeding, fetal distress, type of labor, approximate gestational age.

- *Newborn history*: General condition at birth, need for resuscitation, Apgar score, vital signs, evaluation during transition period.
- *Physical examination*: Nutritional state, presence and distribution of cyanosis. Acrocyanosis or distal cyanosis in feet and hands are common findings within the first days of life. However, central cyanosis is always abnormal, and it is evident when deoxygenated hemoglobin exceeds 3 g/dl, and this suggests the presence of hypoxemia. Cyanosis from crying is possible because a short circuit is caused by the Valsalva maneuver through the foramen ovale. Paleness may suggest shock, vasoconstriction, anemia, and obstruction of the cardiac outflow tract. Polycythemia may be suspected if the child looks plethoric; if the child has meconium stains, then meconium aspiration is suspected, and if there is exanthema or a bad smell, it must be considered that the cause of the breathing difficulty is a pneumonia. Nasal flaring shows the newborn's need for air. The shape of a barrel chest suggests a volume increase, and a bell-shaped chest suggests a volume decrease (Table 36.3). Extremely preterm newborns (<1000 g) have a very compliant thoracic wall. During normal breathing a negative interpleural pressure is created, but it goes even further when the lung is sick, causing an evident intercostal and xiphoid retraction, with a tendency to collapse. This collapsing and protruding of the abdominal content, caused by the diaphragm moving downward, are the factors that cause "swing" or paradoxical breathing, which is typical of the severe breathing difficulty syndrome. Tachypnea is considered when the newborn has more than 60 breaths per minute and is the most sensible sign. Normal premature and term newborns will present a respiratory pattern called periodical breathing, which consists of shallow breaths followed by the cease of respiratory efforts or short apneas, which lasts from 5 to 10 s. It is important to notice the height of the tip of the heart, as it will be displaced if there are pulmonary masses, pneumothorax, or pulmonary hypoplasia. A scaphoid abdomen is typical of diaphragmatic hernias, where part of the abdominal content is placed in the thoracic cavity, which does not allow an adequate development of abdominal cavity, but it looks similar to the abdomen of a child who has eliminated meconium in the uterus. Abdomen distension can be seen when there is a tracheoesophageal fistula, especially when positive pressure has been used. If the belly button moves toward one side during inspiration or presents a "belly button dance" sign, it may be a sign of diaphragmatic paralysis in the side to which it is moving. When there is pulmonary hyperinsufflation, the liver and spleen can be easily palpated.

Table 36.3 Causes of changes in thoracic volume

Bilateral	
Volume increase	Transient tachypnea, meconium aspiration syndrome, pulmonary hypertension, cystic lung diseases
Volume reduction	Hyaline membrane disease, pulmonary hypoplasia, thoracic wall restricted
Unilateral	
Low-volume disease	Atelectasis, unilateral pulmonary hypoplasia
High-volume disease	Pneumothorax, unilateral interstitial emphysema, pulmonary cystic disease, Diaphragmatic disease, chylothorax

Considering lung sounds, grunting is the most characteristic. It is caused by the opposition of vocal cords at the end of the expiration phase. Grunting causes positive pressure toward the end of the expiration, which keeps the small airways open and improves ventilation distribution.

- Stridor suggests an obstruction of large airways. If the obstruction is extrathoracic, stridor will be greater at inspiration, although it can be heard in both inspiration and expiration when the obstruction is severe. Pulmonary murmur can be evaluated according to its intensity, length, symmetry, presence of crepitus, ronchi, or wheezing, although these alterations are less frequent in newborns.

- *Laboratory tests*
  - *Chest X-rays*: Very useful in the differential diagnosis of respiratory and nonrespiratory diseases. Lateral and anteroposterior projections are essential for a good evaluation of pneumothorax, catheter position, and pleural tubes. Bones, soft tissues, and the visible portion of the abdomen must be systemically evaluated before focusing on the heart and lungs. Also, each chest X-ray film must be used to reevaluate the position of tubes and catheters because they usually migrate.

    The trachea is easily curved because of its great flexibility, and it can even seem to have a mass effect, through its compression by other abnormal structures (Table 36.4).
  - *Cell blood count and cultures*: Infections must be actively sought, because of what a prompt treatment involves and also because of the difficulty of making a differential diagnosis, especially when differentiating from hyaline membrane disease.
  - *Pulmonary function test*: Initially it was only performed under investigative conditions, but today many ventilators are equipped with sensors that allow measuring this function. It is very useful to determine tidal volumes (if they are not increased) and pulmonary overdistension signs, which can contribute to neonatal lung damage.
  - *Blood gases*: One of the most useful tests to determine the physiopathology of the disease. It can also be used for treatment, as there are different goals, depending on the gestational age and the type of disease.
  - *Hyperoxy test*: Hypoxemia is considered when extrapulmonary short circuits from right to left are suspected (congenital heart disease and pulmonary hypertension). Oxygen is provided at 100% and gases are controlled. If the disease is pulmonary, PaO_2 increases significantly.
  - *General tests*: Hematocrit must be controlled, because polyglobulic conditions may cause hypoxemia, and acute anemia may cause difficulties in starting spontaneous breathing during resuscitation. In every pathological process glycemia must be controlled because of the immaturity of the regulation systems, which is related to a greater energetic expenditure and reduced intake.

Table 36.4 Common findings and variants in neonatal chest X-ray

Normal findings	Normal variants
Uniform lung fields	Pleural fissures
Less prominence of pulmonary hilums	Tracheal twisting and indentation
8–9 ribs expansion	Mediastinal lines
Tracheal deviation to the right	Pseudohyperlucid lung
Air bronchogram	Apical or intercostal hernia
Cardiac silhouette <60% of thorax	Radiolucency of the suprasternal space

Classification of the Respiratory Problems of the Newborn

I. Respiratory problems caused by perinatal asphyxia.
II. Respiratory problems related to immaturity and lung liquid reabsorption.
III. Respiratory problems related to lung circulation. Respiratory problems conditioned by lung circulation diseases.
IV. Respiratory infections in the newborn: pneumonia.
V. Respiratory problems caused by congenital alterations of the airway and lungs.

Respiratory Problems Related to Perinatal Asphyxia

Cardiorespiratory Depression at Birth

As many as 10% of newborns requires some kind of support to start breathing spontaneously. It is crucial to anticipate this situation by determining which childbirths may produce depression at birth. Because of this, it is important to have at each childbirth at least one qualified person who may provide the initial resuscitation steps, and another person who may perform advanced resuscitation. The action flowchart is taught at the Neonatal Resuscitation Program, which is regulated by the American Academy of Pediatrics and the American Heart Association.

During childbirth the fetus may be exposed to periods of temporary hypoxia, caused by the decrease of the placenta blood flow. The fetus adapts to these periods by redistributing the blood flow to favor the brain, heart, and adrenal glands. During hypoxic periods, the respiratory system has adaptation mechanisms that are not efficient in either the fetus or the newborn: this is called paradoxical response to hypoxia. It happens when the fetus and newborns who have suffered hypoxia increase their respiratory rate and respiratory effort (tidal and minute volume increase), but this is transitory, and it rapidly progresses into apnea. Therefore, it is not uncommon to face a perinatal hypoxia sign consisting of no respiratory effort at birth, which will require resuscitation techniques to start spontaneous breathing. Depending on how long the fetus has been hypoxic, the apnea may be primary or secondary. Secondary apnea implies a greater time suffering hypoxia, wherein compensatory vascular mechanisms have been overwhelmed, and this is reflected in the fall of arterial pressure. When resuscitating a child with secondary apnea it is crucial to provide ventilation with effective positive pressure, and, less frequently, to use cardiac massage and drugs.

Perinatal Asphyxia and Respiratory Distress Syndrome Caused by Meconium Aspiration

Respiratory distress syndrome caused by aspiration of meconium is a common complication of perinatal asphyxia, and sometimes it is a serious one; this is frequently found in a postterm newborn. Its prevention depends on good control and perinatal management.

Intrauterine asphyxia stimulates gastrointestinal motility and the relaxation of the anal sphincter, which allows the meconium to enter the amniotic fluid, but this is uncommon before 37 weeks of gestation. If the fetus is younger than 34 weeks, the anal sphincter does not relax during asphyxia. Hypoxemia also causes the fetus to initiate deep breathing efforts, and so the fetus aspirates the amniotic fluid containing meconium. During birth the risk of meconium aspiration is greater, as a consequence of the first breaths. Meconium impacts different levels of the thinner airways, which causes an obstructive respiratory disease with entrapped air, and alteration of alveolar stability, along with its inflammatory reaction. Entrapped air is one of the causes of the high rate of pneumothorax in this disease. In almost 50% of the cases, respiratory failure is related and complicated by an important degree of pulmonary hypertension. Ventilatory mechanics are altered: airway resistance is increased, functional residual capacity is also increased because of the entrapped air, pulmonary distensibility is reduced, and there is compromise of the ventilation/perfusion ratio. The result is a respiratory distress situation with hypoxemia and hypercarbia.

Generally, the patient is a term or postterm newborn. Sometimes they are small considering their gestational age, with a history of perinatal asphyxia, which has been certified through the presence of meconium in the amniotic fluid, as well as alteration in the fetal heartbeat and cardiorespiratory depression at birth, which requires resuscitation. There can be meconium in the umbilical cord, and the skin of the newborn may have meconium impregnations. Polypnea and respiratory distress signs appear early: chest retraction, grunting, and nasal flaring. The thorax curves outward, with increased anteroposterior diameter. There is a noticeable cyanosis, which, at the beginning of the clinical presentation, usually responds to an increase in the oxygen inspired fraction, unless there is a serious pulmonary hypertension. During auscultation there can be a reduction of the pulmonary murmur and crackles. Other concomitant complications caused by asphyxia, and which may require specific treatment, must be investigated, such as hypoxic-ischemic encephalopathy, renal impairment, cardiogenic shock, and alterations of the coagulation process.

If the aforementioned clinical history and signs are considered, diagnosis is generally clear. The aim of the laboratory examinations is to corroborate the diagnose of meconium aspiration, evaluate the presence of other complications from asphyxia, and for follow-up.

The following examinations must be done:

- *Anteroposterior and lateral chest X-ray.* X-rays will show irregular opacities as nodules or cords, following the distribution of the bronchial tree next to hyperinsufflation zones. The diaphragm is sometimes flat. It is important to rule out the presence of pneumothorax (Fig. 36.2).
- *Arterial gases.* Arterial gases will show the degree of respiratory failure. These measures must be serially controlled every 48 h, as needed. This information will be key for delivering a prompt and adequate treatment, to evaluate its efficacy as well as the progression of the disease.
- *Cell blood count and blood culture.* These tests are important to obtain hematocrit values and detect a possible infection. Meconium is a good culture medium.

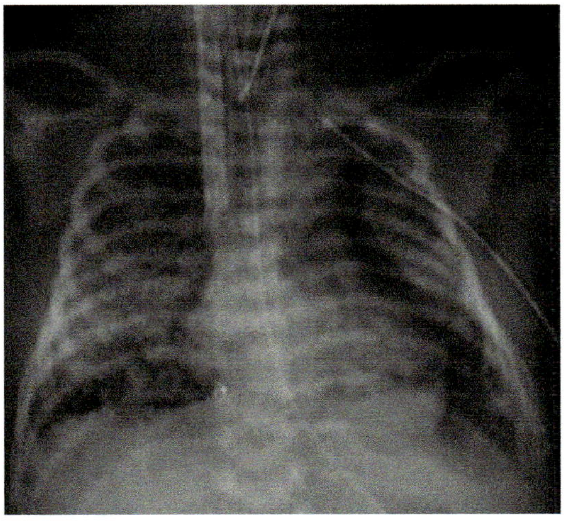

Fig. 36.2 Meconium aspiration syndrome. Chest X-ray of a term newborn combines alveolar interstitial shadows with slightly collapsed areas with pneumothorax to the left side, partially leaking with the insertion of a chest tube. Patient is intubated and connected to venoarterial extracorporeal membrane oxygenation (ECMO)

Depending on the additional problems and the evolution of the patient who has undergone asphyxia and meconium aspiration, other examinations may be necessary if there is suspicion of an important pulmonary hypertension: glycemia, calcemia, cardiac and brain isoenzymes, coagulation tests, brain ultrasound, and echocardiography, when an important pulmonary hypertension is suspected.

Prevention includes good pregnancy control and newborn attention at birth. Meconium aspiration from the trachea, using endotracheal intubation when the newborn is hypotonic, is a common practice, although it has not been validated. Management consists of adequate oxygenation, ventilation support as needed, antibiotics use until an infection is ruled out, and management of complications such as pneumothorax, pulmonary hypertension, and other issues related to asphyxia and sepsis. It has been proven that the administration of diluted surfactant reduces the need of extracorporeal membrane oxygenation and the risk of death.

Respiratory Problems Related to Prematurity and Lung Fluid Reabsorption

Hyaline Membrane Disease

Hyaline membrane disease (or respiratory distress syndrome, RDS) is a respiratory disease characteristic of the premature newborn, caused by pulmonary surfactant deficiency. Surfactant is produced in the type II pneumocytes. It is composed of phospholipids with small quantities of neutral fat, cholesterol, and proteins. The primary active molecule is saturated dipalmitoyl phosphatidylcholine, but phosphatidylglycerol and unsaturated phosphatidylcholine are also present. Surfactant reduces superficial tension, adhering to the alveolar surface and displacing water molecules. It has four proteins: A, B, C, and D. Protein A is more abundant and it is hydrosoluble. It has a key part in the surfactant recycling process and some capacity to protect the lung. Protein B intervenes in the surfactant recycling process. Protein C increases surfactant reabsorption and production. Protein D has a defensive function in the lungs. Type II pneumocytes appear in the lung from 20 to 24 gestational weeks. Steroids and thyroid hormones increase the transcription and synthesis rate of limiting enzymes. The function of the pulmonary surfactant is to reduce the superficial tension in the alveoli to maintain pulmonary stability and volume during exhalation. It is crucial to have an adequate amount of surfactant in the liquid–air interface to sustain alveolar stability. As a result of surfactant deficiency, there is a tendency to alveolar collapse, which causes a progressive atelectasis, with an intrapulmonary blood flow short circuit that evolves into an increasing hypoxia. Functional alterations characteristic of hyaline membrane disease are reduction of pulmonary distensibility and of the functional residual capacity, accompanied by an alteration of the perfusion–ventilation ratio. This alteration of pulmonary mechanics originates a global respiratory failure with hypoxemia and hypercarbia, which is worsened by the fatigue of the respiratory muscles. Hypoxemia and acidosis increase pulmonary vascular resistance, which worsens the condition.

Hyaline membrane disease is the main cause of respiratory morbidity and mortality in the premature newborn. Its incidence is estimated in about 50% of children who are younger than 29 weeks of gestational age and only about 5% of those older than 34 weeks. In the South American region, an incidence of 74% has been found among newborns whose weight is less than 1500 g at birth. Related risk factors have been described (Table 36.5).

Table 36.5 Risk factors related to hyaline membrane disease (HMD)

Increased risk	Reduced risk
Masculine sex	Female sex
White race	Black race
L/E < 2.0 for premature newborns	L/E > 2.0[a]
Previous brother with HMD	Maternal preeclampsia
Maternal diabetes (A, B, C)	Maternal diabetes (D, F, R)
Maternal hypotension	Maternal drug abuse
Cesarean section without labor	Antenatal steroids
Third-trimester hemorrhage	Chronic abruption
Second twin	Prolonged membrane rupture
Fetal hydrops	Intrauterine growth retardation
Neonatal depression	Vaginal childbirth

[a]Lecithin/sphingomyelin

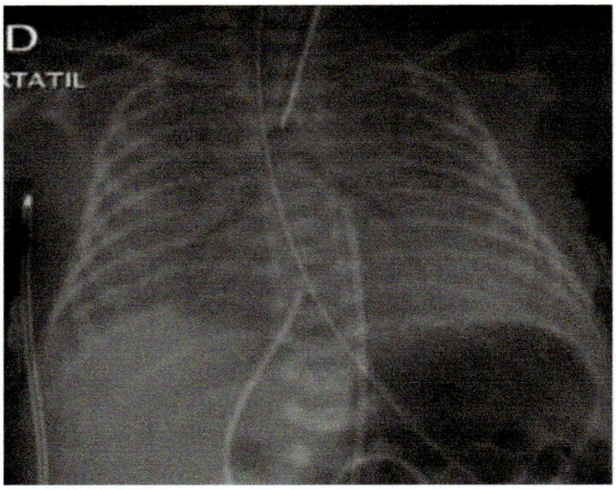

Fig. 36.3 Hyaline membrane disease. Chest X-ray in newborn whose lung volume is lightly reduced (because the newborn has undergone intubation and receives positive pressure), frosted glass sign, and air bronchogram

Hyaline membrane disease is characterized by an early-onset progressive respiratory difficulty, usually starting at birth or during the first 6 h of life. It causes a respiratory grunting, usually audible, nasal flaring, retraction, polypnea, and FiO_2 requirements that increase rapidly. Vesicular murmur tends to be reduced during auscultation. Anteroposterior thoracic diameter is reduced. In severe cases, breathing can become paradoxical or in "swings." There is generally edema and reduced diuresis.

Chest X-ray is essential for the diagnosis. The radiological image is characteristic, but not pathognomonic, showing a homogeneous increase of pulmonary density, described as a frosted glass on which air bronchogram images can be seen (Fig. 36.3).

Blood gases show oxygen requirements that need to be addressed rapidly with fraction of inspired oxygen (FiO_2) above 30–40%. Depending on the seriousness of the case, there may be respiratory or metabolic acidosis.

The most important and difficult differential diagnosis is conatal pneumonia produced by group B streptococcus. The clinical and radiological findings may be identical. Perinatal history is important for making a differentiation, and in the case of pneumonia, a fast progression with a greater tendency to cardiovascular compromise. During the first hours it can also be confused with transient tachypnea of the newborn. The benign course and good lung volume of this last disease differentiates the two.

Prevention of hyaline membrane disease is essentially perinatal: diversion of risk pregnancies to specialized centers, prevention and management of premature labor, determination of fetal lung maturity depending on the case, and the acceleration of fetal pulmonary maturity.

Following the pioneer study done by Liggins and Howie in 1972, several investigations have confirmed that antenatal steroids are related to a significant reduction in the presentation of hyaline membrane disease. In the same way, it has been demonstrated that antenatal steroids reduce mortality and the incidence of intraventricular hemorrhage. Therefore, beyond traditional usage recommendations for the fetus who is 24–34 weeks of gestational age and at risk of premature birth, in many centers steroids are used before the 24 weeks. Their administration between 34 and 36 weeks is currently under study, given the impact of the currently named "late-term premature newborns." In all cases, the benefits obtained surpass the potential risks of steroid usage, although repeated cycles must only be used for investigation protocols, given the association with a worse neurological outcome. Treatment consists of 2 doses of 12 mg IM betamethasone, with a 24-h difference, or 6 mg dexamethasone IM with a 12-h difference. Optimal benefits start 24 h after initiating therapy and persist up to 7 days after.

These children must be admitted to the intensive care unit. Ideally, they are born in a specialized perinatal center, or at least they are promptly taken to a tertiary neonatal center.

Therapy with exogenous surfactant is, without doubt, the most significant therapeutic advance for hyaline membrane disease. The therapy has changed the natural progression of the disease, making it shorter, and significantly improving the survival rate. There are natural and artificial surfactants: the first are extracted from the amniotic fluid of animals and the second are synthesized, which mainly includes surfactant phospholipids, but not its proteins. A range of studies have shown that both natural and artificial exogenous surfactants significantly reduce morbidity and mortality rate in this disease. Other recent studies do not show significant differences when using different kinds of natural surfactant, which are those most used currently. The most effective approach is the early administration of the surfactant, before 2 h of life. It has also been used as prophylaxis in the higher-risk groups, such as those younger than 30 weeks. Nevertheless, it is becoming increasingly common to use it with nasal continuous positive airway pressure (CPAP) for the initial respiratory stabilization in very low weight premature newborns, which seems to be a more appropriate approach than the prophylactic use of surfactant. The INSURE technique has been widely incorporated into clinical practice: this is INtubation-SURfactant-Extubation, with nasal continuous positive airway pressure. During recent years several studies have administered surfactant to the airway, through a fine tube, but results have not been conclusive.

Respiratory assistance includes the prophylactic or early use of continuous nasal positive pressure, which reduces the need of mechanical ventilation, as well as INSURE. The use of noninvasive nasal ventilation through nasal devices that avoid the use of tracheal intubation is still being studied. Regarding oxygen administration to the premature newborn, current experts recommend to start resuscitating with a FiO_2 of 21–30% to avoid oxidative damage. The saturation goal for respiratory distress syndrome is to keep it between 90% and 95%.

Other diseases have been related to hyaline membrane disease, such as alveolar rupture, infection, persistent arteriosus ductus, intraventricular hemorrhage, and pulmonary hypertension. It is possible that with an adequate treatment or prevention for the hyaline membrane syndrome, all these diseases can be prevented or made less stressful.

The chronic disease most usually related to hyaline membrane disease is bronchopulmonary dysplasia. In the long term, newborns who survive this disease seems to have a greater frequency of respiratory diseases during the first years of life.

We must note that congenital surfactant deficiency does exist. SP-B deficiency is the first known cause of genetic neonatal respiratory distress, and it is usually an autosomal recessive disorder. It is usually presented as a respiratory difficulty syndrome in a term newborn who does not respond to any therapy, with progression is death.

The deficiency of transport protein ABCA3 (ATP-binding cassette member A3) has also been described, which is related to the transcellular transport of surfactant and the assembly of lamellar bodies. ABCA3 gene mutations have an autosomal recessive transmission. SP-C congenital deficiency has also been described. These two can appear during neonatal age, and later during childhood, as chronic respiratory disease.

In these conditions, the diagnosis is through determination of the protein content in the surfactant, which has been collected from the fluid obtained in the bronchoalveolar lavage, DNA genetic testing oriented to identify blood mutations, electron microscopy, and immunohistochemical dying for surfactant proteins on an available tissue sample.

There is no treatment for these congenital surfactant deficits. Lung transplant does not present encouraging results, and the hope for the future may lie in gene therapy.

Newborn Apnea

Newborn apnea consists in the absence of an airflow in the respiratory airway during a period of at least 20 s. It can be fewer than 20 s if bradycardia or cyanosis is present. It must be differentiated from periodic breathing, as already described.

Neonatal apnea especially compromises the premature newborn, and it is present in 50% of children of gestational age less than 32 gestational weeks. According to etiology, the classification is as follows:

- *Primary or idiopathic newborn apnea.* It is the most common one. Its origin is unknown but it is probably related to immaturity in the central and peripheral mechanisms of breathing control. Its onset is usually between the second or third day of life, and it disappears when the newborn is 34–35 weeks of adjusted age, although 2% of premature newborns with very low birth weight at birth can continue to present apneas beyond 40 weeks of gestational-adjusted age.
- *Apnea secondary to other disease.* It can appear in premature and term newborns. The most common triggers are metabolic problems (hypoglycemia, hypocalcemia, hyponatremia), neurological alterations (intracranial hemorrhage, asphyxia, seizures), infections, respiratory distress conditions, bronchopulmonary dysplasia, persistent ductus arteriosus, hypothermia, and anemia. The most important action is to treat the triggering cause.

According to their presentation, apneas are classified as follows:

- *Central apnea:* Absence of airflow and stopping of breathing movements.
- *Obstructive apnea:* There are respiratory movements, but no airflow.

(It must be considered that this type of apnea is not detected by the respiratory monitor. This diagnosis must be suspected in newborns with bradycardia crisis and/or cyanosis with no apparent etiology.)

- *Mixed apnea.* During the same episode, both presentations are mixed. Generally, it appears as an obstructive apnea that stops breathing efforts through hypoxemia.

With the intention of an early diagnosis, it is recommended to routinely monitor every newborn who is younger than 34 weeks, given the high risk of apnea. It is important to consider that newborn hypoxemia, especially if the child is premature, has a depressing effect on the respiratory center.

When the diagnosis of premature newborn idiopathic apnea has been established, the following therapeutic measures must be taken: cardiorespiratory monitoring and permanent O_2 saturation, keep the neck in a neutral position, aspire secretions, keep body temperature as stable as possible, close to the lower point of thermoneutrality, correct hypoxemia, and use methylxanthines, because they stimulate the respiratory center and improve the diaphragm contraction capacity. Theophylline has been the treatment most used for premature newborn apnea, with very good results. As an alternative, caffeine may be used, which has fewer adverse effects, and higher doses can be administrated. In this way, other tools have been used for the treatment of apneas, such as proprioception and olfactory stimuli.

In those cases of serious apnea that do not respond to the previous measures, and that by their intensity produce an important decline in the child's condition, an option is to use nasal continuous positive pressure in higher airflows. If there is no improvement, mechanical ventilation must be started.

Transient Tachypnea of the Newborn

Transient Tachypnea of the Newborn is a clinical condition caused by a temporal alteration of the neonatal breathing adaptation. It presents as a respiratory distress disease, characterized mainly by tachypnea, usually with a benign course, short, and self-limited. It is more frequent in the term or near-term newborns, as well as those delivered by a cesarean section.

It is thought that this disease is caused by a delay in the lung fluid reabsorption that is normally present during fetal life. The relationship to a cesarean delivery, especially when this has been an elective procedure, is caused by the fact that labor would stimulate lung liquid reabsorption, probably mediated by catecholamines secretion.

Even though there are clinical and radiological facts that characterize neonatal transient tachypnea, this entity is an exclusion diagnosis. The main differential diagnosis is hyaline membrane disease, pneumonia, post-asphyxia situations, and cardiovascular problems. If the baby was born through vaginal birth, this diagnosis must be reconsidered, and pneumonia must be suspected.

The respiratory distress clinical presentation mainly consists in tachypnea. Oxygen requirements are usually low, and they are important for the differential diagnosis. When they are higher than 0.40 FiO_2, the diagnosis must be reconsidered; this is a crucial element to differentiate it from a hyaline membrane disease. The chest has an increased or regular anteroposterior diameter. Auscultation may be normal, or the pulmonary murmur may be slightly reduced. Progression usually tends to the improvement of the situation during the first 24–48 h. In some cases, progression may take more time.

The chest X-ray may be normal or show vascular congestion and liquid at the fissures, and sometimes in the pleural space (wet lung) (Fig. 36.4).

Oxygen is administered to maintain a normal PaO_2 according to the requirements determined by the blood gases. pCO_2 is slightly increased. While the FiO_2 is close to 0.40 and the respiratory frequency has a rate of 70/min, there should be no oral intake.

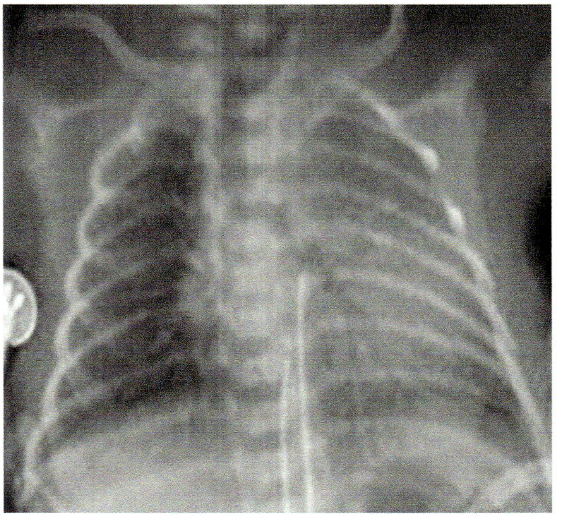

Fig. 36.4 Transient tachypnea of the newborn. Chest X-ray in newborn, where good pulmonary volume is highly visible, with vascular congestion and visible fissure, at the right side

Respiratory Problems Conditioned by Pulmonary Circulation Diseases

Persistent Pulmonary Hypertension

Persistent pulmonary hypertension (PPH) is characterized by an alteration in the evolution from fetal to neonatal blood flow. The pressure of the pulmonary artery and pulmonary vascular resistance are maintained at high values, as happens during the fetal period, which translates in pulmonary hypoperfusion and short circuits from right to left through the ductus and oval foramen. Clinically, this presents through cyanosis and hypoxemia that do not respond to increase of the fraction of inspired oxygen. This problem can present as an isolated condition (idiopathic PPH), but more frequently it is related to other diseases, particularly asphyxia, pneumonia, and meconium aspiration.

Reduction of the resistance and pressure of the pulmonary artery during the hours immediately after birth is central to the conversion from fetal to newborn blood flow. There are predisposing factors for this situation: chronic and acute hypoxia, acidosis and hypercarbia, prenatal maternal use of prostaglandin inhibitors, insufficient anatomical development in the cases of pulmonary hypoplasia, as happens with diaphragmatic hernia or Potter syndrome; and respiratory difficulty syndromes, especially as caused by meconium aspiration.

Pathological analyses of lungs from children with persistent pulmonary hypertension (PPH) show a thickening of the medium muscular layer of the pulmonary arterioles as well as an abnormal extension of the muscular layers in the intra-acinar arteries. This fact has been presented as an explanation for the great lability and sensitivity of the pulmonary vasculature present in these children when faced with hypoxia, acidosis, and other factors that affect it. Some mild hypoxemia episodes can be translated as important changes in the pressure of the pulmonary artery and oxygen requirements (Fig. 36.5).

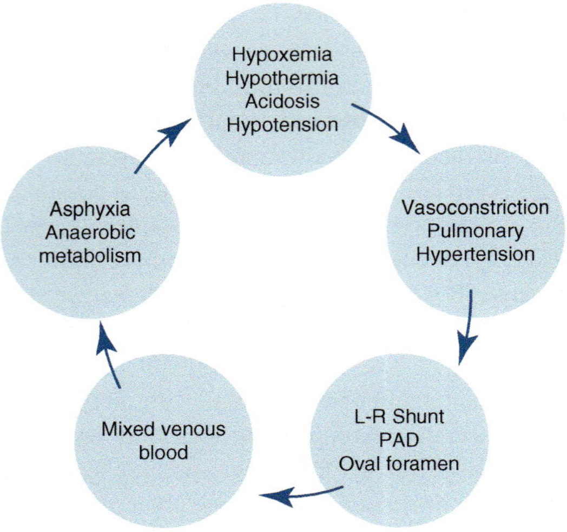

Fig. 36.5 Cycle of events that perpetuate persistent pulmonary hypertension (PPH)

The cardinal clinical sign is cyanosis that does not improve when oxygen is administrated. Considering parenchymal disease, there is a disproportionate hypoxemia and weak oxygenation. There is an important brittleness in PaO_2, even when FiO_2 has not significantly changed. Small reductions in this may be difficult to recover. Other signs that may be present are those typical of heart failure and a systolic murmur with a reinforcement in the second sound.

Signs are not specific, and it can be difficult to evaluate when there is other related respiratory disease. In some cases, especially in the idiopathic presentation, it is essential to consider the differential diagnosis of congenital heart disease. In 50% of newborns, there will be saturation differences greater than 20% between the preductal territory (left arm) and the post-ductal territory (other limbs).

The chest X-ray will show particular signs of the associated disease. In its idiopathic presentation, free and darker lung fields can be seen because of the pulmonary flow reduction. When there is a left ventricular failure, pulmonary venous congestion will be present.

Doppler echocardiography is the most important diagnostic exam. It shows the short circuits from right to left through the ductus and oval foramen, and in most cases, it will exclude heart structural abnormalities, which is the most important differential diagnosis. If there is a tricuspid failure, the pressure of the pulmonary artery can be estimated.

Prevention must consider all the factors that increase pulmonary resistance and blood flow pressure, before and after the birth. Fetal hypoxia treatment must be avoided, and no anti-prostaglandins should be used when facing early labor symptoms. During the postnatal period, a good resuscitation must be done at birth. Meconium aspiration must also be prevented, as well as hypoxemia and acidosis. Hypoglycemia, hypocalcemia, and polyglobulia must be identified and corrected. Room temperature must be neutral, and an adequate arterial pressure must be maintained. These measures are preventive, but once the persistent pulmonary hypertension state has settled in, they must be considered as part of the treatment.

Further, treatment requires the use of measures that will cause pulmonary vasodilatation Oxygen is a potent vasodilator, and therefore therapy must try to keep a PaO_2 within the high range of the normal numbers and a pH around 7.40, to have a better oxygen delivery at tissue level, always considering the hemoglobin dissociation curve. Different means of mechanical ventilation have been used with some success. It does not matter which mode is used: the goal is to achieve a sufficient mean airway pressure (MAWP) and adequate ventilation. Often this is achieved with high-frequency ventilation. It is recommended to use inhaled nitric oxygen (iNO), which produces a selective vasodilatation in the pulmonary vascular territory, when the oxygenation index (IO) is greater than 20 ($IO = MAWP \times FiO_2 \times 100/PaO_2$). Transferring the patient to a center with iNO capacity is recommended to avoid any risks for the patient: it is recommended to transfer the patient when IO reaches 15 and does not improve. iNO response is variable when there is a persistent pulmonary hypertension related to malformations, such as a diaphragmatic hernia. Methemoglobin may be present, as this complication has been described when iNO has been used at high ranges during prolonged periods. A recent multi-centric study in Chile proved that mortality rate is reduced through the administration of endotracheal surfactant, in relation to the use of iNO in newborns whose IO was greater than 20 (González et al.).

Sedation has proven to be of great help because the fight against the ventilator, as painful stimuli, affects oxygenation much more than in other disease. It is worth noting that with this treatment we do not have the ability to estimate the compromise related to the underlying disease and the prolonged hypoxia.

It may be necessary to deliver volume or use vasoactive drugs to keep systemic pressure over the estimated pulmonary pressure. Required doses and drugs must be titrated to keep enough systemic pressure to revert the extrapulmonary short circuit without causing vasoconstriction because of drug excess.

Since 1980 the use of extracorporeal membrane oxygenation (ECMO) has been described as being especially efficient in pulmonary conditions related to persistent pulmonary hypertension in newborns. Chile has had this resource since 2003. With this therapy the lungs are left resting during a few days while blood is being oxygenated through an external membrane. By avoiding pulmonary injure during mechanical ventilation, PaO_2 improvement and the underlying disease recovery time, the pulmonary vasoconstriction is reduced by the end of 5 to 10 days, allowing obtaining a survival rate greater than 85% for patients with no related malformations. It is a highly complex procedure, and costly, and it does entail risks. It is indicated for patients with a high probability of death (IO >40 and/or $PaO_2 \leq 40$). This procedure has technical limitations (indicated for children who are past 34 weeks gestational age and weigh more than 2 kg) as well as ethical limitations (neurological conservation). To improve the efficacy of this therapy, it is recommended to transfer the patient 4 to 6 h before the onset of serious persistent pulmonary hypertension.

Persistent Arteriosus Ductus

Persistent arteriosus ductus (PAD) is a blood vessel that is characteristic of fetal blood flow, which communicates the pulmonary trunk with the descending aorta. During fetal life, it allows most of the cardiac output from the left ventricle to go to the aorta, because the pulmonary artery pressure is greater. This function is normal and essential for fetal blood flow.

The finding of a persistent ductus arteriosus in a term newborn is generally related to an anatomical defect, which may or may not be linked to other heart malformations or genetic syndrome.

In the premature newborn, the persistent arteriosus ductus is fundamentally related to immaturity, with an inversely proportional increase in consideration to gestational age. Ductus sensibility to produce a strong contraction when facing PaO_2 is lowered as the gestational age decreases, and its vasodilatation is greater with prostaglandins. Persistent arteriosus ductus alters pulmonary mechanics as well as the gas exchange, which results in a left-sided heart failure.

Generally, the clinical history corresponds to a preterm newborn whose weight is very low. And notably, during the improvement stage in relationship to hyaline membrane disease, when the pulmonary vascular resistance decreased, a systolic ejection murmur appeared. This murmur is rarely continuous, and it can be better auscultated in the left infraclavicular region and the left superior parasternal border, commonly radiating to the side. Its intensity can vary in a short time, and sometimes it is not perceived during auscultation. The onset of the persistent arteriosus ductus may be accompanied by hyperactive precordium, tachycardia, and jumpy pulses in the postductal region. Sometimes the heartbeat can be perceived in the palm of the hand of the newborn. Mean arterial pressure drops at the beginning according to the diastolic pressure, which produces differential pressures (PS-PD) > 25–30 mmHg. Tachypnea is also present, along with an increase in the apnea pattern and general worsening, with an increase of oxygen requirements, ventilation support, and even including the use of vasoactive drugs. Hypoxemia can be seen in the blood gases, and respiratory or metabolic acidosis may be present, if the ductus is present with systemic hypoperfusion.

Chest X-ray can show cardiomegaly and pulmonary congestion signs (Fig. 36.6). Bidimensional Doppler echography is used to confirm the diagnosis and allows calculating approximately the degree of hemodynamic impact, according to the size of the ductus at the pulmonary end, the magnitude of the blood flow through it, and, to a lesser degree, the relationship between the size of the left atrium and the aorta.

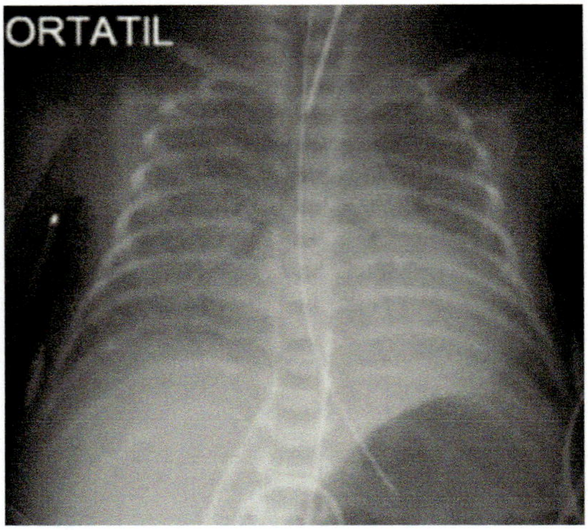

Fig. 36.6 Persistent arterial duct. Chest X-ray of a 31 weeks newborn who, at 10 days of life, presents with respiratory worsening related to a hemodynamically important ductus

In preterm newborns whose weight is less than 1000 g, it is necessary to be careful in ductus detection as it would be easier for this condition to impact the hemodynamic system.

Treatment considers keeping an adequate oxygenation and ventilation support, hematocrit between 40% and 45%, fluid restrictions, a high suspicion of concomitant infection, and pharmacological closure using prostaglandin inhibition, such as indomethacin or ibuprofen. The use of oral or IV paracetamol is still experimental. When these measures fail and hemodynamic compensation persists, surgical closure is performed to avoid secondary pulmonary damage.

Respiratory Infections of the Newborn: Pneumonia

The lung is the organ most frequently affected by infections developed during the first 24 h of life: 90% of fatal infections involve respiratory compromise. Conatal infection is usually ascendant, related to the rupture of membranes, but it tends to happen with intact membranes when they are contaminated by the maternal genital or anal flora at childbirth, and less frequently, transplacental. The other common cause of infections of the airway is the nosocomial in hospitalized newborns, especially preterm newborns.

Because of their immunity limitations and anatomical features, newborns are greatly susceptible to developing lung infections. The most frequent microbial agents are these:

- *Conatal bacterial infections*: Group B *Streptococcus* (GBS), *Escherichia coli*, and *Listeria:* also, *Streptococcus pneumoniae*, *Haemophilus influenzae*, and *Salmonella*, among others.
- *Conatal viral infections*: Herpes simplex, cytomegalovirus, rubella, influenza virus, adenovirus, and echovirus. After the first days, nosocomial bacteria appear, such as *Klebsiella*, *Pseudomonas*, *Enterococcus*, *Staphylococcus*, and *E. coli*. Cytomegalovirus, type II herpes, *Ureaplasma*, and *Pneumocystis jirovecii* (previously known as *P. carinii*) have been identified as causal agents in late pneumopathies, which may produce clinical presentations similar to those of bronchopulmonary dysplasia.

Candida albicans affects premature newborns who receive parenteral feeding and broad-spectrum antibiotics, or who have undergone intestinal surgery.

Chlamydia trachomatis is an organism that can frequently cause neonatal conjunctivitis, and it can also cause a late-onset pneumonia (2–12 weeks of life), in spite of its perinatal acquisition. Its main symptoms are polypnea, grunting, and cyanosis, which rapidly worsen when they are not treated. Early apneas suggest conatal infection. Crackles and abolished pulmonary murmur, which are a particular characteristic of the breastfeeding baby, are not usually found in the newborn. The presence of metabolic acidosis with no clear etiology, as well as a tendency to shock, suggest an infection.

Chest X-ray may reveal areas with pulmonary infiltration, condensations and/or pleural effusions. Nevertheless, it is common to see atelectasis and air bronchogram that cannot be distinguished from hyaline membrane disease.

Culture of airway secretions provides guidance relative to the etiological agent. Cultures must be performed early through tracheal aspiration during the progress of the infection. Positive hemocultures and an altered chest X-ray confirm the diagnosis. A complete blood count (CBC) may show leukocytosis or leucopenia, as well as a deviation to the left. These changes may also appear in cases of perinatal asphyxia or other stressful situations. After the first week of life, changes in the CBC give better signs of infection. C-reactive protein is more useful in nosocomial infection situations. Procalcitonin has also been used as an acute-phase reactant in infections with a good correlation.

These children require treatment in intensive care units. Their treatment includes general control measures of vital signs and internal medium stability: blood gases, glycemia, calcemia, and hematocrit. Many of them require breathing and hemodynamic support with vasoactive drugs. A serious complication is the aforementioned lung hypertension. Specific treatment must be chosen in accordance to the causal agent.

When a conatal bacterial infection is suspected, antibiotic treatment must be implemented early, right after the samples for culture are taken. If the child is referred to a specialized unit, the antibiotic treatment must start immediately after the samples for culture are taken and before the transfer. The scheme used, in accordance to the most frequent infections, is ampicillin and one aminoglycoside, which will be modified if it is necessary when the agent has been identified or depending on the clinical response.

Given the high frequency and severity of the infections caused by group B *Streptococcus* (GBS), some preventive strategies have been developed. The most effective one is to identify mothers who are GBS carriers through perineal culture at 35 to 37 weeks of pregnancy. For them, antibiotic prophylaxis during childbirth is indicated. If this previous information is not known, a prophylaxis treatment is indicated for the pregnant women who are at risk because of their clinical history, such as previous children with GBS infections, chorioamnionitis, membranes ruptured after 18 h, or preterm birth.

Respiratory Problems Caused by Congenital Alterations of the Airway and Lungs

There are several types of malformations. Because these are extensive, and because this text is only one chapter about the issue, we only mention them (Table 36.6). Regular maternal ultrasound has allowed us to determine or suspect the diagnosis before childbirth, and in some selected cases, these malformations can even be treated during the prenatal phase. Nuclear magnetic resonance has been more frequently used during the past decade to obtain further details, especially about malformations related to the central nervous system, lungs, heart, and kidneys. In these situations, the suggested approach is to refer the mothers to high-volume specialized centers and to diagnostic and fetal therapy centers.

Table 36.6 Malformations that can compromise the respiratory system

Congenital malformations of the upper airway	Choanal atresia, Pierre Robin sequence, macroglossia, velopalatal insufficiency, laryngomalacia, vocal cord paralysis, laryngeal tumors, esophageal atresia combined with tracheoesophageal fistula, tracheal agenesis, congenital tracheal stenosis, tracheobronchomalacia, vascular rings, laryngeal cysts and membranes, laryngeal atresia, cervical tumors causing external compromise (e.g., teratomas).
Congenital malformations related to the lung parenchyma	Congenital lobar emphysema, bronchogenic cyst, neurentenic cyst, cystic adenomatoid malformations, lung sequestration, arteriovenous fistula, congenital pulmonary lymphangiectasia, alveolar capillary dysplasia, pulmonary aplasia or agenesis, pulmonary hypoplasia, congenital diaphragmatic hernia.
Congenital malformations related to the diaphragm and thoracic wall	Congenital diaphragmatic hernia, sternum deformities, thoracic deformations, muscular weakness, skeletal dysplasias.

When there is no prenatal information, the clinical presentation, thoracic radiography, tomography, IRM, and endoscopic studies help us to a precise diagnosis and the actions to be taken. In some cases, only pathological anatomy will give us a precise diagnosis. When a breathing tree malformation is confirmed, it is necessary to determine if this is associated with other malformations or if they are part of a specific syndrome.

Some of these lung and airway malformations can be treated in very specialized university centers for fetal therapy, where successful in utero interventions using fetoscopy tracheal occlusion have been performed to treat diaphragmatic hernias; cystic adenomatoid malformations, when they cause hydrops, with thoracoamniotic shunting or radiofrequency ablation. These therapies are still under evaluation in multicenter research protocols, so they are not yet standard therapies. During childbirth, fetal therapies centers have collaterally developed procedures such as EXIT (ex utero intrapartum treatment), which is currently used in patients suspected of having a non-open airway at birth (cervical teratomas, cystic hygroma, bronchogenic cyst, laryngeal atresia, etc.), whose main principle is to maintain placental blood circulation during the 30 to 45 min while the airway is being secured using intubation assisted through laryngoscopy or tracheostomy.

Sources

Bahadue FL, Soll R. Early versus delayed selective surfactant treatment for neonatal respiratory distress syndrome. Cochrane Database Syst Rev. 2012;11:CD001456.

Committee on Fetus and Newborn; American Academy of Pediatrics. Respiratory support in preterm infants at birth. Pediatrics. 2014;133:171–4.

Fehlmann E, Tapia JL, Fernández R, Bancalari A, Fabres J, D'Apremont I, García-Zattera MJ, Grandi C, Ceriani Cernadas JM, Grupo Colaborativo Neocosur. Impacto del síndrome de dificultad respiratoria en recién naci-dos de muy bajo peso de nacimiento: estudio multicéntrico sudamericano. Arch Argent Pediatr. 2010;108(5):393–400.

Finer NN, Carlo WA, Walsh MC, et al. SUPPORT Study Group of the Eunice Kennedy Shriver NICHD Neonatal Research Network. Early CPAP versus surfactant in extremely preterm infants. N Engl J Med. 2010;362(21):1970–9.

González A, Sosenko Y, Chandar J y cols. Influence of infection on patent ductus arteriosus and chronic lung disease in premature infants weighing 1000g or less. J Pediatr. 1996;128:470.

González A, Fabres J, D'Apremont I, Urcelay G, Avaca M, Gandolfi C, Kattan J. Randomized controlled trial of early compared with delayed use of inhaled nitric oxide in newborns with a moderate respiratory failure and pulmonary hypertension. J Perinatol. 2010;30(6):420–4.

Grupo Colaborativo Neocosur. Very low birth weight infants outcome in 11 South American NICU's. J Perinatol. 2002;22:2–7.

Hahn S, Choi HJ, Soll R, Dargaville PA. Lung lavage for meconium aspiration syndrome in newborn infants. Cochrane Database Syst Rev. 2013;4:CD003486.

Halliday HL, Sweet D. Endotracheal intubation at birth for preventing morbidity and mortality in vigorous, meconium-stained infants born at term. Cochrane Library. 2003;1:CD000500.

Henderson-Smart DJ, Steer PA. Caffeine versus theophylline for apnea in preterm infants. Cochrane Database Syst Rev. 2010;1:CD000273.

Ministerio de Salud Chile. Guía Clínica AUGE, Síndrome de dificultad respiratoria del recién nacido. Garantías Explícitas en Salud. Noviembre 2011. www.supersalud.gob.cl.

Murphy KE, Hannah ME, Willan AR, et al. MACS Collaborative Group. Multiple courses of antenatal corticosteroids for preterm birth (MACS): a randomised controlled trial. Lancet. 2008;372:2143–51.

NIH Consensus Conference. Effect of corticosteroids for fetal maturation on perinatal outcomes. JAMA. 1995;273(5):413–18.

Porta NF, Steinhorn RH. Pulmonary vasodilator therapy in the NICU: inhaled nitric oxide, sildenafil, and other pulmonary vasodilating agents. Clin Perinatol. 2012;39(1):149–64.

Rojas-Reyes MX, Morley CJ, Soll R. Prophylactic versus selective use of surfactant in preventing morbidity and mortality in preterm infants. Cochrane Database Syst Rev. 2012;3:CD000510.

Tapia JL, Urzúa S, Bancalari A, Meritano J, Torres G, Fabres J, Toro CA, Rivera F, Céspedes E, Burgos JF, Mariani G, Roldán L, Silvera F, González A, Domínguez A. Randomized trial of early bubble continuous positive airway pressure (CPAP) for very low birth weight infants. J Pediatr. 2012;165:75–80.

Vento M. Oxygen supplementation in the neonatal period: changing the paradigm. Neonatology. 2014;105:323–31.

Weisman LE, Hansen TN. Contemporary diagnosis and management of: neonatal respiratory diseases. 3rd ed. Newton: Handbooks in Health Care; 2003.

Weisz DE, McNamara PJ. Patent ductus arteriosus ligation and adverse outcomes: causality or bias? J Clin Neonatol. 2014;3(2):57–75.

Bronchopulmonary Dysplasia

37

Alberto Toso Milos, Jorge Fabres Biggs,
and Pablo Bertrand

Contents

Introduction

Advances in neonatal intensive care have contributed to an increase in the survival rate of premature patients, and also in an increase in the prevalence of their complications. One of these, bronchopulmonary dysplasia (BPD), has a significant impact in the morbidity and mortality of this population. Its management, follow-up, and prognosis have great economic costs. Thus, research is crucial to have a proper approach that may prevent complications which, in the end, cause deterioration in the quality of life of these patients.

BPD is a term used for the first time in 1967 by Northway, who described the clinical, radiological, and anatomo-pathological characteristics of premature newborns that had developed severe

A. Toso Milos · J. Fabres Biggs
P. Bertrand (✉)
Department of Pediatrics, School of Medicine,
Pontificia Universidad Católica de Chile,
Santiago, Chile
e-mail: jfabres@med.puc.cl; pbertrand@med.puc.cl

P. Bertrand, I. Sánchez (eds.), *Pediatric Respiratory Diseases*,
https://doi.org/10.1007/978-3-030-26961-6_37

hyaline membrane disease, requiring mechanical ventilation and supplementary oxygen. These newborns did not present the usual progression of improvement within days, and started to present a chronic disease course, with radiological and histopathological changes in the lower airways. In its original description, the disease was related to the use of mechanical ventilation with high positive pressures and exposure to high concentrations of oxygen.

Since then, BPD has been described as a prolonged neonatal respiratory failure in children requiring mechanical ventilation and oxygen dependence for more than 28 days of life, or after 36 weeks of corrected gestational age, associated with the persistence of radiological alterations.

Epidemiology

BPD is the most frequent cause of chronic pulmonary disease with sequelae in infants, with an incidence rate between 5% and 50% in premature babies who also suffer hyaline membrane disease, although it is variable among different neonatal units, and clear correlations cannot be established. The prevalence of BPD is inversely related to weight at birth, which increases from 5% in children within the range of 1250–1500 g to 46% in children within the range of 500–750 g. In spite of the advances in the "gentle" neonatal ventilation management, the use of prenatal and postnatal steroids, and the incorporation of surfactant, the incidence of BPD has not diminished during the past years. Incidence has been stable or it has increased, because there has been an increase of the extreme premature newborn population during the past 20 years.

Physiopathology

The pathogenesis of BPD depends on many elements and is the result of the coincidence of many factors, with clear lesions and tissue damage in the lung, with its posterior healing and fibrosis. The originating factors can be divided as in the following.

Oxygen/Mechanical Ventilation Providing high oxygen concentrations favors the development of oxidative stress in the lung tissues, which causes inflammation, fibrosis, alteration of alveolar permeability, formation of hyaline membranes, proliferation of alveolar capillaries, atelectasis, hemorrhages, necrosis, among others. Volutrauma is the main damage described, caused by mechanical ventilation in animal models, which is different from what was previously thought to be barotrauma. Other damaging agents are atelectrauma, caused by use of low ventilation pressures and the damage related to poor humidification and warming of the inspired air, and the mechanical damage to the endotracheal tube, which causes necrosis in the epithelium and alteration of ciliary transport.

- *Prematurity*. Prematurity and low weight at birth favors the development of BPD. Maturation factors, alveolar and pulmonary vascularity (endothelial alterations) development, are important factors that are absent or altered in premature newborns, especially for infants under 32 weeks of gestational age or less than 1500 g at birth.
- *Infections*. Many studies have proven that BPD is related to the increase of inflammatory and fibrotic products in the newborn, even before birth, because they are already present in the amniotic fluid. This inflammatory damage, attributed in a great extent to mechanical ventilation and oxygen therapy, is also importantly related to the presence of chorioamnionitis and conatal infection (example, *Ureaplasma urealyticum*), and also postnatal infection related to healthcare attention.
- *Nutrition*. BDP has been related to amino acid deficiency, micronutrient deficiency, and is also strongly associated to vitamin A deficiency. Besides this, the relationship between malnutrition and the inadequate development of pulmonary tissue, low production of surfactant, and mechanical respiration immaturity includes factors that justify the importance of

nutrition in the development of this disease. Excessive hydric support has also been related to a greater incidence of this disease.

- *Persistent arterial duct*. The presence of persistent arterial duct causes pulmonary hyperflow, which causes pulmonary edema, and consequently, pulmonary damage. It is related to prematurity and infection, so either one of those conditions favors its appearance, thus contributing to the different factors for the development of the disease.
- *Other factors*. Masculine gender has a greater relation to BPD. Besides this, it has been linked to endocrine factors, such as basal cortisol deficit during the first days of life or deficit in the protein related to parathyroid hormone produced by type II alveolar cells to maintain alveolar hemostasis. Recently, there has been greater interest in the search for hereditary and predisposing factors in the molecular pathways of development and healing of pulmonary tissues, which opens new areas of investigation to intervene in these pathways, thus preventing the development of BPD. In this same way, the eventual presence of predisposing factors for premature childbirth is also interesting, because these factors could also intervene.

Diagnosis

During the past 20 years, by the development of intensive neonatal care and the improvement of the survival rate in very low weight newborns, two types of BPD have been identified: the "classic" type, typical of the pre-surfactant era, which is present in premature newborns who survive hyaline membrane disease and who have high requirements of mechanical ventilation and oxygen concentrations (Fig. 37.1). These patients show persistent hypoxemia and hypercarbia, besides radiological alterations progressing from frosted glass appearance to cystic chronic lesions and interstitial densities. At tissue level there is a pronounced damage of the airway with diffuse fibrosis, inflammation, hypertrophy of the mucosal glands, and alveolar destruction, with reduced alveolar multiplication.

Besides this, there is the "new" BPD that appears during the surfactant period, in premature newborns who have a very low or extremely low weight at birth, who recover from the first respiratory distress, or simply do not present it as such. These diseases progress with a grace or "honeymoon" period, in which their additional oxygen requirements importantly decrease, but the newborns then again develop respiratory difficulty and persistent hypoxemia, which requires oxygen, but has a more benign progression than the classic presentation, along with subtler changes in the X-rays, such as diffuse interstitial infiltrations and pulmonary edema (Fig. 37.2).

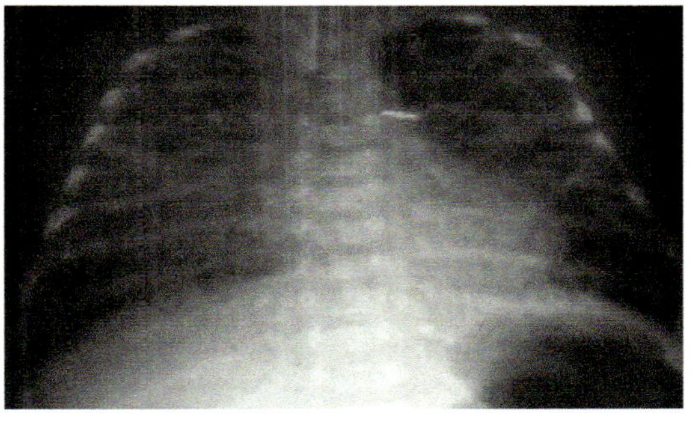

Fig. 37.1 Classic bronchopulmonary dysplasia. Anteroposterior chest X-ray shows interstitial images, with diffuse cystic shadows in a 50-day-old child, a 34-week premature newborn whose weight at birth was 1980 g. Patient did not receive surfactant and underwent permeable ductus surgery

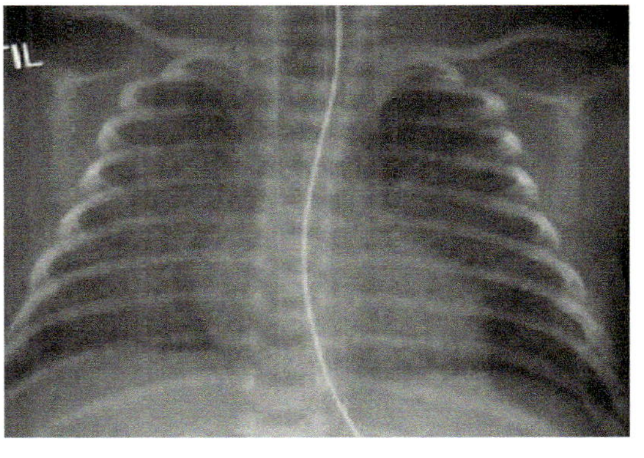

Fig. 37.2 New bronchopulmonary dysplasia. Anteroposterior chest X-ray shows subtle and diffuse interstitial images in a 60-day-old child, who was a 27-week premature newborn, with birth weight 1280 g, and received surfactant treatment

Table 37.1 Main differences between classic and new bronchopulmonary dysplasia (BPD)

	Classic BPD	New BPD
Initial respiratory distress	Severe	Mild-moderate
O_2 initial requirements	High	Low
Mechanical ventilation requirements	High positive pressure and invasive support	Low positive pressure and noninvasive support
Pulmonary lesions	Metaplasia, inflammation, fibrosis, and alveolar distortion	Arrest of pulmonary development and mild fibrosis
Pulmonary hypertension	Frequent	Occasional
Air scape	Frequent	Minimum
Mortality rate	Variable	Low
Presence of sequelae	Frequent	Occasional
Oxygen dependence	Prolonged	Brief

The changes at tissue level show the arrest of alveolar development, with simplified and enlarged air spaces, as well as a general reduction in the alveoli quantity, with less compromise of the central airway (Table 37.1).

Along with this, in 2001 Jobe and Bancalari published the results of the National Institutes of Health (NIH) consensus, creating the new definition and classification of BPD, considering gestational age, oxygen requirements, and ventilation support. With this, they classify it as mild, moderate, and severe (see Jobe and Bancalari 2001).

Complications and Treatment

BPD appears with variable clinical manifestations, depending on how severely the parenchyma is affected.

Respiratory

Respiratory clinical symptoms can be present during the first 4 weeks of life, and they are related to multifactorial lung injury, but they also appear after the maintenance period, being related to the healing process when there already is pulmonary damage.

During the acute period, gentle ventilation management has substantially improved the results obtained in high-risk patients. Adequate ventilatory management includes the following recommendations, which can be modified according to each patient:

- Early CPAP and early surfactant must be considered [the possibility of performing the Insure procedure (intubate–surfactant–extubate must be assessed], thus avoiding mechanical ventilation. (The use of surfactant does not reduce BPD incidence, but it does reduce mortality rates and changes the "classic" BPD for the "new" one, which has a more benign progression.)
- Synchronized ventilation and low ventilation pressures with VT at 4–5 ml/kg, PEEP 4–5 cm of water, short inspiration time (0.3–0.4 s), high RF 40–60 x′, to reach O_2 saturations around 90%.
- Ventilation support with permissive hypercapnia, tolerating pCO_2 up to 60 mmHg so long as pH is maintained above 7.25 to avoid hyperventilation, which increases the risk of BPD and central nervous system compromise.
- Early extubation, using transition ventilation support with CPAP to increase the chances of having a successful procedure.

The use of supplementary oxygen, avoiding hyperoxia, is fundamental to prevent the development of BPD during the immaturity phase of the premature infant. The optimal goals for these patients have been studied relative to pulse arterial saturation, which may avoid retinopathy onset, and at the same time decrease neonatal mortality as well as obtaining a good neurological result. Currently, the recommendation is to look for a safety range of oxygen supply that reaches a SaO_2 range of 88–94%.

During the maintenance phase, the already damaged pulmonary parenchyma starts a healing process that is related to pulmonary fibrosis and active pulmonary growth. In this stage the ventilation support must be modified and a more adequate ventilation for the child must be determined, using longer inspiratory times and greater pressures. When doing this, it is important to keep in mind that the main objective is to suspend the support as soon as possible. At the same time, the goal of oxygen therapy is to avoid hypoxemia, but the scenario changes once the child has acquired a certain retinal maturity, which decreases the probability that complications related to hyperoxia appear; on the contrary, the oxygen supply will yield evident benefits for alveolar growth. Therefore, the objective is to reach SpO_2 levels within the range of 90–94%. Hypoxemia tolerance must not be so permissive, because the periods of SpO_2 fall may be prolonged, which may directly impact the neurological growth and development, besides producing an increase of pulmonary vascular resistance, with the corresponding progression to persistent pulmonary hypertension.

During the transition to the patient's home, it is very important to analyze the oxygen requirements by performing a SpO_2 study for 8 h continuous, wherein the objective condition of the patient can be evaluated. The requirements may vary when facing situations that increase oxygen consumption, such as feeding times or crying, and it can be reduced in resting periods and during sleep. The objective for patients presenting pulmonary hypertension should be individualized, but clearly the goal is to reach SpO_2 levels within a range greater than 93% and 96%.

The most common cause of respiratory acute worsening is the crisis of BPD, with acute respiratory distress episodes, great irritability and agitation, progressing to cyanosis. In some cases, positive-pressure ventilation is required by the presence of apneas and bradycardia. This crisis is the result of several incidents that take place as a result of irritation or painful stimulation. In the beginning, the patient develops anxiety and a sudden change in intrapleural pressures, which causes the obstruction of the proximal airway, usually of the trachea and major bronchus, with secondary hypoventilation. As the child sustains the effort and tries to overcome the obstruction, evident dyspnea appears, along with cyanosis, muscular fatigue, and after this, apnea is also present. These episodes can be easily confused with pulmonary edema (secondary to left or global heart failure), pulmonary hypertension episodes (secondary to shunt increase caused by a permeable ductus or an open oval foramen by the sudden increase of pulmonary artery pressure), and accidents to the airway such as obstruction, or endotracheal tube or tracheostomy tube displacement.

Patients with severe BPD have a greater risk for ventilation support during the first months of life, and some of them cannot be weaned from the mechanical ventilation because of global respiratory failure, or the attempts to extubate are not successful because the airway is unstable, mainly caused by tracheomalacia. In those cases, the decision to perform a tracheostomy for prolonged ventilation must not be delayed to facilitate the improvement of the global development related to early stimulation in these children. Once this stability has been achieved, the transition to the patient's home may be planned under strict vigilance, called domiciliary hospitalization.

In patients with BPD, congestive heart failure and hydric overload may cause pulmonary edema with hypoxemia and respiratory mechanical alterations. Generally, its management is through hydric restriction, with VT, about 130–150 ml/kg/day, and diuretics. The diuretics most commonly used are loop-acting diuretics, such as furosemide. It has been confirmed that furosemide reduces pulmonary resistance and increases pulmonary compliance in patients with BPD, but it has a short-term effect, and therefore the adverse effects, such as hydroelectrolytic disorders and metabolic alkalosis, must be assessed and considered. Besides this, furosemide can cause hypokalemia and hypercalciuria, causing nephrocalcinosis, and also it can intensify metabolic bone disease in the premature newborn. Because of this, its recommended use is for acute episodes during 2 to 3 days.

These patients may present some feeding difficulties, which are related to episodes of aspiration, and which can cause recurrent bronchospasm, pneumonia, and wheezing. In patients with BPD and persistent or recurrent wheezing, particularly in children with neurological damage, a swallowing disorder must be ruled out, and the significance of gastroesophageal reflux may have be assessed.

The use of postnatal systemic steroids to reduce the risk of BPD is controversial. During the first weeks of life, studies have shown that 10 patients at risk must be treated to reduce 1 case of BPD, but with the risk of developing neurological sequelae. Thus, it is not recommended universally. It has been confirmed that after the first 4 weeks of life steroids improve the clinical condition and pulmonary function, thus reducing the time of use of mechanical ventilation without modifying the mortality rate. For selected cases, the short-term use of steroids may be considered for the aforementioned reasons, considering the adverse effects.

For the chronic stage of these patients, chest physiotherapy management is important to correctly handle secretions, avoid atelectasis, and improve respiratory musculature.

Cardiovascular

Persistent pulmonary hypertension, which is the classic cardiovascular complication of BPD, is produced by structural changes in pulmonary vasculature. Remodeling is caused by stimuli such as hypocapnia, hypoxia, and acidosis, which generates an increase in pulmonary vascular resistance, with its corresponding overcharge of right cavities (cor pulmonale) and can progress to a congestive heart failure. Given the great pulmonary vascular reactivity, persistent pulmonary hypertension usually appears as a chronic condition, with crisis episodes in relation to diverse stimuli or infections. Management and follow-up must be done with strict medical vigilance of the clinical and laboratory parameters. It is recommended to check the management of permanent hydric restriction at 130–150 ml/kg/day. Further, oxygen must be supplied according to the requirements, tolerating greater saturations to favor oxygen effect in pulmonary vasodilation. Chronic use of vasodilators with calcium blockers, such as nifedipine, can be considered for severe persistent pulmonary hypertension cases, as well as sildenafil for acute management as well as chronic. The already mentioned use of diuretics requires caution, but without doubt it is one of the pillars of the management of persistent pulmonary hypertension, especially when there is congestive heart failure.

During an acute crisis of persistent pulmonary hypertension, sedation has a fundamental role in the management to reduce vascular reactivity as well as mechanical ventilation and the use of inhaled nitric oxygen. Nevertheless, the effectiveness of chronic inhaled nitric oxide use as a regulator of pulmonary vasculature and angiogenesis has not been confirmed.

If right ventricular hypertrophy and pulmonary hypertension are not resolved within 3 to 6 months, a heart evaluation must be performed, with a search for the cause of hypoxemia, as we already pointed out. Systemic arterial hypertension tends to be present in these patients, and it appears during the first 6 months of life. A non-minor group, about 50%, will require pharmacological control and treatment for arterial hypertension.

Metabolic: Nutritional

Adequate nutritional support is one of the keys in the treatment of the child with BPD, in such a way that an inadequate weight gain is a marker of the severity of the disease. The somatic growth of the body develops in parallel to growth and maturity of the respiratory system; therefore, a close follow-up of weight gain is a good measure of pulmonary growth and directly related to neurological growth. An inadequate weight gain may reflect a scarce nutrient supply, increase of the energetic demand because of respiratory work, and/or silent hypoxia that causes inefficient cell metabolism in anaerobic conditions. It may be related to a short intestine, swallowing disorder, etc.

The caloric supply for a child with BPD must be between 120 and 140 kcal/kg/day, which is adjusted according to the weight gain. In patients who present with hydric restriction or poor tolerance to the 130–150 ml/kg/day supply, the maternal milk must be optimized by fortifying it using appropriate infant formulae. In this scenario, the additional carbohydrate supply generates a greater CO_2 production in comparison to lipid-based feeding support. This change can be reflected in the increase of chronic respiratory acidosis, and therefore the lipid-based feeding support is preferred. Protein intake must be at least 3 g/kg/day, and micronutrients must also be provided. The use of intramuscular vitamin A in doses of 5000 IU three times per week, during the first month of life, has shown to have a protective effect relative to BPD, but its use is not universal.

The preferred feeding method is through oral suction, but frequently premature patients present with swallowing disorders during the first months of life, which forces the use of nasogastric tubes and, sometimes, to avoid aspiration, desaturations, and apneas, besides easing the feeding process. Sometimes, antireflux surgery with fundoplication is needed.

Metabolic alterations are common in patients with BPD, because of the use of drugs and nutritional intake using minerals in high concentrations. Thus, it is mandatory to be vigilant about the appearance of alterations in bone metabolism as well as metabolic alterations, such as metabolic alkalosis, hypokalemia, hypochloremia, and hypercalciuria.

Neurological

Patients who develop BPD suffer the usual neurological injuries present in premature newborns. Intraventricular hemorrhage, hydrocephalus, and periventricular leukomalacia can be present. More severe neurological complications are related to a greater pulmonary compromise, and vice versa. Generally, this disease has been identified as a statistical risk factor, independently of the psychomotor development compromise these patients may have in the future. In the long term, they show poorer motor and cognitive functions. These patients also develop attentional deficit, as well as language and learning disorders. The prognosis of these children is directly linked to the access to neurorehabilitation, besides programmed sessions with occupational therapists and the training of the parents for constant work.

Follow-Up Plan

The follow-up plan for a patient with BPD begins when the patient has reached a clinically stable stage in the neonatal unit and is moving to the patient's home. In this moment, the specialist in respiratory diseases is involved in the treatment of the child with BPD and plans, along with the neonatology specialists, the ambulatory follow-up.

As a general rule, the follow-up plan includes monthly visits to the specialist in respiratory diseases while the ventilation support or oxygen therapy continues, and then every 2 months until the child reaches the first year of life. After this, the follow-up must be annual until the child is 6 years old.

Nutrition

Nutritional support must be optimal for the child with BPD to achieve an adequate growth and avoid further complications. As has been previously established, the mentioned requirements must be pursued in the long-term follow-up with insistence and precision to obtain an adequate somatic growth. Generally, this means providing a generous amount of calories. However, it has recently been established that an excessive weight gain during the first years of life in premature children without BPD is related to recurrent wheezing and asthma during a 4-year follow-up, which could even be more notable in patients with BPD.

An unsatisfactory weight gain during the first months of life is a scenario that must approached with a multidisciplinary focus, because its consequences can be devastating. The follow-up involves different specialists: neonatologist, nutritionist, speech and swallow therapist, and bronchopulmonary physician. Individually, the caloric intake must be adjusted and the energetic consumption must be reduced, starting with enteral feeding progressing to ventilation support that allows for breathing rests.

Oxygen Therapy

During the first few weeks at home the child will need assistance in her/his environment, and therefore it is recommended to maintain oxygen support and closely monitor SpO_2 during resting periods, as well as during feeding and sleep. After verifying that the patient continues to be clinically stable and has an adequate weight gain for at least a month, it is possible to start reducing oxygen supply during the day under strict SpO_2 vigilance. After suspension of oxygen supply during the day has been well tolerated and accomplished, progress to the suspension of oxygen during the night is allowed. It is recommended to perform a continuous SpO_2 study during 8 h during a night. Recommendations for oxygen withdrawal are variable according different centers. In our University Hospital we have agreed that a normal SpO_2 study should result in an average SpO_2 of 93%, and the maximum total time of SpO_2 levels below 90% must be less than 3%.

The average length of oxygen therapy for patients with BPD in our center is 3 months after discharge from the neonatal unit, although it may be extended depending on the severity of the disease, respiratory exacerbations, and SpO_2 goals proposed.

Precautions and Prevention Measures for Respiratory Infections

As happens in the neonatal unit, at home the precautions for respiratory contact and isolation, when needed, are fundamental measures for patients with BPD. These measures must include universal washing of hands, contact precautions for the parents and therapists when there is suspicion of viral infection, but also general measures such as avoiding going outside, limiting home visits, and eliminating every source of indoor pollution, such as kerosene heaters and tobacco smoke exposure.

Patients with BPD present a high probability of hospitalization caused by respiratory infections during the first and second year of life. This likelihood makes it mandatory to use protection strategies, such as protecting the family and caretakers with vaccines against influenza and *Bordetella pertussis*; the use of monoclonal antibodies against the syncytial respiratory virus must also be considered. Administration is variable, because the reality in different countries in relationship to several factors must be assessed, such as the degree of prematurity of the child and the extent of the virus epidemic. In Chile an immunization plan has been implemented, consisting of palivizumab (15 mg/kg/month) during the winter epidemic for all patients younger than 32 weeks of gestational age and with BPD during the first year of life.

Respiratory exacerbations often compromise the small airway, obstructing bronchi and bronchioles. Although the evidence for using bronchodilators and systemic steroids is poor, it is reasonable to perform a therapeutic test during the course of a bronchiolitis episode, and this information will be relevant in the later follow-up when facing new episodes.

When facing respiratory exacerbations, it is still possible to find some compromise of the larynx and trachea, mainly in the subglottic space, caused by intubation injuries: subglottic stenosis, larynx cysts, granulomas, and laryngeal membranes. Although these complications may appear as a failed endotracheal tube weaning in the neonatal unit, they can also appear triggered by respiratory infections.

Recurring Wheezing and Asthma

The general characteristics of the lung in a child with BPD may vary, from a restrictive disease, caused by pulmonary hypoplasia, to an obstructive disease caused by the compromise of the small airways, although generally there is a combination of both components. Studies of pulmonary function in infants with BPD show that even when there is recovery of the pulmonary distension early in life, analysis shows obstruction of the airway during the first 2 years of life, even though these patients suffered from the "new" type of BPD. Up to 30% of these patients show a reversible response to bronchodilators, imitating patients with asthma, but with a lesser degree of atopy and persistent inflammation of the airway. In all the studies of pulmonary function in children aged from 6 to 19 years old, in which children with BPD are compared to control patients, FEV_1 is consistently reduced in children with BPD, with no difference if early treatment with surfactant and gentle ventilation was used in comparison to conventional treatment. This evidence suggests that obstructive disease that presents itself with wheezing episodes in infants with BPD can be explained, mainly, as a structural change in the smaller airway.

Respiratory infections will be the main triggers of the wheezing episodes, caused by the increase of inflammation and hypersecretion, along with accumulation of cellular detritus. Some patients may benefit from the use of bronchodilator therapy.

Patients with BPD may present a dynamic obstruction of the proximal airway, as a consequence of prolonged ventilation and the immaturity of the airway, which is called tracheomalacia and bronchomalacia, depending on the predominant site of the obstruction. In these patients, wheezing tends to be present in every moment of agitation, because the stability of the airway depends of the intra-chest pressure changes. Some of these patients have a paradoxical reaction to the use of bronchodilators, because the stability of the airway depends mainly on the muscular structure, which relaxes with the use of these drugs.

Pulmonary function is an objective and noninvasive follow-up method to check the growth of the airway in children with BPD, and it is desirable to perform this routine evaluation in the follow-up plan of these children until they reach adolescence.

Prolonged Mechanical Ventilation

A small percentage of patients with severe BPD or serious alterations of the proximal airway, mainly tracheomalacia or subglottic stenosis, will need a tracheostomy. This intervention determines a high-risk scenario that must be managed to progress to its transition to the patient's home. Caretakers of these children must train themselves in the routine management of the tracheostomy tube, but especially, they must be aware of their complications. Progress in the long term tends to be very satisfactory, and allows most children to be completely weaned from artificial ventilation as the somatic growth of the new pulmonary parenchyma and stabilization of the proximal airway develop. Those with a fixed alteration of the proximal airway, such as subglottic stenosis, may require balloon dilation or reconstructive surgery, whichever is needed.

Sources

Bancalari A. Actualización en presentación y patogénesis de la displasia broncopulmonar. Rev Chil Pediatr. 2009;80:213–24.

Bancalari E, Claure N. Definitions and diagnostic criteria for bronchopulmonary dysplasia. Semin Perinatol. 2006;30:164–70.

Baraldi E, Filippone M. Chronic lung disease after premature birth. N Engl J Med. 2007;357:1946–55.

Carlo WA. Gentle ventilation: the new evidence from the SUPPORT, COIN, VON, CURPAP, Colombian network, and Neocosur network trials. Early Hum Dev. 2012;88(suppl 2):S81–3.

Gien J, Kinsella J. Pathogenesis and treatment of bronchopulmonary dysplasia. Curr Opinion Pediatr. 2011;23:305–13.

Jobe AH. The new bronchopulmonary dysplasia. Curr Opin Pediatr. 2011;23:167–72.

Jobe A, Bancalari E. NICHD/NHLBI/ORD workshop summary. Bronchopulmonary dysplasia. Am J Respir Care Med. 2001;163:1723–9. https://www.atsjournals.org/doi/pdf/10.1164/ajrccm.163.7.2011060.

Linares M. La nueva displasia broncopulmonar desde el punto de vista del neumólogo pediatra. Neumol Pediatr. 2015;10(3):111–7.

Mandy G, Malkar M, Welty S, Brown R, Shepherd E, Gardner W, Moise A, Gest A. Tracheostomy placement in infants with bronchopulmonary dysplasia: safety and outcomes. Pediatr Pulmonol. 2013;48:245–9.

Meyer S, Kronfeld K, Gräber S, Butzer R, Wahl H, Gortner L. Vitamin A to prevent bronchopulmonary dysplasia: the NeoVita A trial. J Matern Fetal Neonatal Med. 2013;26(5):544–5. https://doi.org/10.3109/14767058.2012.745499. Epub 2012 Nov 28.

Ministerio de Salud. Guía Clínica Displasia Broncopulmonar del Prematuro. Santiago: MINSAL,

2009. http://web.minsal.cl/portal/url/item/721fc45c974a9016e04001011f0113bf.pdf.
Northway WH Jr, Rosan RC, Porter DY. Pulmonary disease following respiratory therapy of hyaline membrane disease: bronchopulmonary dysplasia. N Engl J Med. 1967;276:357–68.
Saugstad OD, Aune D. Optimal oxygenation of extremely low birth weight infants: a meta-analysis and systematic review of the oxygen saturation target studies. Neonatology. 2014;105:55–63.
Stevens TP, Finer NN, Carlo WA, et al. Respiratory outcomes of the surfactant positive pressure and oximetry randomized trial (SUPPORT). J Pediatr. 2014;165(2):240–9.

Allergic Diseases, from the Infant to the Adolescent

38

Mario Calvo Gil and Fernando Iñiguez Osmer

Contents

Definition

Allergic diseases are in general adverse reactions to substances that are innocuous to most people. These diseases are characterized by their high complexity and are denominated hypersensitivity. They are the most common chronic diseases during the pediatric age.

M. Calvo Gil
Department of Pediatrics, School of Medicine, Universidad Austral, Valdivia, Chile
e-mail: mclavo@uach.cl

F. Iñiguez Osmer (✉)
Department of Pediatrics, Hospital de Puerto Montt, Puerto Montt, Chile

Epidemiology

Allergic diseases constitute a global health issue, affecting hundreds of millions of people all around the world, and it is one of the most common causes for primary health care attendance. According to the Global Initiative for Asthma (GINA), 20% of the population would be affected by a disease mediated by immunoglobulin E (IgE). Its incidence has increased during past decades, especially in developed countries, which has led to the creation of the name "noninfectious epidemic." The Worldwide Health Organization (WHO) estimates that by 2020 the cases will double in developed countries, and it will increase

P. Bertrand, I. Sánchez (eds.), *Pediatric Respiratory Diseases*,
https://doi.org/10.1007/978-3-030-26961-6_38

even more in undeveloped countries, where most of the world population lives.

It has not been possible to determine the exact causes of this increase in allergic diseases, but a complex interrelationship among several factors that causes its manifestation has been confirmed. Such factors include the genetic constitution of the person who is affected by this disease, a type Th_2 inflammatory response, environmental factors within the pediatric age, factors related to the antigen, such as modulators and adjuvants, solubility in the microenvironment, size of the sensitizing particle, permeability of the respiratory mucosa, viral infections, and a greater or lower capacity of the effector cells to liberate mediators. Other factors to be considered are environment pollution, exposure to tobacco smoke, lifestyle, and hygiene habits.

The advances in genetic medicine have allowed us to understand better this group of diseases, but there is no unique genetic structure. Different genes have been proposed as candidates, and the manifestation of the disease differs according to the genotype of each of these pathologies: food allergy (FA), atopic dermatitis (AD), bronchial asthma (BA), and allergic rhinitis (AR), each with different phenotypes. They are characterized by a polygenic dominant inheritance, with a large number of genes that predispose to suffering the disease. These genetic determinants can be shared by some of them, for example, AD and BA. It is possible that in the future a specific locus will be determined for each disease. Currently, the genes that predispose to bronchial hyperreactivity (BHR) have been described, and other genes have been identified for their capacity to produce IgE specific to *Dermatophagoides*, and specific loci for eczema, bronchial asthma, allergic rhinitis, positive skin test, etc.

Etiology and Physiopathology

The etiology of this kind of disease changes according to the age in which it manifests, and the same mechanisms can have different clinical progressions depending on the onset age.

The first manifestations of allergy in the infant are FA and AD; BA is less frequent. During the school period, FA manifestations tend to decrease, AD tends to maintain the same level, and the frequency of BA increases. In the schoolchild the most common manifestations of allergy are respiratory signs, such as BA and AR. In the teenager, AR is predominant over BA. Each of these is analyzed in further detail in relation to the clinical manifestations according to age group (Fig. 38.1).

From the physiopathological aspect, the syndromes are characterized by the capacity of the

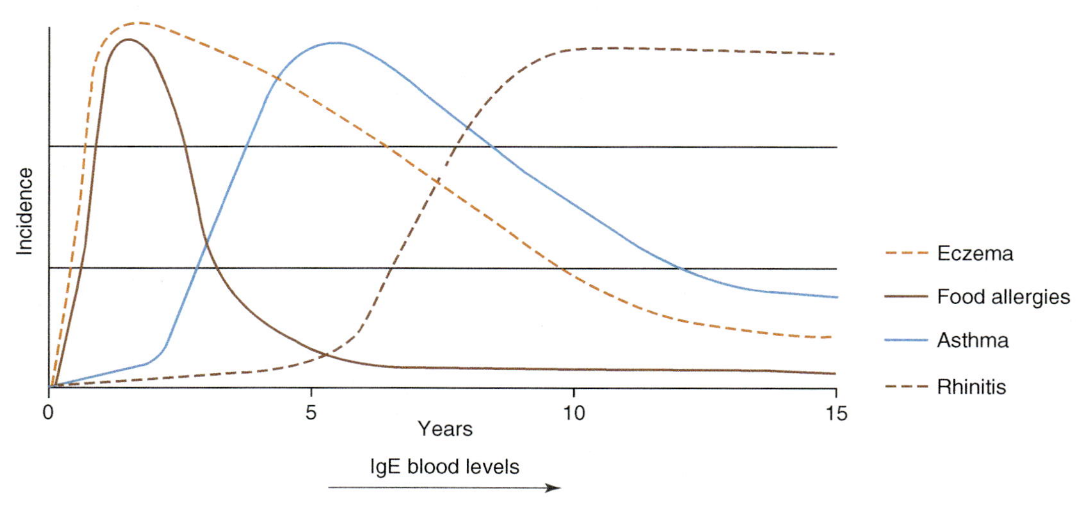

Fig. 38.1 Atopic march

affected person to manifest an allergic hypersensitivity, whether it is mediated by IgE or not. This capacity has a strong genetic basis, which allows the person to respond to different antigens that are common environmental proteins.

IgE-mediated allergy develops by interaction with proteins that have the potential to cause sensitization. An allergen is absorbed by the mucosa (gastrointestinal, cutaneous, respiratory) through a disruption in the affected epithelium and is then recognized by the antigen-presenting cell (APC). The most important cells of this kind are the dendritic cells, which migrate with the allergen toward the lymphatic tissue. These cells present small peptide fragments, resulting from processing to the class II major histocompatibility complex with native LT CD4+. Depending on the type of cytokines present in the initial interaction with the APC, native CD4 cells can be differentiated in five effector cells subgroups: Th1, Th2, Th17, Th22, and Treg. In allergic diseases, the presence of interleukin (IL)-4 promotes the differentiation from T cells to Th2 cells, which are specific for allergens and produce great quantities of IL-4, IL-5, and IL-13, along with no or a minimum amount of interferon-gamma (IFN-γ). IL-4 is the greatest change factor that makes B cells synthesize IgE. The presence of IL-12 and IL-17 favors the differentiation to Th1 cells, which produce large quantities of IFN-γ, which is a potent antagonist of IL-4 and inhibits the differentiation to Th2 cells. IgE-mediated diseases appear by a Th2 predominance because of the lack of regulation that Th1 and Treg must accomplish, which is a high production of IgE-specific antibodies for the antigen that caused the process, which bond to its high-specificity receptor (FcεRI), from different effector cells, such as mastocytes and eosinophils. A new union between the specific antigen and two IgE molecules fixes these effector cells, causing the release of several chemical mediators, such as histamines, leukotrienes, brachinine, platelet activation factor, and others, which migrate to the tissue where the allergic inflammation process has started. The release of an important group of chemical mediators is the cause of early signs of allergic reaction: rhinorrhea, sneezing, and pruritus in the nasal cavities, bronchoconstriction, and erythema, along with skin itching. Cellular infiltration, activated by the release of these mediators and its persistent action, explains late signs, such as persistent nasal obstruction, bronchial hyperreactivity, and remodeling (Figs. 38.2 and 38.3). The union of the IgE allergenic complex to low-affinity receptors (FcεRII, CD23), expressed in lymphocytes, monocytes, macrophages, and platelets, stimulates the lymphocyte activity, thus increasing the allergic response by promoting a greater Th2 response. The predominance of Th2 lymphocytes originates the abnormal synthesis of IL-4, IL-5, IL-9, and IL-13, which are closely related to IgE synthesis, and the immediate and late allergic reaction, with bronchial hyperreactivity eosinophilia and remodeling of the airway.

Clinical Manifestations

Allergic diseases can appear at any time in the life of a child, and the clinical manifestation depends on the age of the patient. A chronological analysis of these manifestations follows.

Newborn Period

Allergic reactions in a child under 1 month old are very uncommon, and when they are present they can be FA (cow's milk proteins) or AD, which are further analyzed in the infant stage section. During intrauterine life, in the maternofetal interface, the period of response to specific antigens begins between the fourth to seventh month of pregnancy. It has been confirmed that the fetus may produce specific IgE from the 11th week of intrauterine life. Reactivity to different allergens in the blood of the fetus is seen by week 22 of gestation, when IL-4 and INF-γ are already present. At 16–17 weeks, IL-10 predominates over INF-γ in the human amniotic fluid, which predisposes to a Th2 response. The tissues of the fetus that are more exposed to the antigens present in the amniotic fluid are the skin and the intestine,

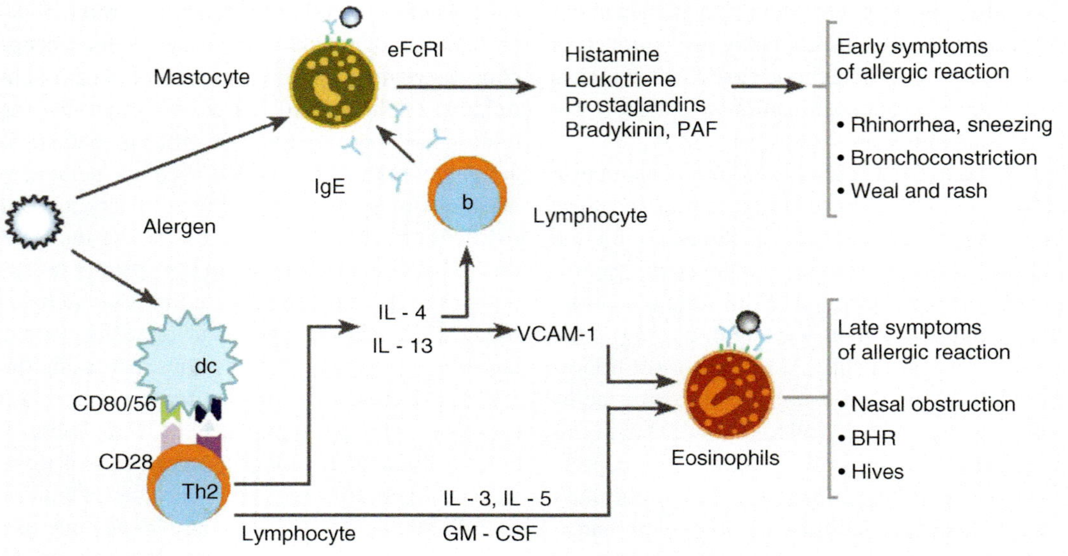

Fig. 38.2 Allergic reaction

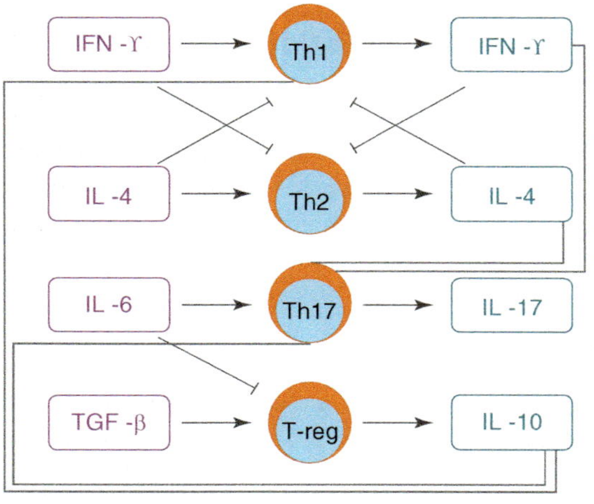

Fig. 38.3 Interregulation among the different subgroups of T-CD4+ cells

and secondarily the respiratory system, which would explain why the first allergic manifestations of extrauterine life are in these organs.

Infant Period

As already mentioned, FA and AD are the earliest manifestations of allergies, constituting the first clinical elements that allow us to suspect atopy in a patient. At 2 years old, 50% of the atopic patients present with symptoms of FA and AD, and at 5 years old, 60% of them; in this same age group, 40% of the atopic patients have symptoms of BA and 25% of AR.

FA has an early onset during the first months of life, beginning an important decrease, depending on the problematic food, between 2 and 3 years old. Its prevalence is greater during the first years of life, around 6% in patients who are under 3 years old. It is infrequent in patients over 5 years old, and its frequency continues to be low until adolescence.

Food allergy FA is the immunological reaction mediated by IgE or another hypersensitivity mechanism to one or more components of a food, and it must be differentiated from the adverse reactions to certain foods, which is the abnormal clinical response caused by some food or additive, caused by nonimmunological mechanisms. Its clinical manifestations are characterized by a wide variety of symptoms and signs, which may be localized or systemic. In infants the most common signs are irritability and gastrointestinal symptoms, such as nausea, vomiting, recurring abdominal pain such as colic, diarrhea, and eventually blood in the stools. It may be present along a stationary growth curve, or show weight loss, in most severe cases. The foods most likely to cause food allergy are the following.

- *Milk*: Milk contains several potentially allergen proteins, and the manifestations of the allergy are presented in about 2.5% of infants; about 85% achieve tolerance when the patient is between 3 and 5 years old. These patients have more than 50% of possibilities to develop other allergies, and more than 80% of chances of developing allergies to inhaled allergens later in life.
- *Egg*: The manifestation frequency of egg allergy in infants is estimated as 2.5%; it contains the most allergen proteins, mainly in the egg white, and its tolerance is achieved around the third year of life. As happens with milk, sensitization to egg is related to an increased risk of developing allergies to inhaled allergens.
- *Peanut*: In countries where the consumption of peanut begins early (incorporated into other foods or as butter), an allergy frequency of 0.6% is reported, and this tends to last during several years, or even for the lifetime. Its tolerance is described as less than 20% at the second year of life.
- *Less frequent*: Soy (0.3–0.4%), wheat, fish, fruits, and vegetables, which are more frequent later in life and during adulthood.

Allergy to cow's milk generally remits at the third year of life, and allergy to egg usually remits before puberty, although if it severe it may last for the lifetime. Allergies to fish, crustaceans, nuts, and peanuts may not totally improve, but they can be less severe later in life.

Atopic dermatitis AD is a recurrent chronic skin disease characterized by reddish lesions, intense pruritus, and usually patches of dry skin in different parts of the body. These lesions usually present at first in the cheeks, and after that they may expand to the forehead, ears, scalp, chest, genitals, and limbs. Later in life the lesions tend to be drier and to be located in skin folds (retroauricular fold, neck, wrists, cubital fossa, and popliteal fossa). Atopy in the family background may or may not be present. Food allergy to the aforementioned foods is one of the frequent causes of AD. The NICE clinical guide includes the signs for its clinical diagnosis, diagnostic criteria, and evaluation of degree of seriousness.

Different follow-up prospective studies have determined the risk factor these pathologies may have in the posterior development of BA or AR. So, if an infant with AD at 3 months has the background of one of the parents or a sibling having atopy, this patient has a more than 50% chance of presenting BA when he is 5–6 years old and about 75% of suffering from this disease during the school years.

AR and AB, along with anaphylaxis, are less common symptoms in infants. Even though they can be present in infants, these symptoms tend to appear later in life.

Bronchial asthma It begins early in the life of the atopic child, who can manifest respiratory symptoms during this stage of life, although it tends to be predominant later in life. Traditionally the groups of symptoms and signs these patients present are classified as wheezing, polypnea, retraction of soft parts, and prolonged exhalation, during periods that can be related or not to viral conditions, such as an acute wheezing episode. A group of these infants (about 25–30%) have bronchial asthma, and although pulmonary tests are not routinely performed to confirm the diagnosis, clinical and laboratory criteria provide orientation in the diagnosis, even during the infant period. The asthma predictive index (API) (published by J.A. Castro-Rodríguez, then modified by T. Gilbert) is detailed in Table 38.1. Following the criteria of the first, it is known that if an infant has more than three acute wheezing episodes within a year and positive (+) API, it is possible to affirm that there is a 77% chance that this child will be affected by BA during the school-age years (6–13 years old). On the contrary, with a negative (−) API, we can affirm, with 68% certainty, that the condition of this child will tend to disappear in time and the child will not have bronchial asthma in the future. In other words,

Table 38.1 Asthma predictive index (API)

Original API[a]	Modified API[b]
Major criteria	Major criteria
Asthma family history	Asthma family history
Medical diagnosis of AD	AD
	Sensitizing to (Björkstén 1999) 1 air allergen
Minor criteria	Minor criteria
AR medical diagnosis	Sensitivity to milk, peanut, or egg
Wheezing without flu	Wheezing without flu
Hematic eosinophilia (Björkstén 1999), 4%	Hematic eosinophilia (Björkstén 1999), 4%

Castro-Rodríguez JA. J Allergy Clin Immunol. 2010;126: 212–6

Guilbert TW, et al. J Allergy Clin Immunol. 2004;114: 1282–7

AD Atopic dermatitis, *AR* allergic rhinitis

[a]A positive index is defined when recurring wheezing episodes are reported within the last years with two major criteria or two minor criteria

[b]A positive index is defined when four or more wheezing episodes are reported, at least confirmed by a doctor, and one major criteria or two minor criteria

infants with a positive API have a sevenfold increase in their risk to suffer from bronchial asthma during their school age in comparison to those who are API negative.

The importance of diagnosing and differentiating these patients lies in the anticipation and adequate prognosis for the family, by enforcing adequate therapeutic measures. About 80% of patients with BA begin to wheeze during the first years of life, usually before 4 years old. The greatest risk factors are atopy and BHR. Infants with atopic BA are born with a normal pulmonary function, and then experience a significant worsening in the function during the first 6 years of life, which is maintained until they reach 18 years of life, and it is not recovered during adulthood. In these patients early sensitizing increases the risk of inflammation of the airway.

Allergic rhinitis Its presentation is less common in infants and its diagnosis is more difficult. About 25% of atopic patients develop AR symptoms during this period. It must be suspected when the infant has some of the already mentioned atopic manifestations, has a family background, and presents clear rhinorrhea, sneezing, nasal pruritus, and nasal obstruction, although this condition is less frequent during this age. See Pérez el al. and Mullol et al. for the backgrounds and symptoms that suggest the existence of allergic rhinitis and its classification according to its seriousness.

Preschool Period

In this transition period, sensitivity to foods tends to decrease or disappear according to the food, as was previously described. AD usually decreases, but present lesions become less humid and tend to be localized in flexion areas.

During this period the greatest recurrence of respiratory symptoms appears, with or without previous sensitization (for example, to foods), or if they are in tolerance stage. The main predominance in the atopic child is, first, BA, and some years later, AR. It is useful to remember that within this age group there are children with non-atopic bronchial asthma, usually triggered by acute viral infections, and even when they have BHR, clinical background and laboratory indexes show that they are not suffering from atopy. This group also includes the infants who, even though they do not suffer from atopy, presented with severe bronchiolitis caused by respiratory syncytial virus, and afterward they manifested symptoms of BHR, which tends to persist until before adolescence. Generally, the children with non-atopic BA symptoms have a better prognosis than children with atopic BA, because in a greater percentage, the clinical manifestations will disappear, and their quality of life will improve as they progress in development into adolescence. In this age, besides family and personal background, the pillars of the diagnosis are the laboratory tests, especially cutaneous tests, and by this age most of them can perform pulmonary function tests, such as the exercise test and spirometry.

School Period

Patients who reach school age with FA and AD will maintain their clinical conditions during the rest of their lives, although with few symptoms. The most important manifestations for the atopic child within this age group are BA and AR. The group of patients with non-atopic BA symptoms start to experience an important decrease in their symptomatology and, by the end of this period, or during the beginning of their adolescence, they tend to be symptom free. This is specially the case for children who previously had BHR, with a background of severe bronchiolitis caused by respiratory syncytial virus and who did not suffer from atopy.

During this period a new phenotype may appear in a group of patients with symptoms of BA. Usually they are schoolgirls who present with obesity between 6 and 11 years of age. This group has a sevenfold increase in the possibility of presenting BA in relationship to eutrophic children. It has been demonstrated that obesity precedes and predicts BA, but there is no inverse relationship; this means that BA does not cause obesity. Even though the relationship between obesity and bronchial asthma is causal, there is still no confirmed relationship between obesity and allergic disease.

Adolescence Period

Most atopic children present with their symptoms localized mainly in the respiratory system, with manifestations such as AR and BA. Besides these symptoms, those manifestations of FA and AD can also be added, in the few patients who could not overcome this. The patient who before adolescence was obese and had bronchial asthma will maintain those respiratory symptoms during adolescence, although the patient may no longer be obese.

As happens in every age group, the evaluation of allergic diseases requires a global approach, and in this age it is focused on the two most frequent manifestations, acute rhinitis and bronchial asthma, which must be treated as indicated in the guidelines. The education of the allergic patient and her/his family is one of the therapeutic pillars, because it is a low-cost measure proven to reduce the use of medications. The same situation is faced with environmental control, which as an isolated measure does not modify the evolution of the disease, but it allows controlling the symptomatology in a better way with fewer therapeutic resources. Preventive pharmacotherapy, although it does not modify the natural progression of the disease, significantly reduces its manifestations, prevents sequelae, and improves the quality of life of the affected patient. Immunotherapy has precise indications, according to its clinical indication and the cost–benefit relationship.

Therapy

The specific treatment for each one of these pathologies is detailed in the corresponding section. Below, we present some general concepts that, although they do not modify the natural progression of the disease, reduce the symptoms and lead to a reduced use of medication for controlling the disease.

The first principle is to avoid contact with the antigen, when possible. If sensitization to certain foods is identified, a crucial part of the treatment is the suppression of the causative food. Inhaled antigens are difficult to avoid, but even in this situation, environmental measures must be taken to avoid contact with the most common antigens: *Dermatophagoides* (house dust mites) and pollen.

The WHO has favored every effort that promotes the use of primary prevention in risk patients. This strategy consists in a group of measures destined to currently healthy population, but who are at risk of developing the disease, and it includes measures to be implemented before any atopic sensitizing is manifested, along with perinatal interventions. These measures must be applicable to all the population, have a low cost, and be free of risks:

- Avoid smoking habits and passive exposure to cigarette smoke during pregnancy and first childhood (A-B Evidence).
- Control humidity conditions at home and reduce in-house contaminants (C Evidence).
- Exclusive breastfeeding until 4–6 months (A Evidence) with no special diet for the breast-feeding mother.
- Reduce inhaled allergens in high-risk children, specially house dust mites, cockroaches, and pets (B Evidence).

Relative to dietary measures during pregnancy, even though some reports indicate a certain beneficial effect when reducing the sensitization frequency of some food and skin atopy, most of them indicate that frequency is kept at similar levels, even when the mother suspends, during pregnancy and breastfeeding, certain foods which may be potentially sensitizing. Categorically, in follow-up studies covering 10 years, there is no effect in reducing the frequency of the positive skin test, asthma symptoms frequency, and atopy frequency in general. According to this, there is currently no evidence that may justify special diets for the mother during her pregnancy, and her adequate nutrition must always be protected. In spite of the controversial role of exclusive breast-feeding in relation to atopy disease, according to the most recent evidence, it is safe to state that most studies assign it a protective effect in the development of food allergy, and atopic dermatitis, but this is not true for the reduction of incidence of bronchial asthma. It must be considered that this beneficial effect may decrease in time.

It has been observed that the use of probiotics (for example, *Bifidobacterium lactis* and *Lactobacillus* GG) has some part in preventing and improving AD in children previously breast-fed. It has been confirmed that probiotics increase the IgA and IL-10 levels, and also suppress TNF-α. Also, probiotics modify intestinal flora to prevent antigen capture through the intestinal barrier, and increase the IFN-γ levels in peripheral blood mononuclear cells, favoring immune deviation to Th1. A recent meta-analysis indicates that early life probiotic administration is effective in reducing IgE levels, as well as reducing the risk of atopy sensitization in small children, but this does not apply to asthma or wheezing.

Secondary prevention strategies are the group of measures aimed at children who do not have a defined allergic phenotype, but who nevertheless possess markers indicating a high risk of manifesting the disease later. These measures must be implemented after the sensitization to allergens has taken place and before the disease becomes evident. These strategies are indicated during the first years of life:

- Treat AD in the infant and child to prevent respiratory allergies (Evidence D).
- Treat acute rhinitis to reduce the risk of developing asthma (Evidence D).
- In small children already sensitized to pets, dust mites, or cockroaches, reduce exposure to prevent the progression of the allergic disease (Evidence B).
- Remove from their workplace those patients who have developed symptoms caused by allergic occupation sensitization (Evidence C).

Subcutaneous immunotherapy with allergens is still a controversial subject, but in patients with acute rhinitis, it significantly reduces the percentage of patients who afterward develop BA in relationship to the control group, and it is one of the preventive measures highlighted by the expert panel on immunotherapy at the WHO, which has been newly considered in recent publications. Immunotherapy in BA with mite allergens, according to different meta-analyses, showed an improvement of 2.7 fold for asthma symptoms, 4.2 fold for medication reduction, and 13.7 fold for BHR. The patient must be carefully selected when indicating immunotherapy, which should be considered for patients whose symptoms are mainly induced by an allergen, mono-sensitized. Immunotherapy can also be considered for patients whose symptoms have been present for a prolonged time, as long as pharmacotherapy, or when therapy produces a serious adverse effect. In the case of acute rhinitis, it is indicated if the patient presents persistent symptoms, and for BA, it must be persistent or moderate, along with normal pulmonary function.

Tertiary prevention is defined as the group of measures taken to suppress the symptoms and the progression of the disease once the disease has manifested. These measures are enforced when the allergic disease is already present:

- For infants who are allergic to cow's milk, avoid its proteins and/or use hypoallergenic formulas (Evidence B).
- For patients with BA, AR, or AD sensitized to house dust mites, cockroaches, or pets, the allergens should be eliminated or the exposure to them should be reduced to have a better control the symptoms and avoid exacerbations (Evidence A-B).
- Pharmacotherapy is indicated to treat the inflammatory underlying process (Evidence A).
- Avoid acetylsalicylic acid and other nonsteroidal antiinflammatories in patients who are sensitive to these drugs (Evidence C).

For AD, the continuous and permanent indication of antihistamines is used to try to suppress or reduce the pruritus, one of the most common symptoms and that which most alters the quality of life of the patients and their parents. Oral steroid therapy is reserved for short periods in the situations of greater intensity. For local treatment, the use of creams or humectant lotions, immunomodulators such as tracrolimus or pimecrolimus, and local steroids in the affected area for short periods, have been proven useful.

For BA, in addition to the environmental control and avoiding indoor pollutants, especially tobacco smoke, preventive pharmacological therapy has a fundamental role in improving the quality of life of the patient and the patient's family.

For acute rhinitis, in addition to the same environmental measures used for BA, pharmacological therapy with antihistamines is recommended: instillation of physiological saline solution for the nose during the periods of greater symptomatology and the use of topic nasal steroids.

Summary

Allergic diseases constitute a group of very prevalent pathologies whose frequency is increasing. The mortality rate is very low, but the diseases severely affect the quality of life of the patient and the patient's family. This disease is becoming more and more common as the result of various environmental factors, so the general practitioner must be capable of recognizing them and starting preventive and treatment measures. Current therapeutic options, although they do not modify the natural progression of the disease, allows the patients suffering from allergic disease to have a normal life.

Sources

Asher M, Montefort S, Björkstén B, and the ISAAC Phase Three Study Group, et al. Worldwide time trends in the prevalence of symptoms of asthma, allergic rhinoconjuctivitis and eczema in childhood: ISAAC phases one and three repeat multicountry cross-sectional surveys. Lancet. 2006;368:733–43.

Björkstén B. The intrauterine and postnatal environments. J. Allergy Clin Immunol. 1999;104:1119–27.

Calderon M, Alves B, Jacobson M, Hurwitz B, Sheik A, Durhan S. Allergen injection immunotherapy for seasonal allergic rhinitis. Cochrane Database Syst Rev. 2007;1:CD001936.

Calvo M. Particularidades de la alergia en la infancia: implicancias diagnósticas y terapéuticas.. En: Guzmán M, editor. Alergias. Guía Clínica; 2012. p. 140–8.

Castro Rodríguez J. The asthma predictive index: a very useful tool for predicting asthma in young children. Allergy Clin Immunol. 2010;126:212–6. https://www.jacionline.org/article/S0091-6749(10)01034-1/fulltext

Castro-Rodríguez J, Holberg C, Wright A, Martínez F. A clinical index to define risk of asthma in young children with recurrent wheezing. Am J Respir Crit Care Med. 2000;162:1403–6.

Castro-Rodríguez J, Holberg C, Morgan W, Wright A, Martínez F. Increase incidence of asthma-like symptoms in girls who become overweight or obese during the school years. Am J Respir Crit Care Med. 2001;163:1344–9.

Chapmann J, Bernstein L, Lee R, et al. Food allergy: a practical parameter. Ann Allergy Asthma Immunol. 2006;96:S1–S68.

De Benedictis D, Bush A. The challenge of asthma in adolescent. Pediatr Pulmonol. 2007;42:683–92.

Ebisawa M, Ikematsu K, Imai T, Tachimoto H. Food allergy in Japan. Allergy Clin Immunol Int. 2003;5:214–7.

Elazab N, Mendy A, Gasana J, Vieira E, Quizon A, Forno E. Probiotic administration in early life, atopy and asthma: a meta-analysis of clinical trials. Pediatrics. 2013;132(3):e666–76.

Global Initiative for Asthma (GINA). National Institutes of Health. Revisado 1 diciembre 2013. www.ginasthma.org.

Guilbert T, Morgan W, Zeiger R, et al. Atopic characteristics of children with recurrent wheezing at high risk for the development of childhood asthma. J Allergy Clin Immunol. 2004;114:1282–7.

ISAAC Steering Committee. Worldwide varations in the prevalence of symptoms of asthma, allergic rhinoconjunctivitis and atopic eczema. Lancet. 1998;351:1225–32.

Jones C, Miles E, Warner J. Fetal peripheral blood mononuclear cell proliferative responses to mitogenic and allergenic stimulae during gestation. Pediatr Allergy Immunol. 1996;7:109–16.

Kondo N, Kobayashi Y, Shinoda S. Reduced INF gamma production by antigen stimulated cord blood mononuclear cells is a risk factor for allergic disorders: 6 year follow up study. Clin Exp Allergy. 1998;28:1341–4.

Mullol J, Valero A, Alobid I, Barta J, Navarro AM, Chivato T, Khaltaev N, Bousquet J. Allergic Rhinitis and its Impact on Asthma Update (ARIA 2008). The Perspective from Spain. http://www.jiaci.org/issues/vol18issue5/2.pdf.

NICE: Atopic eczema in under 12s: diagnosis and management. NICE clinical guideline 57, 2007. https://www.nice.org.uk/guidance/cg57.

Passalacqua G, Durham S. (GA2LEN). Allergic rhinitis and its impact on asthma update: allergen immunotherapy. J Allergy Clin Immunol. 2007;119:881–91.

Pérez J et al. y Grupo de Vías Respiratorias. Protocolo de rinitis alérgica (publicación P-GVR-6, 2009) Available at: http://www.respirar.org/index.php/grupo-vias-respiratorias/protocolos.

Skripak J, Matsui E, Mudd K, Wood R. The natural history of IgE-mediated cow's milk allergy. J Allergy Clin Immunol. 2007;120:1172–7.

Subbarayal B, Geroldinger-Simic M, Bohle B. Birch pollen-related food allergy: an excellent disease model to understand the relevance of immunological cross-reactivity for allergy. In: Pereira C, editor. Allergic diseases. Highlights in the clinic, mechanism and treatment. 2012. p. 141–4.

Wood R. The natural history of food allergy. Pediatrics. 2003;111(6 pt 3):1631–7.

Yssel H, Groux H. Characterization of T cell subpopulations involved in the pathogenesis of asthma and allergic diseases. Int Arch Allergy Immunol. 2000;121:10–8.

Latin America Asthma Epidemiology and Related Risk Factors

39

Viviana Aguirre Camposano, Manuel Soto Martínez, and Manuel Soto Quirós

Contents

Introduction

Asthma is the most common chronic disease in children worldwide. Its high heterogeneity makes it a very complex disease, in which several risk factors, protector factors, and the genetic predisposition of the patient interact to express the disease in different ways and at different times. During the past decades an important increase in the prevalence of this disease has been observed, as well as for other allergic diseases such as allergic rhinitis, rhinoconjunctivitis, eczema, and even food allergies.

V. Aguirre Camposano
Department of Pediatrics, School of Medicine, University of Santiago, Santiago, Chile

M. Soto Martínez
Department of Pediatrics, School of Medicine, University of Costa Rica, San José, Costa Rica

M. Soto Quirós (✉)
Department of Pediatrics, Hospital San José, San José, Costa Rica

The World Health Organization (WHO) and the Global Initiative for Asthma (GINA) estimate that asthma affects around 200 million people in the world. It causes a considerable amount of lost schooldays and workdays, besides the worsening of the quality of life, particularly in those patients who are poorly controlled. The disease is costly to the public health, because in many cases treatment must be continued for years, and patients may present with exacerbations requiring multiple visits to the emergency room or hospital admissions.

The greatest limitation of asthma epidemiological studies, as happens with other allergic diseases, lies in the methods obtained for the diagnosis, which are based mainly on questionnaires, with limited studies using more objective measures such as pulmonary function tests, allergy studies, or allergen determination.

The most important investigation relative to asthma prevalence in children is the International Study of Asthma and Allergies in Childhood (ISAAC), in which the same questionnaire was

P. Bertrand, I. Sánchez (eds.), *Pediatric Respiratory Diseases*,
https://doi.org/10.1007/978-3-030-26961-6_39

applied to children from 6 to 7 years old or adolescents from 13 to 14 years old, worldwide, with their respective translations to the local language. Phase I of the ISAAC featured questionnaires including questions about the presence of symptoms related to asthma, rhinitis, and eczema. In Phase II of ISAAC, which followed Phase I by about 5 years, the main objective was to examine the variation within the tendencies of these diseases, but it also included an environmental questionnaire.

Phase II of ISAAC was developed with the intent to prove certain hypotheses that were generated during the analysis of Phase I. Nevertheless, this second phase included a smaller number of participants from Latin America.

At the same time, besides the epidemiological studies about disease prevalence, several investigations appeared relative to possible risk factors associated with asthma development and other allergic diseases such as rhinitis and eczema. Many of these studies determined that atopy family history is among the main risk factors for developing asthma, rhinitis, and eczema, in addition to the presence of multiple environmental factors, which are considered key factors influencing the expression of the disease.

Asthma in Latin America: Phase I and Phase III ISAAC Studies

In Phase I of ISAAC, a questionnaire was used to determine the prevalence and severity of symptoms that suggest the presence of asthma and other allergic diseases, such as rhinitis and eczema. This phase involved about 257,800 children who were between 6 and 7 years old, distributed around 91 centers in 38 countries, and 463,801 children between 13 and 14 years of age, distributed in 155 centers in 56 countries around the world.

The prevalence of respiratory symptoms that suggested the presence of asthma and other allergic diseases in children in the region was very high and very similar to the prevalence rates reported by developed countries. There was great variability in the prevalence rates of asthma reported by several countries, with a greater tendency rate in countries with tropical weather.

Five to 10 years after the phase I of ISAAC was implemented, Phase III of ISAAC was executed. In Phase III, a total of 1,187,496 children participated from 237 centers in 98 countries. Approximately 85% of the countries that participated in Phase I also participated in Phase III. The design of the study was very similar, but it also included an environmental questionnaire.

The change in the average of prevalence rates of wheezing within the past 12 months between Phase I and Phase III was 11.1% to 11.6% for children who were from 6 to 7 years old (0.13% increase per year), and 13.2% to 13.7% in children who were 13 to 14 years old (0.06 increase per year) (Table 39.1). In Latin America, as in many other regions in the world, there was an increase in the prevalence rate of the disease for both age groups (+0.07% and +0.32%, respectively) (Table 39.2.). It is worth mentioning that independently of the ISAAC phase, most of the centers in Latin America reported the highest prevalence rates of the disease in the world.

There was a worldwide increase in the symptoms for at least two diseases. In the group of 6- to 7-year-olds there was an increase in the proportion of the three diseases from 0.8% to 1.0%, and in the group of 13- to 14-year-olds the change was 1.1% to 1.2%.

Phase III of ISAAC, and other epidemiological investigations, show very clear increasing tendencies in the asthma prevalence rate in children worldwide. It is also important to consider the increase in the prevalence rate of symptoms of eczema and rhinoconjunctivitis, which was even greater than the increase of asthma symptoms. This finding presents a new hypothesis relative to potential modification and risk factors for the appearance of these diseases.

Anther factor to consider was the variability prevalence rate for asthma and other allergic diseases in Latin America, where some countries reported the highest disease proportions at the worldwide level (Costa Rica), and other countries reporting very low prevalence rates (Mexico). The most interesting issue is that this variability has yet no explanation, because in the results of ISAAC it is observed that this is

Table 39.1 Asthma prevalence information within the past 12 months

	Years between phases	Number of children	Phase I of ISAAC (%)	Phase III of ISAAC (%)	Change per year	SD
6–7 years old						
Africa (English speaking)	7.0	2,396	4.8	5.6	0.10	0.19
Asia-Pacific	6.3	43,403	10.0	8.9	−0.06	0.09
Eastern Mediterranean	6.3	13,990	6.8	11.7	0.79	0.08
Indian subcontinent	7.5	18,877	6.2	6.8	0.06	0.17
Latin America	7.1	21,112	19.9	21.4	0.07	0.12
North America	7.5	4,014	16.8	19.1	0.32	0.12
North and East of Europe	6.4	21,984	9.7	9.6	0.05	0.06
Oceania	9.4	13,841	24.3	21.8	−0.21	0.06
West of Europe	7.2	53,787	8.1	9.7	0.20	0.03
GLOBAL TOTAL	7.1	193,404	11.1	11.6	0.13	0.04
13–14 years old						
Africa (English speaking)	6.6	17,686	13.5	15.4	0.18	0.15
Africa (French speaking)	6.0	10,711	7.7	10.2	0.15	0.40
Asia-Pacific	6.4	57,389	8.7	8.8	0.07	0.07
Eastern Mediterranean	6.3	19,887	12.0	11.6	−0.10	0.13
Indian Subcontinent	7.1	20,767	6.7	6.4	0.02	0.14
Latin America	6.9	44,550	17.8	18.8	0.32	0.10
North America	6.5	4,920	19.7	21.5	0.12	0.24
North and East of Europe	6.9	32,608	8.1	11.6	0.26	0.09
Oceania	9.0	13,317	29.7	26.7	−0.39	0.13
West of Europe	7.4	82,844	15.4	15.2	−0.07	0.10
GLOBAL TOTAL	7.0	304,679	13.2	13.7	0.06	0.05

SD Standard deviation

Data taken from Asher et al. Worldwide trends in the prevalence of symptoms of asthma, allergic rhinoconjunctivitis, and eczema in childhood: ISAAC Phases One and Three repeat multicountry cross-sectional surveys. *Lancet* 2006;368(9537):733–743

independent of weather, geographic, cultural, ethnical, or language factors. These results are probably more related to the environment, such as humidity and flora, in addition to outdoor and indoor pollutants.

In general, not only for the region, children in the 6- to 7-year-old group had a greater incidence of respiratory symptoms in comparison to the 13- and 14-year-old group. In relationship to gender, boys 6 to 7 years old had a greater prevalence of wheezing and asthma within the past 12 months than did girls, although girls had a greater prevalence of respiratory symptoms in the group from 13 to 14 years old. The presence of wheezing during the past 12 months was more common in urban areas for the group 6 to 7 years old; in contrast, in the group 13 to 14 years old this risk was greater if they lived in areas with temperatures below 20 °C and at an altitude over 1000 m. Living in a rural area with a weather temperature above 20 °C increased the risk of dry cough and respiratory symptoms in this same age group.

There are multiple hypotheses about the increase of the prevalence of this disease in many countries. It is possible that the asthma increase is caused by an improvement in diagnosis. Nevertheless, high levels of risk and sensitizing factors have been reported, which influence the appearance and poor control of the disease, for

Table 39.2 Asthma prevalence information within the past 12 months (Latin America)

	Years between phases	Number of children	Response (%)	Phase I of ISAAC (%)	Phase III of ISAAC (%)	Change per year	SD
6–7 years old							
Brazil	7.0	3,047	68.2	21.3	24.4	0.44	0.20
Chile (3)	7.0	9,310	88.9	18.2	17.9	−0.06	0.12
Costa Rica	8.0	3,234	80.9	32.1	37.6	0.69	0.20
Mexico	8.0	2,579	84.3	8.6	8.4	−0.03	0.11
Panama	6.0	2,942	92.5	23.5	22.7	−0.13	0.20
13–14 years old							
Argentina	5.0	3,445	99.4	11.2	13.6	0.48	0.24
Brazil (5)	7.4	15,681	91.5	22.7	19.9	−0.42	0.17
Chile (3)	6.7	9,175	89.3	10.2	15.5	0.84	0.13
Costa Rica	8.0	2,436	69.6	23.7	27.3	0.46	0.24
Mexico	8.0	1,431	85.9	6.6	11.6	0.63	0.13
Panama	6.0	3,183	92.9	17.6	22.9	0.88	0.19
Paraguay	5.0	3,000	99.3	19.4	20.9	0.31	0.32
Peru	6.0	3,022	99.2	26.0	19.6	−1.06	0.57
Uruguay	8.0	3,177	90.8	19.0	17.9	−0.13	0.20

Data taken from Asher et al. Worldwide trends in the prevalence of symptoms of asthma, allergic rhinoconjunctivitis, and eczema in childhood: ISAAC Phases One and Three repeat multicountry cross-sectional surveys. *Lancet* 2006;368(9537):733–743
SD Standard deviation

example, passive and active smoke tobacco exposure during pregnancy, and genetic as well as nutritional factors, outdoor and indoor pollutants, and respiratory infections during the first years of life.

Risk Factors

There are many published studies aimed to identify asthma risk factors, and many times the results are contradictory. Factors that have been proven to be protectors for this disease in other countries, especially in developed countries, include the high number of children per family, high percentage of viral respiratory infections, gastrointestinal parasitosis, and lack of hygiene. However, these factors do not seem to have a significant role in Latin America. On the contrary, these factors appear to be risk factors in Latin America, which suggests that socioeconomic status may be a factor. Nevertheless, correlation analyses in several countries of South America did not find a significant variation.

Available information about asthma risk factors, which comes from several studies conducted in countries in all the regions of the world, describes the following:

- *Genetics*. The studies conducted in families and twins establish that asthma has a genetic predisposition, although the genes involved in its pathogenesis are many and can vary according to different ethnic groups. Information gathered from the different studies has identified at least 18 genomic regions and more than 100 genes associated with asthma and allergies in 11 different populations. Besides the genes that predispose to suffering from asthma, there are others related to treatment response. The genetic characterization of asthma has been difficult, and there is still much to be discovered because of the extensive heterogeneity of the genetic base of asthma and its wide interaction with the environment.
- *Obesity*. Asthma is more frequent and more difficult to treat in obese patients. Although

the obese patient has a reduced pulmonary function and a higher comorbidity, obesity is usually present before asthma, and the existing studies suggest maternal obesity during pregnancy has a role. Although the mechanism through which obesity is a risk factor is not completely understood, it has been proposed that it may result from a combination of several factors, such as the development of a pre-inflammatory state caused by the release of cytokines and mediators through adipocytes, or a respiratory pattern that may alter the plasticity and function of the smooth muscle in the airway. All these factors must be considered besides a genetic, hormonal, or neurogenic influence.

- *Gender*. During childhood, the asthma prevalence rate in boys is almost double the rate in girls. As the child grows, this difference is reduced, and during adulthood it is inverted, with women having a greater prevalence rate for asthma. The reasons for this are not very clear, although at birth male lung size smaller than that of women, but during adulthood the lung of men is larger.
- *Aeroallergens*. Atopic sensitizing to inhaled allergens, especially permanent ones, is an important risk factor related to asthma. Although it is clear that both outdoor and indoor allergens cause asthma exacerbations, their role for asthma appearance is not clear. Sensitizing to room dust, cat and dog hair, cockroaches, and *Aspergillus* are risk factors for asthma symptoms during the first 3 years of life. Relative to cats and dogs, the epidemiological studies are contradictory.
- *Infections*. Current knowledge is contradictory. Interest about the impact of bacterial products and its relation to asthma development has produced the hygiene hypothesis, which suggests that infections during the early stages of life help the child's immunological system to develop through a nonallergic path, therefore reducing the risk for asthma and other allergic diseases. This hypothesis would explain the reduced asthma risk in the long term for children exposed to situations that increase the possibility of infection, such as having older siblings, attending daycare, living in an agricultural environment, and having contact with pets and farm animals. However, this hypothesis does not explain the observed increase of asthma prevalence rate in underdeveloped countries with poor hygiene conditions.

  Early infection by rhinovirus and respiratory syncytial virus has been related to the onset of the asthma phenotype. It has been described that up to 40% of the children hospitalized because of respiratory syncytial virus continue to present with wheezing or asthma during childhood. Nevertheless, there is also evidence that certain early infections such as measles, tuberculosis, and even respiratory syncytial virus may protect against asthma.

  The interaction between atopy and viral infection is complex because the atopic state may influence the viral response of the lower airway, and at the same time, the viral infection may influence the development of allergy sensitization. Also, the interaction between these two factors may occur when the individual is exposed simultaneously to allergens and virus. Although in general parasite infections do not protect from asthma, ancylostomiasis may reduce the risk.
- *Antibiotics*. The use of antibiotics during the first year of life has been related to a greater asthma risk, but the results are controversial, and the current recommendation is to avoid the use of broad-spectrum antibiotics during early childhood.
- *Tobacco*. Exposition to tobacco smoke during pregnancy and after birth is related to a greater risk of developing asthma symptoms during the first years of childhood. Tobacco use during pregnancy is related to alterations in pulmonary development. The children of mothers who smoke have a fourfold-increased risk to present with wheezing during their first year of life.
- *Indoor and outdoor pollution*. The role of outdoor pollution as a cause of asthma can be discussed, although it clearly is a trigger of asthma exacerbations. The role of indoor pollutants is also controversial, such as smoke

and gas vapors, as well as combustible biomass used for heating and refrigerating, and the same exacerbations occur with the presence of fungus and cockroach infestations.

Recent information suggests that the immune response of the child may be altered if the mother was exposed to environmental pollution during pregnancy and during the first years of childhood; this would increase the appearance of asthma and allergies.

- *Diet*. Infants fed with breast milk have a lower incidence of wheezing disease during early childhood, in comparison to patients who have been fed with cow's milk or soy milk, although there is not enough evidence to support its protective effect in the development of asthma during childhood.

  Even though there is information suggesting that the Occidental diet may have contributed to the increase of asthma and atopic diseases in general, there is still not enough evidence to support the protector effect of some kind of diet during pregnancy or lactation to avoid asthma development. Recently, it has been described that vitamin D deficiency is related to a increase in the risk for asthma appearance, and ongoing studies using supplements of vitamin D will confirm this in future.
- *Social factors and inequity*. Generally, there is a positive relationship between poverty and greater asthma morbidity, but the relationship to a greater prevalence rate can be discussed, probably from the presence of many covariables related to this condition, such as ethnic group, age of the mother at birth, maternal breastfeeding, attending daycare, urban/rural environment, obesity, and maternal and environmental stress. Studies that originated from ISAAC in relationship to environmental factors associated with asthma, rhinitis, and eczema found a positive relationship between these three diseases and the geographic gross product of each country, although the prevalence rate of severe asthma was inversely correlated.
- *Other factors involved*. A greater asthma risk has been described for children born by urgent cesarean section, particularly for children with the following risk factors: parent allergies, paracetamol consumption during pregnancy and during the first year of the child's life, presence of jaundice during the neonatal period, and environmental stress surrounding the child during the first year of life. However, all these factors must be confirmed in future studies. It is important to highlight the asthma risks described for infants with recurring wheezing episodes. In these patients, the family history of parents with asthma, the presence of eczema, allergic rhinitis, wheezing episodes not related to colds, and peripheral eosinophilia above 4% during the first 3 years of life are greater risks to suffer asthma during childhood.

After many epidemiological studies, we recognize that asthma and allergic diseases in Latin America are a great public health problem for most countries, with a high morbidity, complexity in treatment and follow-up, and high health costs, and carrying a significant alteration in the quality of life of the patients. Although many risk and protection factors have been recognized, there is a great degree of variability in Latin America, which makes it difficult to place highly effective preventive measures.

Asthma Epidemiology in Chile

Studies about asthma prevalence symptoms in Chile mainly derive from the reports of the ISAAC, and they oscillate between 17.9%, for schoolchildren within the age group of 6 to 7 years old, and 15.3% for schoolchildren 13 to 14 years old (0.84% on average per year). These numbers locate Chile in an intermediate position relative to asthma in Latin America, and above the average prevalence at world level. For the group of infants, the most recent information comes from the International Study of Wheezing in Infants (Estudio Internacional de Sibilancias en Lactantes, EISL), which indicates that in Chile the prevalence of recurrent wheezing (three or more episodes) is 21.6% in those under 1 year old, with 57% of severe episodes, 70% of visits to urgency services, and 29% of hospitalization because of wheezing.

Although the hospitalization rate from asthma is low (0.68% of the total of hospital admittances for those under 20 years old) and mortality is practically nil, the use of medical resources represents a significant cost in healthcare. During 2012, 26.8% of all the medical consultations related to respiratory diseases within the primary attention services corresponded to wheezing and asthma for those under 15 years old, which represented 4.4% of all emergency consults of those under 15 years old during 2011. These numbers are probably underestimated, because they do not consider asthma exacerbations, which may be within the diagnoses of pneumonia, influenza, bronchitis, and acute upper tract respiratory infection, for those patients suffering from asthma.

Studies about the risk factors for asthma in children are scarce. Boneberger et al. recently published a study of rural population children in which they described that the precedent of attending daycare within the first year of life and regular contact with farm animals was related to a lower asthma risk, whereas the precedent of pneumonia and fungus/humidity at home was related to a greater risk.

To conclude, according to the reports delivered by the Chilean Ministry of Health, the Public Health Care Network keeps a follow-up (information dated December 2013) of 192,717 children who are under 15 years old. These children have moderate or severe asthma and are incorporated to the program of explicit guarantees in health (garantías explícitas en salud, GES). The evaluation of the impact of this public policy is still pending, although there has been a progressive reduction in the number of patients with severe asthma.

Sources

Antó JM. Recent advances in the epidemiologic investigation of risk factors for asthma: a review of the 2011 literature. Curr Allergy Asthma Rep. 2012;12:192–200.

Asher MI. Recent perspectives on global epidemiology of asthma in childhood. Allergol Immunopathol (Madr). 2010;38(2):83–7.

Asher MI, Montefort S, Björkstén B, Lai CK, Strachan DP, Weiland SK, et al. Worldwide time trends in the prevalence of symptoms of asthma, allergic rhinoconjunctivitis, and eczema in childhood: ISAAC Phases One and Three repeat multicountry cross-sectional surveys. Lancet. 2006;368(9537):733–43.

Asher MI, Stewart AW, Wong G, Strachan DP, García-Marcos L, Anderson HR, et al. Changes over time in the relationship between symptoms of asthma, rhinoconjunctivitis and eczema: a global perspective from the International Study of Asthma and Allergies in Childhood (ISAAC). Allergol Immunopathol (Madr). 2012;40(5):267–74.

Beasley RW, Beasley RW, Clayton TO, Crane J, Lai CK, Montefort SR, Mutius E, et al. Acetaminophen use and risk of asthma, rhinoconjunctivitis, and eczema in adolescents: International Study of Asthma and Allergies in Childhood Phase Three. Am J Respir Crit Care Med. 2011;183(2):171–8.

Boneberger A, Haider D, Baer J, Kausel L, Von Kries R, Kabesch M, Radon K, Calvo M. Environmental risk factors in the first year of life and childhood asthma in the Central South of Chile. J Asthma. 2011;48(5):464–9.

Brehm JM, Celedón JC, Soto-Quiros ME, Avila L, Hunninghake GM, Forno E, et al. Serum vitamin D levels and markers of severity of childhood asthma in Costa Rica. Am J Respir Crit Care Med. 2009;179(9):765–71.

Chong Neto HJ, Rosario NA, Sole D, Latin American IG. Asthma and rhinitis in South America: how different they are from other parts of the world. Allergy Asthma Immunol Res. 2012;4(2):62–7.

Huang L, Bao Y, Xu Z, Lei X, Chen Y, Zhang Y, Zhang J. Neonatal bilirubin levels and childhood asthma in the US collaborative perinatal project, 1959–1965. Am J Epidemiol. 2013;178(12):1691–7.

Lai CK, Beasley R, Crane J, Foliaki S, Shah J, Weiland S, International Study of Asthma and Allergies in Childhood Phase Three Study Group. Global variation in the prevalence and severity of asthma symptoms: phase three of the International Study of Asthma and Allergies in Childhood (ISAAC). Thorax. 2009;64(6):476–83.

Ly NP, Soto-Quirós ME, Avila L, Hunninghake GM, Raby BA, Laskey D, et al. Paternal asthma, mold exposure, and increased airway responsiveness among children with asthma in Costa Rica. Chest. 2008;133(1):107–14.

Mallol J, Solé D, Asher I, Clayton T, Stein R, Soto-Quiroz M. Prevalence of asthma symptoms in Latin America: the International Study of Asthma and Allergies in Childhood (ISAAC). Pediatr Pulmonol. 2000;30(6):439–44.

Mallol J, Aguirre V, Aguilar P, Calvo M, Amarales L, Arellano P, Palma R. Cambios en la prevalencia de asma en escolares chilenos entre 1994 y 2002. Rev Méd Chile 2007;135:580–6.

Mallol J, García-Marcos L, Solé D, Brand P, the EISL Study Group. International prevalence of recurrent wheezing during the first year of life: variability, treatment patterns and use of health resources. Thorax. 2010;65:1004–9.

Odhiambo JA, Williams HC, Clayton TO, Robertson CF, Asher MI, Group IPTS. Global variations in prevalence of eczema symptoms in children from ISAAC Phase Three. J Allergy Clin Immunol. 2009;124(6):1251–1258. e23.

Pedersen SE, Hurd SS, Lemanske RF Jr, Becker A, Zar HJ, Sly PD, Manuel Soto-Quiroz M, Wong G, Bateman EED. Global strategy for the diagnosis and management of asthma in children 5 years and younger. Pediatr Pulmonol. 2011;46:1–17.

Soto-Quiros ME, Silverman EK, Hanson LA, Weiss ST, Celedón JC. Maternal history, sensitization to allergens, and current wheezing, rhinitis, and eczema among children in Costa Rica. Pediatr Pulmonol. 2002a;33(4):237–43.

Soto-Quiros ME, Soto-Martinez M, Hanson LA. Epidemiological studies of the very high prevalence of asthma and related symptoms among school children in Costa Rica from 1989 to 1998. Pediatr Allergy Immunol. 2002b;13(5):342–9.

The International Study of Asthma and Allergies in Childhood (ISAAC) Steering Committee. Worldwide variation in prevalence of symptoms of asthma, allergic rhinoconjunctivitis, and atopic eczema: ISAAC. Lancet. 1998;351(9111):1225–32.

Evaluation of Asthma Risk in Infants and Preschoolers

40

José Antonio Castro-Rodríguez

Contents

Recent cohort studies have provided important information about several issues: natural progression of wheezing during the first years of life, risk factors for asthma development, and the efficacy of different preventive strategies.

The most representative of these studies is the Tucson Children's Respiratory Study (TCRS), which began in 1980, including 1246 newborns who were enrolled shortly after birth, in Tucson, Arizona, United States of America. This study was designed as a prospective cohort to obtain information about potential risk factors related to lower respiratory tract disease. Participants completed questionnaires at 1, 3, 6, 11, and 16 years of life and were evaluated with periodic allergic cutaneous skin tests, E immunoglobulin (IgE), and eosinophil count, with pulmonary function and lung function tests. Using this information, three wheezing phenotypes were described during the first years of life, besides correlating the presence of wheezing with variables linked to genetics, immunology, physiology, and environmental factors.

Another cohort study started in 1989 was conducted in 1456 children born in the province of Wight Island, United Kingdom. This study used questionnaires to recollect clinical information at 1, 2, 4, 10, and 18 years of life. Further, allergy cutaneous skin tests were conducted at 4, 10, and 18 years of life, with total IgE level, lung function tests, and bronchial challenging tests at 10 years of life. New wheezing phenotypes were described. The Multicenter Allergy Study (MAS) that started in Germany in 1990 included 1314 children. Participants were followed and evaluated at 1, 3, 6, 12, 18, and 24 months of life. After this, the follow-ups were done yearly until the participants reached 13 years of age. This study recollected information through questionnaires, specific IgE against food and inhaled allergens (at 1, 2, 3, 5, 7, and 10 years of life), besides

J. A. Castro-Rodríguez (✉)
Department of Pediatrics, School of Medicine, Pontificia Universidad Católica de Chile, Santiago, Chile
e-mail: jcastro@med.puc.cl

P. Bertrand, I. Sánchez (eds.), *Pediatric Respiratory Diseases*,
https://doi.org/10.1007/978-3-030-26961-6_40

lung function tests (at ages of 7, 10, and 13). Thus, this study gathered information about the relationship between allergic sensitizing during early childhood and wheezing.

In 1995, the Manchester Asthma and Allergy Study (MAAS) was started in the United Kingdom, including 1186 infants who were afterward evaluated through the use of respiratory questionnaires at 1, 3, 5, and 8 years of life. Additionally, lung functions tests were done at 3, 5, and 8 years of life, with allergy cutaneous tests and IgE levels at 1, 3, 5, and 8 years of life. The atopic state of the participants was specified in further detail: early, multiple, multiple late, related to house dust mites, and not related to house dust mites. There was a significant association between early multiple atopic state and persistent wheezing. These associations described related type and number of allergens as well as the age when allergic sensitizing takes place.

The Avon Longitudinal Study of Parents and Children (ALSPAC) investigation studied 14,062 children born in the province of Avon, United Kingdom, in 1991. Clinical information was collected annually using respiratory questionnaires between 1 and 7 years of life, as well as conducting pulmonary function and allergy cutaneous tests when the participant reached 7 to 8 years of life.

The Prevalence and Incidence of Asthma and Mite Allergy (PIAMA) started in the Netherlands in 1996, with 3963 children 1 and 8 years old. The authors interviewed their caretakers annually and conducted serum measures for specific IgE when the participants were 4 to 8 years old. When the participants were 8 and 9 years old, lung function and bronchial challenge tests were conducted.

The trials mentioned included similar variables in their analyses, but differences in their reported results may be explained by the differences between employed methodology, number and moment of assessment of the participants, and size samples. Nevertheless, all these studies could determine several types of wheezing phenotypes during the first years of life.

Wheezing Phenotypes and Their Risk Factors

The existence of several wheezing phenotypes and their distinctive characteristics offer a glimpse of asthma development and its natural progression, as well as showing that asthma is a complex disease with multiple physiopathological mechanisms. The identification of these phenotypes is important to study the ways in which asthma progresses, as well as the mechanisms underlying the disease. This information can help to decide which is the most adequate therapy and how to predict the clinical progression of the patients.

The TCRS classified patients in four wheezing phenotypes: "transient early wheezing," "persistent wheezing," "late-onset wheezing" and non-wheezing. Children who presented with one or more wheezing episodes, but improved before 6 years of life, were classified as transient early wheezing. Those who presented with wheezing episodes after 3 years of life and persisted until 6 years of life were classified as suffering from late-onset wheezing. Finally, children who presented with wheezing episodes before 3 years of life that persisted until 6 years of life were classified as persistent wheezing. Some risk factors were identified for each one of the phenotypes: maternal tobacco exposure was related to the phenotype of transient early wheezing, and maternal asthma, being of masculine sex, and the presence of allergic rhinitis within the first year of life were related to late-onset wheezing. Maternal asthma, maternal use of tobacco, and presence of allergic rhinitis and atopic dermatitis during the first year of life, with being of masculine sex, were predictors for persistent wheezing. The fact that each one of the phenotypes has different risk factors suggests that each phenotype reflects different physiopathological entities.

After conducting cutaneous allergy tests at 6 years of life, the TCRS created an additional classification of the wheezing phenotypes, which consisted of three categories: transient early wheezing, non-atopic, and asthma/wheezing related to IgE, based on the results of the methacholine challenge test, the variation of maximum expiratory flow during the daytime, and the answers to a questionnaire inquiring about the presence or absence of wheezing/atopy.

The study conducted in Wight Island and the MAS and MAAS studies adopted similar classifications to those used in Tucson, but the age criteria were different: the study in Wight Island conducted evaluations at 4 and 10 years of life, the MAS study conducted evaluations 3 and 7 years of life, and the MAAS study did so 3 and 5 years of life. The predictors for persistent wheezing were family history of asthma, recurrent respiratory infections at early ages, and allergic sensitization. The presence of wheezing in late childhood was used as the criterion to classify participants. In the study conducted at Wight Island, the patients who still presented with wheezing episodes at 10 years of life were subclassified as suffering from atopic wheezing and non-atopic wheezing, each with different risk factors. The presence of asthma in brothers, atopic dermatitis during the first year of life, rhinitis at 4 years of age, and masculine sex were the most prevalent features in atopic patients suffering from wheezing, whereas maternal asthma with recurrent respiratory infections at 2 years of life were the most prevalent features in non-atopic patients suffering from wheezing. In the MAS study, the presence of wheezing at 13 years old was used to subclassify the patients; it was related to atopy in parents and in patients, high levels of IgE at early ages, and excessive exposure to indoor allergens. The MAAS study included the measure of specific airway resistance (sRaw) at early ages, and it was included as a risk factor for persistent wheezing at 5 years of life.

In the ALSPAC and PIAMA studies, the authors used the classification system used in the TCRS, but with longitudinal latent class analyses, and they added other subgroups. The ALSPAC study phenotypes described were "prolonged early wheezing" (related to maternal asthma, reduced pulmonary function, mild bronchial hyperreactivity, with no atopy), and "intermediate-onset wheezing" (associated with atopy, severe bronchial hyperreactivity, and greatly reduced pulmonary function). The PIAMA study only added the phenotype of intermediate onset. In these two studies, each phenotype had similar features, not only in relation to prevalence rates, but also relative to atopic sensitization, lung function tests, and bronchial hyperreactivity.

These studies have increased knowledge about the mechanisms and natural progression of wheezing during the first years of life, and risk factors for persistent asthma symptoms, as well as predicting lung function test. Nevertheless, in daily clinical practice it is very difficult, if not altogether impossible, to classify an identified patient with recurrent wheezing in one of those phenotypes,. Recently, a new classification system based on symptoms has been proposed in a consensus about wheezing in preschoolers, conducted by the European Respiratory Association (ERS). This tool divides preschoolers with wheezing into the categories episodic viral wheeze (EVW) and multiple trigger wheeze (MTW). According to this definition, the EVW phenotype corresponds to children whose exacerbations are exclusively triggered by respiratory viral infections, without symptoms between episodes. In contrast, the MTW phenotype corresponds to children who present wheezing in response not only to respiratory viral infections, but also to other triggers, such as allergens, physical activity, weather changes, or exposure to tobacco smoke.

At first, this classification was conceived as pragmatic and useful in daily clinical practice for preschooler patients with recurrent wheezing. This tool involved some potential therapeutic proposal, such as low doses of inhaled steroid continuously for children with the MTW phenotype, but not for children with the EVW phenotype, besides continuous or intermittent therapy with montelukast and high intermittent doses of inhaled steroids, which may have some usefulness for children with the EVW phenotype. However, it has been recently criticized for several reasons. There is scarce evidence supporting the idea that these two phenotypes are related to longitudinal patterns of wheezing or to different pathological patterns. This classification has not been objectively validated with lung function tests or markers of airway inflammation. Therefore, it is unknown if EVW and MTW phenotypes represent different conditions with different pathogen mechanisms, or if they are simply degrees of seriousness of the same disease, despite the MTW phenotype having inferior lung function compared to the EVW phenotype.

Finally, this classification does not allow separation of wheezing episodes by other respiratory symptoms, such as cough, cold episodes, or chest congestion. These two phenotypes appear to be unstable in time, as it has been shown that an important proportion of patients (close to 50%) move from one phenotype to the other after a 1-year follow-up. Therefore, it is currently thought that there is little evidence for the EVW/MTW classification system.

Asthma Predictive Indexes

The identification of preschoolers with recurrent wheezing that will present as asthma in the future makes possible setting prevention actions, as well as therapeutic strategies for those patients. To help with the identification of these preschoolers at greater risk of suffering from asthma, several predictive indexes have been developed. The Asthma Predictive Index (API) is currently the most used predictive tool. API combines simple clinical and laboratory parameters that are easy to perform. An identified patient is considered to have a positive API if she/he has had more than three recurrent wheezing episodes during the first 3 years of life, in addition to having one of these major criteria (medical diagnosis of atopic dermatitis, wheezing not related with cold-like episodes, and eosinophilia in peripheral blood greater than 4%) (Table 40.1). The TCRS cohort determined that in comparison to children who had a negative API, children with a positive API had a probability 2.6 to 13 times greater of having asthma between 6 and 13 years of life. The sensitivity, specificity, and positive and negative predictive value of API to predict asthma between 6 and 8 years of life were 22%, 97%, 77%, and 90%, respectively, and the positive and negative likelihood ratios were 7.3 and 0.80, respectively.

Table 40.1 Asthma Predictive Index (API)

Major criteria	Minor criteria
Father or mother with asthma diagnosed by a medical doctor.	Allergic rhinitis diagnosed by medical doctor
Eczema diagnosed by medical doctor.	Wheezing episodes not related to colds
	Eosinophilia in peripheral blood (>4%)

Recurrent wheezing (>3 episodes/year) during the first 3 years of life

A modified API (mAPI) was used in a randomized clinical study that involved 285 participants, included allergic sensitization to one or more allergens as another major criterion, and allergic sensitizing to milk, eggs, or peanuts as a minor criterion, which replaced the medical diagnosis of allergic rhinitis from the original API. Other predictive indexes were developed to predict persistent wheezing.

In 2003 Kurukulaaratchy et al. developed a predictive index using the information gathered from 1456 participants of the Wight Island study. This study found that having a family with a background history of asthma, positive cutaneous allergy tests at 4 years of life, and lower respiratory tract infections at 2 years of life were related to an increase in the probability of presenting with asthma symptoms at 10 years of life. Sensitivity, specificity, and positive and negative predictive ratio were 10%, 98%, 83%, and 64%, respectively, and the positive and negative likelihood ratios were 7.9 and 0.91, respectively. However, external validation studies are still needed to confirm this information.

In 2009, Caudri et al., using the information gathered from 3963 children from the PIAMA study, developed a predictive index named risk score PIAMA, based on eight clinical parameters easily obtained in daily clinical practice (masculine sex, birth after term, educational level of the parents, parent use of inhaled medications, frequency of wheezing episodes, wheezing not related to cold-like episodes, number of infections of the respiratory airway, and diagnosis of atopic dermatitis). When this index was used for the cohort in the PIAMA study, the participants with a score of 30 or greater had a 40% probability of developing asthma at 7 to 8 years of life.

Predictive asthma indexes, especially API, have been questioned. The indexes have been used in clinical practice without having a validation procedure in different populations (external validation). They have not been probed to predict long-term wheezing, the most severe wheezing episodes in children. They have also been found relatively complex with no real benefit over using more simple prediction rules based only on the frequency of wheezing episodes. Nevertheless, recently the API index and PIAMA risk score have been validated in independent populations (Colombia, 130 children; England, 1954 children). The API is a broad-use predictive index easily obtainable in any health center. API has been used with several purposes, such as a criterion of high-risk asthma development in randomized clinical trials, as well as a guide in clinical practice for the treatment of preschoolers with recurrent wheezing. API has been included in the most important guidelines for asthma management in the world, such as the Global Initiative for Asthma (GINA) and the proposal made by the National Institutes of Health (NIH) of the United States of America.

A recent study designed to validate the modified PIAMA risk index (term-born was replaced by prematurity as a criterion, and the infections in the respiratory system were eliminated) in a multiethnic cohort in the Netherlands (R Generation) showed that it has an acceptable discrimination rate and a good calibration in comparison with the original PIAMA cohort. It was also noted that it was independent of different ages and the ethnic origin of preschoolers. In comparison to the original PIAMA, the modified index had a discrete better negative value prediction, a poorer positive value prediction, and a similar positive and negative likelihood ratio (97% versus 95%, 74% versus 76%, 2.4 versus 2.5, and 0.5 versus 0.5, respectively). The Clinical Asthma Prediction Score (CAPS) followed 711 Danish preschoolers who sought primary attention for cough, wheezing, or respiratory distress. These children were followed up until they reached 6 years of age, when the diagnosis of asthma was based on the clinical combination, use of antiasthma medication, and pulmonary function (methacholine hyperreactivity, or bronchial reversibility by spirometry). This study showed a negative and positive predictive value of 0.74 to 0.78, respectively, but external validation studies are needed.

It is important to highlight that the best parameter to determine the use of a diagnostic test is the probability or coefficient variation (positive likelihood ratio), which for API is 7.3. Thus, for a population at low, moderate, or high risk of suffering from asthma during school age (for example, 10%, 20%, and 40%), if a child is evaluated for recurrent wheezing, API application increases the probability of asthma prediction by 4.3 to 2 fold, respectively. In other words, the asthma pretest frequency will change from 10% to 42%, from 20% to 62%, and from 40% to 80%, respectively. Additionally, the most useful feature of the API is its ability to estimate the probability that preschoolers with recurrent wheezing continue to have asthma symptoms during school age. Therefore, the use of API and other indexes of asthma prediction are valid within the clinical context to reduce morbidity in preschoolers with recurrent wheezing who are at a greater risk of developing asthma. All these measures are intended to avoid the unnecessary prescription of follow-up therapies in children who tend to have only transient conditions instead of asthma.

There are three important reasons to diagnose asthma in children under 5 years old who have recurrent wheezing along with a positive predictor index. First, about 80% of patients with asthma present symptoms during the first 5 years of life. Second, the greater reduction in pulmonary function happens before reaching 5 years of life. Third, even in developed countries, the population of children with the poorest asthma control are children less than 5 years old. Therefore, it is probable that parents will adhere better to determined prolonged follow-up treatment if they know that the cause of recurrent wheezing their child presents is a chronic disease called asthma, instead of a disease with a milder-sounding name as sometimes mentioned ("allergy" or "bronchial hyperreactivity," "recurrent bronchitis," "asthma-like bronchitis," "obstructive bronchitis," "pre-asthma," or "principles of asthma"). We know that adherence, measured by electronic dosimeters, to inhaled steroids when treating chronic asthma in children is only about 50%. Poor adherence to preventive treatment is one of the most important risk factors for uncontrolled asthma and hospitalization.

Sources

Brand PL, Baraldi E, Bisgaard H, et al. Definition, assessment and treatment of wheezing disorders in preschool children: an evidence-based approach. Eur Respir J. 2008;32:1096–110.

Castro-Rodriguez JA. The Asthma Predictive Index: a very useful tool for predicting asthma in young children. J Allergy Clin Immunol. 2010;126:212–6.

Castro-Rodriguez JA. The necessity of having asthma predictive scores in children. J Allergy Clin Immunol. 2013;132:1311–3.

Castro-Rodriguez JA, Holberg CJ, Wright AL, et al. A clinical index to define risk of asthma in young children with recurrent wheezing. Am J Respir Crit Care Med. 2000;162:1403–6.

Garcia-Marcos L, Martinez FD. Multitrigger versus episodic wheeze in toddlers: new phenotypes or severity markers? J Allergy Clin Immunol. 2010;126:489–90.

Guilbert TW, Morgan WJ, Zeiger RS, et al. Atopic characteristics of children with recurrent wheezing at high risk for the development of childhood asthma. J Allergy Clin Immunol. 2004;114:1282–7.

Guilbert TW, Morgan WJ, Zeiger RS, et al. Long-term inhaled corticosteroids in preschool children at high risk for asthma. N Engl J Med. 2006;354:1985–97.

Hafkamp-de Goren E, Lingsma HF, Caudri D, et al. Predicting asthma in preschool children with asthma-like symptoms: validating and updating the PIAMA risk score. J Allergy Clin Immunol. 2013;132:1303–10.

Henderson J, Granell R, Heron J, Sherriff A, Simpson A, Woodcock A, et al. Associations of wheezing phenotypes in the first 6 years of life with atopy, lung function and airway responsiveness in mid-childhood. Thorax. 2008;63:974–80.

Kurukulaaratchy RJ, Matthews S, Holgate ST, Arshad SH. Predicting persistent disease among children who wheeze during early life. Eur Respir J. 2003;22:767–71.

Lau S, Nickel R, Niggemann B, Gruber C, Sommerfeld C, Illi S, et al. The development of childhood asthma: lessons from the German Multi-centre Allergy Study (MAS). Paediatr Respir Rev. 2002;3:265–72.

Leonardi NA, Spycher BD, Strippoli MP, et al. Validation of the Asthma Predictive Index and comparison with simpler clinical prediction rules. J Allergy Clin Immunol. 2011;127:1466–1472, e6.

Lowe LA, Simpson A, Woodcock A, Morris J, Murray CS, Custovic A, et al. Wheeze phenotypes and lung function in preschool children. Am J Respir Crit Care Med. 2005;171:231–7.

Martinez FD, Wright AL, Taussig LM, Holberg CJ, Halonen M, Morgan WJ. Asthma and wheezing in the first six years of life. The Group Health Medical Associates. N Engl J Med. 1995;332:133–8.

Morgan WJ, Stern DA, Sherrill DL, Guerra S, Holberg CJ, Guilbert TW, et al. Outcome of asthma and wheezing in the first 6 years of life: follow-up through adolescence. Am J Respir Crit Care Med. 2005;172:1253–8.

Rodriguez-Martinez CE, Sossa-Briceno MP, Castro-Rodriguez JA. Discriminative properties of two predictive indices for asthma diagnosis in a sample of preschoolers with recurrent wheezing. Pediatr Pulmonol. 2011;46:1175–81.

Savenije OE, Granell R, Caudri D, Koppelman GH, Smit HA, Wijga A, et al. Comparison of childhood wheezing phenotypes in 2 birth cohorts: ALSPAC and PIAMA. J Allergy Clin Immunol. 2011;127:1505–12.

Schultz A, Brand PL. Episodic viral wheeze and multiple trigger wheeze in preschool children: a useful distinction for clinicians? Paediatr Respir Rev. 2011;12:160–4.

Schultz A, Devadason SG, Savenije OE, et al. The transient value of classifying preschool wheeze into episodic viral wheeze and multiple trigger wheeze. Acta Paediatr. 2010;99:56–60.

Simpson A, Tan VY, Winn J, Svensen M, Bishop CM, Heckerman DE, et al. Beyond atopy: multiple patterns of sensitization in relation to asthma in a birth cohort study. Am J Respir Crit Care Med. 2010;181:1200–6.

Sonnappa S, Bastardo CM, Wade A, et al. Symptom-pattern phenotype and pulmonary function in preschool wheezers. J Allergy Clin Immunol. 2010;126:519–26.

Van der Mark LB, van Wonderen KE, Mohrs J, et al. Predicting asthma in preschool children at high risk presenting in primary care: development of a clinical asthma prediction score. Prim Care Respir J. 2014;23:52–9.

Asthma: Clinical and Diagnosis Approach

41

Guido Girardi Briere

Contents

Definition

Asthma is a chronic inflammatory disease of the airway that is caused by multiple interactions among cells in the epithelium and those that promote inflammation through the liberation of inflammation mediators, specially mastocytes, eosinophils, and lymphocytes. This disease mainly affects the small airways, but it also compromises the central airway. It has been thought that persistent inflammation may progress to irreversible structural changes in the airway, currently named "remodeling"; nevertheless, its relationship with the severity of the disease has been questioned.

Asthma is characterized by recurrent episodes of cough, wheezing, and dyspnea, which especially appear during the night and at sunrise. Asthma presents variable degrees of reversible bronchial obstruction. The presence of bronchial hyperreactivity (BHR) when facing different stimuli in genetically predisposed subjects determines an exaggerated response and is a pillar in the diagnosis procedure.

Asthma is a multifactorial condition, and it is mainly caused by the interaction of genetic and environmental factors. The genetic factors involved in asthma have been known from a long time. Multiple genes have been described in different chromosomes that codify diverse proteins

G. Girardi Briere (✉)
Faculty of Medicine, Universidad de Chile, Santiago, Chile

P. Bertrand, I. Sánchez (eds.), *Pediatric Respiratory Diseases*,
https://doi.org/10.1007/978-3-030-26961-6_41

involved in the airway inflammation. Nowadays it is not possible to identify an exact relationship between the described genes and a particular phenotype. Some population studies have shown the importance of the parents in relationship to the risk of developing asthma, which is three times higher when one of the parents has asthma.

Also, there are several environmental factors involved. The Western lifestyle explains some of these factors that favor the appearance of atopic asthma. In this situation there is scarce exposure to endotoxins, which require adequate lymphocytes and CD14 levels to facilitate the formation of interferon-γ. This situation also involved an exaggerated use of antibiotics that destroys the intestinal flora, besides a low occurrence of infections that would stimulate a protective TH_1 response, such as hepatitis and measles. It has been described also that an early exposition to allergens may facilitate sensitization and atopy with a Th_2-lymphocyte response.

In developed countries, atopy, a hypersensitivity state mediated by elevated IgE titers, is the main predisposing factor for suffering from asthma. However, the atopy prevalence rate (30–50%) in the general population is significantly lower than the asthma prevalence rate.

Other factors such as low weight at birth, exposure to maternal tobacco, severe viral infections during the infancy period, environmental pollution, and being overweight, increase the risk of suffering from asthma and allergic sensitizing.

For non-atopic asthma, factors related to poverty are considered, such as overcrowding, infections, indoor pollution, maternal use of tobacco, and humidity. Differences relative to asthma prevalence rate and gender tend to disappear during puberty.

Exposure to tobacco smoke during the intrauterine period, or after birth during the pulmonary growth phase, also has an important influence. Atmospheric contaminants, such as environmental pollution, are also an influence, although there is less evidence about this.

Airway sensitization depends mainly on inhaled allergens. Among allergens, some are worth highlighting: house dust mites, house dust, animal dandruff or hair, pollens, and fungus. Tobacco and the possibility of indoor pollution facilitate the sensitization process. Even though there is no evidence that viruses cause asthma, they are important agents for its genesis at an early age or in its recurrences, as well as being the main triggers of asthma episodes.

A recent publication showed that when two countries, England and Scotland, applied anti-tobacco laws, the risk of hospitalization caused by acute asthma episodes was lowered.

Etiopathogenesis

The inflammation of the airway is the result of the interaction of different effector cells and pro-inflammatory mediators. In patients with atopic asthma, the predominance of type Th2 lymphocytes produces a proinflammatory state, with the participation of dendritic neuronal cells and release of cytokines such as interleukin (IL)-3, IL-4, IL-5, and IL-10, which affect local cells, including epithelial cells, but also affect recruited cells, such as eosinophils. Other cells, such as macrophages and mastocytes, interact to boost this permanent state of inflammation. The release of second mediators such as leukotrienes, histamines, and prostaglandins produces the most common epithelial alterations of a patient with asthma, such as bronchoconstriction, hypersecretion, and epithelium disruption. In a preferably eosinophilic inflammation environment, the enlargement of the reticular layer in the basal lamina, and hyperplasia of mucosal glands as well as smooth muscle and vascular tissues, increase the width of the bronchus wall, which makes the bronchi more rigid and reduces the transversal section of the airway: this causes a reduction of pulmonary function and a greater unspecific BHR. These changes in the airway structure would be responsible for the most serious presentation of the disease and of its chronic condition. These mechanisms explain that the disease may be reversible when treated, or it will only be partially reversible because of the damage caused. Therefore, there are multiple mediators involved in promoting the inflammation and

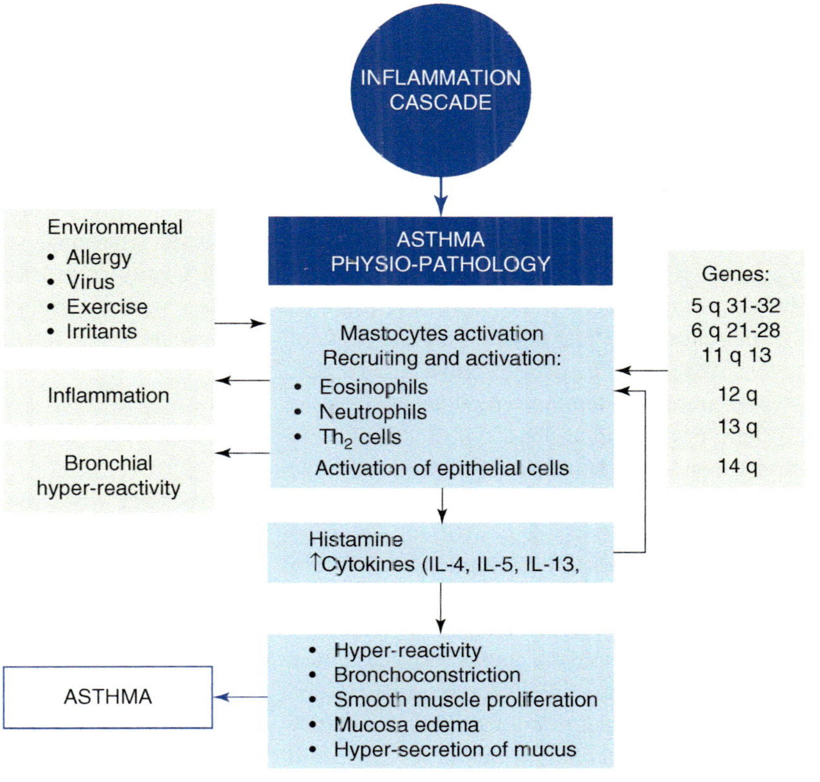

Fig. 41.1 Inflammation physiopathology

obstruction of the airway, although their relative importance is difficult to determine (Fig. 41.1).

Physiopathology

The main asthma mechanism is caused by the reduction of the caliber of the airway. Factors that may contribute to this are enlargement of the bronchial wall caused by edema and cellular infiltration. Every time a major inflammation trigger appears (as it happens when there is a viral infection), the reduction of the bronchial caliber will increase the resistance of the airway, with a reduction in the expiration flow and air entrapment with pulmonary hyperinflation. These changes are related to the increase of respiratory work, altering the ventilation/perfusion ratio, and according to the severity, hypoxemia in the beginning. Only if the obstructive phenomenon progresses until it surpasses the capacity of the respiratory muscles does it cause fatigue and alveolar hypoventilation with global respiratory failure.

The degree of BHR is related to the degree of present inflammation and the enlargement of the bronchial wall. Respiratory infections are the most frequent trigger of asthma crisis for all ages, especially in children that present with episodic disease. In infants and preschoolers, respiratory syncytial virus, rhinovirus, and parainfluenza virus are the most common triggers.

Clinical Aspects

Asthma is a chronic disease with one of the highest prevalence rates in childhood, and it is the most important cause of school absenteeism and frequent hospitalizations, with a corresponding high cost for health systems.

Because of the edema, bronchospasm, and increase of bronchial secretions, the most common symptoms of asthma appear: cough, chest whistle and rhonchus, chest oppression, and various degrees of respiratory failure. If symptoms progress, the patient will present an acute asthma crisis that will be proportional to the degree of airway obstruction. To measure the intensity of the compromise of the airway, clinical scores have been designed, plus pulse oximetry.

A complete clinical evaluation is always important, with a detailed anamnesis and a good physical examination. Laboratory tests can be useful because they help determine the severity of the obstruction. In the periods between episodes, the patient may present no symptoms or signs.

There is no unique phenotype for asthma in children, and therefore the initial symptoms may be unspecific. During the first years, asthma can be presented as a crisis of cough and wheezing that are indistinguishable from infant transient or early wheezing. Nevertheless, the diagnosis of asthma can be suspected if there is also a persistent rhinitis, an atopic dermatitis, asthma family history, and a good clinical response to inhaled salbutamol. A predictor index (API+) can certify an atopic asthma, although this is not as useful for non-atopic asthmatics.

Children may only present with persistent cough, which may be dry or productive, and in the lung examination a prolonged exhalation along with rhonchus, without wheezing. Sometimes it is recommended to manually compress the chest during exhalation to evidence the presence of wheezing that is not perceptible during auscultation. In children who are under 3 months old, a small airway obstruction may produce crackles instead of the expected wheezing, which can still be treated with inhaled salbutamol.

If the child has no symptoms, the appearance of cough and/or wheezing during playtime, laughing, crying, cold, smoke exposure, and excitement is a strong indicator of a diagnosis based on bronchial hyperreactivity, and it constitutes a good parameter for treatment efficacy. It is convenient to ask if there is a seasonal prevalence, specially during spring, which would indicate pollen allergy.

Allergic rhinitis signs tend to coexist and are usually underrated, but they will increase their intensity as the child grows. Allergic conjunctivitis may also be present.

During an asthma crisis the child is usually agitated, has difficulty speaking and feeding, with orthopnea, anguish, chest oppression, feeling of lack of air or suffocation, tachypnea, intense chest retraction, hyperresonant chest, easily heard wheezing, sometimes crackling from small airway obstruction, and reduction of pulmonary murmur in the most severe cases, along with cyanosis and alteration in consciousness.

Asthma Clinical Spectrum

- Recurrent wheezing syndrome in infants or preschoolers, or atopic or non-atopic persistent wheezing, which can be reversed with the use of inhaled beta-agonist.
- Recurrent obstructive acute laryngitis in infants and preschoolers, alternating with episodes of recurrent wheezing.
- Classic asthma, with its cough and chest wheezing exacerbations. Respiratory distress may be absent or present.
- Exercise-induced asthma in teenagers as the only symptom, as the consequence of BHR (characteristic feature of more severe asthma), and night asthma caused by greater fluctuations of the peak expiratory flow (PEF), along reduction of pulmonary function during early morning.
- Chronic cough, recurrent tracheitis that is alarming to the family. Methacholine test may be positive, which helps confirm the diagnosis.
- Allergic chronic rhinitis, chronic rhinosinusitis, recurrent hoarseness from posterior discharge, which in a child may cause oral breathing. Snoring may also be present.
- Recurrent pneumonia (pneumonia or pseudopneumonia, atelectasis).

A 4-year follow-up in newborns showed that among children who did not present with wheezing only 11% was complicated with pneumonia; in contrast, 78% of the children who had persistent wheezing presented with pneumonia.

Differential Diagnosis

If the patient's asthma does not respond to treatment, among other matters it is convenient to confirm the diagnosis and rule out other causes that may secondarily cause an obstructive bronchial syndrome, such as cystic fibrosis, foreign body aspiration, heart disease, bronchopulmonary dysplasia, ciliary dyskinesia, voice cord malfunction, or malformations of the airway that may go unnoticed if there is no clinical suspicion.

Diagnosis

In children, asthma diagnosis is mainly clinical, especially if the child is under 5 years old, although it can be suspected in an infant. Diagnosis is based on the presence of at least three episodes with a suggestive clinical condition: cough crisis, wheezing, and chest rhonchus with spontaneous improvement, or if a good response to inhaled salbutamol is confirmed. In the older child, paleness, allergic shiners, presence of the Morgagni fold, rough skin, and hyperkeratosis in the extension surface of limbs, with allergic rhinitis, are seen. The functional diagnosis can benefit from laboratory tests that may confirm the clinical suspicion, such as spirometry and flow measurement, which show the reduction of the exhalation flow rates, especially for FEV_1, Tiffeneau (FEV_1/FVC) under 70%, and a significant response to salbutamol. Bronchial challenge tests, such as the exercise test, must also be considered if they show drops more than 15% in the PEF and more than 10% for the VEF_1. Chest X-rays may also be useful, as they can rule out complications and support the differential diagnosis.

The severity of the crises in infants and preschoolers can be measured with a clinical score, as the one presented in Table 41.1, which has a lineal correlation with oxygen saturation. Table 41.2 can be used for schoolchildren and adolescents.

Diagnosis Rationale

– *Reversibility of bronchial obstruction:* Total or partially reversible spontaneously (confirmed by history or flow measure), or after

Table 41.1 Clinical score in infants and preschoolers

Score	Respiratory frequency		Wheezing	Cyanosis	Use of accessory muscles
	<6 m	>6 m			
0	<40	<30	No	No	No
1	41–55	31–45	Expiration only	Perioral with crying	+
2	56–70	46–60	Inspiration and expiration	Perioral at rest	++
3	70	>60	Inspiration and expiration at distance	Generalized at rest	+++

Severeness classification: low, 0–4; moderate, 5–8; severe, 9–12

Table 41.2 Clinical score in schoolchildren and adolescents

Parameter	Low	Moderate	Severe
Dyspnea	Walking	Speaking	Resting
Speaking	Long phrases	Short phrases	Only words
Consciousness	Anxious	Agitated	Very agitated
Respiratory frequency	Normal or small increase	Increased	Very increased (>30 × min)
Heart rate	<100 × min	100–120 × min	>120 × min
Accessory muscles	No	Chest retraction +	Chest retraction ++/a +++
Wheezing	End of exhalation	Inspiration–expiration	Easily heard
PEF post B2	>80%	60–80%	<60%
O_2 saturation	>95%	9195%	<90%

the use of inhaled salbutamol (confirmed by history, physical examination, and flow measurement). Relative to laboratory results for pulmonary function, reversibility corresponds to a 12% improvement in the exhalation volume of VEF_1 after a bronchodilator. A 30% improvement in the PEF 25–75, and 15% of the PEF, are highly compatible with asthma.

- *Bronchial hyperreactivity to different stimuli*: Several triggering events can be found in the history of the patient: exercise, laughter, crying, emotion, and irritating allergens such as tobacco smoke. The bronchial exercise challenge test is very specific, but its sensitivity is poor. In contrast, the bronchial challenge test with methacholine is highly sensitive, but its specificity is poor. However, if it is negative, the asthma diagnosis can be reasonably ruled out.
- *Variability*: It is suggestive of asthma to determine a variability greater than 20% in the spirometry, although this is not definitive of diagnosis.
- *Inflammation*: Inflammation markers such as nasal and bronchial eosinophils, eosinophil cationic protein, and exhaled nitric oxide are useful to measure inflammation. Along with this, nasal or bronchial eosinophils obtained by bronchoalveolar lavage or induced sputum are highly dependent on the operator who performs the counting, where more than 10% suggests a positive diagnose. All the other laboratory methods are still not well standardized for all population groups, and they are usually reserved for investigation studies.
- *NO* (*exhaled nitric oxide*): This substance has shown a great specificity for eosinophilic inflammation, which is not always available.
- *Atopy*: Laboratory tests for atopy identification are very useful in allergic asthma, but it is not a criterion for its diagnosis besides the family and personal background. Skin tests identify the allergens involved in the specific sensitization of each patient. It is important to remember that in undeveloped countries the skin test may yield a positive result in no more than 50% of the cases.

Classification

During the past few years, it has been preferred to classify asthma as controlled, partially controlled, or uncontrolled (Table 41.3), which has the advantage of measuring the response to pharmacological therapy, which can be gradually increased or reduced as required by the situation.

Asthma Control Levels

During these past years we have observed what may be a different phenotype of labile asthma. These patients do not seem to have a severe disease, and therefore the pharmacological therapy as well as medical follow-ups are insufficient, and the patients present with sudden crises that evolve in few hours, requiring hospitalization in special care units, sometimes with ventilation

Table 41.3 Levels of asthma control

A. **Evaluation of current control (past 4 weeks)**			
Characteristics	Under control	Partially under control	Uncontrolled
Daily symptoms	None (2 or fewer/week)	More than 2 times/week	Three or more characteristics of partially controlled asthma
Activity limitations	No	Any	
Night symptoms	No	Any	
Rescue medications are needed	No (2 or fewer/week)	More than 2 times/week	
Pulmonary function (PEF/FEV1)	Normal	<80% predictive value or better personal value	
B. **Evaluation of future risks (exacerbation risks, instability, quick reduction of pulmonary function, adverse effects)**			

support. The patients usually have a background of previous hospitalizations in critical care units.

Strangely, there is sparse literature about this issue. In our experience and to a certain extent, this presentation of asthma has replaced what is considered as severe asthma, relative to hospitalizations.

The most common complications can be reduced to the following scenarios:

- Partial or hypoxemic respiratory insufficiency: This is the most frequent complication of mild, moderate, or severe exacerbation.
- Global respiratory failure (hypoxemia and hypercarbia): It is caused by exhaustion and hypoventilation, which will require assisted ventilation besides pharmacological treatment.
- Pneumonia: It is a quite common complication, and therefore chest X-rays are important If there is no clear explanation, it can be related to immunological mechanisms that have not been determined yet, and also to a possible slower motion in the mucociliary clearance.

Psychological problems, being more frequently caused by overprotection, anguish, fear, or self-esteem problems. As a consequence, the family dynamics is altered.

- Pneumothorax. Described in severe cases. Atelectasis is more common.
- Bronchiectasis, secondary to atelectasis with recurrent bacterial overinfection. This condition is unusual nowadays, and it may have other explanations such as cystic fibrosis, ciliary dyskinesia, or sequelae from adenovirus infection.

Sources

Braun-Fahrlander C. Pets and childhood asthma: how should the pediatrician respond to new information that pets may prevent asthma? Pediatrics. 2003;112:974–6.

Castro-Rodriguez JA, Wright AL, Taussig LM, Martinez FG. A clinical index to define risk of asthma in young children with recurrent wheezing. Am J Respir Crit Care Med. 2000;162:1403–6.

Castro-Rodríguez JA, Ramírez AM, Toche P, Pavón D, Pérez MA, Girardi G, et al. Clinical and functional and epidemiological difference between atopic and non-atopic asthmatic children from a tertiary care hospital in a developing country. Ann Allergy Asthma Immunol. 2007;98:239–44.

Garate I, Girardi G. Perfil epidemiológico y clínico de niños que se hospitalizan por exacerbación asmática en un hospital pediátrico, Santiago, Chile. 2012; Libro de Resúmenes VII Congreso Sociedad Latinoamericana de Neumología Pediátrica (Solanep en vías de publicación).

Girardi G. Programa Nacional de Infecciones Respiratorias Agudas y SBO en Chile. Cuadernos Médicos Sociales. 2011;51(4):225–33.

Girardi G, Astudillo P. El programa de IRA en Chile: hitos e historia. Rev Chil Pediatr. 2001;72:292–300.

Girardi G, Quezada A, Zúñiga J, Arriagada A. Asma bronquial en el niño menor de 2 años. Vol Hosp Infant México. 1979;26:679–87.

Magnusson JÖ, et al. Early childhood overweight and asthma and allergic sensitization at 8 years of age. Pediatrics. 2012;129:70.

Mallol J, Sole D. Prevalence of asthma symptoms in Latin America. Pediatr Pulmonol. 2001;32:263–4.

Martinez FD. Development of wheezing disorders and asthma in preschool children. Pediatrics. 2002;109:362–7.

Millett C, Tayu Lee J, Laverty A, et al. Hospital admissions in childhood asthma after smoke-free legislation in England. Pediatrics. 2013;131:e 495.

Morgan WJ, Stern DA, Sherrill DL, Guerra S, Holberg CJ, Guilbert TW, Taussig LM, Wright AL, Martinez FD. Outcome of asthma and wheezing in the first 6 years of life: follow-up through adolescence. Am J Respir Crit Care Med. 2005;15(172):1253–8.

Pavon D, Castro-Rodriguez J, Rubilar L, Girardi G. Relation between pulse oximetry and clinical score in children with acute wheezing in children less than 24 months of age. Pediatr Pulmonol. 1999;27:423.

Riedler J, Braun-Fahrlander C, Eder W, et al. Exposure to farming in early life, pets and childhood asthma development of asthma and allergy: a cross-sectional survey. Lancet. 2001;358:1129–33.

Von Mutius E. The burden of childhood asthma. Arch Dis Child. 2000;82:112–5.

Asthma: Treatment

42

Pablo Bertrand and Andrea Beckhaus Faccin

Contents

Introduction

Asthma is the most common chronic respiratory disease during childhood, and it is associated with a major burden in health costs. It has been shown that adequate treatment controls asthma symptoms, and reduces asthma exacerbations, which increases the quality of life for the patients. Thus, every time that a patient with asthma is evaluated, it is necessary to outline the general objectives of the treatment, which must be in line with the expectations of the child and his family. For many parents and patients, the persistence of symptoms during the regular activities of the child may be seen as a great disability, although patients and family have different perceptions of the disease. It is important to discover those critical aspects of the child's regular life to obtain the maximum potential for every individual without letting the treatment be a heavier load than the disease itself.

In general terms, all guidelines are focused on symptoms and exacerbations control that meets the expectations of the family.

This chapter describes the global treatment of asthma, for both exacerbations and chronic con-

P. Bertrand (✉) · A. Beckhaus Faccin
Department of Pediatrics, School of Medicine, Pontificia Universidad Católica de Chile, Santiago, Chile
e-mail: pbertrand@med.puc.cl

P. Bertrand, I. Sánchez (eds.), *Pediatric Respiratory Diseases*, https://doi.org/10.1007/978-3-030-26961-6_42

trol. In both situations there are different aspects to consider, which are listed with the current level of evidence for each one.

Treatment

Treatment of a chronic disease such as asthma involves different aspects, seeking control of the symptoms in the long term. Recommendations must be oriented for each patient, highlighting different times of the day and the seasons of the year, as well as different activities. For treatment to be successful, parents must have some general knowledge of asthma, as well as the measures that may contribute to reducing symptoms and avoiding exacerbations.

Nonpharmacological Treatment

The ideal objective of asthma treatment is to avoid its appearance or favor its disappearance. With this objective in mind, many investigators have tried to intervene before the onset of the disease (primary prophylaxis) or after the diagnosis has been made (secondary prophylaxis), although there are no known measures that consistently reach this objective.

Primary Prophylaxis

There is an association between early exposure to common allergens and allergic sensitization; however, this is not sufficient to prove that early exposure to allergens predisposes to asthma onset. There is evidence to recommend maternal breastfeeding as a protective action in asthma development, especially in children with an atopic family background. Diet modifications, such as modified formula use, fish oil, dietary supplements, late introduction of solid foods, and use of probiotics (both for the child and for the mother during pregnancy) have shown contradictory results. Nevertheless, there are studies that have found a direct relationship between some interventions and asthma reduction in some patients. Therefore, it is only a matter of identifying this particular population.

Further, exposure to tobacco smoke during pregnancy and after childbirth involves a greater risk for the child to suffer from wheezing episodes and asthma, as well as presenting with decreased lung function during the first years of life. It is strongly recommended to avoid tobacco smoke exposure for both the expectant mother and the child. This prohibition should be maintained until adulthood to avoid the consumption of tobacco during adolescence.

Secondary Prophylaxis

Universal nonpharmacological measures for all patients do not seem to be relevant in the control of the disease, although they may be of great importance for patients who are already sensitized to a specific agent.

It is important to identify and avoid specific triggers such as allergens (Evidence D) and nonspecific triggers such as tobacco smoke (Evidence A), and the risk factors, because they can cause or increase inflammation in the airway. Effective control interventions for *Dermatophagoides* are to reduce the relative humidity of the room to less than 50%, use barrier covers in the bed, eliminate articles that may favor mite growth (carpets, plush toys, etc.), and clean carpets with vacuum cleaners with high-efficiency particulate air filters. To avoid allergies triggered by an animal, all contact must be avoided. It is recommended to effectively control fungus exposure, using special solutions and adequate painting, besides constant cleaning and ventilation. Seasonal allergies are variable in different latitudes and weathers, so additional interventions should be guided by the local situation of each patient. Avoiding inhalation of allergens when the specific index is high is useful, especially when there is a correlation between the clinical history and testing of the child. Tobacco and wood combustion smoke are especially irritant to the airway. To avoid exposure to these agents, it is recommended to avoid smoking in any circumstance, inside the house or in the car, as well as avoiding contaminating heating options such as wood-burning and kerosene heaters. In the same way, it is important to consider that atmospheric contamination, especially during winter months, may combine its action with viral infections. In this scenario, it is recommended to avoid leaving the house with minor infants if it is not necessary, as well as suspending physical activities when the pollution indexes are high.

If a limited sensitization to allergen has been confirmed, the possibility of a specific immunotherapy may be considered (Evidence D), whether it is subcutaneous or sublingual, in a specialized center.

Dietary modifications aiming to reduce weight do improve the control of the disease in the long term, but specific measures such as the administration of fish oil, antioxidants, magnesium, and the use of probiotics have not shown to be useful when treating asthma. Patients who suffer from difficult-to-control asthma could benefit from family therapy. Complementary measures such as acupuncture, ionizers, homeopathy, relaxation therapies, and Chinese herbs have not shown consistent results in asthma.

Asthma Education

Aiming to improve the control of the disease, the creation of education programs has been proposed. These programs would include information about asthma treatment, clinical monitoring, and triggers. Asthma education facilitates an alliance between attending physicians and the patient and her/his family. This bonding is crucial for the implementation and success of the therapeutic plan (Evidence A-B). It is important to emphasize the significance of an adequate adherence to recommendations, even when there are no symptoms. Also, educating parents and children so that they can recognize the symptoms and signs of an acute exacerbation is basic for adequate asthma control. Knowing this, caregivers may proceed commensurately to the severity of the symptoms. Self-monitoring and self-control is a core part of the process (Evidence A), and involves recognizing asthma exacerbation, but also avoiding triggers, such as infections and allergens, besides other environmental factors such as tobacco smoke exposure. It should also be considered that measurement of peak expiratory flow (PEF) has been validated as a method for management in a difficult-to-control asthma situation (Evidence B), especially for adolescents and adults.

Teaching instruments such as brochures, games, and interactive sites on the Internet with educative content are useful. Monitoring through simple clinical cards, such as the asthma control test (ACT) and the asthma control questionnaire (ACQ), have been validated to objectively report the degree of control of the disease, which eases the decision-making process. Training in the use of the inhalers with spacer is important to improve drug deposition in the lower airway and to avoid deposition in the mouth, which carries potential adverse effects. Drug formulation is always changing, so it is crucial to maintain the proper training for each device (Figs. 42.1, 42.2, 42.3).

Pharmacological Treatment

Treatment of Acute Asthma Exacerbations

Treatment of an exacerbation starts with the recognition of symptoms by the patient or his/her caregiver. Appearance of cough, dyspnea, and, frequently, easily audible wheezing are specific markers of an exacerbation. Along with a good knowledge of the self-care guideline, the patient can start with a written plan for the appearance of the symptoms. Respiratory distress may be objectively evaluated at home using a PEF monitor, but only by patients who have been properly trained and can cooperate. When self-care indications have failed, the patient is forced to seek attention. The evaluation of this patient must include a complete clinical history of her/his diagnosis, maintenance treatment, and therapeutic interventions performed. After this, the information must be completed with a complete physical examination.

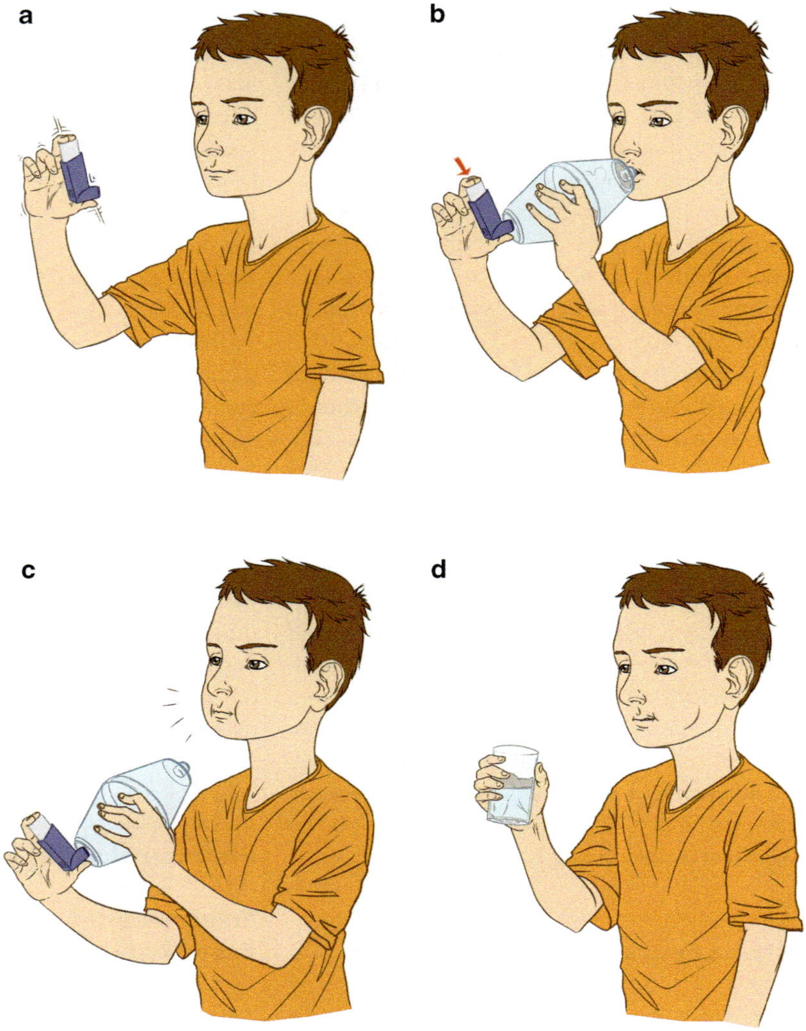

Fig. 42.1 Inhalation technique using salbutamol (MDI) and spacer with mouthpiece

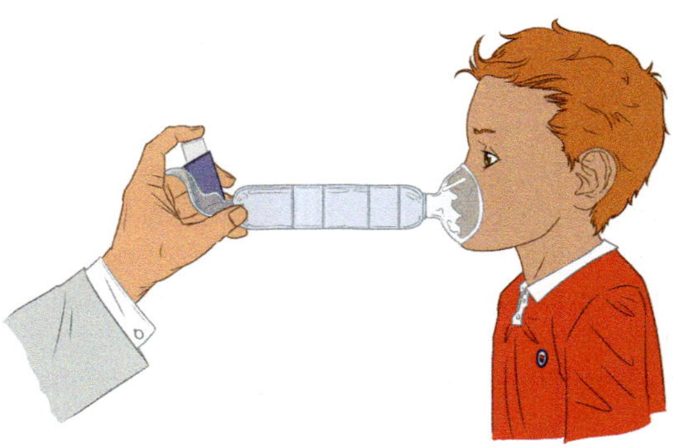

Fig. 42.2 MDI and spacer with mask inhalation technique. The spacer must be placed in the child's face in such a way that it covers mouth and nose. The MDI device is shaken well and then activated, waiting for the child's spontaneous breathing, at least three times.

Using a clinical score (Table 42.1), the severity of the crisis can be quantified to determine the action course to take during the first hours (Fig. 42.4). It is important to consider two situations that are warnings of greater severity: respiratory fatigue that appears as reduction of the respiratory rate, reduction of the sternal retraction and thoracoabdominal asynchrony, and severe hypoventilation manifested as silent chest during auscultation or when the patient cannot speak.

Oxygen

The administration of oxygen is the easiest and most efficient intervention to reduce hypoxemia during an acute asthma exacerbation. It can com-

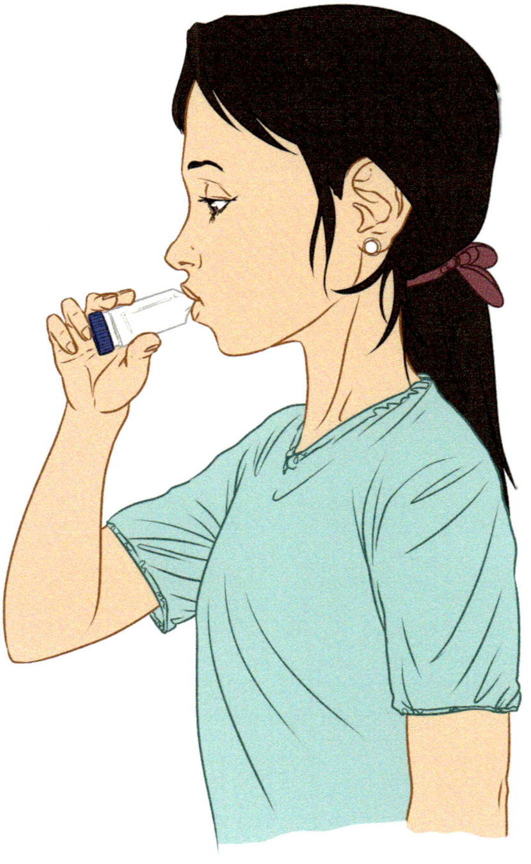

Fig. 42.3 Inhalation technique with a DPI. The dry powder inhaler (DPI) must be active according to the manufacturer's recommendation, because its use technique may vary. A deep inhalation is done with the device placed in the mouth, then the breath must be held, followed by a normal exhalation. It is recommended to rinse the mouth after the inhalation.

pletely correct respiratory insufficiency in most patients, only excepting those with severe hypoventilation. Oxygen is administered through a nasal tube, non-rebreathing mask, or Venturi mask system, according to the need and tolerance of each patient.

Medical oxygen is a dry gas that must be humidified to avoid problems related to drying of the respiratory mucosa when high flow is used. The objective of oxygen administration is to avoid hypoxemia, which can be indirectly measured through pulse oximetry (SpO_2), aiming for a value >93% (Evidence C). Those patients requiring supplementary oxygen at the time they are evaluated in the emergency room should be hospitalized. Patients with a moderate score or those who have respiratory distress when they seek medical attention should be evaluated again after 24–48 h, even if they responded adequately to the treatment used in the first hours of the medical visit, especially those patients who are difficult to follow up, have poor treatment adherence, or have a previous history of hospitalizations caused by asthma.

Bronchodilators

Short-acting beta-2 agonists (SABA) inhaled bronchodilators, such as salbutamol, fenoterol, and terbutaline, are the first-line treatments for acute asthma exacerbation (Evidence A). Administration of inhaled salbutamol (MDI) with a spacer with valve is just as effective as the nebulization of the same drug, and saves time and reduces the need of professional supervision in the emergency room. Additionally, the use of inhaled salbutamol with a spacer causes fewer adverse effects. Salbutamol should be administered proportionally to the seriousness of the crisis, and the clinical effect should be closely monitored and recorded. It is recommended to perform two to eight inhalations each time, and repeat them during the first hour of treatment until the desired clinical response has been achieved. Salbutamol administered in frequent intervals is more efficient, although it is important to assess for adverse effects, which also allows us to guide the adequate doses and frequency for each patient. For those patients with high oxygen requirements (FiO_2 > 30%) the administration of nebulized bronchodilators should be considered. In these cases, it is recommended to use a dose of 2.5–5 mg (standard dose) each time, using the same principle of dosage titling. For serious crises, continuous nebulization has been described as a more effective way of bronchodilator treatment until a clinical response is achieved.

Anticholinergic bronchodilators (ipratropium bromide) in repeated doses add their effect to those of beta-2 agonists in the treatment of moderate and severe exacerbations (Evidence B). Combination with SABA has been associated with a lower risk of hospitalization. They are available combined for both inhalation and nebulization.

Table 42.1 Evaluation of asthma exacerbation

Parameter	Mild	Moderate	Severe
Dyspnea	When walking; it can also be present when lying down	When speaking, prefers to be sitting Crying low and short in infants, has difficulties when feeding.	When resting, the infant cannot be fed
Speaks in	Long sentences	Short sentences	Isolated words
Consciousness	Patient can be agitated	Usually agitated	Usually agitated
Respiratory frequency	Increased	Increased	Very increased
<2 min: <60			
2–12 min: <50			
1–5 to <40			
6–8 to <30			
Heart rate	<100 bpm	100–120 bpm	>120 bpm
2–12 min: <160 bpm			
1–2 to <120 bpm			
2–8 to <110 bpm			
Accessory muscles	No use, generally	Yes	Yes
Wheezing	Moderated: only at the end of exhalation	Intense	Usually intense
Pulsus paradoxus	Absent: <10 mmHg	May be 10–25 mmHg	Present 20–40 mmHg
PEF post β2[a]	>80%	60–80%	<60%
SaO_2 (FiO_2: 21%)	>95%	91–95%	<90%

[a]PEF is conducted only in children who can cooperate and if the procedure does not delay treatment administration

Steroids

Systemic steroids are the preferred antiinflammatory treatment for acute asthma exacerbations (Evidence A). Early use is recommended to reduce the risk of hospitalization. The treatment should be administered over 3 to 5 days, which in most cases is enough to control the crisis. Oral administration of steroids is as effective as their intravenous administration, and therefore the oral option is recommended for its availability and reduced cost. The only exceptions are those patients who must receive the intravenous drug because their condition is serious. Every patient with moderate or severe asthma exacerbations must receive systemic steroids within the first hour of treatment in the emergency room. Those patients with a mild crisis and who have used bronchodilators, but with a poor response, should also receive steroids as a central part of their treatment.

The administration of inhaled or nebulized steroids for the acute asthma crisis is still being evaluated when they are used in combination with bronchodilators. Systematic reviews have shown that the therapeutic effect would be comparable to using oral steroids; nevertheless, its use must be part of a supervised treatment plan to avoid confusion or abuse of the drug. Currently, there is no strong recommendation about this issue.

Other Therapies

Nebulized magnesium sulfate could reduce the hospitalization risk in patients who have serious acute asthma exacerbations that do not respond to bronchodilators. There is no strong evidence to recommend its use in mild to moderate crises (Evidence A). IV magnesium sulfate may be considered for serious asthma crises, when the patient is hospitalized in the intensive care unit (Evidence B), as this medication must be supervised by specialists in intensive care.

Aminophylline and salbutamol can be used in the management of severe and acute exacerbations, but under strict supervision in critical patients as an additional therapy. The effects of

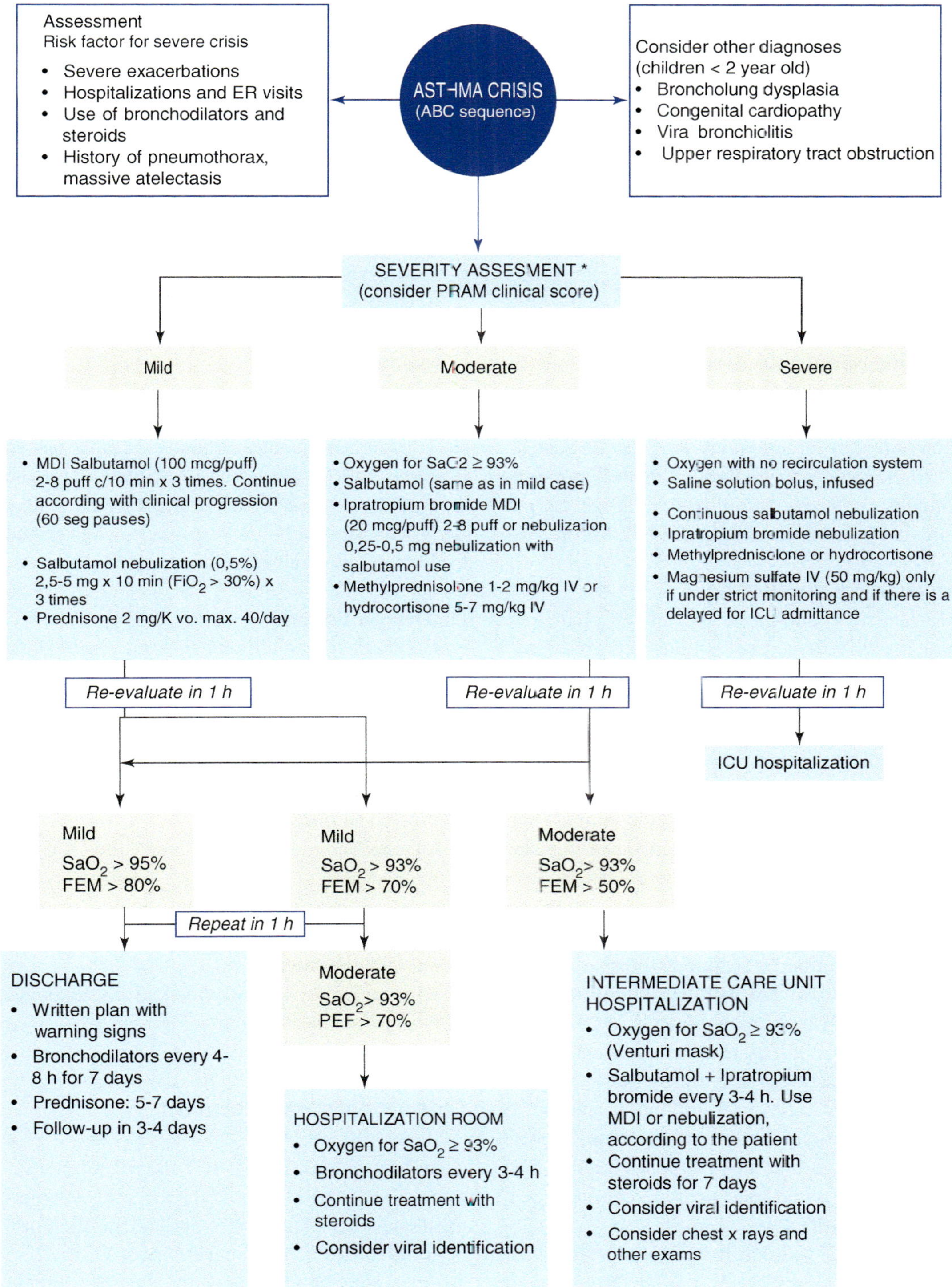

Fig. 42.4 Treatment algorithm for asthma crises

both treatments have been compared, and no differences have been found in their clinical efficacy (Evidence B).

In severe and acute exacerbations, helium in different concentrations mixed with oxygen can be used to gain some time while other measures are being placed to avoid the progression of respiratory distress. Even so, there is no high-quality evidence to recommend its use (Evidence B).

There is no clinical evidence to use IV leukotriene inhibitors in the treatment of acute asthma exacerbations.

There is no evidence to recommend the use of chest physiotherapy during acute asthma exacerbations, and some maneuvers, such as chest percussion or forced compressions, are contraindicated.

In the same way, antibiotics, as well as antihistamines, sedatives, and mucolytic drugs, have no role in the treatment and their use is discouraged.

Mechanical Ventilation

Mechanical ventilation is an alternative in patients with a severe asthma exacerbation in respiratory failure. Indications for its use are based on clinical criteria, although there are absolute indications, such as severe hypoxemia, compromise of consciousness, and cardiopulmonary failure. Preliminary evidence suggests the use of noninvasive ventilation for patients who can cooperate to avoid development of muscular fatigue. This therapy is not an alternative to invasive ventilation; it is only a previous step aiming to avoid endotracheal intubation. In those patients requiring ventilation support, pressure-limited delivery and low flow volumes should be used. The suggested baseline parameters are tidal volume (TV) 8–12 ml/kg, inspiratory time (TI) 0.7–1.5 s, and maximum inspiratory pressure (MIP) 40 cm H_2O. Alveolar ventilation should be optimized with an increase in the time constant, but at the same time favoring prolonged exhalation times to avoid auto-positive end-expiratory pressure (PEEP).

Mechanical ventilation in patients with asthma exacerbation is a therapy that can trigger some complications arising from the high pressures required, such as barotrauma and hemodynamic alterations. If it is necessary to sedate patients undergoing mechanical ventilation, use of morphine and muscle blockers is discouraged.

Hospitalization Criteria

Recurrent clinical evaluation after interventions is critical to make decisions about admissions to the hospital (Fig. 42.4). Some factors to be considered are these:

- Progressive dyspnea and/or increased work of breathing
- Signs and symptoms of moderate or severe exacerbations
- Poor response to treatment after 2 h

Treatment of acute asthma exacerbations in hospitals follows the same principles as for the emergency room, although drug prescription may vary, because the clinical response can be verified by frequent clinical supervision.

Discharge Criteria

- Good general conditions. Feeding can be done normally.
- $SpO_2 \geq 93$ during 8–12 h without additional oxygen support.
- Maintenance treatment with verified administration (specifically for administration of inhaled steroids).
- Discharge plan with clear and written instructions to follow up: warning symptoms, monitoring with peak expiration flow (PEF), and the drugs to be used and their adequate doses.
- Clinical follow-up with treating physician has been scheduled.

Chronic Asthma Treatment

Long-term asthma treatment must be commensurate with the seriousness of the disease, considering the severity of the symptoms and the alteration of lung function. In general terms, controlling asthma includes environmental control, patient education, and pharmacological treatment. To achieve this objective, it is necessary to fulfill the following criteria:

- Educate about the disease.
- Educate about adherence and provide training relative to appropriate inhalation technique.
- Identify individual triggers of asthma exacerbations and teach how to avoid them.
- Propose a treatment plan for asthma exacerbations.
- Set a treatment proportional to asthma seriousness.
- Monitor the clinical response to pharmacological treatment based on the use of rescue medications, appearance of symptoms, and lung function.
- Modify the treatment scheme based on the clinical response.

In general terms, the disease can be classified from the mildest degree, with intermittent symptoms, to the most severe degree, presenting symptoms that are persistent and incapacitating. Although the evaluation of severity is useful for each patient, especially when diagnosing, categorization may vary in time, and therefore the recommendations must be adjusted according to how much the disease has been controlled. Currently, national and international guidelines suggest a level-based pharmacological approach (Table 42.2), according to how well the disease has been controlled. To make the right decision to increase or reduce treatment, it is necessary to categorize asthma as controlled, partially controlled, or noncontrolled.

Asthma shows different presentations according to the age of the patient, ranging from infancy until adolescence, so many considerations are important when a treatment is proposed for patients who are so different. The recommendations stated in this chapter are not applicable to patients under 2 years old who present wheezing episodes related to viral infections; their management is explained in detail in a corresponding chapter.

If asthma presents in episodes, and the main characteristic is the presence of crisis between normal intermediate periods, treatment must be oriented to exacerbations and controlling the triggering factors. Pharmacological treatment will depend on the recurrence and severity of the asthma exacerbations. The guidelines of the Global Initiative for Asthma (GINA) recommend beginning regular therapy when there are one or more risk factors for exacerbations, even when intercritical symptoms may not be present. Among these factors we can mention the abnormal lung function (FEV <60% of predictive value), severe exacerbation requiring steroids use during the last 12 months, admittance into an ICU because of asthma exacerbations, symptoms of noncontrolled asthma, and frequent use of rescue treatment (Evidence D). For those patients with none of these conditions, the use of rescue medication as needed is recommended. The medication most strongly recommended is salbutamol. The clinical response to ipratropium bromide, by itself or combined with fenoterol, as

Table 42.2 Chronic treatment of asthma

Reduction		Stages of the treatment		Increase
Stage 1	Stage 2	Stage 3	Stage 4	Stage 5
		Asthma education		
		Environmental control		
Fast-acting B2 as needed		Fast-acting B2 as needed		
Options for asthma-controlling treatment	Select one	Select one	For stage 3, select one or more	For stage 4, add one alternative
	Low doses of ICS*	Low doses of ICS + long-acting B2	Medium or high doses of ICS + long-acting B2	Oral steroids (low doses)
	Leukotriene modifier**	Medium or high doses of ICS	Leukotriene modifier	Omalizumab
		Low doses of ICS + leukotriene modifier		

*ICS inhaled corticosteroids
**Receptor antagonist or synthesis inhibitors

rescue treatment has been evaluated, and no differences have been found relative to clinical score, lung function, or hospitalizations.

In other scenarios, if a patient requires more than one salbutamol canister per month, or more than 12 inhalations per day, the patient must be assessed and considered for regular treatment. For those patients with frequent exacerbations (six or more episodes per year) or who have a persistent symptoms profile, that is, asthma symptoms and signs for prolonged periods, treatment must be oriented to symptoms and exacerbations control, whose minimal initial period is between 3 and 6 months.

It is common to observe clear deterioration in the quality of life of a patient with a persistent asthma, which may limit the normal development of the child. In most patients the disease is controlled using one medication, but there is a percentage of patients who require more than one medication, known as combined therapy. Available medications for asthma control are supported by a large number of clinical trials and systematic reviews that validate their use. The election of one or another drug must utilize the best possible evidence which, along with the particular characteristics of each patient, will point to the best therapeutic choice in each case.

Steroids

It has been well established that treatment with inhaled corticosteroids (ICS) is the treatment of choice for most patients who have a persistent asthma (Evidence A). ICS choice is based on the characteristics that each has, such as strength, bioavailability, and cost, but the treatment should be individualized to obtain the best efficiency. The usefulness of ICS has been confirmed using multiple clinical parameters such as symptom improvement, reduction of rescue medications, and reduction in the number of exacerbations; it is also based on functional methods such as FEV_1 volume, improvement of morning peak expiratory flow (PEF), as well as improvement in challenge tests. Systematic review evidence supports their use for asthma, strongly recommending these methods for patients between 2 and 18 years old, in comparison to placebo. Its dosage depends on the age of the patient and the severity of the disease. For this purpose, a dosage guideline has been created (Table 42.3) that considers low, intermediate, and high doses for pediatric patients. It is recommended to start with a budesonide dosage of 200 μg per day; fluticasone 100 μg, or its equivalent, for children under 5 years old; and for older children, budesonide 400 μg per day, fluticasone 200 μg per day, mometasone 200 μg, ciclesonide 80 μg, or its equivalent. ICS are available as MDI or dry powders in their different dosages. Their adverse effects depend on the doses used and generally appear when using 800 μg budesonide per day or its equivalent. Adverse effects to be considered are growth delay, adrenal suppression, and osteoporosis. All these effects that have been described when using high doses and the medication has been used for a long time. It is important to keep in mind local adverse effects such as the appearance of oropharyngeal candidiasis and hoarseness. These symptoms have a low frequency because of the widespread use of a spacer, which reduces the drug deposit in the pharynx (Figs. 42.1, 42.2, 42.3). Most medications have been approved to be used two times per day from the beginning of the treatment; nevertheless, there are currently some medications available (mometasone, ciclesonide) that are administered once per day.

Table 42.3 Comparison of inhaled steroids for children

Drug	Low dose	Medium dose	High dose
Beclometasone	100–200 μg	200–400 μg	>400 μg
Budesonide	200 μg	200–400 μg	>400 μg
Fluticasone	100–200 μg	200–500 μg	>500 μg
Ciclesonide	80–160 μg	160–320 μg	>320 μg
Mometasone	200–400 μg	400–800 μg	>800 μg
Triamcinolone	400–800 μg	800–1200 μg	>1200 μg

Most inhaled steroids achieve a drug deposit in the airway of about 8% to 15% of the total administered using good technique and a proper

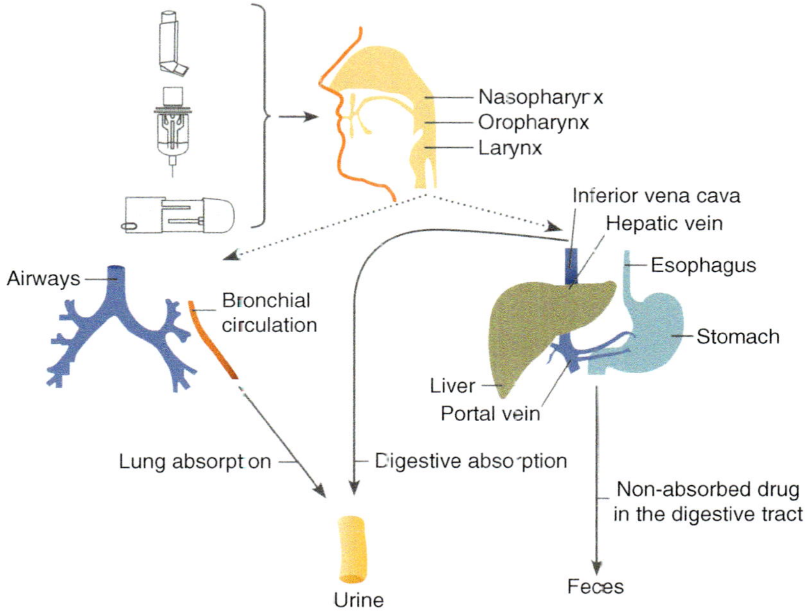

Fig. 42.5 Distribution of the inhaled drug

spacer. Nevertheless, there are new formulations and new drugs (beclomethasone HFA and ciclesonide) that achieve a better airway deposit, which may even reach 50% of the total, mainly the result of the size of the particle, delivery speed, and temperature when delivering the drug. Most have a very low oral bioavailability (budesonide, fluticasone, mometasone), which increases their security profile before use. An additional advantage to inhaled steroids such as a prodrug (ciclesonide) is that it activates once it reaches the airway, and also it is rapidly metabolized when it enters the systemic blood flow (Fig. 42.5).

Studies conducted to assess the daily use of inhaled steroids, when compared to the intermittent use of the same drug, favor the continuous use when considering PEF improvement, number of symptom-free days, need of rescue medications, and fraction of exhaled nitric oxide (FENO). Even so, there are no significant differences for the risk of suffering exacerbations. Currently, the intermittent use is based on sparse and low-quality evidence in relation to relevant clinical parameters, and therefore it has not been standardized in the treatment of asthma with persistent symptoms.

Long-Acting Beta-Agonists

The usefulness of the long-acting bronchodilators (LABA) salmeterol, formoterol, and vilanterol in combination with steroids has been verified as an alternative in the combined treatment for asthma. Formoterol works faster than salmeterol, which improves treatment compliance. In the past, the use of these bronchodilators was aimed at managing the symptoms of the disease, and it was commercialized as monotherapy. Nevertheless, recent evidence forced its suspension as monotherapy, because it contributed to asthma mortality, apparently because of tachyphylaxis in the adult population caused by the drug. Guidelines recommend its use as first-line additional therapy besides inhaled corticosteroids (ICS) for persistent asthma, both moderate and severe, when asthma control has not been achieved with doses of 400 μg budesonide or an equivalent. The efficacy of combining ICS with LABA, versus the sole use of high doses of ICS in children with uncontrolled disease, lies in the changes of lung function and morning flow measurement, but there are no significant differences in the risk of suffering asthma crises, use of oral steroids, hospitalization, or symptom-free days. Nevertheless, patients using a combined treatment need rescue medications less frequently and have a better growth rate in the long term. It is important to consider that there is little evidence and information about security related to the use of long-acting bronchodilators in combined treatment for those patients under 5 years old, so the specialist is encouraged to closely monitor these children and use this treatment with extreme caution.

Leukotriene Inhibitors

The use of these drugs has been increasing during past years. They are effective in improving symptoms and lung function and preventing exacerbations (Evidence A). Nevertheless, the evidence obtained during the past years shows that their strength is less when compared with inhaled steroids, particularly in relation to the measures of lung function, and some studies show a relationship with a poorer protection against exacerbations (Evidence A). For patients with frequent or persistent asthma, its use is recommended as monotherapy when inhaled steroids cannot be used, particularly for those patients with exercise-induced asthma, Its greatest utility lies in excellent chronic treatment adherence in patients under 5 years old. There is preliminary evidence about the intermittent use of leukotriene inhibitors in children under 12 years old, but currently it is still not possible to recommend their use. The use of leukotriene inhibitors as an additional therapy, in addition to inhaled steroids, has shown that, in comparison with long-acting bronchodilators, there are no differences in the risk of exacerbations that require oral steroids. The evidence is stronger in the adolescent population, showing better results when bronchodilators are used with inhaled steroids.

Chromone

Chromones are airway antiinflammatories whose usefulness has been well proven for the treatment of frequent episodic asthma and mild persistent asthma in children and infants. These drugs have an excellent security profile, and adverse effects have been rarely reported. Nevertheless, its limitations lie in the frequency of their administration (3–4 times per day) and their discrete strength in comparison to inhaled steroids.

Theophyllines

Today, the use of theophyllines in the management of chronic asthma is quite individualized (Evidence B). The multiple potential adverse effects should be considered and monitored. Even though theophyllines are administered orally, use may be considered for patients with poor adherence to the chronic treatment, or for those patients who almost exclusively present symptoms during the night, when it could be as effective as using steroids.

Monoclonal Antibody Against IgE

The specific monoclonal antibody against immunoglobulin E, omalizumab, is now available, and it has been shown to be effective in reducing the levels of circulating IgE in selected patients, with associated clinical benefits.

Systemic reviews in the adult and pediatric population have shown that those patients treated with omalizumab are at a lower risk of suffering asthma exacerbation after receiving treatment with inhaled steroids, long-lasting bronchodilators, and leukotrienes inhibitors (Evidence B).

Systemic Steroids

In patients with severe or moderate asthma, when the disease has not been steadily controlled with two or more drugs, and who require frequent use of steroids, its permanent use should be considered. However, the physician must keep in mind the adverse effects that this indication implies, such as hypertension, diabetes mellitus, osteoporosis, and cataracts. The objective is to control the disease with the minimum dosage, aiming to suspend the administration of the drug as soon as possible. To achieve this, the recommendation is to gradually replace the dosage of 1000 μg budesonide, or its equivalent. It is also possible to combine leukotrienes inhibitors, long-lasting beta-2 agonists, and theophyllines for 6 weeks until the changes have been verified.

Exercise-Induced Asthma

In most patients, the appearance of bronchoconstriction induced by exercise is only an indicator of a poor control of the disease. This is the best argument to name this condition as exercise-induced bronchospasm (EIB) instead, to avoid confusion in its origin. EIB must force the physician to review control therapy and its administration mode before considering changes. Initial treatment consists of short-acting beta-2 agonists before exercising. This intervention has shown reduction of the FEV_1 rate when compared to placebo, with quality evidence. When the rescue treatment does not work, the use of a maintenance treatment can be considered, as happens with uncontrolled asthma. For this purpose, inhaled steroids, leukotrienes inhibitors, long-acting beta-agonists, theophyllines, and chromones may be used. The selection of the drug will depend on the individual characteristics of each patient.

Sources

Beckhaus AA, García-Marcos L, Forno E, Pacheco-Gonzalez RM, Celedón JC, Castro-Rodriguez JA. Maternal nutrition during pregnancy and risk of asthma, wheeze and atopic diseases during childhood: a systematic review and meta-analysis. Allergy. 2015; https://doi.org/10.1111/all.12729.

Beckhaus AA, Riutort MC, Castro-Rodriguez JA. Inhaled versus systemic corticosteroids for acute asthma in children. A systematic review. Pediatr Pulmonol. 2014;49(4):326–34.

Bonini M, Di Mambro C, Calderon MA, Compalati E, Schünemann H, Durham S, Canonica GW. $Beta_2$-agonists for exercise-induced asthma. Cochrane Database Syst Rev. 2013;10:CD003564.

British Thoracic Society; Scottish Intercollegiate Guidelines Network. British guideline on the management of asthma. Thorax. 2014;69((suppl 1)):1–192.

Burke H, Leonardi-Bee J, Hashim A, Pine-Abata H, Chen Y, Cook DG, Britton JR, McKeever TM. Prenatal and passive smoke exposure and incidence of asthma and wheeze: systematic review and meta-analysis. Pediatrics. 2012;129(4):735–44.

Castro-Rodriguez JA, Rodrigo GJ. A systematic review of long acting β2-agonists versus higher doses of inhaled corticosteroids in asthma. Pediatrics. 2012;130:e650–7.

Castro-Rodriguez JA, Rodrigo GJ. The role of inhaled corticosteroids and montelukast in children with mild-moderate asthma: results of a systematic review with meta-analysis. Arch Dis Child. 2010;95:365–70.

Castro-Rodriguez JA, Rodrigo GJ. Efficacy of inhaled corticosteroids in infants and preschoolers with recurrent wheezing and asthma: a systematic review with meta-analysis. Pediatrics. 2009;123:e519–25.

Castro-Rodriguez JA, Rodrigo GJ, Rodriguez-Martinez CE. Principal findings of systematic reviews for chronic treatment in childhood asthma. J Asthma. 2015;52(4):407–16.

Chauhan BF, Chartrand C, Ducharme FM. Intermittent versus daily inhaled corticosteroids for persistent asthma in children and adults. Cochrane Database Syst Rev. 2013;2:CD009611.

Chauhan BF, Ducharme FM. Addition to inhaled corticosteroids of long-acting beta-2-agonists versus anti-leukotrienes for chronic asthma. Cochrane Database Syst Rev. 2014;(1):CD003137. https://doi.org/10.1002/14651858.CD003137.pub5.

Chauhan BF, Ducharme FM. Anti-leukotriene agents compared to inhaled corticosteroids in the management of recurrent and/or chronic asthma in adults and children. Cochrane Database Syst Rev. 2012;(5):CD002314. https://doi.org/10.1002/14651858.CD002314.pub3.

DiFranza JR, Aligne CA, Weitzman M. Prenatal and post-natal environmental tobacco smoke exposure and children's health. Pediatrics. 2004;113(4 suppl): 1007–15.

Ducharme FM, Ni Chroinin M, Greenstone I, Lasserson TJ. Addition of long-acting beta-2-agonists to inhaled corticosteroids versus same dose inhaled corticosteroids for chronic asthma in adults and children. Cochrane Database of Systematic Reviews 2010a;(5): CD005535. https://doi.org/10.1002/14651858.CD005535.pub2.

Ducharme FM, Ni Chroinin M, Greenstone I, Lasserson TJ. Addition of long-acting beta-2-agonists to inhaled steroids versus higher dose inhaled steroids in adults and children with persistent asthma. Cochrane Database Syst Rev. 2010b;(4):CD005533. https://doi.org/10.1002/14651858.CD005533.pub2.

From the Global Strategy for Asthma Management and Prevention, Global Initiative for Asthma (GINA). 2015. Available at: http://www.ginasthma.org/.

Griffiths B, Ducharme FM. Combined inhaled anticholinergics and short-acting beta-2-agonists for initial treatment of acute asthma in children. Cochrane Database Syst Rev. 2013;8:CD000060.

Guyatt GH, Oxman AD, Vist G, Kunz R, Falck-Ytter Y, Alonso-Coello P, Schünemann HJ. For the GRADE Working Group. Rating quality of evidence and strength of recommendations GRADE: an emerging consensus on rating quality of evidence and strength of recommendations. BMJ. 2008;336:924–6.

McDonald N, Bara A, McKean MC. Anticholinergic therapy for chronic asthma in children over two years of age. Cochrane Database of Systematic Reviews. 2003;(3):CD003535. https://doi.org/10.1002/14651858.CD003535.

Ni Chroinin M, Lasserson TJ, Greenstone I, Ducharme FM. Addition of long-acting beta-agonists to inhaled corticosteroids for chronic asthma in children. Cochrane Database Syst Rev. 2009;(3):CD007949. https://doi.org/10.1002/14651858.CD007949.

Normansell R1, Walker S, Milan SJ, Walters EH, Nair P. Omalizumab for asthma in adults and children. Cochrane Database Syst Rev. 2014;1:CD003559.

Nurmatov U, Devereux G, Sheikh A. Nutrients and foods for the primary prevention of asthma and allergy: systematic review and meta-analysis. J Allergy Clin Immunol. 2011;127(3):724–733. e1-30.

Papadopoulos NG, Arakawa H, Carlsen KH, Custovic A, Gern J, Lemanske R, et al. International consensus on (ICON) pediatric asthma. Allergy. 2012;67(8):976–97.

Parsons JP, Hallstrand TS, Mastronarde JG, Kaminsky DA, Rundell KW, Hull JH, Storms WW, Weiler JM, Cheek FM, Wilson KC, Anderson SD, American Thoracic Society Subcommittee on Exercise-induced Bronchoconstriction. An official American Thoracic Society clinical practice guideline: exercise-induced bronchoconstriction. Am J Respir Crit Care Med. 2013;187(9):1016–27.

Powell C, Dwan K, Milan SJ, Beasley R, Hughes R, Knopp-Sihota JA, Rowe BH. Inhaled magnesium sulfate in the treatment of acute asthma. Cochrane Database Syst Rev. 2012;12:CD003898.

Rank MA, Hagan JB, Park MA, Podjasek JC, Samant SA, Volcheck GW, Erwin PJ, West CP. The risk of asthma exacerbation after stopping low-dose inhaled corticosteroids: a systematic review and meta-analysis of randomized controlled trials. J Allergy Clin Immunol. 2013;131:724–9.

Rodrigo G, Rodrigo GJ, Neffen H, Castro-Rodriguez JA. Efficacy and safety of subcutaneous omalizumab vs. placebo as add-on therapy to corticosteroids for children and adults with asthma: a systematic review. Chest. 2011;139:28–35.

Singh M, Jaiswal N. Dehumidifiers for chronic asthma. Cochrane Database Syst Rev. 2013;6:CD003563.

Watts K, Chavasse RJ. Leukotriene receptor antagonists in addition to usual care for acute asthma in adults and children. Cochrane Database Syst Rev. 2012;5:CD006100.

Primary Ciliary Dyskinesia

43

Nils Linus Holmgren Palmen,
Ximena Fonseca Arrieta,
and Sergio González Bombardiere

Contents

N. L. Holmgren Palmen
Department of Pediatrics, Clínica Alemana and Universidad del Desarrollo, Santiago, Chile

X. Fonseca Arrieta
Otorhinolaryngology, Pontificia Universidad Católica de Chile, Santiago, Chile

S. González Bombardiere (✉)
Pathological Anatomy, Pontificia Universidad Católica de Chile, Santiago, Chile
e-mail: sgonzale@med.puc.cl

Definition

Primary ciliary dyskinesia (PCD) is a term used to describe the diseases that directly result from congenital defects in the cilia. It is a hereditary autosomal recessive defect in the cilia ultrastructure. This definition includes Kartagener syndrome, immotile ciliary syndrome, ciliary dysmotility, and primary ciliary orientation problems. Kartagener syndrome is composed of the triad of situs inversus, chronic sinusitis, and

P. Bertrand, I. Sánchez (eds.), *Pediatric Respiratory Diseases*,
https://doi.org/10.1007/978-3-030-26961-6_43

bronchiectasis. Situs inversus is present in 30% to 50% of all patients with PCD, and 6% present with heterotaxia.

Epidemiology

The incidence of the disease has been estimated to be between 1/10,000 and 1/20,000 per live births.

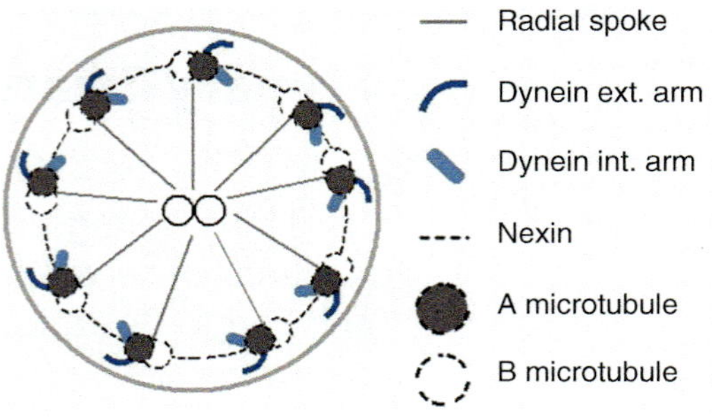

Fig. 43.1 Ciliary structure

Etiology and Physiopathology

Cilia

Cilia are organelles that are structurally related to the flagellum in the protozoa. They are classified according to their microtubule composition: motile (9 + 2) and primary (9 + 0). Motile cilia have nine pairs of peripheral microtubules and two central pairs. In contrast, primary cilia have nine peripheral pairs, but lack the central pair.

Motile cilia have a great inherent capacity to beat at variable frequencies, and they are in all the respiratory epithelium, uterine tubes in the female genital tract, ductus deferens in the masculine genital tract, ependymal canal in the brain, and spermatozoa.

Primary cilia can be subdivided into sensory cilia and nodal cilia. Sensory cilia do not move; they are in most vertebrate cells, and function as mechanoreceptors or antennas that communicate with the extracellular environment. They are present in the lumen of the kidney tubule, retinal rods and cones, ciliary cochlear cells, canals, and olfactory sensory neurons. Additionally, nodal cilia are those cilia with movement and are present in the embryonic node. These cilia determine organ laterality in mammals. Their alteration causes anomalies in rotation, such as situs inversus.

Cilia Structure

Cilia are composed of more than 200 different types of polypeptides. Each cilium has a pair of central microtubules and nine pairs of peripheral microtubules, which are connected by other structures (Fig. 43.1). Each pair of peripheral microtubules is constituted of alpha- and beta-tubulin heterodimers, which are grouped in 13 protofilaments in the A tubule and 11 protofilaments in the B tubule. They are oriented toward the adjacent central cilium, which is important for the production and coordination of the cilia wave beat. Each microtubule at the central pair is composed of 13 protofilaments that contain 23 polypeptides, which are unique and differ in their function and biochemistry. Other very important proteins are the microtubule-associated proteins (MAP), which constitute the internal and external arms of dynein. Dyneins are ATPases. External dynein binds to the A microtubule at one end through an alpha-tubulin, and the other end binds to the B microtubule of the adjacent pair through a beta-tubulin. ATP hydrolysis determines the movement of the dynein head through the axis of the B microtubule, defining the coordinated action of all the microtubules that the cilium bends. Other microtubules include nexin, which connects the peripheral microtubules among each other, and the radial spokes, which connect the peripheral microtubules to the central microtubules. An interflagellar transportation system of protein particles maintains and assembles the cilia structure. Anterograde flow is determined by the kinesin II complex, and the retrograde flow is determined by the dynein cytoplasmic complex (Fig. 43.2).

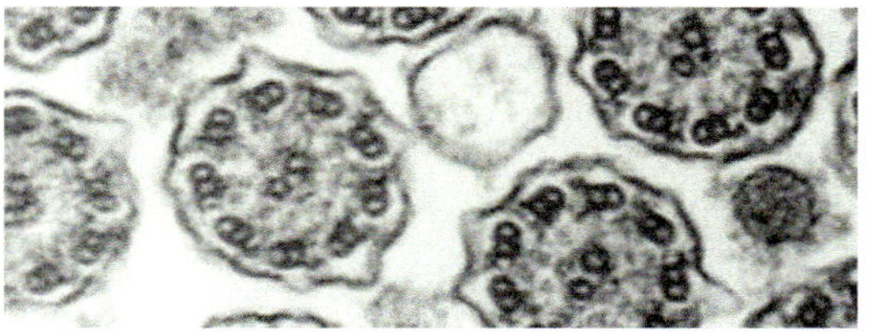

Fig. 43.2 Normal cilia. Cross section of normal cilium and primary ciliary dyskinesia (PCD). Uranyl acetate and lead citrate. ×100,000

Ciliary Function

A cylindrical pseudostratified mucosa covers the respiratory epithelium, which ensures mucociliary transport. This structure is one of the most important first-line defenses of the airway, for both the lower tract and upper tract, including the paranasal sinus and middle ear. Thus, the entrance of particles and infection agents is avoided, protecting the person. This function is the so-called *mucociliary clearance*. Impairment of this system may cause infections in the respiratory tract.

The movement of the microtubule doublets determines the ciliary beat. The external arm of dynein controls ciliary frequency, and the internal arm of the dynein directs the shape of the wave. Radial spokes, which are related to the central pair of microtubules, are in charge of activating the dynein arms. The central pair/radial spoke complex is the regulating key for the activation of the dynein arms.

Cilia have a rhythmic beat. Each cycle has two active components: one movement during which the cilium is completely extended perpendicularly relative to the cellular surface, and a recovery movement in which the inclined cilium moves parallel to the cellular surface, toward its original position. The duration of this phase depends on the frequency of the ciliary beating.

Cilia in adjacent cells are coordinated to beat simultaneously and at the same time. In this way, an effective cilia motility is caused, which expels the mucus. The frequency of the ciliary beat oscillates between 13 and 27 Hz in the respiratory mucosa. It is known that multiple factors affect ciliary motility, such as neural control, external factors (temperature, humidity), and pharmacological effects.

To have an efficient motility and effective mucociliary clearance, it is crucial to conserve the ciliary structure intact, besides keeping an adequate amount and quality of secretions that allow good movement, as well as a good synchronization in the ciliary motility with a correct frequency of ciliary beat.

Age has no impact on the frequency of ciliary beat, which is similar for patients between 3 months old and 74 years old.

Ciliary function can be affected by external factors, such as bacterial toxins and inflammation mediators, which cause ultrastructural cilium alterations and ciliary dysfunction.

Alterations in Ciliary Structure

The ciliary structure may sustain different types of morphological alterations, such as the absence of internal and external dynein arms, alteration of the radial spokes, and cilium fusion.

Anomalies of the cilium ultrastructure may be divided into primary defects, which are those observed in PCD, and secondary defects, which are caused by infections, cigarette smoke, or pollutants. These secondary alterations are different from those found in PCD, and they consist mainly of defects in the microtubules and composed cilia, affecting up to 10% of cilia in normal patients, and when challenged by severe respiratory infections, up to 17% of the cilia may be affected.

Structural anomalies known to cause ciliary dyskinesia are described in Table 43.1.

In one phenotype of PCD, the ultrastructure is normal, but the cilia are not normally oriented in relation to other cilia. This orientation disorder may be primary, but it may as well occur secondary to an infection.

Analysis using a scanning electron microscope shows the number of studied cilia that present a specific anomaly. In this way, the percentage and type of alterations present can be classified. Most authors consider 20% or more of absent dynein internal and/or external arms as significant to classify the case as a PCD. Some examples can be seen in Figs. 43.3 and 43.4.

Table 43.1 Primary ciliary dyskinesia (PCD) structural abnormalities

A. *Dynein arms*	
	Absence or reduction of the number of internal and external arms
	Absence or reduction of the number of internal arms
	Absence or reduction of the number of external arms
B. *Radial spokes*	
	Absence
C. *Microtubules*	
	Defects on the peripheral microtubules
	Absence of the central pair with the transposition of a peripheral pair to the center
D. *Complete ciliary aplasia*	
E. *Orientation defect*	

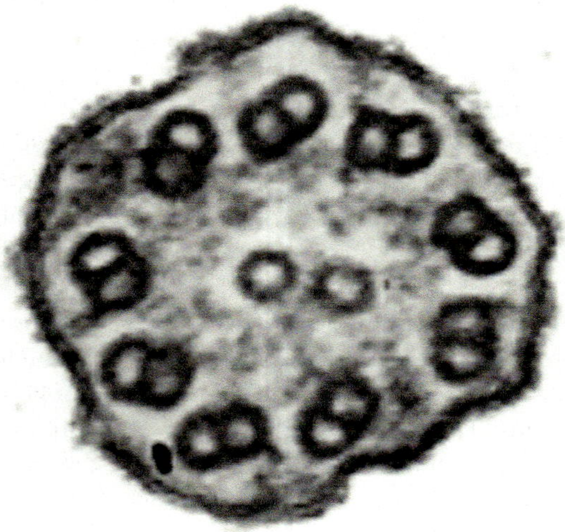

Fig. 43.3 Ciliary dyskinesia. Cross section of cilium showing complete absence of dynein external and internal arms in peripheral microtubules. Uranyl acetate and lead citrate. ×120,000

The most frequent ultrastructural findings, as published in several studies, are the absence of both dynein arms (range, 24–57%), absence of only the external dynein arm (range, 2.9–43%), absence of only the internal dynein arm (range, 29–37%), and anomalies of the central microtubules (4%).

Ultrastructural diagnosis requires trained and experienced specialists, as well as the strict application of morphological and diagnostic criteria. Diagnosis is more reliable when samples have been optimally obtained and processed. Up to 40% of the samples can be labeled as useless, as they do not contain ciliary cells in adequate numbers and lack preservation quality.

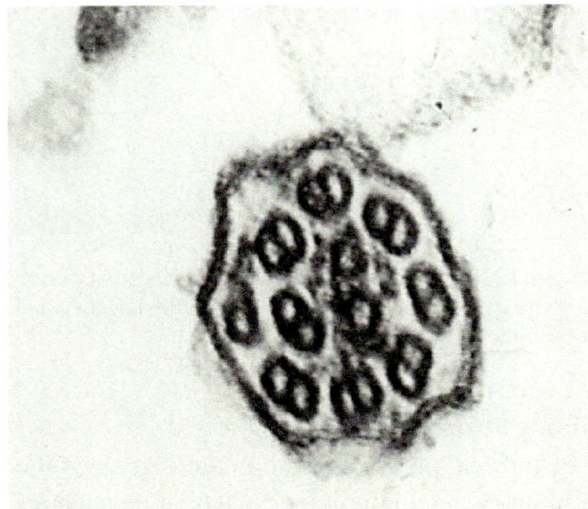

Fig. 43.4 Ciliary dyskinesia

Clinical Condition

Clinical characteristics in PCD depend on the age of the patient.

Antenatal manifestations

- Situs inversus or heterotaxia in antenatal echography
- Mild brain ventriculomegaly in antenatal echography

Neonatal manifestations

- Respiratory distress in term newborn, without risk factors for transitory tachypnea or neonatal pneumonia
- Permanent nasal congestion since the first day of life
- Situs inversus or dextrocardia
- Complex congenital heart disease related to laterality disorders (heterotaxia)
- Biliary atresia
- Hydrocephalus

Infancy and childhood manifestations

- Persistent wet cough
- Atypical wheezing that does not respond to steroids therapy

- Recurrent pneumonia
- Bronchiectasis of unclear etiology
- Frequent rhinosinusitis
- Otitis media with chronic effusion
- Persistent otorrhea after the insertion of ventilation tubes
- Situs inversus associated to sinusitis and bronchiectasis
- Severe gastroesophageal reflux

Manifestations during adulthood

- The same manifestations as present during school-age period
- Greater percentage of ectopic pregnancies and reduced fertility in women
- Greater percentage of infertility in men
- Chronic mucopurulent bronchorrhea
- Digital clubbing
- Nasal polyposis/halitosis
- Function tests show mixed or obstructive pattern

The clinical manifestations most commonly published in the different series are recurrent sinusitis (77%), persistent rhinitis (76%), neonatal respiratory distress syndrome or tachypnea (20–67%), recurrent otitis media (57%), recurrent pneumonia (46–56%), difficult-to-control asthma (26%), bronchiectasis (8.6–24%), and situs inversus (18–69%). The average age at diagnosis is 4 years, but with a high clinical suspicion it can be diagnosed earlier, even within the first month of life.

Diagnosis

The diagnosis of PCD is based on a combination of clinical evaluation and analysis of the ciliary ultrastructure and function, and it can be difficult to determine this diagnosis in some patients. The clinical phenotype is wide and overlaps with other chronic diseases of the airway.

The patient must be thoroughly studied to rule out other pathologies (allergies and immunological studies, X-rays, gastroesophageal reflux, sweat test, etc.) that may be responsible for the clinical condition.

The screening and diagnosis methods for ciliary dyskinesia are detailed next.

Screening Methods

Screening methods measure the speed of mucous transportation, from the nostrils to the pharynx (by saccharine test or technetium-99 m-labeled colloid albumin), or by nasal fractional exhaled nitric oxide (nasal FENO).

a. *Saccharine test:* A piece of saccharine placed in the lower part of the nostril will migrate toward the pharynx by the ciliary movement. The patient should be able to perceive the taste in the mouth before 30 min. The precision of this test is poor; it depends on several variables, and it has no value in children under 10 years old. The result is considered to be openly abnormal if the patient needs 60 min or more in perceiving the saccharine taste.
b. *Technetium-99 m-labeled colloid albumin test*: 50 mCi technetium-99 dissolved in 2.5 μl saline solution is placed in the lower part of the nostril, 1 cm deep. The migration of the tracer is measured with a gamma camera. The result is abnormal if there is no tracer movement within 10 min. It can be used in children under 10 years old. Sensitivity is 100%, but it has a moderate specificity. It has a low positive predictive value but perfect negative predictive value.
c. *Fractional exhaled nitric oxide (FENO) measure*: Very low levels of exhaled nitric oxide have been measured in the nasal mucosa of these patients. This finding is not exclusive of this pathology, but the diagnosis of PCD should be reconsidered if there are high nitric oxide levels. It is very unlikely that the patient has PCD if the value of NO exceeds 105 ppb. Other clinical conditions that tend to be accompanied by low FENO are cystic fibrosis, panbronchiolitis, complete nasal blockage, and nasal polyposis. Each center should have its own reference values.

Diagnosis Methods

Diagnostic procedures should be used in those patients with a positive screening test, or in those patients who could not undergo the screening tests because of their age or availability. A bronchoscopic brush is used to take samples of the respiratory epithelium through a nasal brushing. No sedation is required. Sometimes it is complemented with bronchial lavage and/or biopsy of the nasal and bronchial mucosa. To avoid false-positives, the patient must be free of any respiratory infection in the upper respiratory tract for at least 4–6 weeks.

The diagnosis is confirmed if the patient presents alterations in both ciliary motility and ultrastructure. If only one of these tests is positive, then the diagnosis is only presumptive.

a. *Measuring the frequency of ciliary beat with a light microscope*: Few centers in the world conduct this test. A fresh sample of the respiratory epithelium is needed. A normal ciliary motility discourages a PCD diagnosis. Abnormal beat patterns include rotation movements, independent movement in each cilium, and complete absence of ciliary motion.
b. *Measuring the frequency of ciliary beat after ciliogenesis:* This test involves analyzing a section of mucosa that has been previously cultured for this purpose. The frequency of the beat after ciliogenesis may show the real frequency value of the ciliary motility, because it is not influenced by the external conditions causing secondary ultrastructural and functional alterations.
c. *Study of respiratory mucosa cells:* Study of ciliary ultrastructure and orientation with the electronic microscope suggests ciliary dyskinesia (whether it is primary or secondary) if 20% of the studied cilia lack dynein arms. Some centers consider 10% as abnormal. An adequate sample must be obtained, with at least five good cross sections of cilia, including at least 10 different and nonadjacent cells.

In the cases of PCD there is one type of identical anomaly in all the cilia, whereas secondary anomalies usually present a variety of defects. If the patient has an abnormal cilia motility and a few cilia available for examination, then the biopsy should be repeated to rule out radial spoke pathology or a defect in the transposition of the microtubules.

Some patients have a normal ultrastructure and primary ciliary disorientation. Ciliary disorientation has recently been described as a possible variant of PCD. These patients present a normal structure, as well as a normal, or almost normal, beat frequency; but their cilia lack efficiency because their beat direction is disarranged. These patients have disorientation rates of 20% to 25%; between 10% and 15% is considered normal. Ciliary disorientation can be seen more frequently as a part of secondary ciliary alterations, and therefore if there are doubts, it is recommended to take another sample after the infection and inflammation of the patient have been treated.

Other Studies

Genetic study will probably be a useful tool in the future. The cilium contains more than 200 different types of proteins, and therefore multiple genes could be involved. It has been demonstrated that the disease is genetically heterogeneous, even when it presents the same ultrastructural alterations, which makes it difficult to investigate related genetic alterations. Currently, there are several recognized mutations: DHAH5, DNAI1; DNAH11, TXNDC3, DNAI2, KTU, LRRC50; RPGR, OFD1, RSH9, RSPH4A, CCDC39, and CCDC40. The details of approximated frequency, clinical phenotype, chromosomal location, and ultrastructural findings can be seen in Table 43.2. Currently, it is not recommended to conduct a genetic study on a routine basis for the diagnosis procedure, although it can be done if some of the mutations that are present with a greater frequency (DnAH5 and DNAI1) are suspected because of the phenotype and ultrastructural findings. These tests can also be offered to family members to provide genetic advice.

In the future, the development of marked antibodies (immunofluorescence) against the dependent proteins of the most common mutations will make possible identifying abnormal proteins in the cells of the respiratory epithelium.

Table 43.2 PCD mutations

Gene	Locus	Structural defect	Phenotype	Total of patients with mutations (%)
DNAH5	5p15	AEDA	PDC + KS	28
DNAI1	9p21-p133	AEDA	PDC + KS	7.5
DNAH11	7p15:3-21	Normal	PDC + KS	?
TXNDC3	7p14,-1	AEDA	KS	?
DNAI2	17q25,1	AEDA	PDC + KS	?
KTU	14q21,3	AEDA+ AIDA	PDC + KS	?
LRRC50	16q24,1	AEDA+ AIDA	PDC + KS	?
RPGR	Xp21,1	Variable	PDC + RP	?
OFD1	Xp22	Unknown	PDC + MR	?
RSPH9	6p21	CP	PDC	?
RSPh4A	6q22	CP	PDC	?
CCDC39	3q26,33	AEDA + CP	PDC + KS	?
CDCD40	17q25,3	AEDA + CP	PDC + KS	?

AEDA Absence of external dynein arm, *AIDA* absence of internal dynein arm, *CP* central pair defect, *PCD* primary ciliary dyskinesia, *RP* retinitis pigmentosa, *MR* mental retardation, *KS* Kartagener syndrome

Diagnostic Approach

Those patients who have a clinical condition that is compatible with PCD, after other secondary causes have been ruled out, should be studied first with a mucociliary clearance test (saccharine test or technetium-99 m-labeled colloid albumin test) or nasal FENO. The study of ciliary beat with an electronic microscope is reserved for those cases in which screening tests yield abnormal results. If any of these methods is not available or cannot be used because of the age of the patient, a direct sample of the respiratory mucosa must be taken (Fig. 43.5).

Evaluation and Treatment

The objective of the therapy is to prevent pulmonary complications, such as the appearance of chronic lung damage and bronchiectasis, as well as reducing sinus and ear complications.

There are no properly designed studies evaluating the effectiveness of different types of therapy for the different patients affected by PCD. Most recommendations are based on the opinions of experts, besides extrapolations done considering other diseases such as cystic fibrosis.

These patients require a multidisciplinary assessment, including general pediatricians as well as pulmonologists, otorhinolaryngologists, respiratory physiotherapists, and psychologists.

Respiratory Treatment

Patients must be checked every 2 to 3 months. This evaluation should include monitoring of respiratory frequency, O_2 capillary saturation, and spirometry. Chest X-rays must be taken when there are respiratory exacerbations. A sputum culture is recommended every 3 months to determine what organisms are colonizing the airway. If bronchiectasis is being suspected, it should be confirmed with a computed tomography (CAT) scan; however, it is not recommended to serialize this study in the follow-up. The patient and their family must be educated about the disease, the importance of avoiding exposure to environment pollutants, especially tobacco smoke, and to seek early medical follow-up when there is clinical worsening, even if it is minimal. Yearly vaccination against influenza is recommended, as well as vaccination against *Streptococcus pneumoniae*, if the patient has not yet been vaccinated.

The two therapeutic columns are chest physiotherapy and the intensive use of antibiotics for respiratory exacerbations.

Adequate secretion clearance can be achieved through chest physiotherapy, consisting of bronchial drainage and repeated deep inspiration tech-

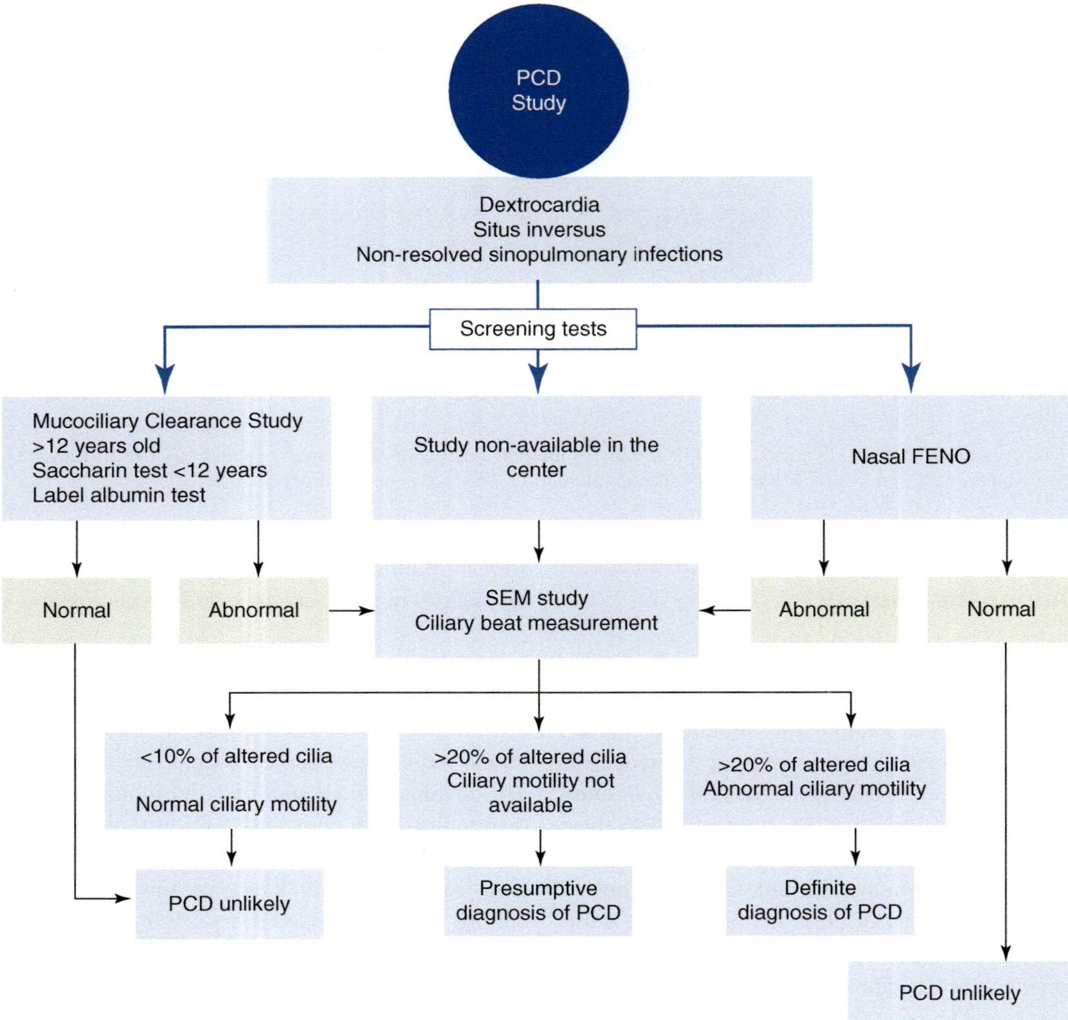

Fig. 43.5 PCD study algorithm

niques, in combination with chest percussion. At least 20 min, twice per day, is recommended. Using β_2-agonists may be useful, but ideally the response to this drug should be documented with spirometry before and after using the bronchodilator. Exercise determines the improvement of expiratory flows in the spirometry in a much better way than β_2-agonists. Ideally, the patient should engage in some kind of physical activity before chest physiotherapy sessions, to promote a greater clearance of the secretions. The use of Flutter or Acapella has not been studied, but they can be considered for older children.

The organism that usually infects these patients is *Haemophilus influenzae* (80%), followed by *Staphylococcus aureus* (13%) and *Streptococcus pneumoniae* (10%). Infection caused by *Pseudomonas aeruginosa* occurs in as many as 20% of the pediatric population. In adult patients it has been isolated in 25% of cases, and in 15% of cases atypical mycobacteria were present. For episodes of cough and sputum, an intense and prolonged antibiotic therapy must be started (>14 days), using antibiotics adequate for the agents involved. An initial ambulatory treatment in high doses is recommended. The use of IV antibiotics must be reserved for patients who do not respond to oral therapy, who are infected by *Pseudomonas aeruginosa*, are hospitalized because of great respiratory distress, or need oxygen.

There is no evidence to support the chronic use of nebulized rhDNAse, nebulized hypertonic serum, *n*-acetylcysteine, or macrolides.

Otorhinolaryngology Treatment

Hearing evaluation must be done in series, through audiometry and impedance audiometry. These patients have a very high rate of otitis media with effusion, which alters hearing and affects language development.

There is controversy relative to what treatment should be used in patients with hearing loss because of otitis media. Some authors do not recommend the use of ventilation tubes, because persistent otorrhea may appear after their implanting. For those patients who have lost 40 decibels or more, hearing aids may help the child to acquire proper language; but persistent otitis media along with effusion may cause a retraction of the posterior tympanic membrane, which will have consequences in the future. Of 33 patients at the Hospital Clínico de la Universidad Católica de Chile who were assessed between 1993 and 2003, tympanostomy tubes indicated for 19. The follow-up of these patients while they had the tubes implanted showed that 13 of them improved satisfactorily without otorrhea episodes, 2 had at least one episode of otorrhea, and 4 presented with three or more episodes. Currently, considering the level of evidence, both the conservative option of using hearing aids as the surgical option are viable treatment alternatives for this group of patients who have suffered hearing loss.

Ideally, for patients with chronic otorrhea caused by *Pseudomonas aeruginosa*, topical antibiotics should be used, and sometimes IV antibiotics therapy is recommended, which should be prolonged for rebel cases.

Chronic rhinosinusitis is present in more than 90% of the patients. Routine sinus X-ray evaluation is not recommended. A CAT scan is suggested if a complication is suspected or if a surgery is planned. The recommended treatment is lavage with high volumes of saline solution, whether it is isotonic or hypertonic ("nasal shower"), twice as a day as a routine, with the intention of creating a mechanical flushing of the secretions. If the patient does not respond to the nasal lavage, then topical nasal steroids are generally recommended. For those patients who do not respond to the aforementioned therapies, antibiotic therapy should be considered, and eventually, surgery.

Future Perspectives

Chhin showed that, using a lentivirus as a vector, a normal (therapeutic) gene could be transferred to human nasal mucosa cells. After this, the transferred gene could be transcribed and expressed, thus reestablishing ciliary ultrastructure and function in those cells. The importance of this study lies in the fact that it is possible to insert therapeutic genes in the cellular genome and thus it offers new perspectives for the treatment of PCD.

Prognosis

Prognosis is generally good, with a normal life expectancy. If treatment is not adequate, however, there may be some serious complications secondary to recurrent infections and iatrogenic complications. The appearance of these complications will depend on the ultrastructural alteration type, how early the diagnosis was made, if there was bronchiectasis or lung damage when the diagnosis was done, and the therapy received. From the reproductive aspect, subfertility occurs in both men and women, and they should be referred to fertility clinics for counseling and treatment. In patients with severe lung damage and dependent on oxygen, lung transplant is a valid option to extend and improve lifespan.

To summarize, early diagnosis and the right treatment yield an adequate survival rate, a better quality of life, and fewer complications in these patients.

Sources

Barbato A, Frischer T, Kueinni CE, Snijerds D, et al. Primary ciliary dyskinesia: a consensus statement on diagnostic and treatment approaches in children. Eur Respir J. 2009;34(6):1264–76.

Busquets RM, Caballero-Rabasco MA, Velasco M, Lloreta J, García-Algar O. Discinesia ciliar primaria: criterios clínicos de indicación de estudio ultraestructural. Arch Bronconeumol. 2013;49(3):99–104.

Chhin B, Negre D, Merrot O, Pham J, Tourneur Y, Ressnikoff D, et al. Ciliary beating recovery in deficient human air-way epithelial cells after lentivirus ex vivo gene therapy. PLoS Genet. 2009;5:e1000422.

Chodhari R, Mitchison H, Meeks M. Cilia, primary ciliary dyskinesia and molecular genetics. Paedit Respir Rev. 2004;5:69–76.

Corbelli R, Brigolf-Isler B, Amacher A, Sasse B, et al. Nasal nitric oxide measurements to screen children for primary cliary dyskinesia. Chest. 2004;126(4):1054–9.

Coren M, Meeks M, Morrison I, Buchdal RM, Bush A. Primary ciliary dyskinesia: age at diagnosis and symptom history. Acta Paediatr. 2002;91:667–9.

De Boeck K, Proesmans M, Mortelmans L, Van Billoen B, Jorissen M. Mucociliary transport using 99m Tc-albumin colloid: a reliable screening test for primary ciliary dyskinesia. Thorax. 2005;60:614–7.

Eley L, Yates L, Goodship J. Cilia and disease. Curr Opin Genet Dev. 2005;15:308–14.

Hjeij R, Loges NT, Omran H. Immunofluorescence microscopy (IFM) analysis of primary ciliary dyskinesia (PCD) patients with suspected inner dynein arm defects (IDA). Cilia. 2012;1(suppl 1):23.

Iñiguez R, Fonseca X, Hernández J, González S, Sánchez I. Disquinesia ciliar: diagnóstico ultraestructural, evolución clínica y alternativas de tratamiento. Rev Med Chile. 2007;135:1147–52.

Mener DJ, Lin SY, Ishman SL, Boss EF. Treatment and outcomes of chronic rhinosinusitis in children with primary ciliary dyskinesia: where is the evidence? A qualitative systematic review. Int Forum Allergy Rhinol. 2013; https://doi.org/10.1002/alr.21227.

Noone PN, Leigh MW, Sannuti A, Minnix SL, et al. Primary ciliary dyskinesia. Diagnostic and phenotypic features. Am J Respir Crit Care Med. 2004;169:459–67.

Steinkamp G, Seithe H, Nublein T. Therapy of primary ciliary dyskinesia. Pulmonologie. 2004;58:179–87.

Cystic Fibrosis: Clinical and Diagnosis Approach

44

Claudio Castaños, Lilien Chertkoff, and Luis Gravina

Contents

Introduction

Cystic fibrosis (CF) is a multi-systemic and autosomal recessive disease that affects the respiratory, digestive, and reproductive systems. It is caused by a mutation in the gene called cystic

C. Castaños (✉) · L. Chertkoff · L. Gravina
Hospital Garrahan, Buenos Aires, Argentina
e-mail: ccastanos@garrahan.gov.ar; lgravina@garrahan.gov.ar

P. Bertrand, I. Sánchez (eds.), *Pediatric Respiratory Diseases*,
https://doi.org/10.1007/978-3-030-26961-6_44

fibrosis transmembrane conductance regulator (CFTR).

From the first descriptions of CF by Andersen in 1938, more than 50 years passed until a responsible gene could be identified in 1989. From this moment on, important advances in the medical knowledge of the disease have greatly affected the diagnosis procedure and its treatment. During these years an improvement of the clinical situation of these patients was achieved, which has yielded a better life expectancy in developed countries, currently reaching 40 years of age. In Latin America the life expectancy is lower, although there are only isolated data from some countries. Even so, every year more patients reach adulthood. Because of the advances achieved during the last decades, currently CF should be considered a chronic disease, of which the progression can be favorably modified if early therapeutic interventions are implemented.

Epidemiology

CF is the lethal hereditary disease most frequent in the white population, with an incidence of around 1:3200 newborns. In non-Caucasian populations, such as Afro-Americans and Asians, the incidence is substantially lower. Even though there are no definitive data for Latin America, the Hispanic population in the United States of America presents an incidence of 1 in 9000 newborns. In Argentina, where neonatal screening has been carried out since 1995, the reported data indicate an incidence of 1 in 7000 newborns. This number is likely related to the ethnic characteristics of this population, caused by the integration within the native population of different European-Caucasian immigration flows.

From the genetics aspect, the distribution of mutations in the CFTR gene also varies greatly according to the ethnic origin and the geographic localization of each group of people. About 2000 mutations have been reported for the CFTR gene, which have been systematically registered in an open access database (Cystic Fibrosis Mutation Database, http://www.genet.sickkids.on.ca). The most frequent mutation is a phenylalanine deletion in position 508 (DF508 or p.F508del according to current nomenclature), which is present in two thirds of the CF alleles in the world.

Studies conducted in different Latin American countries have shown a wide spectrum of CFTR gene mutations: about 100 different mutations have been described. The allele sequence of mutation DF508 varies among the countries in Latin America: Venezuela-Cuba-Ecuador-Chile (29–34%), Mexico-Colombia-Uruguay (40%), Brazil (40–48%), and Argentina (56–60%). This variability reflects the different ethnic backgrounds between Latin American countries depending on the greater or smaller predominance of European immigration.

The second most common mutation is G542X, present in about 5% among them all. The frequency of 15 other mutations (N1303K, W1282X, 1717-1G>A, 3849+10KbC>T, R334W, G85E, DI507, 2183AA>G, 2789+5G>A, 1811+1, 6Kb A>G, R1162X, R553X, R1066C, 621+1G-T, and 3120+1G>A) is about 1%.

Pathophysiology

CF is an autosomal recessive disease caused by mutations in the gene CFTR, localized in the long arm of chromosome 7 (7q31,2), which is 250 kb and composed of 27 exons. It codifies a protein made of 1480 amino acids, composed of two transmembrane domains, two union and two ATP-binding and hydrolysis domains, and one phosphorylation regulation domain (Fig. 44.1). In normal conditions, this protein is present in the apical membrane of the cells in the exocrine epithelium, where it mainly acts in active chloride ion transportation, and it seems to be capable of regulating the function of other ionic channels. The presence of mutations in the CFTR gene causes a defective epithelial ionic transport.

From the functional aspect, mutations are grouped in five classes (I–V). Most of these cause complete channel failure, whether they affect the biosynthesis of the protein (class I), its maturity process (class II), or its function (class III). In contrast, in class IV and V mutations, the proteins produced retain certain residual activity. Generally, class I, II, and III mutations are related to serious manifestations of the disease,

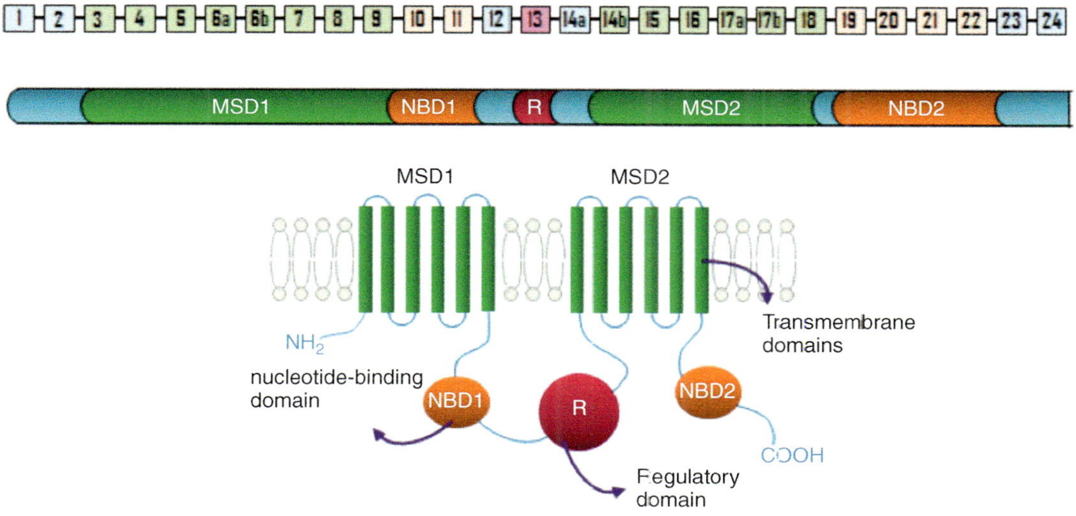

Fig. 44.1 Cystic fibrosis transmembrane conductance regulator (CFTR) gene and protein

which include pancreatic insufficiency, whereas class V mutations present mild manifestations, or even oligo-symptomatic (traditionally named nonclassic presentations, and currently named diseases related to CTFR), such as the congenital bilateral absence of the vas deferens (CBAVD), idiopathic chronic pancreatitis, and bronchiectasis, among others.

Understanding of the physiopathological nature of the disease at the molecular level has improved during the past years. This knowledge prompted the development of new therapeutic strategies oriented to correct the gene dysfunction. Thus, genotyping patients with CF also became important for determining specific treatments according to the mutation class (allele-specific therapies).

Diagnosis

The disease is diagnosed using clinical criteria and laboratory methods. The presence of two or more of the following clinical criteria suggest the disease: chronic pulmonary disease, chronic sinus disease, malabsorption, obstructive azoospermia in males, family history of cystic fibrosis, and salt-wasting syndrome.

Diagnosis confirmation is through these means:

- Two positive sweat tests
- Presence of two mutations in the CFTR gene
- An abnormal transepithelial membrane potential

Nevertheless, a percentage of patients do not have complete expression of the disease, and the physician must be aware to determine the diagnosis (Table 44.1).

According to the International Cystic Fibrosis Association (ICFA), these factors favor delayed diagnosis:

(a) Poor knowledge about the disease among health professionals
(b) Lack of information for timely diagnosis within the first health attention levels
(c) Diagnosis inaccessibility, given difficulties to conduct the sweat test at a location near the patient's domicile

Clinical Manifestations

Lung Compromise

The onset age of respiratory symptoms is variable, and some symptoms can appear even during the neonatal phase, although they always appear during the first years of life. The symptoms may

Table 44.1 Important clinical elements for diagnosis

Respiratory
Upper airway
Nasal polyps
Chronic sinusitis
Lower airway
Persistent tachypnea and retraction
Wheezing with persistent hyperinflation
Chronic cough
Sputum culture positive for *Haemophilus influenzae*, *Staphylococcus aureus*, or *Pseudomonas aeruginosa*
Recurrent pneumonia
Bronchiectasis
Hemoptysis
Chest X-rays
Bilateral air trapping
Persistent atelectasis (particularly in the right upper lobe)
Gastrointestinal
Meconium ileus
Prolonged neonatal jaundice
Malabsorption–steatorrhea
Rectal prolapse
Cirrhosis and portal hypertension
Other
Growth failure
Positive family history
Salty sweat
Edema and hyponatremia
Digital clubbing
Azoospermia and absence of vas deferens
Metabolic alkalosis

be nonspecific, but the pediatrician must suspect and consider CF.

Respiratory disease causes greater morbidity and mortality rates. More than 95% of the patients with CF present with respiratory symptoms, and with malabsorption, it is the most common clinical presentation.

The CFTR protein defect causes an alteration in the mucociliary clearance, where there is inadequate depuration of the respiratory secretions, which tend to be thick, thus favoring bronchial obstruction and chronic infection of the airway. Because of this defect, the clinical presentation during this stage of life may include these:

1. Recurrent or prolonged bronchiolitis
2. Recurrent or persistent atelectasis
3. Chronic bronchitis, with cough and mucopurulent expectoration

Older children may present with bronchial obstruction, cough, and expectoration, which vary according to the compromise of the patient. CF must be considered and ruled out for children with asthma symptoms who do not respond to the treatment.

When the disease has progressed because of the persistence of infections and chronic obstruction, bronchiectasis may be observed, with or without hemoptysis.

Extrapulmonary signs of chronic lung disease may be observed, such as increase of chest anteroposterior diameter and digital clubbing.

> CF must be ruled out in every child with asthma symptoms who does not respond to treatment with bronchodilators or shows failure to thrive.

A characteristic of the disease, granted by the basic genetic alteration, is infection of the airway, which in many cases ultimately causes a chronic infection. In the first stages of CF, the most frequent agents are nontypeable *Haemophilus influenzae* (HI) or *Staphylococcus aureus* (SA). As the disease progresses and the patients become older, *Pseudomonas aeruginosa* (PA) is the main agent.

> The physician should suspect the disease when there is persistence of bronchial secretions in patients who are positive for nontypeable *Haemophilus influenzae* (HI) or *Staphylococcus aureus* (SA), and who have not received mechanical ventilation support. If *Pseudomonas aeruginosa* appears on the cultures, CF must be ruled out.

At first, the chest X-ray may show hyperinflation, but it then progresses to bronchitis with patchy areas with consolidations. These changes

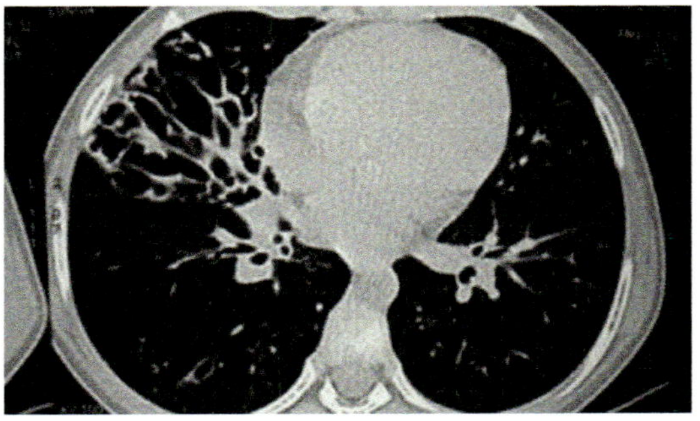

Fig. 44.2 Bronchiectasis. Computerized axial tomography of a 16-year-old patient shows bronchial enlargement and cystic deformations, mainly in the middle lobe

are gradual and increase with the progression of the disease.

In chest computerized axial tomography, cylindrical bronchiectasis can be observed during the beginning of the disease, which afterward progress to a varicose and then to a saccular type (Fig. 44.2).

The presence of cylindrical bronchiectasis, mainly in the superior lobes, is suggestive of the disease, which must be ruled out with a sweat test.

Lung compromise is also observed in lung function tests, which can be present even in the early stages of the disease.

Upper airway
Compromise of the upper airway is caused by the hyperreactivity of the mucus secretion glands. This, with the alterations in mucociliary transport, causes hypertrophy and edema in the mucosa membranes, as well as obstruction of sinus ostia.

Almost all patients with cystic fibrosis present with opacification in the paranasal sinus X-rays, and many have chronic sinusitis symptoms, which may cause infectious exacerbations in the lower airway. More than 25% of all patients with CF have nasal polyps.

> If there are nasal polyps and the cause has not been established, CF must be ruled out.

Intestinal Obstruction

Meconium ileus Meconium ileus appears in 10–15% of patients with CF, and it is the most common manifestation during neonatal age. It occurs secondary to water reduction in the intestines, and most of these patients also have pancreatic insufficiency.

Starting from the 18th week of gestation, it can be recognized through echography. This condition may also appear after childbirth, with abdominal enlargement and scarce stools with mucus, or no defecation at all, as well as biliary vomiting. The obstruction is usually located in the small intestine proximal to the ileocecal valve. Encapsulated meconium peritonitis appears in more than 50% of the patients with meconium ileus.

In the abdominal X-rays, the intestine can appear enlarged, with areas of air mixed with dehydrated meconium, usually in the abdomen right lower quadrant. Calcifications images may also appear.

> The presence of meconium ileus in a newborn is almost synonym for CF, and it should be ruled out. The existence of duodenal atresia has also been related to CF in more than 50% of the patients, and therefore any type of intestinal obstruction in an infant is suggestive of CF, which must be ruled out.

Equivalent of meconium ileus Also called distal intestinal obstruction syndrome, this can be an important complication in some patients, particularly in adolescents. It is characterized by constipation, vomiting, abdominal pain, recurrent colic, and palpable fecal matter in the right iliac fossa, or in the right side.

Gastrointestinal Alterations

Prolonged jaundice Neonatal cholestatic jaundice can appear in patients with meconium ileus (50%), but it can also appear in newborns without meconium ileus.

Exocrine pancreatic insufficiency (intestinal malabsorption) Between 85% and 90% of the patients with cystic fibrosis present with pancreatic insufficiency at birth.

The clinical presentation is abundant fetid stools, with fat presence characteristics (lack of color, shiny, oily). Malabsorption is confirmed using the stool elastase test, or with the collection of 72 h of stools and analyzing the fat contained, named the Van de Kamer test.

About 10% to 15% of the patients have pancreatic sufficiency with some degree of residual pancreatic activity. Given that these patients do not suffer from malabsorption, diagnosis is difficult and it usually takes longer.

> Patients with pancreatic sufficiency may develop pancreatic insufficiency as the disease progresses, and therefore elastase must be controlled annually.

In older patients or in adults, persistent or recurrent pancreatitis of unknown cause is suggestive of CF.

Rectal prolapse It can be present in about 20% of the patients who are under 5 years old and who have never been treated for CF. This sign is secondary to the lack of treatment for intestinal malabsorption.

Liver disease Around 5% of the patients with CF develop liver disease. The process is characterized by focal or diffuse cirrhosis, and the complications include splenomegaly, varicose veins, and bleeding: this is the cause of death of 1–2% of patients with cystic fibrosis.

Another complication related to liver disease is biliary lithiasis, which has a greater incidence in patients with CF.

Growth Delay

These patients frequently present with a delay in growth, which is caused by a combination of several factors: (a) increase of calorie intake; (b) chronic lung disease; (c) poor digestion, with corresponding intestinal malabsorption; and (d) low appetite, caused by active lung inflammation.

Intestinal malabsorption can be confirmed observing the increase in depositions, with abnormal stool color and consistency. Malabsorption, especially of fats, also involves a deficiency in the absorption of liposoluble vitamins.

Sweat Glands

CFTR causes the sweat glands to be the only ionic channel capable of reabsorbing sweat chloride; therefore, the patient with CF has a chloride concentration in the skin five times greater than that of normal patients, which is almost the same as the plasmatic concentration. This abnormality is the base of the diagnostic test of the disease.

The sweat of the affected patients tends to be salty, and the loss could be so important that salt crystals could appear in the hair line. Salt loss during heat waves can be serious and cause hyponatremic dehydration, as well as serious hypochloremic alkalosis, which require immediate intervention. This loss could be the first presentation of the disease.

Vas Deferens

Even though the testicles of males with CF are normal, the epididymis either cannot be palpated or is reduced, and the vas deferentia are absent in almost every patient.

Up to 95% of males who suffer from CF are infertile because of azoospermia, caused by the congenital bilateral absence of a vas deferens. Women may be sterile because of thickening of the cervical mucus or nutritional state.

Diabetes Mellitus

Changes in the glucose mechanism of CF patients were described in 1938, but the relationship between cystic fibrosis and diabetes was described later, in 1953. The cause of diabetes is the progressive fibrosis of the pancreas, which in principle is only present in the exocrine pancreas and then extends to the endocrine portion of the gland.

Reported incidence in different studies is quite variable, with a range between 21% and 75%. The range is so wide that it may be caused by dissimilar criteria used for different studies.

Edematous Ascitic Syndrome

In children under 6 months of age, about 5% of CF patients may also present edema, anemia, and hypoproteinemia. These patients need to be nutritionally recovered before conducting the sweat test, to avoid the possibility of false-negatives.

> The triad edema, anemia, and hyponatremia is considered to be a CF until it been ruled out.

Family History of CF

A family history of CF it is very useful when CT is suspected.

Other less frequent clinical presentations Arthropathy, with arthritis and vasculitis, can be detected. Amyloidosis can be a complication of the chronic inflammation activity caused by an infection. Autoimmune processes and malignant diseases have also been described.

Laboratory Methods

Sweat Test

Quantitative measures of electrolytes in sweat excretion is still the most important test to confirm the clinical suspicion of this disease.

To perform this test correctly and obtain valid results, it is important to apply the procedure using a standardized methodology, in centers where an adequate number of tests are being carried out, to have a good quality control. The test consists in the stimulation of sweat glands through pilocarpine iontophoresis, the sweat collection in gauze or in filter paper (Gibson and Cooke), and the concentration of electrolytes (chloride, or chloride and sodium), is quantified. A Macroduct device can also be used.

- The minimal weight of accepted sweat is 75 mg, and the sweat rate must be more than 1 g/m²/min.
- The results of the sweat test must always be evaluated considering the clinical presentation and the age of the patient, and it should not be the only element in the diagnosis, because false results may be obtained.
- The reference values for the sweat test are shown in Table 44.2.
- Those patients with uncertain results must be reevaluated until a diagnosis can be confirmed.
- Some data state that for children under 3 months of age a concentration greater than 30 mmol/l is highly suggestive of CF.

Warning No technique of direct reading, whether by conductivity or by the specific or selective ion electrode system, chloride indicator patch, osmolarity measure, etc.; may be used as a confirmation method, nor they should be used as the base for a definitive diagnose of cystic fibrosis.

The sweat conductivity test measures the electric conductivity of the ions; uses the Macroduct device for collecting and the Wescor Sweat-Chek

Table 44.2 Reference values for sweat test

	Under 6 months old	Over 6 months old
Normal	≤29 mmol/l	≤39 mmol/l
Intermediate or uncertain	30–59 mmol/l	40–59 mmol/l
Pathologically compatible with CF	≥60 mmol/l	≥60 mmol/l

analyzer. It is a screening method, which must be confirmed by the Gibson and Cooke method.

Practical considerations for the sweat test:

- Test must be done in stable patients.
- It is recommended to apply it for asymptomatic children older than 2 weeks of life and whose weight exceeds 2 kg. For symptomatic patients (for example, meconium ileus), it can be done when the patient has reached 48 h of life.
- The site of choice for the recollection of sweat is usually the forearm; in some circumstances the sweat can be collected from the thigh.
- Samples from different parts of the body must not be added to obtain the minimum amount of sweat.
- Chloride or chloride and sodium concentrations are assessed; when only one ion is quantified, chloride is the one considered. The simultaneous determination of chlorides and sodium, particularly, may be useful when dealing with limit values in the test results.
- In patients with CF the concentrations of both ions should be proportionately elevated, and the difference between them should be no more than 15 mmol/l.
- Values above 160 mmol/l are not physiologically possible and should be considered as mistakes in the test.
- Around 98% of the patients have a chloride concentration greater than 60 mmol/l, and 2%, who present atypical phenotypes, may present with normal or limit values.
- Most people with normal tests have chloride values less than 30 mmol/l.

Factors affecting the concentration of electrolytes in sweat:

- The main reasons for obtaining false-positive or false-negative-results are generally related to nonstandardization issues as well technical mistakes.

Pathologies that may be related to high electrolytes levels in sweat

- Fucosidosis
- Glycogen storage disease type I
- Mucopolysaccharidosis
- Untreated hypothyroidism∗
- Nephrogenic diabetes insipidus∗
- Adrenal insufficiency∗
- Familial hyperparathyroidism∗
- Eczema∗
- Protein and calorie malnutrition∗
- Ectodermal dysplasia
- Prostaglandin E-1 infusion
- Anorexia nervosa∗
- Autonomic dysfunction
- Glucose-6-phosphatase deficiency
- Mauriac syndrome
- Pseudo-hypoaldosteronism∗
- Familial cholestasis

∗Sweat test yields normal results when condition has been resolved.

1. False-negative sweat test
    - Technical tests: Low sweat rate
    - In patients with cystic fibrosis:
        - Edema and hypoproteinemia∗
        - Some mutations that yield "uncertain" chloride results:
            - R117H (7T)
            - 3849+10kb C-to-T
            - G551S
            - D1152H
            - A455E
            - IVS8-5T

    ∗Repeat the test when the situation has been corrected.

Sweat test must be repeated if:

- The test is positive
- The result falls in the uncertainty range
- Clinical evolution is not as expected

Malabsorption Test

Malabsorption tests can show the loss of fats through stools or chymotrypsin deficit in the duodenum. The test can be very simple or very complex.

The most common used ones are these:

- Van de Kamer test: Normal values are less than 2.5 g fat per day. It is the study of choice to confirm malabsorption.

- Steatocrit
- Globules of fat
- Chymotrypsin in stools
- Elastase in stools

Semen Analysis

Obstructive azoospermia is strong evidence of CF, and therefore semen analysis may be important to diagnose patients who are monosymptomatic.

Membrane Potential

The respiratory epithelium, including the nasal epithelium, regulates the composition of the fluid that bathes the surface of the airway, transporting sodium and chloride. This active transportation creates an electric transepithelial potential difference, which can be measured in vivo.

Abnormalities in ionic transportation in the respiratory epithelium of patients with CF are related to a characteristic pattern of potential difference in comparison to the normal epithelium: basal potential tending to negativity, greater changes when exposed to amiloride, and null or poor response when the mucosa is perfused with free chloride solution.

It is very important to have standard techniques and methods before interpreting test results. Measurement must not be carried out in patients with rhinitis, polyps, or tubes which may erode the nasal epithelium. The test may have diagnostic utility in atypical cases.

Molecular Diagnosis

Currently, molecular characterization uses commercial kits developed to detect the most common mutations for the Caucasian population in Europe and in the United States. These tests generally include the aforementioned mutations. However, the rate of detection of these kits in Latin American countries will vary depending on the ethnic predominance of each population. As a consequence, their use should be evaluated according to the mutation range of each population to ensure adequate sensitivity levels (≥70%).

Although most of the mutations described in the CFTR gene are punctual substitutions as well as small deletions or insertions, during recent years different large deletions have been described in the CFTR gene that may involve from only one exon to the complete gene, which affects the activity of the protein, totally or partially. These rearrangements escape detection in the conventional methods routinely used in molecular biology laboratories, and therefore the real frequency may be underestimated. The development of techniques that may establish the extent of the involvement in a determined region of the genome has eased the detection of these extensive rearrangements.

To reach greater levels of sensitivity, it is possible to create a sequence of all the CFTR gene exons, using a procedure that is quite complex and expensive, besides being time consuming. For this reason, in most populations this method is only used where there is a high clinical suspicion that could not be confirmed using other methods. Also, complete sequencing identifies all kinds of alterations in the CFTR gene, ranging from mutations that cause the disease to mutations related to mild or monosymptomatic manifestations, besides alterations whose pathological consequences may not be well defined. Thus, in some cases interpretation of the results may be complex. During past years new sequencing technologies (next-generation sequencing) have been developed, which simultaneously analyze millions of fragments, executing a quick sequencing of large DNA extensions. Although accessing these new technologies is difficult, it is expected that sequencing costs will be reduced within the coming years, and so sequencing of the CFTR gene will be a possible diagnostic method for most countries within the region.

To interpret the consequences of a certain mutation, an open access database named CFTR2 project (Clinical and Functional Translation of CFTR, http://www.cftr2.org) can be helpful. The objective of this project is to provide complete clinical and functional information that is up to date and has been reviewed by experts, relative to a large group of CFTR mutations: it gathers all the clinical and molecular data from 40,000 patients worldwide.

Indications for a Molecular Study

- Confirmation of suspicious cases (limit or unclear chloride values in the sweat test)
- Diagnosis in newborns with suggestive symptoms
- Presymptomatic diagnosis in newborn and infants where CF is suspected because of family history or positive neonatal screening
- Confirmed genotypical definition of patients with CF and detection of asymptomatic carriers in the family, to provide them with adequate genetic counseling
- Diagnosis of atypical manifestations
- Prenatal diagnosis through amniocentesis or biopsy of chorionic villi
- Preimplantation diagnosis

Knowing the genotype is also useful to predict certain phenotypical characteristics, such as pancreatic function (genotype–phenotype correlation), as well as categorizing the patients for the implementation of future therapeutic strategies.

CF Neonatal Screening

In the beginning of the decade of the 1980s, Crossley et al. described measuring immunoreactive trypsin (IRT) in dry blood stains as a simple method for screening newborns for CF. From this point on, the first programs of Newborn Screening for Cystic Fibrosis (NSCF) were developed in New Zealand and Australia. Currently, these programs exist in diverse countries in Europe, North America, Oceania, and, to a lesser extent, in Latin America.

The early detection of CF through these screening programs has made possible the delivery of preventive care measures to improve nutrition, growth, and pulmonary function, as well as reducing hospitalizations. As a result of these preventive and attention measures, in the United States of America the life expectancy of the patients with CF increased from 27 years old in 1985 to 38 years old in 2010.

Screening Strategies

Although developed countries have managed to implement CF screening effectively for more than 30 years, and guidelines and recommendations have been published, there is still no unique analytic protocol that has been universally accepted.

The different strategies that have been implemented during these years share, as a first step, the determination of IRT on dry blood stains on paper. Nevertheless, an IRT isolated measurement has a low specificity and low positive predictive value (PPV). Therefore, the diagnostic performance should be improved by combining IRT study with other tests, as for example, the same IRT in a second sample, the detection of mutations in the CFTR gene (DNA), and measuring the pancreatitis-associated protein (PAP). The different described protocols combine the mentioned studies, which differ in their sensitivity, specificity, positive PPV, recall rate, complexity, and costs. The following are the main strategies:

- IRT/IRT
- IRT/DNA
- IRT/DNA/IRT
- IRT/IRT/DNA
- IRT/PAP

Depending on the strategy followed, if the first sample yields a positive IRT result, there are three alternatives that can be followed:

1. Obtaining a second sample before the first month of life to do a second IRT determination. This option is used in the IRT/IRT and IRT/IRT/DNA strategies. In the IRT/IRT strategy, if an abnormal result is repeated in the second sample, the patient is recalled and a sweat test is indicated to confirm or rule out CF. In contrast, the IRT/IRT/DNA

strategy, when facing a second positive sample, uses the same IRT sample to search for mutations in the CFTR gene. The presence of two mutations confirms the diagnosis. If the molecular study yields no definitive diagnosis, the newborn is scheduled for a sweat test (Fig. 44.3).

2. Molecular studies using the same sample obtained for the initial IRT test. IRT/DNA and IRT/DAN/IRT strategies are used. If the molecular analysis is not conclusive (presence of a mutation or a high IRT value with no identifiable mutation), the patient is recalled for a sweat test (IRT/DNA strategy), or a second sample is requested to perform a second IRT (IRT/DNA/IRT strategy). After this point, the strategy is more similar to the IRT/IRT (Fig. 44.4).
3. PAP measurement in relation to the same sample obtained for the initial test. In this strategy, which is known as IRT/PAP, if the result of the PAP also yields an increased result, then the sweat test is indicated.

The decision of what strategy to use will depend on several factors: the ethnic composition of the population to be screened, the frequency and distribution of the mutations in the CFTR gene, the infrastructure of the laboratory, and the availability of ideal staff who can handle more complex techniques. In the same way, it is crucial to consider the costs and consider the objective of the program, which is to know if the aim is to detect individuals who carry the gene and mild forms of cystic fibrosis, which are generally not considered objectives within a screening program (Table 44.3).

Although currently many programs still use the IRT/IRT strategy, this technique has a lower sensitivity, specificity, and PPV thresholds relative to the other techniques. For these reasons, most of the protocols applied in Europe, North America, and Oceania include the analysis of mutations in the CFTR gene, aiming to obtain a better balance between false-negative and false-positive results.

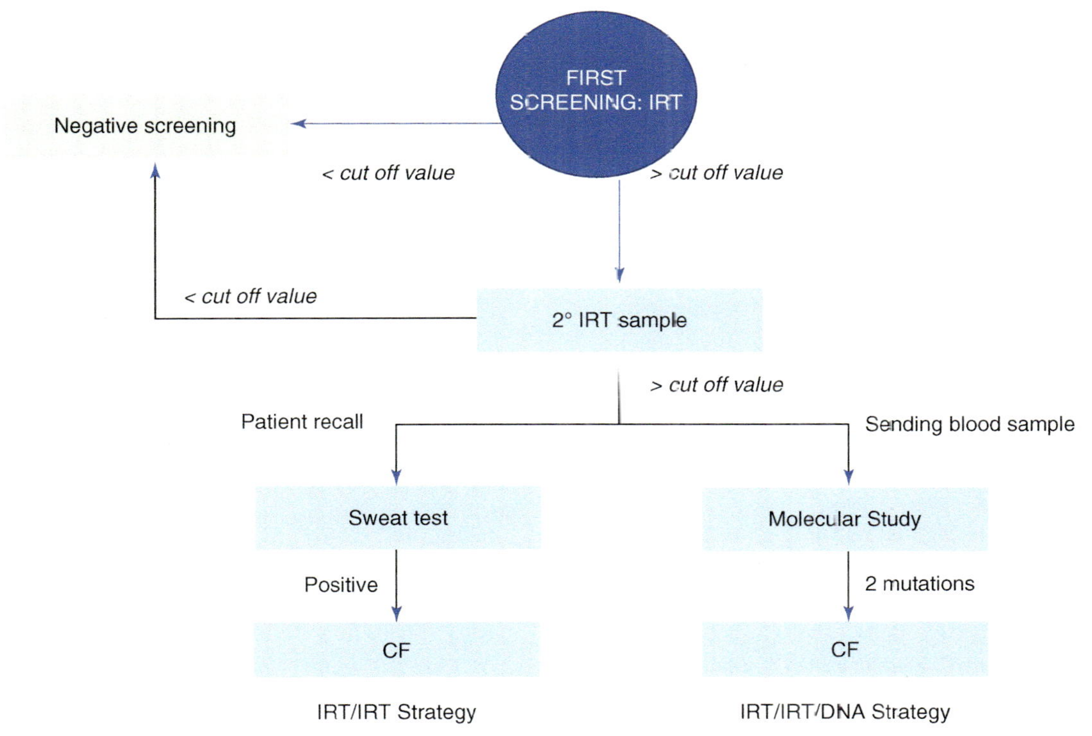

Fig. 44.3 Algorithm for screening: IRT/IRT and IRT/IRT/DNA strategies

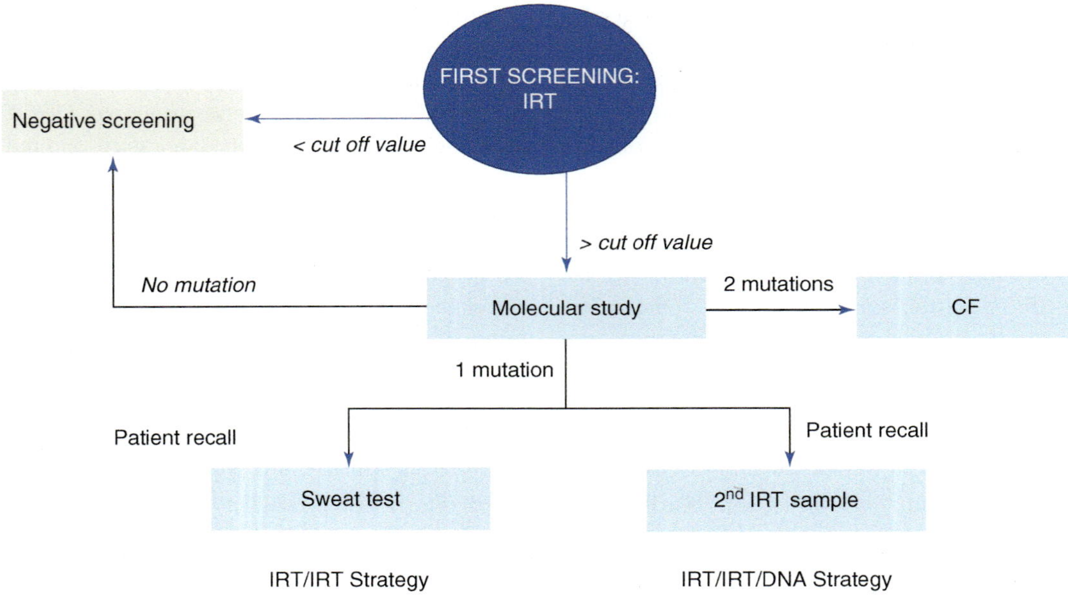

Fig. 44.4 Algorithm for screening: IRT/IRT and IRT/DNA/IRT strategies

Table 44.3 Advantages and Disadvantages of Strategies

	IRT/IRT	IRT/DNA	IRT/DNA/IRT	IRT/IRT/DNA	IRT/PAP
Sensitivity	<	>>	>	<	>
Specificity	<	>>	>>	>	>
Positive predictive value	<	>>	>>	>	>
Patient follow-up	Yes	No	Yes	Yes	No
Detection of carriers	No	Yes	Yes	Yes	No
Detection of mild forms	No	Yes	Yes	Yes	No
Time needed to make a diagnosis	>	<<	<	>	<<
Sweat test requirements	+++	++	+	++	+
Cost	+	+++	+++	++	+

Screening with negative double-trypsin does not rule out the disease. The sweat test is indicated if there is suspicion of CF.

Sources

Andersen DH. Cystic fibrosis of the pancreas and its relation to celiac disease: a clinical and pathologic study. Am J Dis Child. 1938;56:344–99.

Aranzamendi RJ, Breitman F, Asciutto C, Delgado N, Castaños C. Deshidratación y alcalosis metabólica: presentación inusual de un niño con fibrosis quística. Arch Argent Pediatr. 2008;106(5):443–6.

Castellani C, Southern KW, Brownlee K, et al. European best practice guidelines for cystic fibrosis neonatal screening. J Cyst Fibros. 2009;8:153–73.

Comité de Neumonología, Nutrición,Gastroenterología e Infectología. Sociedad Argentina de Pediatria. Arch Arg Ped (en prensa).

De Boeck K, Derichs N, Fajac I, et al. New clinical diagnostic procedures for cystic fibrosis in Europe. J Cyst Fibros. 2011;10(suppl 2):S53–66.

Farrell PM, Rosenstein BJ, White TB, Accurso FJ, Castellani C, Cutting GR, et al. Guidelines for diagnosis of cystic fibrosis in newborns through older adults: Cystic Fibrosis Foundation consensus report. J Pediatr. 2008;153:S4–S14.

Gibson L, Cooke R. A test for concentration of electrolytes in sweat in cystic fibrosis of the pancreas utilizing pilocarpine iontophoresis. Pediatrics. 1959;23: 549–63.

Guía de diagnóstico y tratamiento de fibrosis quística. Actualización 2013.

Kerem B, Rommens J, Buchanan J. Identification of the cystic fibrosis gene: genetic analysis. Science. 1989;245:1073–80.

Knowles M, Stutts J. Spock y cols. Abnormal ion permeation through cystic fibrosis respiratory epithelium. Science. 1983;221:1067–70.

Lay-Son G, Puga A, Astudillo P, Repetto GM, Collaborative Group of the Chilean National Cystic Fibrosis Program. Cystic fibrosis in Chilean patients: analysis of 36 common CFTR gene mutations. J Cyst Fibros. 2011;10(1):66–70.

Massie RJ, Curnow L, Glazner J, Armstrong DS, Francis I. Lessons learned from 20 years of newborn screening for cystic fibrosis. Med J Aust. 2012;196(1):67–70.

Quinton P. Missing Cl conductance in cystic fibrosis. Am J Physiol. 1986;251:C649–52.

Rowntree RK, Harris A. The phenotypic consequences of CFTR mutations. Ann Hum Genet. 2003;67: 471–85.

Sontag MK, Wright D, Beebe J, Accurso FJ, Sagel SD. A new cystic fibrosis newborn screening algorithm: IRT/ IRT1 upward arrow/DNA. J Pediatr. 2009;155(5):618–22.

The Cystic Fibrosis Genetic Analysis Consortium (CFGAC). Disponible en http://www.genet.sickkids.on.ca/cftr.

The National Committee for Clinical Laboratory Standards. Sweat testing: sample collection and quantitative analysis; approved guideline.

Cystic Fibrosis: Treatment

45

Felix Ratjen and María Ester Pizarro Gamboa

Contents

General Considerations

Cystic fibrosis (CF) treatment requires a health team that includes patients and parents as active members. Thus, once the diagnosis has been established, the parents and the patient (if the patient can cooperate) must be educated by the multidisciplinary team.

F. Ratjen (✉)
The Hospital for Sick Children, University of Toronto, Toronto, ON, Canada
e-mail: felix.ratjen@sickkids.ca

M. E. Pizarro Gamboa
Pediatrics, Respiratory Diseases, Associate Asociado, School of Medicine, Pontificia Universidad Católica de Chile, Santiago, Chile
e-mail: mepizarr@med.puc.cl

The follow-up of the patients must be carried out regularly in a center specialized in CF, which needs to have adequate resources to ensure high-quality attention. There must be a multidisciplinary team of health professionals who are trained and experienced in CF. This administrative aspect has been an important factor in realizing better clinical results.

All patients with CF must routinely receive immunizations according to the regular agenda, besides vaccines for hepatitis A and B, influenza, and anti-pneumococcal vaccination.

Nutritional support is crucial for all patients. It is important to intervene early to normalize the nutritional state, especially during the first year of life. Each clinical visit must record weight, size, and cranial circumference (in infants), using

P. Bertrand, I. Sánchez (eds.), *Pediatric Respiratory Diseases*,
https://doi.org/10.1007/978-3-030-26961-6_45

adequate curves, and register the body mass index (BMI), for infants, schoolchildren, and adolescents.

Exocrine pancreatic function must be established when the diagnosis is made through clinical evaluation and stool elastase measurement. Those patients with normal pancreatic function must be reassessed when it is clinically indicated.

The standard follow-up for clinical visits recommends to regularly evaluate lung function using spirometry starting at 5–6 years of life, as it gives guidance for treatment decisions.

In many centers an annual chest X-ray is taken, although its clinical usefulness has not been well established. Chest computerized tomography is more sensitive for detecting early changes in lung disease, but it is currently reserved for specific indications in most CF centers.

Microbiological vigilance is crucial in clinical attention, which is controlled by a sputum sample or pharynx swab on each ambulatory visit and on each pulmonary exacerbation. It is recommended to have a microbiological laboratory with the capability to isolate specific agents of CF using selective media. Currently there is no evidence supporting the routine use of bronchoalveolar lavage (BAL) for the diagnosis and treatment of lung infection in children with CF, but its use is recommended in those patients who do not respond to antibiotic therapy.

It is important to avoid cross-infections among patients in CF centers, and so contact precautions are recommended, besides standard precautions for all the patients with cystic fibrosis, because cross-infection outbreaks of *Burkholderia cepacia* complex, as well as epidemic strains of *Pseudomonas aeruginosa* and *Mycobacterium abscessus*, have been described. This precaution is also valid for the ambulatory setting and for hospitalized patients infected by the *Burkholderia cepacia* complex. Generally, the contact between patients with cystic fibrosis must be limited to avoid the transmission of potential pathogen agents, whether it is through droplets, indirect or direct contact, or even for those patients who have a negative culture for pathogenic agents that are typical of this disease, or when no cultures are available.

As part of the follow-up, it is important to rule out related complications, such as allergic bronchopulmonary aspergillosis through IgE and diabetes by annual checks, using an oral glucose tolerance test, starting from 10 years of age.

The transition to adult care must use a close management plan, and a network for the patient's attention must be available, because only some CF centers will have all the services available (for example, lung transplant).

Minimum Standard of a Cystic Fibrosis Center

A center specialized in the care of patients with cystic fibrosis must have adequate infrastructure and resources to receive patients for ambulatory care and for hospitalization. Also, the patient must have access to the center 24 h/day. A specialized CF center must have at least 50 patients with cystic fibrosis, including adults and children, but the universal recommendation is to have at least 100 patients.

The multidisciplinary team must include the following professionals:

- Pulmonologist/pediatrician: As the professional must keep pace with the current new information, it is recommended that this professional devotes at least 50% of his time to CF patients.
- Infectious disease/pediatrician: This professional should have specific knowledge of CF, besides having a close working relationship with the microbiological laboratory, participating in the diagnostic and treatment of infections as well as the development of their prevention measures.
- Specialized nurse: This nurse should have the necessary knowledge to educate and support patients in the different stages of the disease, such as diagnosis procedures, hospitalizations, use of IV antibiotic treatment in the domicile, diagnosis of comorbidities, transition to the adult attention scheme, gynecological problems

related to pregnancy, transplants, and palliative care. The nurse must be in direct contact with the patients and parents.

- Respiratory physiotherapist: Must lead the attention of the patient in relation to respiratory physiotherapy, exercise, and inhalation therapy. This professional must be capable of taking care of the follow-up of the patients through lung function tests and have experience in the management of patients with non-invasive ventilation and lung rehabilitation.
- Nutritionist: Must lead the optimization of the nutritional state of the patient, including educating them in this area.
- Psychologist/psychiatrist: Must provide support for the patients and their families, ensuring that they have an adequate emotional support network.
- Social assistant: Must have specific knowledge about the disease and the different health systems, besides knowing about the government programs and funding systems, to deliver the best economic support for the families.
- Pharmacist: In charge of maximizing the effect of different treatments, assessing treatment adherence and administration of the medications; besides minimizing the risks of adverse effects related to the therapy and monitoring adverse effects. Finally, the pharmacist is in charge of optimizing the resources spent in the treatment for this group of patients.
- Geneticist: Collaborates in the genetic diagnosis of the disease, advising the family and the patient about reproductive issues. Also, the professional creates a database of the mutations found in the patients.
- Administrative staff and coordinator of a database: Collect complete and organized information to have a better understanding of the progression of the disease, along with evaluating the results of each center, at national and international levels.

Besides this, when needed, the center must have access to other specialists, such as gastroenterology/hepatology (with experience in endoscopy procedure and esophageal varices ligation), diabetes expert, endocrinology, ENT, and interventional radiology (with experience in emergency bronchial artery embolization).

The staff caring for hospitalized patients must have experience in the management of the disease, allowing for a space for the parents to accompany the patients during hospitalization, as well as educational support. Also, there must be resources and available personnel for the administration of IV antibiotic treatments in their home.

A microbiological laboratory must be available. This facility must be capable of adequately processing sputum samples, and performing live blood analysis and pharyngeal culture, as well as correctly identifying *Burkholderia* spp. and *Pseudomonas aeruginosa*, as well as infections caused by fungus and mycobacteria.

Centers who attend pediatric patients must focus in preventing the progression of the disease, and communication and teamwork with the adult centers is very important, even before the transition is made.

Communication between different centers, at both national and international levels, is crucial. In this way, together we can improve the knowledge of this condition.

Nutritional Support and Enzyme Supplements

Nutritional support is based on a high-calorie and high-protein diet, with a supply of pancreatic enzymes, vitamins, and minerals. To maintain a good nutritional state, it is important to control other aspects of the disease, as happens when facing respiratory infections, diabetes, etc.

Good nutritional state positively influences both life quality and patient survival. The recommendation is to administer a diet with 120–140% of the daily calories recommended, not restricting fats or other ingredients, as well as rich in calories and salt. Caloric requirements fluctuate among patients, and calorimetry may help to clarify individual intake needs.

When weight gain and growth are insufficient, it is recommended to increase the nutritional support (±20% on average), and if the nutritional compromise persists, then the support must be more aggressive; a nasogastric tube may be recommended, or a gastrostomy for continuous night enteral feeding if the weight/stature relationship is below the 90% ideal, or if there is a clear reduction in the growth curve.

The use of pancreatic enzymes in patients with pancreatic insufficiency is considered standard care. The common preparations are made from pig pancreatic enzymes, which are coated microspheres resistant to gastric pH, and they are dissolved in the duodenum. Nevertheless, ingesting high concentrations of pancreatic enzymes is a risk factor for the development of fibrosing colonopathy, and therefore it is not recommended to exceed the dose of 10,000 units of lipase/kg/day. Patients who are not well controlled with sufficient enzyme doses must be evaluated for other malabsorption causes and the benefit of adding gastric acid inhibitors in the therapeutic regime verified.

Replacement therapy of pancreatic enzymes must be tailored and adapted to each meal. Depending on how long each meal will last, the enzymes are administered at the beginning of the meal, or they are divided in one half or two thirds at the beginning of the meal, and the other half or third at the end of the meal. Capsules must not be chewed, as the enzymes would be released in the oral cavity, where they may harm the mucosa. If it is necessary to open the capsules, they can be administered with juice, water, or apple puree, avoiding alkaline liquids.

Supplementing with taurine and ursodeoxycholic acid to prevent the progression of hepatic anomalies in patients with CF is controversial, because although these often improve liver function, it is not clear there is positive impact in the progression of the disease.

Patients with CF tend to lose significant salt quantities in their sweat, specially infants in warm weather, and so they should receive salt supplements. Because of pancreatic insufficiency and fat malabsorption, liposoluble vitamins (ADEK) intake is reduced, and supplements are considered standard care in all patients with pancreatic insufficiency. The role of other supplements, such as antioxidant and omega-3 fatty acids, is still very unclear.

Treatment of Lung Disease

It is possible to classify the different therapies and their correlation with the physiopathology of lung disease in the following way (Fig. 45.1).

Gene Therapy and Pharmacotherapy

Gene therapy involves the insertion of a DNA copy that codifies a normal cystic fibrosis transmembrane conductance regulator (CFTR) protein within the defective respiratory cells, using different vectors. Adenovirus have been shown to be efficient vectors in single-dose studies, but it has also been shown that they induce an inflammation in the host when higher doses are used, which limits their clinical application. At the same time, viral vectors induce an immune response that limits the efficiency of repeated doses. Other vectors such as cationic liposomes have shown to be safer, but less efficient, achieving thus a partial correction of the defective CFTR, without improving all the aspects of the disease related to CFTR, such as sodium hyperreabsorption. Although some transient effects on CFTR expression and function have been achieved, no study has been able to show a long-term effect. Even though studies of gene replacement are currently being performed, the main focus of the treatment of CF nowadays is directed to pharmacotherapy.

The objective of pharmacotherapy is to improve CFTR traffic, expression, or function. For patients who have class I mutations, the treatment with ataluren, a compound that promotes early reading through truncated codons in the CFTR mRNA, has proven to increase CFTR expression. Nevertheless, phase 3 clinical trials have shown benefits in only a subgroup of patients.

For patients with G551D mutation (class III), Ivacaftor was approved by the FDA in 2012 to be used in children over 6 years old. Ivacaftor is a

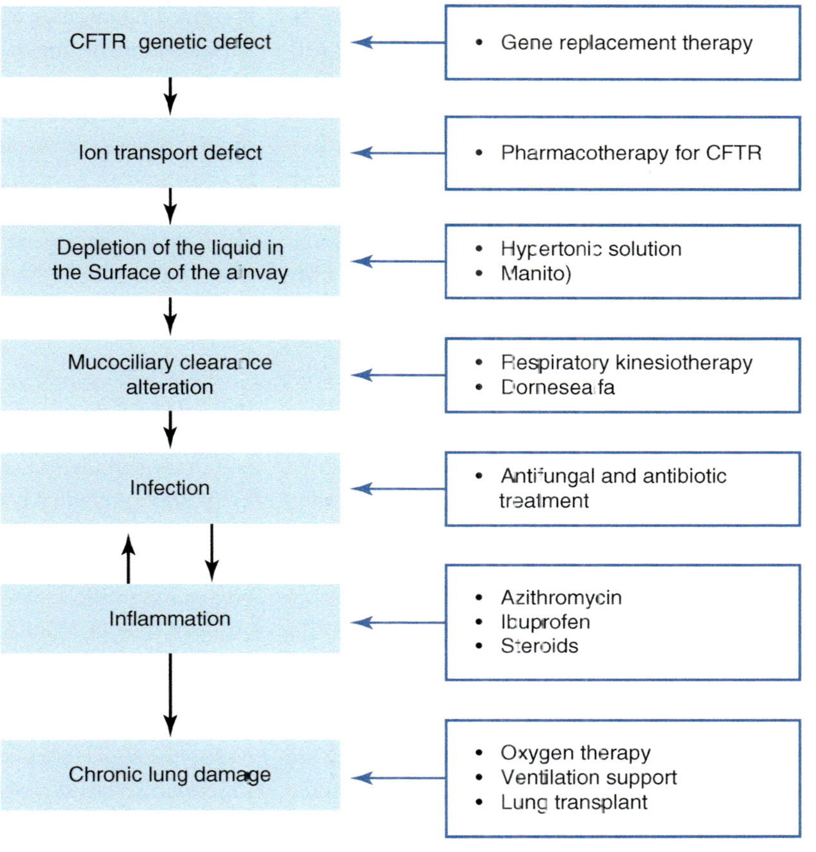

Fig. 45.1 Treatment for cystic fibrosis

function potentiator, which activates the defective CFTR in the cellular surface. In clinical studies, patients who carried at least one copy of the G551D mutations received ivacaftor orally; lung function improved, lung exacerbations were reduced, and weight gain and improvement of respiratory symptoms were associated. It was also observed that it significantly reduced sweat chloride concentrations in treated patients, which reflects the impact of the medication in the basic defect of CF. No important safety issues have been reported in treated patients, but long-term experience is still limited. Some recent studies have shown a similar efficacy in patients with other class III mutations. Their use is recommended for the patients who are carriers of at least one copy of the G551D gene.

For patients with the F507 mutation, lumicaftor, a CFTR "corrector," has been designed to move the CFTR defective protein to the correct place in the airway cell membrane, as well as improving the function as a chloride channel. It has been shown that this provides a limited benefit in the patients with CF, but preliminary studies in association with ivacaftor have shown an improvement in lung function. Currently, two phase 3 clinical trials are ongoing.

Elimination of Airway Secretions

Respiratory Physiotherapy: Physical Exercise

Aerobic exercise is recommended for patients with CF as an adjuvant treatment to clear the airway and improve general health. Physical training is designed to increase physical performance, cardiovascular function, and muscle strength; thus lung function is preserved, by reestablishing sputum elimination and reducing residual volume.

Good adherence to physical training contributes to relief dyspnea, improves exercise tolerance, and is related to a lower reduction of the forced expiratory volume during 1 s (FEV_1). It also stimulates the appetite and contributes to a more positive body image. Besides this, exercise may delay the appearance of osteoporosis by preventing reduction in bone mineral density. Other benefits of physical training are reduction of anxiety and depression, increased feelings of well-being as well as improved performance at work, besides improving recreational activities. It is not clear how much training is required to achieve these benefits, or what combination of aerobic and anaerobic exercise is necessary.

Respiratory physiotherapy is recommended for all patients with CF to improve secretion clearance in the airway, as well as for maintaining lung function. Many techniques have shown benefits in the short term, but the efficacy of long-term information is still very limited. Current practice starts with respiratory physiotherapy soon after the diagnosis.

Different techniques are available (Table 45.1). Some of them can be self-administered by the patient, whereas others require the help of a trained therapist, or a caregiver. The preferred techniques are those that can be self-administered by the patients when they are old enough to do so. There is still no solid evidence to prove that a certain technique is superior to others, but a recent study showed that the positive expiratory pressure (PEP) mask was better than the high-frequency chest wall oscillation (HFCWO) vest regarding pulmonary exacerbations. Respiratory physiotherapy should be tailored according to age and the preference of the patient.

Dornase Alfa

Inflammation in the airway attracts neutrophils, and their degradation increases the DNA content in the sputum, which contributes to an increase in the viscosity of bronchial secretions. It has been proven that administering nebulized dornase alfa breaks down the DNA and reduces sputum viscosity. Clinical studies with dornase alfa have shown an improvement in lung function in patients with moderate and serious disease, besides reducing lung exacerbations. In children within the 6–10 years old range with normal lung function, it was also shown that the rate of lung exacerbations was reduced. An improvement in lung function was also observed.

Table 45.1 Respiratory physiotherapy techniques (RKT)

Conventional RKT	Postural drainage, percussions, huffing, and cough
Active cycle of breathing technique (ACBT)	Self-administered technique that combines respiration control with chest expansion and the technique of forced exhalation.
Positive expiratory pressure (PEP) mask	Breathing with a positive expiratory pressure of 10–25 cm of water. This technique can be self-administered, but it requires a device.
High PEP (HPEP) mask	Complete forced expiration against a fixed mechanical resistance, with pressures from 40 to 100 cm of water This technique can be self-administered, but it requires a device.
Oscillating devices	Includes flutter, cornet, acapella, and intrapulmonary percussive ventilation. This technique can be self-administered, but it requires a device.
Autogenic drainage (AD)	Self-administered respiration technique that uses expiratory optimal flow rates in different pulmonary volumes to move mucus and avoid blockage of the airway.
High-frequency chest compression devices	VestTM and the Hayek oscillator provide external compression of the chest wall. This technique can be self-administered, but it requires a device.
Resistive inspiratory maneuver (RIM)	Includes inhalation and exhalation against a resistance after forced exhalation, as well as repeated inhalations in 80% of the maximum inhalation pressure sustained. This technique can be self-administered, but it requires a device.
Physical training	Aerobic training involves continuous exercise period at an objective intensity (bike or running) Anaerobic training involves exercise of high intensity during a short period (weights or resistance training or speed races)

Long-term therapy has shown decreased inflammation of the respiratory airway, as well as a reduction in the loss of lung function in time. Currently there is solid evidence to recommend it for patients that need to improve lung function or reduce lung exacerbations. The adverse effects include voice alterations, pharyngitis, and facial edema, which are transient in spite of maintenance of the treatment.

Hypertonic Saline Solution and Manitol

Nebulized hypertonic saline (HS) solution acts as an osmotic agent and increases salt concentration in the luminal side of the respiratory epithelium, which attracts water, thus increasing the fluid in the surface of the airway, and hydrates the mucus, which improves mucociliary depuration. Manitol, a sugar prepared as a dry powder formulation, has a similar action mechanism.

For patients who are 6 years and older, nebulized hypertonic saline solution at a 7% concentration, used twice per day, has shown modest improvements in FEV_1, along with a reduction in the rates of lung exacerbations. Studies in children under 6 years old have failed to reduce the exacerbation rate, but a pilot study showed a reduction in the index of lung clearance in this group. Studies have shown that nebulized hypertonic saline solution is well tolerated and safe, even in infants and small children, with adverse effects in less than 10% of the patients. These adverse effects include bronchospasm, salty taste, nauseas, dyspnea, and chest pain. A pretreatment with bronchodilator is required to reduce the risk of bronchospasm. It is currently recommended to reduce exacerbations and improve lung function, with a level of moderate evidence.

Manitol as an inhaled dry powder has been tested in concluded phase 3 studies, and it is available for adults in Europe and Australia, but the FDA has not yet approved its use in the USA. Research has shown improvement in lung function, but hemoptysis rates increased in children, which is currently being studied. One of its advantages when compared to nebulized hypertonic saline solution is that it requires less time for its administration.

Treatment of Infections in the Airway

During the past decades, intensive treatment of respiratory infections has been the main cause of the increase in survival rate for the patients with CF. Respiratory infections in these patients are quite complex, and treatment strategies have been developed for traditional bacteria in CF, such as *Staphylococcus aureus* and *Pseudomonas aeruginosa*, which has led to the appearance of other emerging bacteria, which are treated separately.

Antibiotics therapy may be used with different objectives in CF:

- Treatment of the first bacterial isolation
- Treatment of acute respiratory exacerbations
- Chronic suppressive therapy
- Prophylactic treatment

Treatment of the First Bacterial Isolation

Currently, all guidelines strongly recommend treating the first isolation (eradication) of *Pseudomonas aeruginosa* with nebulized antibiotics (tobramycin or colistin) or in combination with oral antibiotics (ciprofloxacin). When using tobramycin, studies have not shown additional benefits if oral ciprofloxacin is added. There are not similar data available for inhaled colistin.

One of the main problems when managing *Staphylococcus aureus* and other bacteria that colonize the superior airway tract, such as *Haemophilus influenzae*, is that a significant proportion of healthy individuals carry these bacteria in their oropharynx, and therefore a positive culture, specially a pharyngeal swab, does not necessarily indicate an infection of the lower tract airway. In the case of methicillin-sensitive *Staphylococcus aureus* (MSSA), its impact in the long term is not clear, and therefore its eradication is not considered standard care. Some authors recommend treating the first positive culture with oral treatments such as flucloxacillin for 2–4 weeks. In the same way, some authors use amoxicillin/clavulanic acid for 2–4 weeks for the first positive culture of *Haemophilus influenzae*.

Treatment of Acute Respiratory Exacerbations

There is clear evidence showing the importance of early and intensive treatment in acute respiratory exacerbations in patients with CF, recommending a low threshold for the beginning of the treatment and orientating the treatment through the presence of nonspecific symptoms and clinical signs (Table 45.2). The presence of fever and leukocytosis is rare and it is a late sign, so these entities should not be considered to start the treatment. Antibiotic choice and administration procedure are based on the sensitivity of bacteria isolated in the most recent sputum cultures, the functional condition of the patient, and previous clinical history. If there is no information about the bacteria, antibiotic treatment should be aimed to the characteristic pathogens in CF. More serious lung exacerbations tend to be treated with IV antibiotics; oral therapy is used for less severe situations. These patients present with differences in the clearance rate of the antibiotic, and they require doses approximately 50% greater than those used in patients without CF. The antibiotic treatment should last from 14 to 21 days.

Treatment for patients infected by *Pseudomonas aeruginosa* combines two classes of antibiotics, associating an aminoglycoside with a third-generation cephalosporin, or a semisynthetic penicillin, which optimizes clinical efficacy and reduces the development of bacterial resistance. Thus, oral ciprofloxacin is reserved for less serious exacerbations.

Studies comparing the use of aminoglycoside once versus three times per day have not shown significant differences between the groups relative to efficacy. Also, creatinine changes favored the once per day treatment in children.

There is no evidence supporting the idea that inhaled antibiotics are an adequate alternative to IV antibiotics for lung exacerbations. Further, systemic therapy has a more homogeneous antibiotic distribution in poorly ventilated areas, which is an important aspect of serious lung disease. However, when IV therapy is challenging and hospitalization or treatment at home with IV antibiotics cannot be done for social reasons, an oral quinolone (such as ciprofloxacin) and a nebulized antibiotic can be an alternative. If there is an adequate support system, IV therapy at home is safe, reduces social disruption, and may be cost effective. Home IV antibiotic administration must be made according to the individual situation, considering comorbidities, how serious is the exacerbation, and local resources. It is recommended to start IV antibiotic treatment in the hospital.

There is some evidence supporting the use of long IV catheters instead of short IV lines, relative to how long the line can be used and patient satisfaction. Patients with CF and recurrent exacerbations, requiring regular and frequent IV antibiotic treatments, often lose their peripheral vein access, and some of them require a central venous catheter, such as a Port-a-cath system device.

Table 45.2 Symptoms and signs of a lung exacerbation

Symptoms	Physical signs	Laboratory findings
Increase of cough frequency, duration, and intensity	Increase of respiratory effort, intercostal retractions, and use of accessory muscles	10% or more FEV_1 reduction in comparison with the best value in 6 previous months
Sputum appearance or production increase	Increase of respiratory frequency	Increase of air trapping or new infiltration in chest X-ray
Sputum change	Appearance or increase of crackles in chest examination	Leucocytosis
Hemoptysis appearance or increase	Increase of air trapping	Reduction of oxygen saturation (SaO_2)
Appearance or increase of dyspnea, reduction of exercise tolerance	Fever	
Compromise of the general condition, fatigue increase, weakness, lack of appetite	Weight loss	

In the case of infants and preschoolers with frequent viral infections, the clinical progression must be closely monitored, and if the symptoms persist or they are more severe than expected, they should be treated as a bacterial exacerbation and include antibiotic therapy, considering the results of the last cultures.

Chronic Suppression Treatment

The objective is to reduce bacterial load in the lung and in this way reduce toxins produced by these bacteria, reducing inflammation and lung damage. This objective reduces the worsening rate of pulmonary function as well as the frequency of exacerbations. Several inhaled antibiotics have proven to be efficient, achieving high sputum concentrations and minimizing systemic toxicity. The drugs currently most used are tobramycin, aztreonam, and colistin; others are being developed, such as inhaled liposomal amikacin, levofloxacine, vancomycin, and ciprofloxacine.

Therapy has been investigated and focused on patients with chronic infection caused by *Pseudomonas aeruginosa*, which is the most common pathogen agent in the airway of older patients with CF. Mucoid presentation of this disease is related to a faster reduction of lung function and a decreased survival rate. Inhaled therapy is considered standard care for these patients. A Cochrane review showed a better lung function (FEV_1) and fewer exacerbations in the group treated with inhaled antibiotics, and no hearing loss or kidney failure was found. At the moment there is no concluding evidence to support the use of regular IV or oral antibiotic treatments in these patients.

The use of inhaled tobramycin for the treatment of moderate to severe lung disease ($FEV_1 < 70\%$) in children older than 6 years has shown to increase FEV_1, reduce lung exacerbations, and improve the quality of life. In patients with mild disease ($FEV_1 > 70\%$), use has also shown a significant reduction of exacerbations (11% versus 25.6%), a discrete improvement of pulmonary function, a reduction of days using antibiotics (17% versus 48%), and a reduction in antibiotic courses (1.4% versus 2.8%). Since 2013, tobramycin is also available as a dry powder inhaler, which allows a faster and more comfortable administration.

Inhaled aztreonam, when compared to placebo in patients with moderate to severe disease ($FEV_1 < 70\%$), also showed FEV_1 improvement, extended the time until the next exacerbation, reduced hospitalization days, and improved quality of life. Nevertheless, in patients with mild disease ($FEV_1 > 70\%$), only a small improvement for FEV_1 and quality of life was shown.

European and US guidelines recommend using tobramycin and aztreonam in patients with chronic infection caused by *Pseudomonas aeruginosa*. The therapeutic effect is greater in those patients with moderate to severe disease, in comparison to those who have preserved lung function.

A comparative study for inhaled tobramycin and aztreonam confirmed the efficacy for this treatment. Both have been studied during cycles including 28 days of use and 28 days of rest, and therefore many physicians have started to use both treatments in alternate months for patients with severe disease to avoid worsening of the condition during the resting period. More studies are needed to determine the optimum approach to start and continue the increasing inhaled antibiotic spectrum to improve lung function and reducing secondary effects to a minimum.

Prophylactic Treatment

In the United Kingdom, anti-staphylococcal prophylactic antibiotics (flucloxacillin) currently are indicated from the diagnosis to patients up to 3 years old, which has caused a lower isolation rate of *Staphylococcus aureus*. Nevertheless, the clinical importance of this finding is uncertain. The United States Cystic Fibrosis Foundation does not recommend its use, as some studies have shown that it can increase *Pseudomonas aeruginosa* colonization.

Emerging bacteria

- Although methicillin-resistant *Staphylococcus aureus* (MRSA) is an important emerging pathogen in CF, there is no consensus for its management. Children with persistent infection require more IV antibiotic cycles. Adults

show a greater worsening of lung function, along with higher mortality rates. The results of several nonrandomized studies suggest that it is possible to eradicate it, but the clinical impact would be uncertain. Different protocols have been developed to eradicate the first MRSA isolation without establishing a unique regime of treatment. Rifampicin with fusidic acid and inhaled vancomycin have been successfully used. The decision to treat this chronic infection must be made in accordance with the clinical condition of the patient.
- Infection caused by the *Burkholderia cepacia* complex is associated with a worse prognosis. It is inherently resistant to colomycin and is frequently resistant to aminoglycosides and beta-lactamics. Further, a specific efflux pump may cause resistance to quinolones, chloramphenicol, and timethroprim. Multidrug resistance is common in vitro, and 50% of the bacteria are resistant to the ten most common antibiotics used in CF. For patients with chronic infections, trimethoprim/sulfamethoxazole (TMP-SMX) or doxycycline are efficient in treating mild exacerbations, but for more serious infections the treatment is meropenem in association with ceftazidime or chloramphenicol, or TMP-SMX IV, plus high doses of inhaled tobramycin. Eradication is possible in a few cases, and most of the time the infections remain as a chronic condition. Treatment of exacerbations caused by the *Burkholderia cepacia* complex may require prolonged antibiotic therapy (weeks or months) before a clinical response can be obtained.
- *Stenotrophomonas maltophilia* is one of the most common multiresistant organisms infecting patients with CF, and its prevalence is on the rise. It has been isolated in about 8% to 10% of CF patients in North America and about 4% to 30% in Europe. Risk factors for its isolation in the respiratory tract are the use of IV antibiotics and oral quinolones. It has been recently shown that chronic infection caused by *Stenotrophomonas maltophilia* independently predicts acute lung exacerbations associated to hospitalization and use of IV antibiotics. The treatment of an acute pulmonary exacerbation caused by *Stenotrophomonas maltophilia* always includes two antibiotics, oral or IV, according to the sensitivity of the cultures. For the treatment of less serious pulmonary exacerbations, oral TMP-SMX, levofloxacin, and doxycycline can be used.

Nontuberculous mycobacteria (the most common ones are *Mycobacterium avium* and *Mycobacterium abscessus*) are isolated in the respiratory tract in about 5% to 20% of the patients with CF. In some cases, they are commensals and have no significant impact on the respiratory function or the nutritional state, but in other cases they cause lung disease, which quickly reduces lung function and even causes death. Of all the mycobacteria, *Mycobacterium abscessus* is most probably related to important lung disease, as well as being the most difficult to treat. Antibiotic choice depends on the species that has been isolated. Generally, lung disease caused by *Mycobacterium avium* is treated with a combination of a macrolide (clarithromycin or azithromycin) and rifampicin or rifabutin and ethambutol. *Mycobacterium abscessus* is more resistant to antimicrobial agents, so the recommendation is to use a combined therapy of clarithromycin, amikacin, and cefoxitin or imipenem. Antibiotic treatment of lung infections caused by nontuberculous mycobacteria can potentially improve lung function, reduce the frequency of lung exacerbations, and eradicate infections, but there is no information about the efficacy of early antibiotic treatment to eradicate nontuberculous mycobacteria or about antimicrobial chronic suppressive treatment to avoid the worsening of lung function in patients with CF. Recently, inhaled amikacin has shown promising results as a possible maintenance therapy for patients with persistent infection.

Antiinflammatory Treatment

Cystic fibrosis is characterized by an intense neutrophil inflammation, and lung destruction is the result of the vicious cycle of infection and inflammation. This inflammatory process happens early in life, which is documented in a recent study that showed that 4-month-old infants presented with inflammation. Besides this, the studies have demonstrated that the inflammatory response can be detected even in the airway of those patients who present with a clinically mild disease. There is a hypothesis that proposes that prolonged use of antiinflammatory therapy may prevent progressive lung damage and respiratory morbidity. The challenge is to achieve inflammation reduction without fettering the response of the host against chronic infections.

Steroids

Oral steroids in doses of 1–2 mg/kg prednisolone on alternate days seem to slow lung disease progression in patients with CF who also present with chronic infection caused by *Pseudomonas aeruginosa*, but they should not be used because of the high risk of related important adverse effects, such as glucose intolerance, alteration in growth, arterial hypertension, oral candidiasis, and less frequently, cataracts and osteoporosis. Short treatments have been used during acute exacerbations, according to the degree of airway obstruction, but a pilot study showed that this is not related to a better treatment response.

Inhaled steroids (IS) are not related to these adverse effects, but a sustained effect in relationship to the inflammation of the airway and lung function has not been proven. Approximately 40% of patients with CF use IS although there is no evidence supporting their use, and studies with treatment interruption have not shown any change in the clinical parameters for the patients who do not have asthma. It is necessary to confirm bronchial hyperreactivity (BHR) with a FEV_1 increase of at least 12% after the use of a bronchodilator, or a positive methacholine bronchial challenge test, to justify the treatment, which happens in about 25–49% of patients with CF.

Azithromycin

Different mechanisms have been proposed to explain the action of azithromycin in CF, such as the effect of expression and liberation of epithelial cell mediators in the airway, reducing the adhesion and migration of neutrophils, thus accelerating their apoptosis, reducing virulence factors that increase the activity of *Pseudomonas aeruginosa*, such as the production of a mucus biofilm, altering the conversion of nonmucoid strain to mucoid and interrupting the method through which bacteria interact with one another. Modulation of chloride alternative channels has also been described, as well as effects in the production of nitric oxide and the increase of antioxidant activity. At the same time, azithromycin achieves great tissue concentrations, long half-life, and can be used three times a week, which is attractive for patients with CF.

Patient with chronic infection caused by *Pseudomonas aeruginosa* and treated with azithromycin for 6 months showed a consistent improvement in their FEV_1 indexes, and they were twice as likely to be free from lung exacerbation, besides showing a significant reduction in the use of oral antibiotics, with a greater increase in their weight.

According to several studies, when treatment is provided, pediatric patients not infected by *Pseudomonas aeruginosa* did not show an improvement in lung function, but basal lung function was normal for most of these patients, and similarly, in patients infected with *Pseudomonas aeruginosa*, a reduction of more than 50% was observed in lung exacerbations, as well as a reduction in the inflammation markers.

Adverse events were uncommon, and the treatment was associated with a reduction of *Staphylococcus aureus* in the cultures, along with a significant increase of macrolides resistance.

The American Cystic Fibrosis Foundation recommends the chronic use of azithromycin for all patients older than 6 years, for those who have *Pseudomonas aeruginosa* as well as for those who do not have *Pseudomonas aeruginosa*, to reduce exacerbations.

Ibuprofen

High doses of ibuprofen would reduce the influx of neutrophils to the airway, probably through a mechanism mediated by LTB4. However, animal studies suggest that low serum levels of ibuprofen would increase neutrophil migration. Because of this, it is key to maintain an ibuprofen concentration between 50 and 100 mg/ml, for which serum level control is needed. In a study in only one center, which considered children under 12 years old, high ibuprofen doses significantly reduced the annual reduction rate of the pulmonary flow according to FEV_1, with forced vital capacity (FVC) and forced expiratory flow between 25% and 75% (FEF 25–75%). It was also related to a reduction in the use of IV antibiotics, improvement in chest X-rays, as well as nutritional condition. No adverse effects were reported, but the power of the study was too low to identify them, and significant gastric hemorrhage appeared in selected cases. A multi-centric study did not show improvement on FEV_1, but a tendency to improvement was observed in FVC. A further analysis of the study suggests that the treatment could positively affect the worsening of the lung function. Although some guides have recommended this treatment, its use is still uncommon.

Other Therapies

Bronchodilators

Approximately 25–40% of patients with CF have bronchial hyperreactivity, which is defined by a positive bronchodilator response. This phenotype is not constant in time, and therefore it is important to evaluate the patients in regular intervals. β_2-agonists have a direct effect in smooth muscle relaxation and increase the frequency of ciliary beat, but their effect in the reduction of the fluid in the airways may reduce its potential benefit in the patients with CF.

When compared to placebo, short-acting β_2-agonists increase FEV_1 in the short term and PEF in the long term for patients who present with bronchial hyperreactivity or respond to bronchodilators. For short-term results, when compared to placebo, long-acting β_2-agonists increase FEV_1 and (FEF 25–75) in patients who have a positive response to the bronchodilator, but they yield inconsistent results in long-term trials. A short-acting anticholinergic had no additional consistent effect in the lung function tests, whether for the long term or the short term.

Bronchodilators are widely indicated in CF for different reasons, including relief of symptoms caused by asthma, as a complement of respiratory physiotherapy to improve sputum elimination, and before using nebulized therapies (for example, tobramycin), to prevent symptoms such as bronchoconstriction, as well as allowing a better deposit of the drug. Their use is recommended before exercise and respiratory therapy.

Oxygen and Ventilation Support

Oxygen is used in patients with CF and advanced lung disease along chronic hypoxemia (Fig. 45.2) to relieve the symptoms of dyspnea and fatigue and to retard the appearance of *cor pulmonale*. If oxygen saturation is low during a lung exacerbation, it is important to reevaluate the condition during a stable period, using pulse oximetry at night, and if the saturation is still low (saturation <90%, >3% of the time), then night oxygen in the domicile should be considered. In these cases, the morning CO_2 must be controlled, as it can increase with oxygen therapy.

Some recent studies have shown that noninvasive mechanical ventilation (NIMV) reduces

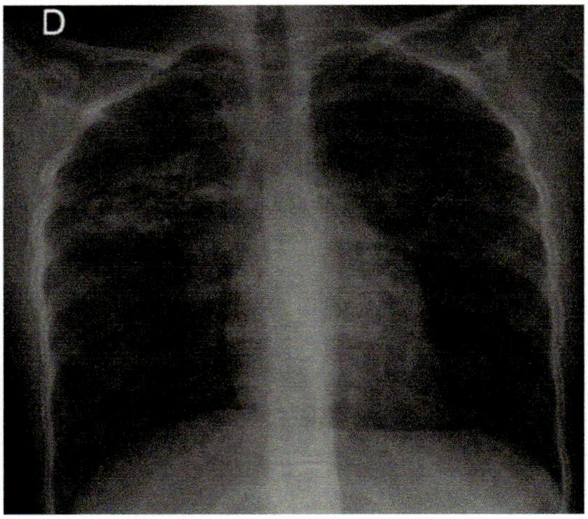

Fig. 45.2 Severe lung disease. Chest X-ray of 14-year-old girl with CF presenting with dyspnea and chronic hypoxemia. Air trapping can be observed along linear and cyst images. Bilateral bronchiectasis, condensation, and bullae at the apex of the right lung

muscular fatigue and increases muscle performance, alveolar ventilation, and gas exchange. NIMV has been used in CF as a treatment for hypercapnic respiratory failure, in night hypoventilation, or as a bridge to lung transplant. It can also be used as a complement to respiratory physiotherapy and to ease exercise. Preferably it should be used during sleep, because hypoventilation tends to occur during REM sleep. Some patients experience a significant improvement in their quality of life, although the long-term effect in relation to survival or sleep quality has not been thoroughly studied yet.

Lung Transplant

When therapy aimed at improving or maintaining pulmonary function fail, double-lung transplant becomes an option. Depending on the center and the waiting times for the transplant, the indications include short life expectancy (between 6 and 24 months), FEV_1 < 30%, relative to the baseline condition, PaO_2 <55 mmHg, or $PaCO_2$ >50 mmHg, and lung hypertension Contraindications will vary according to the centers: Some centers do not admit patients who are carriers of the *Burkholderia cepacia* complex, whereas other centers have confirmed a survival rate benefit, even for this high-risk population.

During 2010, the International Society for Heart and Lung Transplantation (ISHLT) reported that 26% of all lung transplant patients had CF. According to the information of the United Network for Organ Sharing (UNOS), among the pediatric transplants done during the period 2008–2009, graft failure rate was 3.4% at 6 months, 13.6% after a year, and 19.8% at 3 years. For lung transplants performed during the 2006–2007 period, graft failure at 5 years was 51.4%, and for lung transplants done in the 2000–2001 period, graft failure at 10 years was 68.6%.

It is important to recognize that even though lung transplant improves the quality of life for most patients, complication rates are high, and although the results have improved, they are still below the success rate of other transplants. ISHLT reported the survival rate in all the receptors of bilateral lung transplant from January 1994 until June 2012, the median of which was 7.5 years in the patients with CF. Graft rejection causes 56% of deaths within the first 60 days, infections cause 40% of deaths during the first year after the transplant, and finally, obliterative bronchiolitis causes 67% of late deaths.

Treatment of Complications

Allergic Bronchopulmonary Aspergillosis (ABPA)

ABPA is a type TH_2 hypersensitivity response to *Aspergillus fumigatus* that appears in 7–9% of the patients with CF. ABPA is characterized by acute or subacute clinical worsening that cannot be explained by other causes, along with serum IgE concentrations greater than 1000 IU/ml, positive skin prick test, specific antibodies for *Aspergillus fumigatus*, positive precipitins or IgG for *Aspergillus fumigatus*, and alterations in the chest X-rays or CAT scan with no response to regular therapy.

The treatment is aimed to control the acute episode and avoid chronic worsening. Steroids therapy quickly reduces eosinophilic infiltrates and the associated symptoms. The drug of choice is prednisone, starting with 2 mg/kg/day for 1 week, followed by 1 mg/kg/day for another week. After this, the dose is gradually reduced until reaching a dose of 0.5 mg/kg/ in alternate days, which is maintained for 3 months. In this period the patient must be closely monitored, checking the symptomatology, performing clinical examinations, IgE levels, and chest X-rays; and if there is a relapse, the prednisone dose should be increased again.

Antifungal treatments, such as itraconazole, should be considered as adjunct treatment for the steroids therapy, helping reduce their dose.

Omalizumab use may be considered as an adjunct, but there are not enough controlled and randomized studies to ensure its security and efficacy.

Sources

Borowitz D, Robinson KA, Rosenfeld M, Davis SD, Sabadosa KA, Spear SL, Michel SH, Parad RB, White TB, Farrell PM, Marshall BC, Accurso FJ. Cystic Fibrosis Foundation evidence-based guidelines for management of infants with cystic fibrosis. J Pediatr. 2009;155:S73–93.

Conway S, Balfour-Lynn IM, De Rijcke K, Drevinek P, Foweraker J, Havermans T, et al. European Cystic Fibrosis Society Standards of Care: framework for the Cystic Fibrosis Centre. J Cyst Fibros. 2014;13(suppl 1):S3–S22.

Döring G, Flume P, Heijerman H, Elborn JS. Treatment of lung infection in patients with cystic fibrosis: current and future strategies. J Cyst Fibros. 2012;11:461–79.

Flume PA, Mogayzel PJ Jr, Robinson KA, Goss CH, Rosenblatt RL, Kuhn RJ, Marshall BC. Cystic fibrosis pulmonary guidelines. Treatment of pulmonary exacerbations. Am J Respir Crit Care Med. 2009;180:802–8.

Flume PA, Robinson KA, O'Sullivan BP, Finder JD, Vender RL, Willey-Courand DB, White TB, Marshall BC. Cystic fibrosis pulmonary guidelines: airway clearance therapies. Respir Care. 2009;54(4):522–37.

Heijerman H, Westerman E, Conway S, Döring DT. Inhaled medication and inhalation devices for lung disease in patients with cystic fibrosis: a European consensus. J Cyst Fibros. 2009;8:295–315.

Kerem E, Conway S, Elborn S, Heijerman H. Standards of care for patients with cystic fibrosis: a European consensus. J Cyst Fibros. 2005;4:7–26.

Mogayzel PJ Jr, Naureckas ET, Robinson KA, Mueller G, Hadjiliadis D, Hoag JB, Lubsch L, Hazle L, Sabadosa K, Marshall B. Cystic fibrosis pulmonary guidelines, chronic medications for maintenance of lung health. Am J Respir Crit Care Med. 2013;187(7):680–9.

O'Sullivan BP, Freedman SD. Cystic fibrosis. Lancet. 2009;373:1891–904.

Sinaasappel M, Stern M, Littlewood J, Wolfe S, Steinkamp G, Heijerman HG, Robberecht E, Doring G. Nutrition in patients with cystic fibrosis: a European Consensus. J Cyst Fibros. 2002;1:51–75.

Smyth AR, Bell SC, Bojcin S, Bryon M, Duff A, Flume P, et al. European Cystic Fibrosis Society Standards of Care: best practice guidelines. J Cyst Fibros. 2014;13(suppl 1):S23–42.

Stern M, Bertrand DP, Bignamini E, Corey M, Dembski B, Goss CH, et al. European Cystic Fibrosis Society Standards of Care: quality management in cystic fibrosis. J Cyst Fibros. 2014;13(suppl 1): S43–59.

Pulmonary Aspergillosis

46

Claudio Castaños, Verónica Aguerre,
and Verónica Giubergia

Contents

Epidemiology

Clinical presentations are determined by the susceptibility of the host. Immunocompromised patients may present with saprophytic or invasive aspergillosis. Immunocompetent patients tend to present with hypersensitivity, and sometimes saprophytic disease. Although these entities are well defined, some patients present with characteristics of more than one disease, and the disease could progress from one presentation to another.

C. Castaños (✉) · V. Aguerre · V. Giubergia
Hospital Garrahan, Buenos Aires, Argentina
e-mail: ccastanos@garrahan.gov.ar;
vaguerre@garrahan.gov.ar;
vgiubergia@garrahan.gov.ar

Etiology and Physiopathology

Although more than 200 species of *Aspergillus* have been identified, the most common pathogen associated with respiratory disease is *Aspergillus fumigatus* (AF). *Aspergillus niger*, *A. terreus*, *A. nidulans*, and *A. flavus* have also been related to pulmonary disease, but to a much lesser extent.

In most cases, *Aspergillus* enters the respiratory system after the inhalation of spores as an opportunistic mycosis. The integrity of the host defense mechanisms is important to prevent the disease. In the lungs, alveolar macrophages are the first line of defense against the conidia. Toll receptors, dectin-1 and mannose, bind to lectin, and participate in fungus identification and in the recruiting of neutrophils that set the immune response in motion.

P. Bertrand, I. Sánchez (eds.), *Pediatric Respiratory Diseases*,
https://doi.org/10.1007/978-3-030-26961-6_46

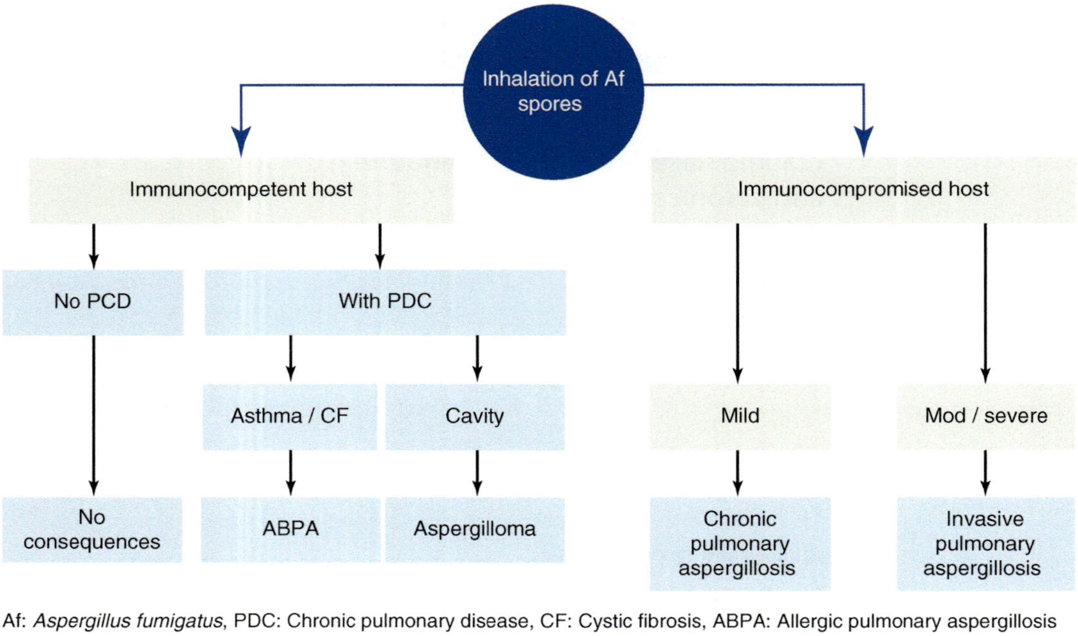

Fig. 46.1 Clinical presentations of pulmonary aspergillosis. *AF Aspergillus fumigatus*, *PDC* chronic pulmonary disease, *CF* cystic fibrosis, *ABPA* allergic pulmonary aspergillosis

Clinical presentations include invasive pulmonary aspergillosis, chronic pulmonary aspergillosis, and allergic pulmonary aspergillosis (Fig. 46.1).

Invasive Pulmonary Aspergillosis

The greatest risk factors for invasive pulmonary aspergillosis (IPA) in the pediatric population are the presence of neutropenia, chronic steroids therapy, immunosuppression therapy, neoplastic disease, and acquired immunodeficiency. Use of chemotherapy and immunosuppressive agents has increased the rate of aspergillosis during the past decades. In a study examining the autopsies of immunocompromised patients between 1978 and 1992, the rate for invasive aspergillosis varied between 0.4% and 3%, with a rate increase between 17% and 60% in the autopsies performed during the past years. The mortality rate exceeds 50% for neutropenic patients, and it may reach 90% in receptors of bone marrow transplant.

Aspergillus enters the lower respiratory tract through spore inhalation, and less frequently, the infection can initiate in other locations, such as the paranasal sinus, digestive tract, or the skin. The most frequent presentation forms of IPA include pulmonary and upper airway disease, both with a high mortality. Clinically, its presentation is nonspecific: febrile syndrome, productive cough, and dyspnea. Pleura pain may be present, as well as hemoptysis, associated with vascular microthrombosis and small areas of pulmonary infarction. IPA is one of the most common causes of hemoptysis in neutropenic patients, and it may be associated with cavity appearance during neutrophil recovery. From the radiological aspect, early findings are also nonspecific, with rounded opacities tending to appear, besides pleural base infiltrations that may suggest lung necrosis and cavitated lesions.

Hematogenic dissemination to other organs is possible, fundamentally to the central nervous system, developing meningitis, epidural abscess, brain stroke, etc.

A significantly lower percentage of patients have presented tracheobronchitis caused by *Aspergillus*, which is the isolated invasion of the tracheobronchial tract. Three presentations have been described for this disease: obstructive, pseudomembranous, and ulcerative.

The diagnosis of IPA is based on the presence of risk factors, signs, symptomatology, chest X-ray findings, histopathological findings, and the development of *Aspergillus* in the culture.

Its diagnosis is difficult in immunocompromised patients. It is necessary to keep a high suspicion index when working with higher-risk groups. Definitive diagnosis is based on the histopathological identification of hyphae invading the lung tissue, along with a positive culture for *Aspergillus* in the same site. Histopathological findings and the type of local antiinflammatory reaction will depend on the immunological condition of the host.

The steps to follow after *Aspergillus* has been isolated in the sputum will depend on the condition of the host. Generally, immunocompetent patients will present a colonization with no clinical consequences, and thus antifungal therapy would not be indicated, but IPA should be ruled out. In contrast, when *Aspergillus* has been isolated in immunocompromised patients, it has a high positive predictive value for this infection. Nevertheless, negative sputa do not rule out IPA.

Early chest computed tomography (CT) helps to have a prompt *Aspergillosis* diagnosis, although no pathognomonic signs may be present. Multiples nodules, early presence of the halo sign (area of attenuation secondary to hemorrhage surrounding the nodule) and late presence of the half-moon sign (hyperlucid area secondary to necrosis in the original nodule region) are characteristic and suggest the diagnosis (Fig. 46.2).

Bronchoalveolar lavage (BAL) may be useful, although *Aspergillus* recovery percentages in the fluid obtained are very variable. It can be used to search for anti-*Aspergillus* antibodies and rule out other infections.

Recently, *Aspergillus* antigen detection techniques have been used, such as galactomannan in body fluids. This antigen can be present days before the appearance of symptoms, signs, and radiological alterations. Its main limitations are its low positive predictive power and the possibility of false positives and false negatives.

IPA is associated with high mortality rates. The treatment considers amphotericin B as first line drug, which is associated to nephrotoxicity, hydroelectric alterations, and hypersensitivity. New liposomal presentations of this drugs have less secondary effects, with usually adequate antifungal action. Voriconazole has been approved as first line drug for the treatment of IPA, and is associated to less adverse effects, thus it is more tolerable. Generally, treatments must be indicated for prolonged periods, up to a year. Caspofungin, micafungin, and anidulafungin are therapeutic options for patients with refractory

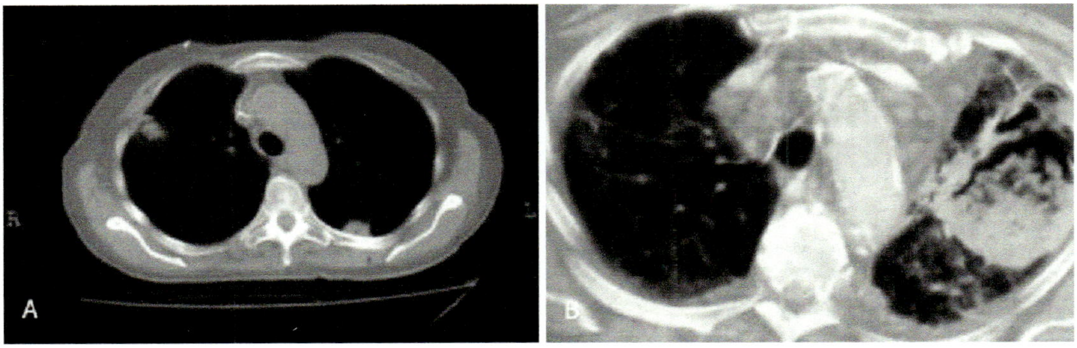

Fig. 46.2 Invasive pulmonary aspergillosis. Chest computed axial tomography of an immunosuppressed teenager presenting with nodular subpleural lesions and halo sign (**a**) and half-moon sign with condensation (**b**)

IPA when the usual treatment has been used, or if the patient cannot tolerate it.

Surgical resection should be considered in the cases of massive hemoptysis, lung lesions close to vital structures (great vessels, pericardium) or residual lesions in patients who are still immunosuppressed.

Chronic Necrotizing Pulmonary Aspergillosis

Chronic necrotizing pulmonary aspergillosis is very infrequent, and there are only isolated cases or case reports for this type of presentation of the disease.

It has been mostly described in adults with alterations of local defense mechanisms associated with chronic pulmonary disease (chronic obstructive pulmonary disease, sarcoidoisis, tuberculosis or radiotherapy history) or with systemic diseases that cause mild degrees of immunosuppression (malnutrition, connective tissue diseases, chronic liver disease, alcoholism, liver failure, etc).

Clinically, it can have a certain degree of overlapping with aspergilloma, and it is characterized by the presence of general symptoms (fever, fatigue, weight loss), productive cough, and hemoptysis. Image studies evidence consolidation, pleural enlargement, and cavitary lesions, which progress slowly. Sputum cultures tend to be positive for *Aspergillus*. The confirmation of the diagnosis is done through the histopathological findings of hifa in lung tissue and positive culture for the fungus. The treatment consists in the administration of antifungal agents such as itraconazole or voriconazole. The surgical option should be used only for completely localized lesions in patients with good respiratory reserve or if the therapy fails.

Aspergilloma

Aspergilloma is the most common lung disease that usually takes place in a preexistent cavity of the lung. An aspergilloma, or fungal ball, is composed of the hyphae of the fungus, inflammatory cells, fibrin, mucus, and remaining tissue. Some cavitating lung diseases such as tuberculosis, sarcoidosis, bronchiectasis, bronchial cysts, and bullas may be complicated by aspergillomas. The fungal ball can move within the cavity, but it does not invade the pulmonary parenchyma or the blood.

In a study conducted on 544 patients with pulmonary cavities secondary to tuberculosis, 11% had radiological evidence of aspergilloma.

Most of the patients are asymptomatic. When there are symptoms, most patients present hemoptysis. Less frequently, cough and dyspnea related to the underlying disease may also appear. Fever is secondary to the underlying disease, or to bacterial overinfection. Poor prognosis risk factors include the seriousness of the underlying pulmonary disease, the increase in the size or the number of the lesions, immunosuppression, the increase of IgG-specific antibody titers, and hemoptysis.

Diagnosis is made considering the clinical and radiographic characteristics showing a mobile intracavity mass, located in a preexistent cavity with a peripheral half-moon space, with microbiological and serological evidence of *Aspergillus* spp. Computerized axial tomography (CAT) confirms the findings. Sputum cultures for *Aspergillus* spp. are positive only in 50% of the cases. IgG antibodies against *Aspergillus* are positive in most cases.

Treatment is considered only when the patients present with symptoms, usually with hemoptysis. There is no agreement about the best treatment. Administration of percutaneous amphotericin B guided by chest CT seems to be efficient, especially in patients with massive hemoptysis. There is not enough knowledge about the use of IV amphotericin B. Itraconazole has a high tissue penetration, and it may be useful in some patients, showing improvements in 50% of cases. The role of voriconazole has not been established.

Surgical removal of the cavity with exeresis of the fungal ball is indicated for patients with recurrent hemoptysis.

Allergic Bronchopulmonary Aspergillosis

This disease is caused by the hypersensitivity of AF antigens. Although this is the main pathogen causing allergic bronchopulmonary aspergillosis (ABPA), there may be other related pathogens involved. In most cases, it affects patients with asthma or cystic fibrosis. It has been estimated that 2% of asthmatic patients, and around 7–14% of asthmatic patients who are steroid dependent have ABPA. Incidence is greater in atopic patients.

In the case of CF, it is variable in relation to different locations, but according to several authors, around 1–5% of patients with CF may develop ABPA at some point. The pathogenesis of ABPA is currently unknown. It has been proposed that inhaled spores are trapped in the mucus of the large airway. The spores may germinate when they develop hyphae, which release antigens and cause the immune response. The hypersensitivity reaction they cause is characterized by IgG and IgE production, as well as specific antibodies for AF. This reaction, combined with the production of cytotoxic metabolites, such as AF proteolytic enzymes, cause a local immunosuppression reaction, phagocytosis inhibition, and flaking of epithelium cells. As a whole, this reaction causes AF colonization and allows for its persistence in the airway, with lung infiltrations, tissue damage, and finally lung tissue destruction.

ABPA tends to be clinically suspected, and it is confirmed through serum tests and chest X-ray. Most patients present with episodic wheezing, sputum expectorations, dark blockages, dyspnea, pleural chest pain, fever, and sometimes hemoptysis that do not respond to the usual therapy.

Chest X-ray can be normal during the first stages of the disease. During exacerbations, brief central lung infiltrations appear in the superior lobes, along with atelectasis. In subsequent stages of the disease, central bronchiectasis and lung fibrosis may appear. Chest CT images can show bronchiectasis in more than three lobes, centrilobular nodules, and mucoid impaction, which all suggest this diagnosis. In CF, chest CT may show lung infiltrations and central bronchiectasis, that are not so useful as in asthma, because they are commonly found as a consequence of the disease.

Lung function tests do not yield characteristic results of ABPA, and show reversible obstructive lung disease, which becomes irreversible in the advanced stages of the disease. Oral steroids are the main treatment, which will vary according to the stage of the disease and if the patient suffers from asthma or CF.

Allergic Bronchopulmonary Aspergillosis in Asthma

Sensitization of AF antigens occurs in 28% of patients with asthma, but ABPA is found in 2% of asthma patients, 7–14% of steroid-dependent asthma patients, and 33% of severe asthma patients. Sensitization to AF antigens may cause severe obstruction of the air flow and therefore greater use of oral steroids.

The criteria for the diagnosis of ABPA in patients with asthma have been standardized, as shown in Table 46.1.

Clinical evolution is divided into five stages, which do not necessarily appear in order. The first four are potentially reversible, with no long-term sequelae.

- *Stage I or acute phase*. Increased IgE, positive antibodies, eosinophilia, lung infiltrations, and AF IgE and IgG. Patients are rarely identified in this stage.

Table 46.1 Diagnosis criteria for ABPA in asthma

Classic	Minimal criteria
Positive specific skin test for AF (prick test)	Immediate skin reactivity to AF antigens
Serum precipitins for AF	Total IgE 1000 UI/ml
Increase of AF-specific IgE and IgG	Increase of AF-specific IgE and IgG
1000 UI/ ml for total IgE	Central bronchiectasis
Current or previous pulmonary infiltrations	
Central bronchiectasis	
Eosinophilia (1000 cells/ml)	

- *Stage II or remission*. IgE may decrease, but it is usually maintained at high levels; there is no eosinophilia, and chest X-ray is normal. AF IgG antibodies may be slightly increased.
- *Stage III or exacerbation*. The findings of phase I are repeated in patients with ABPA diagnosis. IgE doubles from the reference level.
- *Stage IV or steroid dependency*. It appears in patients who suffer from asthma, requiring steroids in high doses. The asthmatic condition is worsened, and X-ray changes can be appreciated, with IgE increase. Frequently, chest CT shows central bronchiectasis.
- *Stage V*. In this stage the disease is irreversible because of lung fibrosis and bronchiectasis. Dyspnea, cyanosis, rhonchus, and *cor pulmonale* may be observed. Fortunately, few patients progress to this condition.

Oral steroids are the principal treatment. The treatment varies according to the stage of the disease. For stage I, oral steroids are indicated for 2 weeks (0.5–2 mg/kg oral prednisone; maximum, 60 mg/day). After the symptoms remit, the oral steroid may be reduced and suspended. For the stage II condition, use 0.5–2 mg/kg/day, alternating the days, during 1–2 weeks, and it can be suspended in 2–3 months. Treatment with itraconazole is indicated for relapses (stage III) or if the patient suffers from steroid-dependent asthma (stage IV).

Although inhaled steroids control asthma symptoms, their effectivity in the treatment of ABPA has not been confirmed.

Serum IgE is a marker of the activity of the disease, and it must be reassessed 6–8 weeks after the start of the therapy, and then every 8 weeks during a year, until the IgE values return to normal levels.

Allergic Bronchopulmonary Aspergillosis in CF

The prevalence of ABPA in CF varies between 0% and 25%, in part because of differences in diagnosis criteria. The European CF Registry shows a frequency of 7.8%, with great variances between countries. Its development is not related to any CFTR genotype in particular.

The diagnosis of ABPA in patients who suffer from CF may be difficult, and is mainly based on immunological evidence, because the lung infiltrations and central bronchiectasis that appear in the chest CT are usually found in patients with CF. The United States Foundation for Cystic Fibrosis proposed the minimum criteria shown in Table 46.2.

In imaging, ABPA cannot be differentiated from the underlying disease. Chest CT shows infiltrations or bronchiectasis that may not appear in the chest X-ray. ABPA bronchiectasis is central, and if there is CF, may be peripheral or central, which makes its diagnosis impossible to differentiate. Varicose and cystic bronchiectasis are more associated with ABPA than with CF.

Worsening of lung function is more acute in those patients with CF and ABPA, and therefore early diagnosis and treatment are very important to prevent severe, and potentially irreversible, lung damage.

Treatment of ABPA in patients with CF is similar to that proposed for ABPA patients with asthma. Patients with CF present particular characteristics, such as vulnerability and toxicity to steroids, altered pharmacokinetics, and a different interaction with the drug. Steroids are the drug of choice for the treatment of ABPA in the patient with CF, at the doses recommended for asthma. They may be used orally or parenterally

Table 46.2 Diagnosis criteria for ABPA when the patient has cystic fibrosis (CF)[a]

Acute or subacute clinical worsening of the condition, which cannot be explained by other causes or exacerbation.
Total IgE > 500 UI/ml (ABPA suspicion, IgE between 200 and 500 UI/ml if the patient receives steroids. In this case, IgE must be repeated every 1–3 months, or when steroids are suspended).
AF-specific skin test (prick test over 3 mm).
AF-specific IgE increase.
New or recent abnormalities in chest X-ray (infiltrations, mucus blockages) or CAT scan (bronchiectasis) that do not improve or disappear with antibiotics.

[a]According to the US Cystic Fibrosis Foundation

(with fewer adverse effects): methylprednisolone in pulses of 10–15 mg/kg/day for 3 days. No benefits have been shown with the use of inhaled steroids.

Itraconazole (5 mg/kg/day; maximum dose, 400 mg/day, using dose in blood) is used in combination with steroids. Recently, oral voriconazole has been used, which has the same activity against AF with better absorption.

Treatment time is variable: it may require 6–12 months. IgE serum levels are used to evaluate treatment response. When these values return to normal levels, treatment may be suspended.

Sources

Agarwal R, Aggarwal AN, Gupta D, et al. Aspergillus hypersensitivity and allergic bronchopulmonary aspergillosis in patients with bronchial asthma: systematic review and meta-analysis. Int J Tuberc Lung Dis. 2009;13:936–44.

Albelda SM, Talbot GH, Gerson SL, et al. Pulmonary cavitation and massive hemoptysis in invasive pulmonary aspergillosis. Influence of bone marrow recovery in patients with acute leukemia. Am Rev Respir Dis. 1985;131:115–20.

Burgos A, Zaoutis TE, Dvorak CC, et al. Pediatric invasive aspergillosis: a multicenter retrospective analysis of 139 contemporary cases. Pediatrics. 2008;121(5):e1286–94.

Curtis AM, Smith GJ, Ravin CE. Air crescent sign of invasive aspergillosis. Radiology. 1979;133:17–21.

De Pauw B, Walsh TJ, Donnelly JP, et al. Revised definitions of invasive fungal disease from the European Organization for Research and Treatment of Cancer/invasive fungal infections cooperative group and the National Institute of Allergy and Infectious Diseases mycoses study group (EORTC/MSG) consensus group. Clin Infect Dis. 2008;46:1813–21.

Greenberger PA, Patterson R. Diagnosis and management of allergic bronchopulmonary aspergillosis. Ann Allergy 1986;56:444–8.

Herbrecht R, Denning DW, Patterson TF, et al. Voriconazole versus amphotericin B for primary therapy of invasive aspergillosis. N Engl J Med. 2002;347:408–15.

Horger M, Hebart H, Einsele H, et al. Initial CT manifestations of invasive pulmonary aspergillosis in 45 non-HIV immunocompromised patients: association with patient outcome? Eur J Radiol. 2005;55:437–44.

Horvath JA, Dummer S. The use of respiratory-tract cultures in the diagnosis of invasive pulmonary aspergillosis. Am J Med. 1996;100:171–8.

Kotloff RM, Ahya VN, Crawford SW. Pulmonary complications of solid organ and hematopoietic stem cell transplantation. Am J Respir Crit Care Med. 2004;170:22–48.

Kousha M, Tadi R, Soubani A. Pulmonary aspergillosis: a clinical review. Eur Respir Rev. 2011;20(121):156–74.

Mastella G, Rainisio M, Harms HK, et al. On behalf of the investigators of the Epidemiologic Registry of Cystic Fibrosis. Allergic bronchopulmonary aspergillosis in cystic fibrosis. A European epidemiological study. Eur Respir J. 2000;16:464–71.

Moss R. Allergic bronchopulmonary aspergillosis, chapter 28. In: Taussig L, Landau L, editor. Pediatric respiratory medicine. 2nd ed: Mosby; 2008.

Moss R. Allergic bronchopulmonary aspergillosis and *Aspergillus* infection in cystic fibrosis. Curr Opin Pulmon Med. 2010;16:598–603.

Patterson K, Strek ME. Allergic bronchopulmonary aspergillosis. Proc Am Thorac Soc. 2010;7:237–44.

Pfeiffer CD, Fine JP, Safdar N. Diagnosis of invasive aspergillosis using a galactomannan assay: a meta-analysis. Clin Infect Dis. 2006;42:1417–27.

Segal BH, Walsh TJ. Current approaches to diagnosis and treatment of invasive aspergillosis. Am J Respir Crit Care Med. 2006;173:707–17.

Spanakis EK, Aperis G, Mylonakis E, et al. New agents for the treatment of fungal infections: clinical efficacy and gaps in coverage. Clin Infect Dis. 2006;43:1060–8.

Post-Infectious Bronchiolitis Obliterans

47

Alejandro Colom, Gilberto Fischer, and Alejandro Teper

Contents

Prevalence

Interest in BO increased with the publication of the first cases related to serious respiratory infection caused by adenovirus in Argentina in 1979. During the past decades, different countries have reported cases, particularly Chile, Brazil, Korea, Turkey, and Argentina (Fig. 47.1). In Europe and in the United States of America, most cases are secondary to bone marrow and pulmonary transplants, but the Southern Cone of South America the cases are mostly secondary to infections, especially those caused by adenovirus (Table 47.1). There are no epidemiological studies determining the prevalence of this disease in the population. Published data allow us to infer a higher prevalence of post-infectious bronchiolitis obliterans (PIBO) in Chile, Brazil, and Argentina.

A. Colom (✉)
Pediatric Pulmonology, Hospital Ricardo Gutiérrez, Buenos Aires, Argentina

G. Fischer
Pediatric Pulmonology, Federal University of Health Sciences of Porto Alegre, Porto Alegre, Brazil
e-mail: gbfischer@ufcspa.edu.br

A. Teper
Faculty of Medicine, Universidad de Buenos Aires and Division of Pediatric Pulmonology, Hospital Ricardo Gutiérrez, Buenos Aires, Argentina

P. Bertrand, I. Sánchez (eds.), *Pediatric Respiratory Diseases*,
https://doi.org/10.1007/978-3-030-26961-6_47

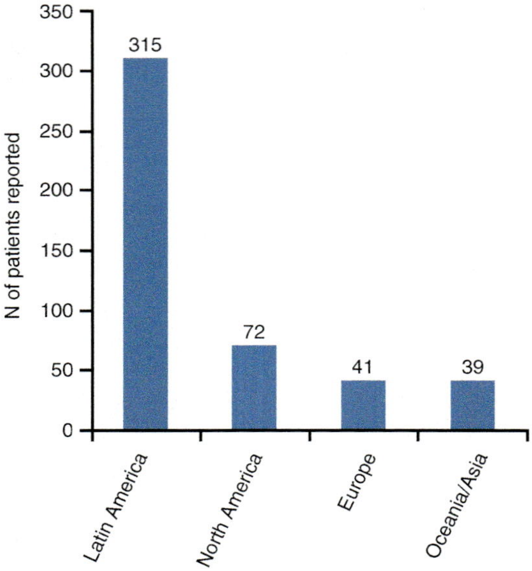

Fig. 47.1 Frequency of post-infectious bronchiolitis obliterans (PIBO)

Table 47.1 Causes of bronchiolitis obliterans (BO)

Transplant	Graft versus host after bone marrow transplant	
	Chronic rejection after lung transplant	
Infections	Virus	Adenovirus: 3, 5, 7h, 21
		Influenza
		Parainfluenza
		Measles
	Mycoplasma	
Other	Collagen disease	
	Toxic inhalation (NH_3, NO_2)	
	Mineral dust	
	Drugs	
	Aspiration	
	Steven–Johnson syndrome	

Pathology

Bronchiolitis obliterans (BO) is characterized by the partial or total occlusion of the terminal respiratory bronchiole space, caused by inflammatory tissue and fibrosis. Pathological findings in their different etiologies suggest that it would be the final process of response to different aggressions to the lower respiratory tract.

From the pathological aspect, BO may be classified in two main categories. The first one corresponds to proliferative BO, characterized by the obstruction of the space in the small airway by polyps caused by granulation tissue. If the granulation tissue extends toward the alveoli, the lesion is named BO with organizing pneumonia (BOOP). The second category is constrictive BO, which is characterized by peribronchiolar fibrosis, with different degrees of narrowing of the bronchial lumen.

Post-infectious BO is mainly characterized by a constrictive BO pattern, with different degrees of inflammation and obliteration of the airway. In these patients the signs of airway disease are frequent, such as bronchiolar inflammation, mucostasis, macrophage accumulation, and bronchiolar distortion and dilation. Bronchiolar dilations are more frequent in patients with post-infectious BO, in comparison to other causes. Histological analysis is limited by the multifocal nature of the disease.

Etiology

Different respiratory viruses, such as influenza, parainfluenza, respiratory syncytial virus (RSV), and especially adenovirus, have been associated with BO. Other infectious etiologies include *Mycoplasma pneumoniae*, measles virus, and human immunodeficiency virus-1. Also, in lung transplant patients, infection caused by cytomegalovirus was associated with the development of BO bronchiolitis.

Adenovirus In 2006 a case-control study conducted in Buenos Aires was published that included 109 patients with bronchiolitis who developed BO and 99 control patients, patients with bronchiolitis who did not progress to BO. Risk factors for developing BO were adenovirus infection (OR 49) and the need for mechanical ventilatory assistance (OR 11). Although mechanical ventilatory assistance was an independent risk factor, the results did not identify if ventilatory support was by itself the cause of the injury or if it was only an indicator of the seriousness of the disease. The main role of the infection caused by adenovirus in the development of BO was widely documented. In our study, 72% of the patients who developed BO presented with adenovirus infection. In 1984 a new adenovirus genotype, 7h, was described as one of the most virulent types, but other adenovirus such as serotypes 3, 5, and 21 can also cause BO.

Adenovirus 7h is responsible for 20% of all the infections caused by this agent, according to publications issued by the World Health Organization (WHO). In the Southern Hemisphere the incidence of the B subgene adenovirus and serotypes 4 and 7 is greater. Epidemiological studies between 1991 and 1994 in children hospitalized for lower acute respiratory infection in Argentina, Chile, and Uruguay identified that 71% of the infections caused by adenovirus where of the B subgene, and 61.2% of them corresponded to the 7h genome.

Other studies have shown that the global prevalence of adenovirus genotypes changes in relationship to time and geographic region, which makes it difficult to develop a vaccine with global effectiveness. In Argentina, during the past decade, a reduction of serious and fatal cases caused by this virus has been observed, which could be explained by a reduction of genotype 7 incidence, besides an increase of genotype 3. A reduction of infections caused by adenovirus has also been observed since 2004, perhaps because of an interference of infections caused by rhinovirus or the A H1N1 influenza pandemic in 2009.

Three different types of epidemics are caused by adenovirus:

1. Epidemics during the winter months among hospitalized infants (generally under 2 years old), which cause a high rate of serious infections and death.
2. Nonseasonal periodic epidemic outbreaks, community-driven, which compromise older children and adults, but cause few and infrequent respiratory sequelae.
3. Epidemic outbreaks of acute respiratory diseases among military recruits.

Patients with a serious infection caused by adenovirus present with immune complex in the lung containing adenovirus antigens, as well as high levels of interleukin (IL)-6, IL-8, and tumor necrosis factor (TNF)-α serum.

Susceptibility to developing BO seems to be related to the geographic origin of human groups. The populations of native children in New Zealand, Canada, Alaska, and South America have a greater incidence of post-infectious BO when compared to the populations of Europe and other regions of America. Recent studies conducted in Argentina in patients with this disease show that the HLA haplotype DR8-DQB1*0302, and native aborigines, determined by the mtDNA markers, are increased in relationship to control groups.

Although the studies are limited, the innate immunological response would have a preponderant role in the seriousness of the adenovirus infection and the development of BO in predisposed populations.

Mycoplasma pneumoniae Infection caused by *Mycoplasma pneumoniae* is a frequent cause of atypical pneumonia in older children. It was identified as an etiology of BO in 1986, although its development in patients with *Mycoplasma* infections is a rare complication. In other areas, such as Malaysia and Korea, it is the second most common etiological agent for BO, after adenovirus infection. In these countries, infection by *Mycoplasma* was present in 20% of the patients with BO, most of these secondary to *Mycoplasma* epidemic outbreaks.

Influenza Up to 20% of influenza patients develop complications, particularly small children (0–4 years old). In spite of this, BO is a rare complication of influenza infection, and few cases in infants and small children have been published.

Measles virus BO is an infrequent complication of measles. Viral load and the initial immunological condition, as well as the virus persistence in the lung parenchyma, probably determine chronic lung damage.

Respiratory syncytial virus This virus circulation has an epidemic pattern during winter months, and it is the most common cause of lower respiratory tract infection. Association between BO and respiratory syncytial virus is rare and it is not clearly defined. Simultaneous infection of syncytial virus and adenovirus can happen. In these cases, it seems more likely that the development of BO is caused by the adenovirus infection.

Clinical Findings

In most cases, the disease starts very early, before the first year of life. However, age has not been confirmed as a risk factor for developing post-infectious BO.

Initially patients start showing symptoms that are not different from those of a regular viral bronchiolitis caused by syncytial virus. Most patients present serious bronchospasm, with hypoxemia, and in many cases they need mechanical ventilation. Physical examination is not specific. Wheezing and rhonchus can be heard bilaterally. If a patient with an adenovirus infection does not improve in 3 weeks, BO should be suspected.

After the clinical condition of the patient becomes stable, tachypnea persists, wheezing and productive cough become permanent, and oxygen saturation is reduced. Some patients with nosocomial pneumonia caused by adenovirus with an important respiratory compromise present a similar progression, requiring long hospitalizations and intensive care.

Diagnosis

The objective of diagnosis methods is to show the obliteration of the small airway, which is an anatomopathological lesion of this disease. Because of this, lung biopsy yields the best results. Lung function tests can show severe and fixed obstruction. Indirect signs of the disease can appear in the lung images.

Chest X-ray images are not specific: air trapping, atelectasis, peribronchial enlargement, and areas with a honeycomb appearance (Fig. 47.2). Some patients present unilateral compromise in one lobe/lung with an area with hyperclarity in a smaller lobe/lung, known as Swyer–James or MacLeod syndrome. These images result from the loss of vascular structure and air trapping. Occasionally these findings may be observed as the only image in patients with a less serious presentation of the disease.

Lung grammagraphy shows perfusion defects, with a subsegmental, segmental, or lobar pattern.

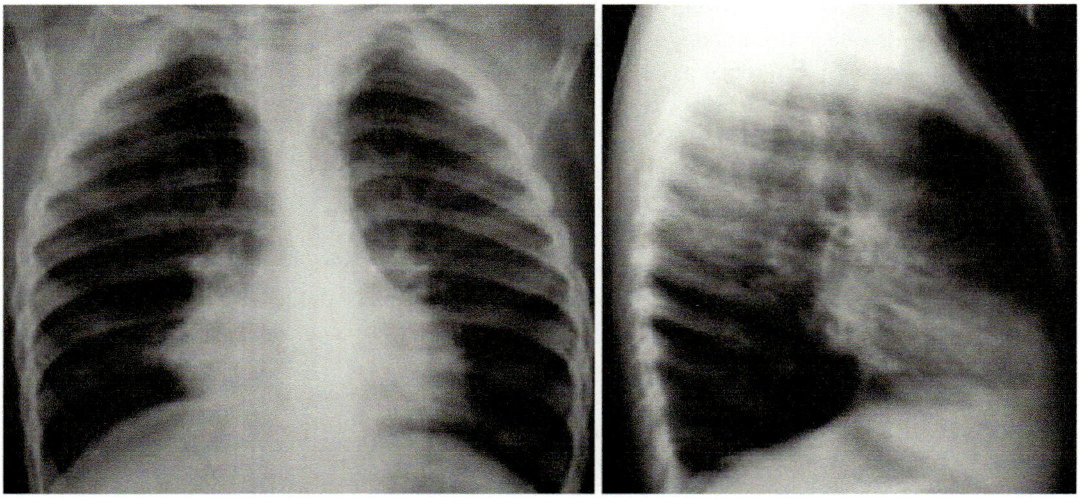

Fig. 47.2 Post-infectious bronchiolitis obliterans (PIBO). Chest X-ray of a 7-year-old schoolchild shows air trapping, atelectasis, and bronchiectasis

When comparing pulmonary perfusion with the chest X-ray, gammagraphy findings correspond to the most affected areas, with bronchial enlargement and bronchiectasis. This technique of pulmonary perfusion may not describe the nature of the bronchopulmonary anomaly, but it does show an objective evaluation of the extension, distribution, and seriousness of the lesion. Its usefulness for diagnosing BO is not relevant.

The most characteristic sign of BO in high-resolution computerized tomography (HRCT) is areas showing a mosaic pattern, caused by air trapping and vascular shunt from the hypoventilated areas toward normal or over-ventilated areas. Perfusion is impoverished in reduction areas of the parenchyma because of the vasoconstriction caused by tissue hypoxia (Fig. 47.3). Other signs include air trapping, especially observed during exhalation, and bronchiectasis. Air trapping can be detected during exhalation in the HRCT. This study method is considered as the most sensitive and early step when BO is suspected, as was described for the first time in relation to a transplant, and which has an important role in the initial diagnostic suspicion. In small patients who do not cooperate, a lateral recumbent position may be useful to identify air trapping in patients who show a reduction mosaic pattern.

Lung function in infants with post-infectious BO was described in 1999 and studied at first using the technique of fast thoracoabdominal compression. In these patients, respiratory mechanics is altered, with an increase of resistance and severe alterations of pulmonary elastic retraction. In the curves of forced partial volume flows it can be observed that the maximum flow at functional residual capacity (V'_{max} FRC) is very reduced and it does not respond to bronchodilator administration. Because V'_{max} FRC is an index used to evaluate the caliber of the airway, we may conclude that the patients with PIBO have an important compromise of the pulmonary function, which manifests itself as a severe and fixed obstruction of the airway. These patients have a more serious compromise of the small airway in comparison to other diseases, such as bronchopulmonary dysplasia or asthma, which in many cases respond to bronchodilators. These findings represent the functional expression of the histopathological damage of BO bronchiolitis (Fig. 47.4).

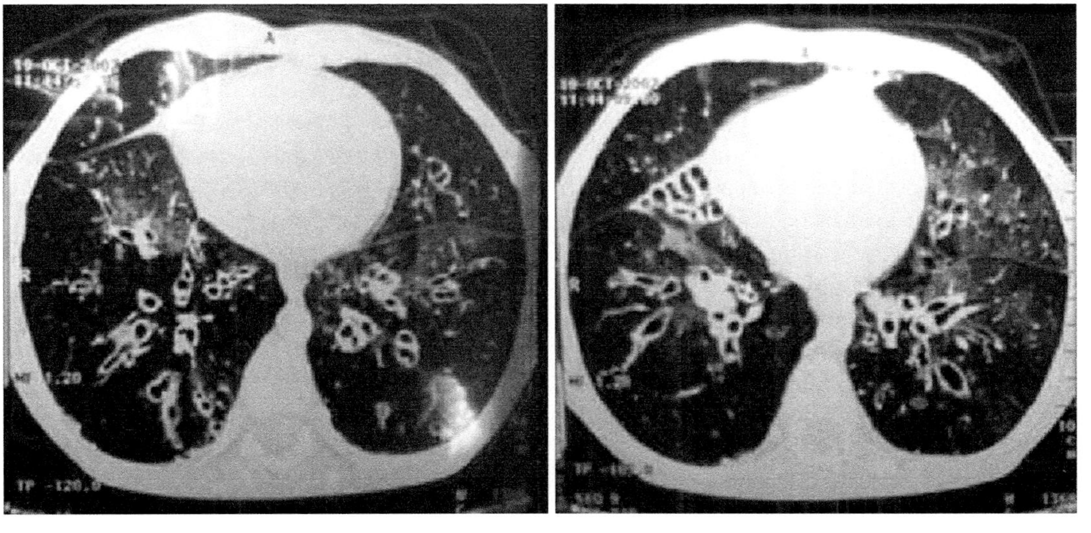

Fig. 47.3 PIBO. Chest computerized tomography of a 14-year-old adolescent shows mosaic pattern areas, atelectasis, and bronchiectasis

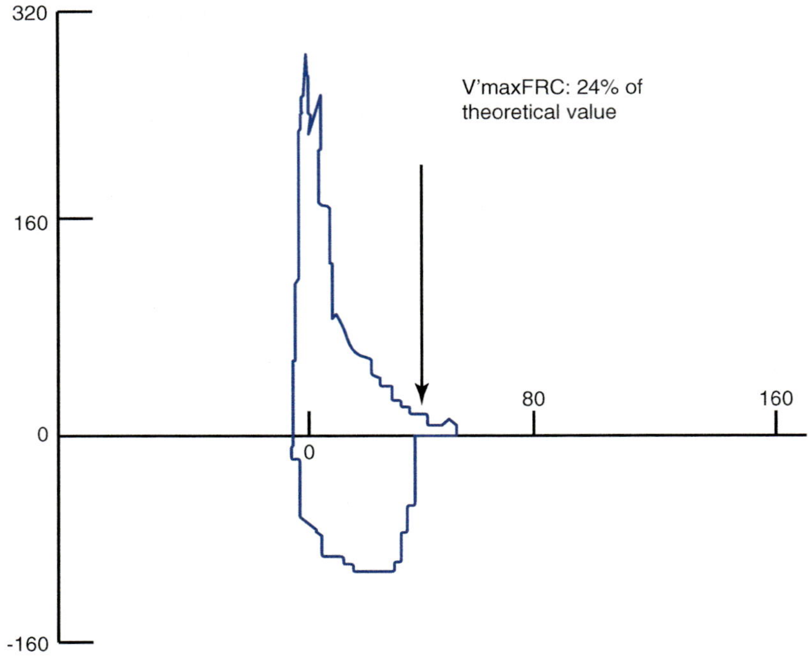

Fig. 47.4 Lung function. A forced partial volume/flow curve, with severe obstruction of the air flow expressed in reduction of the maximum flow level of the residual functional capacity (V'_{max} FRC: 24% of theoretical value) in a 11-month infant with BO caused by adenovirus

Another factor related to BO that may cause deterioration in lung function is gastroesophageal reflux, which is frequent in these patients (54%). Currently, there are no studies of its prevalence in patients with BO.

To summarize, when other causes of chronic pulmonary disease have been ruled out, clinical history, chest X-ray, and HRCT are sufficient in most cases to confirm the diagnosis and differentiate this disease from others. This evaluation should be considered along with pulmonary function. If there are doubts about the diagnosis, a lung biopsy must be considered.

Lung biopsy is the gold standard for the diagnosis of BO. The main difficulty of its application is the clinical condition of the patient. During the diagnosis stage, most of the patients are seriously compromised, and therefore the decision to conduct an open lung biopsy is difficult, because of the associated morbidity and mortality rates. The output of this procedure is limited by the patchy distribution of lung damage. Because of this, lung biopsy is only done for those patients about whom there are still doubts about the diagnosis after having done all the aforementioned procedures.

Radiological Clinical Score (BO Score)

The diagnostic criteria of posttransplant BO have been clearly defined, but they have not been as well defined as for post-infectious BO. Definitive diagnosis of BO is done by lung biopsy, although conducting it on these patients is related to high morbidity and mortality, especially in very seriously ill patients. Lung function has great value because of its characteristic pattern, but this is not available for most pediatric pneumonologists.

A study was developed with the objective to accurately establish diagnostic criteria for post-infectious BO in children under 2 years of age with chronic lung disease. In this study, a scale was created and validated, wherein specificity is favored over sensitivity to make it more reliable in positive cases, and 125 patients under 2 years old with chronic lung disease were evaluated. The following variables were significantly associated with the diagnosis:

- "Typical clinical history" (4 points), defined as previously healthy patient, with a serious episode of bronchiolitis/pneumonia developing chronic hypoxemia (sat $O_2 < 92\%$) for more than 60 days;

- "History of infection caused by adenovirus" (3 points); "HRCT with mosaic pattern" (4 points) (Table 47.2).

A score of 7 or greater predicts the diagnosis of post-infectious BO with a high degree of accuracy (100% specificity and 67% sensitivity). It must be highlighted that a negative score (<7) does not completely rule out the diagnosis of BO, as only very sick patients have been included.

Evolution and Prognosis

Clinical evolution of the patients with post-infectious BO is characterized by a slow and gradual improvement. Most patients require supplementary oxygen. In our series, the median duration of this treatment was 5 months (range. 2–26 months) after discharge. Hospitalizations are frequent and are caused by lower respiratory tract airway infections. The number of hospitalizations and the oxygen requirements progressively decrease during the years in which the disease progresses. Lung function does not change significantly during the first years of age.

Table 47.2 Radiological clinical score

	Value	
Predictor variable	Present	Absent
Typical clinical history	4	0
Infection by adenovirus	3	0
HRCT with mosaic pattern	4	0
Range of score is from 0 to 11		

From the systematic follow-up of the pulmonary function in children and young people between 5 and 21 years old, we could observe that FVC and FEV_1 increase by 11% and 9% per year, respectively, and the relationship FVC/FEV_1 decreases 1.9% per year (Fig. 47.5). The fact that FVC increases more than FEV_1 could be explained by a differentiated growth of the lung parenchyma and respiratory airways, indicating an asymmetrical growth of the lung. In other words, this recovery of pulmonary growth and airways after the initial lesion could be possible in terms of the number of alveoli, called neo-alveolarization. This lung growth could be not so important in relation to the size of the airway. Besides this, although lung function increased in absolute values, the Z score of FVC and FEV_1 were reduced in 0.07 and 0.09 Z score/year, respectively, showing that the degree of lung development is slower than that of the general population of the same age (Fig. 47.5).

In the same way that the values of spirometry parameters increase, plethysmography studies show a reduction of the air trapping (residual

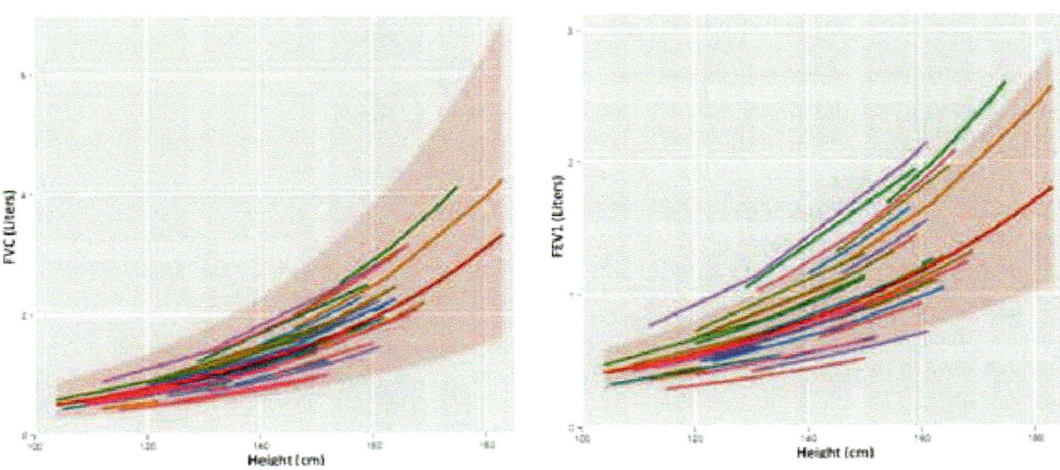

Fig. 47.5 Progression of pulmonary function. Follow-up of pulmonary function (FVC/FEV_1) in 46 patients with BO between 6 and 21 years of age. (*Source:* Thorax 2015;70:169)

volume decreases). Respiratory mechanics measured with forced oscillation technique show a low distensibility and an increased resistance.

In most patients, perfusion defects observed at the beginning of the disease persist, and sometimes they improve.

Cardiopulmonary assessment during exercise shows reduced functional capacity, which has been confirmed by cardiac stress test, or by the 6-min walking test, a simpler test to perform.

Although lung function remains severely compromised, presenting from intense to moderate airway obstruction, during childhood only a few patients require supplementary oxygen. The clinical improvement observed in these patients may be caused by lung growth, and it probably is not a sign of small airway pathology recession.

The mortality rate of post-infectious BO is not known with certainty, and it varies according to the different series published, according to the different grade of impact in the condition of the included patients.

The individual prognosis of a certain patient may be related to different factors, such as time requiring oxygen and the severity of the airway reinfections.

Treatment

Therapeutic interventions aiming to avoid initial damage are based on the suppression of the inflammatory response. Anti-inflammatory treatments, such as steroids, chloroquine, and hydroxychloroquine, have been used in studies involving a few cases with unsuccessful results. Because BO is an infrequent disease, it has not been possible to conduct controlled and randomized studies.

Different cytokines have been identified in the pathogenesis of post-infectious BO, TNF-α and fibroblast production among them. A successful treatment case of BO after bone marrow transplant was published. The treatment involved a TNF-α blocker (infliximab) for an 8-year-old child.

Other studies suggest that a maintenance treatment with macrolides has a potential role, because of its antiinflammatory properties.

When the disease is established, the main treatment consists of support measures, which include bronchodilators, respiratory physiotherapy, antibiotics for acute respiratory infections, and diuretics. Gastroesophageal reflux has been increasingly recognized as a factor that may significantly contribute to patient morbidity, and therefore treatment is mandatory.

Some patients develop chest deformity, which consists of an asymmetrical keel chest, and the most severe cases require surgical correction. These abnormalities would be the result of a combination of bone demineralization and chronic air trapping. It is plausible that these deformities in the chest wall may be clinically harmful because of interference with respiratory mechanics.

In patients with localized bronchiectasis that cannot be adequately controlled with clinical treatment, a lobectomy may be done to improve their quality of life. The indication to perform a chest surgery in these patients must be carefully considered, because complications such as infections, pneumothorax, and bronchial fistulas are common.

Although the evolution of these patients is almost always satisfactory, lung transplant is the last therapeutic option for those patients whose life prognosis is serious.

Sources

Andrade CF, Melo IA, Holand AR, Silva ÉF, Fischer GB, Felicetii JC. Surgical treatment of non-cystic fibrosis bronchiectasis in Brazilian children. Pediatr Surg Int. 2014;30(1):63–9.

Castro-Rodriguez J, Daszenies C, Garcia M, Meyer R, Gonzales R. Adenovirus pneumonia in infants and factors for developing bronchiolitis obliterans: a 5-year follow-up. Pediatr Pulmonol. 2006;41:947–53.

Chang A, Masel J, Masters B. Post-infectious bronchiolitis obliterans: clinical, radiological and pulmonary function sequelae. Pediatr Radiol. 1998;28:23.

Colom AJ, Andrada G, Teper A. Development of a clinical prediction rule to diagnose post-infectious bronchiolitis obliterans in children. Am J Respir Crit Care Med. 2008;177:A703.

Colom AJ, Maffey A, Garcia Bournissen F, Teper A. Pulmonary function of a pediatric cohort of patients with postinfectious bronchiolitis obliterans. A long term follow up. Thorax. 2015;70:169.

Colom AJ, Teper AM, Vollmer WM, Diette GB. Risk factors for the development of bronchiolitis obliterans in children with bronchiolitis. Thorax. 2006;61:503–6.

Fischer GB, Sarria EE et al. Post infectious bronchiolitis obliterans in children. Paediatr Respir Rev. 2010;11(4):233–9.

Gerhardt S, McDyer J, Girgis R, et al. Maintenance azithromycin therapy for bronchiolitis obliterans syndrome. Results of a pilot study. Am J Respir Crit Care Med. 2003;168:121–5.

Linares PM, Meyer PR, Soto GG. Evaluación de la respuesta broncodilatadora en pacientes secuelados de adenovirus. Rev Chil Pediatr. 2004;5:37–44.

Maffey A, Colom A, Kofman C, Vidaurreta S, Teper A. Longitudinal study of pulmonary function in infants with postviral chronic pulmonary disease (PCPD). Am J Respir Crit Care Med. 1996;153:498.

Mattiello R, Sarria EE, Stein R, Fischer GB, Mocelin HT, Barreto SS, Lima JA, Brandenburg D. Functional capacity assessment in children and adolescents with post-infectious bronchiolitis obliterans. J Pediatr. 2008;84(4):337–43.

Nayar E, Saavedra M, Escobar AM, Vidal A. Función pulmonar y calidad de vida en niños y adolescentes con bronquiolitis obliterante por adenovirus. Rev Chil Enferm Respir. 2011;27:191–5.

Teper A, Colom A, Bailliet G, et al. Association between the incidence of bronchiolitis obliterans (BO) in Argentine children and their native-American maternal and paternal lineage. Am J Respir Crit Care Med. 2003;167:998.

Teper AM, Kofman CD, Maffey AF, et al. Lung function in infants with chronic pulmonary disease after severe adenoviral illness. J Pediatr. 1999;134:730–3.

Teper AM, Marcos CY, Theiler G, Colom AJ, Fainboim L. Association between HLA and the incidence of bronchiolitis obliterans (BO) in Argentina. Am J Respir Crit Care Med. 2004;169:382 (abstract).

Vega-Briceño L, Zenteno D et al. Guía clínica para el diagnóstico y cuidado de niños/adolescentes con bronquiolitis obliterante post-infecciosa, 2009. Rev Chil Enferm Respir. 2009;25:141–63.

Yalçına E, Dogrua D, Halıloglub M, et al. Postinfectious bronchiolitis obliterans in children: clinical and radiological profile and prognostic factors. Respiration. 2003;70:371–5.

48 Obstructive Sleep Apnea Syndrome in Children

Asher Tal, Pablo Brockmann Veloso, and Aviv Goldbart

Contents

A. Tal · A. Goldbart
Ben Gurion University of Negev, Beersheba, Israel
e-mail: ashik@bgu.ac.il; avivgold@bgu.ac.il

P. Brockmann Veloso (✉)
Department of Pediatrics, School of Medicine,
Pontificia Universidad Católica de Chile,
Santiago, Chile
e-mail: pbrockmann@med.puc.cl

P. Bertrand, I. Sánchez (eds.), *Pediatric Respiratory Diseases*,
https://doi.org/10.1007/978-3-030-26961-6_48

Introduction

The spectrum of sleep-disordered breathing (SDB) ranges from primary snoring to obstructive sleep apnea syndrome (OSAS). Primary snoring appears during sleep and is associated with a greater respiratory effort, but it does not evidently present micro-awakenings or alterations in the gas exchange. The upper airway resistance syndrome is characterized by brief and intermittent awakenings associated with respiratory events during sleep, with no apneas or alterations in gas exchange. OSAS is characterized by a partial or complete obstruction of the airway that alters ventilation and causes a disruption in normal sleep architecture, with alterations in gas exchange (Fig. 48.1).

Physiopathological mechanisms associated with the described consequences of SDB are fundamentally sleep disruption, intermittent night hypoxemia, and chronic inflammation of the airway.

Epidemiology

The prevalence of sleep-disordered breathing (SDB) is estimated to be about 10–20%, and OSAS prevalence is estimated to be about 1% in children under 15 years old. These numbers fluctuate from region to region, and the prevalence is higher in Afro-American and Hispanic populations. Multiple risk factors affect the prevalence of SDB, and the sociodemographic factor is an important one. These factors are more frequent in children of lower socioeconomic status, premature, and obese. The prevalence of OSAS linearly varies according to the body mass index of the patients studied, and it was present in about 60% of morbidly obese patients. In Chile, studies have shown an SDB prevalence of 18% in the pediatric population.

Physiopathology

To understand the physiopathology and mechanisms involved in OSAS, it is important to consider the following principles:

- Ventilation control that regulates upper airway tone and awakening response; both physiologically decrease during sleep.
- Residual functional capacity decreases and may cause hypoxemia and apnea, which is caused by a reduction of the intercostal muscular and upper airway tone, especially during REM sleep.
- The tone of the upper airway tract is reduced during sleep and causes an increase of its

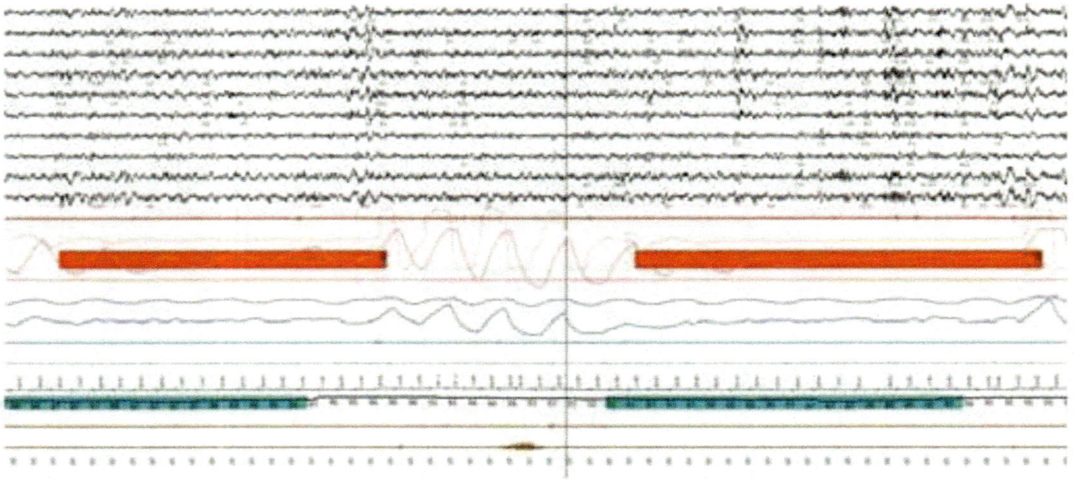

Fig. 48.1 Polysomnography in severe obstructive sleep apnea syndrome (OSAS). *Lines* represent 60 s of sleep N2. Two obstructive events are shown (in *red*). Desaturations (in *green*) can be observed toward the end of the obstructive events

resistance, which at the same time may impact ventilation and gas exchange.

- Progressively, and as a result of the aforementioned phenomena, hypoxemia and hypercarbia will be present during sleep. This physiological phenomenon worsens if it coexists with any other lung or airway disease.

Besides this, children with OSAS tend to have an airway with reduced space. They generally present with a narrowing of the airway related to intermittent hypercarbia and hypoxia. The site of greater obstruction tends to be more distal than in adults, usually including the oropharynx and hypopharynx. Children with this symptom have inspiratory aphasic activity in the muscles of the upper tract of the airway during sleep.

Infants and children normally have a narrower airway than adults. Nevertheless, they usually snore less and show fewer obstructive apneas in comparison to adults, which could be explained by anatomical differences and also by a different muscular tone of the upper airway. Critical pressure reflects the balance between the anatomical structure and the muscle tone of the airway; however, it is very difficult to determine a critical pressure in children as the airway is very resistant to collapse, probably because children have a greater ventilatory drive. Because of this, it is possible that children have greater activation of the muscles of the upper airway when responding to different stimuli.

The upper airway in children with OSAS is more collapsible in comparison to control children without this syndrome, for both awake or sleep and anesthesia periods. A series of mechanisms may create a greater degree of collapsibility in these patients, among which we can mention lower muscle tone, increase of airway distensibility, and increase in the inspiratory pressure, caused by the narrowing of the proximal airway.

A recent study used magnetic resonance imaging to evaluate the changes in the shape and size of the sectional area in the airway during breathing at tidal volume. In this study, it was shown that children with this syndrome have greater fluctuations in the airway when compared to control subjects. The explanations for this can lie in a reduced distensibility or a greater resistance. Studies that have involved the denervated upper airway have shown that lack of muscle tone may cause a greater collapse. It was recently proven that children have active upper airway responses to both negative pressures and hypercapnia during sleep. Healthy children could compensate the small size of the airway by increasing ventilatory command. This compensation mechanism could be reduced or absent in children with this syndrome.

To summarize, a combination of the structure of the airway with neuromuscular control, besides other genetic, hormonal, and metabolic factors, cause the appearance of OSAS in children.

Physiopathological Consequences

Increase of respiratory work This increase could be a factor that causes poor growth in children with OSAS. As a result of the greater diagnosis and consciousness about this syndrome, most children are detected before they can present any lack in their growth, and currently it is very infrequent.

Intermittent hypoxemia Children with OSAS tend to present (Fig. 48.2) with intermittent hypoxemia that can contribute to the increase of lung pressure and the development of *cor pulmonale* in advanced stages. Nevertheless, the most frequent consequence, and probably the one that causes most sequelae in this syndrome, is neurocognitive and behavior problems. The relationship between the duration of hypoxemia and the degree of desaturation versus secondary cognitive damage is still unknown.

Sleep fragmentation Sleep fragmentation is a well-documented consequence of OSAS in adults, but it is not yet fully understood in children. Although micro-awakenings have a protective role in this syndrome, their increase in frequency can cause a disruptive sleep instead of a reparative one. Sympathetic activation, as well as the activation of secondary inflammation

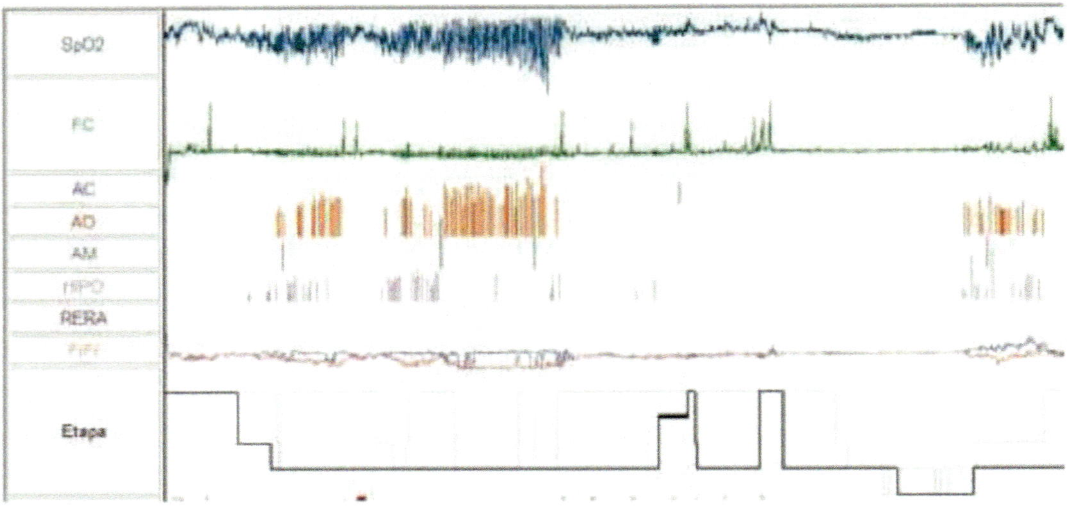

Fig. 48.2 Hypnogram in severe OSAS. Record of 4 h in a 1-year-old patient showing frequent obstructive events (in *red*) and cluster desaturations (in *green*)

mediators, has similar or even worse consequences than intermittent hypoxemia. The identification of micro-awakenings in adults is based on ECG interpretation. In contrast, in children more variables have to be considered, as most micro-awakenings are subcortical and are not necessarily observable through ECG.

Alveolar hypoventilation Associated with OSAS, alveolar hypoventilation is the result of long periods of upper airway increased resistance and hypercapnia, with or without hypoxemia. In the end, this causes long-term effects in the neural tissue and vasomotor tone. CO_2 increase is the main characteristic of this condition.

Table 48.1 Symptoms Related to OSAS in Children

Daytime
Behavioral problems
Hyperactivity
Belligerence
Poor school performance
Lack of appetite
Daytime sleepiness
Poor concentration
Nighttime
Snoring
Respiratory distress
Apnea as reported by parents or caregivers
Nonrestful sleep
Frequent awakenings
Night sweats
Night enuresis

Clinical Presentation

Nighttime Symptoms

Snoring Snoring is the most characteristic symptom of OSAS in children (Table 48.1). Generally, this condition worsens when children have an upper airway infection. Compared to adults, small children can snore in any position, and it does not necessarily worsen with the supine position. Common snoring is not per se a specific symptom of OSAS. Every child who usually snores is a primary snorer, although the child may not present apnea, hypopnea, or oxygen desaturation during sleep. Most children with primary snoring do not progress to this syndrome, and those who do, usually have a mild presentation of it. Nevertheless, some recent studies have shown behavioral and neurocognitive consequences, even when there are no polysomnography alterations to suggest this syndrome.

Respiratory distress during sleep Such distress is a subjective manifestation usually informed by the parents of children with OSAS. Usually, they describe paradoxical respiratory movements in which "the abdomen lowers, while the chest rises."

Apneas Parents frequently describe breathing stops during sleep, and some of them mention that respiratory noises stop for a few seconds, which are followed by a "grunt" or energic breathing.

These three cardinal symptoms are the most consistent ones in children with this syndrome At the beginning of the 1980s, Brouillete et al used these to create the "OSA Score." This score states that those children who snore every night had sleep respiratory distress, and those whose parents have witnessed apneas would have OSAS. Although the predictive positive value was acceptable (50–75%), this was not true for the predictive negative value (25–80%).

Nonrestful sleep Unrestful sleep is the consequence of repeated micro-awakenings during sleep. Parents usually describe a child who moves and has diverse postures during sleep, sometimes with the head in hyperextension.

Frequent awakening Such awakenings are a commonly reported clinical situation. At first, parents may believe that this is related to behavior, hunger, or thirst during sleep.

Night sweats Night sweats are the result of respiratory distress during sleep and micro-awakenings and movements. It can be observed in an important number of children affected.

Enuresis Enuresis has been reported in 8–47% of children with OSAS. A recent study has shown that two thirds of the children with this syndrome have primary enuresis, and one third of them have secondary enuresis. The risk of presenting with enuresis is greater in all children with SBD, even when do not suffer from this syndrome.

Daytime Symptoms

In many children with OSAS, symptoms may be the result of sleep disruption that involves an alteration during the day. In contrast with adults, in which day sleepiness is characteristic, children present this symptom with less frequency. Attentional deficit and clear hyperactivity may be present. Also, these diseases have been associated with poor school performance. Children with adenotonsillar hypertrophy may present as well with mouth breathing, recurrent respiratory infections, and language problems. Morning headaches are infrequent in children with OSA.

Extrapulmonary Clinical Manifestations

Children with OSAS are frequent users of health services. They present recurrent respiratory infections such as pharyngitis, otitis, and bronchitis in greater frequency than in control subjects. After surgery for tonsils and adenoids, visits to health services are significantly reduced.

Growth

Growth failure and delay are classic consequences described during decades in OSAS. The main causes related to these consequences are these:

1. Low caloric intake: Children with tonsillar hypertrophy lack appetite and have dysphagia, which causes a low caloric intake.
2. Increase of energy expenditure because of the respiratory work increase during sleep.
3. Growth hormone (GH) secretion is altered in children with OSAS. Insulin growth factor type-1 (IGF-1) is reduced in these children. After tonsils and adenoid surgery it is common to observe weight gain and the reestablishment of normal GH and IGF-1 values.

Cardiovascular Manifestations

Lung hypertension is one of the most common causes of cardiovascular complications in children. The first cases described in the literature in the 1960s show how nasopharyngeal obstruction caused cardiomegaly, *cor pulmonale*, and severe lung edema. Currently, a reduction in the frequency of these complications has been observed. Diagnosis is done through an echography, where the degree of tricuspid failure can be estimated, as well as a ventricular failure.

Systemic arterial hypertension is also a frequent complication in children with OSAS, and it should be timely diagnosed. According to some reports, diastolic tensional numbers during sleep persist during wakefulness hours in these children. A recently studied group of children showed changes in the left ventricular wall, besides an increase in the afterload. Arrhythmias have also been observed in these children.

Development and Neurocognitive Symptoms

Concentration problems, hyperactivity, and learning difficulties have been consistently documented in children with OSAS. Even from the first reports from the nineteenth century, attention and neurocognitive problems have been related to this syndrome.

There is solid evidence supporting the association between OSAS, respiratory sleep disorders, even primary snoring, with attentional deficit with hyperactivity in children. Although we currently have this evidence, it is not possible to attribute syndrome causality in this association. Children with this syndrome present symptoms suggesting attentional deficit, without having all the criteria for attentional deficit with hyperactivity.

Although daytime sleepiness is more common in children, it has been estimated that many children with hyperactivity or attention problems will afterward develop some degree of sleepiness.

Learning problems and poor school performance are considered as one of the most severe consequences of OSAS. An extremely high prevalence of this syndrome was reported in first-degree students in a study conducted in the United States. Besides this, an important improvement of school performance could be confirmed after adenotonsillectomy. A recent retrospective study suggests that children who frequently snore have a greater risk of developing neurocognitive problems, which do not seem to be completely reversible. In our center, a study has shown an improvement in neurocognitive alterations in long-term follow-up of children between 5 and 9 years old after adenotonsillectomy, showing results which could be compared to those of children who do not snore.

It is likely that both intermittent hypoxemia as well as the disruption in sleep architecture have a role in the pathogeny and neurocognitive consequences associated with this syndrome in children. Studies in adults could show a correlation between blood gases and neurocognitive performance. The degree of night hypoxemia has been positively related to the seriousness of the consequences in attention measurement tests, problem-solving tests, and short-term memory tests. Deficits in executive functions have generally been associated with problems in the prefrontal cortex of patients with this syndrome. In some cases, these alterations would persist despite the treatment.

OSAS in Children with Craniofacial Dysmorphology

Adenotonsillar growth is the main risk factor for the appearance of OSAS in children. Other risk factors are obesity, family predisposition, race, and prematurity. Nevertheless, there are patients with genetic syndromes that have constantly been associated to OSAS. These syndromes include those related to micrognathia and midface hypoplasia.

Pierre Robin sequence Consists in the triad of micrognathia, tongue placed further back than normal, and cleft palate; it is frequently associated to SBD. It usually appears early during life, even in newborns. Infants may develop reflux or stridor related to this condition. Treatment includes jaw distraction, intraoral devices, and eventually continuous positive airway pressure (CPAP).

Treacher Collins syndrome Caused by mutations in chromosome 5 (5q32-32.2), which codifies a treacle protein, this syndrome causes jaw hypoplasia, malar hypoplasia, antimongoloid palpebral fissure, and characteristic fascia Coloboma and ocular alterations may also be present.

Among other causes of midface hypoplasia we can mention the Crouzon, Apert, and Pfeiffer syndrome. In these children, the worsening of OSAS can be invariably observed in different degrees as they grow up.

Achondroplasia is another strongly related condition to OSAS. It is characterized by a dominant skeletal dysplasia, which frequently causes obstruction but also central apneas. Up to two thirds of the patients will required noninvasive ventilation as treatment.

Children with Down syndrome will usually present with OSAS because of their hypotonia, a smaller size of craniofacial structures, and a smaller nose. Also, it has been possible to observe an increase in adenotonsillar tissue in patients with Down syndrome, easing the appearance of OSAS.

Arnold Chiari-type malformations may be associated with a greater risk to suffering from this symptom, because of the compression of the brainstem. Nevertheless, respiratory drive compromise, as well as compromise of the nuclei of the cranial nerves, can cause the appearance of central apneas.

Children with Prader–Willi syndrome, consisting of hypotonia, obesity, hypogonadism, and some degree of cognitive impairment, may very frequently present with OSAS, and therefore they should be considered at risk. At the same time, all patients with mucopolysaccharidosis will present with a narrowing of the airway caused by the deposit of mucopolysaccharides, including tongue, pharynx, trachea, and bronchi. Usually, adenotonsillectomy is not useful, and it may require CPAP or even tracheotomy in selected cases.

Obesity and OSAS

Obesity in children significantly increases the risk to develop OSAS. Its persistence after adenotonsillectomy is significantly greater in obese children in comparison to their non-obese peers. Besides this, there are certain distinct physiopathological mechanisms in this syndrome associated to obesity. Considering these differences, a classification was created: OSAS type I refers to children with adenotonsillar hypertrophy who are not obese, and OSAS type II refers to obese children without adenoid and/or amygdale hypertrophy.

OSAS and Asthma

Asthma and OSAS share several epidemiological risks. Further, patients with asthma tend to have a greater development risk in comparison to those patients who do not have asthma. It seems that asthma and OSAS involve a common inflammatory and physiopathological mechanism. One of the modifiable asthma risk factors in children is precisely SBD. OSAS treatment is related to a stabilization and eventual symptomatic improvement in children with asthma.

OSAS and Inflammation

Some recent studies show that both children and adults with OSAS present local and systemic inflammation. Inflammatory changes found show an activation of different inflammatory paths, such as lipoxygenase, which is involved in other inflammatory conditions in children and adults, such as allergic asthma and rhinitis. In children with OSAS, an increase in local and systemic leukotrienes has been observed. An increase in C-reactive protein in the blood level in children with OSAS is probably the best evidence of systemic inflammation. It has been possible to correlate the levels of C-reactive protein in these patients to the indexes of apnea, hypopnea, desaturations, and micro-awakenings. Several other inflammatory markers have been studied in children with OSAS: interleukin-6, interferon-gamma, interleukin (IL-8), tumor necrosis factor (TNF)-α, and fibrinogen. It is difficult to differentiate between the inflammatory mechanisms that cause a sleep respiratory disorder and those which are secondary to this disease. Therefore, it is not clear if inflammation is the cause or the effect of OSAS. The importance of identifying OSAS-related inflammatory mechanisms lies in the possibility of using antiinflammatory medication as treatment.

Diagnosis

The first step to diagnose OSAS is the identification of high-risk children; for example, those with craniofacial malformations, neuromuscular weakness, and genetic conditions. In healthy children it should be suspected if there is snoring, movements during sleep, awakenings, night sweats, and enuresis. Other symptoms to consider are behavioral problems, school or performance problems, hyperactivity, and concentration problems. It must be clear that clinical history by itself is insufficient to diagnose OSAS, and it is not possible to differentiate primary snoring using only the interview.

Recent recommendations of the American Academy of Sleep Medicine include directly asking about snoring in every well-child care visit. The first stage of physical examination is observation to recognize alterations such as micrognathia, Pierre Robin sequence, or craniofacial dysmorphisms. Genetic diseases, such as Down syndrome, are known risk factors to develop OSAS. In healthy children, body mass index must be calculated, because obesity has been associated to a greater OSAS prevalence. Characteristic adenoid facia and mouth breathing are present in many children with OSAS. It is important to observe and define tonsillar size, which is clinically determined by the occupying space in the oropharynx inspection. Tonsils that occupy about 25% or less of the pharyngeal space are defined as grade 1, <50%, grade 2, <75%, grade 3, and those that touch in the medial line are grade 4 (kissing tonsils).

Laboratory Exams

Night polysomnography is considered the gold standard to diagnose OSAS in children. Nevertheless, other tools and exams can be used for screening.

Lateral neck X-ray could indicate adenoidal hypertrophy. Direct visualization is only possible through nasoendoscopy, which is much more reliable than X-rays. Electrocardiogram and echocardiography may show signs of hypertrophy in the right cavities, and even lung hypertension in advanced stages of the disease. The use of video or audio recordings in the patient's home has been suggested as a diagnosis option with a good positive predictive value (>90%), but with a poor negative predictive value (<30%). Night pulse oximetry is another simple way to detect serious presentations of OSAS. Unfortunately, it is not an acceptable tool, because of its poor negative predictive value (<50%). These observations have been confirmed in adults with OSAS. Besides this, because most events happen during REM sleep, abbreviated polysomnography or nap studies are no longer recommended.

Night polysomnography done in a sleep laboratory is considered the gold standard to diagnose OSAS in children. Nevertheless, the precise sensitivity and specificity of polysomnography have not been stablished with certainty. The recommendation of the American Academy of Sleep Medicine is to conduct polysomnography in children who snore for whom a diagnosis has not been made for clinical or observational reasons. Polysomnography is very useful to determine the degree of OSAS severity based on an index. Polysomnography includes electroencephalography channels to study micro-awakenings and phases of sleep. It also includes electro-oculography, electrocardiography, chin and leg movement electromyography, nasal flow, chest and abdominal movements, $ETCO_2$, snoring, and body position. In very selected cases, pHmetry, intraesophageal pressure, and video recording can be used.

Polysomnography studies in children are done in sleep laboratories, especially adapted and with qualified staff to read the studies in these children. The use of drugs or sedatives to induce sleep is not recommended.

Stages

Wakefulness/sleep and sleep stages can be divided according to the recommendations of Rechtschaffen and Kales in 1968. In 2007 a change was made in the new guidelines of the American Academy of Sleep Medicine. Micro-awakenings should be evaluated with the consensus recommendation of the American Academy of Sleep Medicine. To summarize, they define awakenings as a wakefulness time of more than 15 s in the electroencephalogram. Micro-awakenings and awakenings index is calculated as the number of these events per sleep hour.

Obstructive apneas and hypopneas should be identified according to the consensus of the American Academy of Sleep Medicine. The hypopnea–apnea index is calculated considering all the respiratory events corresponding to apnea or hypopnea divided by the hours of sleep. Average SpO_2 should also be recorded in the polysomnography record. Desaturation index is calculated as the number of desaturation events with 4 or more percentage points per hour of sleep. The consolidated time the child spent under 90% of SpO_2 is also added to the report.

Treatment

Medical Treatment

Medications for OSAS include using of intranasal steroids and leukotriene receptor antagonists. Improvement has been consistently confirmed in the parameters of polysomnography for those patients who use these medications versus placebo. In a noncontrolled study our group could even confirm an improvement in children with mild OSAS. A randomized, controlled, double-blind study conducted by Goldbart et al. showed that a 12-week treatment with daily montelukast reduces OSAS severity and tonsils size. By comparing 23 patients treated with daily montelukast to 23 untreated patients, a reduction in the size of the adenoids, and improvement in the symptoms, as well as in several polysomnography indexes, could be observed. The hypopnea–apnea index was reduced by more than 50% in 65.2% of the children treated. Besides this, its use in children with moderate to severe OSAS requires more evidence before it may be recommended.

Surgical Treatment

Because adenotonsillar hypertrophy is the most frequent and important cause of the OSAS in children, adenotonsillectomy is proposed as the first-line treatment for this disease.

Adenotonsillectomy is a very common procedure with a very low rate of complications, but a possible rate of morbidity and mortality should be considered. Adenotonsillectomy must be as objective as possible, ideally with a previous diagnostic polysomnography. Risk factors for the development of complications after surgery in children with OSAS are age under 3 years, severe OSAS, *cor pulmonale*, growth alteration, morbid obesity, neuromuscular diseases, prematurity, and craniofacial alterations.

Most children with OSAS improve in symptomatology after surgery; thus, their indexes of hypopnea apnea, night hypoxemia, and micro-awakenings are reduced. Studies comparing pre- and post-adenotonsillectomy conditions in children with OSAS have shown an improvement in the right ventricular function, increase in growth factors, improvement in life quality and behavior, reduction of general morbidity, and less need of health services.

A recent multicenter, randomized study compared adenotonsillectomy with a follow-up observation in children with OSAS. Investigators included 464 children, from 5 to 9 years old, to one of the two aforementioned treatments. Polysomnography and neurocognitive test series were evaluated at baseline and 7 months after that. A significant improvement in symptoms was confirmed, but there were no important differences in relation to neurocognitive testing of either group. A detailed analysis showed that more than 50% of non-obese children and more than 50% of non-Afro-American children in the control group (only receiving follow-up without surgery) would not be within the normal values for polysomnography. It has been concluded that medical treatment and very close follow-up may be an option for those patients with a milder form of OSAS.

Also, those children who present symptoms and have a hypopnea index greater than 5.0 should be considered candidates for surgery. In these cases, the suggestion is to conduct a polysomnography evaluation, besides analyzing the clinical symptoms and consequences the patients are presenting. A multidisciplinary team, composed of sleep expert physicians, otorhinolaryngologists, maxillofacial specialists, and respiratory physicians, would be of great help. The surgery to perform is still under debate. Tonsils and adenoids extirpation is suggested, but it should be discussed in randomized future studies. Particularly, the group of smaller children and infants should be studied to find the best treatment possible.

Uvulopalatopharyngoplasty, diversions, tongue surgeries, osteotomy, and hyoid suspensions should be considered only for exceptional cases of children with OSAS, and not as a first-line treatment. In some rare cases, usually related to an underlying disease, tracheotomy is required.

CPAP

Continuous positive airway pressure (CPAP) in children without adenotonsillar hypertrophy and with severe sleep obstructive apneas has been seldom used. In high-risk groups such as children with Down syndrome, morbid obesity, and neuromuscular defects, CPAP is a very effective therapy, and it is an option to adenotonsillar surgery, which in these cases may fail. The use of nasal CPAP is generally safe and well tolerated in children and even in infants with obstructive sleep apneas. The treatment should be long term. It is recommended to do a titer measurement with a polysomnography to evaluate the pressure range at which the respiratory events, such as apneas and hypopneas, disappear.

Oxygen

There are cases in which oxygen can be used as a transition treatment toward a definitive one, but in general its use is not routinely recommended for children with obstructive sleep apnea.

Sources

American Academy of Pediatrics. Section on Pediatric Pulmonology, Subcommittee on Obstructive sleep apnea: Clinical practice guideline: diagnosis and management of childhood obstructive sleep apnea syndrome. Pediatrics. 2002;109:704–12.

American Thoracic Society. Standards and indications for cardiopulmonary sleep studies in children. Am J Respir Crit Care Med. 1996;153:866–78.

Chervin RD, Ruzicka DL, Archbold KH, Dillon J. Snoring predicts hyperactivity four years later. Sleep. 2005;28:885–90.

Friedman BC, Hendeles-Amitai A, Kozminzki E, Leiberman A, Friger M, Tarasiuk A, Tal A. Adenotonsillectomy improves neurocognitive function in children with obstructive sleep apnea syndrome. Sleep. 2003;26:999–1005.

Goldbart A, Greenberg-Dotan S, Tal A. Montelukast for children with obstructive sleep apnea: a double-blind, placebo-controlled study. Pediatrics. 2012;130:e575–80.

Gozal D. Sleep-disordered breathing and school performance in children. Pediatrics. 1998;102:616–20.

Marcus CL, Moore RH, Rosen CL, the Childhood Adenotonsillectomy Trial (CHAT). A randomized trial of adenotonsillectomy for childhood sleep apnea. N Engl J Med. 2013;368:2366–76.

Marcus CL, Omlin KJ, Basinski DJ, Bailey SL, Rachel AB, Von Pechman WS, Keens TG, Ward SL. Normal polysomnogram values for children and adolescents. Am Rev Respir Dis. 1992;146:1235–9.

Tal A, Bar A, Leiberman A, Tarasiuk A. Sleep characteristics following adenotonsillectomy in children with obstructive sleep apnea syndrome. Chest. 2003;124:948–53.

Tarasiuk A, Simon T, Tal A, Reuveni H. Adenotonsillectomy in children with obstructive sleep apnea syndrome reduces health care utilization. Pediatrics. 2004;113:351–6.

Sudden Infant Death Syndrome 49

María Angélica Oyarzún
and Pablo Brockmann Veloso

Contents

Introduction

Sudden infant death syndrome (SIDS) is the main cause of death in children under 1 year old in developed countries. It is defined as such when a child dies before the first year of life and, after an exhaustive physical examination, laboratory exams, autopsy, and inspection of the place where the infant dies, it is not possible to state a definite cause of death.

M. A. Oyarzún (✉)
Pontificia Universidad Católica de Chile, Santiago, Chile

P. Brockmann Veloso
Department of Pediatrics, School of Medicine, Pontificia Universidad Católica de Chile, Santiago, Chile
e-mail: pbrockmann@med.puc.cl

Its diagnosis involves ruling out other possible death causes, and it forces the physician to exhaust all other probable diseases involved in this type of events, justifying the implementation of strict investigation protocols, as well as ruling out differential diagnosis. Detailed necropsies are also needed.

During past decades, countries in the Northern Hemisphere have started prevention campaigns that have demonstrated an important reduction in the mortality caused by this syndrome. One of them is the campaign "back to sleep," in European countries and in North America, recommending that parents place their children in dorsal supine position when sleeping. With this intervention, a great reduction of the number of cases of sudden death has been observed in this group.

P. Bertrand, I. Sánchez (eds.), *Pediatric Respiratory Diseases*,
https://doi.org/10.1007/978-3-030-26961-6_49

Epidemiology

SIDS incidence varies. Some series conducted in the United States of America show an approximate frequency of 0.5/1000 live births: It is more common in black children and less common in Hispanic children. In South America, specifically in Argentina, a review showed an incidence of 0.49 every 1000 live births, and in a more restricted group in the South of Brazil, a rate of 0.55 every 1000 live births was observed.

A recently published Chilean study identified 1442 cases reported as sudden deaths between 1997 and 2009, with a rate of 0.45 every 1000 live births. This rate was similar to the average of developed countries during the 1990s, before prevention campaigns, comparable to those published in neighboring countries, but still very distant from the rates of Netherlands and Japan, with 0.1 and 0.16 every 1000 living births, respectively.

A recent publication (Hauck and Tanabe) gathered information about sudden death in 13 countries and showed a generalized reduction, with ranges oscillating between 40% and 87%. This decrease may be related to the implementation of educational campaigns since 1990, which informed the general population about sudden death and its prevention. One of these campaigns was the already mentioned "back to sleep," through which a significant reduction was achieved, once that it was established as a public health policy. In Chile, a decrease of 25% has been recorded in a period of 13 years, which is a lower reduction rate than those experienced in the mentioned countries. Although in our countries there is a general knowledge about the recommendation of the dorsal decubitus position, massive health campaigns are still not in place. Another factor that could contribute to the reduction in the rates of sudden death is the increase of other causes of unexpected sudden deaths of children. This factor is explained by the advances and optimization for investigating the cause of deaths, recognizing other child deaths related to sleep, such as asphyxia mortality, accidental suffocation or strangulation in the bed, and poorly defined or unspecified deaths, which are usually related to prone positions, co-sleeping, and using soft surfaces/cushions for sleeping.

Etiology

For years, multiple studies have approached sudden death, which has increased the knowledge about related factors. Nevertheless, its etiology is still not clear. SIDS is a multifactorial polygenic condition, whose main factors are genetic, environmental, and sociocultural. The "triple risk model" proposed by Wedgwood in 1972, and supported by studies conducted afterwards by Kahn et al., explains this phenomenon according to three factors: (1) inherent patient risk; (2) risk age; and (3) predisposing condition.

A sudden alteration in the awakening threshold has recently been proposed as the main mechanism in sudden death. Anomalies in the serotonin receptors in the ventral medulla have been reported, possibly because of a dysfunction in the cardiorespiratory responses to excitation/awakening. Also, some studies have shown a greater frequency of certain polymorphisms of a gene of the serotonin transport protein in infants who died because of sudden death. Polymorphisms in the gene of the sodium channel have also been described, which is associated with a prolonged QT interval, as well as genes that affect the development of the autonomic nervous system. Therefore, certain children may have a genetic predisposition that manifests when certain triggers are present, such as tobacco exposure or prone decubitus position.

Risk Factors and Clinical Presentation

There are multiple risk factors related to SIDS. The triple risk model proposes that this is caused by an inherent vulnerability, age, and exogenous damage. Age is considered as one the most important factors involved, as most of the cases correspond to children between 3 and 5 months of life (90% happens before 6 months).

Among the factors described as part of this inherent vulnerability are the alterations in the awakening when certain stimuli, such as hypoxemia and hypercarbia, appear. Awakening control would be less developed in some patients, particularly in premature babies. This particular vulnerable situation may be worsened by external factors, such as prone position while sleeping, respiratory infections, smoking at home, excessive blankets, and co-sleeping. In the national study it was confirmed that almost 25% of the cases would be premature babies. As it was shown in previous publications, boys have a greater rate than girls, and the reason for this is unknown. Besides this, several parameters related to low socioeconomic level were notably present, such as the educational level of the mother. This information corroborates what has been found in international studies that have associated low socioeconomic level and overcrowding with sudden death.

Other noticeable characteristics of sudden death in Chile are the distribution of cases within the year, showing an increase during winter months (Fig. 49.1), and geographic distribution, which shows an increase in the southern parts of the country (Fig. 49.2). The reasons for this geographic difference could be several, as, for example, a different prevalence rate of respiratory diseases, different sleep habits, or a greater accuracy in the notification of the disease. Nevertheless, these hypotheses must be confirmed in future studies.

Pacifier Several studies, including two meta-analysis, have supported the use of a pacifier as a protective factor with an OR adjusted 0.39–0.48. The mechanism through which its use would reduce sudden death rate is not clear, and a reduction in the excitation threshold, or autonomic response during the sleep transition to awakening, have been proposed as explanations. In this age group, it has been confirmed that using a pacifier does not cause breastfeeding or odontological problems. The American Academy of Pediatrics recommends the use of the pacifier as a strategy to reduce the risk of SIDS, and it should be introduced once breastfeeding has been well established, after 2–4 weeks of age.

Smoking Maternal smoking increases the risk of SIDS up to 40 fold. Both prenatal and postnatal smoking have been associated. Besides this, there are studies relating in-home smoke of any family member with sudden death. This habit is one of the preventable factors most strongly related to the disease.

Vaccines There is no current evidence relating sudden death to vaccines and immunizations.

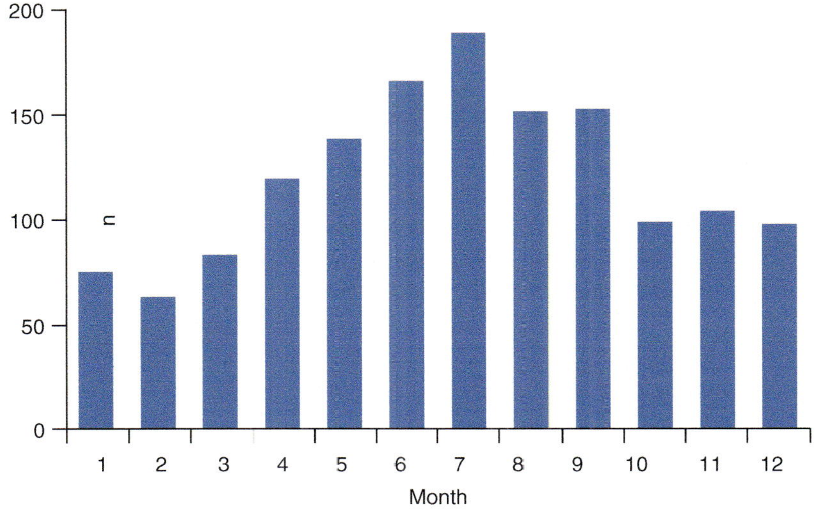

Fig. 49.1 Sudden infant death (SID) in Chile (1997–2009) (n = 1442): seasonal distribution of 1442 SID in Chile

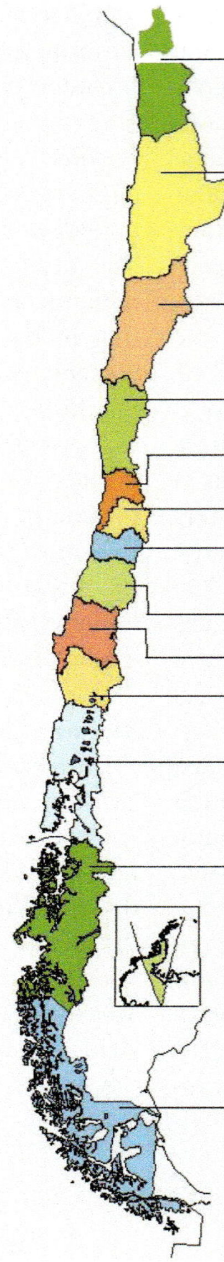

Fig. 49.2 Sudden infant death rate

There are reports relating cases of diphtheria, tetanus, and pertussis vaccine to sudden death, although there is no information supporting this statement. A meta-analysis published in 2007 showed that immunization reduced the risk of SIDS in 46%.

Maternal breastfeeding The protective role of maternal breastfeeding has been discussed over the years, but the experts have still not issued a consensus. Some recent reports, including a meta-analysis in 2011, show a protective effect of maternal breastfeeding against SIDS, with an approximate reduction of 50% when the child is breastfed, and this effect would be greater when the child is exclusively breastfed. Physiological studies have shown that breastfed infants have a lower awakening threshold in comparison to their peers who received formula, which could support the argument of the protection of breastfeeding against sudden death. Other possible reasons for this protective effect include the prevention of infectious diseases and global immune benefits.

SIDS and ALTE The association between sudden death and an apparent life-threatening event (ALTE) is still controversial. Although it is the main cause of death of children suffering from an ALTE, only 3% to 7% of infants who died of sudden death have had a previous ALTE episode. There is still not enough evidence sustaining such an association.

Prevention and Approach

Reducing sudden death risk lies in controlling and eliminating the risk factors already mentioned, and therefore recommendations for "safe sleeping" have been published (Fig. 49.3).

1. *Promote supine position for sleeping infants.* An association between prone position and an increase of SIDS rate has been confirmed. After the massive introduction of the campaign "back to sleep," a reduction in the rate of sudden infant death could be observed in the countries that applied it. It has been shown that sleeping in lateral position has increased the number of death cases caused by sudden death, and therefore it should not be recommended as an alternative.
2. *Avoid prone and decubitus lateral positions.* As it has been previously pointed out, all other positions, with the exception of supine decubitus, are dangerous, and should be avoided. Prone and lateral position have shown a reduction in the micro-awakening thresholds.
3. *Avoid having too soft surfaces where the infant sleeps.*
4. *Avoid soft objects such as plush toys, blankets, and similar items in the crib of the infant.* Suffocation caused by any soft item near the infant must be avoided.
5. *Suspend maternal tobacco use and postnatal exposure to tobacco.* Tobacco use is the main modifiable factor to prevent sudden death. Both prenatal and postnatal tobacco exposure have been related to an increased chance of SIDS.
6. *Suggest that the infant sleeps close (in a crib) to the parents.* It is not recommended that infants and parents sleep in the same bed. Co-sleeping is not recommended.
7. *Do not use excessive blankets during sleep.*
8. *Do not use a cardiorespiratory monitor as a preventive method for sudden death.* It should only be indicated when it is really justified.

No known study has confirmed a real prevention of SIDS when using cardiorespiratory monitors. "Apneas" as the sole mechanism are not convincing as a reliable cause of sudden death. The Collaborative Home Infant Monitoring Evaluation (CHIME) 26, which included more than 1000 patients in California, showed similar

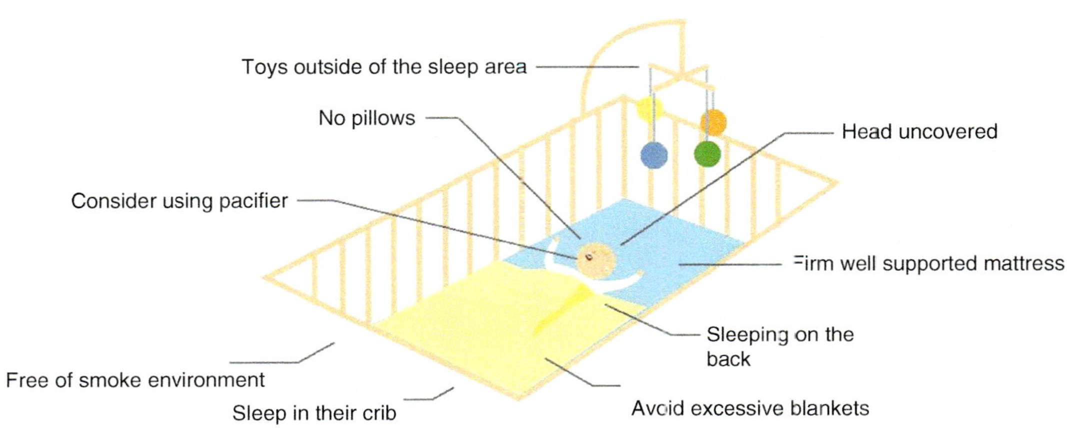

Fig. 49.3 Recommendations for "safe sleeping"

sudden death rates in groups with and without cardiorespiratory monitors. Further, it is well documented that patients correctly connected to a cardiorespiratory monitor have died.

9. *Consider using a pacifier when sleeping.* However, its use must not be forced once the child lets go of it.

Conclusions

Although reduction in its rate has been confirmed, sudden infant death syndrome is still one of the main causes of death in this age group. As a health team, we must know about its existence and the factors associated to the population. Delivering consistent messages and use of public health campaigns are crucial to reduce the generalized feeling that these deaths are unavoidable.

Sources

Ball HL, Volpe LE. Sudden infant death syndrome (SIDS) risk reduction and infant sleep location—moving the discussion forward. Soc Sci Med. 2013;79:84–91.

Beckwith JB. Defining the sudden infant death syndrome. Arch Pediatr Adolesc Med. 2003;157(3):286–90.

Brockmann P, Oyarzún MA, Villarroel L, Bertrand P. Sindrome de muerte súbita del lactante: prevalencia y cambios en los últimos años en Chile. Rev Méd Chile. 2013;141:589–94.

Brockmann PE, Abara S, Campos C, et al. Consenso sobre el manejo de eventos de aparente amenaza a la vida del lactante (ALTE). Comisión de Sueño de Sochinep, 2013. Rev Chil Pediatr. 2014;85(3):378–87.

Carpenter RG, Irgens LM, Blair PS, England PD, Fleming P, Huber J, et al. Sudden unexplained infant death in 20 regions in Europe: case control study. Lancet. 2004;363(9404):185–91.

Franco P, Szliwowski H, Dramaix M, Kahn A. Decreased autonomic responses to obstructive sleep events in future victims of sudden infant death syndrome. Pediatr Res. 1999;46(1):33–9.

Guntheroth WG, Spiers PS. The triple risk hypotheses in sudden infant death syndrome. Pediatrics. 2002;110(5):e64.

Hauck FR, Tanabe KO. International trends in sudden infant death syndrome: stabilization of rates requires further action. Pediatrics. 2008;122(3):660–6.

Hauck FR, Thompson JM, Tanabe KO, Moon RY, Vennemann MM. Breastfeeding and reduced risk of sudden infant death syndrome: a metaanalysis. Pediatrics. 2011;128(1):103–10.

Horne RS, Sly DJ, Cranage SM, Chau B, Adamson TM. Effects of prematurity on arousal from sleep in the newborn infant. Pediatr Res. 2000;47(4 pt 1):468–74.

Kahn A. Sudden and unexplained infant death. Bull Mem Acad R Med Belg. 1983;138(3):225–35.

Leach CE, Blair PS, Fleming PJ, Smith IJ, Platt MW, Berry PJ, et al. Epidemiology of SIDS and explained sudden infant deaths. CESDI SUDI Research Group. Pediatrics. 1999;104(4):e43.

Mitchell EA, Blair PS, L'Hoir MP. Should pacifiers be recommended to prevent sudden infant death syndrome? Pediatrics. 2006;117(5):1755–8.

Moon RY, Fu L. Sudden infant death syndrome: an update. Pediatr Rev. 2012;33(7):314–20.

Sawaguchi T, Namiki M. Recent trend of the incidence of sudden infant death syndrome in Japan. Early Hum Dev. 2003;75(suppl):S175–9.

Task Force on Sudden Infant Death Syndrome, Moon RY. SIDS and other sleep-related infant deaths: expansion of recommendations for a safe infant sleeping environment. Pediatrics. 2011;128(5):1030–9.

Vennemann MM, Höffgen M, Bajanowski T, Hense HW, Mitchell EA. Do immunisations reduce the risk for SIDS? A metaanalysis. Vaccine. 2007; 25(26):4875–9.

Wedgwood R, editor. Review of USA experience. Sudden and unexpected death in infancy (cot deaths). Bristol: Wright; 1972.

Willinger M, James LS, Catz C. Defining the sudden infant death syndrome (SIDS): deliberations of an expert pan-el convened by the National Institute of Child Health and Human Development. Pediatr Pathol. 1991;11(5):677–84.

Primary Immunodeficiencies and Immune Diseases

50

Eduardo Talesnik Guendelman
and Cecilia Méndez Rivera

Contents

E. Talesnik Guendelman (✉) · C. Méndez Rivera
Pediatrics, Immunology and Rheumatology, Pontificia
Universidad Católica de Chile, Santiago, Chile
e-mail: etalesni@med.puc.cl

P. Bertrand, I. Sánchez (eds.), *Pediatric Respiratory Diseases*,
https://doi.org/10.1007/978-3-030-26961-6_50

Introduction

Immunodeficiencies are a heterogeneous group of diseases caused by one or more alterations in the immune system. The most common clinical manifestation tends to be a predisposition to infections. Immunodeficiencies may be primary, associated with genetic disorders, or acquired immunodeficiency diseases of the immune system.

Clinical history and physical examination are key in the differential diagnosis of the different predisposing causes of recurrent respiratory infections, secondary immunodeficiencies, and primary immunodeficiencies (PID). Predisposing factors of recurrent infections are more frequent than secondary immunodeficiencies, and these are more common than PID (Table 50.1).

Recurrent viral respiratory infections are common in children under 2 years old, whose immune system is still maturing, and they are caused by exposure to infectious agents at home or at daycare. Six or more high respiratory tract infections during the first years of life are considered normal. Tobacco exposure is also a relevant predisposing factor for recurrent respiratory diseases.

Recurrent lung suppurative infections in the same site suggest malformation, obstruction, or foreign object in the airway. In contrast, aspiration related to oropharyngeal incoordination, gastroesophageal reflux, cystic fibrosis, ciliary dyskinesia, and alpha-1-antitrypsin deficiency, as well as PID and secondary immunodeficiencies (SID), should be considered in patients who have a history of recurrent multifocal pneumonia.

Allergy is a common predisposing factor for recurrent respiratory infections, and inadequate treatment in patients with asthma and allergic rhinitis has been associated with pneumonia and recurrent sinusitis, respectively.

Table 50.1 Recurrent respiratory infections

A. Predisposing factors
Immune system development in children under 2 years old
Lack of maternal breastfeeding
Family exposition to infections (number of brothers)
Daycare attendance
Passive smoking
Allergy
B. Secondary immunodeficiencies
Diseases with anatomical compromise: Adenoid hypertrophy, airway malformations, foreign body, bronchiectasis, ciliary dyskinesia, congenital heart diseases, splenectomy, aspiration associated with oropharyngeal incoordination, gastroesophageal reflux, etc.
Diseases with systemic compromise: Cystic fibrosis, alpha-1-antitrypsin deficiency, malnutrition, neoplasia, systemic lupus erythematosus, nephrotic syndrome, HIV infection, measles, etc.
Drugs and immune reconstitution: Bone marrow transplant, steroids, immunosuppressors, etc.
C. Primary immunodeficiencies
Innate immunity
Acquired immunity

In children and adolescents with recurrent respiratory infections, the possible association of two or more causes should be considered; for example, allergic rhinitis and asthma, both related to adenoid hypertrophy, or alterations in antibody immunity, such as polysaccharide antibody deficiency.

Considering the wide differential diagnosis in children and adolescents with recurrent infections, the clinical and imaging studies, besides the laboratory tests to be requested, depend on the clinical orientation of each individual case.

Primary Immunodeficiencies (PID)

More than 200 PID have been described, and most of them have been identified as to the causative gene. Diagnosis should be done under high suspicion, as delays in diagnosis are frequent and are related to greater morbidity and mortality. PID are characterized by a greater susceptibility to infections, but there is also an increased risk for autoimmunity, and less frequently, cancer. Incidence has been estimated as 1 in every 10,000 live births to 2 in every 20,000 live births, although relative incidence is variable. Some are frequent, such as IgA deficiency, with incidence up to 1 in 700, and most are very infrequent, such as severe combined immunodeficiency, with an incidence estimated as 1 in 100,000. Onset age spans from newborn to adult life, but the clinical manifestations of most of these diseases begin during childhood. Some of their presentations may be transient during childhood, and others develop as the patient grows.

PID may be monogenic or polygenic and may compromise one or more of its components (innate immune response, antibody adaptive immune response, cellular immunity, phagocytes, or complement system).

Essential genes for immune function are distributed along the genome; nevertheless, a dominance of immunodeficiency is associated to the X chromosome, as a result of homozygosity in males, but also from frequent and new spontaneous mutations of these genes related to the X chromosome. PID have also been recognized as autosomal recessive, as autosomal dominant, and others that do not have an evident inheritance pattern. Different clinical syndromes may be caused by different mutations in the same gene, and the same syndrome may be caused by different genetic causes. PID by chromosomal deletion have been described, such as 22q11,2, with a DiGeorge syndrome phenotype.

Clinical history suggesting PID:

- Consanguineous parents
- Family history of serious infections in small children or deaths caused by infections in children, adolescents, or young adults.
- PID diagnosed in siblings or family, where there are no clinical symptoms.
- Lung, sinus, and otic recurrent suppurative bacterial infections: four or more episodes of acute otitis within 1 year, two or more episodes of acute sinusitis within 1 year, two or more episodes of pneumonia within 1 year.
- Lung, sinus, and otic chronic infections.
- Infections caused by opportunistic agents.
- Need to use IV antibiotics to treat infections.
- Persistent infections with poor or no response to antibiotic treatments.
- Recurrent cutaneous or organ abscess.
- Failure to thrive.
- Recurrent lung infections associated to persistent or chronic diarrhea, intestinal malabsorption, chronic sinusitis, bronchiectasis, neutropenia, or skin abscess.
- Recurrent infections associated with autoimmunity: among these, autoimmune cytopenia, thyroiditis, or rheumatological diseases.

- Two or more serious infections or sepsis
- Early-onset autoinmune diseases
- Adverse reactions to vaccines: paralytic polio, CGB dissemination
- Persistent ganglionar suppuration
- Recurrent or persistent candidiasis, oral or cutaneous
- Graft-versus-host reaction
- Combination of eczema and thrombocytopenia (Wiskott–Aldrich syndrome), ataxia and telangiectasia (ataxia-telangiectasia syndrome), delayed umbilical cord detachment, and soft tissue infections (leukocyte adhesion deficiency type 1), oculocutaneous albinism (Chediak–Higashi syndrome)

The respiratory system is one of the main organs targeted by infections in patients with PID. Besides the susceptibility to specific infections, the clinical presentation depends on the area of the immune system that has been compromised (Table 50.2).

Antibody PID is more frequent, followed by well-defined PID syndromes, PID combined cellular and antibodies, and phagocytes. The relative PID frequency can be observed in Table 50.3.

Table 50.2 Association between primary immunodeficiencies (PID) and infections

Infection immunodeficiency	
Cellular	Virus, fungus, gram-negative bacteria, protozoans, *Pneumocystis jirovecii*,
	Candida albicans, Calmette–Guérin bacillus (CGB)
Antibodies, complement: classic and alternative path, lectins, and C3 IRAK4	Extracellular bacteria: *Staphylococcus aureus*, *Streptococcus pneumoniae*, *Haemophilus influenzae*
Combined cellular and antibody	Opportunistic germs, extracellular bacteria
Phagocytes	*Staphylococcus aureus*, *Serratia*, *Nocardia*, *Aspergillus*
Complement terminal components: C5–C9	*Neisseria gonorrhoae* and *Neisseria meningitidis*
Cytokines: IFN-γ, IL-12	Mycobacteria, Calmette–Guérin bacillus (CGB, *Salmonella*)
Toll-like receptors (TLR) TLR-4	Meningococcus, pneumococcus, septic shock

Table 50.3 PID Frequency

PID antibodies	53.2
PID combined cellular and antibodies	9.5
PID defined syndromes	22.65
PID phagocytes	8.6
PID complement	2.8
Immune regulation alterations	3.3

Source: Registro Latinoamericano IDP (LAGID). 3321 patients

Antibody Immunodeficiencies

Antibody PID, also called humoral PID, are usually related to otic, sinus, or lung recurrent infections. The most useful laboratory exams for the quantitative study of antibodies are serum immunoglobulins IgG, IgA, IgM, as well as the IgG subclasses (IgG1, IgG2, IgG3, IgG4), considering both reference tables for each age group. Qualitative response is measured through isohemagglutinins, preferring antibody response to vaccines, for instance, tetanus toxoid (diphtheria toxoid) to evaluate the response to protein antigens, and polysaccharide pneumococcal vaccine to evaluate the response to polysaccharide antigens. If the patient has one of the more serious presentations of PID, quantification of total B lymphocytes and B memory lymphocytes with isotopic changes is needed to conduct an advanced study.

Antibody immunodeficiencies are caused by development alterations of B lymphocytes. Figure 50.1 shows different stages of B-lymphocyte development, until the production of serum immunoglobulins.

X-linked agammaglobulinemia This immunodeficiency is related to the X chromosome. Its origin is the lack of development of B lymphocytes, caused by Bruton tyrosine kinase deficiency (Btk), which is essential for the development of B lymphocytes (Fig. 50.1). It is predominant in males starting at 6 months of life, without lymphatic ganglion and bacterial pyogenic recurrent infections caused by *Pseudomonas*, *Mycoplasma*, and enteroviral meningoencephalitis. Predominant infections are located in the upper and lower airway. As many as 50% of the patients develop chronic lung disease, bronchiectasis, atelectasis, and enlargement of the bronchial wall. Lymphocyte B count is very low or nonexistent, as well as serum immunoglobulins and antibody response to vaccines. Septic arthritis and gastrointestinal infections are also frequent.

Common variable immunodeficiency Common variable immunodeficiency (CVID) is the most common form of humoral PID, requiring monthly IV gamma globulin. It appears in children older than 2 years of age when alterations in the final stages of B lymphocytes develop.

Approximately 20% of the patients with CVID have a family history of PID, and specific genetic mutations have been found in 10% of these: transmembrane activator and CAML interactor (TACI), inducible costimulatory (ICOS), B-cell activating factor receptor (BAFF-R), and CD 19 (superficial molecule of B lymphocytes; binds to receptor antigen for B lymphocytes).

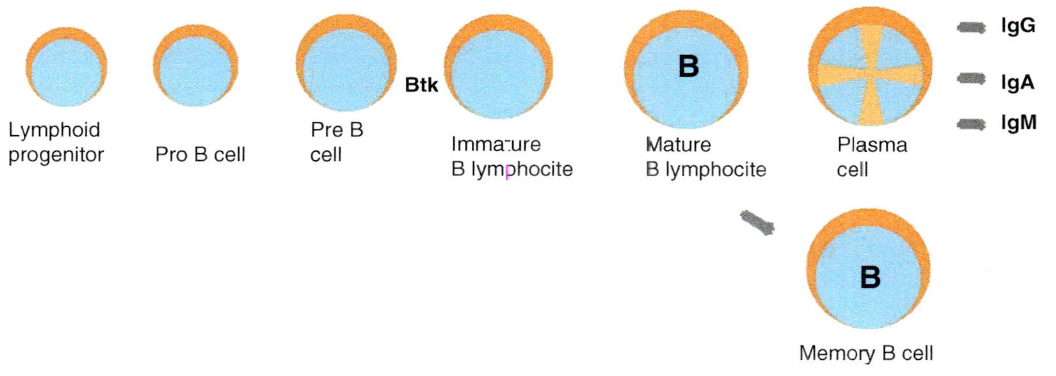

Fig. 50.1 Lymphoid cell development

More than 95% of the patients present with sinus and lung infections caused by non-typifying *Haemophilus influenzae* and *Streptococcus pneumoniae*. Infections caused by *Moraxella catarrhalis* and other *Streptococcus* sp. are less common. Infections caused by *Mycoplasma* have also been described. Recurrent bronchitis is the usual clinical presentation; this initially responds to antibiotics but may progress to bronchiectasis. Persistent sinusitis progresses to a chronic condition. Intestinal infections caused by *Giardia lamblia* and *Campylobacter jejuni*, as well as arthritis and meningoencephalitis caused by enterovirus, may also appear. Approximately 20% present with autoimmunity manifestations, and among these, cytopenia is the most common. Also, autoimmune thyroiditis, primary biliary cirrhosis, and rheumatological diseases have been found in the pediatric population. At the same time, these patients have a greater susceptibility to present with adenopathy, splenomegaly, lymphocytic interstitial pneumonia, gastrointestinal lymphoid hyperplasia, and lymphoreticular neoplasia.

The diagnostic criteria are IgG and IgA < 2 SD, usually related to IgM < 2 SD, considering age, absence of isohemagglutinins, poor response to vaccines composed of protein antigens (tetanus toxoid), and polysaccharide (polysaccharide pneumococcal vaccine, 23-valent), excluding the secondary causes of hypogammaglobulinemia. Lymphocyte B count is normal or low.

IgA deficiency This deficiency is the most common PID, occurring in 1 in 700 (1 in 396 to 1 in 2000) live births, and it is characterized by an IgA serum level less than 7 mg/dl, with normal IgG and IgM levels, in children over 4 years old. Most patients are asymptomatic, and some present with recurrent respiratory and gastrointestinal infections, in whom IgG2 deficiency and specific antibody deficiency should be studied. A greater frequency of chronic allergies and autoimmune diseases has been described, such as systemic lupus erythematosus, juvenile idiopathic arthritis, and rheumatoid arthritis.

IgG subclasses deficiency This deficiency is characterized by lack of IgG2, IgG3, or both, with a normal value for total IgG. IgG2 is a heterogeneous group of alterations, ranging from transient to persistent presentations, isolated or in combination with IgA deficiency or specific antibody deficiency. It appears with recurrent sinus and lung recurrent infections, otitis media, and disseminated infection caused by *Streptococcus pneumoniae*. Patients with IgG3 have the same type of infections, but these infections tend to be moderate and transient.

Specific antibody deficiency This is a frequent PID in children over 2 years old, characterized by a deficient specific response to polysaccharide antigens, with normal levels of serum immunoglobulin. In some patients, the immune response to pneumococcal conjugate vaccines is normal. Its pathogeny is unknown, and it has been estimated that it corresponds to 55% to 10% of children referred by recurrent infections. Specific antibody deficiency can be associated to other PIDs such as IgA deficiency, IgG2 subclasses, Wiskott–Aldrich syndrome, and deletion 22q11,2, DiGeorge syndrome phenotype.

Specific antibody deficiency has been found in children with their complete scheme of conjugate pneumococcal vaccines (with four doses at 2, 4, 6, and 12 months of life, or with three doses at 2, 4, and 12 months, in Chile), and also in patients with an initial adequate response to polysaccharide vaccines, whose antibody titers are progressively reduced.

Patients present with recurrent bacterial infections: otitis, bronchitis, sinusitis, and recurrent pneumonia caused by *Streptococcus pneumoniae*. Infections caused by *Haemophilus influenzae*, *Branhamella catarrhalis*, and *Staphylococcus aureus* have also been reported. Most patients respond to the usual antibiotic treatment.

Polysaccharide vaccine 23-valent is recommended to study these patients through the determination of specific antibodies to pneumococcus (14 serotypes in the United States, 10 serotypes in Chile), 4–6 weeks after the vaccine, which is therapeutic in a large percentage of these patients. About 80% and 90% of those who do not respond to the polysaccharide vaccines do respond to a conjugate vaccine dose.

The molecular defect of specific antibody deficiency has not been found, and some of the most serious presentations have a deficiency of memory B lymphocytes.

The serum level considered as protective for pneumococcal antibodies after the administration of 23-valent pneumococcal vaccine is ≥1.3 μg/ml or a fourfold increase in 50% of the basal level for 10 studied serotypes in children from 2 to 5 years old; 70% of these serotypes are present in older children (Table 50.4).

Transient hypogammaglobulinemia of infancy This deficiency is defined by the accentuation and prolongation of physiological hypogammaglobulinemia observed between 3 and 6 months of life, with IgG levels <2DS, in comparison with normal values per age, and it has been associated with a reduction in immunoglobulin isotypes. It has been found in younger children, with no history of infections, who have relatives with PID, and with recurrent infections: otitis media, recurrent bronchitis, and bacterial meningitis. This is a transient disease and does not require treatment with gamma globulin in most cases, but 10% to 20% may develop CVID or other dysgammaglobulinemia.

Table 50.4 Poor response to pneumococcal vaccines

Failure severity	IgG antibodies after vaccination	IgG antibodies after vaccination
	2–5 years old	≥6 years old
Severe	No protection level in any serotype	No protection level in any serotype
Moderate	Protection level	Protection level
	≤50% serotypes	≤70% serotypes

Cellular and Combined Immunodeficiency

Hyper-IgM syndrome This syndrome is an heterogeneous group of genetic diseases with alterations in the change of immunoglobulin isotypes. The most common form is deficiency of the CD40 ligand linked to the X chromosome. CD40 is one of the receptors of tumoral necrosis factor (TNF), expressed by B lymphocytes, dendritic cells, and macrophages (Fig. 50.2). Its activation is fundamental for the proliferation of B lymphocytes and immunoglobulin production, which occur as a result of the union to its natural ligand CD154 or CD40, expressed on the activated T lymphocytes. Another form is autosomal recessive caused by CD40 deficit, associated with antibody immunodeficiency.

The hyper-IgM syndrome is caused by a mutation in genes CD154 (HIGM1), bound to the X chromosome or CD40 (HIGM3), respectively. This syndrome is characterized by very low levels of IgG, IgA, and IgE, with normal or elevated IgM. The predominant clinical manifestations are viral and bacterial respiratory infections

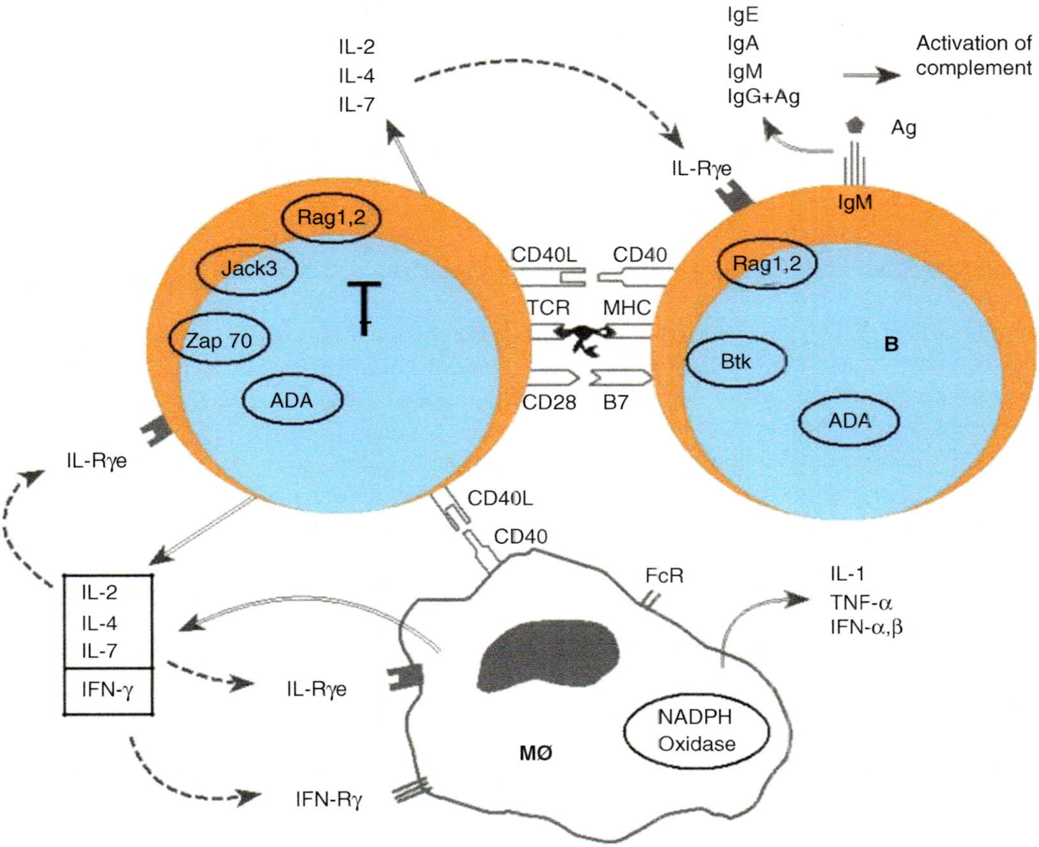

Fig. 50.2 Mediators involved in immunodeficiencies. Schematic representation of T and B lymphocytes, macrophages, and their soluble mediator interaction. Several immunodeficiencies mentioned in the text are caused by genetic defects that alter the expression of some patients, which are present in the diagram. (*Source:* Carrión F, Figueroa, F, Rodríguez C. La inmunología clínica: una perspectiva molecular. Rev Méd Chile. 2000; 120: 650–568. Creative Commons License)

in both the high and lower airways. In patients with CD40 linked to the X chromosome, interstitial lung infection caused by *Pneumocystis jirovecii* can be found. Infections related to humoral deficiency and diarrhea caused by *Cryptosporidium parvum* can also appear. Sclerosing colangitis, and aplastic anemia induced by parvovirus, are also found.

Severe combined immunodeficiencies This group of genetic diseases is characterized by the absence and dysfunction of T and B cells, and in some situations, of natural killer (NK) cells. The frequency of severe combined immunodeficiencies (SCID) has been estimated to be about 1 in 75,000 and 1 in 100,000. A series of molecular effects have been identified, the most common one related to the X chromosome in 50% to 60% of the cases, located at the γ-chain of the interleukin-2 receptor (IL-2R γc), IL-4, IL-7, IL-9, IL-15, and IL-21.

Clinical manifestations present after the neonatal period or during the first months of life, and are characterized by oral candidiasis, persistent diarrhea, failure to thrive, BCG vaccine dissemination, eczema, skin abscess, meningitis, hepatitis, and cholangitis, as well as systemic infections caused by cytomegalovirus or Epstein–Barr virus. Higher and lower respiratory tract infections are very common: otitis media, sinusitis, chronic bronchitis causing bronchiectasis and pneumonia caused by common bacteria, as well as interstitial pneumonia caused by *Pneumocystis jirovecii* and serious or deadly respiratory infections caused by adenovirus, respiratory syncytial virus, and type 3 parainfluenza. Most patients present with lymphopenia, and their levels of serum immunoglobulin are low or undetectable. T-lymphocyte count is reduced, in combination with low counts of B lymphocytes or NK cells, according to the CVID type. During past years a neonatal screening method has been developed for its early diagnosis, through the detection of an early precursor in the development of T lymphocytes: the T-cell-receptor excision circle (TREC).

DiGeorge Syndrome (DGS) This syndrome is characterized by compromise in the development of facial, heart, parathyroid, and thymus structures, caused by defects in the formation of the 3rd and 4th laryngeal pouch. Up to 90% of these patients present a microdeletion in the chromosomal region 22q11,2. In most patients, cell immunodeficiency is mild to moderate, with T-lymphocyte function in order. Less than 5% presents with cellular immunodeficiency with quantitative and functional compromise of T lymphocytes, along with a risk of opportunistic infections. Patients present with facial dysmorphia, micrognathia, palatine fissure, low implantation ears, short philtrum, and hypertelorism, along with conotruncal heart disease and hypocalcemia secondary to hypoparathyroidism.

Malformations of the airway have been described from the supraglottis to the segmental bronchi. Malformations in the larynx and laryngeal membrane have been associated with recurrent respiratory distress. Laryngomalacia and tracheomalacia, and bronchomalacia combined with conotruncal congenital heart disease, have been observed in patients with recurrent lung infections.

Velocardiofacial syndrome, also related to microdeletion of the chromosomal region 22q11,2, presents with velopharyngeal failure.

A specific antibody deficiency to polysaccharides has been described in about 50% of the patients who have a 22q11,2 deletion.

Phagocytes Immunodeficiencies

Chronic granulomatous disease This disease is present in 1 in 125,000 live births, and it is caused by a failure in the production of superoxide radicals, oxygen peroxide, and other oxygen radicals that are fundamental for the intracellular death of microorganisms, where a specific b-cytochrome of phagocytes and NADPH oxidase are required. Chronic granulomatous disease (CGD) may be caused by mutations in any of the four structural genes of NADPH oxidase. In 65% of the cases, the disease is associated to the X chromosome where a mutation of the gene that codifies the 91-kDa chain (gp 91 phox) has been found. Three other mutations are autosomal recessive. Clinical presentation appears during the first years of life with suppurative adenitis, granulomas, or skin, liver, lymph nodes, and lung infections caused by *Staphylococcus aureus*, *Burkholderia cepacia*, *Serratia marcescens*, and *Nocardia* and *Aspergillus* species. Lung compromise is very frequent, including hilar lymphadenopathy, pneumonia, empyema, and lung abscess. Diagnosis is made through the respiratory burst test using flow cytometry with dihydrorhodamine. Lung image study reveals chronic condensation, pleural retraction, interstitial enlargement, and hilar or mediastinal adenopathy. Diagnosis is confirmed with the test of respiratory burst and genetic study.

Clinical Case

A 15-year-old male was diagnosed with chronic granulomatous disease at 10 months when he presented with episodes of suppurative adenitis caused by *Serratia marcescens*. The nitroblue tetrazolium test and respiratory burst test were 0%, the gp 9 phox mutation. The patient was on cotrimoxazole and itraconazole with no important infections until 12 years of age, when lobar pneumonia with cavitation appeared in the left upper lobe. He was started on ciprofloxacin, vancomycin, and voriconazole with partial clinical and radiological response. Interferon gamma was added, three times a week, with significant clinical and radiological improvement (Fig. 50.3a, b).

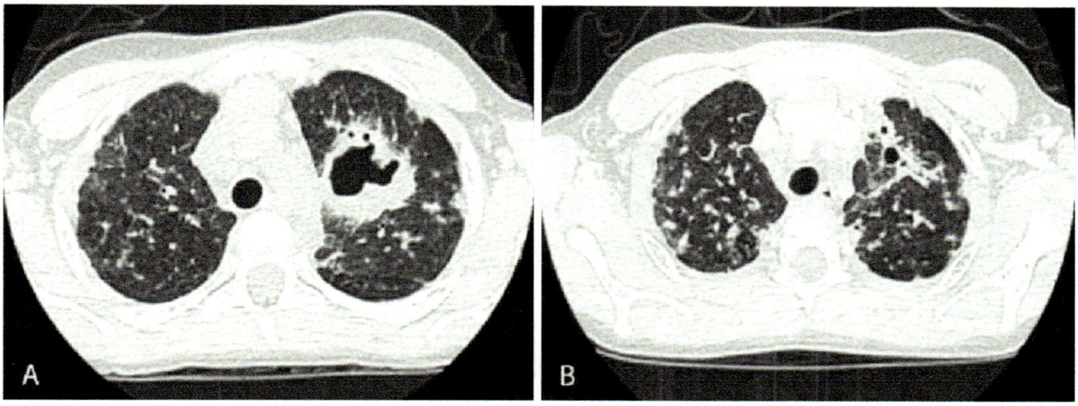

Fig. 50.3 Chronic granulomatous disease. Chest computed axial tomography shows cavitation pneumonia of the left upper lobe (LUL) of the lung before the beginning of treatment with interferon-γ (**a**) and after 6 months treatment (**b**) in a 15-year-old child with chronic granulomatous disease

Complement Immunodeficiencies

Complement deficiencies Complement deficiencies correspond to 2% and 3% of PID. This deficiency of the initial components of the complement cascade is characterized by recurrent infections caused by encapsulated bacteria, *Hemophilus influenzae* b and *Streptococcus pneumoniae*, and it can be associated with autoimmunity clinical manifestations. C3 is a relevant opsonin, and the clinical presentation of its deficiency is similar to those of hypogammaglobulinemia. C2 deficiency is the most frequent one and it has been related to autoimmune diseases, as with other early components of the classic pathway from C1 to C4. Component deficiency from C5 to C9 is associated to a greater susceptibility to infections caused by *Neisseria*.

Non-classified PID

Hyper-IgE syndrome This syndrome is an infrequent PID characterized by recurrent skin abscesses, recurrent pneumonia with lung abscesses, and pneumatocele caused by *Staphylococcus aureus*, high IgE levels, >2000 UI/ml, and poor lymphocyte response to diverse antigens. Infections by fungi, *Haemophilus influenzae* b, and *Streptococcus pneumoniae* have also been found. During the newborn phase, skin lesions can be similar to those of atopic dermatitis. Coarse facies, scoliosis, delay in the appearance of primary dentition, ligamentous laxity, and recurrent fractures have also been found. Many cases are sporadic, but families with dominant recessive and autosomal inheritance have been reported. Some patients present a mutation in STAT3.

Clinical Case

A 6-year-old female presented with history of suppurative skin lesions and persistent rhinitis and sinusitis starting the first year of life. She was admitted to the hospital with complicated pneumonia caused by a *Staphylococcus* abscess (Fig. 50.4).

Hyper-IgE syndrome was suspected because of some findings: coarse facies, double set of temporary and permanent teeth, hypermobility, and scoliosis. Diagnosis was confirmed with IgE level = 2000 UI/ml and a mutation in the STAT3 gene.

Wiskott–Aldrich syndrome This early-onset PID is characterized by eczema, thrombocytopenia with microplatelets, and recurrent infections. It is associated with the X chromosome, and it is caused by a defect in the WASP protein, which is responsible for the polymerization of cytoskele-

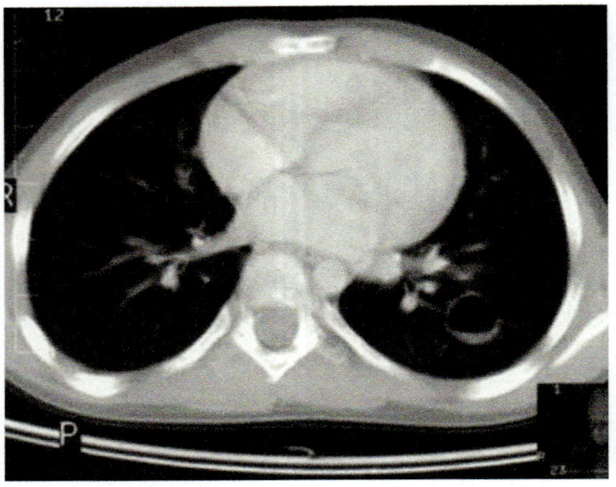

Fig. 50.4 Hyper-IgE syndrome. Chest computed axial tomography in a 6-year-old child with hyper-IgE syndrome shows an abscess in the LUL of the lung

tal actin. Levels of IgA and IgE are high, IgM is reduced, and IgG quantification is variable. Nevertheless, the patients have a diminished response to polysaccharide antigens and a moderate response to protein antigens. They also present with recurrent infections in different organs and lung infections caused by *Streptococcus pneumoniae*, herpes, and *Pneumocystis jirovecii*.

Alterations of IL-12 pathway and interferon-γ Alterations in the IL-12 pathway and interferon-γ present through infections caused by specific microorganisms. Disseminated infections caused by tuberculous mycobacteria or infections caused by herpesvirus or *Salmonella* have been reported.

Patients with PID may present lung sequelae secondary to infections, pneumatoceles, abscesses, and empyema.

Noninfectious lung complications have been also described in PID secondary to chronic inflammation and associated autoimmunity. Findings are air trapping, enlargement of the chest wall, atelectasis, and bronchiectasis. Some patients may present with bronchial obstruction, interstitial lymphocyte infiltration, or lung granulomatous disease.

Bronchiectasis is associated with some PID, such as X-linked agammaglobulinemia and common variable immunodeficiency. These diseases have been related to diagnosis delay and starting the treatment with IV gamma globulin, which involves a poorer patient prognosis.

Lung interstitial disease appears late in the variable common immunodeficiencies, and its frequency in children and adolescents is low.

PID treatment Early diagnosis and treatment of infections is relevant in all PID. IgA deficiency, and some transient PID such as childhood hypo-gammaglobulinemia, do not require specific treatment.

Preventive antibiotic treatment with cotrimoxazole and itraconazole is mandatory in granulomatous disease, as well as cotrimoxazole for PID with reduced CD4 lymphocyte count. In the case of antibody diseases with poor response to IV gamma globulin, amoxicillin, or cotrimoxazole and azithromycin, can be suggested.

Patients with PID should not receive live virus vaccines, nor the BCG vaccine. Patients with IgA deficiency and transient immunodeficiencies can receive these vaccines.

IV gamma globulin treatment is absolutely indicated in agammaglobulinemia linked to the X chromosome, hyper-IgM syndrome, variable common variable immunodeficiency, and severe combined immunodeficiencies while waiting for bone marrow transplant. The recommended dose is 400–600 mg/kg every 4 weeks, and the objective of the treatment is to reduce the frequency of the infections and avoid complications such as bronchiectasis and worsening of lung function, maintaining IgG levels above 500 mg/dl.

Bone marrow transplant is the treatment of choice for severe combined immunodeficiency, and the prognosis has been related to how early the therapy is executed, with a high percentage of immune reconstitution. In Wiskott–Aldrich syndrome the transplant of hematopoietic cells has been successful. For other PID, such as chronic granulomatous disease, protocols are being developed.

Genic therapy is still a treatment in investigation. Advances have been reported for lentiviral genic therapy for severe combined immunodeficiency with deficit of adenosine deaminase, Wiskott–Aldrich syndrome, and chronic granulomatous diseases.

Immunological Diseases

Connective tissue disease represents a group of diseases characterized by the presence of abnormalities in the immune system, whose most usual clinical manifestations are caused by acute and chronic musculoskeletal inflammation, blood vessels, and skin. It can compromise different organs. Vasculitis are characterized by the immunologically mediated inflammation of blood vessels, with a wide range of compromised vessels and clinical manifestations. Some of these diseases may present lung and airway compromise, but this is uncommon during childhood.

Lung compromise usually appears at the same time or after the beginning of the disease. Besides lung compromise, it can affect the higher airway and the pleura. Pleural effusion can be the first clinical manifestation of diseases such as systemic erythematous lupus.

Laboratory studies include CBC, sedimentation rate, biochemical profile, creatinine, and urine test. In several of these diseases, the directed study of antibodies is essential, as well as factors of the C3 and C4 complement; and in some patients, study of the functional system of the complement CH50. Image studies in these diseases include chest X-ray and computer axial tomography. Bronchoalveolar lavage is relevant for the study of some of these diseases, as well as for lung function study.

Table 50.5 shows the pediatric rheumatological diseases that most frequently involve lung compromise.

Etiopathogenesis

The etiology of most of these diseases is unknown, but several environmental and genetic factors are combined.

Table 50.5 Immunological Diseases with Lung Compromise

Systemic erythematous lupus
Systemic juvenile idiopathic arthritis
Dermatomyositis juvenile
Systemic esclerodermia
Kawasaki disease
Polyarteritis nodosa
Schönlein–Henoch purpura
Wegener granulomatosis
Churg–Strauss vasculitis
Microscopic polyangiitis
Connective tissue mixed disease
Goodpasture syndrome
Sjogren syndrome

Diverse immunological mechanisms have been proposed as involved in lung damage of rheumatological diseases: the damage can be allergic, mediated by IgE. Gell and Coombs damage type II is mediated by antibodies and has been observed in vasculitis associated with ANCA(+) and neonatal lupus. The damage type III mechanism is caused by the immune complex in systemic erythematosus lupus (SLE), as well as T failure and presence of antibodies for this disease. Damage type IV mechanism has been related to the formation of granulomas observed in sarcoidosis.

Vasculitis and Lung Compromise

Several rheumatological diseases in children and adolescents are associated to lung vasculitis, which is characterized by a compromise of small arterioles, venules, and capillaries.

Henoch-Schonlein Purpura

Henoch-Schonlein purpura is a vasculitis with generalized small vessel compromise, affecting skin, joints, intestines, and kidneys. It is one of the most common vasculitis in childhood. A subclinical lung compromise with lung interstitial disease and alteration of gas exchange has been reported. Lung hemorrhage with respiratory failure has been observed in adolescents and adults, but is uncommon before puberty.

Kawasaki Disease

Kawasaki disease is a multi-systemic vasculitis that compromises median vessels and has a particular predilection for the coronary arteries. It preferentially affects children under 5 years old. Respiratory compromise is infrequent in Kawasaki disease. In children under 6 months, and in the atypical presentation, tachypnea, dyspnea, cough, and acute rhinitis have been reported. Lung consolidation has been reported in patients during the febrile phase of this disease showing reticulogranular and interstitial pattern, pleural effusion, and atelectasis.

Polyarteritis Nodosa

Polyarteritis nodosa is a systemic necrotizing vasculitis, which can affect the medium-sized and small arteries. It may compromise any muscular arteria, and therefore it compromises a wide variety of organs: skin, lymph nodes, muscles, central nervous system, eyes, kidneys, testicles, heart, gastrointestinal tract and, lungs. This disease begins with unspecific constitutional symptoms, such as fever, weight loss, headache, abdominal pain, arthralgias, and myalgias.

Lung compromise is infrequent and is manifested by cough, dyspnea, pleuritis, interstitial pneumonia, lung infiltrations, and lung hemorrhage.

It has been associated with hepatitis B and C. Laboratory exams reflect a systemic inflammation, and alterations in the urine test, such as proteinuria and hematuria, can also be observed. Biopsy of compromised organs using an angiographic study is important for the diagnosis.

Systemic Vasculitis Associated to Anti-neutrophil Cytoplasmic Antibodies

Anti-neutrophil cytoplasmic antibodies (ANCA) are associated to several systemic vasculitis syndromes with kidney and lung damage. Its presence has been considered as a pathogenic factor in these diseases. Children and adolescents present vasculitis associated to positive anti-neutrophil cytoplasmic antibodies, including these:

1. Granulomatosis with polyangiitis (Wegener granulomatosis)
2. Microscopic poluangiitis (MPA)
3. Churg-Strauss vasculitis

Granulomatosis with Polyangiitis (Wegener Granulomatosis)

Granulomatosis with polyangiitis, previously known as Wegner granulomatosis, corresponds to a necrotizing vasculitis, with predominance in the small vessels, which is characterized by granulomatosis inflammation of the upper and lower respiratory airway, associated to pauci-immune crescentic glomerulonephritis. It is a rare disease in the pediatric population. During childhood, subglottic stenosis may appear and predominate in females. Airway compromise is present in around 80% of the patients, and the most common clinical manifestations are sinusitis, epistaxis, and less frequently, oral ulcers, acute otitis media, nasal ulcers, sensorial-conductive deafness, nose shaped as a saddle, subglottic stenosis, and nasal septum perforation.

Nasal disease appears as a mucus discharge and nasal obstruction, nasal ulcers, and septal perforation. Laryngotracheal disease can appear without symptoms and clinical presentation includes from snoring to stridor with airway obstruction. Lung compromise is very frequent, and the most common symptoms are cough, pleuritis, and hemoptysis. Lung hemorrhage is a serious emergency of this disease.

A localized presentation of this disease compromising the airway has been described: it is characterized by the formation of granulomas in the upper or lower airway, with no systemic compromise or constitutional symptoms, and it is completely different from polyangiitis granulomatosis (Wegner granulomatosis), because of the lack of systemic vasculitis.

Most common chest X-ray findings are pleuritis and nodule lobes, which usually have multiple and bilateral presentations, and can be cavitated. Observing granulomatous inflammation in the biopsy is relevant. The most useful laboratory exams are the altered urine test and the presence of c-ANCA, directed against proteinase 3 (PR-3), which appears in about 85% of the patients. Positive rheumatoid factor is present in about 60% of the patients, as well as anticardiolipins, and lupus anticoagulant.

Microscopic Polyangiitis

Microscopic polyangiitis is a necrotizing vasculitis of the peripheral vessels, without granulomas, which affects capillary, venules, and arterioles, but middle-sized vessels can also be affected. It appears with unspecific symptoms such as fever, myalgias, arthralgias, and high respiratory tract symptoms. The most common clinical manifestation is focalized severe glomerulonephritis segmentation, which can be associated with lung compromise, particularly lung hemorrhage. Most common respiratory symptoms are cough, dyspnea, and hemoptysis. It is characterized by the presence of p-ANCA, with myeloperoxidase reactivity. This is a serious disease, with a significant risk of chronic kidney failure, besides mortality by lung compromise.

Churg-Strauss Syndrome

Churg-Strauss syndrome is a very rare vasculitis during childhood. The first phase, or prodromes of the disease, appears with allergic rhinitis or asthma symptoms, which can persist for several years. The second phase is characterized by worsening of the asthma symptoms, peripheral eosinophilia, and lung infiltrations. In the third phase the systemic vasculitis appears along weight loss, fever, arthralgias, myalgias, nodular exanthema, and neuropathy, besides a regression of the symptoms of asthma. Antineutrophil cytoplasmic antibodies (ANCA) directed against PR-3 and MPO have been found. Biopsy of affected tissues is usually diagnostic, with perivascular eosinophilic infiltrations and, occasionally, extravascular granulomas.

Connective Tissue Diseases and Lung

Systemic Erythematosus Lupus

Systemic erythematosus lupus (SLE) is a multisystemic disease caused by immune dysregulation at different levels of the production of antibodies. Criteria from the American College of Rheumatology are used for its diagnosis. It is more frequent in females, and the estimated incidence in patients under 19 years old is 6 and 18.9 cases per 100,000.

Lung compromise is common in children and adolescents with SLE, about 25–75% of patients. The presentation varies from asymptomatic to lung function compromise, presence of pleural pain, or lung hemorrhage, which is infrequent, but its prognosis is poor and its mortality is high (between 50% and 90% of the cases). Compromise of the upper airway has also been described.

Clinical presentations are pleuritis, interstitial disease, acute lupus pneumonitis, secondary acute infectious pneumonia, lung hemorrhage, lung hypertension, and pneumothorax. Less frequent manifestations are diaphragmatic compromise or shrinking lung syndrome, lung vasculitis, and lung thrombosis.

Airway compromise involves ulcers in the larynx, edema, and vocal chords paralysis. Subglottic stenosis and epiglottitis may also be present and both are severe.

The most common lung manifestation of SLE is unilateral or bilateral pleuritic. Patients present with chest pain and variable degrees of respiratory compromise. SLE affects about one third of the patients at the beginning of the disease, and approximately 40% during its progression. Pleural fluid is an exudate with low LDH, normal pH, and glucose. Mild pleuritis can be treated with nonsteroidal antiinflammatory drugs, but generally the use of steroids is required.

Parenchymal compromise is infrequent. Lung hypertension, interstitial disease, which can be exacerbated by a lupus crisis, and thromboembolic disease, associated to anticardiolipin and lupus anticoagulant, have been described. Lung hemorrhage and acute lupus pneumonitis constitute medical emergencies with an acute initial phase with cough, dyspnea, hypoxemia, and progressive respiratory distress. In lung hemorrhage, hemoglobin and hematocrit levels are reduced. In contrast, acute lupus pneumonitis can be associated with fever. Considering its seriousness, diagnosis must be considered, and early treatment for these complications should be administered.

Chest computerized axial tomography and bronchoalveolar lavage must be done early, to establish the diagnosis and determine if the respiratory compromise is caused by the autoimmune disease, by an opportunistic agent if immunosuppressed, or by the immunosuppression treatment.

The initial study and the follow-up of laboratory exams such as CBC, VHS, complete urine tests, biochemical profile, creatinine, C3, C4, and autoantibodies (ANA, DNA, ENA profile, anticardiolipin, lupus anticoagulant) are relevant when studying SLE in children and adolescents.

Mixed Connective Tissue Disease/ Undifferentiated Connective Tissue

Mixed connective tissue disease is characterized by the combination of different manifestations of the several connective tissue diseases. Its frequency is low: the Kasukawa diagnostic criteria have been used in pediatric presentation:

- Raynaud syndrome, finger inflammation, or both
- Positive RNP antibodies

Compromise of at least one of the following:

(a) Systemic lupus erythematosus signs or symptoms
(b) Juvenile systemic sclerosis signs or symptoms
(c) Dermatomyositis signs or symptoms

Lung compromise has been found in about 40% of the patients with mixed connective tissue disease. Interstitial lung diseases, pleural effusion, and pulmonary hypertension have been described. The most frequent clinical manifestations are exercise dyspnea and persistent cough. Chest pain may also be present. Nevertheless, some patients with mixed connective tissue disease and lung compromise may not present clinical symptoms.

The following have been reported:

1. Restrictive lung disease in about 35% of patients
2. Reduction in CO diffusion in 24–42% of patients
3. Lung fibrosis in up to 30% of patients
4. Pulmonary hypertension in 6–9% of patients

Lung compromise must be ruled out in mixed connective tissue disease, even when there are no clinical symptoms, through the study of images and lung function.

Juvenile Dermatomyositis

Juvenile dermatomyositis (JDM) is an inflammatory vascular disease that mainly affects muscles and skin, but it can also compromise the airway and lungs. Weakness of respiratory muscles and diaphragmatic dysfunction with secondary lung compromise has been reported in up to a third of the patients. Infrequent complications of JDM reported are exercise dyspnea from aspiration, interstitial fibrosis, vascular lung damage caused by lymphoproliferative compromise of arterioles and small muscular arteria, and damage to the small airway, causing cryptogenic organizing pneumonia (previously named bronchiolitis obliterans with organizing pneumonia, BOOP). Reduction in ventilatory capacity is frequent in patients suffering from JDM without respiratory symptoms.

Juvenile Systemic Sclerosis

Juvenile systemic sclerosis (JSE) is a multisystemic chronic disease that greatly compromises the microvascular and vascular tissue, characterized by the enlargement of the skin and fibrosis of diverse organs such as esophagus, intestine, heart, kidneys, and lungs. Its appearance during childhood is infrequent.

Respiratory compromise is an important cause of morbidity and mortality in the systemic presentation of scleroderma, but it is not observed in the localized presentation. Lung compromise without clinical symptoms is frequent, and it can be observed in lung function studies. Patients may present with dry cough and exercise dyspnea: the rates of presentation are 15% of the patients at the beginning of the disease, and 40% during progression. Initial interstitial lung fibrosis in the base of the lungs, which progresses, is a complication with a poor prognosis, but its frequency is low during childhood. Pulmonary hypertension may appear secondary to lung fibrosis, but it can be observed alone. It has been described in later stages of constriction diseases, caused by the enlargement of the skin in the chest wall.

In juvenile systemic sclerosis, lung compromise must be directly sought, even when there are no clinical symptoms, with imaging studies as well as examination of lung function. High-resolution chest computerized axial tomography may show lung disease, even when the chest X-ray is normal, and therefore it is the study of choice in lung parenchyma evaluation for patients with juvenile systemic sclerosis. The most frequent findings are ground glass appearance, subpleural micronodules, linear opacity, and honeycomb images.

Lung diffusion study and spirometry are sensitive tools to assess lung compromise in juvenile systemic sclerosis. Echography is an important test for the early confirmation of pulmonary hypertension, dilation of the right ventricle, and arterial pressure in the lung artery.

Juvenile Idiopathic Arthritis

Juvenile idiopathic arthritis (JIA) is a group of diseases characterized by chronic arthritis in children under 16 years old. Pleural compromise is present in 4–8% of children with the systemic presentation of this disease. Pleural disease is more common than lung parenchyma compromise. Some cases of transient interstitial lung infiltration have been reported, with hyperplasia of the bronchial-associated lymphoid tissue, and lymphocytic interstitial pneumonia. Some of the less frequently reported complications in patients with juvenile idiopathic arthritis are lung hemosiderosis and lipoid pneumonia.

Goodpasture Syndrome

This syndrome is characterized by glomerular nephritis associated with the appearance of lesions, lung hemorrhage, and antibodies against the glomerular basal membrane. Lung compromise appears as hemoptysis, anemia, and lung infiltrations in chest X-rays, as well as an increase in lung diffusion, caused by the presence of hemoglobin in the alveoli.

Autoinflammatory Diseases of the Lung

Autoinflammatory diseases are a group of disorders of the innate immune system, characterized by inflammation episodes, with no evident cause, and with no relationship to autoantibodies or to a specific T-cell response. Monogenic periodic fevers have been described, with Mendelian inheritance, but also with polygenic inheritance and noninherited. The range of these diseases has been broadened to include Behçet's syndrome and systemic juvenile idiopathic arthritis.

Most autoinflammatory diseases do not have lung compromise. The TNF receptor-associated periodic syndrome (TRAPS) presents fever episodes every 1–4 weeks, as well as synovial, cutaneous, and serosal inflammation, peritonitis, pericarditis, or pleuritis. Deficiency of the interleukin-1-receptor antagonist (DIRA), which has a low frequency, appears during the first weeks of life with pustulosis, aseptic otitis, and periostitis without fever. Half the reported patients present with pulmonary compromise, interstitial pulmonary disease, and pulmonary fibrosis. A vasculopathy caused by a mutation in the TMEM173 gene, which codifies for the interferon gene stimulator, which has been recently reported as STING syndrome, presents with fever, cutaneous compromise, distal vessels compromise (finger or toe gangrene), nasal septum perforation, and lung compromise, characterized by interstitial lung disease, lung fibrosis, paratracheal adenopathy, and alteration of lung function.

Sources

1. Athreya BH, Doughy RA, Bookspan M, Schumacher HR, Sewell EM, Chattew J. Pulmonary manifestations of juvenile rheumatoid arthritis. Clin Chest Med. 1980;1:361–74.
2. Barron K, Athreya BH, Kastner D. Periodic fever syndromes and other inherited autoinflammatory diseases. In: Textbook of pediatrics rheumatology. Philadelphia: Saunders; 2011. p. 642–60.
3. Belostotsky VM, Shah V, Dilon MJ. Clinical features in 17 paediatric patients with Wegener granulomatosis. Pediatr Nephrol. 2002;17:754–61.
4. Benseler SN, Silverman E. Systemic lupus erythematosus. Pediatr Clin N Am. 2005;52:443–67.
5. Buckley RH. Pulmonary complications of primary immuno-deficiencies. Pediatr Respir Rev. 2004;5(S):225–33.
6. Carrión F, Figueroa F, Rodríguez C. La inmunología clínica: una perspectiva molecular. Rev Méd Chile. 2000;120:650–8.
7. Casanova JL, Fieschi C, Bustamante J, Reinbenbach J, Remus N, von Bernuth H, Picard C. From idiopathic infectious diseases to novel primary immunodeficiencies. J Allergy Clin Immunol. 2005;116:426–30.
8. Dedeoglu F, Sundel RP. Vasculitis in children. Pediatr Clin N Am. 2005;52:547–75.
9. Gómez L, Bonilla G. Manifestaciones pulmonares de las enfermedades del colágeno. Arch Bronconeumol. 2013;49:249–60.
10. Jesenak M, Banovcin P, Jesenakowa B, Babosikova E. Pulmonary manifestations of primary immunodeficiency disorders in children. Front Pediatr. www.frontierssin.org July 2014/Vol 2/Article 77.
11. Jon'czyk-Potoczna K, Szczawin'ska-Popłonyk A, Warzywoda M, Brn'borowicz A, Pawlak B. Hyper IgE syndrome (job syndrome, HIES): radiological images of pulmonary complications on the basis of three cases. Poland J Radiol. 2012;77:69–72.
12. Parvaneh N, Casanova JL, Notararangelo LD, Conley ME. Primary immunodeficiencies: a rapidly evolving story. J Allergy Clin Immunol. 2013;131:314–23.
13. Perez E, Sullivan K. Chromosome 22q11,2 deletion syndrome (DiGeorge and velocardiofacial syndromes). Curr Opin Pediatr. 2002;14:678–83.
14. Poli MC, Sorensen R. Inmunodeficiencias primarias y sistema respiratorio. In: Quezada A, Zenteno D, editors. Alergia e inmunología respiratoria. Santiago: Editorial Mediterráneo; 2013. p. 201–14.
15. Saukkonen JJ, Center DM. Immunologic lung diseases. In: Rich RR, editor. Clinical immunology. St. Louis: Mosby Year Book; 1996. p. 1551–78.
16. Sorensen RU, Paris K. Selective antibody deficiency with abnormal immunoglobulins. http://www.uptadate.com/.
17. Al-Herz W, Bousfiha A, Casanova JL, Chatila T, et al. Primary immunodeficiency diseases: an update on the classification from the International Union of Immunological Societies Expert Committee for Primary Immunodeficiency. www.frontiersin.org April 2014 | Volume 5 | Article 162 | 1.
18. Woroniecka M, Ballow M. Office evaluation of children with recurrent infection. Pediatr Clin NA. 2000;47:1211–24.

Acquired Immune Deficiency Syndrome

51

Anamaría Peña Donati and Marcelo Laufer

Contents

Introduction

The human immunodeficiency virus (HIV) is an RNA virus enclosed by a dual capsid. It is a member of the genus *Lentivirus*, family Retroviridae, with two serotypes, HIV-1 and HIV-2. Its main characteristic is an enzyme-labeled reverse transcriptase that enables it to synthesize DNA by integrating its RNA into the host cell. HIV was discovered in the 1980s in the blood serum of humans who suffered from acquired immune deficiency syndrome (AIDS). It has a lengthy incubation period, after which its characteristic symptoms appear: immune system deterioration, opportunistic infections, and nervous system damage. HIV binds to specific receptors present in many parts of the body, such as the hematopoietic system and brain, skin, intestine, bone, and lung tissue. It can cause damage directly or as a result of infections derived from the immune suppression that it produces.

Lung diseases are common in children with HIV and tend to be the first manifestation of these infections. Recurrent respiratory infections in a child who also suffers from dermatitis, generalized lymphadenopathy, chronic parotid compromise, hepatomegaly, splenomegaly, growth deficit, chronic diarrhea, or psychomotor development retardation must also raise suspicions of an HIV infection.

Lung infections represent 65% of the diseases associated with AIDS and are the main cause of morbidity and mortality in children with AIDS in

A. Peña Donati (✉)
Pontificia Universidad Católica de, Santiago, Chile
e-mail: anapena@med.puc.cl

M. Laufer
Pediatrics, Infectious Diseases, Nicklaus Children's Hospital, Miami, FL, USA

P. Bertrand, I. Sánchez (eds.), *Pediatric Respiratory Diseases*,
https://doi.org/10.1007/978-3-030-26961-6_51

developing countries. In this chapter, we describe both the infectious and noninfectious lung manifestations of HIV infection.

Epidemiology

In 2013, UN/AIDS estimated that 35 million people are infected with HIV globally, with 2 million being adolescents and 3 million under 15 years of age. Most of the infected children live in Sub-Saharan Africa (92%) and the Asia-Pacific region (6%). Data from 2013 indicate that 240,000 children acquired the infection during that year, which amounts to 1 child infected every 2 min. Similarly, 1.3 million infected women gave birth to 199,000 infected newborns (vertical transmission rate = 16%).

Perinatal transmission is still the most common cause of infections in children, despite the positive impact of the program for detecting infections in pregnant women. Transmission to newborns can occur in utero (35%), during childbirth (65%), or in the postpartum stage during breastfeeding (14–29%). Maternal viral load is directly related to the likelihood of transmission to the child, although the use of antiretroviral drugs during pregnancy and childbirth cause a significant reduction. When used during pregnancy and childbirth, zidovudine (AZT) can achieve a reduction in transmission rates ranging from 8% to 26%.

Currently, pregnant women benefit from highly effective antiretroviral regimes (HAART) combined with cesarean sections (in childbirths lasting more than 12 h) and maternal breastfeeding suppression, all of which reduces transmission risk to less than 1%. In developed countries, vertical transmission causes fewer HIV cases in people under 18 years old than sexual transmission.

Physiopathology

HIV produces cellular and humoral immunodeficiency. The selective loss of CD4+ T lymphocytes occurs because they are the main target cell. HIV infects these cells and then becomes part of their genome to destroy them. Thus, newborns with an HIV infection display a marked reduction in their total number of CD4+ T lymphocytes during their first 2 years of life.

From an immunological point of view, classification depends not only on the absolute number of CD4+ T lymphocytes, but also on their relative percentage. Absolute number varies with age and is higher during a person's first years of life. Percentage is a better predictor of progression to AIDS or death in children under 1 year old, whereas absolute count is more appropriate for children over 6 years of age. The immunological classification described in Table 51.1 is important because it enables practitioners to make a more accurate estimation of opportunistic infection risk in children infected with HIV, which is higher when immunological deterioration is severe.

The virus also infects monocytes, macrophages, and dendritic cells, but the destructive effect on them is not as strong as on CD4+ T lymphocytes; therefore, these cells become a repository for the virus and enable it to be distributed throughout the rest of the body. When these cells are infected, phagocytosis, chemotaxis, and antigen presentation are affected. These anomalies increase susceptibility to infections.

HIV produces an overstimulation of B lymphocytes, which results in polyclonal hypergammaglobulinemia mainly based on IgG, which appears earlier than the selective loss of CD4+ T lymphocytes. This polyclonal hypergammaglobulinemia is inefficient and behaves as functional

Table 51.1 Immunological classification

Immune category	Age: <12 months CD4/µl (%)	Age: 1–5 years CD4/µl (%)	Age: 6–13 years CD4/µl (%)
No immunosuppression	≥1500 (≥25)	≥1000 (≥25)	≥500 (≥25)
Moderate immunosuppression	750–1499 (14–24)	500–999 (14–24)	200–499 (14–24)
Severe immunosuppression	<750 (<15)	<500 (<15)	<200 (<15)

hypo- or agammaglobulinemia, leading to a high infection rate from encapsulated bacteria and an insufficient response to antibodies, which explains the recurrence of infections and the deficient response to immunization.

In lung tissue, as in the peripheral bloodstream, the virus also infects lymphocytes and causes a reduction in CD4+ T lymphocytes; in addition, there is an increase in CD8+ T lymphocytes that infiltrate interstitial and alveolar spaces.

Clinical Aspects

Respiratory diseases secondary to HIV infection can be infectious or noninfectious in nature and have a wide range of clinical presentations. Some of these resemble those observed in healthy children, which are caused by common bacteria or viruses, whereas others are atypical, being caused by opportunistic agents. Both can have a progressive and severe development, causing acute and chronic morbidity, sequelae, and death (Table 51.2).

The etiology of lung infections as well as their severity, development, and outcome depend on the patient's immunosuppression level. In two thirds of the children infected perinatally, who are neither diagnosed nor treated with antiretroviral drugs in a timely fashion, viral load increases rapidly during the first months of life. Afterward, the absolute count of CD4+ T lymphocytes drops sharply, which leads to the development of severe opportunistic infections with a high mortality. These patients are known as rapid progressors. Another patient subgroup has a slower and more benign progression, with lower viral loads and relatively high CD4+ T-lymphocyte counts that prevent the development of opportunistic infections. They develop bacterial infections that are similar to normal children, but recurrent. These cases are referred to as slow progressors. In a third group, progression is intermediate.

Unfortunately, no reliable markers have been identified earlier than 24 months of age that would enable clinicians to identify the progression and behavior of the virus in each individual.

Table 51.2 Respiratory system compromise

Infections not suggestive of AIDS
Persistent or recurrent upper acute respiratory infections (otitis, sinusitis)
Acute pneumonia, pleuropneumonia (1 episode in 1 year)
Bronchial infections, lung infections from herpes simplex virus (in <1 month of life)
Bronchial infections, lung infections from cytomegalovirus (in <1 month of life)
Lung infection caused by *Mycobacterium tuberculosis*
Infections suggestive of AIDS
Bacterial pneumonia (2 or more episodes in 2 years)
Pneumonia from *Pneumocystis jirovecii*
Pneumonia from cytomegalovirus (in >1 month of age)
Bronchitis, pneumonitis from herpes simplex virus (in >1 month of age)
Pneumonia from *Candida*
Disseminated or extrapulmonary infection caused by *Mycobacterium tuberculosis*
Lung infection fromto non-tuberculous *Mycobacterium* (*M. avium* complex and others)
Noninfectious causes
Chronic lung disease
Lymphoid interstitial disease/lymphoid interstitial pneumonitis
Bronchiectasis
Immune reconstitution syndrome
Tumors

Therefore, the current recommendation is to initiate antiretroviral treatment in all children under 1 year of age with a confirmed infection to prevent immunological deterioration.

Infectious Complications

Infections in HIV-positive children can have a bacterial, viral, or fungal etiology. In general, they present with rapid-onset respiratory symptoms, increased breathing effort, fever, usually with a clear chest X-ray; in contrast, noninfectious complications are characterized by progressive and slow starting respiratory symptoms with chest X-ray shadows.

Bacterial Infections

Upper airway bacterial infections (sinusitis and otitis media) are more common in children with HIV and can be classified as clinical stage A or mildly symptomatic. Recurrent respiratory bacterial infections must cause clinicians to suspect an HIV infection when they are associated with other unspecific manifestations such as adenopathy, chronic parotid swelling, hepatomegaly, or splenomegaly.

Among the severe bacterial infections, bacterial pneumonia is the most frequent infectious entity in all stages of the disease, even without immune deterioration, and especially during the first 12 months of life.

During the AIDS stage, there is a high risk of complications that is directly proportional to the viral load and inversely proportional to the absolute count and percentage of CD4+ T lymphocytes. Its incidence has been reduced from 11 to 2 per 100 children-year with HAART and immunizations (especially the conjugate *Streptococcus pneumoniae* and *Haemophilus influenza* type b vaccines), but it remains the most prevalent infection in this group. The etiology of bacterial pneumonia is diverse. Even though it is not easy to make an etiological diagnosis, authors have described infections caused by gram-positive, gram-negative, and mixed bacteria.

The main cause of bacterial infection is *Streptococcus pneumoniae*, although *Staphylococcus aureus* now is more important given the high levels of oxacillin (50%) and clindamycin resistance (22–30%). The most common gram-negative bacteria are *Haemophilus influenzae* (encapsulated and non-encapsulated), *Escherichia coli*, *Salmonella* non-typhi, and *Pseudomonas aeruginosa*. Other agents that cause lower respiratory infections include *Mycoplasma pneumoniae* and *Chlamydophila pneumoniae*.

In patients with HIV, bacterial pneumonia can lead to concomitant bacteremia and suppurative complications such as empyema and necrotizing pneumonia (Fig. 51.1). Long-term complications in patients who have had severe and recurrent lower respiratory infections include bronchiectasis, which was much more common before HAART. Its clinical behavior was similar to that observed in patients with cystic fibrosis colonized by organisms such as *Klebsiella* sp. and *Pseudomonas* sp.

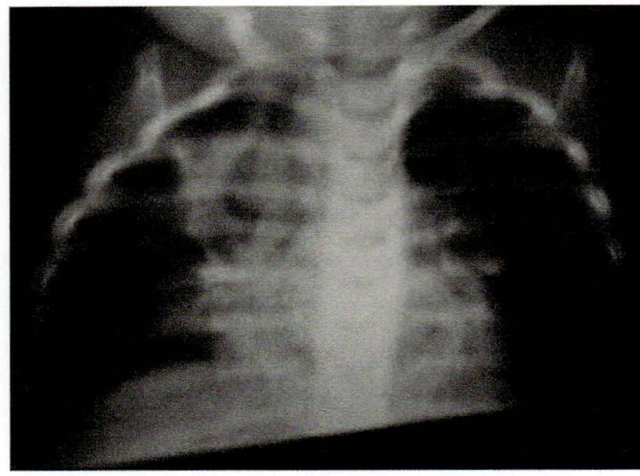

Fig. 51.1 Necrotizing pneumonia. Chest X-ray of 2-year-old girl shows a bilateral condensation pattern with a right apical abscess. *Streptococcus pneumoniae* was isolated in the bronchoalveolar lavage and hemoculture

Any episode of pneumonia or confirmed bacterial pleuropneumonia indicates clinical stage B or moderate symptomatology, and two or more episodes over a 2-year period indicate clinical stage C or severe symptomatology.

Treatment Treatment for bacterial pneumonia is similar to that recommended for the general pediatric population. All guidelines propose using amoxicillin as an initial antibiotic therapy associated with macrolides when clinical or radiological signs suggest the presence of an *Mycobacterium pneumoniae* or *Chlamydia pneumoniae* infection. In the case of *Haemophilus influenzae* (encapsulated or non-encapsulated) and *Moraxella catarrhalis*, the use of clavulanic acid or sulbactam is recommended.

Prophylaxis Primary prophylaxis involves immunizations and the administration of intravenous immunoglobulin for patients with absolute (IgG <400 mg/dl) or functional hypogammaglobulinemia (insufficient IgG production in response to specific immunizations).

Secondary prophylaxis is conducted with intravenous immunoglobulin or trimethoprim sulfamethoxazole (TMP-SMX) in patients with more than two confirmed episodes of severe bacterial infections.

The conjugate pneumococcal vaccine has caused a 60-fold reduction in invasive pneumococcal disease in this population versus a 15-fold reduction in normal children. Patients who do not receive HAART display a marked decrease in anti-pneumococcal titers over a period of 2 to 4 years; therefore, periodic reinforcement is recommended. It is useful to conduct an anti-pneumococcal antibody titer test in patients with a history of frequent or severe pneumonias to indicate the reinforcement of the 13-valent conjugate vaccine, followed by the administration of the 23-valent polysaccharide vaccine 6–8 months later in children with low titers. The conjugate *H. influenzae* type B vaccine, included in immunization programs, has had a positive impact on the incidence of invasive disease in these patients.

Mycobacterium Infections

The global reemergence of tuberculosis (TB) resulting from the AIDS epidemic, among other factors, is currently followed by WHO as a global emergency. TB/HIV coinfection, manifested as either latent tuberculous infection or as active tuberculous disease, is a major public health problem. Estimates suggest that, in 2009, 1.1 million new coinfections had occurred globally and 24,000 in the Americas. Because of its high prevalence, every time a TB case is diagnosed, it is necessary to rule out HIV infection, and vice versa. In HIV-positive children, it is generally a primary infection transmitted by an adult with an active infection. High risk results from the reduction in T1 lymphocytes, the subsequent limited production of interferon-gamma (IFN-γ), and the functional alteration of the macrophage systems, all of which constitute the basic defenses of the body against *Mycobacterium tuberculosis*. As cellular immunodeficiency affects patients with HIV, the infection is poorly controlled, which fosters its progression to TB disease, its dissemination, the development of extrapulmonary forms, its recurrence, and its high fatality rate (causing the death of up to one third of patients with AIDS). In addition, the reservoir that these patients constitute increases the risk of transmission to the community. TB bacillus induces the macrophage to produce tumor necrosis factor and interleukins 1 and 6, proinflammatory substances that foster the replication of HIV in infected areas, thus increasing viral load and accelerating the progression to AIDS and death. In this patient group, more treatment failures are observed because of the increasing multiresistance of the TB bacillus (resistance to rifampicin and isoniazid).

TB can appear at any point of the HIV infection in children, either in the non-AIDS stage (lung compromise) or in the AIDS stage (disseminated or extrapulmonary compromise), and either with or without immunological deterioration.

Latent TB infection occurs when the tuberculin test (PPD) or the interferon-γ test are reactive in an asymptomatic patient, with a negative bacillus smear and normal chest X-rays. Active TB disease occurs when the patient is symptomatic, sputum cultures are positive, and chest X-rays are abnormal. In addition, PPD can be positive.

Clinical presentation in HIV-positive children is atypical and severe, depending on the level of immunosuppression. Miliary compromise and extrapulmonary manifestations are more common than in HIV-negative children. In general, they appear in children with a history of contact with TB or diagnosed TB and symptoms such as fever, major weight loss, sweating, tachypnea, and unsolved condensing or interstitial pneumonia with persistent X-ray signs despite the treatment administered.

Diagnosing TB in children is hard, especially in HIV-positive children. If the treating physician suspects TB, it is essential to obtain samples to confirm its etiology through bacteriology.

Laboratory tests:

- Tuberculin test (PPD): Only 10–35% of HIV-positive patients infected with the bacillus have a positive PPD. Also, given that miliary and meningeal infections in children under 2 years of age usually yield a negative PPD, this test is normally unhelpful for diagnosis. In HIV-positive patients, an induration of 5 or more mm is considered to be positive.

Tests that rely on interferon-γ (QuantiFERON and T Spot) have the advantage of being objective thanks to the use of positive and negative control tests, which makes it possible to differentiate tuberculin-positive patients caused by a recent BCG vaccination, and do not identify positive cases resulting from the booster effect of frequent PPD in vaccinated patients. Current US guidelines recommend using QuantiFERON as soon as HIV is diagnosed. Patients infected perinatally require a first test between 3 and 12 months of age and an annual test if the first one is negative.

- Bacillus smear: At least six sputum samples preceded by nebulizations with hypertonic saline solutions must be obtained. Other useful samples include bronchoalveolar lavage (80–90% positivity), ganglion tissue, urine, cerebrospinal fluid, or other sterile fluids.
- Koch culture in a Loewenstein-Jensen medium, observed for at least 8 weeks, or in radiometric liquids that shorten observation to 10 days. Cultures are more useful when bacillus smears are negative.
- Semiautomatic hemoculture through lysis-centrifuge procedure automated through a radiometric method in disseminated presentations.
- Polymerase chain reaction (PCR) (Xpert MTB /RIF [Xpert]), which makes it possible to quickly identify the bacillus and determine the presence of markers of resistance to isoniazid and other drugs.
- Chest X-ray: Persistent radiological images caused by lymphoid interstitial pneumonitis or bronchiectasis secondary to HIV infection can confound diagnosis. In patients with tuberculosis, X-rays can be normal or reveal unspecific images, with multifocal diffuse interstitial infiltrates, similar to those produced by other opportunistic agents. Lymphadenopathies are often observed, with pleural effusion also being possible, but X-rays tend to be normal in cases of advanced AIDS.
- Other imaging resources: Ultrasound and abdominal CT scans can reveal intraabdominal adenopathies and necrotic visceral lesions in extrapulmonary presentations. In meningeal tuberculosis, brain CT scans reveal atrophy and ventricular compromise.
- Ganglion biopsy: Histology reveals granulomas and caseous necrosis.

Treatment Anti-tuberculosis therapy entails several difficulties and must be tailored for each patient. It is necessary to select drugs whose metabolism does not interfere with the metabolism of antiretroviral drugs. Rifampicin, being a cytochrome P450 inducer, can interact with nevirapine (a reverse-transcriptase inhibitor) and with protease inhibitors. The ideal course of action is to use two nucleoside analogue reverse-transcriptase inhibitors as antiretrovirals, plus a non-nucleoside reverse-transcriptase inhibitor.

Initial anti-tuberculosis treatment must include these four drugs: isoniazid, rifampicin, pirazinamide, and ethambutol or streptomycin; when the bacillus is confirmed to be susceptible to the first three, the fourth can be suspended. After the first 2 months of induction therapy, isoniazid and rifampicin are used for 7 additional months.

When HIV is diagnosed, soon before or after tuberculosis, and HAART has not yet been initiated, the decision to start administering it depends on the patient's immunological status and the clinical stage, because this can lead to an immune reconstitution syndrome in patients with AIDS and severe immunological deterioration. If there is no immunological deterioration or if it is mild and the patient has not entered the AIDS stage, anti-tuberculosis treatment must be initiated and even completed before starting HAART. If the patient has entered the AIDS stage and immunological deterioration is moderate or severe, HAART must be delayed for as long as 2 to 4 weeks after the start of anti-tuberculosis therapy, or at least until the induction phase has been completed. If an HIV-positive patient is diagnosed with tuberculosis, HAART should be suspended; alternatively, dosage adjustments should be implemented or a regime without rifampicin be adopted.

HIV-positive patients are more likely to become infected with isoniazid-resistant bacilli or even with bacilli resistant to various agents. In such cases, treatment must include three drugs with no resistance for 12 months. Options are streptomycin, cycloserine, ethionamide, clarithromycin, azithromycin, ciprofloxacin, or linezolid.

Prophylaxis Patients with latent tuberculosis receiving monotherapy (isoniazid) have a significantly lower risk of progression to TB. The WHO recommends prophylactic isoniazid in HIV-positive children under 1 year of age in high-prevalence areas for up to 3 years, regardless of their PPD results. Isoniazid is also recommended for 6 to 9 months, regardless of PPD, in HIV-positive patients who have been in contact with confirmed tuberculosis cases once the active disease has been ruled out. The bacillus Calmette–Guérin (BCG) vaccine is contraindicated in HIV-positive children and must be delayed in perinatally exposed newborns until a normal CD4+ T-lymphocyte count is observed.

Non-tuberculosis *Mycobacterium* infections are less frequent in children. This group includes the *Mycobacterium avium* complex (MAC), of which two species are known: *M. avium* and *M. intracellulare*, slow-growing (10–21 days), acid/alcohol-resistant, non-chromogenic coccobacilli. These microorganisms are widely distributed in the environment—water, soil, plants, and animals—and their pathogenicity depends on the host immunity as they do not cause diseases in immunocompetent patients.

With respect to the *Mycobacterium avium* complex, infections, manifestations, and prognosis are CD4+ and T-dependent. It can manifest itself as a localized disease (cervical adenitis, pneumonia, hepatitis, splenomegaly, or local abscesses) or as a generalized disease (fever of unknown origin, weight loss, chronic diarrhea, and pancytopenia). Cervical lymphadenitis is more common in children aged 1–4 years. It is generally unilateral, has an insidious presentation, and evolves toward fistulization and chronic suppuration. Lung infection usually coexists with other opportunistic infections and may disseminate. Chest X-rays reveal nodular or cavitary opacities and bronchiectasis (Fig. 51.2).

Diagnosis

- Bacillus smear: Reveals acid/alcohol-resistant bacilli, but it does not differentiate them from tuberculous bacilli.
- Culture: Blood, sputum, bronchoalveolar lavage, lung tissue, ganglion tissue, bone marrow, or any sterile fluids. It is recommended to conduct an automated hemoculture, reseeding in a Loewenstein-Jensen medium, and performing a final diagnosis after 4–12 weeks.
- Specific tests: Amplification of specific DNA sequences, high-performance liquid

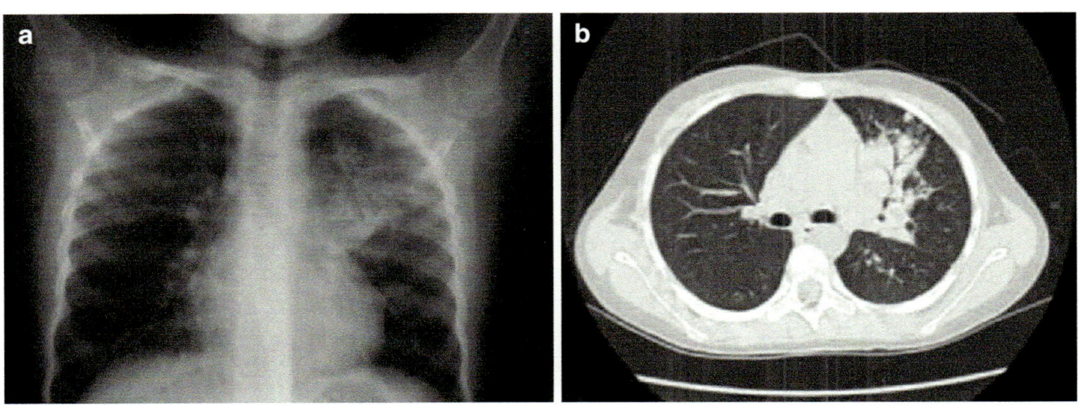

Fig. 51.2 Pneumonia caused by *Mycobacterium avium* complex (MAC). Chest X-ray of a 12-year-old girl recently diagnosed with HIV displays a condensation pattern and atelectasis in the left upper lobe. MAC was confirmed through a PCR test of lung tissue biopsy (**a**). Chest CT scan of the same patient displays condensation and atelectasis of the left upper lobe (**b**)

chromatography, and hybridization probe assays for identifying species and genotype.

Prophylaxis *Mycobacterium avium* complex infection usually is a disseminated infection and mortality is inversely proportional to CD4+ T-counts. Infection occurs in advanced stages with severe immunosuppression (CD4+ T < 100 cells/μl). Primary prophylaxis with a macrolide is recommended, considering patient age and CD4+ T count (<1 year: CD4+ <750/μl; 1–2 years: CD4+ <500/μl; 2–6 years: CD4+ <75/μl; >6 years: CD4+ <50/μl). It can be interrupted when the patient has received HAART and has achieved immune recovery for a 6-month period.

Treatment Localized forms are treated with at least two drugs (a macrolide and ethambutol) to prevent or delay resistance. In cases of disseminated disease, one or two antibiotics are added (rifampicin, rifabutin, ciprofloxacin, amikacin, or clofazmine). It is recommended to conduct a susceptibility test to rule out resistance. Treatment is considered to have failed if no clinical response is observed and if bacteremia persists 8–12 weeks after therapy. Treatment is ineffective when not complemented with HAART, because the infection becomes fatal if no immune recovery is achieved.

Viral Infections

Upper and lower respiratory tract infections of a viral origin have the same incidence as in normal children but tend to be severe. The pathogens involved can be common viruses affecting children such as the respiratory syncytial virus (RSV), adenoviruses, parainfluenza (PI), influenza, metapneumovirus, and rhinovirus; in cases of systemic diseases, they can include varicella zoster (VZ), herpes simplex (HS), Epstein–Barr, and cytomegalovirus (CMV), which can cause extensive and necrotizing pneumonias. Viral excretion last longer than in normal children, up to 30 days for parainfluenza, 90 days for RSV, and several months for adenovirus. Chest X-rays show interstitial pattern, multifocal condensation, and pleural effusion. A quick diagnosis can be made by examining respiratory samples with immunofluorescence, short culture, or PCR, as well as by using PCR in blood for cases of systemic infection.

Cytomegalovirus is among the opportunistic agents that most commonly infect HIV-positive children. Infection risk is greater than in healthy children, either via congenital acquisition (because of the high level of coinfection in HIV-positive pregnant women) or via postnatal infection (usually during the first years of life). Cytomegalovirus infection risk is higher in cases of severe immunosuppression (CD4+ T <50 cells/μl). It causes high morbidity; its fatality rate can reach 30% in HIV-positive children, and represents 8–10% of AIDS-indicating diseases. It is often the first manifestation of an HIV infection and is associated with a faster progression of the disease and greater central nervous system compromise. The most common presentation is interstitial pneumonia, which can progress to respiratory failure or respiratory distress or become part of a systemic disease (Fig. 51.3). It occurs often as a coinfection with opportunistic agents such as *Pneumocystis jirovecii*, tuberculosis, and *Candida*, among others. Therefore, it is necessary to demonstrate the presence of viral replication in lung samples to confirm a cytomegalovirus disease.

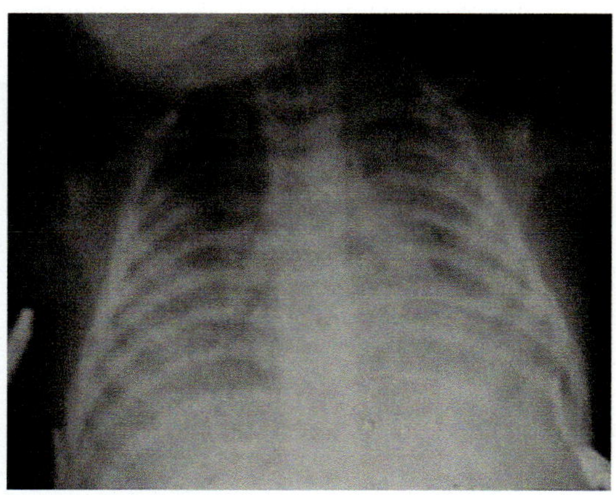

Fig. 51.3 Pneumonia caused by *Cytomegalovirus*. Chest X-ray of 5-month-old infant with a multifocal pattern and fast progression to acute respiratory distress. Cytomegalovirus was isolated from bronchoalveolar lavage

Prophylaxis Administration of influenza vaccine from 6 months of age onward is one of the few preventive measures available. The prophylaxis of cytomegalovirus can be considered in special cases (serum antibodies IgG and CD4+ T <50 cells/μl) as well as in the maintenance period after the completion of the daily treatment phase and until the patient has received HAART for 6 months with immune recovery (TCD4+ ≥500 cells/μl or ≥15% [1–5 years]; ≥200 cells/μl or ≥15% [≥6 years].

Treatment Early treatment with antivirals makes a difference in the evolution of viral infection. Oseltamivir, when administered within the first 72 h after symptoms begin, can reduce the severity of the disease and its complications. It is the treatment of choice even in vaccinated patients and can be used as a prophylactic measure in patients who have been exposed. Oral acyclovir oral has a deficient absorption level (20%); therefore, parenteral administration is recommended in severe cases of HS or VZ disease. Intravenous ganciclovir is the drug of choice for cytomegalovirus, in association with immunoglobulin IV. Valganciclovir has a 50–60% oral absorption rate and is a viable alternative for maintenance therapy. Foscarnet must be used in resistant cases.

Fungal Infections

Pneumocystis jirovecii

An agent currently categorized as a fungus, it was the most common cause of atypical pneumonia in HIV-positive children, with an incidence rate of up to 42%. This entity, classified as an AIDS-indicating disease, can progress quickly with no treatment, even leading to respiratory failure with a fatality rate of up to 50%, especially when associated with cytomegalovirus. It affects children under 1 year old, particularly before 6 months of age, and can mark the beginning of an HIV infection even if the CD4+ T-lymphocyte count is normal; however, in children over 1 year old incidence is inversely proportional to the CD4+ T-count, with risk increasing when immunosuppression is severe.

P. jirovecii adheres to alveolar walls and proliferates in the extracellular, causing epithelial cell shedding followed by the generation of an exudate that fills the alveoli and prevents oxygen exchange. It can have an insidious or abrupt manifestation with dry cough, fever, tachypnea, intercostal retraction, and hypoxia. Auscultation can be normal in the beginning but, as the disease progresses, a generalized reduction in air intake and rhonchi or crackles are heard. Laboratory tests confirm hypoxemia; also, the value of lactate dehydrogenase (LDH) is very high. Chest X-rays can be initially normal or display hyperaeration and diffuse interstitial images. As the disease progresses, interstitial images and bilateral alveolar filling can be observed, with a "ground glass" or granular reticle appearance. It is less frequent to observe condensation, pneumatocele, pneumothorax, or pleural effusion (Fig. 51.4).

Diagnosis Pathogen identification must be confirmed, either via silver stain, identification of the antigen with a monoclonal antibody, or PCR of bronchial fluid obtained through bronchoscopy or lung biopsy. Sputum induced by hypertonic serum or nasopharyngeal aspirate have less sensitivity, although they can be used to identify the pathogen while avoiding invasive methods.

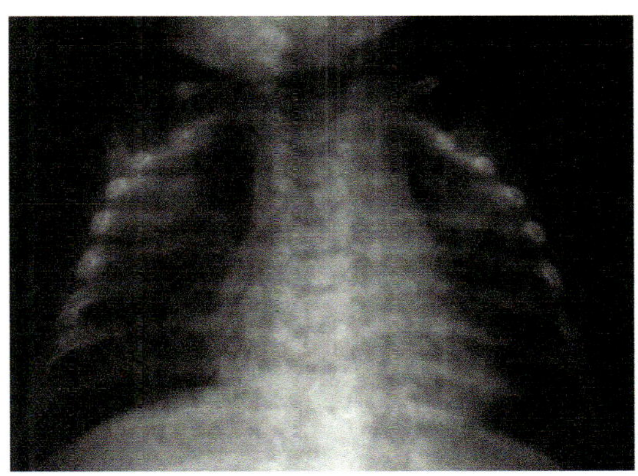

Fig. 51.4 Pneumonia caused by *Pneumocystis jirovecii*. Chest X-rays of 6-month-old infant with a nodular reticle pattern and "ground glass" image associated with hypoxemia. *P. jirovecii* was confirmed in a sample of bronchoalveolar lavage

Treatment The therapy of choice is intravenous TMP-SMX, even in patients receiving prophylactic treatment with this antimicrobial drug. Therapeutic alternatives are pentamidine, atovaquone, dapsone, or primaquine in combination with clindamycin. This antimicrobial drug must be combined with steroids (prednisone or equivalent; 2 mg/kg/day divided into two doses, followed by decreasing doses over the next 7–14 days) during the first 5–7 days.

Prophylaxis Prophylaxis is effective and is recommended in all children under 1 year old, both infected or undergoing tests (undetermined status), in those with perinatal exposure regardless of CD4+ T-count, and in children over 1 year old with severe immunosuppression (immunological stage 3) or at clinical stage C. Prophylaxis can be suspended in newborns not fed with breast milk after ruling out infection from perinatal exposure and in infected children who have received HAART for ≥6 months with immune recovery (CD4+ (≥500 cells/μl or ≥15% [1–5 years]; ≥200 cells/μl or ≥15% [≥6 years]. In younger children, it must be maintained until the child reaches 12 months of age, regardless of HAART length and immune recovery. The prophylactic drug of choice is TMP-SMX three times per week. Alternatives are dapsone, oral atovaquone, and nebulized pentamidine.

Other fungi that affect the respiratory system are *Candida* sp., *Cryptococcus neoformans*, *Histoplasma capsulatum*, *Coccidiodes immitis*, *Penicillium marneffei*, and *Aspergillus*.

These infections often produce invasive and disseminated diseases with general symptoms such as fever, appetite loss, depressed mood, and weight loss.

Cryptococcosis is usually complicated with meningitis. *Histoplasma*, a dysmorphic fungus whose mold form in nature can enter the lung through inhalation, commonly causes pneumonia first, but dissemination to other organs is very frequent. Etiological diagnosis is made using cultures (blood, bone marrow, and lymph, lung, or liver tissue). *Histoplasma* can be detected by measuring the antigen in urine or blood. *Candida* tends to infect the gastrointestinal rather than the tracheobronchial system; however, dissemination can follow infection in any of these two locations. *Aspergillus* infection is uncommon, but it occurs in late states of the disease with severe immunosuppression and can affect the paranasal sinuses, the nasal cavity, and the lung, producing necrotic lesions. Diagnosis is made with PCR, galactomannan measurements (both of which can be used as follow-up strategies), and chest CT scans suggestive of infection.

Treatment Prognosis for these infections has changed given the multiple therapeutic alternatives currently available. Polyenes (amphotericin and combinations with various lipophilic vehicles) have been replaced by two types of anti-mycotics: azoles (fluconazole, itraconazole, voriconazole, and posaconazole, with the latter three targeting molds and yeasts) and echinocandins (micafungin, caspofungin, and anidulafungin).

Noninfectious Complications

Chronic Lung Disease

This entity is relatively frequent in the pediatric population infected with HIV, especially in children who do not receive HAART. Previous to this therapy, up to one third of children under 4 years of age displayed chronic chest X-ray changes associated to low CD4+ T count and high viral load: persistent consolidation for ≥3 months (8%), nodular changes for >3 months (8%), or reticular changes and increase in bronchovascular marking lasting ≥6 months (14%). These patients present with clubbing, persistent crackles, tachypnea, hypoxemia, and exercise intolerance.

The following conditions include the spectrum of manifestations described in these patients whose clinical and radiological presentation is juxtaposed:

- Lymphocytic interstitial pneumonia
- Chronic bacterial infections
- Bronchiectasis
- Interstitial pneumonia

Lymphocytic interstitial pneumonia (LIP) is the most common of these entities. This is the only B-category condition that classified the patient as having AIDS, but they have become uncommon after HAART. It is important to remember it when working with patients who have not started HAART or who have displayed poor treatment adherence. It is a noninfectious radiological entity. Its etiology is unknown and probably multifactorial, although it has been suggested that it related to a lymphoproliferative response, with hyperproduction of cytokines against HIV and other agents such as Epstein–Barr virus.

LIP commonly starts during the second year of life, although some chest X-ray changes have been described before 12 months in asymptomatic patients. It presents with cough, tachypnea, and exercise intolerance, progressing to respiratory failure with cyanosis, clubbing, dyspnea, and progressive hypoxemia. It is accompanied by the same lymphoproliferative response in lymph nodes, liver, spleen, and parotid glands, manifested by adenopathy, hepatomegaly, splenomegaly, and parotid hypertrophy. Chest X-rays show bilateral reticulonodular interstitial infiltrate with or without perihilar adenopathy that persists despite treatment. Patients have hypergammaglobulinemia with IgG levels over 2000 mg/dl. Definitive diagnosis is achieved by histology of a lung biopsy showing interstitial, diffuse, and peribronchiolar infiltration of lymphocytes and plasma cells, but generally, diagnosis be could be based on the observation of persistent chest X-ray images despite antimicrobial treatment for 2 months and the absence of a detectable agent. All chest X-ray changes described can respond to HAART and patients who display undetectable viral loads for over 6 months improve significantly. Patients who have been unable to benefit from HAART require support treatment: oxygen therapy, bronchodilators, and sometimes antimicrobial agents.

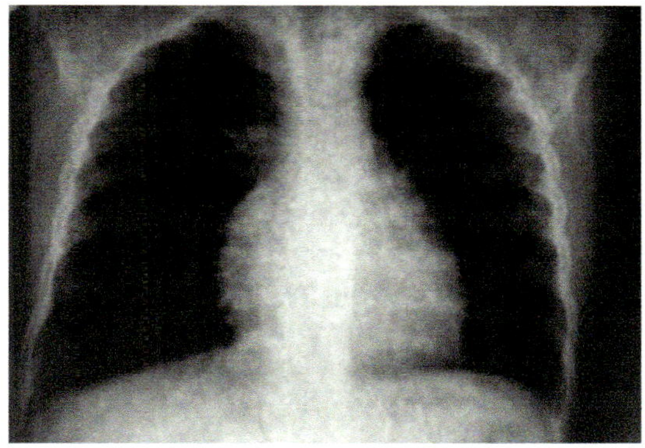

Fig. 51.5 Lymphocytic interstitial pneumonia. Chest X-ray of 5-year-old girl with a persistent reticulonodular pattern, no response to treatment, and negative etiological tests

Bronchiectasis can occur as a sequela of recurrent bacterial pneumonia, lymphocytic interstitial pneumonia, infection from *Pneumocystis pneumoniae*, and non-tuberculosis *Mycobacterium* disease, among other diseases. Chest X-ray changes persisting for over 6 months, including small cystic lesions, opaque areas, atelectasis, and loss of volume from lung destruction, should cause clinicians to suspect bronchiectasis (Fig. 51.5). High-resolution CT scans reveal bronchial dilation, thickening of the bronchial wall from fibrosis, and air entrapment.

Immune Reconstitution Syndrome

Immune reconstitution syndrome is a paradoxical state of clinical deterioration that follows the start of treatment for an opportunistic infection concomitant with antiretroviral therapy. It results from the patient's immunological recovery, which causes an exaggerated inflammatory response to certain antigenic stimuli. This clinical entity can occur in patients who have suffered multiple opportunistic infections that have been treated or before subclinical and atypical infections neither diagnosed nor treated. It has been described in infections produced by mycobacteria, cytomegalovirus, herpes simplex and zoster. *Cryptococcus neoformans*, lung capillary wedge pressure, among others. In patients with tuberculosis, it manifests itself through the appearance or worsening of symptoms that had initially receded: Fever, lung infiltration, skin lesions, peripheral and mediastinal adenopathies, and serous gland and central nervous system damage, all of which are potentially severe symptoms. PPD also becomes positive.

Immune reconstitution syndrome appears during the first 3 months after the start of antiretroviral therapy, generally during the first 15–21 days. It is self-limited and can last for up to 40 days. Etiological tests yield negative results. In some cases, it is necessary to administer steroids to control the patient's symptoms.

Diagnosis is clinical and requires ruling out treatment failure, adverse effects of the medications, associated infections, or tumors. Also, it must meet the following conditions: temporal connection with the start of antiretroviral therapy, severe immunosuppression when starting antiretroviral administration, and good immunological and virological response to this therapy. To prevent the appearance of the immune reconstitution syndrome, it is necessary to rule out the presence of opportunistic infections before administering antiretrovirals; also, infections must be treated adequately some weeks before initiating antiretroviral therapy.

Neoplasia

Although neoplasias are infrequent in children affected by HIV, their incidence is higher than in normal children. After being diagnosed with AIDS, 2.5% of these children develop malignant tumors. The most common neoplasms are non-Hodgkin lymphoma, Kaposi's sarcoma, leiomyosarcoma, and Hodgkin's lymphoma. Neoplasms tend to be highly undifferentiated.

These tumors can start in the lung or spread to it. Clinical presentation is similar to that of pneumonia with cough, fever, hemoptysis, and exercise intolerance. Because lymphatic tissue is abundant in the airway, lymphatic proliferation is common in HIV infection, and pseudolymphomas are usually detected.

Sources

Centers for Disease Control and Prevention. Revised surveillance case definition for HIV infection-United States, 2014. MMWR. 2014;63(RR-3):1–10.

CDC. Guidelines for the use of antiretroviral agents in pediatric HIV infection 1994 revised classification system for human immunodeficiency virus infection in children less than 13 years of age. MMWR. 1994;43(RR-12):1–10.

CDC. Guidelines for prevention and treatment of opportunistic infections among HIV-exposed and HIV-infected children. MMWR. 2013;62(44):889. http://aidsinfo.nih.gov/contentfiles/lvguidelines/oi_guidelines_pediatrics.pdf

Coinfección TB-VIH. Guía clínica, versión actualizada 2010. Washington DC: Organización Panamericana de la Salud (OPS); 2010.

Dankner W, Lindsey J, Levin M, Pediatric AIDS Clinical Trials Group Protocol Teams. Correlates of opportunistic infections in children infected with the human immunodeficiency virus managed before HAART. Pediatr Infect Dis J. 2001;20(1):40–8.

Graham SM. Non-tuberculosis opportunistic infections and other lung diseases in HIV-infected infants and children [State of the Art]. Int J Tuberc Lung Dis. 2005;9(6):592–602.

Kilborn T, Zampoli M. Immune reconstitution inflammatory syndrome after initiating highly active antiretroviral therapy in HIV-infected children. Pediatr Radiol. 2009;39(6):569–74.

Nachman S, Gona P, Dankner W, Weinberg A, Yogev R, Gershon A, et al. Rate of serious bacterial infections among HIV-infected children with immune reconstitution who have discontinued opportunistic infection prophylaxis. Pediatrics. 2005;115(4):488–94.

Panel on Antiretroviral Therapy and Medical Management of HIV-Infected Children. Guidelines for the Use of Antiretroviral Agents in Pediatric HIV Infection. http://aidsinfo.nih.gov/contentfiles/lvguidelines/pediatric-guidelines.pdf. Accessed on July 15th of 2015; table 7, page F-9.

Peña A, Larrañaga C, Luchsinger V, Villarroel J, Chávez A, Wu E y Comité Nacional de SIDA Pediátrico, Sociedad Chilena de Pediatría. Enfermedad por citomegalovirus (CMV) en niños chilenos infectados por el virus de la inmunodeficiencia humana (VIH). Rev Chil Infectol. 2007;24(6):477–84.

Theron S, Andronikou S, George R, du Plessis J, Goussard P, Hayes M, Mapukata A, Gie R. Non-infective lung disease in HIV-positive children. Pediatr Radiol. 2009;39(6):555–64.

UNAIDS. The Gap report. Acceso 24 de octubre de 2014 http://www.unaids.org/en/resources/campaigns/2014/2014gapreport/gapreport.

Sickle Cell Disease

52

Ofelia Álvarez and María Angélica Wietstruck

Contents

Definition

Sickle cell disease (SCD) is a type of recessive autosomal hemoglobinopathy. It is caused by a specific mutation in the gene that codifies the globin beta-chain in the hemoglobin (Hb) molecule, which results in a substitution of glutamic acid by a valine in the 6th position of the chain, thus creating HbS. This Hb is polymerized in the red blood cell, causing an alteration in its shape and hemolysis, which causes acute events and progressive damage in different organs. In 1910 James Herrick was the first to describe the characteristic shape of the red blood cell (drepanocytes, sickle cell, from the Latin *falx, falcis*: "sickle shape"). Subsequently, Pauling et al. identified electrophoresis anomalies in HbS, and proposed the term "molecular disease" in 1949, thus demonstrating for the first time that the

O. Álvarez (✉)
Clinical Pediatrics, University of Miami,
Coral Gables, FL, USA
e-mail: oalvarez2@med.miami.edu

M. A. Wietstruck
Pediatrics, Oncology, Pontificia Universidad Católica
de Chile, Santiago, Chile
e-mail: mwietstr@med.puc.cl

P. Bertrand, I. Sánchez (eds.), *Pediatric Respiratory Diseases*,
https://doi.org/10.1007/978-3-030-26961-6_52

production of an abnormal protein could be the cause of a genetic disorder.

There are several genotypes of the disease, causing different clinical manifestations. The concept of sickle cell anemia refers to the most usual presentation, in which the patient inherits HbS from both parents, thus being homozygote for the disease (HbSS); those who inherent an S-gene and another causing alteration in the β-chain will have other presentations of sickle cell disease, such as HbSC or HbS/β thalassemia (β^0 when there is no production of β chains; β+ when there is partial production). In all of these, HbS represents the greatest proportion of Hb in the erythrocyte. Heterozygous patients inherent only one allele from their parents: the other allele is normal (HbA), and they are named carriers (HbAS), and have what is known as "sickle cell trait." Carriers are usually asymptomatic.

Epidemiology

The distribution of HbS in the world indicates two factors: migration and the selection of individuals who are HbS carriers because of their resistance to malaria in endemic regions. The greatest prevalence of SCD is in tropical Africa. It has been estimated that every year 230,000 children affected by this disease are born in this region (0.74% of all live births), in comparison to the 2,600 children born in the United States, and 1,300 in Europe. Migrations have spread the disease in America, not only in the African population, but also in their descendants. Diagnosis is confirmed with Hb analysis through electrophoresis or chromatography.

Etiology and Physiopathology

The physiopathological manifestations of SCD are hemolysis and vaso-occlusion (Fig. 52.1). When red blood cells flow in microcirculation, Hb deoxygenation is caused, which involves a change in the composition of the molecule. HbS is less soluble in a deoxygenated environment (which can also be caused by stress, hypoxia, or acidosis), and therefore Hb is polymerized within the red blood cell, and its membrane is distorted, originating a rigid cell with poor deformability. Hb polymers trigger a cascade of events within the cell:

a. Activation of transport channels, with potassium loss and cellular dehydration.
b. Disruption of the red blood cell membrane, thus exposing it to membrane components, such as band 3 protein, which binds to specific antibodies, promoting erythrophagocytosis caused by macrophages.
c. Liberation of hemoglobin in the plasma, with Fe^{3+}, which promotes oxidative damage in the microenvironment.

Vaso-occlusive crises are caused by erythrocyte and leukocyte entrapment in the microcirculation, originating vascular obstruction and tissue ischemia. Although this process requires HbS polymerization, the trigger event for vascular obstruction is a type of inflammation. This inflammation results from an interaction between the erythrocyte and vascular endothelium, causing obstruction and ischemia episodes, which are followed by a restitution of the vascular flow, causing tissue damage mediated by reperfusion. Then, oxidative stress is triggered, which causes adhesion molecule overexpression, increasing inflammatory cytokines synthesis and leukocytosis. Hemolysis also contributes to vaso-occlusion. Hemoglobin liberation in plasma, caused by intravascular hemolysis, generates superoxide radicals and hydroxyl, which are potent inhibitors of nitric oxide (NO). This compound is produced under normal conditions in the endothelium and regulates the basal vasodilator tone, inhibits platelets, hemostatic activation, and the expression of adhesion molecules dependent on the nuclear factor kβ (FNkβ). Hb release into the plasma also causes endothelial dysfunction and NO resistance. Hemolysis also liberates arginase-1 in the erythrocyte, which metabolizes arginine into ornithine, exhausting the substrate required to synthesize NO. All of this helps to maintain hypercoagulability, with an increase in the platelet activation and the levels of procoagulant factors in the blood.

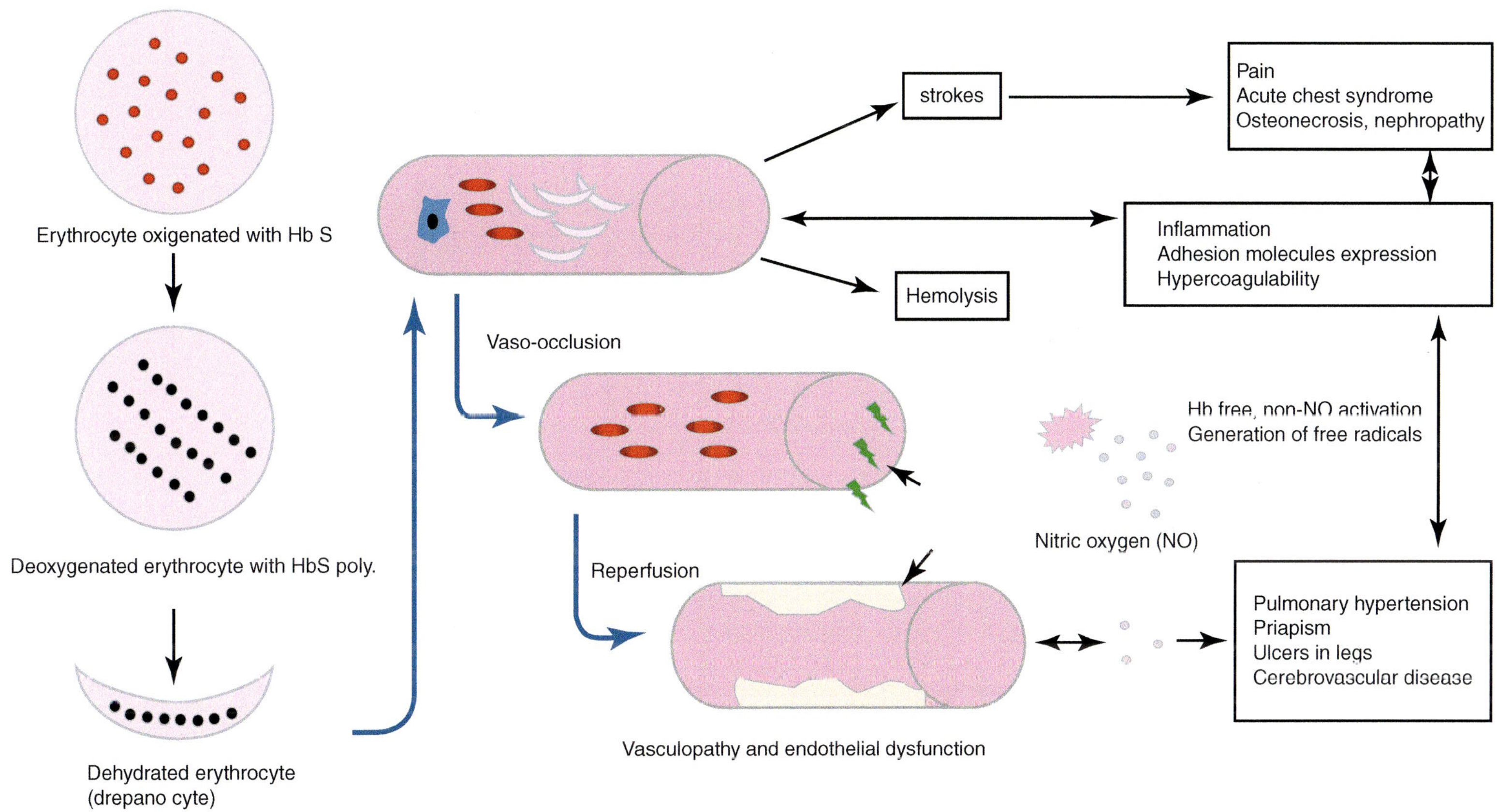

Fig. 52.1 Physiopathology of sickle cell anemia. (*Source:* Adapted from Rees DC et al. *Lancet*. 2010;376:218–222)

It is important to note that acute and chronic inflammatory events happen in the lung because erythrocytes are exposed to relatively low O_2 tensions, as well as the slow flow of the cells. The airway and vascular system are in close connection, which eases the transference of inflammatory mediators among each other.

Clinical Manifestation of Sickle Cell Disease

SCD has considerable phenotypical heterogenicity, influenced by genetic and environmental factors. Hb of fetal concentration (HbF), coexistence of other hemoglobinopathies, and certain types of polymorphism in simple nucleotides modulate the risk of certain complications. Among environmental factors, environmental humidity, cold, and pollution negatively influence the patient, and particularly by increasing vaso-occlusive events.

Complications worsen with age. In infants, dactylitis (painful inflammation of the fingers and toes), anemia, hyperbilirubinemia, splenomegaly, and infections in the respiratory tract are common. Among other complications, children may present growth and puberty delay, cognitive alterations, and cerebrovascular accidents. Adults tend to have articular pain, chronic ulcers in the legs, kidney failure, and neurocognitive disorders.

Sickle cell anemia complications can appear in any organ, and some of them can be very serious. In this chapter we only present the pulmonary complications (Table 52.1).

Table 52.1 Respiratory problems associated with sickle cell anemia

Pulmonary manifestation	Respiratory symptoms	Causes
Acute chest syndrome	Hypoxemia and dyspnea Crackles Sound reduction in lung fields	Multifactorial
Asthma	Wheezing Dyspnea	Airway hyperreactivity
Alterations in lung function	Asymptomatic Hypoxemia	Restrictive and obstructive lung disease
Obstructive sleep apnea	Flow oximetry reduction during sleep Apnea	Increase of lymph tissue in Amygdale and adenoids
Day hypoxemia	Hypoxemia Dyspnea	Hemoglobin desaturation Pulmonary fibrosis
Pulmonary hypertension	Hypoxemia Dyspnea Exercise intolerance	Hemolysis Endothelial dysfunction

Respiratory Clinical Manifestations, Diagnostic Approach and Treatment

Acute Chest Syndrome

Acute chest syndrome (ACS) is a symptom of sudden pulmonary damage, defined as an infiltration of new consolidated alveoli in chest X-rays, with no evidence of atelectasis, and which involves at least a whole lung segment. Generally, the patient presents with chest pain, fever, tachypnea, wheezing, cough, and hypoxemia. The Cooperative Study of Sickle Cell Disease (CSSCD) reported an incidence of 29% (12.8 episodes for 100 patient-years) in patients with sickle cell anemia type SS. Almost half the patients with sickle cell anemia will present with one episode of acute chest syndrome, which is the second cause of hospitalization, after vaso-occlusive crisis (VOC). This may be the initial presentation, although it can also appear after the first 3 days, in 10% to 20% of the cases during their hospital stay. Children between 2 and 4 years of age have the greatest incidence (25.3 years per patient).

Risk factors for this complication involving having HbSS or HbS/β0, thalassemia, asthma, chronic hypoxemia, low HbF, tobacco smoke exposure, general anesthesia, and surgery, mainly abdominal, and during the winter season. There are multiple causes for ACS. The National Acute Chest Syndrome Study Group (NACSSG) studied the causes in 671 episodes presented in 538 patients. Infections were the main cause in 29% of the cases. It is thought that respiratory infections promote an inflammatory response in the lung. Pneumonia caused by *Chlamydia* was the most common cause, followed by the pneumonia caused by *Mycoplasma*, viral pneumonia, and bacterial infections last.

Another cause for the acute chest syndrome is fat embolism. During a bone ischemic event, a piece of the marrow or bone that is detached because of a bone marrow stroke migrates through the blood flow to the lungs. As a consequence, sudden inflammation appears. This syndrome caused by fat embolism tends to have a severe clinical presentation, and it tends to appear with pain, neurological symptoms, thrombocytopenia, and increase in transaminases.

Activation of the secretory phospholipase A2 hydrolyzes the fat emboly in sn-2 position, creating free fat acids and lysophospholipids, which cause lung damage. When arachidonic acid is caused by this hydrolysis, a series of inflammation mediators appear, such as thromboxane, leukotrienes, and prostaglandins. Secretory phospholipase A2 increases (336 ± 209 ng/ml; basal level 10 ± 8.4 ng/ml) during an acute chest syndrome presentation, and this increase can predict the disease within the following 24–48 h. Nevertheless, this analysis is still not commercially available, and it has to be validated as a diagnostic test.

A third mechanism of the ACS is pulmonary strokes. This phenomenon has not been carefully studied, and it could be an exclusion diagnosis. Recently, it has been observed that patients may have pulmonary artery thrombosis. This etiology was discovered in 17% of the cases using multidetector computed tomography (CT). Most of the positive findings (81%) in the study by Mekontso Dessap et al. were partial defects in blood vessels. Patients received anticoagulation treatment. Risk factors involved were thrombocytosis and less evidence of hemolysis.

The clinical presentation of the ACS fluctuates in severity. The physician must be alert to detect the beginning of this process. The typical clinical presentation is characterized by chest or limb pain, and fever, followed by hypoxemia and dyspnea. Sometimes the patient has yellow sputum, probably related to fat embolism. Lung examination may reveal crackles, wheezing, and reduction of lung sounds. It is common to find a reduction of hemoglobin levels of 0.7 g/dl on average, and sometimes thrombocytopenia is also present. Thrombocytopenia is an independent risk factor to suffer from multilobe ACS, as well as for needing assisted ventilation. Although most patients can be treated without problems, 13% may require assisted ventilation. CSSCD investigators reported a mortality of 1.1% of children and 4.3% in adults. Other studies have reported a rate of almost 9% in adults.

During an episode of vaso-occlusive crisis, it is recommended to constantly monitor the oximetry. If the patient develops hypoxemia (oximetry <95%), or if during auscultation symptoms or signs compatible with acute chest syndrome appear, a chest X-ray will be required. The diagnosis is confirmed by the finding of a new consolidation in the chest X-ray. Consolidations are more common in lower and medial lung fields (Fig. 52.2). There may be pleural effusion, usually sterile. This infiltration is long lived, usually continuing between 10 and 12 days, especially if an infection is involved. Computerized tomography gives a better view of hyperfusion, reduced number of arterioles and venules, and areas with ground glass presentation.

It is recommended to repeat the hemogram to diagnose anemia and thrombocytopenia, as well as obtaining a crossed histocompatibility test, in case a transfusion is needed. Obtaining a gasometric analysis will be of use during the treatment, particularly if the patient presents with a case of respiratory distress. If fever is present, a blood culture is required, to identify the bacterial agent in a reduced number of patients (3.5%). The following are not routine tests: sputum culture, D-dimer exam, and computerized tomography.

Bronchoscopy is not necessary for diagnosis and it is not recommended. Nevertheless, in special cases, if the patient's condition worsens considerably in spite of the treatment, it could help to find a cause such as plastic bronchitis. This complication consists of a mucus blockage caused by bronchial secretions that worsens the hypoxemic state and lung condensations. In this case, the procedure improves the patient's condition, both clinically and radiographically. Secretion block-

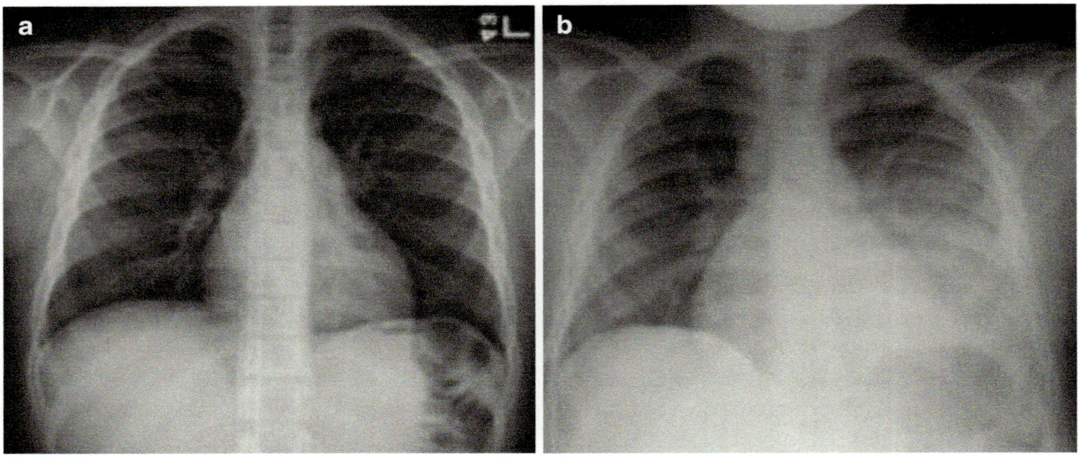

Fig. 52.2 Acute chest syndrome (ACS) shown in chest X-ray in 12-year-old schoolchild with ACS (**a**) at admittance caused by coronavirus (CoV), and (**b**) after ACS has been established

ages can be removed with saline washing and continuous suction of the blockage, which is then attached to the tip of the bronchoscope; after this, the bronchoscope is removed, with the blockage of the airway attached to it.

Figure 52.3 summarizes the algorithm of diagnosis and management of ACS. One of the most important measures to avoid in this syndrome is directed spirometry with 10 maximum inspirations every 1–2 h when the patient is awake. Small children who do not know how to use the equipment may blow soap bubbles. Another important measure is to adequately manage pain, without oversedation. Maintenance hydration is important during the vaso-occlusive process, because patients with SCD do not concentrate urine correctly and tend to dehydrate. Nevertheless, excessive liquids should be avoided, as this promotes lung edema.

A combination of an IV cephalosporine, such as cefuroxime, with a macrolide such as oral azithromycin, is the standard care. As an alternate regime, in case of allergies, a quinolone or a macrolide with a beta-lactam antibiotic is recommended. Oxygen must be supplied to keep the saturation over 95%. Blood transfusion must not surpass a maximum of Hb 10–11 g/dl to avoid increasing viscosity. This precaution may prevent ACS worsening, and is are recommended for severe anemia or persistent hypoxemia. Transfused red blood cells must be S negative. Blood replacement is recommended for the cases when the initial hemoglobin is high (Hb $\geq$ 10 g/dl) and the patient requires transfusion. Other indications for blood replacement are severe hypoxemia in spite of oxygen therapy, patients who need an artificial respirator, multilobe ACS, and also if there is no improvement after a simple transfusion.

An echocardiography is recommended for patients who need intensive care to detect lung hypertension. If this is the case, patients must receive intensive treatment with blood replacement.

Because of airway hyperreactivity in SCD, some investigators propose the routine use of bronchodilators, although others only use it for treating wheezing or prolonged expiration.

Use of steroids such as IV dexamethasone 0.3 mg/kg every 12 h at four doses may shorten hospitalization time, but it is associated to relapses in up to 25% of the patients once the treatment is interrupted, and therefore its use is controversial. Although NO seems to be related to the pathology of the hemolysis, as well as improving ACS in preliminary trials, it did not reduce the duration of the vaso-occlusive crisis. Therefore, it had no impact on the development of this syndrome in clinical trials done afterward.

ACS morbidity is wide, both in the short and long term. This syndrome may be conditioned to

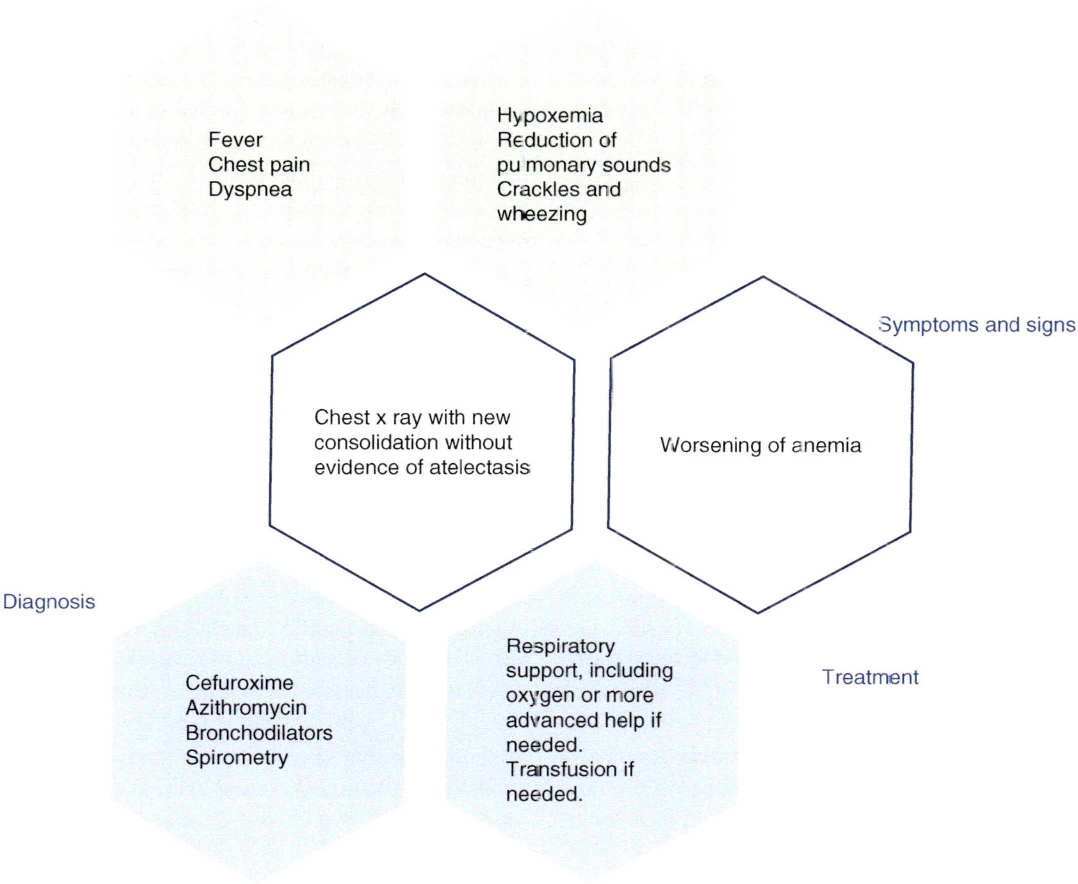

Fig. 52.3 Algorithm of diagnosis and management of ACS

the development of chronic lung disease, acute lung hypertension during the episode (specially in adults), and respiratory failure (13% of NACSSG patients). Wide lobal affectation, platelets <200,000/mm^3, and a history of heart disease are independent prognosis factors for respiratory failure. For difficult cases of respiratory failure that do not respond to conventional treatment, high-frequency oscillator and extracorporeal membrane oxygenation (ECMO) have been used.

Neurological events are other complications during ACS, appearing in 11% of the patients. The most common events are alterations of the mental state, convulsions, and neuromuscular abnormalities. A platelet count under 200,000 mm^3 is a risk factor for neurological complications.

The prevalence of acute kidney damage increases with the severity of the chest syndrome. Patients with this syndrome may develop multiple organ failure. Hydroxyurea, a drug that has the capacity to increase HbF, or a chronic regime of monthly transfusions could reduce the recurrence or severity of the episodes. Patients who continue to experiencing episodes even when treated with hydroxyurea or transfusions are candidates for bone marrow transplant, especially if they have a histocompatible sibling.

Pulmonary Function Tests

Spirometry, lung volume, diffusing capacity, or t transfer factor of the lung for carbon monoxide

Table 52.2 Lung function

↓Functional residual capacity (FRC)
↓Forced expiratory volume in 1 s (FEV_1)
↓Forced vital capacity (FVC)
↓Peak expiratory flow (PEF)
Normal FEV_1/FVC
No change when using bronchodilator
↓Peak expiratory pressure (PEP)

(DLCO), corrected for hemoglobin, and reactivity measures of the reversible airway with bronchodilator are routine lung function tests for patients with SCD. The methacholine parasympathetic agonist challenge test is not done routinely, because of the low risk to induce vasoconstriction and vaso-occlusion.

These patients suffer from lung dysfunction (Table 52.2). During childhood, obstructive ventilatory dysfunction may appear in 35% to 37% of the cases, and restrictive ventilatory dysfunction may appear in 8%. The Wedderburn study, which included children with SCA who were 5–16 years old, concluded that functional residual capacity (FRC), forced expiratory volume in 1 s (FEV_1), vital forced capacity (VFC), and peak expiratory flow (PEF) are lower in comparison to healthy children, but the FEV_1/VFC proportion is the same. These differences persist after receiving a bronchodilator, which suggests a mild restrictive disease. After the 10 years of age, 14% of the patients had restrictive or obstructive alterations. Children with sickle cell anemia may lose 3% of FEV_1 and 2% of total capacity per year.

Besides this, patients with SCA have a reduced percentage of peak expiratory pressure (PEP), in comparison to peak inspiratory pressure (PIP), which is the inverse proportion of normal adults and children. This PEP deficiency may contribute to a reduction in lung volume, as well as atelectasis. Changes in expiratory muscle force are caused by the fact that abdominal and internal intercostal muscles are supplied by epigastric and intercostal arteries, which do not have extensive collaterals. On the contrary, the diaphragm contributes to inspiration, and it is supplied by several arteries, and therefore is more resistant to ischemic processes.

As patients age, lung function worsens. Only 10% of the adults with sickle cell disease have a normal lung examination according to the CSSCD analysis, which was conducted before the general use of hydroxyurea. Generally, adult patients showed a reduced lung cavity of about 70 ± 15% on average in relationship to the expected value, with restrictive pattern and a DLCO adjusted for 64 ± 20% expected value of hemoglobin. Spirometry was within normal, with FEV_1 and FVC values about 83% and 84% of what was expected, respectively.

Therefore, a yearly evaluation of lung function in children who can cooperate and adults is important to detect changes. The exam must be preferentially done when the patient is stable, and at least 2 weeks after a painful episode. Although hydroxyurea reduces the number of ACS events in both adults and children, there is currently not enough information to know if it will modify the changes in lung function. The study BABY HUG Follow Up II, sponsored by the National Institute of Health in the United States, will evaluate if this drug preserved lung function after 10 years, in comparison to those children who have not received hydroxyurea.

Airway Hyperreactivity and Asthma

Airway hyperreactivity, measured after bronchodilator use or subfreezing air hyperventilation, is more common in children with SCD than in control patients, particularly for younger children. Prevalence of such hyperreactivity may be as high as 85% in children with SCD and asthma, and 64% for SCD patients without asthma. Hyperreactivity detected after methacholine is 78% in patients with SCD, in comparison to 18% in children in the general population.

As a comparison, Valdivia et al. pointed out that there was a 9% prevalence of asthma, and 20% of wheezing, during the last 12 months before the study in Chilean schoolchildren. In the United States, 16.8% of 291 children with SS hemoglobin, who were followed as part of the multi-centric observational study of the CSSCD, had bronchial asthma. This prevalence is similar to the asthma prevalence among Afro-Americans.

It is important to point out that asthma patients have a two- to four fold risk to develop acute chest syndrome during a hospitalization for a vaso-occlusive crisis, as well as having long hospitalizations, and to be readmitted 3 days after they were discharged. Also, asthma is associated to a double death risk among patients with SCD.

It is not clear why asthma may complicate SCD. The explanation may lie in common mechanisms, such as leukotrienes. Leukotrienes are lipids derived from arachidonic acid that mediate inflammation. Phospholipase A2 releases arachidonic acid from the cellular membranes and causes the production of A4 leukotriene. Leukotriene B4, which is produced in this process, is involved in the activation and chemiotaxis of neutrophils and cysteine leukotrienes, causing bronchoconstriction, smooth muscle proliferation, mucus production, and airway edema; these may be associated to pain pathogeny.

The clinical record must include questions about the onset of respiratory distress and wheezing, exercise intolerance, and family history of asthma. Patients can be evaluated at the same time with questionnaires to detect asthma. Controlling environmental factors and the possibility of other conditions, such as gastroesophageal reflux, sinusitis, and obstructive sleep apnea, must be considered.

A patient with asthma and SCD must be treated as any other, following the recommendations for asthma diagnosis and treatment summarized by a group of experts at the National Institute of Health (NIH) in the United States, which are also available on the Internet. Although there is some evidence that systemic steroids may exacerbate a vaso-occlusive crisis, the benefit of asthma control exceeds the risks. Therefore, inhaled or systemic steroids should be administered if they are needed. If a beta-3 agonist is needed, it may be necessary to have an electrocardiogram to evaluate the QTc interval, because such agonists may increase morbidity in patients who have a prolonged QTc.

Hypoxemia

Hypoxemia is defined as a hemoglobin saturation in the oximetry under 95%. Hemoglobin desaturation in sickle cell anemia is in part caused by the movement to the right of the hemoglobin dissociation curve, due to HbS properties and the effects of chronic anemia through biphosphoglycerate 2.3. A retrospective analysis reported by Quinn, which involved 585 children under 20 years old, with an average age of 9 years old, found that patients with SS or S/β0 thalassemia had an average pulse oximetry saturation (Sat O_2) of 96.3%; 33% presented with a saturation <96%, and 2.8% presented a saturation under 90%. When compared to the patients who had HbSC or S/β+ thalassemia, they had an average O_2 saturation of 98.7%; 3.6% had a saturation level <96%, and 0.5% at <90%. A good saturation was correlated with higher Hb, reticulocyte count, and lower age in the patients with SS/Sβ0.

It is recommended to control O_2 saturation during the follow-up of these patients. It is also important to check those patients who received IV opioids during pain exacerbations to prevent a prolonged hypoxemia. Oxygen administration in hypoxemic patients with sickle cell disease is a safe treatment that does not increase anemia.

Sleep Obstructive Apnea

Snoring prevalence during sleep tends to be increased in patients with sickle cell disease (37%), and the same happens for sleep obstructive apnea (19%), because of the increase in the lymphatic tissue of amygdale, adenoids, and retropharyngeal nodes, which may increase because of the functional asplenia. At the same time, apnea/hypopnea and night hypoxemia are related to priapism, pain exacerbations, and cerebrovascular events. Clinical history must include questions about sleep disorders, and if there is a suspicion of such, a polysomnography must be requested.

Obstructive sleep apnea can be treated through amygdalotomy or adenoidectomy, if there is hyperplasia in these structures. For resistant cases, oxygen should be administered, with or without a BiPAP machine.

Table 52.3 Stages of chronic lung disease

Categories	Stage 1	Stage 2	Stage 3	Stage 4
Chest pain	Substernal pain and chronic cough	Pain increase considering stage 1	Severe pain in medial line	Severe and prolonged pain with resting dyspnea
Arterial gases	O_2 normal saturation	O_2 normal saturation	Basal hypoxia with O_2 partial pressure of 70 mm Hg	Basal hypoxia with O_2 partial pressure of 60 mm Hg
X rays	Reduced distal vascularity, hyperinflation, evidence of increased interstitial marks	Fine and diffuse interstitial fibrosis in all lung lobes	Lung fibrosis	Severe lung fibrosis
Lung function	FVC, FEV_1, TLC, and FEV_1/FVC in 80% of the expected value	FVC, EFV_1, TLC, DLCO, and EFV_1/FVC in 60% of the expected value	FVC, VEF_1, TLC, DLCO, and FEV_1/FVC in 40% of the expected value	Patient has difficulties to complete the test because of hypoxia
ECG and ECO	Left ventricle hypertrophy	Biventricular hypertrophy	Right ventricle hypertrophy and enlargement of the right atrium. Progressive increase in heart size	Severe hypertrophy of the right ventricle and right atrium. T-ischemic waves in V_1 and V_2 and lung pressure
Lung arterial pressure	Normal	Normal	Normal or minimum increase normal	Increase with lung hypertension

Thromboembolism

Patients with sickle cell disease are not free from suffering from venous thrombosis and lung embolism, because anemia is a procoagulant condition, and if this is added to the bedridden condition of pain exacerbations, the risk increases. Doppler ultrasound tests of the limbs and chest helicoidal computerized tomography are useful to detect lung embolism. The management of these complications is the same as for any other type of patients.

Chronic Pulmonary Disease

Although advanced chronic pulmonary disease is rare in children with sickle cell disease, this disease is related to acute and recurrent events of vascular etiology, such as acute chest syndrome, lung edema, and chronic fibrosis. Fibrosis can be observed mainly in the bases of the lung, and it can be detected through high-resolution tomography or chest X-ray. Chronic lung disease tends to be progressive, worsening hypoxemia, dyspnea, and reducing the parameters for lung function. A patient with a corrected DLCO for Hb under 40% has a severe lung disease. Sometimes, different levels of chronic lung disease are referenced in sickle cell anemia (Table 52.3).

Lung Hypertension

Lung hypertension is defined as media lung arterial pressure (mPAP) $\geq$25 mm Hg, determined through heart catheterization, and it is responsible for the death of 30% of adults with SS:

It is thought that lung hypertension is caused by hemolysis and NO reduction, as was discussed in the physiopathology section. Both NO and endothelin-1 are opposing vaso-active factors that regulate lung vascular tone. Endothelin-1 and the plasminogen activator inhibitor-1 (PAI-1) are increased by the effect of hypoxia-inducible factor 1-alpha (HIF-1α) subunit in endothelial cells of lung microvasculature. At the same time, HIF-1α is produced by the placental growth factor, which is a pro-angiogenic factor, produced by sickle cells. Plasma hemin may also contribute to the activation of the immune system and inflammation. Other clinical factors that contribute are chronic lung disease, hypercoagulability condition of the sickle cell anemia, such as low levels of C and S protein, and a previous history of splenectomy.

The American College of Cardiology Foundation and the American Heart Association recommend a yearly evaluation for the patients under risk of developing lung hypertension, such as patients with sickle cell anemia. Echocardiograms may be used as a test of adverse prognostic if tricuspid regurgitation rate (TRR) is ≥2.5 m/s, which is the value of two standard deviations above the median. At the same time, TRR is used to calculate mPAP. mPAP is estimated using a modified Bernoulli equation: mPAP = 0.61sPAP + 2, where sPAP is the systolic pressure of the lung artery, which is estimated through the formula sPAP = 4 × TRR(Kanter and Kruse-Jarres 2013) + right atrium pressure. TRR prevalence at ≥2.6 m/s is present in 11% of the children. In adults, 30% will have a TRR ≥ 2.5 m/s, but only 6–10% have lung hypertension because of catheterization.

Besides the echocardiography evaluation, N-terminal pro-b-type natriuretic peptide (NT-proBNP), the 6-min walk test, and use of a catheter are steps in the diagnostic process (Fig. 52.4).

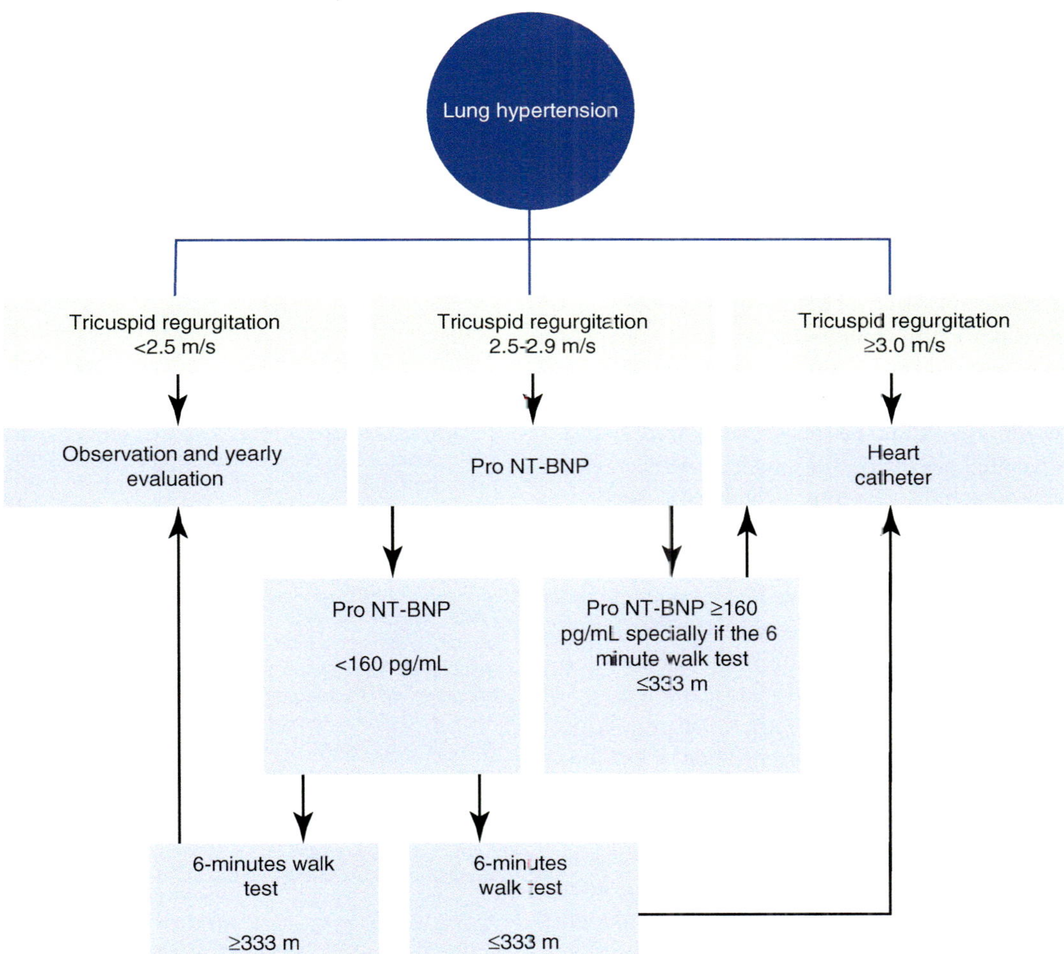

Fig. 52.4 Diagnostic algorithm of lung hypertension

Lung hypertension can be arterial, venous, or mixed: 50% of patients with lung hypertension have the arterial presentation (mPAP ≥25 mm Hg) and lung capillary pressure (PCP ≤15 mm Hg), which means that the vasculopathy is mainly located in the arterial lung system. Further, 50% of patients have venous-lung hypertension with mPAP ≥25 mm Hg, and besides this, the diastole final pressure of the left ventricle is >15 mm Hg, or there is evidence of diastolic failure. If the transpulmonary pressure gradient is <12 mm Hg, lung hypertension is venous; and if it is ≥12 mm Hg, it is mixed.

Lung hypertension therapy in SCD is divided into therapies aimed to anemia, such as hydroxyurea and blood transfusions to keep HbS under 20%. Relative to therapies directed to lung hypertension, the Walk PHaSST double-blind clinical study "Treatment: Progression of pulmonary hypertension and sickle cell anemia with sildenafil treatment" was designed to treat those patients with a tricuspid regurgitation rate >2.7 m/s with sildenafil. There were 483 participants, 52 of them (10.8%) were 12–20 years old, and most of them were adults. Unfortunately, the study ended early, because the adverse events reported for the patients treated with sildenafil had a twofold increase, particularly in relationship to pain, in comparison to those who received placebo. No differences in efficiency were found.

Another alternative for lung hypertension is to use endotelin-1 receptor antagonists, such as bosentan and ambrisetan. Nevertheless, double-blind studies ASSET-1 and -2, which studied bosentan in patients with sickle cell anemia and lung hypertension, were closed because of lack of enrollment. Therefore, information about these drugs in relation to these patients is limited.

In patients with systemic arterial hypertension or diastolic disorder, pressure should be controlled, and antidiuretic treatment should be started if there is heart failure. Prostanoid analogues are effective to treat lung hypertension. Epoprostenol administration reduces lung arterial pressure and lung vascular resistance, as well as increasing the cardiac output in patients with sickle cell anemia and lung hypertension. However, the chronic treatment of these patients has not been reported. An adolescent with sickle cell anemia and lung hypertension, which was resistant to sildenafil, bosentan, and treprostinil, who continued with severe symptoms, underwent a bilateral lung transplant successfully after 1-year follow-up.

Sources

Adekile AD. What's new in the pathophysiology of sickle cell disease? Med Princ Pract. 2013;22:311–2.

Kanter J, Kruse-Jarres R. Management of sickle cell disease from childhood through adulthood. Blood Rev. 2013;27:279–87.

Klings ES, Wyszynski DF, Nolan VG, Steinberg MH. Abnormal pulmonary function in adults with sickle cell anemia. Am J Respir Crit Care Med. 2006;173:1264–9.

Knight-Madden J, Forrester TS, Lewis NA, Greenough A. Asthma in children with sickle cell disease and the association with acute chest syndrome. Thorax. 2005;60:206–10.

Machado RF, Barst RJ, Yovetich NA, Hassell KL, Kato GJ, Gordeuk VR, et al. Hospitalization for pain in patients with sickle cell disease treated with sildenafil for elevated TRV and low exercise capacity. Blood. 2011;118:855–64.

MacLean JE, Atenafu E, Kirby-Allen M, MacLusky IB, Stephens D, Grasemann H, et al. Longitudinal decline in lung volume in a population of children with sickle cell disease. Am J Respir Crit Care Med. 2008;178:1055–9.

Mekontso Dessap A, Deux JF, Abidi N, Lavenu-Bombled C, Melica G, Renaud B, et al. Pulmonary artery thrombosis during acute chest syndrome in sickle cell disease. Am J Respir Crit Care Med. 2011;184:1022–9.

Miller AC, Gladwin MT. Pulmonary complications of sickle cell disease. Am J Respir Crit Care Med. 2012;185(11):1154–65.

Minniti CP, Sable C, Campbell A, Rana S, Ensing G, Dham N, et al. Elevated tricuspid regurgitant jet velocity in children and adolescents with sickle cell disease: association with hemolysis and hemoglobin oxygen desaturation. Haematologica. 2009;94(3):340–7.

Morris CR. Asthma management: reinventing the wheel in sickle cell disease. Am J Hematol. 2009;84:234–41.

Odievre MH, Verger E, Silva-Pinto AC, Elion J. Pathophysiology insights in sickle cell disease. Indian J Med Res. 2011;134:532–7.

Ong BA, Caboot J, Jawad A, McDonough J, Jackson T, Arens R, et al. Respiratory muscle force and lung volume changes in a population of children with sickle cell disease. Br J Haematol. 2013;163:112–7.

Paul RN, Castro OL, Aggarwal A, Oneal PA. Acute chest syndrome: sickle cell disease. Eur J Haematol. 2011;87(3):191–207.

Quinn CT, Ahmad N. Clinical correlates of steady-state oxyhaemoglobin desaturation in children who have sickle cell disease. Br J Haematol. 2005;131(1):129–34.

Rees DC, Williams TN, Gladwin MT. Sickle cell disease. Lancet. 2010;376:218–31.

Strauss T, Sin S, Marcus CL, Mason TB, McDonough JM, Allen JL, et al. Upper airway lymphoid tissue size in children with sickle cell disease. Chest. 2012;142(1):94–100.

Sylvester KP, Patey RA, Milligan P, Dick M, Rafferty GF, Rees D, et al. Pulmonary function abnormalities in children with sickle cell disease. Thorax. 2004;59:67–70.

Valdivia G, Caussade S, Navarro H, Cerda J, Pérez E, Aquevedo A, et al. Influencia del nivel socio-económico (N SE) en el asma bronquial y cambios en su prevalencia en población escolar en un periodo de 6 años. Rev Méd Chile. 2009;137:215–25.

Vichinsky EP, Neumayr LD, Earles AN, Williams R, Lennette ET, Dean D, et al. Causes and outcomes of the acute chest syndrome in sickle cell disease. National Acute Chest Syndrome Study Group. N Engl J Med. 2000;342:1855–65.

Wedderburn CJ, Rees D, Height S, Dick M, Rafferty G, Lunt A, et al. Airways obstruction and pulmonary capillary blood volume in children with sickle cell disease. Pediatr Pulmonol. 2013; https://doi.org/10.1002/ppul.22845.

Congenital Malformations of the Airway

53

Ilse Contreras Estay, Luis Enrique Vega-Briceño, and Ignacio Sánchez

Contents

Epidemiology

Congenital malformations of the airway include a wide list of diseases that are generally infrequent in occurrence but that can have a very relevant repercussion. It is one of the groups with the greatest mortality, only surpassed by cardiovascular and neurological mortality. Its exact incidence is unknown. Clinical approximations yield 1 case in 5,000 to 50,000 newborns for laryngeal and tracheal malformations, or malformations associated to high tracheal impact, such as esophageal atresia.

There is no consensus in relation to its classification, and different proposals have been made based on anatomical factors, pathogenesis, and association with malformations of other systems. Because of this, it is even more difficult to estimate its frequency.

Clinical Presentation

Patients with airway congenital malformations have no healthy periods between exacerbations, so they present symptoms permanently and their symptoms increase with exacerbations, which are usually common respiratory infections during childhood. Depending on the anatomical level of the airway obstruction, symptoms will be related to respiratory distress and transmission noises

I. Contreras Estay
Department of Pediatrics, Hospital Padre Hurtado, Santiago, Chile

L. E. Vega-Briceño (✉)
Faculty of Medicine, Universidad del Desarrollo, Santiago, Chile
e-mail: levega@udd.cl

I. Sánchez
Department of Pediatrics, School of Medicine, Pontificia Universidad Católica de Chile, Santiago, Chile

P. Bertrand, I. Sánchez (eds.), *Pediatric Respiratory Diseases*, https://doi.org/10.1007/978-3-030-26961-6_53

caused by the lumen airway obstruction. At the same time, the cardinal sign will be stridor when extrathoracic compromise is dominant, and wheezing will be the cardinal sign when the compromise is intrathoracic.

Laryngomalacia

Laryngomalacia (LM) is the most frequent cause of congenital stridor as well as the most common congenital laryngeal anomaly, corresponding to up to 75% of congenital stridor. It is more frequent in males, in a 2:1 ratio. LM is caused by a laryngeal obstruction in the supraglottis, secondary to flaccidity of cartilage or muscle arytenoid structures, arytenoid epiglottic folding, or a combination of these (Fig. 53.1). It has been proposed that probable mechanisms are (1) anatomical causes, such as omega epiglottis, short aryepiglottic ligaments, and redundant arytenoids; (2) histological causes, because of a degree of cartilage immaturity, such as an intrinsic weakness and tendency to collapse during inspiration; and (3) neurological causes, because of muscle control immaturity, which would be associated to generalized hypotonia in the muscular support of the larynx. This last theory proposes that the relaxation of the interior concomitant esophageal sphincter would explain the presence of gastroesophageal reflux as a primary cause, but this relationship has not been confirmed.

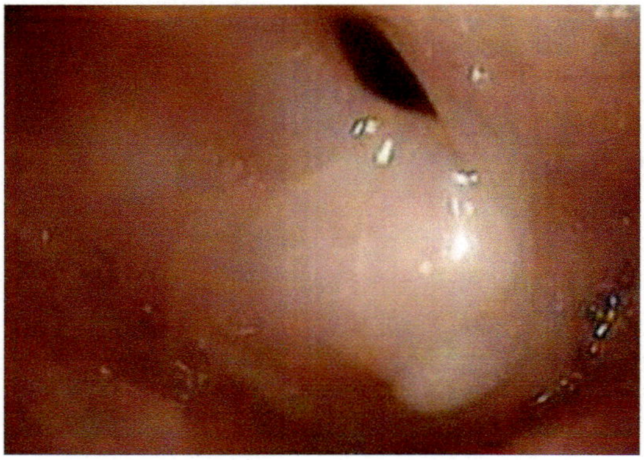

Fig. 53.1 Laryngomalacia. In laryngeal endoscopic visualization, the collapse of the arytenoid cartilage can be appreciated, occluding the lumen of the airway, in infant with persistent stridor

The characteristic inspiratory noise has a high tone, and it is intermittent. It is usually not present at birth, but it appears within the first 2 weeks of life, increases in intensity up to 6 months of life, and then it gradually disappears. In general, at 18 months most patients have no stridor, although it can persist for years in a small percentage of the patients. Typical stridor is exacerbated during effort situations, such as crying, agitation, feeding, and when in supine position. Stridor tends to be reduced with cervical extension and prone position. Most severe cases may present with respiratory difficulties, as well as cyanosis and apneas exacerbations. These symptoms are associated to alterations in feeding, gastroesophageal reflux, and lack of growth. Usually, stridor is not associated with cough, wheezing, or significant respiratory distress, and some degree of retraction may be observed. Stridor intensity is not necessarily correlated with the degree of collapse. LM severity has been classified in several ways, according to different anatomical and clinical findings (Table 53.1). Airway endoscopic evaluation is indicated if there is extreme anxiety on behalf of the parents, doubts about the diagnosis, stridor persistence after 9 to 12 months, or stridor increase after 6 months. The most common associated morbidity in LM is gastroesophageal reflux, which is present in 65% to 100% of the cases. Nevertheless, a systematic review of 27

Table 53.1 Laryngomalacia severity scale

Severity level	Respiratory symptoms	Feeding symptoms
Mild	Inspiratory stridor when crying Saturation 98–100% at rest	Occasional cough or regurgitation
Moderate	Inspiratory stridor Saturation ~96% at rest	Frequent regurgitation or feeding disorders
Severe	Inspiratory stridor at rest Cyanosis, apnea, retraction Saturation ~90% at rest	Aspiration or poor growth increase

studies that evaluated the relationship of these two diseases concluded that there is limited evidence to indicate a casual relationship. The presumptive diagnostic is clinical if the complete history and physical examinations yield the classical results of inspiratory stridor progression, and this does not require a routine endoscopic examination. The X-ray study is usually normal, but the definitive diagnosis is made through endoscopic study of the airway in 88% of the cases.

A complete airway study is recommended in patients with LM associated with other serious symptoms, such as severe respiratory distress, growth impairment, cyanosis crises, apneas, possible deglutition or aspiration disorder, recurrent wheezing or pneumonias, and those patients with an underlying condition. In these cases, an association with another lower airway abnormality can be found in as many as 15% of the cases.

For those patients with LM and hypotony, neuromuscular disorders, or genetic syndromes, it has been suggested to complete the study with polysomnography, because of the increase in central apneas (in 46%), and echocardiography for those who also have heart congenital diseases, or suspicion of hypoxemia related to LM. Prognosis is good, and therefore a great percentage requires only clinical observation to support a spontaneous improvement in 75% of the cases, and an additional 15% to 20% improve when they reach 18 months of life. Those with persistent stridor at 2 years of age should also be endoscopically assessed. Up to 5% to 15% of cases may present serious obstructive symptoms and require surgery. Supraglottoplasty is the technique of choice, as well as an arytenoepiglottoplasty, to avoid chronic hypoxemia and eventual *cor pulmonale*. In surgery cases it is suggested to associate treatment to block acid reflux. Currently, tracheotomy has been displaced, and its indication is only when supraglottoplasty fails, or for an underlying condition.

Use of noninvasive ventilation would be an option for children with severe LM and respiratory distress, as well as obstructive sleep apneas waiting for a definitive surgical resolution.

Tracheomalacia/Bronchomalacia

Tracheomalacia5 is a weakness of the tracheal wall caused by an alteration in the elastic fibers in the membrane or cartilage support. It is more frequently located at intrathoracic level, and therefore its main symptoms are present during expiration, as the lumen size is reduced. This alteration may be localized or diffuse, and compromise the cartilage support of the first- or second-generation bronchi, being called bronchomalacia (BM). Its appearance may be primary or secondary. A reduction in tracheal diameter of one third during expiration is considered mild, a reduction of one half is moderate, and a reduction that compromises three fourths of the airway is considered severe (Fig. 53.2).

Primary or congenital tracheomalacia, the most common congenital tracheal alteration, appears with a greater incidence in premature newborns. This alteration is attributed to tissue immaturity, but it is also associated to some genetic syndromes, or to disease that causes some alteration of the cartilage matrix or collagen fibers, such as mucopolysaccharidosis. TM is present in all the patients who have a tracheo-esophageal fistula, or different degrees of esophageal atresia.

Because this is a defect in embryonic development, it would still be significantly present even

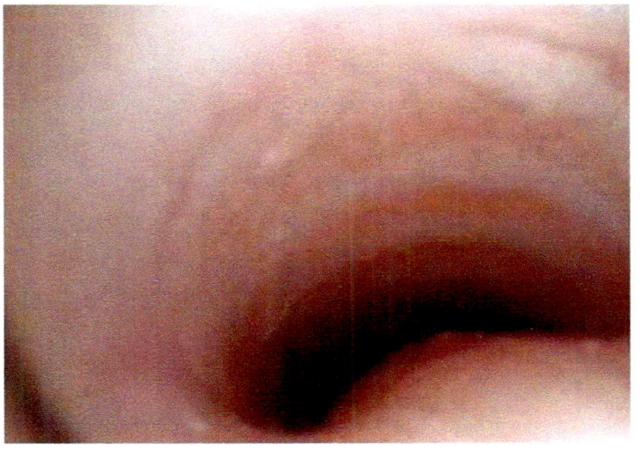

Fig. 53.2 Tracheomalacia. Endoscopic visualization of the intrathoracic trachea shows the collapse of the posterior wall moderately occluding the lumen (>60%), in an infant with Down syndrome, heart disease, and recurrent wheezing

after surgical repair. In primary cases not related to other diseases, the evolution of tracheomalacia is self-limited, normalizing close to the second or third year of life. Secondary TM is more frequent than the primary presentation, and it is predominant in males. It appears following a degeneration of the tracheal cartilage, because of prolonged intubation, tracheotomy, local injury (oxygen-caused toxicity, infections, ulcerations, or necrosis caused by local damage), or extrinsic prolonged compression (vascular rings, hypertrophy of the left atrium).

Its pathogeny is not clear, but it has been proposed that the following could be predisposing factors: genetic alteration in genes such as Sox9 and Shh, alteration in type I collagen, which is involved in the formation of the airway; or type II, which intervenes in the tension of the cartilage.

In histopathological terms, it has been observed that there is an imbalance between muscle and cartilage structure; the first one is predominant, whereas the second one is scarce. TM incidence is estimated as 1 in 1500–2500 children; this number would increase significantly if we only considered premature newborns. The most usual symptoms of TM are respiratory stridor and croup cough, which generally appear during the first weeks of life, and sometimes, in the mild cases, it is only present when there are viral infections. Stridor appears frequently, because of the collapse of the proximal area, when there is an increase in the pressure gradient caused by obstruction. Feeding disorders may appear, as well as increase of secretions in the lumen, or reflex apnea, in those patients in whom there is vascular compression. In TM and BM, a clinical history of recurrent wheezing, and atelectasis and recurrent ipsilateral pneumonias, are frequent. In severe TM and BM, airway obstruction may appear, as well as cyanosis during exacerbations. The most important action for the diagnosis is clinical suspicion after a careful anamnesis and physical examination, differentiating it from asthma, foreign body aspiration, and atelectasis caused by a different entity, among other possibilities. If the newborn is premature, or there are genetic syndromes, heart diseases, or neuromuscular disorders, this entity must be suspected.

Imaging studies can be very useful, as, for example, the evaluation using contrast agents in fistulas, esophageal atresia, or vascular rings. In tracheomalacia, high-resolution computerized tomography (HRCT) can show slides and reconstruction of the airway, as well as showing the defect. Ideal diagnosis is done through a dynamic evaluation of the airway under pseudo anesthesia and spontaneous breathing, with a bronchial endoscopy. In older children, suspicion starts when a spirometry has a fluctuant obstruction in the air flow, namely in the flow/volume curve (inspiratory or expiratory branch, depending of the case). In an important percentage of patients with TM and BM, the disease spontaneously progresses to its resolution during the first 2 years of life. The recommendation is to avoid viral infections and inappropriate treatments. Chest physiotherapy is suggested for patients with ineffective cough, atelectasis, or abundant secretions. Use of bronchodilators is controversial, as a reduction in the muscle tone would favor airway collapse, although the role that the bronchospasm may have in the airway must be considered.

In the most severe cases, or those who do not improve, according to the experience of the centers, they can be managed with continuous positive pressure in the airway (CPAP), tracheotomy, and mechanical ventilation. A surgical treatment can also be considered for those who have presented vital risk or no resolution, such as aortopexy, tracheopexy, resection, and tracheal reconstruction with cartilage implants. Use of stent support tracheal devices (metallic or silicone) has been shown to be effective, and they would be useful in the short term, but they are related to other important complications: granulomas, tearing, bleeding, etc. The stents are indicated after other techniques have failed, and it has been suggested to use preferentially those that are auto-expandable and thermoplastic.

Tracheal Stenosis

Tracheal stenosis is a very infrequent disease. The trachea is characterized by the presence of approximately 20 cartilages along its length, which can range from 5.5 to 8 cm, from birth to 2 years of life. These cartilages support the lumen of the respiratory airway, but they are not complete in the posterior tracheal segment, where the membranous section is located. Tracheal stenosis is characterized by a reduction in the tracheal lumen in diverse diameters and lengths, caused by the presence of complete tracheal rings and the absence of the membranous section in the smooth muscle fibers, which may be congenital or acquired. Three types of lesions have been described: segmental stenosis with variable length, hourglass stenosis, and funnel stenosis, as well as generalized tracheobronchial hypoplasia. It is difficult to estimate its incidence, and it varies among different centers. It has been reported that the congenital tracheal stenosis rate is about 10% and the rate of acquired stenosis is 90%, secondary to prolonged intubation (75–90%), trauma, connective tissue diseases, neoplasia, or idiopathic causes. Clinical manifestations are variable and depend on the degree of severity, newborn respiratory distress, cyanosis, persistent or recurrent inspiratory stridor with prolonged progression, recurrent wheezing, atelectasis, and pneumonia. In other cases, the diagnosis has been suspected in children who have undergone an early surgery in their life and weaning has not been successful.

Recently, a review of approximately 310 children showed that there is predominance in the masculine gender and that almost half the children affected have some associated comorbidity. The most common comorbidities were pulmonary artery ring, defects in the ventricular septum, defects of the atrium septum, persistent arteriosus ductus, lung agenesis, Fallot tetralogy, and aortic restriction. A minority had associated genetic syndromes. This diagnosis is proposed for children with persistent wheezing, or 'seal cough' associated with compatible X-rays. Definitive diagnosis is through tracheal endoscopy, which allows visualizing the obstruction, its diameter, and degree of compromised length. Chest HRCT with airway reconstruction gives a better characterization of the lesion and helps to decide the type of corrective surgery. In some cases, if other malformations are suspected, a magnetic resonance image (MRI) may be requested as a complement. In older children, a spirometry presenting a fixed obstruction in the intrathoracic airway in the flow–volume curve strongly suggests tracheal stenosis.

Treatment may be conservative for mild or moderate cases, where there is no early respiratory distress, extubation failure, or poor growth, and the follow-up can be made through endoscopy during the first 2–3 years of life, but its resolution is usually surgical. Tracheoplasty may be considered, resecting the stenosis area and using end-to-end anastomosis for small lesions. However, in children with tracheal compromise, in whom more than 50% of tracheal length is compromised, a slide tracheoplasty may be needed, as well as the interposition of cartilage, thus widening the tracheal lumen in critical situations.

Vascular Rings

Vascular rings (VR) are congenital anomalies of the aortic arch and its branches that cause tracheal or esophagus compression, or both. They are infrequent, and their incidence is not clear, but they have been estimated to be about 1–3% of the congenital cardiovascular anomalies. They are classified as complete and incomplete VR. The most common ones are the complete ones, which in almost 90–95% of the cases are represented by the double aortic arch (DAA) and its subtypes (right dominant arch, left dominant arch, balanced arch), and right aortic arch (RAA) and its subtypes (RAA and left aberrant subclavian artery, and RAA+ and mirror vessels pattern). The most frequent complete ring is DAA, at about 75–90% of all, and second in place is RAA, at about 12–25%. Incomplete vascular rings do not form a complete ring around the trachea and the esophagus, but they do compress them. These rings are represented by innominate artery compression, pulmonary artery ring, and left aortic arch (LAA), with right aberrant subclavian artery. It is thought that this last entity is subdiagnosed or its diagnosis is done late, as it tends to be asymptomatic. In 38% of cases it is related to Down syndrome. An aberrant innominate artery represents 10% of the VR, and compresses the trachea through its anterior surface; it presents more symptoms if it is related to tracheomalacia or esophageal atresia, when there is no dysphagia. A pulmonary artery ring is commonly associated with a full cartilage ring, which determines the greatest cause of mortality caused by VR, and it is related to tracheobronchial alterations, such as TM, hypoplasia, or tracheal stenosis, as well as being related to heart diseases such as persistent arteriosus ductus, or ventricular or atrial communications. Sometimes VRs have been reported as associated with other congenital malformations, such as kidney (agenesis, ectopy, horseshoe kidney), tracheoesophageal fistula, hiatal hernia, diaphragmatic eventration, imperforated or ectopic anus, PHACE syndrome (posterior cranial fossa alteration, facial hemangioma, alteration of brain, cardiovascular, and eye arteries), and some genetic syndromes, such as trisomy 21, deletion 22q11.

VRs frequently present symptoms early in life, which depend on the type and degree of compression of the clinical manifestations. Usually VR appear with stridor, persistent cough, respiratory distress, or dysphagia, especially with solid foods (late symptom). Cough has been described "like a seal," or tracheal, with a metallic tone, and it is very noticeable when there are unimportant respiratory infections. Stridor is generally biphasic, but it can appear as only one sound during expiration, which is monophonic and persistent and should be called wheezing. All symptoms tend to increase with crying, feeding, playtime, or respiratory infections. Respiratory symptoms are present in 70% to 97% of all the children, according to several studies, and they may cause a poor growth. Less frequently, and only when there is a significant tracheal compression, it may appear during the newborn period with respiratory distress, suprasternal and costal retraction, tendency to cervical hyperextension, cyanosis, reflex apnea, and extubation failure. The VRs that present more symptoms are the DAA and the RAA, caused by early tracheal compression, although the aberrant subclavian artery may also be evident, because of the posterior esophageal compression, which appears later.

Diagnosis must be done through clinical suspicion in those patients with persistent symptoms, prolonged progression of the disease or poor response to usual treatments, because they share symptoms with other more common diseases, and tend to be confused with asthma. It appears between 2 and 18 months of life, but in some cases it has been diagnosed in patients more than 50 years old. A cervical X-ray shows the relationship between the trachea and the aortic arch (DAA, RAA, and LAA), besides indentations, retro-tracheal opacity, hyperinflation, and T-shaped trachea. A barium esophagogram is the exam of choice and it is very useful to show a VR, where an indentation is observed in the trachea/esophagus level in more than 90% of the cases, but a normal exam does not rule it out. It is requested when feeding symptoms are present. An image of indentation posterior suggests an aberrant subclavian artery, whereas a bilateral indentation image suggests a double aortic arch (Fig. 53.3), and if the image shows a reduction in the anterior pulse caliber using lateral projection, it suggests a ring of the pulmonary artery.

Evaluation of the airway with flexible bronchoscopy is important in the study of stridor and persistent wheezing for the differential diagnosis, where an anterior or lateral pulsatile external compression can be observed. If there is a strong suspicion of a VR, the study should be completed with angio-CAT or angio-MRI to differentiate it from other extrinsic compressions, such as bronchogenic cysts, hemangiomas, or mediastinal tumors, thus defining the specific alteration and its path and to plan the surgical approach. Both exams are very good, and there is no clear consensus about which one offers the best performance. The angio-CAT availability is wider, and it requires less time, and therefore it only requires sedation or pseudo-anesthesia. Besides this, it allows for the reconstruction of the airway and virtual bronchoscopy. The advantage of MRI is that it can picture more accurately the relationship between the structures, the presence of heart anomalies, as well as ventricular function and heart flow function, and it does not present irra-

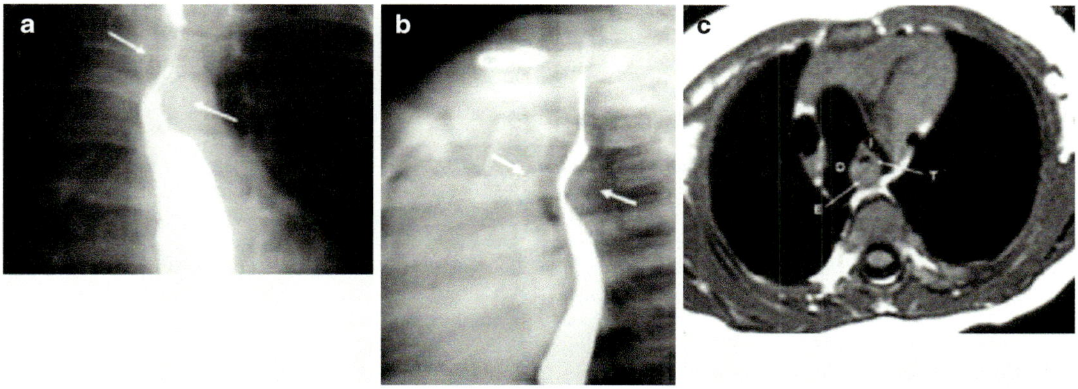

Fig. 53.3 Double aortic arch. Anteroposterior X-ray (**a**) and lateral projection (**b**) show indentation caused by the double aortic arch (DAA) (*arrows* show level of indentation); in axial slice at the aortic arch level, nuclear magnetic resonance in sequence T1 (**c**) shows a DAA (D, *right*; I, *left*) compressing the esophagus (E) and trachea (T)

diation. The great disadvantage is that it is not so readily available and it has a greater cost, and as it takes more time, it requires anesthesia for smaller children.

Cardiological evaluation (ECG and Doppler echocardiogram) must be done if there is a VR diagnosis because heart disease is present in 12–30% of cases. Lung function evaluation with spirometry may be done from preschool age in children with respiratory symptoms and an obstructive pattern that does not respond to bronchodilator use, as these are signs which can be observed when there are VRs. This fixed obstruction of the airway appears as a reduction in the expiratory flows, and a plateau at the beginning of the expiration flow–volume curve can be observed. When this defect appears in the inspiratory phase, both respiratory times are compromised. During past decades, with the improvements in fetal ultrasonography studies and specialized centers, the diagnosis of some VRs can be done early, through visualization of the origin and flow of the vessels.

Treatment will depend on the clinical condition and the type of anomaly. In children with mild or intermittent symptoms, management is conservative, avoiding respiratory infections or treating them when they are present, using physiotherapy if needed. Most of the cases in which the innominate artery is compressed spontaneously remit during the first and second year of life. Many VRs can be asymptomatic for long periods of time, so there would be no mandatory indication of a surgery. Surgical management is reserved for those cases with serious symptoms, such as cyanosis or apneas, extubation failure, with more than 50% of airway compression, or when there is no response to conservative management. Surgical technique varies according to the type of ring, arteriopexia in some types of rings in the pulmonary artery or ligament sections when they are the complete components of the rings. Operation may be through open thoracotomy or by video-assisted thoracoscopy (VATS). In general, the prognosis is very good, with a low index of complications if it is not related to a complex heart disease or underlying disease. Those patients with significant external tracheal compression may afterward progress to variable degrees of tracheomalacia and respiratory symptoms.

Sources

Contreras I, Roza G, Navarro H, Bertrand P, Cuevas M, Sánchez I, Caussade S. Estridor en el paciente pediátrico: estudio descriptivo. Rev Chil Pediatr. 2004;75:247–53.

Digoy GP, Burge SD. Laryngomalacia in the older child: clinical presentations and management. Curr Opin Otolaryngol Head Neck Surg. 2014;22:501–5.

Dobbie AM, White DR. Laryngomalacia. Pediatr Clin N Am. 2013;60:893–902.

Kir M, Saylam GS, Karadas U, Yilmaz N, Çakmakçi H, Uzuner N, et al. Vascular rings: presentation, imaging strategies, treatment, and outcome. Pediatr Cardiol. 2012;33:607–17.

Licari A, Manca E, Rispoli GA, Mannarino S, Pelizzo G, Marseglia GL. Congenital vascular rings: a clinical challenge for the pediatrician. Pediatr Pulmonol. 2015;50:511–24.

Pan W, Peng D, Luo J, Liu E, Luo Z, et al. Clinical features of airway malacia in children: a retrospective analysis of 459 patients. Int J Clin Exp Med. 2014;7:3005–12.

Perillán J. Traqueobroncomalacia en niños. Neumol Pediatr. 2012;7:6–12.

Sittel C. Pathologies of the larynx and trachea in childhood. GMS Curr Top Otorhinolaryngol Head Neck Surg. 2014;13:1–15.

Thompson DM. Laryngomalacia: factors that influence disease severity and outcomes of management. Curr Opin Otolaryngol Head Neck Surg. 2010;18:564–70.

Thorne MC, Garetz SL, et al. Paediatr Respir Rev. 2015;s1526-0542(15):00009–3.

Ywaquin R, El-Hakim H. Congenital tracheal stenosis managed conservatively: systematic review of the literature. J Otolaryngol Head Neck Surg. 2012;41:288–302.

Zgherea D, Pagala S, Mendiratta M, Marcus MG, Shelov SP, Kazachkov M. Bronchoscopic findings in children with chronic wet cough. Pediatrics. 2012;129:e364–9.

Congenital Lung Malformations 54

Juan Carlos Pattillo Silva, Sergio Zúñiga Rocha, and José Vuletin Solís

Contents

Embryology

To know the details of the origin of these malformations, it is necessary to study the embryology and development of the respiratory system. This process is directed by a finely tuned interaction between the mesenchyme (vessels) and the epithelium, which controls the time and space expressions of multiple regulatory elements needed for the creation of the lung (transcription factors, growth factors, and their cellular receptors, extracellular matrix proteins, and adhesion molecules).

Multiple exogenous and endogenous factors can affect this process, originating changes in growth, maturation, and lung function. The development of the lung in the human, which starts with the embryonic phase, has its origin in the anterior primitive intestine, and begins toward the end of the third month of gestation, with an invagination in the surface of this primitive intestine, which originates the laryngotracheal groove. In the caudal end of the invagination a bifurcation appears: lung or bronchial buds, which by separating from the esophagus or primitive anterior intestine, migrate toward the caudal end, introducing themselves in the mesoderm. Mesenchymal cells that surround these buds will

J. C. Pattillo Silva · S. Zúñiga Rocha
J. Vuletin Solís (✉)
Pediatric Surgery, Pontificia Universidad Católica de Chile, Santiago, Chile
e-mail: jpattill@med.puc.cl; zuniga@med.puc.cl; fvuletin@med.puc.cl

P. Bertrand, I. Sánchez (eds.), *Pediatric Respiratory Diseases*,
https://doi.org/10.1007/978-3-030-26961-6_54

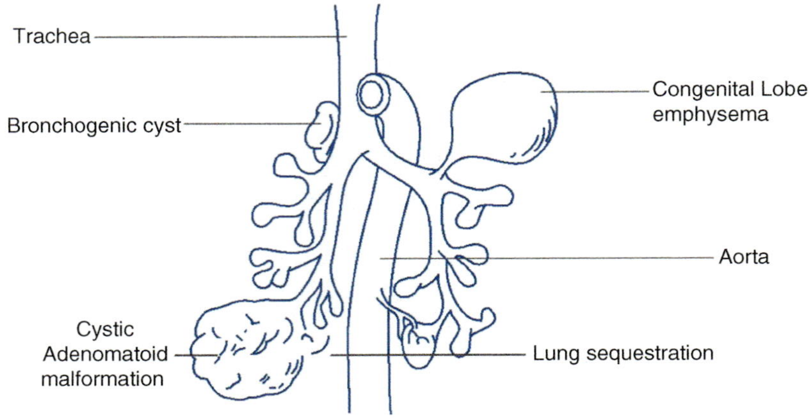

Fig. 54.1 Origin of the different bronchopulmonary malformations

generate the tracheal and bronchial walls. Then, after the fifth week, secondary buds appear. The adjacent mesoderm begins to differentiate in the parenchyma of each lung lobe. Tertiary bronchi appear during the seventh week, and so the divisions continue until reaching 17 at the moment of birth. This second stage, characterized by rapid bronchial proliferation that happens between the fifth and seventeenth week, is named the pseudoglandular phase. Most bronchopulmonary malformations take place in one of these two initial stages, after the canalicular phase begins (weeks 16–26), and then the saccular phase (weeks 24–38), when all the lung structure is developed. Starting at week 24 and until week 28, the cuboidal epithelium of the terminal air sacs starts to transform into a flat structure; this originates alveolar cells type I and type II, which will produce surfactant. By continuing the differentiation, the appearance of the lung tissue changes, from a glandular one to a highly vascularized picture, such as the alveolar organ, which will reach maturity toward the end of week 28. Finally, after birth and up to 2 to 3 years of life, the lung goes through a phase of microvascular maturation.

Anomalies in this development process may have different presentations (see Stocker). In this way, we may observe a congenital lobe emphysema (CLE), caused by the alteration in the development of a lobar or segmental bronchi, bronchogenic cysts (BC), or more appropriately, cysts of lung buds, caused by an eventual previous origin before bronchi formation: they may be related to esophagus, lung sequestration (LS), early genesis in embryonic development, before the separation of aortic and lung circulations, and cystic adenomatoid malformation (CAM), which is probably the product of the bronchial maturation arrest, along with the growth of mesenchymal elements (Fig. 54.1).

Epidemiology

It has been difficult to estimate the precise incidence of lung malformations, and because they are asymptomatic lesions, many authors consider that their frequency may be undervalued. In 2008, the European Record for the vigilance of congenital malformations (Eurocat) estimated an incidence rate of congenital chest malformations at 3.5 per 10,000 live births. The estimated incidence of cystic adenomatoid malformation was 0.7 per 10,000 live births.

Congenital Malformations of the Lung

Cystic Adenomatoid Malformation

The first case of cystic adenomatoid malformation described was published by Ch'in and Tang in 1947. In 1975, Garret conducted the first antenatal diagnostic report of a cystic adenomatoid malformation using echography. Today, almost

90% of these malformations are diagnosed before birth, and correspond to small lesions that are almost always asymptomatic, at least during the neonatal period.

These malformations are cystic lesions that are circumscribed to a segment or lung lobe in more than 95% of the cases, and any lobe may be compromised. Bilateral lesions are rare (<3%) and have a poor prognosis. Histology reveals a proliferation of terminal bronchioles, which form communicated cysts covered in respiratory epithelium with different degrees of differentiation, as well as a reduction in the number of alveoli. There is no cartilage and there is an increase of the elastic fibers. The exact cause of cystic adenomatoid malformation is unknown, and there are arguments to sustain that its different types can originate in different stages of the lung development process. Bronchiolar types (type 1, 2, and 3) may develop during the pseudo-glandular phase, while those of the acinar-alveolar type (type 4) may be the consequence of a late injury in the saccular stage. It has been proven that in cystic adenomatoid malformations there is an increase in the proliferation and a reduction of apoptosis. All these details give strength to the hypothesis of a localized interruption during lung maturation.

At first, Stocker classified them in three types based on postnatal histology. Afterward, he added types 0 and 4, which correspond to infrequent forms of cystic adenomatoid malformation. Type 0, or acinar dysplasia, refers to a tracheobronchial defect characterized by hard and small lungs connected to a tracheobronchial path, whereas type 4 corresponds to an alveolar defect located in the periphery of the lung. Only types 1 and 3 are adenomatoid, and types 1, 2, and 4 are cystic. Stocker himself has proposed to change the name of cystic adenomatoid malformation to congenital lung airway malformation, which has become popular, although it has not been universally adopted (Table 54.1, Fig. 54.2).

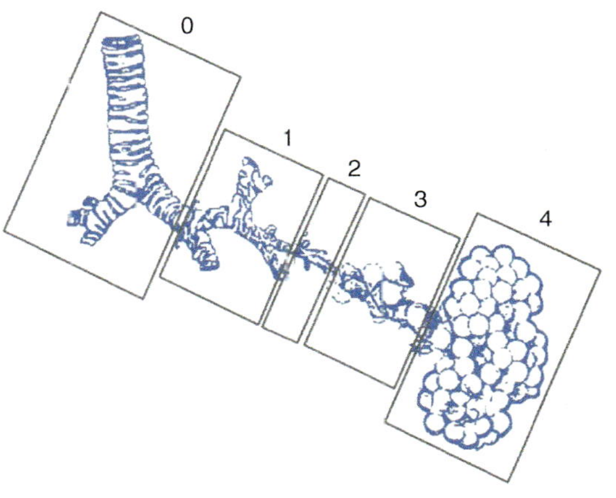

Fig. 54.2 Congenital malformation of the lung airway. Classification of the congenital malformation in the lung airway or cystic adenomatoid malformation, according to the supposed origin during lung development

Table 54.1 Classification of congenital lung malformations in the lung airway

	Incidence	Size of cysts	Histology	Notes
0	Infrequent		Complete failure of development after pseudo-glandular phase	Congenital acinar dysplasia (lethal)
1	Frequent 50%	>2 cm, may be multiple	Dilated alveolar structure, with scarce to minimum adenomatoid component. Ciliated pseudostratified columnar epithelium, with interposition of mucosal cells	
2	Frequent 40%–45%	Multiple cysts, small, "sponge"	Dilation of structures with bronchial appearance, with interposition of the alveolar parenchyma. Occasional presence of striated muscle.	Associated with genitourinary and gastrointestinal malformations
3	Infrequent 5%	Solid (cysts <3 mm)	Bronchiolar structures separated by small air spaces covered by the cuboidal epithelium, similar to late fetal lung	
4	Very infrequent	Large cysts	Peripheral cysts with alveolar or bronchial epithelium on elastic mesenchymal tissue	Related to type pleuropulmonary blastoma

The clinical presentation forms of cystic adenomatoid malformation are variable. During the antenatal period, large cystic lung lesions may cause mediastinal deviation, poor venous return, hydrops, and fetal mortality during the third trimester. During the first months of life, respiratory distress, caused by compression or pneumothorax because of the rupture of a cyst, can be an early indication of surgery in about 20% of the cases. Older children tend to be asymptomatic, and the infection of the anomalous tissue will cause recurrent pneumonias. The median for the development of the symptoms caused by infections is 10 months. The treatment is surgery, which consists of resecting the affected lobe or segment (Fig. 54.3).

Lung Sequestration

Lung sequestration is defined by the presence of lung tissue inside or outside the visceral pleural (intra- or extralobar sequestration), with no connection to the normal tracheobronchial path, and characterized by an anomalous blood delivery in the systemic veins. Venous drainage of intralobar sequestration runs toward the pulmonary veins, while the extralobar sequestration runs to the azygous vein. It has been estimated that lung sequestration is a consequence of an anomalous accessory lung bud, which was created in the primitive intestine that descends toward the caudal along with the esophagus. Extralobar sequestration may be related to other esophageal and bronchial malformations, as well as diaphragmatic defects. Most lung sequestration cases do not present symptoms during the neonatal period, and they present as an incidental image in a routine chest X-ray. They are usually located in the inferior lobes: 70% are in the left inferior lobe; 10% are under the diaphragm; and in 20% of the cases arterial irrigation comes from the infradiaphragmatic aorta. In infants, the most frequent presentation form of lung sequestration is the presence of recurrent pneumonia, which may cause localized bronchiectasis, and a particular complication is congestive heart failure, which is not present in cystic adenomatoid malformation, and is caused by the presence of aberrant circulation, and in some cases, by a significant shunt.

Lung sequestration may be diagnosed through echography and Doppler, but computerized axial tomography with contrast agent is the examination of choice, for planning and studying the surgical treatment of these lesions. This treatment consists of resection of the pathological tissue with anomalous vasculature control (Fig. 54.4). There is a superposition between cystic adenomatoid malformation and lung sequestration in several surgical series of lesions that do not exactly fulfill some of the previous categories and that are classified as mixed:

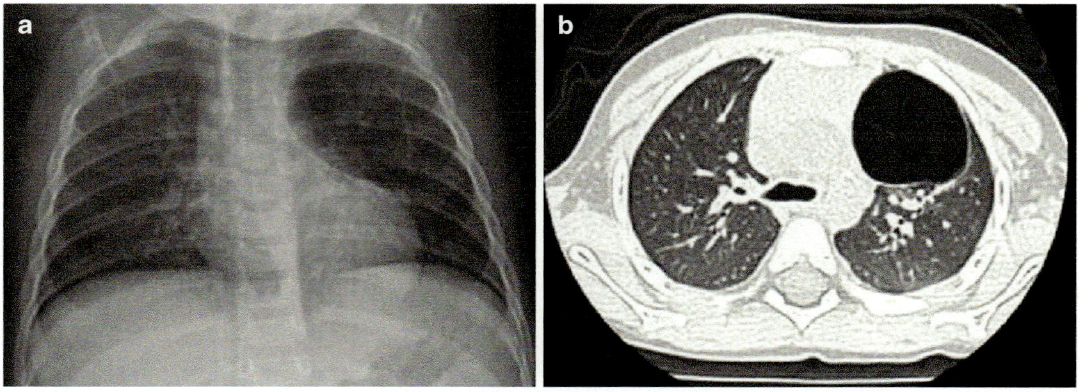

Fig. 54.3 Cystic adenomatoid malformation. (**a**) Chest X-ray of 1-year-old infant with persistent cough shows a radiolucent region in the superior left lobe. (**b**) Complementary study of the patient with computerized tomography shows a unique cystic lesion, with fine septations

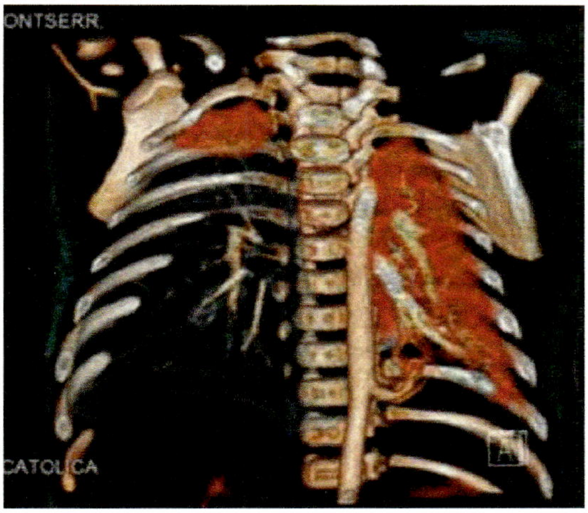

Fig. 54.4 Lung sequestration. Three-dimensional (3D) reconstruction of computerized tomography of patient with an antenatal diagnosis created when the patient was 6 months old to plan lesion extirpation. Emergence of the aberrant vessel is directly from the chest aorta

- Anatomical extralobar sequestration, but with cystic adenomatoid malformation histology
- Extralobar sequestration and cystic adenomatoid malformation in the same patient
- Cystic adenomatoid malformation in one lobe, but with systemic irrigation

Congenital Lobar Emphysema or Congenital Lobar Hyperinflation

Congenital lobar emphysema (CLE) or congenital lobar hyperinflation is the overinflation of one or more lung lobes. As this lobe increases in size, it compresses and displaces mediastinal structures and the rest of the lung. The most common cause is the presence of a valve type of bronchial obstruction, followed by the intraluminal obstruction caused by secretions or granulation tissue. Poor development of the cartilage that supports the bronchi of the affected lobe is found in only half the cases. The left upper lobe is the most commonly affected. It is more frequent in males, and it is related to congenital heart disease in 15% of the cases (ventricular septal defect, patent ductus arteriosus).

Clinical presentation includes bronchial obstruction and respiratory distress (tachypnea, costal retraction, cyanosis), which will depend on the degree of hyperinflation of the affected region. Children with CLE usually have no symptoms at birth and start to present symptoms during the first years of life: 50% of the patients present symptoms around the first month of life, and almost all of them present symptoms around 6 months of life. The development of respiratory distress may be sudden in some patients, but in others the progression is insidious. A chest X-ray helps in the diagnostic approximation, showing a lobe with fewer grids and mediastinal displacement toward the contralateral section, besides diaphragmatic flatness and compression in the rest of the lung parenchyma. The diagnostic study may be completed with a computerized axial tomography or magnetic resonance scan. Routine echocardiography evaluation is recommended to rule out associated heart diseases.

When there is doubt, flexible bronchoscopy is useful to rule out other diseases that may appear as a congenital lobe emphysema (foreign body, localized bronchomalacia).

Once the diagnosis has been confirmed, treatment consists of resecting the affected lobe. Recovery is fast and without sequelae, with lung re-expansion and early relocation of the mediastinum after the operation. Some patients with late clinical presentation or with few symptoms may be followed and treated with surgery if there are repeated infections or progression of the respiratory failure (Fig. 54.5).

Bronchogenic Cyst and Esophageal Duplication Cyst

Duplication cysts of the anterior intestine are lesions that emerge during the embryonic period (week 4–8) from the esophagus, known as enteric cysts, or from the upper airway, known as bronchogenic cysts (BC). A third way of duplication is that one caused by neurenteric cysts. As a group, these lesions are responsible for 20% of the mediastinal masses, half of them corresponding to bronchogenic cysts. Localization of bronchogenic cysts depends on the moment of development where the separation

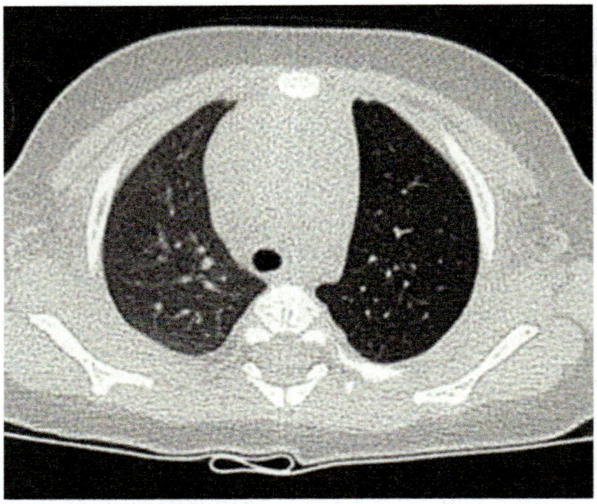

Fig. 54.5 Congenital lobe emphysema. Computerized tomography of 10-month-old infant with congenital lobar hyperinflation. Left upper lobe is more radiolucent than the right upper lobe because of the amount of air in the lung parenchyma

of the bronchial path took place; if it was early in the development, it will be located in the mediastinum; if it was late in the development, it will be located in the lung parenchyma. Bronchogenic cysts have a thin wall; they are covered by ciliated pseudostratified columnar epithelium and usually contain elements of tracheobronchial structure, such as cartilage, smooth muscle, and bronchial glands. In general, these cysts are unique, unilocular, and round. The size varies between 2 and 10 cm. According to their location, they are classified as mediastinal cysts or lung cysts. Most of the bronchogenic cysts are located at the same level as the carina, in the superior part of the trachea, where they compress the airway. They can also be paratracheal, hiliar, or paraesophageal.

The presentation of bronchogenic cysts is variable, and mainly appears during childhood, although some cases in adults have also been described. Diagnosis can be made during the antenatal period using echography. In about one third of the children this is a finding in an asymptomatic patient: 50% have respiratory symptoms associated, 10% present gastrointestinal problems, and 5% may have chest pain. Among the respiratory symptoms, respiratory distress is included, in different degrees of severity or intermittent, wheezing, stridor, and cyanosis, which worsen when crying and feeding. Another presentation mode of bronchogenic cysts is the recurrent infection, characterized by fever, cough, and pneumonia. Lung examination is usually normal, but hypersonority and signs of bronchial obstruction may be found.

A chest X-ray is useful at the beginning: It shows round or oval lesions, with uniformed density, and hydro-aerial levels can be observed. Mediastinum cysts are generally located at subcarinal level; lung cysts appear in the periphery. Computerized axial tomography (CAT) scan or magnetic resonance images (MRI) are used to define the anatomy of bronchogenic cysts, as well as their delimitation and relation with adjacent organs, to plan the surgical resection (Fig. 54.6).

Surgical resection is the treatment of bronchogenic cysts, as these cysts have a tendency to become malignant, present infections, and compromise the airway (Fig. 54.7). If the cyst cannot be completely removed, it is recommended to fulgurate the mucosa.

Esophageal duplication cysts are caused by an error in the esophagus vacuolization during embryonic development. Other malformations may be associated, such as esophagus atresia, other duplications, and vertebral anomalies. They are more common in men than in women, and tend to be present in the right hemithorax, toward the inferior esophagus. The cysts may be attached or be a part of the esophageal wall, and in up to 10% of the cases they are communicated through their lumen. It may be discovered as an asymptomatic finding, or appear with respiratory compromise, dysphagia, increase of localized volume in the neck, or enlargement of the mediastinum, in association with epigastric or retrosternal pain.

Such cysts can be suspected in the chest X-ray by the enlargement of the mediastinum, which may be deviated, or tracheal compression. A barium study may show the effect of the mass on the esophagus. Computerized tomography and magnetic resonance are the options for further study of these entities. These cysts should be operated. If there is communication with the esophagus lumen, a primary reparation may be done.

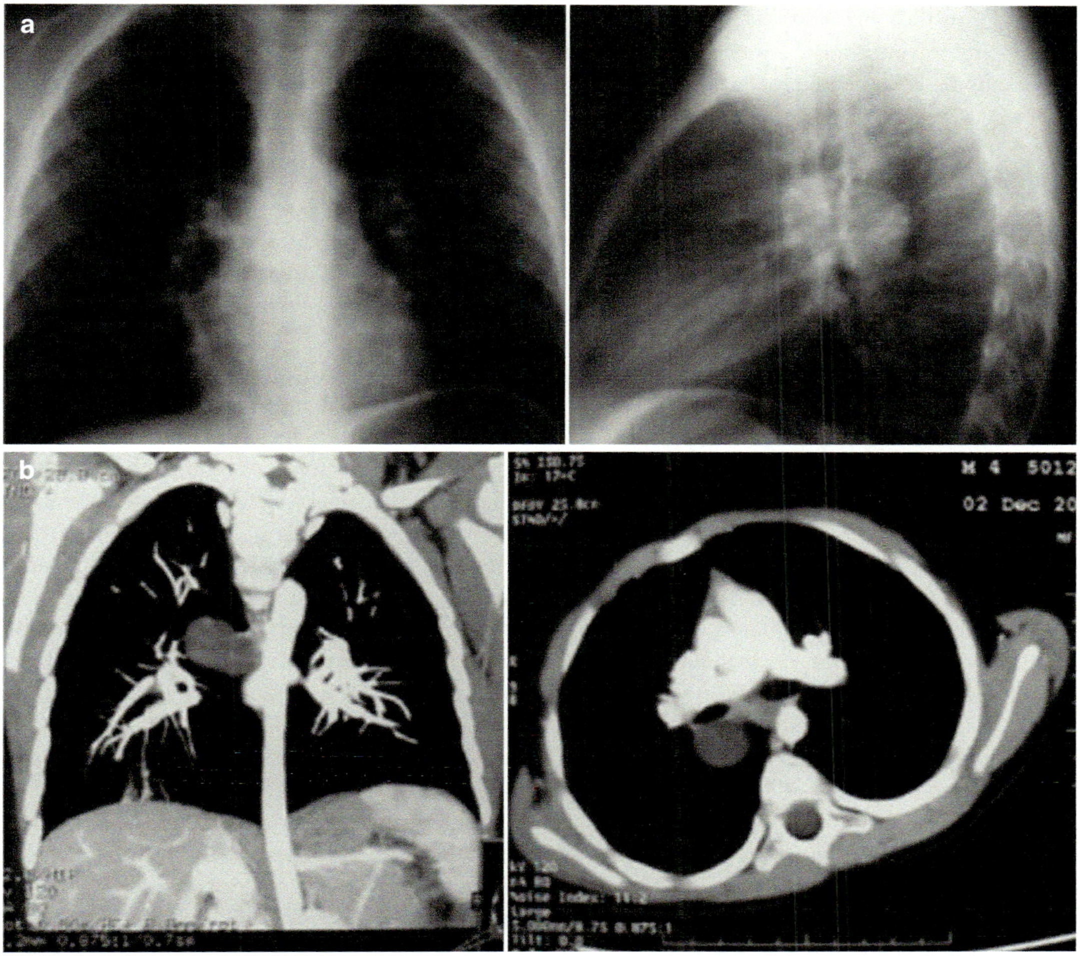

Fig. 54.6 Bronchogenic cyst. (**a**) Anteroposterior (AP) and left chest X-ray in an adolescent shows a circumferential lesion, well delimited in the posterior mediastinum. (**b**) Chest computerized tomography confirms the presence of a cystic lesion in the posterior mediastinum

Lung Agenesis, Aplasia, and Hypoplasia

Agenesis refers to the total absence of lung, vascular, and bronchial tissue. Aplasia consists of a rudimentary pouch, and hypoplasia is characterized by a reduction in the number and size of the airway, alveoli, and lung vascular structures. Agenesis and aplasia re caused by an event during the embryonic period, affecting only one lung, and generally the contralateral lung presents a compensatory hyperplasia. It may be associated to other congenital malformations, such as heart or gastrointestinal malformations. Clinical presentation includes

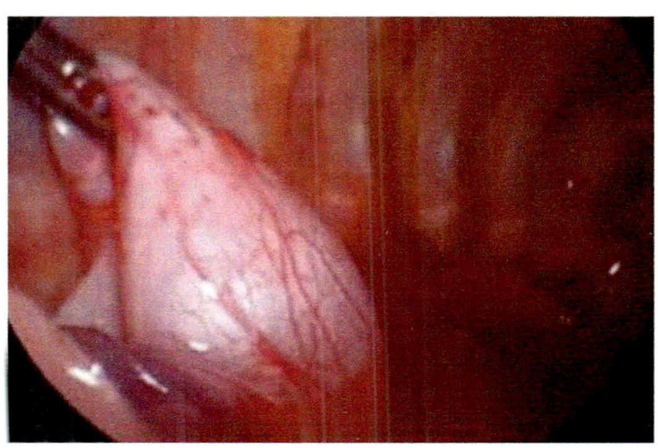

Fig. 54.7 Bronchogenic cyst in image captured in video thoracoscopy with patient in lateral decubitus position. The bronchogenic cyst is easily identified, and its resection is conducted manually

respiratory distress in variable degrees and recurrent respiratory infections. Absence of the right lung may be a serious situation, as the compensatory growth of the left lung may displace the heart toward the right side, as well as causing sudden death by compression of the great vessels. Chest X-rays show a homogeneous density in the affected side, with no lung web. The mediastinum is deviated and the healthy lung presents hernias. Computerized tomography confirms the absence of blood vessels and lung parenchyma. Lung agenesis may be confirmed through flexible bronchoscopy where there is no carina.

Medical treatment consists of chest physiotherapy to avoid respiratory infection, bronchodilators, and antibiotics. Lung hypoplasia is more frequent than the other entities, and half the cases are related to heart and genitourinary malformations, or congenital diaphragmatic hernia. Chest X-rays show poorly ventilated lung tissue, ascended diaphragm, and mediastinal deviation. Management is medical, and surgery is only proposed for those patients with localized hypoplasia or to correct a diaphragmatic hernia as a determinant factor.

Diagnosis

As previously mentioned, the wide use of obstetric echography has made the discovery of antenatal congenital lung lesions more common. In part, this has helped the study of the natural history, although as it happens in intrauterine life, these are not always single lesions. Echography is quite precise to detect lesions such as cystic adenomatoid malformations, represented in the characteristic way through echogenic lung images. This test also makes it possible to evaluate the lesion size, presence of mediastinal deviation, hydrops, and polyhydramnios. The presence of sequestration or mixed lesions can be suspected when there are systemic circulation vessels entering the lung. When the differential diagnosis is uncertain, a fetal magnetic resonance study may be used.

The antenatal progression of a cystic adenomatoid malformation is highly variable, and it is known that even large lesions can disappear. They reach a growth plateau at 28 weeks of gestation, and after this they are reduced in size, probably the result of apoptosis. Cases of hydrops resolution after this period have been reported. If, on the contrary, the hydrops progresses, some kind of fetal treatment can be proposed, such as conducting a thoracentesis, or a pleuroamniotic shunt. When handling microcystic lesions of a considerable size, open fetal surgery may be proposed. For patients who are not candidates for fetal surgery, or if this alternative is not available, the use of maternal steroids is suggested, which would advance the plateau in lesion growth.

Lung sequestration appears in echography as echo-dense masses, well defined, and homogeneous, with systemic circulation. It is important to look for associated malformations, particularly those in the heart. Antenatal management of a fetus lung sequestration with hydrops will depend on the gestational age: a 30-week-old fetus may be a candidate for thoracoamniotic shunt.

It is important to highlight that although an antenatal management may be successful, these patients require important extrauterine ventilation support, and they may even need extracorporeal membrane oxygenation (ECMO). Therefore, the birth should be planned in centers with adequate neonatal support and pediatric surgery available.

Treatment

There is a consensus that patients with symptoms with postnatal diagnosis of a lung lesion should be urgently operated for treatment. For a cystic adenomatoid malformation, lung lobectomy is the resection technique of choice; however, in selected cases a segmental resection may be sufficient. For lung sequestration, surgery is relatively simple, once the vascularization of aberrant vessels has been controlled. If there are heart decompensations, it is possible to perform selective embolizations as a definitive treatment or in combination with the previous surgical resection.

Any congenital lung lesion that presents symptoms because of an infection should be adequately treated before performing a surgical resection.

Even in those patients who do not present symptoms, or in whom an echography regression of an antenatally diagnosed lung lesion is suspected, a computerized tomography scan will be needed after birth. Some authors perform it early, between 4 and 6 weeks of life; others wait until 6 months if the lesion is not visible in the chest X-ray. If the lesion does not appear in computerized tomography, the patient can be followed up, and a new study can be considered if there are respiratory infections. Care must be taken when labeling as cystic adenomatoid malformation the lesions of antenatal diagnosis that "disappear," because often a histological diagnosis is done through an echography lesion, and these lesions may correspond to other types of lesions, such as mucus blockages or neuroblastomas, for example.

Development of lung infections is, without doubt, the most common manifestation of congenital lung lesions in children beyond the neonatal period. They can be often confused with a cystic adenomatoid malformation with a residual pneumatocele after an infection. Bronchiectasis or hemoptysis may be observed in older patients.

Neoplasia is a well-documented fact of lesions attributed to lung congenital cysts, such as pleuropulmonary blastoma (infants and small children). In a recent series of lung tumors in infancy, 8.6% of these were associated with a previously existent lung malformation. There is a clear association between cystic adenomatoid type 1 malformation and bronchoalveolar carcinoma.

Other secondary complications attributed to congenital cysts or lung sequestration include the possibility of pneumothorax, sudden enlargement of the lesion, hemoptysis, and lesion stroke.

Because of the risk of developing infections and malignancy, surgery in these patients should take place during childhood. We propose conducting a computerized tomography scan before the first 6 months of life (depending on the X-ray findings), and planning the surgery at some point in time between 6 months and 1 year of life. The reason for this delay is waiting for the patient to reach an adequate weight and size to undergo a minimally invasive surgery.

Sources

Azizkhan RG, Crombleholme TM. Congenital cystic lung disease: contemporary antenatal and postnatal management. Pediatr Surg Int. 2008;24(6):643–57.

Chen HW, Hsu WM, Lu FL, Chen PC, Jeng SF, Peng SS, Chen CY, Chou HC, Tsao PN, Hsieh WS. Management of congenital cystic adenomatoid malformation and bronchopulmonary sequestration in newborns. Pediatr Neonatol. 2010;51(3):172–7.

Davenport M, Warne SA, Cacciaguerra S, Patel S, Greenough A, Nicolaides K. Current outcome of antenally diagnosed cystic lung disease. J Pediatr Surg. 2004;39(4):549–56.

Kotecha S, Barbato A, Bush A, Claus F, Davenport M, Delacourt C, Deprest J, Eber E, Frenckner B, Greenough A, Nicholson AG, Antón-Pacheco JL, Midulla F. Antenatal and postnatal management of congenital cystic adenomatoid malformation. Paediatr Respir Rev 2012;13(3):162–70.

Laberge JM, Puligandla P, Flageole H. Asymptomatic congenital lung malformations. Semin Pediatr Surg. 2005;14(1):16–33.

Stocker JT. Cystic lung disease in infants and children. Fetal Pediatr Pathol. 2009;28(4):155–84. Available in https://www.tandfonline.com/doi/full/10.1080/15513810902984095.

Gastroesophageal Reflux and Respiratory Diseases

55

María Francisca Jaime Méndez,
José San Martín Prieto,
and Juan Cristóbal Gana Ansaldo

Contents

Introduction

Gastroesophageal reflux (GER) occurs when gastric content goes back to the esophagus, sometimes even reaching the mouth. GER is a physiological event in most cases and may appear during all ages in life, but it is more frequent before the first year of life, usually for a brief period of time during the postprandial period. GER may present as a disease when it causes symptoms or complications directly related to this phenomenon, whether they are esophageal or extraesophageal.

Laryngopharyngeal reflux or extraesophageal reflux occurs when the gastric content passes to

M. F. Jaime Méndez · J. San Martín Prieto
J. C. Gana Ansaldo (✉)
Pontificia Universidad Católica de Chile, Santiago, Chile
e-mail: mjaime@med.puc.cl; jsanmart@uc.cl

P. Bertrand, I. Sánchez (eds.), *Pediatric Respiratory Diseases*,
https://doi.org/10.1007/978-3-030-26961-6_55

the pharynx and larynx, and it can even get into the nasal cavity, middle ear, and airway (trachea, bronchi, lungs).

GER has been related to obesity, neurologic diseases, esophageal atresia history, hiatal hernia, achalasia, prematurity, some chronic respiratory diseases, and lung transplant. In addition, GER has been associated with different respiratory conditions, such as asthma, recurrent bronchitis, chronic cough, swallow disorders, poor growth, persistent dysphonia, acute laryngitis, laryngomalacia, subglottic stenosis, recurrent respiratory papillomatosis, apparent life-threatening event (ALTE) episodes, recurrent otitis media, and persistent rhinosinusitis. Nevertheless, these associations do not imply causality.

In this chapter, we will review the relationship between gastroesophageal reflux and the following respiratory diseases: asthma, chronic cough, swallowing disorders, obstructive sleep apnea, ALTE, subglottic stenosis, laryngomalacia, recurrent laryngitis, and recurrent laryngeal papillomatosis.

Proposed GER Damage Mechanisms in Respiratory Diseases

GER may contribute to extra-esophageal syndromes, whether by a direct mechanism of aspiration (reflux theory) or by an indirect mechanism, mediated by vagal mechanisms (reflex theory).

The presence of gastric fluid may damage the airway, which is not prepared to be in contact with acidic material (or sometimes alkaline material, if it comes from the duodenum), and enzymatic activity. This reflux will cause damage depending on the intensity of exposure (quantity, length of time, frequency), intrinsic resistance of the parenchyma, and the presence of comorbidities or local concomitant alterations.

Within the agents present in the gastric juice, which may be potentially harmful in both the esophageal and extraesophageal mucosa, we may mention gastric acid, pepsin, bile salts, pancreatic proteolytic enzymes, and bacterial reflux content. This last component would be particularly important in patients who use inhibitors of the proton pump. It is important to highlight that using these medications reduces the gastric pH, but it does not affect enzyme secretion, and it does not directly impact gastrointestinal motility.

Pepsin is a protease that has the greatest activity when the pH is around 1.9–3.6 and is inactive when pH is above 6.0. However, it does not naturalize itself, and therefore it has been observed in animal models to cause damage when it adheres itself to the esophageal mucosa, being reactivated at a posterior reflux episode, with a lower pH.

It has been confirmed that bile salts cause direct damage in the esophageal and extraesophageal mucosa, including lungs. In vitro and animal studies have shown damage in the mucosa because of an increase of proton permeability, and even cellular death, at the lung level.

Among pancreatic proteolytic enzymes, we have trypsin and chymotrypsin. Trypsin is active within a pH range of 6.0–10.0, and around 8.0 is the optimum level. In order for trypsin to damage proximal stomach tissue, the pH value must be 2.0, which may be present in patients using proton pump inhibitors.

Recent clinical studies have described an association between acid suppression therapy and an increase in pneumonia risk. It has been proposed that the cause would be a bacterial overgrowth in the stomach, which would be a consequence of the change in the luminal pH.

Asthma

Asthma and GER disease have a high prevalence rate, and therefore the presence of both in the same patient is frequent. A systematic review of 2010, which included 19 studies, described a prevalence of GER disease in asthma patients from 19% to 80%, with a cumulative average of 23%. This high variability reported is explained by the differences in the methodologies used in the study: questionnaires, pH-metry, and endoscopy.

Several potential interaction mechanisms have been described between esophagus and lung:

- Embryonic origin and shared innervation through the vagus nerve. In association with this, bronchoconstrictive vagus reflex has been described. It consists of bronchoconstriction caused when there is acid and esophageal distention. There are also local reflexes where esophageal neurons project axons to the trachea, causing edema in the airway when faced with acid in the esophagus, mediated by tachykinins and substance P.

- Intrathoracic pressure effect: During exacerbations, because of the increase of respiratory work, negative intrathoracic pressure also increases. Under these circumstances, the capacity of the internal inferior esophageal sphincter may be overcome, and reflux episodes can increase.
- Asthma treatment: Medications used for asthma, including theophylline, aminophylline, and β 2 agonists inhaled, may increase GER by causing a reduction in the pressure of the inferior esophageal sphincter. Oral steroids increase the contact time between esophageal mucosa and the acid.

In spite of this, two systematic reviews performed in 2002 and 2009, found no use in reflux treatment for asthma. A randomized study published in 2012 in patients with non-controlled asthma, which used lansoprazole versus placebo, found no improvement, but a greater amount of respiratory infections in the treated group. Other studies suggest that there may be some subgroups that could benefit from the treatment, which are not well characterized yet. These variable results could translate the results of a treatment in a heterogeneous population, and so in some patients GER is a concomitant event, and in other patients GER may have a role in the physiopathology of the disease. Currently, GER treatment is not recommended for patients with difficult-to-control asthma who have no proven reflux.

Chronic Cough

Chronic cough study is one of the more frequent indications for pH-metry. The association between them varies according to different reports, which may be partly determined by methodological problems.

Esophageal reflux may trigger cough through the indirect stimulation of the nerves involved in cough reflex, as it was described for asthma. In adults with chronic cough evaluated through high resolution manometry, it has been described that partial clearing of food in the distal esophagus can stimulate cough reflex.

Use of pH-metry plus impedantiometry has improved the detection of GER episodes, classifying them as "non-acidic" (pH >7), "mildly acidic" (pH 4 a 7) and "acidic" (pH <4). Only the last two are detectable through conventional pH-metry. In a study of patients with chronic cough, in over 78% the association between cough and GER was detected. In infants, a greater relationship between cough and "mildly acidic" reflux was detected, while in preschoolers and schoolchildren a greater relationship with "acidic" reflux was detected.

A Cochrane review updated in 2010, which included 6 pediatric studies, with high heterogeneity, found that the treatment with proton pump inhibitor was not useful for improving respiratory symptoms.

The fact that, in infants, cough is more related to mildly acidic and non-acid reflux could explain the inconstant response to acid block therapy. Nevertheless, more studies with adequate methodology are needed, which may enable us to identify what subgroups of patients will benefit from reflux treatment.

Swallow Disorders

Swallowing is a complex process where different structures and mechanisms intervene to allow the transit of the bolus from the mouth to the stomach, in a safe and effective way. In normal conditions, the food goes from the pharynx to the esophagus, without penetrating the larynx or the distal airway. For this, structural, motor, and sensitive indemnity is required. Pharyngolaryngeal reflux causes a chronic inflammation state in the superior aerodigestive airway, mainly at the oro and hypopharynx, which reduces the sensitivity in the mucosa. Then, transport of food is not timely detected, altering the complex mechanisms ruling swallowing, as well as the airway protection mechanisms. Eventually, food or fluids may enter the larynx, and may be aspirated to the distal airway.

Larynx sensitivity may be studied through the evaluation of the laryngeal adductor reflex, which is triggered by the laryngeal stimulation through an air impulse performed with a laryngoscope. The objective is to determine the threshold to trigger the reflex. A value above 4 mmHg is considered abnormal. In a study of cases with swallowing disorder where this reflex was altered, and patients with other neurological diseases were excluded, it was observed that GER treatment for at least 3 months with acid inhibition improves pharyngolaryngeal sensitivity, and therefore it improves the swallowing disorder. Larynx sensitivity measured by laryngeal adductor reflex improved from 6.3 to 3.7 mmHg after the GER treatment ($p < 0.001$), while the proportion of patients who presented aspiration was reduced from 85% to 14% ($p < 0.001$).

Obstructive Sleep Apnea

As it happens with asthma, both GER and obstructive sleep apnea syndrome (OSAS) are prevalent diseases, and therefore both may be frequently present in the same patient, but not necessarily in a cause–effect relationship. GER could trigger apnea. Prolonged exposure to acid in the respiratory tract causes local edema and an increase in respiratory secretions, which may contribute to cause an obstructive apnea.

There are few studies evaluating the relationship between GER and obstructive sleep apneas in the pediatric population. In a study that included 37 pediatric patients, 21 of them with OSAS and reflux disease were treated with proton pump inhibitors for 4–8 weeks. A variable response was observed: from non-significant changes in the polysomnography in preschoolers, to a complete resolution in schoolchildren with mild OSAS. Nevertheless, the sample for this study was small, and therefore we still cannot have conclusions for usual clinical practice.

Apnea and ALTE

GER has been related to apnea episodes. Around 30–50% of infants who present ALTE are diagnosed with GER disease and are frequently treated with anti-reflux medications to prevent a recurrent event.

Two main mechanisms have been proposed to explain its relationship: first, laryngopharyngeal reflux, which puts fluid from the stomach in contact with the larynx and/or trachea, creates a laryngospasm episode caused by direct irritation. Second, a reflex mechanism is activated by the presence of gastric fluid in the distal esophagus, which also triggers a laryngospasm episode. It does not matter which mechanism causes the spasm, if it is long enough, it can cause severe hypoxemia and eventually infant deaths.

In a study that conducted polysomnography and pH-metry, the diagnosis of GER by a functional study did not affect the risk of ALTE recurrence, and GER treatment did no reduce this risk.

Another study performed in premature patients who were under 33 weeks of age and had recurrent apneas, detected an association between apneas and GER episodes, particularly non-acid reflux, which had not been detected by isolated pH-metry.

The use of proton pump inhibitors, as well as thickened formulas, has not been confirmed to reduce the frequency of apneas related to reflux or ALTE recurrence, and therefore its general use is not currently recommended.

Subglottic Stenosis

Laryngopharyngeal reflux has frequently been associated with subglottic stenosis, and its presence has been estimated to be four times greater in comparison to children without stenosis. Studies in both children and adults have confirmed the presence of GER in up to 80% of these patients. Other more frequently associated factors are trauma and local infection. It has been proposed that laryngopharyngealreflux creates inflammation and mucosa damage, impairing re-epithelization and promoting the increase of connective tissue. Different reports show benefits of treating GER in patients with subglottic stenosis by reducing symptoms. A study that included 25 children with subglottic stenosis who planned to undergo corrective surgery found that GER treatment avoided surgery in nine cases. Patients who will require surgery usually are initiated on GER treatment.

Laryngomalacia

Laryngomalacia is the most common cause of persistent congenital stridor during infancy. This condition is caused by neuromuscular immaturity of the pharynx and by the flaccidity and redundancy of supraglottic structures. It is mainly manifested by inspiratory stridor, which varies in its intensity. Besides this, according to how severe it is, it may cause dyspnea, cough, chocking episodes, swallowing disorders, and it may even impact the nutritional state and growth in infants.

Laryngomalacia is frequently associated with laryngopharyngealreflux. There are studies that show that up to 2/3 of the children with laryngomalacia present GER, and that in cases of moderate to severe laryngomalacia the risk of presenting GER is almost ten times greater. Nevertheless, the causality relationship between these two entities is not clear. In a prospective study published in 2007, a strong correlation between GER treatment and reduction of laryngomalacia symptoms was reported. In this study, patients were separated into three groups: mild laryngomalacia, moderate laryngomalacia, and severe laryngomalacia. Almost 89% of the patients who had moderate and severe laryngomalacia showed improvement after receiving anti-GER treatment for 7 months. Nevertheless, these conclusions have been questioned because improvement of the symptoms may be caused by the natural progression of the disease instead of the therapy. Although there are no more quality studies that actually compare the effectivity of the anti-GER treatment in patients with laryngomalacia, anti-GER treatment is still widely used in these patients, which justifies conducting more quality studies that may define the real usefulness of this therapy.

Recurrent Laryngitis

Laryngopharyngeal reflux has been considered one of the causes of recurrent *croup*. Patients with recurrent laryngitis who underwent pH-metry or endoscopy with esophageal biopsy have been found with GER at a rate around 47–100%. Chronic inflammation of the larynx caused by laryngopharyngealreflux plus viral respiratory infections explains this susceptibility.

Recurrent Laryngeal Papillomatosis

Laryngeal recurrent papillomatosis is a benign infectious disease caused by the human papillomavirus. The number of patients where latent papilloma virus can be found in the laryngeal epithelium is greater than the number of patients who actually develop laryngeal papillomatosis. It is not clear which factors activate the virus and trigger the growth of papilloma, but it has been proposed that laryngopharyngealreflux could be one of them. There are reports of patients where GER treatment in mild to moderate papillomatosis may improve or even cure the disease. For example, in a series of four cases of children with difficult-to-treat laryngeal papillomatosis, who were also diagnosed and treated for GER, a substantial improvement of papillomatosis in all the cases was observed, and two of them had a complete resolution of the disease. Besides this, it has been observed that anti-GER therapy may cause a reduction of secondary complications due to multiple resection surgeries, as happens with anterior scars and laryngeal membranes. Although it is not recommended to use GER treatment as the only measure against laryngeal papillomatosis, it does seem adequate to use it as a coadjutant to minimize consequences or arrest the progression of the disease.

Diagnosis

Diagnosis of GER may be complex, mainly in patients who have presented subtle and/or prolonged symptoms. It should be suspected in children with the above clinical conditions, as well as in those with feeding problems, non-explained airway problems, or who do not respond to other treatments. The process must start with a clinical detailed history with special emphasis in symptoms related to swallowing and the aerodigestive path.

In relation to swallowing (and its eventual disorders), it is crucial to ask for characteristics, such as how long do meals take, stress or uncomfortableness when feeding, signs of respiratory difficulty when feeding (for example, tachypnea, wet voice or crying, increasing nasal congestion, chocking, cough, cyanosis), and growth.

Request for complementary tests must be oriented to the answer of a certain question, for example, does this patient have some anatomical condition that favors GER? How can GER be attributed to the extradigestive symptoms of this patient? Is the patient receiving enough treatment for GER?, etc.

Currently, the consensus reached between the North American Society for Pediatric Gastroenterology, Hepatology and Nutrition (NASPGHAN) and the European Society for Paediatric Gastroenterology Hepatology and Nutrition (ESPGHAN) considers that pH-metry is useful to evaluate the correlation between the symptoms and the presence of GER, as well as those patients with respiratory symptoms where GER could be worsening the clinical condition. Particularly, pH-metry with multichannel intraluminal impedance, detects changes in electric conductivity between electrodes, and so it can assess the pathway for foods, liquids, and even gases; it is considered superior to isolated pH-metry, because impedancemetry can detect acid reflux, mildly acidic reflux, and non-acid reflux, whose relationship with respiratory disease has been previously discussed. Although these two tests are useful, the fact that they take 24 hours makes it difficult to conduct them in children. Besides this, pH normal or basal values for hypopharynx have not been completely defined, and the same happens with children impedance values, which makes it difficult to interpret the results obtained.

In relation to endoscopy studies, gastric and duodenum endoscopy is useful to register esophagitis macroscopic signs, as well as for obtaining histological samples, especially when associated diseases, such as eosinophilic esophagitis, are suspected. Besides this, flexible laryngoscopy is a non-invasive fast procedure, which does not require sedation, and it can be studied at any age through the anatomy of the aerodigestive pathway. In this case, special emphasis must be made on the characteristics of the pharynx and larynx. There are studies showing a correlation between the findings of this exam and the results of the ph-metry. Among the most significant endoscopic findings are arytenoid edema and erythema (RR 2.46), lingual tonsil hypertrophy (RR 2.24), edema and erythema in the posterior laryngeal commissure (RR 3.19), edema in the posterior laryngeal commissure (3.19), vocal cord edema (RR 12.15), and subglottic stenosis (RR 2.5). Nevertheless, the presence of these findings is not pathognomonic of GER.

The tests are summarized on Table 55.1.

Treatment

There are pharmacological and non-pharmacological measures for patients with confirmed disease caused by gastroesophageal reflux. For pediatric patients, the strategy of "empirical treatment" with no clear symptoms of GER has not been confirmed as sensitive or specific for the diagnosis of this disease, and therefore it is not recommended as a diagnosis method.

Use of thick or "anti-regurgitation" formulas, although they reduce the number of regurgitations observed by the caregivers, is not translated in pH-metry improvement. Formula thickened at home with rice cereal increases weight in infants, considering the caloric density it involves.

In older children and adolescents, weight reduction is recommended in children with

Table 55.1 Study in patients with gastroesophageal reflux

Study	Usefulness	Observations
Esophageal pH-metry	Evaluates the presence of acidic fluid Useful to evaluate anti-GER treatment	Does not detect mildly acidic or non-acidic fluids
Esophageal pH-metry multichannel intraluminal impedance	Evaluates the presence of acid, mildly acidic, and non-acid reflux Useful to evaluate the effectiveness of anti-GER treatment and its association with extradigestive symptoms (cough, difficult-to-control asthma, chest pain)	Impedance normal values for pediatric age are missing
Esophagus-duodenum-stomach x ray	Anatomical evaluation when malformations are suspected	Should not be used to diagnose GER or quantity of
Gastric endoscopy	Evaluation of macroscopic signs of esophagitis and taking of histological samples for differential diagnosis of other pathologies (eosinophilic esophagitis)	If no macroscopic alterations are found it may not diagnose GER
Flexible laryngoscopy	Evaluates the anatomy of the aerodigestive way and macroscopic signs of laryngopharyngealreflux	Findings are not necessarily related to GER
Gastroesophageal scintigraphy	Evaluation of postprandial and aspiration GER	Lack standardization technique and normal values for each age

excess malnutrition. Although suspending certain foods a priori is a commonly used strategy, it has not been confirmed that it actually reduces GER episodes. Instead, it is recommended to reduce certain foods according to each case.

It has been shown that prone and lateral decubitus position reduces GER episodes. Nevertheless, these positions have been associated with an increased rate in sudden death syndrome, and therefore supine position is recommended for those patients who are under 1 year of life and also have GER. Prone position can be kept when they are awake and always supervised.

In relation to pharmacological measures, there are medications that have a buffer effect on the acid, a barrier effect on the mucosa, anti-acid secretors, and prokinetics.

Evidence about pediatric use of antacids is limited, and special care must be taken with those drugs containing aluminum, in relation to milk-alkali syndrome. They are generally not recommended for the treatment of GER in children.

Acid secretion inhibitors are ion histamine type 2 receptor agonist (H2RA), such as ranitidine and famotidine, and the proton bomb inhibitors, such as omeprazole, esomeprazole, and lanzoprazole. Proton pump inhibitors are considered to be better than the H2RA in suppressing acid effects, which also present tachyphylaxis after 6 weeks of use, and even reactions like irritability, headache, and sleepiness may be wrongly interpreted as GER worsening. It has been confirmed that proton pump inhibitors are better than histamine receptor inhibitors in treating erosive esophagitis. Nevertheless, it has some difficulties in the dosage and administration, because there is no syrup presentation. In general, the use of costumed preparations is not recommended, as there are few studies supporting the stability and bioavailability of these substances. Besides this, the use of proton pump inhibitors is not risk free, because idiosyncratic reactions may occur, as well as diarrhea, constipation, nauseas, hypergastrinemia with its chronic use, hyperplasia of enterochromaffin-like cells, and in the long term, micronutrients malabsorption (iron and B12 vitamin). In premature babies an increased risk of necrotizing enterocolitis and candidemia was observed. Table 55.2 shows the recommended dosages for H2RA and proton pump inhibitors.

Prokinetics such as cisapride reduce the GER index; nevertheless, its use has been limited by its association with prolonged QTc interval in the

Table 55.2 Gastroesophageal reflux treatment

Type	Medication	Doses	Observations
H2RA	Ranitidine	5–10 mg/Kg/day, divided in 2–3 doses	Tachyphylaxis
	Famotidine	1 mg/Kg/day, divided in 2 doses	Tachyphylaxis
PPI	Omeprazole	0.7–3.3 mg/Kg/day	Formulation: 10 and 20 mg capsules MUPS in 10 and 20 mg
	Lansoprazole	0.7–3 mg/Kg/day	30 mg envelopes 15 and 30 mg capsules Mouth dissolving tablet 15 and 30 mg
	Esomeprazole	0.7–3.3 mg/Kg/day	Formulation: 10 g envelopes. Capsules and tablets of 20 and 40 mg

H2RAs Histamine type 2 receptor agonist
PPI Proton pump inhibitor

electrocardiogram. The efficiency of domperidone, widely used for the treatment of GER, has not been confirmed. It has been observed that metoclopramide reduces the GER index as measured by pH-metry, but its use is limited by its adverse effects, which particularly affects extrapyramidal structures, and in general its use is not recommended.

In those cases where there is documented GER, where the optimal medical therapy has failed, who depend on therapy during prolonged periods or who may have life-threatening complications, surgical treatment can be considered, including open and laparoscopic fundoplication, and even limited experiences through endoscopy. Nevertheless, evidence of its use in pediatrics is limited to retrospective studies, and it presents morbidity–mortality rates, and therefore the risks and benefits must be considered before its indication.

Conclusions

1. Disease caused by gastroesophageal reflux must be differentiated from the physiological gastroesophageal reflux, which is particularly frequent in infants.
2. There is an association between gastroesophageal/laryngopharyngeal reflux and diverse respiratory diseases. Nevertheless, in most of them causality has not been confirmed.
3. Only a minority of patients require additional tests, and these tests should only be requested when there is a specific clinical question. Testing is not for every patient.
4. Currently, there are few studies with a correct methodology that may establish which patients with respiratory symptoms will benefit from anti-GER therapy. In these circumstances, empirical treatment of patients with no symptoms of gastroesophageal reflux is not recommended.

Sources

Chang AB, Lasserson TJ, Gaffney J, Connor FL, Garske LA. Gastro-oesophageal reflux treatment for prolonged non-specific cough in children and adults. Cochrane Database Syst Rev. 2011;(1):CD004823. https://doi.org/10.1002/14651858.CD004823.pub4.

Corvaglia L, Spizzichino M, Aceti A, Legnani E, Mariani E, Martini S, Battistini B, Faldella G. A thickened formula does not reduce apneas related to gastroesophageal reflux in preterm infants. Neonatology. 2013;103(2):98–102.

Ghezzi M, Guida E, Ullmann N, Sacco O, Mattioli G, Jasonni V, Rossi GA, Silvestri M. Weakly acidic gastroesophageal refluxes are frequently triggers in young children with chronic cough. Pediatr Pulmonol. 2013;48(3):295–302.

Hartl TT, Chadha NK. A systematic review of laryngomalacia and acid reflux. Otolaryngol Head Neck Surg. 2012;147(4):619–26.

Holland BW, Koufman JA, Postma GN, McGuirt WF Jr. Laryngopharyngeal reflux and laryngeal web formation in patients with pediatric recurrent respiratory papillo-mas. Laryngoscope. 2002;112(11):1926–9.

Karkos PD, Leong SC, Apostolidou MT, Apostolidis T. Laryngeal manifestations and pediatric laryngopharyngeal reflux. Am J Otolaryngol. 2006;27(3):200–3.

Lightdale J, Gremse D and Section on Gastroenterology Hepatology, and Nutrition. Gastroesophageal reflux management guidance for the pediatrician. Pediatrics. 2013;131:e1684.

Little JP, Matthews BL, Glock MS, Koufman JA, Reboussin DM, Loughlin CJ, McGuirt WF Jr. Extraesophageal pediatric reflux: 24-hour double-probe pH monitoring of 222 children. Ann Otol Rhinol Laryngol Suppl. 1997;169:1–16.

May JG, Shah P, Lemonnier L, Bhatti G, Koscica J, Coticchia JM. Systematic review of endoscopic airway findings in children with gastroesophageal reflux disease. Ann Otol Rhinol Laryngol. 2011;120(2):116–22.

Mittal MK, Donda K, Baren JM. Role of pneumography and esophageal pH monitoring in the evaluation of infants with apparent life-threatening event: a prospective ob-servational study. Clin Pediatr (Phila). 2013;52(4):338–43.

Miura MS, Mascaro M, Rosenfeld RM. Association between otitis media and gastroesophageal reflux: a systematic review. Otolaryngol Head Neck Surg. 2012;146(3):345–52.

McKenna M, Brodsky L. Extraesophageal acid reflux and recurrent respiratory papilloma in children. Int J Pediatr Otorhinolaryngol. 2005;69(5):597–605.

Pearson JP, Parikh S, Orlando RC, et al. Review article: reflux and its consequences-the laryngeal, pulmonary and oesophageal manifestations. Aliment Pharmacol Ther. 2011;33(Suppl 1):1–71.

Rosen R, Nurko S. The importance of multichannel intraluminal impedance in the evaluation of children with persistent respiratory symptoms. Am J Gastroenterol. 2004;99(12):2452–8.

Rudolph CD. Supraesophageal complications of gastroesophageal reflux in children: challenges in diagnosis and treatment. Am J Med. 2003;115(Suppl 3A):150S–6S.

Suskind DL, Thompson DM, Gulati M, Huddleston P, Liu DC, Baroody FM. Improved infant swallowing after gastroe-sophageal reflux disease treatment: a function of im-proved laryngeal sensation? Laryngoscope. 2006;116(8):1397–403.

Thompson DM. Laryngopharyngeal sensory testing and as-sessment of airway protection in pediatric patients. Am J Med. 2003;115(Suppl 3A):166S–8S.

Pneumothorax and Thoracic Trauma

56

Claudia Fuentes Sáez and Raúl Bustos Betanzo

Contents

Pneumothorax

Definition

The pleural space is a virtual space filled with a minimum amount of fluid between the visceral and parietal pleura. When air gets into the pleural space, it is called pneumothorax and it modifies intrapleural pressure and causes partial or total lung collapse. It is classified as spontaneous, traumatic, or iatrogenic. Spontaneous pneumothorax can also be classified as primary or secondary to a preexisting respiratory disease.

C. Fuentes Sáez (✉)
Pediatrics, Respiratory Diseases, Hospital Regional de Concepción, Concepción, Chile

R. Bustos Betanzo
Pediatrics, Intensive Care at Clínica Sanatorio Alemán, Concepción, Chile
e-mail: rabustos@udec.cl

Epidemiology

The incidence of spontaneous pneumothorax in children is from 7.4 to 18 per 100,000 males and from 1.2 to 6 cases per 100,000 females, with a ratio of 2:1. The average age of onset has been reported between 14 and 16 years of age. In general, patients are tall males with decreased body mass index. Mortality is rare.

Although the incidence of secondary spontaneous pneumothorax is not well defined, patients with asthma and cystic fibrosis have the greatest risk. In these patients, the probability of secondary

P. Bertrand, I. Sánchez (eds.), *Pediatric Respiratory Diseases*,
https://doi.org/10.1007/978-3-030-26961-6_56

spontaneous pneumothorax occurrence increases as lung function decreases, with morbidity and mortality being greater due to the reduced lung volumes in an affected lung. In cystic fibrosis, the appearance of pneumothorax is considered a late complication and a sign of poor prognosis. Several studies show that between 16% and 20% of patients with cystic fibrosis older than 18 years will experience a pneumothorax during their lives. Most of them (75%) have a FEV1 <40%, which has been associated with high mortality.

Infectious causes, such as *Pneumocystis jirovecii* pneumonia and necrotizing pneumonia (anaerobes, gram-negative or *Staphylococcus aureus*), are associated with a high incidence of secondary pneumothorax. Patients with connective tissue diseases, such as Marfan and Ehlers-Danlos syndromes, are also at high risk. The most frequent causes of secondary pneumothorax appear in Table 56.1.

When considering pediatric thoracic trauma, pneumothorax may occur in up to a third of patients, most of them associated with extrathoracic and intrathoracic injuries, but one third may present only pneumothorax.

Iatrogenic pneumothorax is a consequence of medical procedures, most of them being performed in the emergency room or intensive care units. The most frequently associated procedures are central venous catheterization, thoracentesis,

Table 56.1 Causes of secondary pneumothorax

Airway disease	Asthma, cystic fibrosis, interstitial emphysema
Postinfectious	*Pneumocystis jirovecii*, tuberculosis, lung abscess, necrotizing pneumonia, HIV, parasites
Connective tissue diseases	Marfan syndrome, Ehlers–Danlos syndrome, juvenile idiopathic arthritis, systemic lupus erythematosus, dermatomyositis, Birt–Hogg–Dube syndrome
Oncological diseases	Lymphoma, pulmonary metastasis
Congenital malformations	Cystic adenomatoid malformation Congenital lobar emphysema
Foreign body aspiration	
Catamenial pneumothorax	Related to menstrual cycle

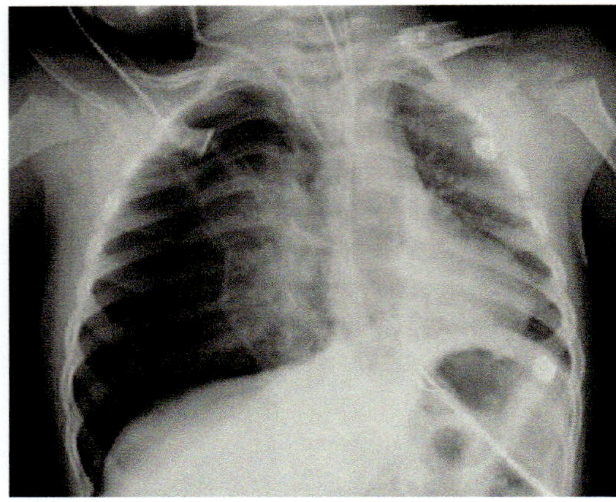

Fig. 56.1 Iatrogenic Pneumothorax. Anteroposterior chest X-ray of a 2-year-old patient on mechanical ventilation due to convulsive status. It shows right-sided pneumothorax secondary to insertion of a central venous catheter into the internal jugular vein on the same side

and positive support by mechanical ventilation (Fig. 56.1). The internal jugular vein and subclavian vein catheterization are procedures with a high-risk for developing pneumothorax. The use of ultrasound techniques has reduced the incidence of pneumothorax by central venous catheterization and thoracentesis in adults. Strategies of protective lung ventilation, with tidal volumes limitation and plateau pressures, have enabled the diminishment of the effects of barotrauma secondary to mechanical ventilation.

Etiology and Pathophysiology

The increase in transpulmonary pressure is the mechanism described in the appearance of spontaneous pneumothorax. This causes alveolar distension, and if the gradient is high enough, alveolar rupture. It can occur secondary to increased work of breathing, a Valsalva maneuver, positive pressure ventilation, and airway obstruction that causes an obstruction ball valve effect, among others.

Once alveolar rupture occurs, air may reach the perivascular space producing pneumomediastinum; if the air pressure increases, it can go to the neck and face (subcutaneous emphysema), advance toward the peritoneal cavity (pneumoperitoneum),

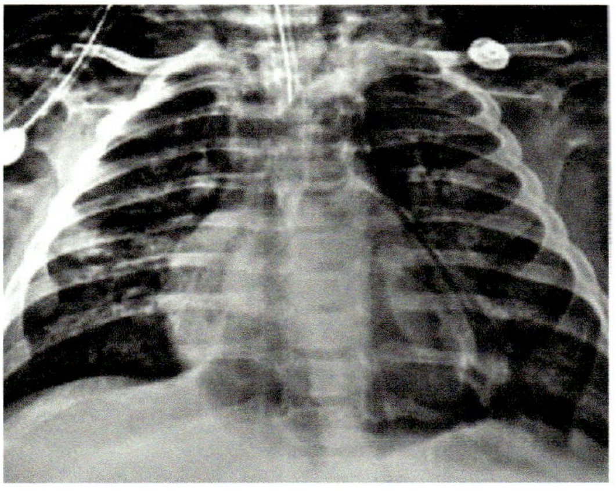

Fig. 56.2 Postinfectious Pneumothorax. Anteroposterior chest x-ray of an 8-month-old patient with severe pneumonia due to adenovirus. It shows pneumothorax, pneumomediastinum, pneumopericardium, and subcutaneous emphysema secondary to mechanical ventilation

or penetrate the pericardium (pneumopericardium) (Fig. 56.2).

Spontaneous pneumothorax seems to occur due to changes in the connective tissue that predispose air leaks from the airways into the pleural space. The mechanisms proposed for both primary and secondary pneumothorax are multiple. Frequently, the existence of subpleural bullae, or bullas, has been associated with the production of primary pneumothorax. In studies performed with computerized axial tomography scans, bullas have been detected in between 28% and 100% of the cases that developed a primary pneumothorax and between 70% and 95% in patients who required video-assisted thoracoscopy surgery (VATS) due to this pathology. In newborns, high transpulmonary pressures during the first breaths contribute to the appearance of primary pneumothorax.

The role of tobacco, both in the development of primary and secondary spontaneous pneumothorax, has also been widely analyzed, especially in adults. Prevalence of smoking in children with primary pneumothorax is between 11% and 14%, while in adults is between 24% and 88%. This supports the theory between time exposure to tobacco and changes in connective tissue and/or chronic bronchiolitis that are observed in adult patients and predisposition to pneumothorax.

A familial form of primary spontaneous pneumothorax has been described, related to a mutation in the folliculin gene, located on chromosome 17, which plays a role in the definition of cell shape, size, and movement. This condition has been associated with the Birt–Hogg–Dube syndrome, in which there is a predisposition to the formation of multiple lung cysts that lead to the development of primary spontaneous pneumothorax.

Secondary spontaneous pneumothorax results in systemic or local inflammation of the lung tissue caused by an underlying disease. In children, asthma and cystic fibrosis are the most commonly recognized chronic respiratory diseases. The mechanism involved in asthma is the chronic inflammation of the small airway, which allows creation of the necessary pressure for the air to escape to the pleural space, although secondary spontaneous pneumothorax has been observed in asthma patients without respiratory exacerbation. The mechanism involved in cystic fibrosis is inflammation and obstruction of the distal airway, due to thick secretions that lead to air entrapment in the alveoli. When the alveolar pressure exceeds the interstitial fluid pressure, the air moves to the interstitium, reaching the hilum, and escaping to the mediastinal pleura. Other mechanisms described are rupture of subpleural bulas at the level of the visceral pleura and *Pseudomonas sp.* or *Burkholderia cepacia* infections (Figs. 56.3 and 56.4).

In newborns, the most common causes of secondary spontaneous pneumothorax are meconium aspiration syndrome (MAS) and hyaline membrane disease (HMD).

Clinical Manifestations

Symptoms and signs of pneumothorax vary according to the patient's age, level of lung collapse and previous lung volumes. Small pneumothoraxes can be asymptomatic and show normal vital signs. Spontaneous pneumothorax occurs mostly at rest, but it may be caused by situations that increase intrathoracic pressure through the Valsalva maneuver (such as lifting objects or stretching).

Acute chest pain and dyspnea are the most frequent symptoms in pediatric spontaneous pneumo-

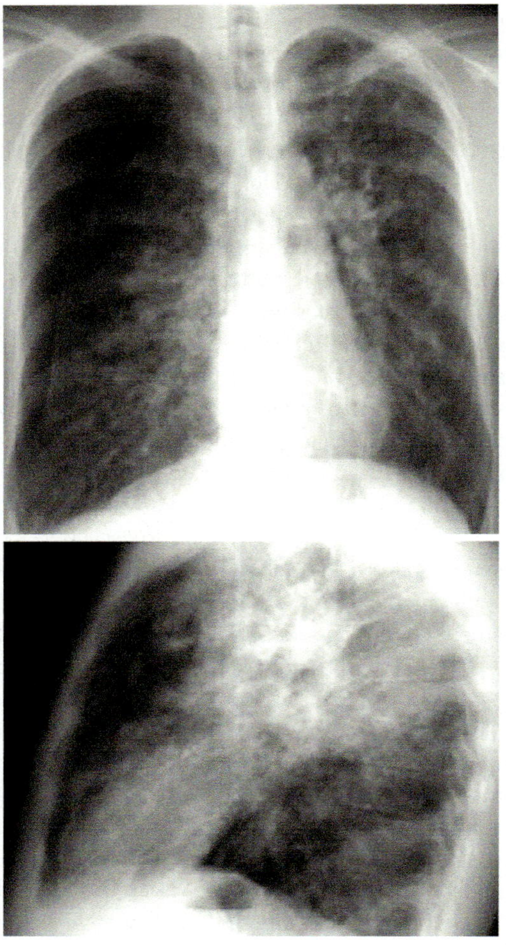

Fig. 56.3 Pneumothorax in Chronic Disease. Anteroposterior and lateral chest X-ray of a 14-year-old patient with cystic fibrosis and advanced lung disease. It shows lateral and anterior pneumothorax on the right side

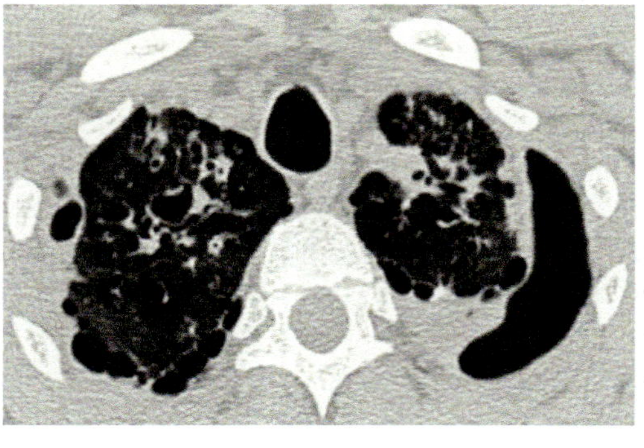

Fig. 56.4 Pneumothorax in Chronic Disease. Chest CAT scan in a patient with cystic fibrosis. It shows left apical pneumothorax and multiple bilateral subpleural bullas

thorax. Even without treatment, the symptoms resolve in 1–3 days; however, pneumothorax persists in most patients. Physical examination findings depend on the size of the pneumothorax. Small ones may not be detected clinically. Clinical signs include decreased pulmonary sounds, dyspnea, tachycardia, hyperresonance on percussion, and decreased vocal fremitus. In a minority of patients it can present itself as tension pneumothorax, with respiratory distress, hypoxemia, tachycardia, and arterial hypotension. The latter is a respiratory emergency and requires immediate intervention.

Diagnostic Approach

Once the pneumothorax diagnosis is suggested by the presentation and clinical examination, it is confirmed with an anteroposterior and lateral chest X-ray. Expiratory X-rays have been suggested for detecting small pneumothoraxes, although low yield has been demonstrated. Chest X-rays in lateral decubitus position may be useful in emergencies or intensive care units. In critically ill patients, when pneumothorax is suspected, most chest X-rays are taken in supine position. In these cases, the air moves toward an anterior or sometimes medial location adjacent to the mediastinum, sub pulmonary or lateral, and the lateral costophrenic angle can be distended to the caudal direction, which causes the so-called deep sulcus sign, showing asymmetry of the lateral costophrenic recesses due to a greater depth and radiolucency of one of them; the angle can even extend to the hypochondrium and adopt a triangular morphology (Fig. 56.5).

Ultrasound In recent studies, chest ultrasound has been used to diagnose pneumothorax in the adult population, having found a sensitivity of up to 95% for diagnosis. It seems that the diagnostic accuracy of ultrasound would be superior to chest X-rays in trauma and critically ill patients. There is not enough evidence to routinely recommend chest ultrasound in children. In addition, the quantification of pneumothorax is difficult with this method and therefore it will hardly replace chest X-rays for diagnosis in children.

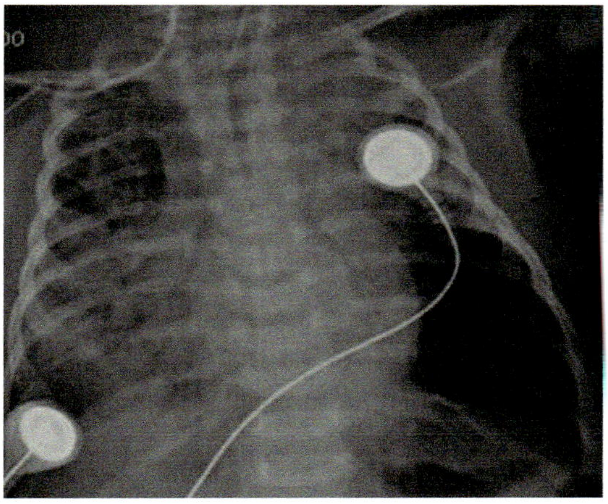

Fig. 56.5 Deep Sulcus Sign. Decubitus anteroposterior chest X-ray in infant with severe pneumonia. It shows left pneumothorax with deep sulcus sign

Computerized axial tomography scan When there is an important clinical suspicion of pneumothorax, with negative chest X-rays, a computerized axial tomography scan could be considered in the diagnosis of subtle pneumothorax. This could be relevant in the detection of secondary pneumothorax in patients with an underlying disease who have low lung volumes, in order to help in a possible evacuation.

In thorax trauma, computed tomography has become the method of choice to identify pneumothorax. Recently, volumetric measurements of the pneumothorax have been used with three-dimensional images through multidetector computed tomography, which have reached 100% sensitivity in diagnosis. On the other hand, in primary spontaneous pneumothorax, it has been described that the detection of bullas by computed tomography could be a predictive sign of recurrent pneumothorax, especially when they are detected on the contralateral side of the pneumothorax.

Quantification of Pneumothorax Size

Different methods to calculate the size of pneumothorax in adults have been applied in children with inconsistent results; thus, currently, there are no validated methods for estimating the pneumothorax volume in the pediatric population. The guidelines of the British Thoracic Society in adult patients with stable clinical condition, define a large pneumothorax as the presence of a visible edge of up to 2 cm between the lung image and the chest wall on an anteroposterior chest X-ray. According to the guidelines of the American College of Chest Physicians, the apical distance must be greater than 3 cm. In children, the definition of large pneumothorax, according to the previously described guidelines, can result in an error, because the thorax size differs in relation to the age and body type of the patient. It is important to consider that when defining the management strategy of spontaneous pneumothorax, clinical status is more important than size estimated by radiology.

Treatment

Scarce evidence in the pediatric population makes it difficult to establish some explicit therapeutic guidelines, so that management follow adult recommendations. Pediatric guidelines for the management of spontaneous pneumothorax do not exist in the scientific literature. The guidelines for the management of spontaneous pneumothorax in adults do not include recommendations for pediatric patients.

Treatment depends on the extent and type of pneumothorax, in addition to the severity of the symptoms. It should be remembered that estimating the magnitude of the pneumothorax can be difficult due to different thorax sizes according to age.

Treatment options for spontaneous pneumothorax in a clinically stable patient include: monitoring on high oxygen concentration administration, single evacuation puncture, small-bore pleural catheter (10–14 F), large-bore catheter (>20 F) or thoracotomy tubes.

There are several reported cases, including adults and children, in which conservative management has been followed. A total of 68 of 82 cases reach a spontaneous remission of primary spontaneous pneumothorax, but they required up to 32 days.

Standard recommendations in adults for the treatment of small primary spontaneous pneumothorax, without respiratory distress and clinically stable, is monitoring for 3–6 hours in the emergency department; after this, clinical follow-up in 12–24 hours or before in the case of worsening symptoms. Not recognizing the deterioration of the patient is one of the risks of this type of treatment.

Administration of oxygen at high concentrations (100%) creates a partial pressure gradient between the pleural cavity and the capillary web; diminished nitrogen partial pressure in the blood produces an increase in the pressure gradient of the gases between the pleura and the venous blood, favoring the absorption of all air.

Management of primary spontaneous pneumothorax in unstable patients involves a fine needle evacuation puncture, which is as effective as the use of a small-bore catheter, and it would reduce hospital days.

For secondary spontaneous pneumothorax, guidelines recommend hospitalization and use of small-bore catheters (10–14 F). An adult study shows similar results regarding the resolution of the pneumothorax when comparing the installation of a pigtail catheter versus large-bore catheters. When the pneumothorax occurs in a patient with cystic fibrosis, clinical guidelines propose hospital admission and thoracotomy tube insertion. In traumatic pneumothorax, the use of traditional pleural drainage catheters is recommended. Iatrogenic pneumothorax, which is associated with barotrauma, will require the insertion of thoracotomy tubes. A study evaluating 70 patients on mechanical ventilation who developed pneumothorax showed that the use of pigtail catheters was beneficial in only 43% of the cases, requiring most of them to change to traditional pleural drainage due to clinical deterioration. An algorithm for treating of pediatric pneumothorax is presented below in Fig. 56.6.

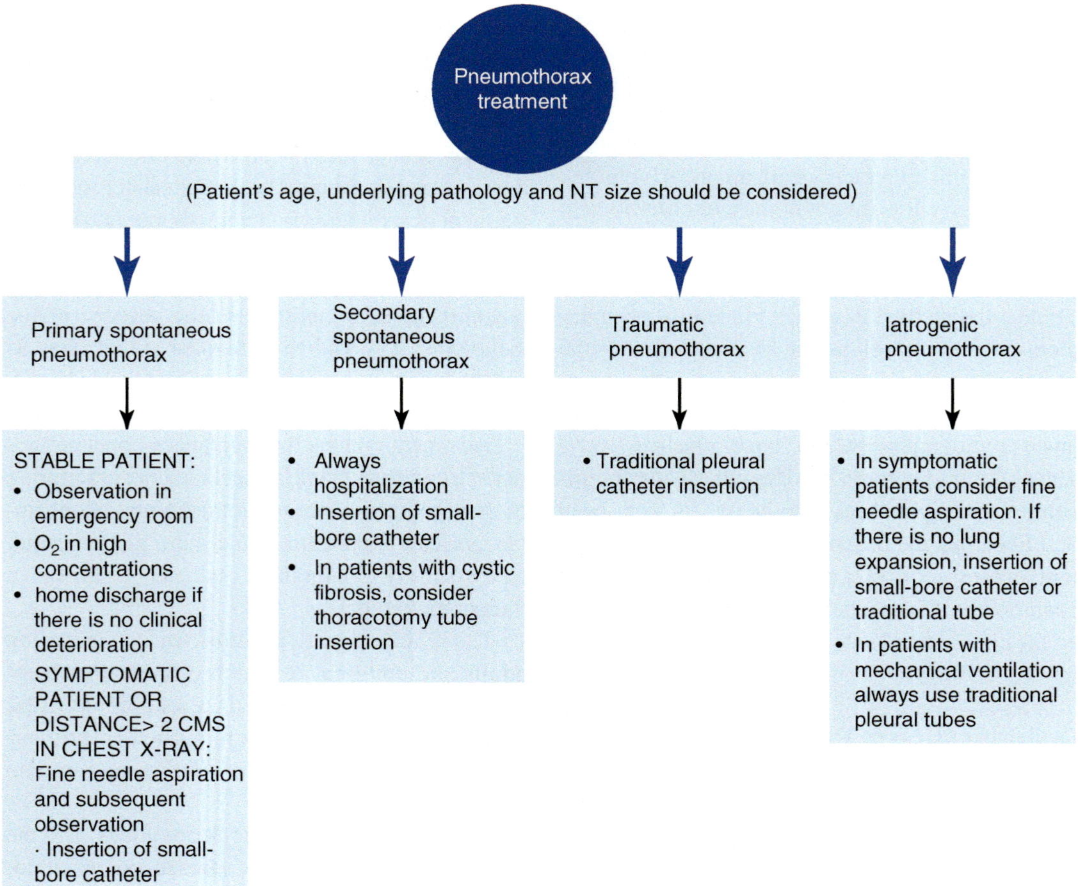

Fig. 56.6 Algorithm for the treatment of pneumothorax

If there is no resolution and the air leak persists (3–5 days), or if there is recurrence, the use of video-assisted thoracoscopy surgery (VATS) should be considered. Reports in the pediatric population indicate a recurrence of pneumothorax up to 60%, but most authors recommend VATS only after the second episode. Some surgical indications of pneumothorax are: ipsilateral pneumothorax (second episode), first contralateral pneumothorax, synchronous bilateral spontaneous pneumothorax, persistent air leak (according to guidelines >4–7 days), failure of lung expansion despite the drainage tubes, spontaneous hemothorax, high-risk professions that have experienced an episode of pneumothorax (pilots), and pregnancy.

Different methods have been used to treat persistent air leaks, including prolonged use of pleural drainage, surgical repair, chemical pleurodesis (via injection of sclerosing agents, such as tetracycline or talcum powder) or pleurodesis with autologous blood patch. Some recent studies support the use of the latter method due to its efficacy, good tolerance, minimal collateral effects, decrease in complications, and shorter hospital stay.

Thorax Trauma

Thoracic trauma corresponds to less than 10% of the traumas in children. Different pediatric series have reported a mortality rate between 8% and 26%. The classification of thoracic trauma is shown in Table 56.2.

Most trauma occur in children during their first decade of life and are secondary to traffic accidents and falls. They are high energy impacts and usually involve other regions of the body; approximately half of the children with chest trauma have lesions in the skull, abdomen, and extremities. The most frequent chest lesions are pulmonary contusions with or without rib fracture; tracheobronchial tree, heart, aorta, esophagus or diaphragm compromise are rarely observed.

Table 56.2 Classification of thoracic trauma

Non-penetrating trauma
Does not involve opening of the chest
Corresponds to 80–90% of cases
Penetrating trauma
Causes an open injury

Pulmonary contusion is the result of the direct application of high energy in the lung parenchyma. After the contusion, anatomical changes appear, including hemorrhage, edema, and consolidation, which reduce pulmonary compliance, leading to ventilation/perfusion alteration, hypoventilation, and hypoxia. Up to 20% of patients develop pneumonia after a pulmonary contusion. If the contusion is accompanied by laceration, air leak and pneumothorax may appear, and sometimes hemothorax as well. If there is a massive pneumothorax secondary to tracheobronchial injuries, air accumulates not only in the pleural space, but also in the mediastinum, neck, and subcutaneous tissue.

Most traumatic lung injuries are treated with respiratory support and pleural drainages. Massive hemothorax requires exploratory thoracotomy. Persistent air leak, which may correspond to a tracheobronchial rupture, requires intubation, endoscopic airway evaluation, and eventual reparative surgery. In the case of open pneumothorax, the defect must be sealed.

Summary

Pneumothorax is the presence of air between the parietal and visceral pleura. It is classified as spontaneous, traumatic, and iatrogenic. Primary spontaneous pneumothorax is an infrequent entity in pediatrics outside the neonatal period. Secondary spontaneous pneumothorax is associated with multiple lung conditions, the most common being asthma and cystic fibrosis. Chest X-ray is the first choice test to confirm diagnosis, although computed tomography is a good alternative to detect subtle pneumothorax and to estimate their magnitudes.

There are no guidelines for the treatment of pneumothorax in pediatrics, so its management in school children and adolescents is based on recommendations for the adult population. In infants and preschoolers, an exhaustive study in search of the etiology is necessary to establish the appropriate treatment. It is important to consider that the estimation of the extension of the pneumothorax in this group of patients can be difficult, due to the differences in the thorax size according to age. The choice of the different therapeutic methods will depend on the type of pneumothorax, age of patient, associated condition, and severity of the clinical picture. Most pneumothorax can be managed conservatively; however, in patients with preexisting pulmonary disease or recurrence, there are more aggressive and definitive treatment options that should be considered (VATS).

Future research is needed to assess the benefit of the various therapeutic interventions available in the pediatric population and to determine if current adult guidelines can be used in children.

Sources

Alrajab S, Youssef AM, Akkus NI, Caldito G. Pleural ultra-sonography versus chest radiography for the diagnosis of pneumothorax: review of the literature and meta-analysis. Crit Care. 2013;17:R208.

Ayres J, Gleeson F. Imaging of the pleura. Semin Respir Crit Care Med. 2010;31:674–88.

Benbow MK, Nanagas MT. Pneumothorax beyond the newborn period. Pediatr Rev. 2014;35:356.

Dotson K, Johnson LH. Pediatric spontaneous pneumothorax. Pediatr Emerg Care. 2012;28:715–20.

Flume PA, Mogayzel PJ Jr, Robinson KA, Rosenblatt RL, Quittell L, Marshall BC, Clinical Practice Guidelines for Pulmonary Therapies Committee, Cystic Fibrosis Foundation Pulmonary Therapies Committee. Cystic fibrosis pulmonary guidelines: pulmonary complications: hemoptysis and pneumothorax. Am J Respir Crit Care Med. 2010;182:298–306.

Flume PA. Pneumothorax in cystic fibrosis. Curr Opin Pulm Med. 2011;17:220–5.

Johnson NN, Toledo A, Endom EE. Pneumothorax, pneumomediastinum and pulmonary embolism. Pediatr Clin N Am. 2010;57:1357–83.

Light RW. Pleural controversy: optimal chest tube size for drainage. Respirology. 2011;16:244–8.

MacDuff A, Arnold A, Harvey J, BTS Pleural Disease Guideline Group. Management of spontaneous pneumothorax: British Thoracic Society Pleural Disease Guideline 2010. Thorax. 2010;65(Suppl 2):ii18–31.

Manley K, Coonar A, Wells F, Scarci M. Blood patch for persistent air leak: a review of the current literature. Curr Opin Pulm Med. 2012;18:333–8.

Robinson PD, Cooper P, Ranganathan SC. Evidence-based management of paediatric primary spontaneous pneumothorax. Paediatr Respir Rev. 2009;10:110–7.

Shaireen H, Rabi Y, Metcalfe A, Kamaluddeen M, Amin H, Akierman A, Lodha A. Impact of oxygen concentration on time to resolution of spontaneous pneumothorax in term infants: a population-based cohort study. BMC Pediatr. 2014;14:208.

Tomà P, Owens CM. Chest ultrasound in children: critical appraisal. Pediatr Radiol. 2013;43:1427–34.

Tovar JA, Vazquez JJ. Management of chest trauma in children. Paediatr Respir Rev. 2013;14:86–91.

Tovar JA. The lung and pediatric trauma. Semin Pediatr Surg. 2008;17:53–9.

Nutrition in Chronic Respiratory Disease

57

Salesa Barja Yáñez

Contents

Introduction

Changes in the epidemiological profile of infant morbidity and mortality has made secondary malnutrition an emerging problem. As a result, infectious diseases have decreased and the survival of preterm children and others with serious illnesses has improved. The nutritional management of these patients is part of the multidisciplinary treatment and is increasingly complex.

The prevalence of malnutrition in Chilean children under the age of 6 in outpatient setting is less than 0.4%, and short stature is 2%; however, in children's hospitals it has been reported between 25% and 30%. This is mainly associated with chronic diseases in patients who require complex, high-cost treatments and whose prognosis is better because of nutritional improvement. The highest proportion is related to chronic respiratory diseases, with 30% of acute malnutrition and up

S. Barja Yáñez (✉)
Pontificia Universidad Católica de Chile, Santiago, Chile
e-mail: sbarja@uc.cl

P. Bertrand, I. Sánchez (eds.), *Pediatric Respiratory Diseases*,
https://doi.org/10.1007/978-3-030-26961-6_57

to 50% of growth delay in the most serious cases. At the opposite extreme, obesity has increased, associated with asthma in childhood and interrelated diseases in its genesis and progression.

Factors that Influence Nutritional Status

Several factors compromise the nutritional status of children with chronic diseases, which are also applicable to chronic respiratory diseases:

- *Type of underlying disease*: Both patients with cystic fibrosis and bronchopulmonary dysplasia in which there is also post infectious lung damage require particular nutritional approaches, as it will affect nutritional recovery and future growth.
- *Age of onset, duration, and severity of the pathology*: Severe, early-onset chronic respiratory diseases will affect further growth. For example, children with bronchiolitis obliterans whose infection occurred before 6 months of age, have greater nutritional deterioration than those patients where the infection occurs afterward.
- *Prevention, early detection of malnutrition, and timely support*: The anticipatory and regular nutritional evaluation by a multidisciplinary team enables them to efficiently prevent and manage problems that must be approached in an integral manner.
- *Drugs*: They can interact with nutrients or modify energy expenditure, bone metabolism, body composition, or decrease growth (Table 57.1).

Mechanisms Involved in Malnutrition

The energy balance results from the difference between the energy that enters the organism (nutrients) and the total daily energy expenditure (TDEE). The latter is the sum of basal metabolic rate (BMR) + diet induced thermogenesis (DIT) + losses + energy for growth + expenditure for physical activity. From this equation we deduce different mechanisms involved in malnutrition in children with chronic respiratory diseases (Fig. 57.1). Often several coexist, the most frequent being the decrease in food intake and the increase in total energy expenditure.

Table 57.1 Interaction Between Drugs and Nutrients

Drug	Nutritional effect
Anticonvulsants:	Folate, Ca, Vit B_{12}, B_6, D, C. Dyslipidemias
Phenytoin	Folate, Ca, Vit B_{12}, B_6, K, C. Dyslipidemias
Phenobarbital	
Anti-inflammatories:	Vit C, Fe
Aspirin	Proteins, fats, glucose, Zn, K, Na, Ca
Corticosteroids	
Antimicrobials:	↓Endogenous Vit K in the bowels
Isoniazid	Vit B6, niacin
Trimethoprim	Folate
Penicillin	K
Cathartics:	Vit A, D, E, K, carotene, Ca
Mineral oil	
Others:	K, Mg, Ca
Digitalis	Zn, Ca, Na, K
Furosemide	Ca, Vit A, Fe, phosphate
Antiacids	B_{12}, Fe
H_2 antagonists	Fe, Ca
Inhibitor b. Protons	Vit A, D, E, K, Ca, fats
Cholestyramine	
Beta-agonists	↑GERD in infants, K

Lower food intake Anorexia caused by chronic diseases can increase with acidosis, drugs, infections, and specific deficits (iron or zinc, the latter producing dysgeusia). Food intake is also affected by infant's fatigue, water restriction in those with bronchopulmonary dysplasia, alteration of swallowing maturation processes due to immaturity and prolonged use of probes, and the development of behavioral disorders. Moreover, frequent hospitalizations are associated with lower intake and even setbacks concerning achieved milestones.

- *Resting metabolic rate (RMR) increase*: It has been demonstrated in children with bronchopulmonary dysplasia, cystic fibrosis, and in those with steroid treatment. Infection,

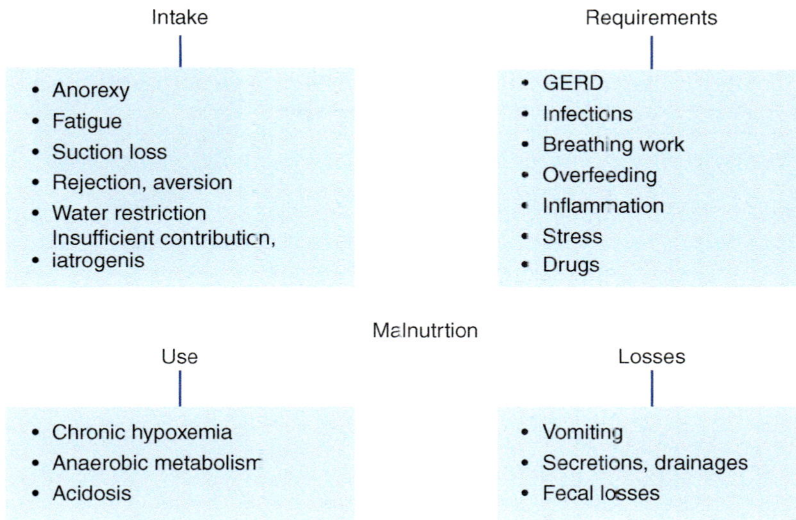

Fig. 57.1 Mechanisms of malnutrition in children with chronic respiratory diseases

inflammation or stress increase energy requirements, anorexia, and low weight. Although the work of breathing constitutes only 2–3% of the BMR, in preterm infants its impact is greater. Excessive inputs can increase TDEE, although normally only 10% corresponds to the DIT. This occurs especially if the excess is protein, whose storage expense is greater than that of carbohydrates (and greater than that of fat). In children with bronchopulmonary dysplasia, a high load of glucose via parenteral administration increases breathing work, with less effect if enterally administered.

- *Anaerobic metabolism*: It has lower energy efficiency; chronic hypoxemia, even mild (during sleep or feeding), affects growth. Moreover, acidosis decreases protein accretion and exacerbates anorexia.
- *Digestive losses*: These increase with vomiting associated with cough, especially in infections or worsening of the disease. Gastroesophageal reflux is common in children with bronchopulmonary dysplasia, neurological diseases, or who are tube-fed. In addition, dysphagia and esophagitis cause a decrease in intake due to pain. In cystic fibrosis there are intestinal losses due to steatorrhea and, also, there may be protein loss through secretions or drainages (bronchiectasis, cystic fibrosis).

Interaction Between Nutrition and Lung Function

The interaction between nutrition and lung function is complex. Chronic respiratory diseases challenge childhood growth and development and malnutrition alters lung growth and development. This interaction has a greater impact during the first 2 years of life, due to lung and respiratory musculature development (Fig. 57.2) with an increase in work of breathing and predisposition to infections. In turn, this increases the requirements and promotes a vicious circle with greater morbidity and mortality. Malnutrition damages the lung defense mechanisms; physical barriers are less efficient and cellular immunity is impaired to a greater degree than humoral immunity.

It has been suggested that in preterm infants malnutrition begins in prenatal life, so it precedes the development of bronchopulmonary dysplasia and interacts later with other factors, decreasing the lung regeneration mechanism, the defense against hyperoxic damage, the response to infections, and lung growth. Nutritional improvement promotes a better evolution of the underlying disease and improvement in lung damage contributes to optimize the nutritional status.

Malnutrition by excess can also affect lung function and defense mechanisms. Although in

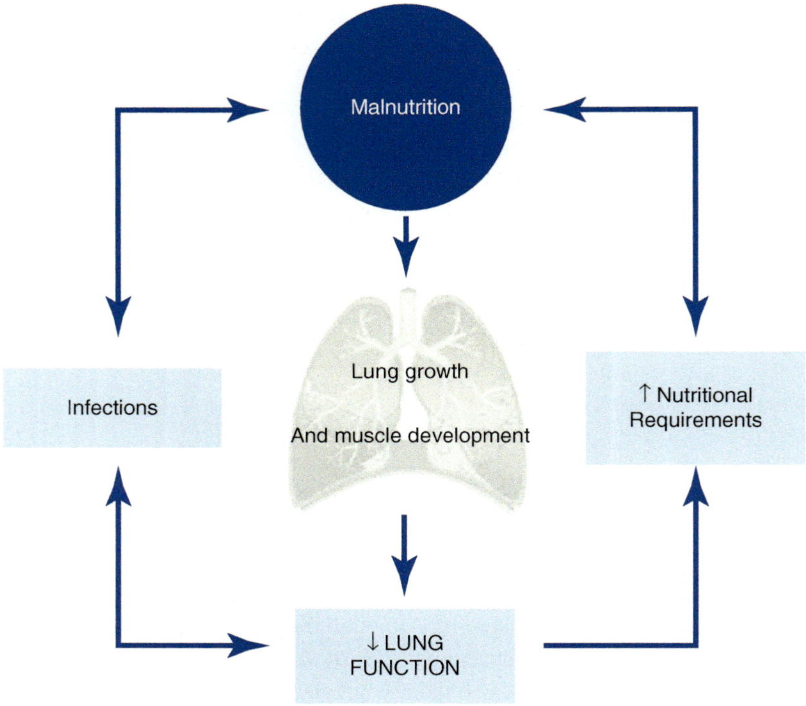

Fig. 57.2 Interaction between nutrition and lung function

children nutritional deficit continues to determine the prognosis, this would be worse in adults with severe obesity who suffer from acute pulmonary infections, as it was demonstrated in the epidemic of influenza A (H1N1).

Specific Diseases

Bronchopulmonary Dysplasia

Preterm patients who develop bronchopulmonary dysplasia are a group at high risk of malnutrition. The factors of prematurity or intrauterine growth restriction are added to those of the disease during a period of high demand and accelerated growth. In the period immediately following neonatal discharge, malnutrition ranges between 30% and 67%. Subsequently, infants have accelerated weight gain until the sixth month, followed by deceleration. At 1 year corrected age, they have a weight-for-age Z-score (ZW/A) of −1.5 and −2.7 (male and female). Regarding height, they progress at a normal rate, but in smaller numbers and reach height-for-age (ZH/A) of −0.8 and −1.5 a year. However, they have lower lean mass and lower total body fat after the sixth month than term infants. The impact of pre and postnatal corticosteroids on height and bone mineral accretion has been recognized, although its use is justified considering the benefit–cost ratio.

The greatest nutritional deficiency in children with bronchopulmonary dysplasia occurs within their first three years of life; in the neonatal period, low nutritional intake is caused predominantly by delay in initiating and achieving enteral supply, high requirements, volume restriction, and comorbidity. These patients usually develop suction–swallowing disorders, gastroesophageal reflux, and subclinical hypoxemia, recurrent infections or obstructive episodes, with repeated hospitalizations. However, long-term growth would be affected to a greater extent by factors derived from prematurity, in comparison to factors related to bronchopulmonary dysplasia.

The prevention of bronchopulmonary dysplasia by nutritional modification or supplementation is controversial and is related to protection against oxidative damage. There is greater evidence of the preventive role of vitamin A, which promotes re-epithelialization and tissue repair. Its use in preterm infants <1000g was linked with a lower occurrence of death or O_2 requirement at 1 month of age (RR 0.75–0.93), a trend similar to 36 weeks of gestational age, with decreased retinopathy. This was not linked with a better long-term prognosis and although other deleterious effects have not been demonstrated, the most effective route is painful and the dose is high (intramuscular, 5000 IU, 3 times per week for 4 weeks). More studies are required, especially if it coexists with corticosteroid therapy that increases plasma levels of retinol. The evidence is scarce for the protective role of vitamin E and polyunsaturated fatty acids, and insufficient for inositol, selenium, and magnesium.

Preterm infants, with or without bronchopulmonary dysplasia, have a higher risk of developing recurrent wheezing. The influence of pre or postnatal factors, within which the development of obesity is found, has been studied. Also, preterm infants have a higher risk of chronic diseases and higher cardiovascular risk in adulthood. It has been suggested that the intrauterine programming of those with low birth weight (in particular, small for gestational age), accentuated by the accelerated gain of postnatal weight, are significant factors that would explain it. For both reasons, it is advisable that once the initial period of nutritional deficit is over, excess contributions are avoided and a healthy diet and an active lifestyle are stimulated, preventing a sedentary lifestyle that is frequent in these patients.

Post-infectious Chronic Lung Damage

Nutritional compromise usually develops later after a variable period of normal growth. However, growth can be significantly affected if malnutrition is premature, leading to a delayed growth in height. Thus, in a group of 18 Brazilian children with post-viral chronic lung damage, oxygen-dependent, 4.5 ± 2.7 years, 47% had short stature (Z-score for H/A ≤2). This is not necessarily irreversible: in a group of 21 Chilean children with severe bronchiolitis obliterans and similar height deficits, it was possible to achieve growth and height recovery with adequate management. However, in those patients in which there is no such recovery and have less physical activity, the development of obesity is also promoted, so that they require adequate follow-up and nutritional advice.

Cystic Fibrosis

Cystic fibrosis constitutes a model of interaction between chronic lung disease and nutritional status. Along with improvement of survival, it has been possible to observe the impact of the nutritional status optimization on the prognosis, without considering malnutrition as an unavoidable condition. The corresponding chapter discusses the multidisciplinary approach that several consensuses have delineated to anticipate and modulate the different nutritional variables that intervene in its treatment.

Asthma

There is controversy about the relationship between obesity and asthma. As both are multifactorial in nature, it is difficult to demonstrate common causality, which is discussed in the corresponding chapter. In clinical and epidemiological studies there is a higher prevalence of obesity in asthma. A balanced diet, decreased sedentary lifestyle, and increased physical activity are the most valuable tools to prevent and treat obesity in these patients.

Patients with Prolonged Ventilatory Support

Children who require chronic ventilatory support have different nutritional problems according to their underlying disease; those with severe chronic respiratory diseases tend to develop protein–caloric malnutrition, and patients with neuromuscular diseases may present malnutrition due to deficit or excess. Malnutrition affects respiratory function, since it reduces muscle mass and contractile force, which results in decreased respiratory effort, endurance, and vital capacity. These effects are, in general, reversible with nutritional improvement. Chronic ventilatory support in infants promotes nutritional progression and, conversely, it is possible to confirm in clinical practice that the withdrawal of ventilatory support may be associated with lower weight development and should be done gradually, monitoring oxygenation, and in parallel to a greater nutritional contribution if required.

Some children with neurological diseases and chronic ventilatory support may have higher caloric expenditure, such as those with hypertonia, severe seizure syndromes or increased movements, but most of them have decreased muscle mass (more active metabolic tissue) combined with less mobility and growth. This determines a lower energy requirement, so that proper contributions for their sex, age, and weight can lead to a greater fat mass deposition in most of them, although not necessarily reflected in the rates of overweight or obesity. This increases immobility, breathing work, loss of bone mass, and impairs motor and respiratory rehabilitation. Thus, energy requirement must be corrected by the muscle tone and degree of physical activity. However, the excessive limitation of the contribution in order to prevent obesity can lead to protein, mineral, and trace element depletion, so there must be monitoring and follow-up by an multi-disciplinary team that including a nutrition specialist.

Nutritional Support In Chronic Respiratory Diseases

The main objective of the nutritional support in children with chronic respiratory diseases is to optimize their growth and development, to promote a better evolution of their disease and quality of life, as well as to prevent the chronic disease of adulthood.

The following describes the nutritional management of children with chronic lung damage in the period after discharge from the neonatal unit, in the case of preterm infants with bronchopulmonary dysplasia. The nutritional treatment during the hospital stay can be reviewed in the references, and that of children with cystic fibrosis or asthma, in the corresponding chapter. Some general principles of nutritional support can be considered first, and specific management measures can be considered later.

Regular Monitoring of Food Intake

Because one of the main causes of poor weight gain in patients with chronic respiratory diseases is low intake, it is important to make a detailed nutritional history, considering the previous and present dietary history: feeding schedules, composition of milk formula and meals, method of preparation, use of supplements, volume offered and received, feeding time, and respiratory and gastrointestinal tolerance. In older children, one should ask for food between meals and general habits. Food records of 2 or 3 days a week provide very useful objective information.

Regular Monitoring of Nutritional Status

It is necessary to monitor growth, since the sequential measurement of the improvement in weight, height, and cranial circumference allows early identification of the deceleration or lack of improvement. It is essential to graph the evolution of the particular patient, which allows clear visualization of the tendency in its growth. In preterm infants it is recommended to adjust the chronological age up to 2 years and in cases of children of less than 28 weeks, up to 3 years.

For children up to age 5, the most appropriate growth reference is the WHO 2006 standard. Children from 5 to 19-years-old use the CDC-NCHS 2000 reference, although WHO 2007 is also available, which corresponds to a reconstruction of the previous one. The following anthropometric indexes are calculated and integrated:

- Weight/age (W/A) is the most sensitive index in detecting malnutrition, being able to overestimate it in those with low genetic or family size.

- Height/age (H/A) is less sensitive than W/A, and it is more strongly affected in periods of rapid growth; indicates long-term nutritional status.
- Weight/height (W/H) is sensitive, although it underestimates the deficit in children with short stature. It indicates an adequacy of the weight for the height, a relation that can also be expressed as Waterlow index (%) = (current weight/ideal weight) × 100.
- Body mass index (BMI) also expresses the harmony between weight and height and it is usually considered after 2 years of life. In cystic fibrosis, a close correlation between BMI and pulmonary function has been demonstrated, which guides the nutritional management.

To evaluate growth in children with neurological diseases, specific growth curves are available for cerebral palsy and some neuromuscular diseases. In them, when height measurement is difficult due to hypertonia or posture, it is possible to approximate it by measuring body segments.

Along with assessing normal staturo-ponderal development, it is important to also consider its quality, that is, the body composition. Because of this and because in older children medical checkups are more spaced in time and can be focused primarily on intercurrent pathologies, it is recommended that these patients be managed by an interdisciplinary team that includes a nutrition specialist. Although it has limitations, clinical estimation of the fat mass by means of skinfold measurement allows the optimization of nutritional management. This prevents overcorrection of the deficit in hypercaloric diets that promote fat mass deposition (not protein accretion), development of obesity, and appearance of chronic diseases in adult life.

Early Nutritional Intervention

Intervening early in children with chronic diseases, in stages in which there is less nutritional compromise, allows the improvement of the growth rates that are affected in a reversible manner. It also makes it possible to use a more physiological diet, potentiates regular feeding, and avoids the inappropriate or excessive use of protein or caloric supplements, which are more expensive and can displace the intake of foods that make up a balanced diet, promoting a greater fat deposition and later eating disorders.

Laboratory Tests

Laboratory tests are sometimes supportive measures, but in general they do not determine the diagnosis of nutritional compromise.

- *Plasma markers*: Albumin is a late marker of protein depletion for its half-life of 15–20 days, and although this is lower for prealbumin, both levels are altered in situations of stress or infections, and have an adaptive preservation in states of chronic depletion. Other more sensitive markers of protein deficiency have no clinical application. The plasma levels of vitamins are useful for specific cases, and as for minerals, cell blood count allows the evaluation of anemia and the plasma ferritin indicates depletion of iron deposits. Zinc status is difficult to measure in clinical practice and is considered only if there is a marginal intake or compatible clinical picture. Finally, the levels of calcium, phosphorus, and alkaline phosphatases make it possible to understand the situation of bone metabolism and the measurement of 25 OH vit D in plasma, the status of vitamin D.
- *Measurement of energy expenditure*: Indirect calorimetry measures the REE and allows, in an objective manner, adjustment of the caloric intake and assess the composition of the diet, with the calculation of the respiratory quotient (RQ = VCO2 produced/VO2 consumed). The RQ is 1.0 for the metabolism of carbohydrates, 0.8 for proteins, and 0.7 for fats. A mixed diet has an RQ of 0.85 (optimal range of 0.8–0.9), if it is <0.7 this indicates undernourishment, lipolysis or oxidation of ketones and if it is >1.0, overfeeding, lipogenesis or excessive production of CO_2.

This test requires careful monitoring in children with ventilatory support systems to avoid failures in the circuit's indemnity and variations in the FIO_2 that can determine greater variability in the results.

- *Measurement of body composition*: It is very useful, especially in patients with chronic ventilation who have decreased physical activity and high risk of demineralization. Bone densitometry allows the evaluation of both body composition (fat and lean mass percentage) and bone mass, but it still has a high economic cost. Although bioelectrical impedance analysis is a simpler and lower cost alternative, it has high variability, does not evaluate bone mass, and it is highly dependent on the degree of hydration.

Specific Measures of Nutritional Management

Energy, Macronutrients, and Water Contribution

The nutritional requirements of reference for calories, volume, macro and micronutrients in preterm infants have been well studied and appear in extensive references, adapted for optimal growth comparable to the intrauterine growth.

In order to calculate the energy required, the REE is estimated in infants and older children using WHO formulas and corrected for different factors (Table 57.2). Children with bronchopulmonary dysplasia are given a contribution of between 120% and 150% of the recommendations for healthy children (Table 57.3), to achieve catch-up growth and to meet the greater demands for their illness. The contribution must be gradual and individualized, considering that the best indicator of its adequacy is a normal growth and height development. In older children who have short stature as a consequence (not recoverable), the achievement of a harmonic weight to size ratio must be considered, particularly in the current context of high prevalence of obesity and the increased risk of chronic diseases in adult life.

General recommendations for protein intake have decreased (Table 57.4), although in preterm and malnourished infants, due to their accelerated growth, these must be greater for the synthesis of new tissues (lean mass): about 3 g per kilogram per day. Finally, the water volume requirement can be estimated according to the weight (Holliday-Segar method) or body surface (Table 57.5).

Contribution of Micronutrients

The updated contributions of vitamins and minerals according to age are available in the references.

Children with severe chronic respiratory diseases, vitamin D deficiency can reach 40%, with short-term effects on lung function as well as being associated with bronchial hyperresponsiveness, immunological disorders, and asthma. This, along with the effect on the bone metabolism of these children who have less sun exposure, justifies daily supplementation with 400 IU of vitamin D, adjusting the dose according to the plasma level of 25OH vitamin D. In addition, up to 20% of children with chronic respiratory diseases may have anemia promoted by their chronic condition, low iron intake, higher losses, and frequent

Table 57.2 Energy contribution for children with chronic respiratory diseases

Components	Age	Male	Female
REE calculation formulas (WHO 1985)	0–3	(60.9 × weight) − 54	(61 × weight) − 51
	3–10	(22.7 × weight) + 495	(22,5 × weight) + 499
	10–18	(17.5 × weight) + 651	(12,2 × weight) + 746
Correction factors (+)	Contribution for food metabolization (10%)		
	Growth (10–25%)		
	Degree of physical activity (10–25%)		
	Weight recovery (5 calories per extra gram daily)		
	Disease severity factor		

Table 57.3 Energy requirements

Age (months, years)	Male (cal/k/day)	Female (cal/k/day)
0–1 m	113	107
1.1–2 m	104	101
2.1–3 m	95	94
3.1–4 m	82	84
4.1–5 m	81	83
5.1–6 m	81	82
6.1–9 m	79	78
9.1–12 m	80	79
1.1–3 y	82.4–83.6	80.1–80.6
3.1–6 y	79.7–74.5	76.5–71.5
6.1–9 y	72.5–68.5	69.3–63.8
9.1–12 y	66.6–62.4	60.8–54.8
12.1–15 y	60.2–55.6	52.0–47.0
15.1–18 y	53.4–50.3	45.3–44.1

Total daily energy expenditure (TDEE) plus the energy required for growth and the average level of physical activity in people older than 1 year is considered. ↓15% for mild physical activity and ↑15% for vigorous physical activity

Table 57.4 Tolerable upper intake level (UL) for protein for children and adolescents

Age (years)	WHO 1985 (g/k/day)	UL 2002 (g/k/day)
0–6 m	2.2	1.8
6 m–12 m	1.6	1.5
1–3 years	1.2	1.1
4–6 years	1.2	0.95
7–10 years	1.0	0.95
11–14 years	1.0	0.8
15–18 years	0.9	0.8

Table 57.5 Water requirements

Method	Weight (kg)	Amount per day
Vol/weight	0–10 kg	100 ml/kg/day
	10–20 kg	1000 ml + 50 cc per each k > 10 k
	>20 kg	1500 ml + 20 cc per each k > 20 k
Vol/body surface[a]	0–70	1500–1700 ml/m^2
Vol/calories	0–70	100 ml/100 Cal metabolized

[a]Body surface = $\sqrt{[\text{Weight (k)} \times \text{height (cm)}]/3600}$

infections. It is recommended to monitor the reserves with plasma ferritin before decreasing plasma hemoglobin or, otherwise, consider prophylactic supplementation with 1–2 mg Fe++ per kilogram per day.

Route of Feeding

If an adequate oral intake is not achieved, either by respiratory or gastrointestinal intolerance, or by rejection; or if, despite achieving it, an adequate improvement is not obtained, it is advisable to use the enteral route through a nasogastric tube if its use is short-term. The use of a nasojejunal catheter is reserved for patients with risk of pulmonary aspiration due to the coexistence of gastroesophageal reflux disease (GERD) or gastric emptying disorders, together with airway protection mechanisms that are insufficient.

In the medium- or long-term, the use of gastrostomy is indicated either as a temporary or definitive measure, according to clinical follow-up of the patient. Gastrostomy is performed simultaneously with a fundoplication when pathological gastroesophageal reflux coexists with aspiration risk, which is common in patients with associated neurological damage. It has been demonstrated that early use of gastrostomy in children with bronchopulmonary dysplasia and malnutrition significantly improves nutritional deficit, and its late indication increases morbidity and mortality.

When the enteral route is a temporary measure, the use of a pacifier should be encouraged and oral stimulation should be maintained, supervised by a specialized team. When these capacities have been lost or not developed, future rehabilitation of swallowing is slower and harder.

Feeding Frequency

The increase in oral feeding frequency is a useful measure, but it must consider fasting periods of at least 3 hours that allow a complete gastric emptying and appetite appearance for the next feeding. When the enteral route is used, bolus feeding, which is more physiological, should be preferred. However, to optimize the absorption of nutrients or respiratory or gastrointestinal tolerance, sometimes continuous infusion is required, always considering short periods of intestinal rest.

Breastfeeding

In infants with bronchopulmonary dysplasia, a low percentage of mothers manage to initiate and maintain breastfeeding through expressed milk, at first, and then directly through the breasts. The composition of the breast milk of mothers of preterm infants differs from those of term infants and needs to be fortified with specific products that increase the caloric, protein, vitamin, and mineral content, to adapt it to the child's greater requirements. An alternative is to add 5–10% of preterm milk formula to the expressed breast milk. If, nevertheless, the child does not have an adequate growth, it can be supplemented with milk formula for preterm infants. Patients with exclusive breastfeeding should be supplemented, as all preterm, with vitamin D (400UI per day), iron (2 mg Fe ++ per kilogram per day), and zinc (3 mg per day), up to 12 months corrected age.

Adapted and Enriched Formulas

Different studies have shown that post-discharge growth in preterm infants with bronchopulmonary dysplasia is enhanced by a formula with a higher protein and mineral content. Compared to a fortified formula for term infants, at 3 months it is associated with better height and weight development, as well as bone mineral and lean mass accretion, but if it is discontinued, the effect is reversed when the child reaches 1 year of age (corrected age). The recommendation is to maintain, until then, preterm infant formulas, with higher energy, protein, and mineral content than formulas for term children (Table 57.6).

If water restriction is required or if there is poor weight development, the concentration of the formula can be increased by 1–2% and fortified simultaneously with 2% maltodextrin and 1% medium-chain triglycerides (MCT oil) or long-chain triglycerides (canola, raps, or sunflower vegetable oil), and if necessary, 0.5% of modular protein. This provides 1 cal/mL without reducing the protein intake or greatly increasing the renal solute load. Tolerance and weight improvement should be evaluated, considering that an excess of glucose polymers can increase osmotic load in the intestine, promoting diarrhea. An excess of lipids can cause steatorrhea, and an excess of MCT oil increases CO_2 production.

Infants with bronchopulmonary dysplasia or chronic lung damage, older than 1 year, who do not progress well, can be maintained with fortified formulas as described above, whether as a continuation or based on cow's milk. Fortification must be balanced: cereal (3–5%), maltodextrin (3–5%) or oil (1.5–2%), together with an increase of 2 to 3% in the formula concentration, with proteins representing between 10% and 15% of total calories, to optimize their accretion.

Another alternative at this stage is the use of liquid or powdered polymeric formulas, which have low viscosity, high caloric density (1 cal/mL), and are isotonic to plasma (±300 mO/l). In proper volumes, they provide the requirements of vitamins

Table 57.6 Composition of macronutrients of different formulas (in 100 mL)

Formula	Energy (Cal)	Proteins (g) P%	Carbohydrates (g)	Lipids (g)
Starter formula (term infant)	67	1.5–1.8 9–10	7.5	3.6
Starter formula (preterm infant)	81	2.3–2.6 10–12	8.6–9.2	3.9–4.4
Preterm formula, modified[a]	105	2.75 10.4	11.7	4.9
Modified continuation formula[b]	94	2.5 10.6	13.8	2.6
Hyperproteic hypercaloric formula[c]	111	3.5 12.6	13.6	4.75
Polymeric formula[d]	100–108	3.0–2.9 12–10.7	11–12.8	5.0–4.9

[a]↑Concentration in 2% + 2% maltodextrin +1% MCT or oil
[b]↑Concentration in 2.5% + 5% cereal +3% maltodextrin
[c]Fortified whole milk at 12.5% + 3% cereal +3% maltodextrin +3% sucrose +1.5% oil
[d]Pediasure® 20%. Abbott Laboratory

and minerals when they are used as a single source of food, particularly for patients enterally fed. Contributions and micronutrients should be monitored to avoid excessive fat deposition.

In adults, there is evidence that specific formulas for lung diseases, with high fat content (±55%) and low in carbohydrates (±28%), decrease CO_2 production and breathing work, which is a favorable effect in patients with CO_2 retention. However, these are not appropriate for infants, due to their unbalanced composition and high protein, osmotic, and solute load. In infants with bronchopulmonary dysplasia receiving parenteral nutrition with high glucose levels, an increase in the O_2 requirement and CO_2 production have been demonstrated. A prospective randomized study in 10 infants with bronchopulmonary dysplasia compared the seven-day effect of a term formula supplemented with glucose polymers (52% of calories) versus an isocaloric formula with high fat content (67% of calories). In those who received the latter, a reduction of 11% and 12% in the CO_2 produced was obtained, without being associated with improvement in lung function. However, patients had greater steatorrhea and lower weight gain. Therefore, more evidence is needed to evaluate the possible benefits versus the long-term deleterious effects of the use of formulas with this composition, in aspects such as growth, gastrointestinal tolerance, impact on the lipid profile and development of organic acidurias due to problems in the long chain fatty acids oxidation. Besides this, the energy increase through carbohydrates is related to a lower protein oxidation reduction, but it is not necessarily related to a better nitrogen balance. A higher CO_2 concomitant production may have physiological repercussions in patients with a CO_2 retention problem, with a $PCO_2 > 55$ mm Hg.

Solid Feeding

In preterm infants with or without bronchopulmonary dysplasia, it is recommended to start solid feeding at 6 months of corrected age, upon reaching sufficient intestinal maturation. Frequently, the use of liquefied food is prolonged, either by slow or late acquisition in food skills, or to optimize the intake. Counseling and periodic follow-up are important in order to avoid exaggerated weight gain, especially at the expense of fat mass in older children. Excessive use of dietary supplements tends to displace the foods that constitute a balanced and healthy diet, so it is preferable to use them complementary to a normal diet. Eating habits and support must be emphasized in those patients who have had enteral nutrition for prolonged periods, to prevent, identify, and treat eating disorders.

Conclusion

Children with chronic respiratory diseases require a special emphasis in the care of their nutritional status. Regular monitoring of their growth pattern allows early detection of abnormalities and timely intervention, which is promoted by a coordinated interdisciplinary team management. Adequate nutrition allows normal growth and development, promotes a better evolution of their disease, and probably decreases the later appearance of eating disorders and other chronic diseases.

Sources

Abrams SA. Chronic pulmonary insufficiency in children and its effects on growth and development. J Nutr. 2001;131:938s–41s.

Ambrosino N, Clini E. Long term mechanical ventilation and nutrition. Respir Med. 2004;98:413–20.

Atkinson SA. Special nutritional needs of infants for pre-vention of and recovery from BPD. J Nutr. 2001;131:942s–6s.

Barja S, Capo E, Jakubson L, Briceño L, Méndez M, Becker A. Anemia y déficit de hierro en niños con enfermedades respiratorias crónicas. Nutr Hosp. 2013;28:787–93.

Barja S, Rebollo MJ. Manejo nutricional de niños y adolescentes con fibrosis quística. Rev Chil Pediatr. 2009;80:274–84.

Barja S, Espinoza T, Cerda J, Sánchez I. Evolución nutricional y función pulmonar en niños y adolescentes chilenos con fibrosis quística. Rev Med Chile. 2011;139:977–84.

Bosa VL, Mello ED, Mocelin HT, Benedetti FJ, Fischer GB. Assessment of nutritional status in children and adolescents with post-infectious bronchiolitis obliterans. J Pediatr. 2008;84:323–30.

Cano N, Roth H, Court-Fortune I, et al. Nutritional depletion in patients on long-term oxygen therapy and/or home mechanical ventilation. Eur Respir J. 2002;20:30–7.

Chateau B, Prado F, Méndez M, Barja S. Nutritional Status of children with Chronic Respiratory Insufficiency. ATS Congress, San Francisco CA, May 2007. Am J Resp Crit Care Med. 2007;175:A722.

Darlow BA, Graham PJ. Vitamin A supplementation to pre-vent mortality and short and long-term morbidity in very low birthweight infants. Cochrane Database Syst Rev. 2011;10:CD000501.

Dumas C, Skaff C, Just J, et al. Body composition of children with chronic lung disease. Pediatr Pulmonol. 1997;16:174–6.

Guimber D, Michaud L, Storme L, Deschildre A, Turk D, Gottrand F. Gastrostomy in infants with neonatal pulmonary disease. JPGN. 2003;36:459–63.

Hendricks KM, Duggan C, Gallagher L. Malnutrition in hospitalized pediatric patients: current prevalence. Arch Pediatr Adolesc Med. 1995;149:1118–22.

Holditch-Davis D, Merrill P, Schwartz T, Scher M. Predictors of wheezing in prematurely born children. J Obstet Gynecol Neonatal Nurs. 2008;37:262–73.

Human Energy requirements. Report of a join FAO/WHO/UNU Expert Consultation. Rome, 17–24 October 2001. FAO, Food and Nutrition Technical Report Series.

Huysman WA, De Ridder M, De Bruin NC, et al. Growth and body composition in preterm infants with BPD. Arch Dis Fetal Neonatal Ed. 2003;88:F46–51.

Loughlin G, Heigen H. Respiratory disease in children, diagnosis and management. In: Barsky DL, Stallings VA, editors. Nutritional Management in Pediatric Pulmonary disease. Baltimore: Williams and Wilkins; 1994. p. 813–28.

Mena P, Llanos A, Uauy R. Nutrición y patología pulmonar en el neonato de bajo peso al nacer. Rev Chil Pediatr. 2005;76:12–24.

Ministerio de Salud de Chile. Estadística nutricional. Programa Nacional de Alimentación Complementaria (PNAC) del Prematuro Extremo. Displasia broncopulmonar del prematuro: guías clínicas. Accedido el 19 de julio de 2014. Disponible en: http://web.minsal.cl/programas_alimentarios.

Moreno M, Maya MJ, Bustos E, Astudillo C, Barja S. Evaluación y evolución nutricional en niños con bronquiolitis obliterante. 53° Congreso Chileno de Pediatría, II Conferencia de actualización en Pediatría, ALAPE. Santiago, Noviembre 2013. Rev Chil Pediatr. 2013;84(S1):91.

Morgan OW, Bramley A, Fowlkes A, Freedman DS, Taylor TH, et al. Morbid obesity as a risk factor for hospitalization and death due to 2009 pandemic influenza a (H1N1) disease. PLoS One. 2010;5(3):e9694. https://doi.org/10.1371/jour-nal.pone.0009694.

Muñoz E, Bustos E, Muños C, Briceño L y Barja S. Status de vitamina D en niños con enfermedades respiratorias crónicas y hospitalización prolongada. VII Congreso Chileno de Nutrición Clínica y Metabolismo. I Congreso Regional Sur, FELANPE. 29 de mayo al 1 de junio 2013. Viña del Mar, Chile.

Pereira G, Baumgart S, Bennett M, et al. Use of high-fat formula for premature infants with bronchopulmonary dysplasia: metabolic, pulmonary, and nutritional studies. J Pediatr. 1994;124:605–11.

Diseases Caused by Pollutants and Tobacco Exposure

58

Lidia Amarales Osorio,
María José Prieto Correa,
and Gabriela Muñoz Gómez

Contents

Introduction

Environmental pollution is an increasing and avoidable risk factor for respiratory disease, which impacts children with greater strength, because they are exposed to a greater effective dose of pollutants per weight kilogram, but also because their respiratory and immune systems are still in the development phase. The anatomical and physiological characteristics of the respiratory system that contribute to this susceptibility are: smaller volume and alveolar surface, greater respiratory frequency, and greater minute ventilation per body mass unit at rest, absence of contralateral ventilation (Kohn pores and Lambert channels), greater resistance of the peripheral airway, lower cough effectivity, and greater difficulty eliminating particles.

Environmental pollution can be divided in atmospheric pollution (AP) or in-house pollution (HP). HP is the main component of environmental

L. Amarales Osorio (✉)
Ministry of Health, Santiago, Chile

M. J. Prieto Correa
Respiratory Kinesiology, Academic at UMCE, UNAB, Santiago, Chile

G. Muñoz Gómez
Faculty of Medicine, Universidad de Chile, Santiago, Chile

P. Bertrand, I. Sánchez (eds.), *Pediatric Respiratory Diseases*,
https://doi.org/10.1007/978-3-030-26961-6_58

pollution and is defined as the atmospheric presence of one or several substances in large enough quantities to cause health problems. HP is the emission of pollutants at home, whether by solid combustibles (gas kerosene) or biomass (firewood or coal), combined with the infiltration of atmospheric contaminants to indoor environments, and/or contamination caused by environmental tobacco smoke (ETS).

The WHO has declared that the global burden of morbidity caused by indoor and outdoor air pollution causes millions of premature deaths, which are associated with tobacco risks, currently represent the greatest sanitary risks around the globe, only surpassed by hypertension and malnutrition. It has been estimated that around 3% of the total world deaths attributed to AP correspond to children under 5 years of age, and this number increases to 13% when considering deaths by HP in this same age group.

Atmospheric Pollution (AP)

AP is presented as an aerosol, with its gas components and particulate material (PM), causing great damage to ecosystems and altering the quality of life of the population. AP has a greater effect on the health of those who already have an underlying disease and in the most vulnerable groups: children, elderly, and poor families with limited access to medical assistance. Children with chronic diseases, such as cystic fibrosis and asthma, are particularly vulnerable to pollutant effects.

Intrauterine and perinatal periods, as well as the first years of life in children, are characterized by a greater vulnerability to pollutants. In these stages the respiratory system is more susceptible to damage, which will damage the lung capacity that will be acquired as an adult, along with an increase in infection susceptibility. There is evidence supporting that this is associated with multiple respiratory morbidity, pulmonary function alteration, and greater incidence of child cancer.

The effects that AP may have in the long and short-term are many, including an increased risk to suffer from acute and chronic respiratory diseases, as well as cardiovascular diseases. The effects are directly related with the effective dose, determined by three factors: time of exposure, concentration of the pollutant per area, and pulmonary ventilation. High-pollutant concentrations, although it may be for short periods of time, cause acute effects and worsen chronic diseases. Up to 80% of premature deaths related to pollution in the exterior air are caused by ischemic cardiopathy and cerebrovascular accident, while 14% are caused by a chronic obstructive pulmonary disease, or acute infection of lower airways, and 6% to lung cancer. AP at the same time has effects later in time, such as mutagenesis and carcinogenesis, which may appear long after the interruption to the exposure and extend to future generations.

During the past decades, AP has become an important and serious global problem, caused by a lack of development planning, which along with the production of the energy and its use, are responsible for the emission of the pollutants. The emission of man-made gases is increasing the atmospheric concentration of those gases that catch energy and heat from the sun, which amplifies the natural "greenhouse effect", which makes life on Earth possible. Of these gases, the one with the greatest concentration is carbon dioxide (CO_2), which comes mainly out of fossil combustibles (coal, oil, gas), which causes an increase in the atmospheric temperature and greatly impacts ecosystems. Nevertheless, the risks to health are also caused by exposure to gases, such as ozone (O_3), nitrogen dioxide (NO_2), and sulfur dioxide (SO_2), whose concentrations are usually high in urban areas of middle and low-income countries.

PM is the pollutant most associated with mortality and morbidity events in the population. PM is defined as solid or liquid particles that are in suspension. We classified them according to size and origin. Thus, particles smaller than 10 μm are called PM_{10}, and those that are smaller than 2.5 μm, $PM_{2.5}$. Considering that the diameter of a human hair is around 60 μm, PM_{10} has almost the tenth part, and the finer particles $PM_{2.5}$ are even smaller and can enter very deeply in the respiratory tract. These particles are difficult to remove and carry with them other chemicals when they settle themselves, such as sulfates, nitrates, carbon, metals, and organic material, while large particles tend to have materials, such as silica, rubber, salts, and pollen.

There is a close relationship between exposure to high concentrations of PM_{10} and an increase in morbidity and mortality. This is true for both daily exposure and the one that persists in time. On the contrary, when there is PM reduction, related mortality is also reduced. Repeated exposures may create greater effects on health than a single exposure. Although the acute and long-term effects are not the total sum of the acute exposure, these are greater, suggesting that they do not correspond to exacerbations but to a progression of an underlying disease. There is also toxicological and clinical evidence of the effect of particles originated during combustion, where short-term exposure (less than 1 hour to a few hours), also carries immediate physiological changes. Biological mechanisms of exposure are related to systemic inflammation, oxidative stress, alterations in heart biomarkers, coagulation effects, and thrombosis increase.

AP affects both developed and undeveloped countries. It has been estimated that it causes the death of almost 3.7 million people in the world, caused mainly by PM $\leq$10 exposure. Up to 88% of these deaths take place in countries with middle and low-incomes, affecting 82% of the population worldwide. The America continent contributes with around 140 thousand deaths. Although older adults have the greatest risk for mortality, the evidence shows that during the postnatal period the risk of death due to a respiratory cause increases.

Deregulated concentrations of both gases and particles affect the health condition. Therefore, pollutant emissions are now thoroughly being studied, and there is also the need to reduce their production. Most of environmental pollutant sources are beyond individual control, and public policies are required in sectors, such as transportation, energy, construction, and agriculture.

Epidemiology in Chile

When estimating the attributed burden per risk factor, the Ministry of Health of Chile (MINSAL) issued the Disease Burden Study, which described that 13 deaths are directly caused by the levels of urban pollution and one of every 11 deaths is directly caused by active smoking (sub-estimated information, without considering the effects in the passive smoker). The relative importance of the risk factors is similar to high-income countries; nevertheless, urban air pollution has an unusually high place in the world ranking, as it would be characteristic of a less developed country.

Concern for the high pollution levels dates from the 1980s, and so a monitoring network was set in place, with daily measures of PM_{10}, $PM_{2.5}$, and other pollutants. This, along with the records of morbidity and mortality, has enabled us to conduct timely studies of the acute effects of atmospheric pollution, where an association has been made between the concentration increase and daily mortality, urgency pediatric visits because of a respiratory cause, and visits for cardiovascular causes.

The main results of Chilean national studies done in the Metropolitan Region refer to a significant increase in the daily risk rate of 4% in the general population. The increase in hospital admittances caused by lower tract respiratory diseases when PM_{10} concentration increases to 50 μg/m^3 is: 4–12% increase for patients under 2 years old, and 3–9% increase for children between 3 and 15 years old. Another study showed that 3 days after a 45 μg/m^3 increase in the daily concentrations average of $PM_{2.5}$, there was an increase of 6.7% in pneumonia cases. In a cohort study including children under 4 months in the South of Santiago, Pino confirmed a 5% increase of the cases of wheezing associated with an increase of 10 μg/m^3 in $PM_{2.5}$. In downtown Santiago (2001–2006) it was determined that the increase of urgent medical visits because of respiratory disease, particularly in children under 1 year, was caused by high $PM_{2.5}$ levels due to vehicle and industrial contamination. Cifuentes et al. showed that there was a 4.2% increase in daily mortality in the Metropolitan Region when $PM_{2.5}$ levels were at 64 μg/m^3 (daily average level of 47.3 μg/m^3).

Respiratory Morbidity Associated with Atmospheric Pollutants

The World Health Organization (WHO 2013) has documented the effects of PM_{10} pollution during pregnancy, for both the fetus and the mother. Pollution can affect the blood pressure of the mother, increasing it, as well as cause changes in the size of the fetus, usually associated with the reduction of some parameters, such as head circumference, size or weight at birth, and also premature childbirth, which are all parameters associated with a poorer health expectancy for the child.

Several national and international studies have shown that there is an association between the level of pollutant concentrations, such as MP, O_3, SO_2, and NO_2, and the incidence of premature deaths and child respiratory morbidity. At the cellular level, environmental pollutants may cause damage, even if the exposure is brief and the pollutant levels are low. Sulfuric acid components may interfere in the mucociliary transport and sulfur dioxide may cause bronchoconstriction if there is asthma. Besides this, O_3 may impair the actions of the immune system against infections, contribute to a persistent infection in the airway, as well as increasing permeability in pneumocytes, easing the access of substances and promoting allergen sensitization. It seems that contaminants interact with other environmental factors, such as allergens, virus, and diet, which would have a role in how pollutants globally affect the respiratory health of children.

There is a correlation between the high levels of pollutants and an increase of acute respiratory diseases requiring hospitalizations, particularly in preschoolers, where admittance caused by wheezing may be tripled. A study conducted in European countries showed that pollution causes more than 290,000 bronchitis cases in children under 15 years old. At the same time, clinical trials studying nasal and bronchial epithelium cells have been conducted. These studies exposed the cells to *Rhinovirus*, and pro-inflammatory activity markers where used to study the response. Thus, evidence was obtained in relation to the mechanisms through which environmental oxidative pollution (NO_2-O_3) may exacerbate viral respiratory infections in vivo. Therefore, exposure to oxidative pollutants (NO_2, among others) has the potential to exacerbate the inflammatory effects of viral infections in the lower tract airway, causing the release of inflammatory mediators, ciliary dyskinesia, epithelium damage, bronchoconstriction, and bronchial hyperreactivity (BHR).

Besides this, there is a correlation between high pollutant levels and an increase in hospitalizations caused by asthma. After periods with high O_3 levels, the frequency of asthma exacerbations can increase up to 40%, and for urgency medical visits, the increase can be of up to 37%.

When facing atmospheric pollution caused by MP, the physiological increase in lung function is impaired, which normally appears as the patient grows. This is an additional factor in critical situations, such as viral infection.

The effects of pollution on children lung function, with its corresponding growth alteration in their spirometry values, can be observed in the Integrated Science Assessment (ISA) 2009 document (see EPA), where the most significant scientific evidence is gathered.

In Chile, toward the end of the decade of 1980, Belmar et al. showed the differences in spirometry values of children living in Santiago city versus Los Andes. Thirty years later, this condition remains the same when spirometry function values are compared to those of healthy children in Cerro Navia (Metropolitan Region). This is a significant worsening of lung function, in comparison to Los Andes.

Strategies and Recommendations

The recently published Encyclical Letter "Laudato si" states that "technology based on the use of highly polluting fossil fuels — especially coal, but also oil and, to a lesser degree, gas —

needs to be progressively replaced without delay". This document proposes that the deterioration of the environment is caused by consumerism and the economic and financial system that smothers the poor.

Chile is not excluded from this analysis, as its strong economic growth and high dependence on natural resources has had a cost in the condition of the environment, particularly in relation to the quality of the air. The use of renewable energy sources is mainly limited to hydroelectric power plants, and the energy needs of the country are, to a large extent, satisfied importing fossil fuels. The mechanisms to promote the adoption of clean technologies are still insufficient.

Because of this, the WHO (2005) has created guidelines that provide a general orientation about the limit thresholds for key atmospheric pollutants, which are related to current health risks. In the ISA study from 2009, as well as in the WHO study from 2013, the range of annual PM10 concentrations that cause health deterioration in the long-term is between 20 and 40 $\mu g/m^3$. According to the estimations made by the WHO, if the median of PM_{10} annual concentration is reduced from 70 to 20 $\mu g/m^3$, a 15% of the mortality rate caused by AP in the long-term can be avoided.

Chile has national-wide quality air norms, which regulate the concentration of the six main types of harmful pollutants: PM_{10}, $PM_{2.5}$, SO_2, NO_2, CO, O_3, and lead (Pb), plus daily and annual norms of PM10, 150, and 50 $\mu g/m^3$, respectively. These values exceed the values of 50 and 20 $\mu g/m^3$ recommend by the WHO, which would be permissive enough to prevent health effects and avoid excesses in mortality rates. Because of this, it is crucial to enforce daily and annual norms and regulations recommended by international organisms and experts in order to improve air quality. The aim of these measures is to control atmospheric pollutants, thus protecting the population against these pollutants and therefore decreasing the morbidity load.

Cities must determine which are the main sources of air pollution and enforce strict policies as well as adequate interventions that will improve air quality. Among these, we can mention promoting power plants that use clean and renewable sources instead of coal, improvements in the energy efficiency of buildings and manufacturing facilities, promoting and improving public transportation and use of bicycles, instead of relying on private cars. At the same time, it is important to raise awareness in the population about relatively simple interventions, such as improving the use of wood and using public transport system, which can help to reduce the AP levels, thus yielding important health improvements.

Effectively following-up the interventions is another important way to increase awareness, as it helps to create norms which will bring health and environmental benefits.

Although significant advances have been made in mega cities, such as Los Angeles, México City, São Paulo, and Santiago, where constant efforts are being made to reduce pollution levels, there is still a lot to do. Several successful cases have been developed and public policies aiming to reduce urban air pollution have been set in place. Public transport integrated systems developed in Curitiba (Brazil) and Bogotá (Colombia) have become a model for other large cities in the region (México City, São Paulo, and Santiago de Chile) as well as in Europe (Bilbao and Sevilla).

Even though many countries in the region have a legal framework to control air pollution, current standing norms vary a lot, some of which do not set limits for some parameters, or consider limits over the ones recommended in the WHO guidelines.

More investment is needed for continuous monitoring of air quality, as well as searching for options to reduce emissions, investigation research associated with the creation of regional norms, and participation of the society to reduce exposure during environmental eventualities.

Indoor Pollution (IP)

IP or household air pollution is also a serious health problem for over 3 trillion people, particularly in underdeveloped countries that still depend on solid fuels. IP can exceed AP in many countries in the world, and so it is the most important environmental risk factor. IP is responsible for 5% of the global load of these diseases, and it is also the highest load in low-income countries. IP causes around 4.3 million early deaths, 81 thousand of them happen in America (2012). Greater equality in energy access at the worldwide level would benefit the development of communities and population health.

In Santiago de Chile, in the households within the extreme poverty band, where parents smoke in over 50% of the households, it was found that the concentration of pollutants (PM, SO_2, and CO) was greater inside of the house than outside of the households, and these concentrations were higher than those defined in the national norms. The carcinogenics found inside of the households was 6.5 times higher than outside of the households. Although all domestic energy sources may have deleterious effects on health, the most important direct risk is the pollution caused by the incomplete combustion of paraffin, petroleum, coal, and other sources used for cooking, lighting, and/or heating.

The Household Environment Observatory studied and compared the different types of heating systems used in Chile. With this information, a value chart was created. This chart showed the emission values for gases and PM. Both traditional and modern paraffin heaters have the greatest pollution indexes for all pollutants. New convective heaters have the lowest pollution levels, whether they are powered by natural gas or liquefied petroleum gas (LPG), although these heaters emit a high level of nitric oxide (NO_x) gases. Coal heaters are the ones with the highest rates of CO emission, which is dangerous (Table 58.1).

Respiratory Morbidity and Mortality Associated with Indoor Pollution

Generally, pollutants cause airway and lung inflammation, thus hindering the immune response and impairing the capacity for oxygen transportation in the blood. SO_2 and NO_x are gases that cause irritation of the airway, reduce lung function, and leave the patient in a vulnerable state, which makes them more susceptible to suffer from diseases, such as colds or bronchopulmonary problems. Although high concentrations of these gases do not cause a swift death as happens with CO, prolonged exposure may cause severe respiratory complications, particularly for children and elderly patients.

In small children, IP exposure, including tobacco smoke, increases mortality rate and the risk of suffering acute respiratory infections. Pneumonia risk in children under 5 years old who are exposed to solid combustibles is 1.8 times higher. In general, PM_{10} exposure quadruples the risk of upper respiratory infections (OR 4.30) and doubles the risk of lower respiratory infections. Besides this, there is an association between the size of the particles and the risk of developing wheezing in children who are under 3 years old (OR) –$PM_{1:}$ 5.9, $PM_{5:}$ 5.5, and $PM_{10:}$ 3.4–. More than 50% of deaths caused by pneumonia in children under 5 years old are related to household air pollution. Women and children, who are the ones who spend more time at home, are particularly vulnerable.

Recommendations

The WHO has generated a series of three guidelines to improve the quality of indoor air: dampness and mold (2009), specific pollutants

Table 58.1 Pollution indexes according to different types of heating sources

	PM	CO	SO_2	NO_x
Traditional paraffin	2.3–3.6	2.3–3.2	3.4–4.0	1.9–2.7
Modern paraffin	2.1–3.1	1.7–2.1	3.4–4.3	7.6–8.0
NG Convective	0.4–1.6	0.4	0	5.7
NG Radiant	1.0–1.2	0.8	0	1.1–2.7
LPG Convective	0.4–1.2	0.3	0	6.5
LPG Radiant	1.2		0	2.7–3.4
Coal		72.9		

Value chart for gases and PM emission

0: Optimum
0–2: Regular
2–10: Poor
>10: Dangerous

(2010), and indoor combustion fuels pollutants (2014).

In poorly ventilated households, the level of $PM_{2.5}$ emissions and other contaminants may be higher than the levels recommended by the WHO. This increase can be up to 100 times over these suggested levels. One of the most effective ways to guarantee cleaner indoor air is controlling the emission of pollutants expelled by the sources of energy used in the households.

Coal must not be used as house fuel, because of the high mortality associated with CO, and also because it is a carcinogen. Besides this, when it has not been processed, it usually contains toxic elements, such as arsenic, fluoride, lead, selenium, and mercury, which is not destroyed when the fuel is burnt. The use of paraffin as home fuel is not recommended, because of the emission of highly harmful pollutants, as well as an increased risk in burnings, fires, and poisoning. Although there are few studies of clean fuels, such as biogas and ethanol, the evidence gathered from emissions tests suggests that these fuels, along with electricity, are the best alternatives to solid fuels. All of this indicates that the practices of energy use at home originate high pollution levels. Nevertheless, considering the prevalence and the importance of deleterious health effects, the main indoor pollutant is cigarette smoke.

Smoking, a Pediatric Disease

Smoking is a pediatric disease, although most of the diseases related to tobacco exposure appear later in life. This is caused by the fact that environmental tobacco smoke (ETS) affects several diseases in each of the pediatric stages of life (fetus, childhood, and adolescence). Besides this, the diseases caused by tobacco use in adults subclinically appear during the first two decades of life, and 90% of the smokers present this addiction before reaching 18 years of life.

More than 5 decades ago, the US Public Health Service presented the first report that showed how tobacco use is harmful for the health of a person, thus beginning the development of several initiatives at the worldwide level to reduce its use, and therefore, the consequences for the general population as well as for the individual patient. In 2009, the WHO declared the *Global Tobacco Epidemic* as a preventable cause of death, which annually takes the lives of more than 5 million people.

During the past years in Chile, the regulation about tobacco use has advanced (Law 20.105, year 2006, and since 2013, Law 20.660), advocating for environments free of smoke in every public place, among other multiple measures recommended by the WHO Framework Convention on Tobacco Control, with a clear benefit for the children. Nevertheless, there is still much to do in relation to cultural changes and tobacco use, particularly in relation to women, in order to reduce its high prevalence and therefore reduce even more second-hand and third-hand pollution. Health teams have some ineludible responsibilities, especially pediatricians and specialists, who should inform the parents about the passive smoker status of their children, thus achieving to eliminate the tobacco use of the parents. In this, the burden of the disease in the family, especially children, will be reduced.

Epidemiology of Smoking in Chile

Tobacco use is the most important preventable risk factor in chronic non-communicable diseases, which is present in children exposed to passive smoking. In Chile, 16,532 people die every year, 45 people die every day, which has an annual cost for the State that is equivalent to 11.5% of the national health budget (MINSAL 2014). Mortality attributed to tobacco use is 25% for diseases, such as sudden death or sudden infant death syndrome (1985–2005). At the national level, the monthly and daily prevalence of tobacco use in the general population is 34% and 21.9%, respectively, which is higher in the lower socioeconomic levels (SENDA 2012). A sustained and significant reduction has been observed since 2006, with the first modification to the Tobacco Law. Until 2008, Chile was first place for smoking prevalence in adolescents

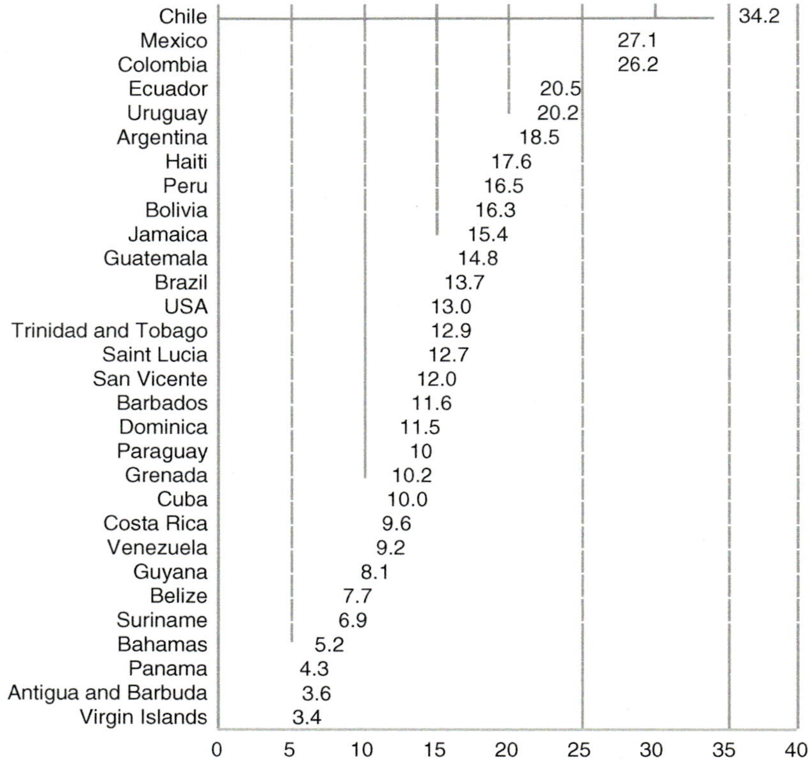

Fig. 58.1 Smoking Prevalence in schoolchildren (13–15 years old)

between 13 and 15 years old at the regional level, which was 34.2%, with significant differences with other countries, which varied between 3.4% up to 27.1% (Fig. 58.1). It also had the first place in the world of smoking prevalence among women: 39.9%, which is even more serious (EMTA 2008).

Currently, monthly and daily tobacco consumption in schoolchildren at the national level (8th grade to last year of high school) is estimated to be 26.7% and 7.3%, respectively. These numbers also show a sustained and significant reduction, associated with a progressive increase in the perception of smoking as a dangerous activity (SENDA 2013).

Chilean adolescents start to smoke very early: among the ones who smoked during the last month, 5.5% start before they are 7 years old, and between 74.6% and 81.7% start before reaching 13 years of age. Among the adolescents who smoke, the risk of being a smoker in 5 years is 8.4 times higher in comparison to non-smokers. Therefore, an early onset is strongly related to dependence and addiction, and nicotine dependence is quickly established during adolescence. Clearly, when parents smoke, it is an important factor in adolescents: Adolescents who smoked are 2.1 times more likely to smoke than those adolescents whose parents do not smoke.

Physiopathology

Tobacco smoke is a complex mixture of chemical products containing over 4000 chemical substances, particles, and gases, including chemical irritants and 70 carcinogens. Each one of them has different deleterious effects in all the organs and systems, including the respiratory system. Its effects range from neuroendocrine stimulation and depression, causing addictions, besides inflammation, humoral and cellular immune alterations, allergic sensitization, increase of bronchial hyper reactivity, carcinogenesis, toxicity related to ciliary genesis, transport alteration, and oxygen use.

Passive Smoking: Second-Hand and Third-Hand Smoking

Second-hand smoking happens when the patient inhales the ETS emitted by other people while smoking. Although the smoke has a similar composition to the one exhaled by the smoker, *the concentrations of toxins and carcinogens are often higher*. Children have no control on their tobacco polluted environment, which has effects in the uterus and particularly during the first years of life, while they eat, play, crawl, or sleep at home.

Several studies show that the children of parents who smoke are passive second-hand smokers. This has been confirmed through the presence of significantly higher levels of mediators—cotinine in the urine and nicotine/cotinine in the hair—in children under 10 years old, particularly in those children under 1 year old, whose parents smoke, in comparison to children whose parents do not smoke. This situation is worsened when the first cigarette is smoked 30 minutes after getting up, as well as when there is partial or no restriction at all to tobacco use at home, when compared to a total restriction. Third-hand smoke exposure is the result of the inhalation, ingestion, and skin absorption of pollutants that remain in the air, dust of the room, surfaces, clothing and hair of the parents, caregivers, care providers, or educators who smoke. Small children are more vulnerable to third-hand smoke, as they are routinely in contact with carpets, floor, furniture, and other contaminated objects, which they usually place in their mouth. It is particularly risky in homes with children who are under 1 year old, and smoking outside of the house reduces, but does not protect, from ETS. ETS exposure and pollution is 5–7 times higher in the homes of smokers who try to protect their children smoking in an open space, when compared to homes of non-smokers. Urine cotinine measured in infants indirectly exposed is 7.5 times higher in comparison to non-exposed infants.

In Chile, the National Health Survey of 2009–2010 showed that smoking was allowed in 30.7% of Chilean homes. At the same time, exposure to tobacco smoke in transport vehicles and/or parks and or entertainment venues are daily situations that increase the frequency or degree of exposure for the child.

Second-hand and third-hand smoke are clearly related and coexist. While second-hand smoke can be reduced ventilating the spaces, pollutants in third-hand smoke may persist in the environment, homes, or cars, for several hours, days, or months after the cigarette has been smoked. There is no safe level of third-hand environmental tobacco exposure, thus causing potentially harmful exposures. The only effective way to protect children from tobacco smoke is to eliminate the parent's tobacco use, particularly tobacco use of the mother and that of caregivers educating the child, besides having the home and cars completely free from tobacco smoke. ETS has been widely recognized as a significant cause of damage, for both short- and long-term, particularly impacting the health of children. Children are particularly vulnerable, as they present a greater risk for several respiratory diseases.

Respiratory Morbidity and Mortality Associated with Tobacco Exposure

Epigenetics

Prenatal exposition to pollutants, such as tobacco smoke and other substances, may active or silence genes related to immunity, with substantial effects in immune programming, thus determining the risk to suffer from several diseases. The epigenetic action from tobacco smoke is translated in the remodeling of pro-inflammation genes, with an increase in the expression of inflammation mediators.

T helper cells differentiation in a Th_1 or Th_2 phenotype is partially directed by the expression or repression of specific genes, and it was the foundation of the *hygiene hypothesis* that appeared some years ago, which regulated Th_1/Th_2, and that explained the increase of asthma and allergic diseases. Currently, it has been confirmed that the development of the immune system is epigenetically regulated, and Th_1/Th_2 differentiation is related to tobacco exposure during pregnancy, activating or silencing these genes, thus altering the balance of the neonatal immune response. Therefore, we may propose that maternal tobacco use, or exposure to ETS, may alter the immune function in the fetus, contributing to a greater risk to suffer respiratory disease, asthma, and allergic diseases in children. This could explain, among other factors, the significant increase of early childhood allergy, wheezing rates, and the appearance of asthma at the worldwide level, with its corresponding national correlation, as confirmed by the International Study of Asthma and Allergies in Childhood (ISAAC).

Fetal Tobacco Syndrome

The description from 1985 summarizes the effect that tobacco has in the pregnant woman and the newborn. This greater fetal risk is caused by maternal anemia, fetal hypoxia, and polycythemia, causing poor perinatal growth and alteration of the brain morphological substrate, which results from the fetal response to hypoxia. Table 58.2 summarizes works that confirm damage that intrauterine tobacco causes. Among these risks we may mention the association between prenatal mother use of tobacco and sudden infant death syndrome, which doubles and almost quadruples this probability. Besides a clear association to prenatal maternal use of tobacco, there is a clear association to several respiratory child diseases, such as early wheezing, recurrent wheezing, visit to emergency room, or hospitalization because of lower respiratory infections and asthma, among others. Studies conducted by Mallol in Chile show that the children of mothers who smoked during pregnancy had a significantly greater risk to suffer from wheezing, acute respiratory diseases, and hospitalization because of pneumonia, in comparison with the children of non-smokers mothers.

Table 58.2 Impact on child health because of exposure to tobacco smoke in uterus

Effects on pregnancy	Evidence
Reduced fetal growth	+++
Premature childbirth	+++
Fissures	++
Effects on the newborn	
Low weight at birth	+++
Sudden infant death syndrome	++
Reduced pulmonary function	++
Effects in infants and school-age children	
Overweight	+++
Reduction of pulmonary function	++
Bronchial asthma	+++
Infections	+
Acute otitis media	++

Evidence: + = Some retrospective studies, or studies for cases and control groups; ++ = several retrospective studies, few prospective studies; +++ = many prospective studies and metanalysis

In relation to the greater risk of acute otitis media, a prospective cohort composed of 8556 pregnant women showed a clear dose–response relationship between the degree of tobacco use by the mother during the 1st trimester of pregnancy and the risk for this affection until the fifth year of life.

Sudden Infant Death Syndrome

A systematic review concluded that after adjusting for confusing factors, such as sleep position and socioeconomic situation, if the mother uses tobacco after birth, the risk for sudden infant death syndrome is doubled. In 59% of the cases, children who were exposed to ETS did so because the mother smoked. Besides this, other studies show that there is a greater nicotine concentration in pulmonary tissue of infants who died because of sudden infant death syndrome, as well as observing that the relationship depends on the dose. The number of cases of sudden infant death syndrome has been significantly reduced in those countries where tobacco use has also decreased.

Child Respiratory Morbidity and Mortality

Passive smoking doubles the risk of respiratory infections in children. The main mechanisms are related to structural and immunological changes. Within the structural changes we can mention the ones related to the anatomical damage caused in the upper and lower airway (inflammation, reduction in mucociliary transport, Eustachian tube blockage, among others) and the increase of bacterial adherence to respiratory mucosa. Nicotine and other products of tobacco smoke favor the microorganism invasion of the middle ear, which colonize the nasopharynx. Immunological changes include inhibition of the phagocytic activity of the neutrophil and alveolar macrophages, as well as altering specific cell and humoral immunity response: Nicotine inhibits cellular Th_1 response, reducing the production of IgG and IgA, as well as stimulating Th_2 response, along with an increase of IgE and eosinophil production.

A common problem in pediatrics, which causes a considerable morbidity, is acute and chronic middle ear disorder. There is a clear association between tobacco use of any of the parents and middle ear infectious pathology. Particularly, chronic middle ear disease is 20–50% more frequent in children exposed to ETS, related to recurrent otitis media, middle ear effusion, or ear surgery, with a positive association between duration of the effusion and the number of smokers at home during the first and second year of life. Sinusitis is also related to ETS: among the children who present sinusitis, 68.8% are exposed to passive smoking at home, according to some investigators.

Children of parents who smoke are at double risk to suffer from a serious respiratory disease during childhood. This risk is greater in children under 2 years old, especially for children with low weight at birth (OR 4.5). Besides this, there is a dose–response correlation for acute respiratory infections depending on the number of smokers in the house and/or quantity of cigarettes smoked by the mother. Bronchiolitis caused by *syncytial respiratory virus*, a frequent respiratory entity in our country, and feared because of its seriousness in infants, presents a greater incidence when it is associated with passive smoking. Cough, one of the most prevalent and frequent symptoms for child visits, is associated with ETS, as well as hypersecretion and respiratory distress. The relationship between infant wheezing and tobacco use has been widely documented, especially when the mother smokes, and it increases when both parents smoke. Besides this, a risk gradient is observed according to the quantity of cigarettes smoked, with a greater gradient if the mother smokes.

In relation to asthma and rhinitis, a study conducted in 27 European countries describes an increase between 7% and 11% in the number of asthma episodes in <14 years-old exposed to ETS. ISAAC (Table 58.3) shows the risk association between passive smoking and asthma and severe asthma symptoms, but especially if the mother smokes during the first year of life of the child in the lower age group. At the same time, a crescent gradient related to tobacco use of each of the parents was described. Association of rhinitis with tobacco use of the parents is certainly weaker, with a greater risk of conjunctivitis in the 6–7 years old age group, a greater risk when the mother smokes, and an even greater risk if both parents smoke, with no relation to dose dependence.

In Punta Arenas city the study conducted by Amarales L. as a collaborator of ISAAC (2001) shows that children who smoke in the older age

Table 58.3 Pediatric morbidity among tobacco exposure

Symptoms	Only mother smokes	Only father smokes	Both parents
6–7 years old	OR (95% CI)	OR (95% CI)	OR (95% CI)
Recurrent wheezing	1.31 (1.22–1.41)	1.13 (1.08–1.18)	1.37 (1.29–1.45)
Recurrent rhinoconjunctivitis symptoms	1.13 (1.04–1.23)	1.07 (1.02–1.12)	1.16 (1.09–1.24)
Asthma	1.28 (1.19–1.38)	1.07 (1.02–1.12)	1.29 (1.22–1.38)
Severe asthma symptoms	1.31 (1.18–1.46)	1.19 (1.11–1.27)	1.46 (1.34–1.59)
13–14 years old	OR (95% CI)	OR (95% CI)	OR (95% CI)
Recurrent wheezing	1.27 (1.19–1.36)	1.13 (1.07–1.18)	1.43 (1.36–1.51)
Recurrent rhinoconjunctivitis symptoms	1.15 (1.08–1.23)	1.12 (1.07–1.17)	1.27 (1.21–1.34)
Asthma	1.16 (1.09–1.23)	1.04 (0.99–1.08)	1.21 (1.16–1.28)
Severe asthma symptoms	1.28 (1.18–1.39)	1.16 (1.09–1.23)	1.57 (1.47–1.67)

group (13–14 years old) significantly presented a greater prevalence of asthma symptoms in relation to non-smoking children (16.8% vs 10.7%), dose-dependence, and a greater prevalence of exercise induced asthma symptoms (19.98% vs 15.07%).

People exposed to ETS inhale a pulmonary carcinogen that metabolizes and is cleared through urine. These urinary metabolites are present in up to 90% of children exposed, with a correlation between the cigarettes smoked per day at home and the urinary levels of those metabolites, clearly showing that in-house smoking is an important source of child exposure to a pulmonary carcinogen. At the same time, 3rd hand exposure to tobacco smoke is genotoxic in human cellular lines.

Diagnostic Approach and Recommendations

Pediatricians and pulmonologists have a strategic and privileged place to avoid tobacco damage. Within the obligations, *prevention and protection to the fetal, child, and juvenile population must be encouraged, particularly for pathologies related to passive smoking. At the same, the onset of active tobacco use must be prevented during pre-adolescence and youth, through sustained actions coordinated with the parents and teachers, besides stimulating parents and family members who smoke to quit the habit. The diagnose of personal (for schoolchildren and adolescents) or familial use of tobacco is crucial, and it should be mandatory in every pediatric visit, particularly with the specialists, as well as treating active tobacco use during the first years of juvenile addiction.* The diagnosis is made in only 33–35% of medical visits, as well as the anti-tobacco counseling in adolescents who smoke.

It is important to consider that parents who smoke are frequently unaware of the damage that ETS cause in their children, or the relationship between tobacco exposure with the corresponding diseases, particularly when these are recurrent respiratory diseases. This is especially true for the 3rd hand smoke, when they argue that they smoke out of the house and minimize the damage. Even so, it is frequent that specialists, when facing recurrent pathologies, start a detailed study to obtain an etiopathogenic diagnose, without having first conducted an exhaustive anamnesis about family tobacco use, which could be an RF in these pathologies.

Informing the parents about the harm that ETS causes in the corresponding pathology may reduce or eliminate tobacco use rates in the parents, therefore reducing the exposure or eliminating children's exposure. Because of this, the American Medical Association has proposed the need for pediatricians to approach the parent's tobacco use. The recommendations of the Treatment of tobacco use in children and adolescents guidelines includes: (a) asking pediatric and adolescents patients about tobacco use, (b) send a strong message about the importance of completely abstaining from using tobacco, (c) have counsel interventions to help them quit smoking, hopefully with written information, (d) promote abstinence and quitting tobacco use for the parents who smoke, along with a brief counseling, and (e) set follow-up visits. Brief counselling made by the physician increases the quitting rate in 66%, in comparison to a lack of intervention. Therefore, pediatric visit must be an opportunity to discuss the risks associated with tobacco use in people of all ages, influence the beliefs of the parents about 2nd and 3rd hand tobacco damage, promote smoke free environments, and quitting tobacco use of both adolescents and parents who smoke.

Lastly, measures will probably be more effective if they are placed within a juvenile tobacco prevention program, framed within an integral program involving population policies, such as the current law in Chile (Free from tobacco smoke), reduction of advertising, and taxes increase (greater taxes and effective inspection); incorporating lack of tobacco as a guaranteed public and private offer, avoiding presenting tobacco use as an "activity for grown-ups", and emphasizing how tobacco industry addresses young people, making them addicted to nicotine from an early age.

Sources

Anderson ME, Johnson DC, Batal HA. Sudden Infant Death Syndrome and prenatal maternal smoking: rising attributed risk in the Back to Sleep era. BMC Med. 2005;3:4. 1–7.

Cebulj D, Vildoso J, Quezada E, Figueroa F, Prieto MJ, Díaz V, et al. Función pulmonar en niños sanos de 7 y 8 años de las comunas de Cerro Navia y Los Andes expuestos a diferentes niveles de contaminación por MP10. Salud Uninorte. 2011;27(2):198–20.

Boldo E, Medina S, Öberg M, Puklová V, et al. Health impact assessment of environmental tobacco smoke in european children: sudden infant death syndrome and asthma episodes. Public Health Rep. 2010;125:478–88.

Cakmak S, Dales RE, Gultekin T, Blanco C, Farnendaz M, Rubio MA, et al. Pollution and emergency department visits in Chile. Arch Environ Occup Health 2009;64(3):148–55.

Cifuentes LA, Vega J, Köpfer K, Lave LB. Effect of the fine fraction of particulate matter versus the coarse mass and other pollutants on daily mortality in Santiago, Chile. J Air Waste Manage Assoc. 2000;50(8):1287–98.

Cook DG, Strachan DP. Summary of effects of parental smoking on the respiratory health of children and implications for research. Thorax. 1999;54:357–66.

Dherani M, Pope D, Mascarenhas M, Smith K, Weber M, Bruce N. Indoor air pollution from unprocessed solid fuel use and pneumonia risk in children aged under five years: a systematic review and meta-analysis. Bull World Health Organ. 2008;86(5):390–8.

Drehmer JE, Ossip DJ, Rigotti NA, Nabi-Burza E, Woo H, Wasserman RC, Winickoff JP. Pediatrician interventions and thirdhand smoke beliefs of parents. Am J Prev Med. 2012;43(5):533–6.

EPA United States Environmental Protection Agency. Integrated Science Assessment for Particular Matter. 2009. Available at: https://cfpub.epa.gov/ncea/risk/recordisplay.cfm?deid=216546.

Franck U, Herbarth O, Röder S, Schlink U, Borte M, Diez U, Lehmann I. Respiratory effects of in-door particles in young children are size dependent. Sci Total Environ. 2011;409(9):1621–31.

Gurkan F, Kiral A. The effect of passive smoking on the development of respiratory syncytial virus bronchiolitis. Eur J Epidemiol. 2000;16:465–8.

Hang B, Sarker AH, Havel C, Saha S, Hazra TK, Schick S, et al. Thirdhand smoke causes DNA damage in human cells. Mutagenesis. 2013;28(4):381–91.

Horak F, Fazekas T, Zacharasiewicz A, Eber E, Kiss H, Lichtenschopf A, Riedler J. The Fetal Tobacco Syndrome – A statement of the Austrian Societies for General- and Family Medicine (ÖGAM), Gynecology and Obstetrics (ÖGGG), Hygiene, Microbiology and Preventive Medicine (ÖGHMP), Pediatrics and Adolescence Medicine (ÖGKJ) as well as Pneumology (ÖGP). Wien Klin Wochenschr. 2012;124(5–6):129–45.

Kakish KS, Mahafza T, Batieha A, Ekteish F, Daoud A. Clinical sinusitis in children attending primary care centers. Pediatr Infect Dis. 2000;19(11):1071–4.

Koutrakis P, Sax SN, Sarnat JA, Coull B, Demokritou P, Oyola P, Garcia J, Gramsch E. Analysis of PM10, PM2.5, and PM2 5-10 concentrations in Santiago, Chile, from 1989 to 2001. J Air Waste Manage Assoc. 2005;55(3):342–51.

Kunzli N, Kaiser R, Medina S, Studnicka M, Chanel O, Filliger P, et al. Public-health impact of outdoor and traffic-related air pollution: a European assessment. Lancet. 2000;356:795–801.

Mallol J, Koch E, Col Y. Prevalencia de enfermedades respiratorias en el primer año de vida en hijos de madres que fumaron durante el embarazo. Rev Chil Enf Respir. 2007;23:23–9.

Martino D, Prescott S. Epigenetics and prenatal influences on asthma and allergic airways disease. Chest. 2011;139(3):640–7.

Matt GE. Households contaminated by environmental tobacco smoke: sources of infant exposures. Tob Control. 2004;13(1):29–37.

Mitchell EA, Beasley R, Keil U, Montefort S, Odhiambo J. The association between tobacco and the risk of asthma, rhinoconjunctivitis and eczema in children and adolescents: analyses from Phase Three of the ISAAC programme. Thorax. 2012;67(11):941–9.

Ostro BD. Conferencia: Análisis de mortalidad y morbilidad en Chile y efectos en el Aparato Respiratorio: Partículas PM10 y PM 2.5 Primera Cumbre Científica: Contaminación del Aire y Efectos en Salud. 2008 Chile.

Ostro BD, Eskeland GS, Sanchez JM, Feyzioglu T. Air pollution and health effects: a study of medical visits among children in Santiago. Chile Environ Health Perspect. 1999;107(1):69–73.

Pino P, Walter T, Oyarzun M, Villegas R, Romieu I. Fine particulate matter and wheezing illnesses in the first year of life. Epidemiology. 2004;15:702–8.

Ruiz P. Informe AMICUS CURIAE sobre la derogación de la norma de MP 10 de concentración anual. Marzo 2014.

Saldías F, Méndez JI, Ramírez D, Díaz O. El riesgo de infecciones respiratorias en el fumador activo y pasivo. Rev Chil Enf Respir. 2007;23:179–87.

Shuk-Mei H. Environmental epigenetics of asthma: an update. J Allergy Clin Immunol. 2010;126(3):453–65.

Thomas JL, Guo H, Carmella SG, Balbo S, Han S, Davis A, et al. Metabolites of a tobacco-specific lung carcinogen in children exposed to secondhand or thirdhand tobacco smoke in their homes. Cancer Epidemiol Biomark Prev. 2011;20(6):1213–21.

Vargas C. Efectos de la fracción gruesa (PM10-2.5) del material particulado sobre la salud humana. Revisión Bibliográfica. Disponible en http://www.sinia.cl/1292/articles-51242_Estudio_cvargas.pdf. VISITADA EL 2 de marzo de 2015.

Nursing Care Education in Chronic Respiratory Diseases

59

Ana Moya Isamitt

Contents

A. Moya Isamitt (✉)
School of Health, Duoc UC, Santiago, Chile

P. Bertrand, I. Sánchez (eds.), *Pediatric Respiratory Diseases*,
https://doi.org/10.1007/978-3-030-26961-6_59

Introduction

Recently, important changes have taken place in life expectancy and quality of life of patients with chronic respiratory diseases, which have created a huge challenge for nursing care to improve attention for our patients, because they are more involved in their healthcare.

A chronic disease is the alteration in the health state that persists in time and requires continuous and permanent care, such as in the case of cardiovascular diseases, diabetes, cancer, respiratory diseases, and AIDS, among several others. Chronic diseases have an important place in the epidemiological profile. They usually cause multisystemic sequels, which generate significant changes in the lifestyle, adding special and specific needs, for both care and self-care, according to the disabilities or limitations that its progression may cause.

A big part of chronic diseases share aspects associated with physical and emotional suffering, which meaningfully affect the person who confronts the disease and the family, with a big impact in life quality, because of the needs and demands of care and support they require.

These diseases have common characteristics:

- They are permanent and irreversible, progressing with residual alterations.
- They are multi-causal and must be confronted from this perspective.
- They require specific training of patients and their family, for securing caregiving, and collaboration of both with the healthcare team.
- They need long periods of caregiving and treatments for their control and counteracting the effects of the disease.
- They carry feelings of loss as a specific and predominant component of any kind of chronic disease.

When a person is diagnosed with, or suffers from a chronic respiratory disease, it affects his/her physical, psychological, family, social, and work aspects, depending on the nature of the disorder and its severity, as well as on individual aspects of the patient. Physical problems, independent of their nature, can be originated from the disorder itself or as consequences of medical treatment. Labor problems directly influence family, which is forced to adapt or completely abandon their work activities, or they have to use prolonged medical licenses. In the family area, the most relevant conflicts are linked to the loss of role of parent and becoming main caregiver (for the most part, mothers). Social problems largely depend on loss of relationships and emotional bonds, the most important being caused by change of status related to job loss, social isolation, free time usage, and quantity and quality of social interactions. The experience is always individual for each nuclear family, where perception and meaning differ from one person to the next, even though they share trigger conditions and their effects, or have the same therapeutic and social resources for their attention.

Development of attention and care strategies demand a continuous effort of the nursing team and others health professionals, through which the approach of physical, biological, psychological, sociocultural, and spiritual dimensions that involve human experience may be approached. A very useful tool that is available for the healthcare team is the education of health contents for patients.

Educational intervention requires the collaboration of teams, so they can act in a coordinated way at the hospital, home, and school, which also applies to the coordination of all available resources and the active participation of parents, since they are the most stable agents in the child's development. Because of that, in these instances, the most important thing is to educate parents and children in consideration to their age.

It is a challenge to advance in pragmatic implementation of nursing theories, but contributes to differentiating it from other health professions involving usage of a distinct professional language. Even then, in this aspect, concepts of person, environment, health, and nursing are used from the perspective of applied theory. Using theories contributes to distancing nursing from the biomedical focus that has predominated for a long time and has influenced care. Healthcare has been identified as the essence of nursing, despite other disciplines, aside from nursing, having approached and described the concept.

The study of healthcare has allowed the understanding of the importance and magnitude of nursing attention for human health, development, and survival. Nevertheless, this is not an exclusive action of nursing, since a large part of activities made around human healthcare are done in a non-professional level, in the scope of everyday life.

Caring refers to those acts of assistance, support, help, and conservation, which allow and make it easy for persons who need to improve their life conditions, to accomplish that, and to anticipate those needs.

Nursing care in chronic patients requires orientation with holistic efforts, and a primary thing—strengthening the care of the person's whole life—to respond to the patient's aspirations and patterns, particularly in relation to a circumstantial dimension of the disease or a limitation provoked by it. The disease by itself does not define the needs of the individual or his/her family, but rather when the disease appears, is resolved, or increases because of the way that the experience is lived. The nurse has a privileged position in the explanation to others about the patient's world, family, and processes that happens within, because they know those universes in a way that none other discipline does.

Among the most used theories nowadays, there is the Dorothea Orem's theory, which conceives the human being as a biological, rational, and thinking organism. Human beings have the ability to reflect about themselves and their surroundings, ability to symbolize what they experience, and to use symbolic creations (ideas, words) for thinking, communicating, and directing efforts for making things that are beneficial for themselves and others. Nursing care helps the individual to accomplish and keep self-care actions for conservation of health and life, recover from the disease, and confront its consequences. The environment is understood in this model as all those physical, chemical, biological, and social factors, whether they are family or community ones, which can influence and interact with the person. Finally, the concept of health is defined as a state in which, for the person, it means different components and changes according to the person's human and biological characteristics (Fig. 59.1). The most important concept is self-care, which is a behavior that exists in particular situations of life, aimed to the persons or their surroundings, for regulating factors that affect their own development and functioning for the benefit of their life, health, and well-being. It is an activity learnt by individuals and directed toward an objective.

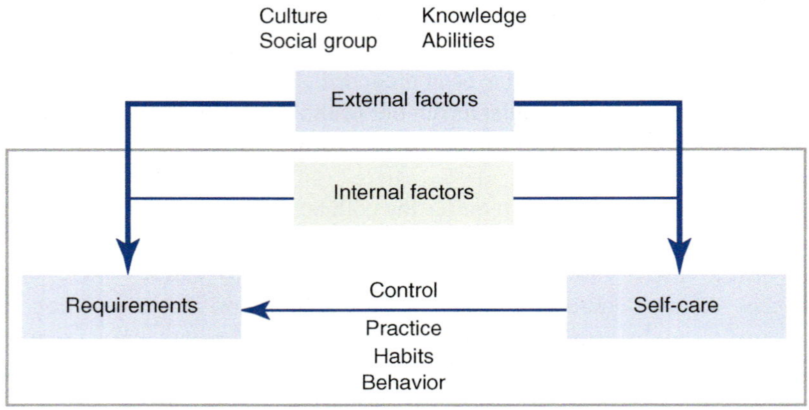

Fig. 59.1 Self-care theory

Nursing Care Management

Management of care involves clinical processes linked to people's healthcare. Management of clinical processes can be seen as the most appropriate for adjusting the criterion of the health team according to the most dominant sanitary criterion in management teams, having links between clinical logic, which has the individual patient as its thrust, and sanitary logic, which considers collective users/patients.

In order to generate an effective management of care, we have to consider available evidence through different updated publications, patient's preferences in relation to what are his/her educational needs, and the environment and available resources.

The new model of global hospital management is based on the integral model of health attention, which is defined as the group of actions that enforce and facilitate efficient, effective, and opportune attention directed not to specific incidents but toward persons considered in their physical and mental completeness, and as social beings belonging to different types of families and communities that are in a permanent process of integration and adaptation to their physical, social, and cultural environment.

Characteristics of a Correct Educational Instance for Self-Care

In the outpatient field, and particularly in a pulmonary function laboratory, the diversity of patients gives a rich educational instance for delivering tools for health self-care. "The self-care agency is the group of powers and abilities within the patient which allows him/her to commit to self-care". This complex ability maintains or enforces the integrity of human structure, its functioning, and promotion of well-being, and it is acquired to satisfy continuous care requirements which regulate different processes.

For all diseases, adherence to treatment is the most important factor, but as it is susceptible of being modified, it compromises the results of treatments.

The diversity of diseases makes educational needs in children with a chronic disease heterogenous, diverse, unstable, shifting, and less predictable than those presented in other children. These special educational needs are of three types:

1. Needs derived from diagnosis and treatment of the disease: adherence to treatments and control of the disease, family, and school environment.
2. Needs derived from emotional and social disorders, for the adapting of parents and children: psychological support to the child and family.
3. Needs related to school curriculum and early attention for favoring an appropriate cognitive, motor, affective, and social development of the child: early attention services, school units of support in hospital institutions, educational domiciliary attention, and school centers of reference.

In early childhood, the objectives of educational attention are:

(a) Adaptation of hospital, family, and school environment to the needs derived from the disease, for eliminating associated risk factors.
(b) Education of parents about how to control the disease and obtaining adherence to treatments. It represents a priority objective in this stage of the development of the child.
(c) Child's control of the disease: management of devices, preparation for diagnostic tests and treatments. This objective is accomplished by incorporating the child to the educational instances.

Since 2009, there has been a program in our institution named "Education for health self-care", where according to the patient's pathology, certain topics are addressed for improving his/her health and to clarify question of his/her parents about basic care or general measures for maintaining good control of the disease.

Objectives of Educational Programs

- Emphasizing the concept of disease;
- Encouraging prevention according to the disease;
- Directing the educational program to target group (depends on age group).

Educational programs have shown that they modify life quality and adherence to treatment.

Characteristics of an Efficient Education

Education must be understood as a continuous and dynamic process, adapted to the patient's needs, for obtaining changes in attitudes and lifestyles of the patient and the family, which will surely produce an improvement in their life quality, allowing self-control and autonomous decision making.

Among the items to consider in an efficient educational instance, there are:

- Education is very important for the child that has a chronic disease.
- Education must involve the patient, his/her family, and school environment.
- Education must start when the diagnosis is made.
- Education is continuous, and it is complemented until accomplishing self-management.
- The main objective of education for self-care is to increase quality of life with no limitations.
- For establishing a good, effective educational plan it is required to previously identify the real educational needs and the core of the disease presented in the child and his/her family.

Learning Areas

When raising educational instances, we must consider three learning areas:

- *Affective*: The main caregiver will recognize the importance of his/her participation in caring activities.
- *Cognitive*: The caregiver can describe the signs of the chronic disease that affects the patient.
- *Psychomotor*: The caregiver is capable of showing through supervised repetition each technique taught in the educational instance.

Evaluation of Educational Instances

They consider learning outcomes, whether the evolution of the disease is beneficial or not, and the way in which the patient, family, tutor, or main caregiver manages his/her everyday life. It is required to determine to what degree each agreed objective has been accomplished, the quality and effectiveness of applied techniques, and the quality of teachers in charge of transmitting the educational plan, and that is why the continuous training of the whole health team is so important. In order to clearly satisfy defined objectives, readjustments in the educational sequence have to be made, considering the learning capacity of the patient, family, or tutor, and their personal peculiarities.

Minimum Contents of an Effective Educational Instance

In a center of reference of respiratory diseases, the health professional is in contact with several diseases, as well as the patients and their families. Asthma, cystic fibrosis, sleep disorders, and food allergies are reviewed in this chapter.

Self-Care in Asthma

It must be highlighted that education is not just informing. Information is necessary, but insufficient. The objective is that the child and his/her family acquire abilities for controlling asthma.

Education must be stepwise, from basic knowledge, to self-control, if possible. In addition, it must be continuous, progressive, and adapted.

Authors themselves say that the use of educational programs generates a decrease in unscheduled medical visits, emergency visits, and hospitalizations, as well as school absenteeism.

Basic Knowledge about Asthma

A simple description, also adapted to the age of anatomical and functional changes that happen in asthma. For that, we count on educational primers, which include some simple data, which are addressed by answering the following questions

- What is asthma?
- What factors influence in the emergence of asthma?
- Rules for avoiding triggering allergens

Treatment Description

Patients and their relatives must know what rescue medications are and how to use them, along with knowing about preventive control medications. Frequent questions presented by parents are about adverse effects of the treatment, tachycardia associated with bronchodilators, and low height gain associated with steroids.

Prescription and Sequence of Utilization

Asthma treatment pursues two objectives: to obtain and maintain control of clinical signs and symptoms, preventing exacerbations, chronic obstruction of air flow, and decreasing mortality.

Pharmacological treatment of asthma is based on controlling inflammation, which is treated by anti-inflammatory drugs (basically, steroids, and in some cases, chromones or leukotriene antagonists), whereas bronchodilator drugs are applied as symptomatic drugs, also named rescue medications.

There is plenty of evidence that shows that patients do not correctly use the inhalation technique and that even the health personnel ignore the technique. It has been described that up to 80% of patients do not know how to use the inhaler, and to avoid this it is important to consider the following elements:

1. Choosing the most appropriate device before prescription, which can be detected by the nursing personnel in the first encounter with the patient for educational instance.
2. As we have seen, verifying the technique in every instance and showing in a physical way the technique and asking to repeat, to know whether both patient and tutor understood the technique.

Techniques for Medication Use

This is put into practice during the time exams are being made, which is the best instance for educating, because the patient stays at least 15–60 minutes with the nurse or nurse technician. In the medical visit, some contents can be reinforced.

Patients must correctly use the inhalation technique, which will be different according to the inhalation system used. An incorrect inhalation technique is equal to not taking the medication. In addition, a high and increasing number of commercial products for inhalation therapy exist:

metered dose inhalers (MDI), holding chambers, dry powder inhaler (DPI), unit doses, multi-doses, auto-trigger systems, among others.

In toddlers, medium doses of MDI and small volume chambers with a mask are favored, whereas in school children (because of capacity), DPI or medium dose of MDI and chambers with a mouth piece are favored. We discourage mouth direct administration of MDI. Assessment of the technique must be a part of every encounter in children with asthma. Families must know how to keep chambers clean, verify the device's correct functioning, know when few doses of the drug are left if it does not have a dose counter, and buccal hygiene rules after its administration.

Educational Factors

For a satisfactory self-control of asthma in children, it is necessary to master what we call self-care abilities:

- Recognizing and avoiding triggering factors
- Ability to monitor symptoms
- Correctly mastering drug inhalation techniques.
- Ability to recognize when asthma is worsening

Knowing how to act pre-emptively before any variation of the process is essential.

Self-care abilities will be applied by families in cases of breastfed babies and infants, and progressively, according to growth, the child will be involved in the control of his/her disease. There has to be room for the child to express feelings about his/her disease and his/her opinion about the treatment, letting him/her choose, as far as possible, his/her inhalation device, as long as the child has a good command of the technique. In many occasions, especially in adolescents, talking to the patient alone is useful, without the presence of the parents. Starting with the information and correct application of the abilities acquired, self-control will be the ability to understand clinical situations and make the right decisions for them.

In order to act in case of deterioration, there has to be a previously made self-treatment plan. On the basis of a control of symptoms or measurement of peak expiratory flow (PEF), there must be a written maintenance treatment: when to use rescue medication, when to increase the dose of anti-inflammatory inhalation medication, when to start a pattern of oral steroids, and when, how, and whom to ask for medical help.

In pediatrics, the strategy for recognizing signs and symptoms of progressive obstruction of the airway and developing a plan depends on factors, such as age, sociocultural level of the family, and also involving the older child or adolescent in the process, the severity of the asthma or whether it is persistent or seasonal.

In breastfed and young children, symptoms registrations are often utilized, as well as in older children who cooperate and in persistent asthma. More rarely, PEF and symptoms registration may be followed using a so-called warning zone or color system (Fig. 59.2).

The importance of peak expiratory flow in self-control of asthma lies in the possibility of home

	No symptoms - No limitation in activities	- PEF between 80 and 100% of normal personal value. - Attend to scheduled consultation.	**Controlled asthma** - Follow usual treatment.
	Daily symptoms - Cough, wheeze, limitation in activities, nighttime awakenings, etc. Rescue medication must be used as per written instructions, variation in undercurrent treatment.	- PEF between 50 and 80% of normal personal value. - Attend to medical control while managing symptomatology.	**Precaution** - Adjust treatment.
	Progressive worsening - Progressive fatigue, cough, wheeze that do not respond to short-acting bronchodilators.	- PEF between 40 and 60% of normal personal value. - Attend emergency department.	**Danger** - Treatment prescribed by a doctor.

Fig. 59.2 Self-control measures (warning system)

use, because the PEF measuring device is small in size and easily transportable, its use is basic, and provides objective and quantifiable values.

Self-Care in Cystic Fibrosis

Cystic fibrosis (CF) is the most frequent autosomal recessive disease in the white race. Commonly, this results in development of chronic obstructive pulmonary disease and secondary malnutrition. Since pulmonary damage flourishes progressively, early diagnosis and focusing on respiratory and nutritional management are crucial for improving the prognosis of these patients.

Medical advances achieved during the last 30 years have increased survival rate, which is now up to 40 years of life. As it is a multisystem and progressive disease, whose treatment includes different daily measures affecting nutrition and the respiratory system, patients and caregivers have a great responsibility in controlling the disease and applying treatment measures, aiming for a better general health condition as well as slowing the progression of the disease. Educational intervention helps patients and families to solve problems, set goals, and plan some changes in their lifestyles in order to better manage the disease.

The role performed by the patient and family members in the active management of their attentions is now considered relevant for increasing the probability of positive health results. Educational programs in cystic fibrosis traditionally provided specific knowledge with the only purpose to fulfill the pharmacological treatment. Currently, educational programs are oriented toward placing patients and their relatives as experts that work collaboratively with sanitary professionals in the treatment of the disease.

The group of professionals dedicated to working with patients with cystic fibrosis has the following objectives:

- Education of the patient and her/his relatives;
- Aforementioned respiratory physiotherapy and muscular training;
- Psychosocial and nutritional control;
- Oxygen therapy teaching and control;
- Non-invasive ventilation teaching and control, in required cases;
- Home assistance.

Throughout the years, parents become specialists in the disease, and the level of response they expect requires a trained health team. Specialist nursing personnel is actively involved in the decision making related to the treatment and monitoring of medical attention in these patients that are with the health team for years.

Nursing personnel must coordinate the attention between patient and family, besides extra-hospital services, both at a practical level and through support and advice. This is accomplished through their function as a teacher, reliable caregiver, advisor, and confidant. Trusting this professional must have a benefit in the good management of acute and chronic symptoms.

Patients have the responsibility of taking the correct doses of the prescribed medications in a timely manner and in the right order. Normally, patients with cystic fibrosis have very complex pharmacological regimes. The clinical pharmaceutical professional can help in educating patients about correct drug reconstitution, inhalation, and the correct order of the drugs.

Education of the patient with cystic fibrosis is considered fundamental, since he/she has to be aware of the disease in all its aspects, because patients that know their problem (progression, treatment to follow, etc.) get much more involved in therapeutic guides, both of medicines and its rehabilitation, and they are more motivated to fight for its healing or relief.

Nurse Specialized in Cystic Fibrosis

He/she has responsibilities with patients, relatives, and personnel involved in medical attention of patients, so he/she has to commit to care for them.

The responsibilities of a nurse in charge of an educational program about cystic fibrosis are:

- Advocating for each patient and having updated information about current treatment practices.

- Maintaining and teaching clinical experience and practice.
- Support and advice.
- Education and investigation.
- Relationship with patients and relatives.

As a chronic disease, with differences in its development, educational stages overlap when working with the patient.

Some of the objectives that must emerge with a patient with cystic fibrosis are:

- Decreasing respiratory symptoms and flare-ups;
- Improving state of mind (increasing motivation);
- Increasing tolerance to efforts (by improving muscular function);
- Decreasing number of hospital admissions;
- Reducing days of hospitalization;
- Prolonging survival.

Hereunder, we deliver some topics as an example to educate family and patient:

Basic Knowledge About the Disease

Cystic fibrosis is an inherited and incurable disease, which mainly affects the digestive tube, lungs, and pancreas. It is one of the most common chronic pulmonary diseases in boys, girls, and young adults. Cystic fibrosis is caused by an abnormal gene that produces a thick and sticky liquid called mucus, which accumulates in airways and pancreas. This causes pulmonary infections that can be complex, as well as digestive problems, and may affect the male reproductive system.

Cystic Fibrosis Signs and Symptoms

Symptoms do not appear simultaneously, but many times they do it gradually. That is why it is important to mention them in each educational instance to make the patient, family, or main caregiver alert for symptoms that can appear in the course of this chronic disease.

Education can be separated by organs, to ease the education process of the parents or tutors, which at the moment of diagnosis can be confusing and generate stress in the patient's environment. A simple way of confronting this is:

- *Upper airway manifestations*: Symptoms and signs of the upper airway according to age.
- *Lower airway manifestations*: Symptoms and signs of lower airway according to age.
- *Respiratory exacerbations*: Most patients have an insidious respiratory worsening, that is characterized by exacerbations of its chronic pulmonary infection. It is taught to parents or tutors to recognize these changes and to have a meticulous registration of pulmonary images, cultures, and lung function tests.
- *Microbiology*: Patients are colonized according to the disease's progression and the accompanying flora varies over the course of the disease, for this purpose, active vigilance during exacerbations is important. In this process, patients and relatives have a leading participation.
- *Pulmonary complications*: They are taught to recognize the presence of atelectasis, bronchiectasis, hemoptysis, and pneumothorax according to the disease's progression.
- *Pancreatic, hepatic, and urogenital complications*: They are taught about signs and appearance of complications according to the disease's advance, in order to detect them in a timely manner.

Fundamental and Permanent Pillars for the Disease

- To obtain an appropriate nutrition status;
- To use medicines against respiratory infections and inflammation;
- To do physical therapy regularly: respiratory physiotherapy, thoracic musculature strengthening exercises to prevent deformities.

Respiratory Physiotherapy

If the patient is aware of the importance of chest physiotherapy there will be much more adherence to it. The same can be said about aerosol therapy (how to execute the sessions correctly, cleaning of the device, etc.) and daily drugs that need to be taken, as well as oxygen guidelines in the case of having home oxygen therapy (how many liters to carry, its risks). If this educational aspect is correctly led, it will have better results in the life quality of the patient.

Inhalation Therapy

- Appropriate inhalation device (or devices) selection;
- Patient or family training in its optimal use;
- Management, cleaning, and necessity of maintenance and substitution of the device;
- Treatments for clearing secretions of the airway.

Physical Activity

Physical activity allows clearing secretions and prevents the appearance of osteoporosis, a pathology with a high incidence in patients with cystic fibrosis. For a design exercise plan, a previous stress test is needed.

The challenge that emerges in this instance is that the team of cystic fibrosis has to work together, and sometimes, a professional acquires prominence at commanding the work oriented toward improving the quality of life.

Self-Care in Sleep Disorders

Sleep is an essential organic function for the appropriate health of the individual, and as every physiological activity, it can present several alterations. The amount of sleep needed for resting varies according to age, going from 12 to 16 hours in breastfed babies and newborns, to an average of 10.5 hours in schoolchildren and preschoolers.

Among entities that affect sleep, we find not only respiratory disorders but also involvement of disorders in all other systems, such as neuroendocrine, metabolic, cardiovascular, etc. These in turn can vary from mild to severe depending on compromise of such alterations, and finally they can involve the family environment and psychological profile of people.

Sleep problems are often a source of stress for parents, as well as learning and behavior difficulties in children, so it is important to confront them and provide appropriate information about all their questions and concerns. At the same time, both parents and children need to learn new behavior patterns, thus obtaining an appropriate management of these disorders that can generate behavior or learning issues in the child.

It must be highlighted that there is important evidence about the effectiveness of educational programs, with a behavior focus that integrates elements of sleep hygiene. These elements have been applied in adult groups, with results that allow having records about factors proven to be effective and which can be extrapolated to the child population.

The optimal thing is to initiate programs for the prevention of sleep disorders, consisting in the creation of advice that is explained and given in writing to the relatives in the health examinations. The ideal thing is to be able to educate in a calm environment, with the child and both parents present.

Those who are part of the pediatric ambulatory team are the professionals who best know the child, adolescent, and his/her family. Thus, they are in a privileged position for establishing preventive or health-promoting measures that controls these issues to a good extent.

Among the topics we must address, there are five relevant points at the moment of an intervention:

1. Wakeup schedules;
2. Bedtime schedules;
3. Activities prior to sleep;
4. Meals prior to bedtime;
5. Comfort in bed.

1. Waking up at the same time, having in mind:
   - Child's age
   - Scheduled day activity
2. Reasonable time for going to bed
   - Awakening hours, number of sleep hours needed for his/her age
3. Relaxing before going to bed
   - Avoiding hectic games 2 hours prior
   - Bath decreases body temperature and helps to relax
4. Light dinner, avoiding:
   - Excess of liquids
   - Stimulating beverages
5. Comfort in bed
   - Temperature between 18 °C and 23 °C
   - Darkness
   - Silence

Depending on age group that we have to assist, we must check the following points, which have to be handed out in writing and spoken with the parents. Ideally, they should be done in health controls of the patient or in nurse interventions in health centers.

Sleep Hygiene during the First Months of Life

Accomplishments in this phase:

Parents have to clearly understand that children learn to fall asleep by themselves, and they must know how to recognize active sleep, so that they do not act incorrectly, and the mother or main caregiver should be able to adapt to the sleep schedule of the child. This is a complex phase for parents, who ask lots of questions, and that is why the reception is important for the delivery of information.

Topics to address in this instance are:

- Children have to learn to fall asleep by themselves.
- Each child set his/her own pace for sleeping. Not every child is the same.
- Do not use strolls or cradlings for getting the baby to sleep; it is possible that, in later phases he/she will have sleep problems.
- Until 2 months of age, after eating, the child starts what we call "active sleep" (the child seems uneasy). This kind of sleep is normal and we don't have to interrupt it, usually lasts for 30–40 minutes where he/she enters in a deeper sleep, which we call "quiet sleep".
- Parents must keep the baby awake while eating; if the baby falls asleep, they must stimulate him/her to wake up before lodging the baby in the cradle.
- After eating, lodge the child in the cradle, while still awake.
- Parents must stay with the baby for soothing him/her but not for sleeping with him/her.
- Starting with the instauration of maternal breastfeeding, a pacifier can be used.
- It is advisable that the main caregiver follows the same sleep schedules as the child.
- Parents must facilitate a proper schedule and place for sleeping.

The objective is that the child recognizes the pleasure of sleeping by him/herself.

Reinforce in this instance:

- Crying is not hunger
- Feeding moments during nighttime must be brief, the child should learn that night is for sleeping.
- When the child wakes up during nighttime to get breastfed, light should not be turned on; breastfeeding must take place silently and with the least possible stimulation.
- The last memory before falling asleep must be the cradle and not breastfeeding. The child has to incorporate the cradle as a familiar, nighttime environment.
- Children take 20–30 minutes to fall asleep. It must be explained to the parents that they must not be present in that time, and must know that, as a minimum, 6% of the time that the child is in the cradle, he/she will stay awake and every child wakes up during nighttime.
- If the child cries when putting him/her in bed, he/she must be comforted, but the parents should try to put him/her in the cradle before falling asleep.

Sleep Hygiene Starting at 6 Months of Age

Accomplishments in this phase:

Parents have to clearly understand that nighttime awakenings are physiological and normal. The child starts to sleep fewer hours and stays awake longer during the day.

Reinforce in this instance:

- DO NOT feed the child if he/she wakes up. In this age, the last feeding is at midnight. Maternal breast or baby bottle are not necessary during nighttime.
- DO NOT turn the lights on.
- DO NOT get him/her out of the cradle.
- Comfort should be through loving words.
- Seek a washable cuddly toy to be his/her partner in the cradle.
- Let the room door be open.

Sleep Hygiene Starting at 12 Months of Age

Accomplishments in this phase:

Parents or main caregivers must avoid long naps in children, 45 minutes of day sleep are enough, in all phases and especially in this one the child has to learn to sleep without help.

Reinforce in this instance

- If the child has tantrums, parents must ignore him/her and leave the room; if the child gets out of bed, he/she must be put into bed quickly, avoiding interaction with the child.
- Same routine must always be followed.
- Parents must transmit the message of teaching him/her to sleep, independently, and that it is not about a punishment or an argument between parents and child.

Sleep Hygiene Starting at 18 Months of Age

Accomplishments in this phase:

Before awaking, parents or main caregivers must provide confidence, so he/she does not gets thrown off balance. Breast, baby bottle, or dummy should not be used as a sleep inducer. Each family has their own level of tolerance and beliefs: there are not good or bad systems, just different ones.

Reinforce in this instance

- Do not self-impose cut-off times for getting the child to sleep. Probably these times will not be met and will generate stress.
- Restrict yourself to follow the rules.
- React calmly when the child wakes up during the night.
- Must transmit the message that the child is able to enjoy sleeping by him/herself. If he/she gets mad, this will only upset him/her even more.
- If there has been a recent change in the life of the child, do not expect that he/she sleeps deeply.
- Allowing the child to sleep outside of bed will not help at all for her/him learning to fall asleep by him/herself. Consider that by sleeping in the same bed as the parents, the child's sleep physiology is altered, in addition to the parent's. Sleep of older children that sleep with their parents is less restful and with a bigger risk of suffocation.
- Breast, baby bottle, or pacifier seem very useful for falling asleep, but the child will end up needing them every time that he/she has to fall asleep and once the child awakes.

Take turns: you will get more rest and the child will not "direct" the night. If not possible, take a break when you notice that you are losing your patience. The important thing is to transmit educational serenity and confidence.

Sleep Hygiene Between 2 and 5 Years of Age

Accomplishments in this phase:

If the child is not able to fall sleep, the parents must keep in mind that this is a good instance for talking some minutes about the events of the day.

Reinforce in this instance:

- During the day, is advisable that children take a nap, as a complement to night sleep, 45 minutes as maximum.

- Parents or main caregiver must not self-impose a cut-off time for sleeping. It will be very hard to meet and it will increase distress and unease.
- The message we want to transmit to the patient is: "you are capable of enjoying sleeping by yourself".
- Do not allow use of electronic games for falling asleep.
- Keep the television out of the room.

Sleep Hygiene from 11 Years of Age

Accomplishments in this phase:

In this phase the sleep pattern is well established, but it is also a period in which it is very probable that sleep disorders may appear because of the type of activities that the patient carries out.

Reinforce in this instance:

- We must inform the parents or caregivers about the changes in adolescence, especially about the physiological delay of sleep start, more need to sleep, and sleep alterations caused by the use of cellphones, internet, etc., before going to bed. It is ideal to turn off these devices.
- Recognize the signs of sleep deprivation: irritability, hard to wake up, recovery during the weekend.
- A family dialogue must be established about sleeping and its importance. Create awareness about the importance of sleeping.
- Encourage a good environment toward the end of the afternoon.
- Importance of the example on behalf of the parent, remember than in this period the parents are role models.

Sleep Hygiene in Adolescence

Accomplishments in this phase:

In this phase, sleep disorders arise again. The child must have regular schedules, even on weekends. Exposure to intense light in the morning will help to regulate the sleep cycle. Parents must encourage sports activities and avoid internet, mobile phones, and videogames before sleeping.

Reinforce in this instance

- Must have regular schedules
- Keep the television out of the room
- Do not take stimulants (caffeine, cola drinks), especially after the midday meal
- Regularity in meal schedules
- Must not fall asleep with TV on (reduces sleep's depth)
- Practice physical exercise regularly
- Do not study during the night

Weekday schedules must be the same as the weekend's, since they start to go out during the night and sleep disorders arise again.

Prevention is effective, reduces medical spending, and improves the quality of life of the child and his/her surroundings. This has allowed decreasing the prevalence of sleep issues in our assisted population.

The final message is to pay attention to sleep issues of these patients with chronic diseases, since a correct diagnosis and appropriate treatment of these problems can have a beneficial effect on psychological, academic, and physiological aspects in the patient. Even more, it can have a favorable impact in other family members and caregivers of the child, thus obtaining a global improvement in the life quality of the patient.

Self-Care in Allergies

Food allergies are a group of diseases where symptoms are produced by an immune response of the organism when confronting an allergen present in some foods. Clinical manifestations mostly affect the gastrointestinal tract, respiratory tract, and skin; gastrointestinal manifestations predominating in breastfed babies and young children.

Of the population, 20% has symptoms of an adverse food reaction during their lifetime. In the last three decades, concern about food allergies in occidental developed societies has increased.

Food allergies are a kind of adverse reaction to food products generated by immune mechanisms.

The main causes of food allergies are cow milk, peanut, nuts, fish, and seafood. They have different levels of severity: from simple itching, inflammation, or urticaria (which are the most frequent), to other more severe reactions with digestive, respiratory, and circulatory symptoms.

Allergy to a food product is frequent in early ages, varies from mild reaction to anaphylaxis, and typically its trigger is accidental or unaware exposure (inhalation, ingestion, contact, etc.) to the allergen.

Eliminating food product or products is the basis of treatment for immediate reactions, especially in cases of anaphylaxis. Most allergies will improve after some years, except the allergy to peanut, nuts, fish, and seafood. The objective of the nurse is to provide continuous education in every chance where there is interaction with the patient.

Basic Knowledge About Physiology of Food Allergies

What Is a Food Allergy?

Food allergies are a high sensitivity reaction (hyper-sensitivity) to external substances called allergens, which are present in food. People that present these kinds of reactions produce a large amount of specific antibodies (proteins), which are called immunoglobulins E (IgE).

What Factors Influence the Onset of Symptoms?

Genetic factors or early contact with the allergens facilitate the appearance of symptoms. For detecting food products, it is essential to record in a log what foods the patient has consumed. In the case of foods with several ingredients, a list of all of them must be made, emphasizing whether there is one of the eight most common allergy-inducing food products, especially milk, egg, or any food that is usual in the environment. It is also required to ask about the kind of cooking of the food, and to discard contact with other likely sources of reaction, such as underlying infectious processes and medications use.

Time period to consider: highly suspicious foods are those consumed within the first 2 hours before the reaction, and those consumed more than 24 hours earlier than the reaction are low suspicious foods. During the first 2 hours, usually the allergy mechanism is IgE mediated, and in later reactions a cellular response may intervene. Late reactions tend to appear with eczema, gastrointestinal symptoms, and probably eosinophilic mediation. It is common to see a patient that has tolerated a suspicious food product during a short period of time and afterward presents a reaction after the contact. This first phase is the phase of sensitization, where the specific immune response is established. For the cases of milk and egg, reactions can occur after the first direct contact, which is occasioned by the child's contact to proteins of these foods through breast milk or by consumption of products that contain milk or egg as ingredients.

Knowing if the patient has tolerated the suspicious food product in new exposures can help to discard an allergy or, in the case of several suspicious ingredients, to refine the diagnosis. It is possible that the patient has generated tolerance to the food. The type of food tolerated must be recorded, since if it is a very cooked product, it cannot be stated that the patient will not react to less cooked versions. Patient's symptoms and reaction time after exposure help to define whether the patient is allergic or not.

Rules to Avoid Triggering Allergens

Initial management consists in a proper education directed toward the complete restriction of the suspicious food product. In case of children under 2 years old, it may be necessary to add a nutritionist's evaluation to avoid disorders in the child's development.

Among the indications, there is one consisting in recording the day when the reaction appeared, what the patient was doing and what she/he ate, in order to detect crossed allergies or foods that match the days that had reactions, and attaching the labels of those commercial made products consumed.

If the food has already been identified, it is important to teach parents to organize where to keep food (out of children's reach).

School plays a fundamental role. Below are some of the tools the school can provide:

Father, mother or legal caregiver is responsible for:

- Informing the educational center, as soon as possible, about diagnosis through a medical report, so they can quickly initiate the required actions for generating a safe environment for the patient.
- Contributing in the elaboration of a customized plan of precautions for the allergic students in the educational center.
- Facilitating a written authorization to the educational center to administrate the medication and educate the child in its administration.
- Providing the educational center with specific material and medication.
- Cooperating with the school in anything needed to control the allergy of son or daughter.
- Identification of students with food allergies.
- Carrying food products from home, since food from school is not advisable, to avoid cross-contamination.

The patient

Students with food allergies, according to their abilities, should:

- Know what the allergy is, why it is caused, what are the symptoms of emergencies that could occur. The rest of the students should also know these matters, and discuss them with teachers with the help and orientation from specialized personnel, who will facilitate the required information (Table 59.1).
- Conduct all tasks appropriate for his/her age and development phase, actively collaborating, in any situation, with teachers, equals, and other members of the educational community, as well as the health professionals.
- Avoid using the allergy as an excuse for distinction or advantage.

Table 59.1 Plan for facing an allergic reaction at school

Step 1: Assessing and treating				
	Symptoms	Major risk	Self-injectable adrenaline	Doctor
1.	Mouth itching, mild rash surrounding mouth or lips, swollen mouth	No	Yes	Yes
2.	Urticaria, welts, rash, itching, or swelling of limbs or other zone of the body	No	Yes	Yes
3.	Nausea, abdominal pain, diarrhea, vomits	No	Yes	Yes
4.	Eye itching, red eyes, tearing, nose itching, repetitive sneezes, abundant white mucus	Yes	Yes	Yes
5.	Closed throat, hoarseness, repetitive cough, swollen tongue/eyelid/lips/ears	Yes	Yes	Emergency
6.	Shortness of breath, repetitive cough, dry cough, lips exhaustion, or bluish skin	Yes	Yes	Emergency
7.	Weak pulse, low blood pressure, fading, paleness, bluish lips or skin	Yes	Yes	Emergency
• In quick progressive reactions, although symptoms are not severe (number 1–4), it is advised to prematurely administrate self-injectable adrenaline to avoid progression to a severe reaction (5–7 symptoms) • In children with severe symptoms (7), it is desirable to keep them lying down with their legs elevated • After administrating adrenaline, it is important to take the patient to the emergency room (ER)				
Step 2: Alerting				
Emergency call				
Never leave the child alone				
Call to ER and state that it is an evolving allergic reaction				
Even if parents/caregivers cannot be contacted, the child must be taken to emergency services				

- Learn and use all available instruments for autonomously controlling the allergy, securing supervision and help from an adult.
- Carry an identification that facilitates recognition of the food-allergic condition.

Description of Different Treatments

The main treatment is avoiding the food product, besides explaining the self-injectable adrenaline. This role must be conducted by specialists and reinforced by the health team in every consultation.

The most important thing is that the patient, when he/she is able to be responsible of the medication, always carries it with him/her, particularly when going to his/her school activities and food consumption cannot be supervised.

Educational Factors

There are special events, such as birthdays or gatherings with friends, where it is important to inform about food allergies. Eating outside of home is also an issue for food-allergic patients, and it is important to ensure that cross-contamination does not take place. On occasions, crises are related to physical exercise. In principle, the person tolerates the food product, but when doing physical exercise after consuming it, an urticaria–angioedema picture appears (face, eyelids, lips, ears swelling) or anaphylaxis (severe allergic reaction).

In relation to the food product, it is important to consider whether its presentation is raw or cooked, because some substances that provoke allergy are thermolabile (they are inactivated with heat) and are tolerated if previously cooked, for example, some fruits and vegetables. Also, it is important whether it is the complete food or just a part of it: skin or pulp, egg-white or yolk, etc. The peels of fruits usually produce more allergies, and some people tolerate pulp and only react when eating the complete fruit or are in contact with the skin.

To avoid allergies:

- Discard meals out of home
- Avoid prepared food
- Precaution in the way of cooking (breading, pre-breaded, sauces)
- Carefully reading food composition before eating it (not all labels contain all components)

Cross-reactions:

They are frequently associated with food groups, for example:

- Cow milk: There is a cross-reaction between proteins of other mammals' milk (goat, sheep). In 20% it also occurs with meat.
- Egg: There is a cross-reaction between eggs from different birds, and between egg-white and yolk.
- Fishes; It is possible that some species can be tolerated, but it must be confirmed.
- Some children react to seafood and crustaceans but have not shown cross-reactions.
- Nuts: The person that is allergic to a type of nut usually presents reactions to other nuts.
- Latex-fruits: Half of people allergic to latex show an allergy associated with certain food products, being the most usual to bananas, kiwis, chestnuts (when they are consumed raw).

Rules of Management of the Disease

- It is a widespread allergic reaction provoked especially by food, insect bites, or medications in people allergic to them. It appears suddenly and puts the person's life in serious danger. In general, it starts with tingling in the mouth, heat, nasal congestion, tearing, and subsequently, bronchospasms, hoarseness, and then respiratory distress, shock, and death.
- Emergency treatment consists in administration in the exterior part of the thigh of adrenaline through a preloaded syringe, according to the patient's weight.
- Education delivered to the patient must be reinforced in every interaction about the

importance of the management of food allergies. School or places where the patient lives must be safe places.
- The role of the nurse team in the communication with the patient, as well as empower the patient.

Food allergies are still an issue that complicate school and home environments, which is why organized teaching, where direct communication with the health professional can take place, would decrease the patient's risk and calm his/her environment.

Conclusions

The evaluation of the nurse in relation to a person with a chronic disease, using theoretical orientation, allows the construction of a profile that clarifies problems related to the patient's health and life where she/he can intervene and where she/he cannot. Besides, it encourages interrelations of the professional team in order to contribute in the consolidation of the professional identity, around the chronic disease's nature, goal, and objective.

Education, a tool incorporated in our professional instruction, helps to decrease sequels of pathologies, to improve quality of life, and to calm the anguish of parents/caregivers, which are our main focus of attention.

Education also involves applying systematic registrations and working experiences, as a possibility for finding practice and academic colleagues from different places, conducting encounters or exchanges of experiences through different communication and socialization media; creating and maintaining networks of information, work, and support that facilitate a better attention for the patient.

Sources

Ayala R, Torres MC, Calco MJ. Gestión del cuidado en enfermería. Santiago: Ed. Mediterráneo; 2009.

Guzmán MA. Alergia, guía clínica. 2ª ed. Santiago: Ed Mediterráneo; 2012.

Herrera AM, León A, Ubilla C, Pérez MA, Lozano J. Utilidad de la educación en asma bronquial infantil: experiencia piloto. Rev Chil Enf Respir. 2014;30:197–202.

Manrique JJ. Higiene del sueño. Acta de Otorrinolaringología & Cirugía de Cabeza y Cuello. 2011;39(3-Suplemento):49–51.

Saieh C, Pinto V. Manual de pediatría ambulatoria. Santiago: Ed. Mediterráneo; 2013.

Sánchez I, Prado F, editors. Enfoque clínico de las enfermedades respiratorias del niño. Santiago: Ediciones Universidad Católica de Chile; 2007.

Valenzuela P, Moore R, editors. Pediatría ambulatoria. Un enfoque integral. 3ª ed. Santiago: Ediciones Universidad Católica de Chile; 2011.

Evidence-Based Medicine for Respiratory Diseases

60

Carlos Ubilla Pérez,
María Angélica Palomino Montenegro,
and José Antonio Castro-Rodríguez

Contents

Introduction

The concept of evidence-based medicine (EBM) has been in medical literature since the1990s, and it basically refers to the adequate integration of research data to clinical decision-making. There is a controversy surrounding the real relevance of evidence-based medicine in clinical practice, and many of these criticisms come from incorrectly highlighting the relevance of clinical skills, patient preference, and health care expenses. Fortunately, we can say that nowadays EBM has been incorporated particularly in internal medicine and progressively in pediatrics and pediatric pulmonology.

Training in EBM techniques is a powerful tool that allows a more comprehensive approach to the increasing medical information, which not infrequently is contradictory or out of date. Not every physician will have the same EBM skills, and EBM will change throughout the lifetime of the physician. However, for a specialist who prefers to remain updated, it is important to learn how to critically assess primary information sources or to accept protocols and guides based on evidence as summarized by the experts.

How to Practice Evidence-Based Medicine

When facing a clinical situation and information is necessary, the steps in Table 60.1 are required.

C. Ubilla Pérez · M. A. Palomino Montenegro
Faculty of Medicine, Universidad de Chile, Santiago, Chile
e-mail: cubilla@med.uchile.cl; mpalomino@med.uchile.cl

J. A. Castro-Rodríguez (✉)
Department of Pediatrics, School of Medicine, Pontificia Universidad Católica de Chile, Santiago, Chile

P. Bertrand, I. Sánchez (eds.), *Pediatric Respiratory Diseases*,
https://doi.org/10.1007/978-3-030-26961-6_60

Table 60.1 Steps for evidence-based medicine practice

Turn the problem into a valid question.
Efficiently locate the best fitting evidence in: Clinical history/physical exam, laboratory diagnoses, publications ("research evidence"), and other sources.
Critically evaluate the evidence regarding its validity (proximity to truth), measure of results, and clinical applicability.
Apply the results of the critical evaluation to regular clinical practice.
Evaluate our performance.

Turn the Problem into an Answerable Question

Often, clinical practice presents questions, many of which are easy to solve. Preparation questions are part of the general knowledge of a certain condition, with available answers in books or journal articles. In the case of action questions for a specific clinical situation during therapy, diagnosis, or prognosis, the clinical problem at hand must be thought of as a question that can find precise answers in the medical literature. Clinical questions are structured in a number of components, summarized by the acronym of PICOT. The aim of this format is to define the problem, identify keywords to assist in the efficient search for information, and define an adequate test design.

Components of a Clinical Action Question

P: Patient, population or problem of interest It entails a brief, but precise description of a patient group by specific characteristics, such as age, sex, severity, etc., matching our group as inclusion criteria or clinically relevant characteristics that may influence the results.

I: Intervention or action This part is essential, with an etiological, prognosis-related, or exposure-related factor, the exactness of a diagnosis test, preventive measures, therapeutic efficiency, or damage. In this step, the formulation of the question must be quite specific.

C: Comparison This element is what we will compare our intervention to, which may be a therapeutic alternative to standard treatment or placebo, allowing no risk of exposure, or diagnosis test considered as the standard of reference.

O: Outcome endpoint This point corresponds to what is observed, measured or expected as an important clinical result of the intervention.

T: Type of study This point identifies the best type of design to answer the question.

For example: In the case of infants suffering from viral bronchiolitis (problem), does hypertonic saline solution treatment (intervention), when compared to physiological saline solution (comparison), shorten hospital stay (outcome)? [Therapy.]

In the case of infants without a family history of asthma or atopy (problem), is respiratory syncytial virus-induced bronchiolitis (intervention) the cause of asthma (outcome)? [Prognosis.] Comparison is not always necessary.

In brief, a structured question constitutes a fundamental step in clearly defining the problem, streamlining the necessary evidence and study design, which enables us to decide if it can be applied to our patients.

Search for Information

From a good clinical question we can extract the necessary information to design a research strategy. Sensitivity and specificity search will be based on the aim and the amount of time we have. By sensitivity search we mean an exploration that covers a wide range of research articles; however, specificity search will only include the more relevant articles, at risk of excluding other important articles. We favor specificity search and faster queries for our action questions.

Relevant databases are available on the internet. Primary sources such as Medline allow comprehensive searches. Secondary sources like Cochrane Library publish systematic literature reviews. High quality clinical guides with the adequate methodology—of which are many for this specialization—are also considered a good source. Meta-searchers, such as Tripdatabase and Epistemonikos, allow fast and specific access to high quality evidence. The advantage of using them is their fast and simultaneous search across the most relevant sites, with a rapid response time for the most pertinent information about the search. The steps to take in our search will be: Choice of database, logically combined keywords, setting boundaries for the search. We do not intend to elaborate further on this topic, but it is doubtlessly necessary to have training in search strategies or having the help of a specialist.

Critical Analysis of the Evidence

Once the research articles have been picked, a critical analysis is due in order to define internal validity or risk of bias, magnitude and precision of the results and, lastly, external validity or applicability to our clinical practice.

How to Analyze a Therapy Article

The optimal design to answer a question regarding the effectiveness of a certain therapy, screening test, or preventive measure is a randomized controlled therapeutic trial (RCT), or even better, a systematic review of trials. The publication of a clinical trial requires a detailed, exact, and clear description of its design, execution, analysis, and results. In 1996, the Consolidated Standard of Reporting Trials (CONSORT) guidelines were published considering 25 indispensable items to be included on every RCT report. This is a type of experimental design were patients are randomized in two groups following a specific time frame. One of the groups is subject to an intervention, whereas the other group undergoes regular therapy or placebo, obtaining by the end of the trial a result or outcome. Its critical analysis requires answering some questions (Table 60.2).

Table 60.2 Therapy article analysis

1. *Are the results valid?*
   (a) Did the experimental and control groups start the study under similar prognostic factors?
   (b) Were patients randomized?
   (c) Was the randomization blind?
   (d) Were base prognostic factors the same?
   (e) Was prognostic balance maintained throughout the study?
   (f) Was group assignment kept blind to patients, health personnel, data collectors, and analysts?
   (g) Were prognostic factors kept at the end of the study?
   (h) Was follow-up completed?
   (i) Was the study stopped early in case it showed benefits?
   (j) Were patients analyzed in the randomized group?
2. *What were the results?*
   (a) How large was the treatment effect?
   (b) How precise was the estimate of the treatment effect?
3. *How can I apply these results to patient care?*
   (a) Were the study patients similar to my patients?
   (b) Were all the relevant outcomes considered?
   (c) Is there a higher probability of benefits than harm and costs?

Are the results valid or with a low risk bias?
During a controlled randomized therapeutic trial, both the experimental and placebo groups must be equal regarding their relevant prognostic factors except at the point of intervention, which must be maintained throughout the trial, including during treatment applied independently from the intervention. This can be achieved by randomly assigning patients to each group. The researcher must distribute every factor or characteristic of the patient, such as sex, age, comorbidities, etc., evenly in both groups. In order to avoid the risk of bias, researchers must randomly assign the participants using a hidden list. This will allow the base prognostic factors to be similar. Patients, health personnel, and data analysts must be blind to the group assignment, something that can be achieved by using placebos. Sometimes a blind study may not be possible, as for instance in surgical treatments. In this case, it must be the clinical output reviewers who are be blind. Follow-up must be comprehensive and with enough time to evaluate the results and avoid the bias that comes from patients leaving a study, either because of a personal decision, death, or adverse effects. Patients must be analyzed on an intention-to-treat basis, that is, according to the group they were randomly assigned to. This is the most recommended form of analysis as it is the closest to clinical practice.

On the other hand, analyses on the basis of protocol are at a higher risk of bias. In addition, something to consider is whether the outcome is relevant, as for instance, asthma exacerbations defined as oral steroid use or emergency consultation vs. average lung function.

- *What were the results?*
  We must consider if the results were relevant and precise. The estimator to measure controlled randomized therapeutic trial results is relative risk (RR), which is obtained by dividing the rate of events (R_1) of the treated group by the rate of events in the control group (R_2). For instance, administering a new asthma treatment to 40 patients, compared to 40 patients who received a placebo, showed asthma exacerbations in 10 patients (R_1 10/40 = 0.25 or 25%) from the treated group compared to 33 from the control group (R_2 of 33/40 = 0.825 or 82.5%). Relative risk, that is, R_1/R_2, is 0.25/0.825 = 0.3. This demonstrates the protective capacity of the new therapy as it showed how it reduced the risk of asthma exacerbations by 70%. Each of these values must be followed by a 95% confidence interval (CI 95%), setting boundaries to the range of the real value of the result 95% of the times. The smaller the CI, the more precise the results will be. Relative risk reduction (RRR) is the difference between the rate of events in the control group and the experimental group, divided by the rate of events in the control group, describing relative results. In our example, RRR = (0.82 – 0.25)/0.82 = 0.57/0.82 = 0.695, rounded up to 0.7 or 70% for practical purposes. A simpler way to calculate it is 1-RR. (RRR = 1 – 0.3 = 0.7 or 70%.) Absolute terms include absolute risk reduction (ARR) and number needed to treat (NNT). Absolute risk reduction (ARR), or risk differences, is the absolute difference between the event rate in the control group (0.82) and the event rate in the experimental group (0.25). The ARR in our example will be 0.82 – 0.25 = 0.57. If we treat 100 patients, 57 would stop having asthma exacerbations because of the treatment when compared to the placebo. The NNT is inversely calculated to ARR and it describes how many patients will need treatment in order to avoid an event. The lower the NNT, the more efficient the drug will be. The relevance of the NNT value will depend on the event being studied. In our example, NNT will be 1/ARR = 1/0.57 = 1.75. Since patients cannot be treated in fractions, we can round that number up and say that two patients will need treatment to avoid an asthma exacerbation.
- *How do I apply these results to my patients?*
  If the study is at a low risk of bias and its results are relevant and precise, we must define whether the intervention can be applied to our own patients. That is why we must consider if our patients are similar to those in the study and if they are at a similar risk of death as the patients of the controlled randomized therapeutic trial by evaluating potential differences of the following type: socio-demographic, other risks, age, sex, etc. Something else to verify is whether all the outcomes were taken into consideration. How will the intervention act in real life? Is it feasible to incorporate it in my environment? What are the expectations or opinions of the patients? An evaluation of the benefits vs. risks or costs must be done in order to reach a final decision.

How to Analyze a Study on Diagnostic Tests

In clinical practice we postulate diagnostic hypotheses, which are relevant when we decide what treatment to apply, establish a protocol and, generally speaking, give quality attention. In cases when the disease is frequent, the physician usually has some level of experience, and the disease appears with its typical presentation, diagnosis tends to be fast and safe. Here the physician makes use of a powerful tool: Pattern recognition, a key element when training physicians. In less frequent diseases or those with atypical presentation, an analytic strategy becomes necessary. In this case more information is called for, with diagnostic tests needed to improve accuracy. There is a growing development of new diagnostic tests, but achieving a high prognostic accuracy

Table 60.3 Analysis of articles on diagnostic tests

1. *Are the results valid?*
(a) Was there diagnostic uncertainty?
(b) Was there a blind comparison with an independent reference standard?
(c) Did the test result affect the decision to perform the reference standard?
2. *What were the results?*
3. What was the likelihood ratio (LR)?
4. *How can I apply these results when treating my patients?*
(a) Can the test be reproduced?
(b) Do the results apply to my patients?
(c) Will the results change how I manage my patients?
(d) Will my patients improve because of the exam?

can be expensive, invasive or simply impossible. To better understand the clinical role before a specific prognostic probability, it is important to understand the concept of decision thresholds.

The therapeutic threshold is given when our diagnostic probability is enough to decide on a treatment without further exams. The diagnostic threshold is the diagnostic probability on which we discard, on a reasonable basis, a disease without further exams. These thresholds are not invariable for different pathologies and will depend on the properties of the diagnostic test, cost, safety, prognosis, effectiveness, and safety of treatment. A critical analysis of an article on diagnostic tests requires us to follow certain steps for a critical reading (Table 60.3).

- *Are the results valid?*

  It is important for the studied group to have diagnostic uncertainty. This means that subjects with the studied condition should have similar symptoms to those without the condition, and there should be an adequate range of clinical manifestation. A blind comparison to an acceptable and independent reference standard is required. This is of the utmost importance for the validity of the study, understanding a reference standard as the best diagnostic method as accepted by the medical community. It is sometimes necessary to combine exams and patient progression in order to define the reference standard. Something else to keep in mind is not to allow the test result to affect the decision of performing a reference standard.
- *What are the results?*

  Once the results are valid, we have to see what the results were and how important they are. A 2 × 2 table should be identified or made. In this way we can get the typical values, such as sensitivity and specificity, fixed values that are intrinsic to the diagnostic test and immutable to prevalence. Predictive values, defined as the probability that in the case of a positive test result the patient will present the disease (positive), or the probability that, in the case of a negative result the patient will not present the disease (negative), are modified with prevalence values, as they provide useful data when the population in the study is similar to our patients. If the pre-test probability of presenting a certain condition is very different to that in the study, these values will not be directly applicable to our situation.

The most useful aspect of a diagnostic test is measured by its capacity to modify a pre-test probability into a new post-test probability. The possibility to cause such a change is evaluated through likelihood ratios (LR). A positive LR refers to how more likely the probability of a positive result will be in patients when compared with healthy individuals. A negative LR refers to how more likely the probability will be of a negative result in healthy individuals when compared with patients. A positive LR of 10 or higher and a negative LR of less than 0.1 are of clinical relevance. However, this is a relative number, as the real benefit of LR comes when either the diagnostic or therapeutic threshold is crossed, moving our position past uncertainty. For a better implementation of LR, we can use Fagan's nomogram (Fig. 60.1). Thus, calculating pre-test probability and knowing the LR values and results of our test, we can infer the post-test probability. For instance, a study to evaluate the usefulness of night oximetry as compared with polysomnography for diagnosing obstructive sleep apnea in children gave a positive LR of 19.4 and a negative LR of 0.58. In this study, the pre-test probability is set at

Fig. 60.1 Fagan nomogram
Draw a line connecting the pre-test probability and the likelihood ratio for the study and extend this line to the post-test probability column to determine the results

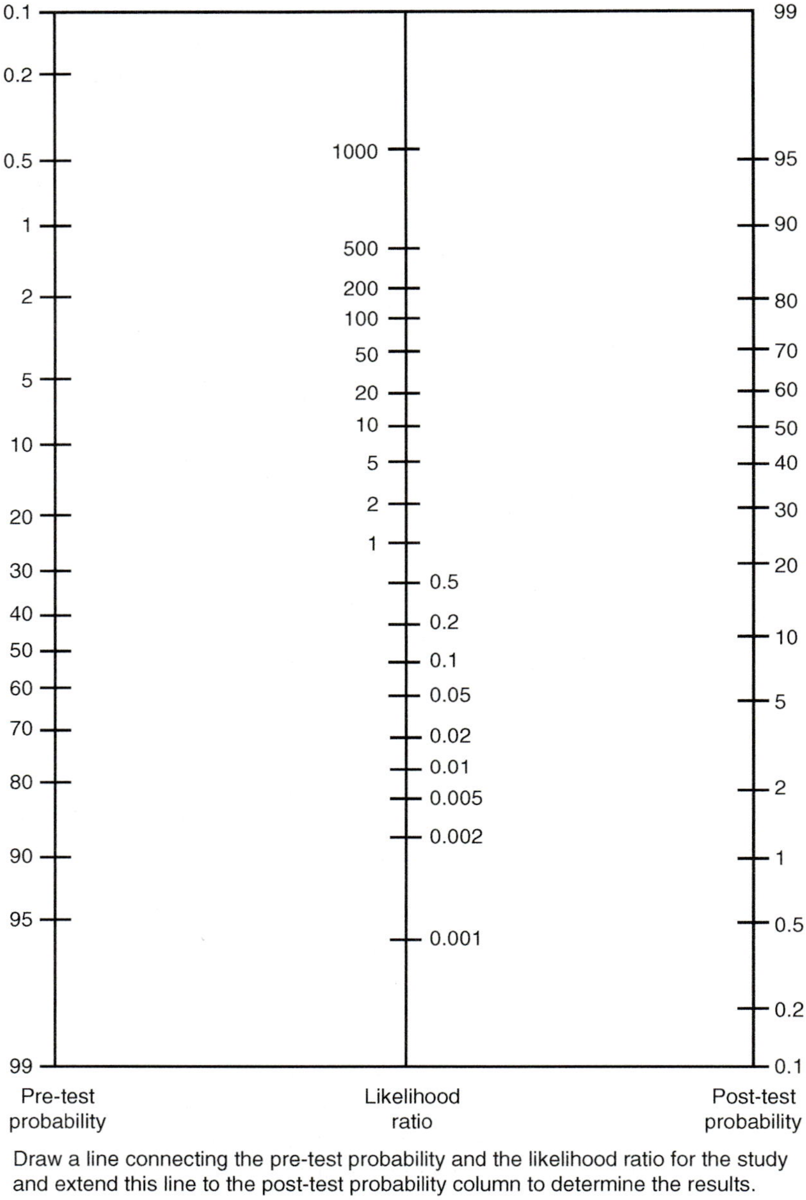

60%. If the test result is positive, it becomes a post-test probability of 97%. If the test result is negative, the probability becomes 47%. It is important to note that the usefulness of these LRs will depend on the validity and accuracy of the results. It is interesting to notice that LRs do not change with disease prevalence, or in other words, it is applicable to different pre-test diagnostic probabilities.

- *How can I apply these results to my patients?* Once the results are valid and relevant, we must evaluate if the diagnostic test is reproducible and applicable to my patients. We must take into account if the studied subjects share similar characteristics with our patients. Finally, we must evaluate if the diagnostic test results will modify our management strategy and if patients will benefit from the exam.

How to Analyze Systematic Reviews and Meta-analyses

Unstructured reviews are useful to get a general view of a clinical condition, but they do not provide us with a certain and impartial answer to a specific clinical question. Systematic reviews (SR), on the other hand, can give us an answer to a specific clinical question in a structured and reproducible fashion. This will usually come together with a meta-analysis, a statistical aggregate of the results of different studies, giving us a unique estimate of the effect.

Individual clinical studies may not be representative of general evidence, or they may be at a risk of bias. On the other hand, collecting and evaluating multiple studies requires time and skills that physicians usually lack. Systematic reviews usually occur with a wider range of patients than an individual study, potentially increasing confidence that the results can be applied to our patients. A meta-analysis can also present the opportunity to explore the reasons as to why there might be inconsistencies between different studies. One of the constraints of systematic reviews and meta-analysis lies in the fact that they only produce trustable estimates when the studies included are trustable themselves.

Systematic reviews have two parts: credibility and confidence in their estimates. Credibility is based on having both design and execution free of wrong results, failure when correctly synthesizing results, or an inadequate literature search. Even if credibility is adequate, results may have low confidence. The most common reasons for this are high bias risk in the studies, inconsistent results or a small sample size in the body of evidence, all of which leads to inaccurate estimates.

Was the methodology of the systematic review credible?

Systematic reviews of treatment questions must be very clear and answer questions as particularly determined by patients, interventions, comparisons, and outcomes.

Was the review exhaustive regarding relevant studies?

Systematic reviews are at risk of bias if they fail to obtain a complete or representative sample of eligible studies. This risk is minimized when searching through at least three databases (Medline, Embase, and Cochrane Central). It is necessary to use multiple synonyms and keywords for each concept. Additional references can be identified by using clinical study registries, reference lists from the studies themselves, conference proceedings, by contacting experts in the area or through the databases kept by the pharmaceutical industry and agencies such as the FDA.

Was the selection criteria and evaluation of the studies reproducible?

The authors of systematic reviews must decide which studies to include, their risk of bias, and what data from the study abstracts is worth covering. And even if there is a standard protocol, some decisions will remain being subjective and thus prone to error. Having two or more reviewers participating in the study will reduce this risk.

Did the reviewers deliver the results ready for clinical application?

A meta-analysis can estimate the proportion of the effect (magnitude of difference between groups). This effect will depend on the nature of the outcome or measured effect (relative risk, odds ratio, risk difference, hazard ratios, standardized mean difference), which will allow the comparison between different studies notwithstanding the different units of measure or scales they may have used.

The results of the meta-analysis are usually displayed as a forest plot. The results of each study are represented by squares with sizes proportional to the weight of the study and horizontal lines representing their confidence interval. More precise studies (shorter confidence interval) will have more weight and higher influence over the combined final result. The total added effect of all the studies, or their pooled estimate, is represented by a diamond, where its width corresponds to its confidence interval. For binary outcomes, accuracy will depend on the number of events and sample size. For continuous outcomes, weight will also depend on the accuracy of the study, sample size, and standard deviation or variability.

Usually, the most frequent meta-analyses are the ones using the information of each study, or "study-level-information". Nevertheless, when the information of each individualized patient included in the study is considered, then the meta-analysis done is called "patient-level-information", which makes it easier to do a more detailed study of, for instance, subgroups or those who are intended to undergo treatment.

Continuous outcomes can also be presented in a more useful manner when relating or comparing them with pre-established clinical scales.

Did the reviewers focus on the confidence on the estimate of the effect?
A well performed systematic review must inform the risk of bias of each study included in it, something that could explain their heterogeneity.

What is the confidence level of the estimate of the effect?
The level of confidence of studies is generally based on the design of the study. Randomized studies are assigned a high level of confidence, but it can decrease in the case of high risk of bias, inconsistencies, inaccuracy, or direct applicability of publication bias. In observational studies, when the impact of the effect is large, its assigned confidence may increase.

How serious is the risk of bias in the body of evidence?
A well done systematic review should inform us of the risk of bias of each study. Differences in risk of bias may explain important differences between results. Less rigorous studies may sometimes overestimate therapeutic effects or preventive interventions. There is no single correct way to face this risk of bias. The Cochrane Risk of Bias Tool is frequently used to evaluate randomized studies.

Are results consistent across studies?
Readers of systematic reviews must judge whether the results differ from one study to the next (variability or heterogeneity). This can be done visually through a forest plot. The bigger the difference between estimated points, or in the case their confidence intervals do not overlap, the more likely it is that results will not be reliable. The most common statistic used to measure heterogeneity is I2. If there is considerable heterogeneity (usually $I^2 > 40\%$), the physician should expect some explanations from the authors, and in this case, there should be subgroup analyses.

How precise are the results?
There are two reasons a study may be deceiving: because of a systematic error or bias and because of a random error. This last type has a bigger impact when sample size is small or the number of events is reduced, giving way to inaccurate results. When results are inaccurate, we lose confidence in our estimate of the effect. Meta-regression does not simply estimate the average of the effect across studies, but it also gives us a confidence interval. That way, physicians can judge the accuracy of the results by checking their minimum value and maximum confidence interval.

Are results directly applicable to my patients?
The best evidence to make decisions comes when interventions are of clinical interest and when they evaluate population and relevant outcomes. If population, intervention, and outcomes in the study are different from those we are interested in, evidence may be taken as indirect.

Is there any problem with reporting or publication bias?
When researchers decide to publish their work on the basis of magnitude, direction or statistical significance of the results, there is a systematic error called reporting bias. This is the hardest kind of bias to solve in systematic reviews. When a study is not reported, the correct term is reporting or publication bias. The magnitude and direction of the results are usually taken as both decisive and the most important part of a publication, even more so than design, relevance or quality of the study. When the authors or sponsored studies only publish outcomes or specific analyses, the term "selective outcome reporting bias" is used. Reporting bias may cause errors in the estimate of the effect. However, detecting publication bias in

Table 60.4 Critical analysis of systematic reviews

1. *Are the results valid?*
   (a) Was there an explicit question?
   (b) Was there a detailed and exhaustive search of relevant studies?
   (c) Was the methodological quality of the primary studies high?
   (d) Were the included studies evaluated as reproducible?
2. *What were the results?*
   (a) Were the results similar across studies?
   (b) What were the global results of the study?
   (c) How accurate were the results?
3. *How can I apply these results to the care of my patients?*
   (a) Were all the relevant outcomes considered?
   (b) Were all the posited effects on the subgroups credible?
   (c) Are the benefits and costs potential risks?

a systematic review is complex. When reviews include a meta-analysis, one thing to check is whether the results of small-scale studies are too different from those of large-scale studies, and the funnel plot graph may also be consulted. Another thing to check is the number of studies included in the review. Empirically speaking, 30 studies should be an adequate amount. Of course, if the systematic review was successful in including unpublished studies, this would work as a solution to overcome this bias (Table 60.4).

- *Is there a reason to increase the confidence value?*
  There are situations that increase the confidence value of the estimated effects from observational studies: When treatment reaches a strong effect in a short amount of time; or in patients with a known condition whose condition would worsen without the intervention, for example, epinephrine when used to prevent mortality in anaphylaxis.

Classification of Quality of Evidence and Strength of Recommendations

One of the beneficial consequences of evidence-based medicine is the development of clinical guides to evaluate the quality of the evidence while also establishing different recommendations. By quality of evidence we mean how reliable the estimate of a certain effect is, and by strength of recommendation we understand how much we can trust that the recommendation will lead to more benefits than risks.

There are multiple evidence classification and recommendation strength systems. A type of classification that has been progressively incorporated by different scientific societies and health institutions is the Grading of Recommendations Assessment, Development and Evaluation (GRADE) system. This system incorporates other relevant aspects beyond study design and potential biases. What this methodology does is categorize relevant outcomes (hospitalizations) and their relative relevance. Then the quality of the evidence is assessed for each of the outcomes, obtaining a global quality of the evidence, and finally the strength of the recommendations is graded. This process is complex and requires training. The clinician—the main user of evidence-based medicine—must understand the implications of this classification.

These are classified in the following way:

- *Quality of evidence*
  High: There is high confidence that the estimator of the effect is very close to the real effect.
  Moderate: There is moderate confidence in the estimator of the effect, and it is likely that it is close to the real effect, but with the chance that there may be substantial differences.
  Low: Confidence in the estimator of the effect is low, and it may be substantially different to the real effect.
  Very low: There is very low confidence in the estimator of the effect, and it is very likely that it will be substantially different from the real effect.
  Strength of recommendations
  Strong: The benefits exceed the risks and costs (or vice versa). It applies to most patients without reservations.
  Weak: The benefits are in close balance with the risks and costs, or they are uncertain. Any alternative may be just as reasonable.

Strong recommendations emerge from high methodological quality, clearly reflecting that the benefits outweigh risks and costs. They point to a sufficient amount of evidence to advise or discourage a specific intervention. On the other hand, weak recommendations come from regular or low-quality evidence, as for instance, observational studies or series of cases, and they do not reflect a sufficient efficacy test. This points to the need for other decision-making criteria, such as costs, risks, availability, or patient preference. A strong recommendation is equivalent to an "always do it" (or never do it) sort of recommendation, whereas a weak recommendation should be taken as a "you may do it, but take into account other factors before making a decision."

Sources

Brouillette R, Morielli A, Leimanis A, et al. Nocturnal pulse oximetry as an abbreviated testing modality for pediatric obstructive sleep apnea. Pediatrics. 2000;105:405–12.

Claro JC, Lustig N, Soto M, Rada G. El primer paso: la pregunta clínica. Rev Méd Chile. 2012;140(8):1067–72.

Guyatt G, Rennie D. User's guides to the medical literature. Essentials of evidence-based clinical practice. The Evidence-Based Medicine Working Group. Chicago: JAMA & Archives Journals/American Medical Association; 2002.

Guyatt GH, Oxman AD, Vist GE, GRADE Working Group, et al. GRADE: an emerging consensus on rating quality of evidence and strength of recommendations. BMJ. 2008;336(7650):924–6.

Higgins JPT, Green S. Cochrane handbook for systematic reviews of interventions. Version 5.1.0 ed. Chichester: Wiley; 2011.

Moher D, Schulz KF, Altman D. The CONSORT statement: revised recommendations for improving the quality of reports of parallel group randomised trials. The CONSORT Group Lancet. Lancet. 2001;357:1191–4.

Moher D, Liberati A, Tetzlaff J, Altman DG, PRISMA Group. Preferred reporting items for systematic reviews and meta-analyses: the PRISMA statement. J Clin Epidemiol. 2009;62(10):1006–12.

Murad MH, Montori VM, Ioannidis JP, et al. How to read a systematic review and meta-analysis and apply the results to patient care: users' guides to the medical literature. JAMA. 2014;312(2):171–9.

Sackett D, Staus SE, Richardson WS, Rosenberg W, Haynes RB. Medicina basada en la evidencia. Cómo practicar y enseñar la medicina basada en evidencias. 2da ed. Madrid: Ed. Harcourt; 2000.

Schünemann HJ, Jaeschke R, Cook DJ, et al. An official ATS statement: grading the quality of evidence and strength of recommendations in ATS guidelines and recommendations. Am J Respir Crit Care Med. 2006;174(5):605–14.

Staus SE, Richardson WS, Glaszious P, Haynes RB. How to practice and teach evidence based medicine. 3rd ed. Edimburgo: Ed. Elsevier Churchill Livingstone; 2005.

Valenzuela L, Cifuentes L. Validez de estudios de test diagnósticos. Rev Méd Chile. 2008;136:401–4.

Inhalation Therapy

61

Fernando Iñiguez Osmer
and Viviana Aguirre Camposano

Contents

Physical Characteristics of Aerosols

Definition An aerosol is a suspension of liquid or solid particles in a gaseous medium. Inhalation therapy is the administration of an aerosol to a patient for therapeutic purposes.

Particle size and mass The size of the particles is a very important physical characteristic when considering the efficiency in the lung deposition of an aerosol. The aerodynamic diameter (d_a) is, by definition, the diameter of a sphere with density of one ($r = 1$), which has the same terminal settling velocity as the particle under consideration. When analyzing the characteristics of the particle, this independent variable can correlate the effect of geometric diameter and particle density, as described in the following equation, with particles greater than 1 μm, where d corresponds to the actual sphere diameter, r to the particle density, and $\rho 0$ to 1 density (of water). Expressed more simply, d_a corresponds to the product of the particle diameter multiplied by the square root of the particle density. The latter is valid for spherical particles in which the shape correction factor is not applied, and so it is registered by multiplying $\rho 0$.

$$d_{ae} = d\sqrt{\frac{\rho}{\rho_0}}$$

F. Iñiguez Osmer (✉)
Department of Pediatrics, Hospital de Puerto Montt, Puerto Montt, Chile

V. Aguirre Camposano
Department of Pediatrics, School of Medicine, University of Santiago, Santiago, Chile

P. Bertrand, I. Sánchez (eds.), *Pediatric Respiratory Diseases*,
https://doi.org/10.1007/978-3-030-26961-6_61

Mass median aerodynamic diameter (MMAD) is a particle size (in microns, μm) that divides the mass in such a way that half of the particles of that aerosol have a larger diameter and the other half a diameter smaller than the diameter of the MMAD. The geometric standard deviation (GSD) is the ratio between the MMAD and the diameter of the particles at a median standard deviation (or 84th percentile). When the GSD is less than 1.22, an aerosol is considered monodisperse; if this value is higher, it is considered polydisperse. The greater the MMAD, the greater the average size of the particles; the greater the GSD, the wider the dispersion of particle sizes in that aerosol. Most aerosols for medical use are polydispersed.

The mass median aerodynamic diameter standardizes the size of the particle to the behavior of a spherical water drop, which by definition has a density of 1. Since medical aerosols never have a uniform diameter, shape, or density, the mass median aerodynamic diameter is determined by inertial impact, laser diffraction or digital image processing methods, among others.

The primary method for defining the diameter of the particles and their distribution is the use of an inertial cascade impactor. For example, the Andersen Cascade Impactor has 8 different stages (collectors), capturing particles from 0.43 to 9.0 μm when operating at a flow rate of 28 L/min. The Next Generation impactor has 7 stages and captures particles from 0.24 to 11.7 μm at 30 L/min. The aerodynamic particle size distribution is determined by the quantities of drug deposited in each collector. The total mass of drug collected is reported as the delivered dose. When the partial mass of drug collected in the smaller diameter collectors is measured, the respirable or fine particle dose is obtained. The limit of this can be set arbitrarily in particles smaller than 6.4, 5.0 or 3.0 μm. Frequently, the fine particle dose includes those with diameters between 1 and 5 μm.

When an aerosol particle increases in size, so does its mass. By doubling the radius of a sphere, the volume grows approximately 8 times ($V = 4 \times k \times r3$). As the volume increases, the mass increases proportionally. When the mass of an aerosol particle increases, gravity will have a greater influence on it, and it will remain suspended for a shorter time.

Physical Nature of the Particles

- *Hygroscopicity*: It is the intrinsic tendency of a material to absorb moisture from its environment. It is influenced by the material crystallinity and the morphology of the particles. Hygroscopic drugs pose a greater risk of physical and chemical instability. For dry powder drugs, moisture gain or loss due to changes in relative humidity can lead to dissolution and subsequent recrystallization, hindering deagglomeration and therefore affecting drug delivery from the device.

  Moisture can be captured within the device prior to delivery (e.g., dry powder inhaler or DPI) or after the dose goes into the airway, where the particle is in a moist and warm environment (37 °C and 99% relative humidity in the carina). The susceptible particle will experience hygroscopic growth, which increases its mass and dimensions. When inhaled, this particle tends to be deposited in the airway in a more proximal location than that of a non-hygroscopic aerosol particle. This is because hygroscopic ones tend to coalesce, creating particles of greater mass and volume that tend to be suspended for less time.
- *Tonicity*: It refers to solute concentration in a solution regarding the concentration in body fluids. When creating an aerosol with a hypertonic solution (>0.9% NaCl) its particles will be hygroscopic, increasing its size. An isotonic solution (0.9% NaCl) will create aerosol particles with neutral affinity for water that tend to remain stable. A hypotonic solution (<0.9% NaCl) will create aerosol particles with a tendency to release water, therefore decreasing in size and mass.
- *Electric charge*: Because of the methods used to create an aerosol, the particles have an electric charge. This phenomenon seems to have little physiological effect on the patient, but it influences the lung deposition since there are interactions between the particles and the walls of the devices used.

Aerosol Deposition Mechanisms

The particles are deposited in the airway when they are definitively removed from the laminar flow that has been created by the inspiratory movement. The knowledge of the processes and factors that influence the deposition of particles in different regions of the airway makes it easier for the clinician to choose the best therapy for their patient. There are five mechanisms by which a particle can be deposited in the airway: inertial impaction, sedimentation, diffusion, interception, and electrostatic precipitation. The first two mechanisms are directly related to the size of the particle, while the third is inversely related to it. Interception depends on the shape of the particle and occurs when two of them meet, which is more common for elongated particles. Electrostatic precipitation is related to the electric charge, when two particles of opposite charges meet. The most relevant mechanisms are the first three.

(a) Inertial impaction Occurs when aerosol particles have sufficient momentum (mass × velocity) to maintain their trajectory despite a change in the air flow direction, thus colliding with the walls of the airway. The probability of inertial deposition increases when the particle is able to travel long distances, which depends on its mobility, mass, and speed. This is expressed in the following equation, where S corresponds to distance, B to mobility (velocity × unit force), m to mass, and v to particle velocity.

$$S = B \cdot m \cdot v$$

The Stokes number (Stk) is dimensionless and describes the airway particle deposition probability by impaction. The greater the number of Stokes, the more likely is the particle deposition by inertial impaction, according to the following equation, where ρ_p is the density of the particle, d its diameter, V is gas velocity, h its viscosity, and R is the radius of the airway.

$$Stk = \frac{\rho_p \cdot d^2 \cdot V}{18 \cdot \eta \cdot R}$$

Large particles traveling at high speed are more likely to impact the airway proximal regions. This mechanism is responsible for the filter role carried out by the upper airway on the inspired air, since particles larger than 10 μm tend to be deposited. Impaction increases dramatically with high inspiratory flows; and it is the predominant mechanism of deposition in the first seven generations of the airway.

(b) Gravitational sedimentation It is a time-dependent mechanism, in which the particles settle by the action of gravity. It is related to particle size and the flow velocity of the inhaled gas. This is the primary deposition mechanism for particles with a MMAD <2 μm, although it can affect larger particles in low flow conditions. This mechanism optimizes lung deposition. Gravitational sedimentation increases when the patient performs an apnea technique; and predominates as a deposition mechanism after the eighth generation of the airway, given the flow decrease and the smaller diameter.

(c) Diffusion Occurs in particles <0.5 μm, less influenced by gravity, in which Brownian motion plays a more important role and favors the coalescence of the particles. This mechanism is influenced by electrical charge. A significant percentage of these particles are exhaled.

General Factors That Affect Airway Aerosol Deposition

Medical aerosols vary not only in the distribution of the particles according to their size but also in other factors that affect the lung deposition: physical state (solid or liquid), density, shape, and speed. In addition, a system of dynamic forces confronts the particle in its journey through the airway, such as gravity, resistance to inspiratory flow, and inertial force. The balance between these forces, influenced by the properties of the aerosol, is what eventually determines the predominant lung deposition mechanism for the aerosol particles. Several factors affect the ability of an aerosol to be deposited in a patient's airway.

Table 61.1 Factors of stability and airway deposition of an aerosol

Physical nature of the particle: size and mass, hygroscopicity, tonicity, electric charge
Aerosol: Particle size, gravity, inertia, gas temperature, and gas humidity
Patient: Age, respiratory pattern, airway anatomy, respiratory mechanics
Equipment: Aerosol generator, type of drug, propellant, holding chamber or spacer device

These factors can be grouped into three categories: Those dependent on the physical characteristics of the aerosol, those dependent on the patient, and those dependent on the equipment used (Table 61.1).

Aerosol-Dependent Factors

Particle size, gravity, and density If the size and mass of the particle increase, the gravitational forces exerted on it have a greater influence and tend to remove it from the suspension. Ideally, most particles should have a mass such that the influence of gravity promotes deposition by sedimentation in the desired place, because when the particles are very small they lean to remain suspended, achieving minimum lung deposition and resulting in that many of them are exhaled. The optimal size for a proper deposition in the respiratory bronchioles ranges from 1 to 5 μm (breathable dose).

A denser particle will have a greater mass median aerodynamic diameter and a larger Stokes number.

- *Inertia*: It is related to the size and mass of the particle. According to Newton, kinetic energy is equal to 50% of the product of the mass times speed squared. When a larger mass particle is set in motion it will have more inertia than a smaller mass particle, even when both move at the same speed. When a particle starts moving, it tends to stay that way unless external forces act on it. Owing to its greater momentum, a particle of large mass tends to travel in a straight line even though there is a change in the direction of the gas flow in which it is suspended. Large particles (>10 μm) tend to be removed in the upper airway, while smaller particles can reach more distal regions.
- *Temperature and humidity*: There is a close relationship between these two factors related to the percentage of aerosol particles that remain in suspension. When the temperature of gas increases and humidity remains stable, particles lose water and decrease in size. By increasing gas humidity and keeping the temperature stable, particles collect water, depending on their hygroscopic capacity, and tend to coalesce and increase their size. For very small particles that are deposited by diffusion, an increase in temperature favors this mechanism due to greater Brownian motion.

Patient-Dependent Factors

- *Respiratory pattern*: This factor has a huge influence on the amount of lung deposition. In spontaneous ventilation, a slow and deep inspiration followed by a voluntary apnea of 6–10 seconds increases the deposition by sedimentation. On the contrary, the cry of an infant prompts an opposite effect, since the inspiration is short and expiration prolonged, minimizing lung deposition. Some elements to consider in this regard are: age, respiratory rate, tidal volume, inspiratory/expiratory time ratio, and aerosol delivery time regarding the respiratory cycle.
- *Anatomy of the airway and respiratory mechanics*: Anatomical alterations influence the deposition fraction (dose deposited/nominal dose) of an aerosol, since they affect gas flow velocity. In areas where the airway bifurcates (bronchial carinae), impaction of the particles may occur, depending on their inertia. In regions with anatomical (bronchial stenosis, mucous plug) or functional (bronchospasm) narrowness, a low deposition fraction may occur. Although it is true that slow flow favors deposition by sedimentation, this

means that the total amount of gas that reaches the distal region is lower, so fewer aerosol particles are available to be deposited. This happens in areas with high resistance to gas flow.

Equipment-Dependent Factors

- *Type of aerosol generating device*: Nebulizers, pressurized metered-dose inhalers (pMDI), and dry powder inhalers (DPI) are available to administer aerosols. Their performances depend on the limitations and advantages of each one of them.
- *Type of drug*: In pMDIs it may be a combination (short-acting beta-2 agonist plus ipratropium, long-acting beta-2 agonist plus steroid) or a single drug (salbutamol, ipratropium, steroid). Certain drugs can only be administered as aerosols when they are nebulized (adrenaline, dornase alfa, mucolytics).
- *Propellant*: The aerosol generating device requires a propulsive energy, which in the case of nebulizers is a source of compressed air (air network, oxygen, balloon) or electrical energy, in pMDIs and in dry powder inhalers the propellant is the patient's own inspiratory effort.

Spacer device Spacers and valved holding chambers are used together with pMDIs to administer drugs to patients with spontaneous ventilation. Volume, type of interface (oral or naso-oral), presence of valves, and static are factors that affect the performance of a chamber.

Advantages and Disadvantages of Aerosol Drug Therapy

Inhalation therapy is so firmly incorporated in clinical practice that there is often little time to reflect on the advantages of this modality when compared with other routes of drug administration, such as oral, intravenous or intramuscular (Table 61.2).

Aerosol Generating Systems

Inhalation therapy considers the delivery of a large number of drugs, such as bronchodilators, steroids, antimicrobials, mucoactive drugs, proteins, peptides, anti-inflammatories, prostacyclin analogs, and analgesics, among others. In pediatric age, the most frequent use of inhalation therapy is focused on the first two drugs mentioned.

Table 61.2 Advantages and disadvantages of inhalation therapy

1. *Advantages*
Dosage: Doses of aerosol drug are usually lower than those of systemic administration.
Onset of action: Faster with inhaled drugs than with oral drugs.
Systemic exposure: The drug reaches the lungs directly, with minimal systemic exposure.
Adverse effects: Less frequent and less severe with inhaled therapy than with systemic delivery (e.g., salbutamol).
Comfort of administration: In general, aerosol therapy is well tolerated, since it is not painful and is usually comfortable for the patient.
2. *Disadvantages*
Deposition fraction: Lung deposition is a relatively low fraction of the total dose delivered (nominal dose)
Influence of multiple variables: There are many variables that influence lung deposition. This increases the possibility of error in therapy
Lack of knowledge of professionals and patients: The correct use of the device that creates the aerosol must be known first by the professional who indicates or uses the therapy, an essential requirement so that they can teach its use to the patient
Different devices confuse the patient: A patient may be confused between the controller drug (steroid) and the reliever drug (salbutamol). If a patient uses two or more types of devices (e.g., DPI plus pMDI), it may be confusing, since higher inspiratory flows are required when using a dry powder inhaler.
Absence of quality technical information on inhalers for clinicians: At present, clinical guidelines on inhalation therapy are not readily available to guide the physician in choosing the most appropriate device for his patient or in educating him about its use.

Aerosol drugs can be generated from pMDIs, nebulizers, and dry powder inhalers. There are advantages and disadvantages for each device, and in recent years, the increase in the variety of these has caused confusion in patients and doctors.

Pressurized metered-dose inhaler This is the most commonly used device because it is small in size, portable, relatively inexpensive, does not require drug preparation, can deliver multiple doses quickly, and its contents are protected from contamination by pathogens. Its great disadvantage is that the dose of drug deposited is highly dependent on the patient's technique.

The design consists of a plastic holder with a cap. In the cap, there is a metal canister with a delivery valve and a sprayer. Inside the canister there is a mixture of the drug, propellant, and excipients in solution or suspension (Fig. 61.1). When used, a fixed dose of this mixture is released at high speed (between 10 and 100 m/s) with particles of varying size, depending on the drug, the propellant used, and the manufacturing conditions of the device. Owing to the high speed with which the particles are released, the size of these particles, their low temperature, and the need for good coordination between shooting and inhalation, the use of a holding chamber (or spacer) is recommended when administering aerosols delivered by a pressurized metered-dose inhaler. This decelerates and divides the expelled particles, warms the mixture, and favors coordination between shot and inhalation.

There are two types of spacers or holding chambers: valved and non-valved. Both can have a facemask or a mouthpiece. In infants and preschoolers, a double-valve holding chamber should be used to separate inhalation from exhalation, thus optimizing lung deposition; in schoolers and adolescents a spacer can be used. Ideally, the device should be metallic to avoid electrostatic charging, although plastic ones specially manufactured to reduce their static charge can be used; or treating them by washing them with detergent. Its maintenance also should include washing them in water with detergent and air drying. Although there is no consensus on the frequency, doing it once a week seems reasonable. Finally, the spacer

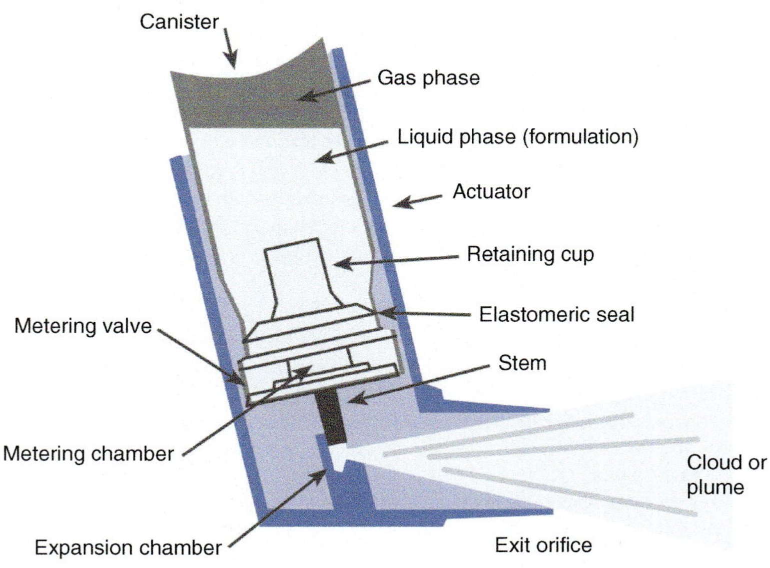

Fig. 61.1 Pressurized metered-dose inhaler (pMDI)

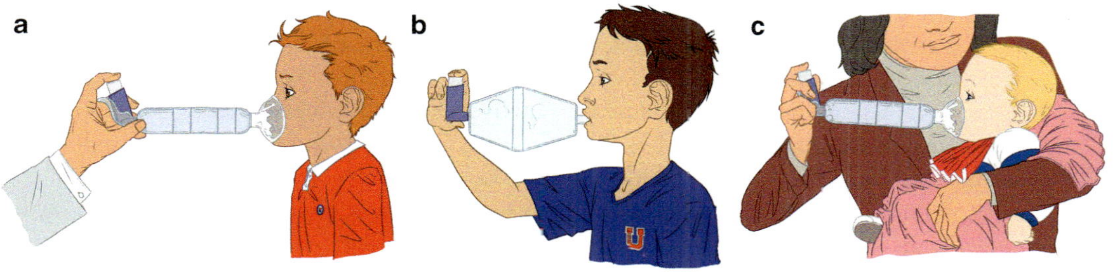

Fig. 61.2 Recommendations for administering a drug using a pMDI. (**a**) Schoolchildren and adults: spacer with mask. (**b**) Preschoolers, schoolchildren and adults: holding chamber with mouthpiece. (**c**) Infants and preschoolers: holding chamber with mask

Recommendations for administering a drug through a pMDI: for (a, b) choose a spacer or holding chamber according to age, shake the pMDI and connect, attach only to the mouth, administer 1 puff and then inhale slowly, from residual volume to total lung capacity; hold your breath for 6–10 seconds; exhale slowly; repeat the same procedure for the following doses. In infants (c) always use an air chamber. With the child sitting in the adult's arms, remove the pMDI cover, shake it vertically and connect it. Attach the holding chamber covering the mouth and nose and trying to avoid leaks. With the holding chamber in horizontal position, press the inhaler once, wait for the patient to complete at least 6–8 respiratory cycles observing the thoracic or valve movements. Rinse or perform oral hygiene after inhalations to prevent caries (salbutamol) and fungi (steroids)

must have a proper length that allows deceleration of the particles (15–18 cm) and a volume according to the age of the patient (Fig. 61.2).

Since the Montreal agreement in 1987, chlorofluorocarbons (CFCs), as harmful propellants for the ozone layer, have been replaced by hydrofluoroalkane (HFA), which generate aerosols with smaller plumes that are warmer and with lower exit velocity compared to pressurized metered-dose inhalers that use chlorofluorocarbons. In the case of solution aerosols (beclomethasone, ciclesonide) with HFA as a propellant, extra fine particles can be generated, which improves lung deposition (~50% of the nominal dose) when compared to ones with chlorofluorocarbons (<20%). The most modern pressurized metered-dose inhalers overcome the coordination problem between the trigger and the inhalation since they are activated by inspiration, requiring a minimum inspiratory flow (around 20–30 L/min) and patient collaboration (Autohaler®, Easibreathe®, K-haler®, MD Turbo®, Xcelovent®, Smartmist®).

Although most pressurized metered-dose inhalers contain a larger number of doses than labeled, once this number is reached the amount of drug released is erratic, which has led the recommendation that all devices have a dose counter. This phenomenon occurs less in HFA-propelled pressurized metered-dose inhalers (more consistent) compared to those propelled by chlorofluorocarbons.

Nebulizers Generally, it should always be preferred to use pressurized metered-dose inhalers or dry powder inhalers, limiting the use of nebulizers to precise indications: administration of drugs in patients with oxygen requirements, high and continuous doses of a bronchodilator, absence of formulation of a drug (e.g., adrenaline, antibiotics, DNase).

There are several types of nebulizers:

- *Jet (or pneumatic) nebulizers*: Use a compressed air source to convert a drug in liquid state into an aerosol and to produce a fine mist using the Bernoulli's principle. According to the aerosol delivery during respiration, jet nebulizers can be classified into: (1) conventional, with constant output through the respiratory cycle; (2) favored by breathing, with constant output but increased during inspiration; (3) triggered by breathing: this only produces aerosol during inspiration, which minimizes aerosol loss.
- *Ultrasonic nebulizers*: Use electricity to vibrate a piezoelectric crystal at very high frequency. This vibration produced is transmitted

to a reservoir containing the solution, creating a series of waves that on the surface will separate particles from the liquid to form an aerosol. There is an increase in the temperature of the solution during its operation, which is why they are not suitable for nebulizing biological products (proteins).

- *Mesh nebulizers*: Use the ultrasonic principle to generate drops that will be impelled through a vibrant mesh (Aeroneb Go®, Aeroneb Pro®, Pari eFlow®, ODEM TouchSpray®, Pfeiffer Michrohaler®) or a static mesh (Omron MicroAir®) to form a plume. Some of these nebulizers include sensors to provide systems that activate or integrate with breathing.
- *Soft Mist Inhaler*: It is a recently developed type of nebulizer (Respimat®) that atomizes the drug solution using mechanical energy that comes from a spring. When the spring is released the solution is forced through a narrow nozzle system, which produces a slow-moving fine mist that has less deposition in the oropharynx and greater lung deposition (39%).

The most commonly used are the conventional jet nebulizers with constant output. These devices are charged with a certain volume of liquid and connected to an air or oxygen flow that will divide the solution drops in small particles whose size will depend on the characteristics of each brand and device in particular. Generally, unless otherwise stated by the manufacturer, the filling volume is 4–5 mL and necessary flow for proper operation is 6–8 L/min, preferring the use of a mouthpiece over the facemask. Nebulizers have the advantage that they do not require coordination with patient inhalation; they also allow the administration of a wide range of products in high doses, and generate particles with lower velocity, so they do not need spacers (only facemasks or mouthpieces). However, they are more expensive, require a management system (nebulizer, compensated flow meter, air or oxygen compressor), and the administration procedure takes more time. In addition, its generating system is less efficient than pressurized metered-dose inhalers. It is not recommended to mix drugs: pentamidine, ribavirin, and tobramycin have been approved for use with specific nebulizers and compressors (e.g., PARI LC® plus with PARI BOY® compressor and tobramycin). New breath actuated nebulizers (AeroEclipse®) or favored by it (iNeb®, AKITA®) have been developed.

Nebulization technique must comply with a series of requirements that ensure a better lung deposition (Fig. 61.3). The use of low-power compressors that do not produce the necessary flow for a proper aerosol generation should be avoided. For its use at home, it is recommended to clean nebulizers after each use with sterile or distilled water and then to air dry it on an absorbent paper. Once or twice a week wash it with soapy water and disinfect it with a mixture of distilled water and white vinegar at 1.25%. In health centers, nebulizers should follow the usual disinfection guidelines.

Inhalation therapy with aerosols generated by pressurized metered-dose inhalers or a nebulizer can also be administered to patients receiving ventilatory assistance, both invasive and non-invasive.

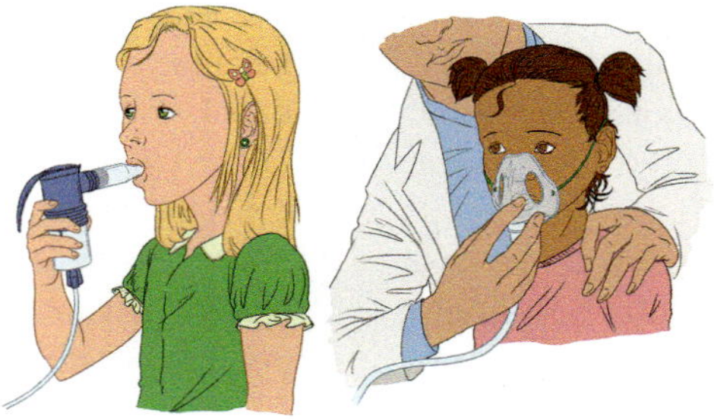

Fig. 61.3 Recommendations for nebulization
Fill with 4–5 mL (drug and saline); use a 6–8 L/min flow, enriched with oxygen only if necessary; 5–7 minutes of nebulization; mask firmly attached to the face and use of mouthpiece in children from 4-years-old; calm breathing at tidal volume; facial cleaning and eye protection with anticholinergic use when mask is used

Table 61.3 Technique for administering a drug through a DPI

1.	Patient sitting or standing.
2.	Verify in the dose indicator that there is drug available.
3.	Prepare the dose according to the manufacturer's instructions. Keep the device in position avoiding putting the mouthpiece down.
4.	Exhale slowly until reaching residual volume and take care not to do it inside the inhaler.
5.	Place the mouthpiece between the lips ensuring a good seal. Do not block the mouthpiece with your tongue.
6.	Aspire quickly, energetically, and continuously to full lung capacity.
7.	In apnea, remove the inhaler. Keep the apnea for 6–10 seconds.
8.	Cap or close the device and store it in its box in a dry place.
9.	Rinse mouth.

Dry powder inhalers Are devices in which the drug has been formulated in pure form or mixed with an inactive excipient such as lactose (transporter). In this powder the crystals are agglomerated, so they must be disaggregated and converted into an aerosol in a complex process known as fluidization, by means of an appropriate inspiratory flow that varies between the different available devices (minimum 30 L/min). These devices can be used for children from 4 to 5-years-old. This system has the advantages of being portable, having a dose counter, being propellants-free, having a lung deposition similar or greater to pressurized metered-dose inhalers, being activated by the inspiratory flow (passive device), and not requiring the use of a spacer. It also allows using single or multiple doses depending on the type of device used. Within its limitations are their high cost and the different forms of use between different types of dry powder inhalers. Currently, there are a number of devices to deliver drugs, both in single doses (Diskhaler®, Cyclohaler®, Spinhaler®, Aerolizer®, Handihaler®) and in multiple doses (Turbuhaler®, Rotahaler®, Diskus®, Clickhaler®, Easihaler ®, Maghaler®, Novolizer®, Pulvinal®, Spiromax®, Twisthaler®, Genuair®, Airmax®, Swinghaler®, Spiros®, Airmax®). The use of a dry powder inhaler must follow certain recommendations (Table 61.3).

Sources

Aguilar P, Mallol J. Flujos inspiratorios máximos en niños de 4–8 años. Implicancias para la inhalación de medicamentos en polvo. Arch Bronconeumol. 2000;36:3.

Amirav I, Newhouse M. Review of optimal characteristics of facemasks for valved holding chambers (VHCs). Pediatr Pulmonol. 2008;43:268–74.

Barrueto L, Aguirre V, Aguilar F. Aerosolterapia. In: Paris E, Sánchez I, Beltramino D, Copto A, editors. Meneghello Pediatría. 6ª ed. Madrid: Editorial Médica Panamericana; 2013. p. 1193.

Carvalho T, Peters J, Williams R. Influence of particle size on regional lung deposition. What evidence is there? Int J Pharm. 2011;406:1–10.

Dhand R. Aerosol therapy in patients receiving noninvasive positive pressure ventilation. J Aerosol Med Pulm Drug Deliv. 2012;25:63–78.

Dolovich M, Ahrens R, Hess D, et al. Device selection and outcomes of aerosol therapy: evidence-based guidelines. American College of Chest Physicians/American College of Asthma, Allergy and Immunology. Chest. 2005;127:335–40.

Geller D. Comparing clinical features of the nebulizer, metered-dose inhaler, and dry powder inhaler. Respir Care. 2005;50:1313–21.

Iñiguez F. Terapia inhalatoria en los pacientes con ventilación mecánica domiciliaria. Neumología Pediátrica. 2008;3:87–99.

Laube B, Janssens H, de Jongh F, et al. What the pulmonary specialist should know about the new inhalation therapies. ERS/ISAM Task Force Report. Eur Respir J. 2011;37:1308–31.

Lavorini F. The challenge of delivering therapeutic aerosols to asthma patients. ISRN Allergy. 2013;2013:17; Article ID 102418.

Myers T. The science guiding selection of an aerosol delivery device. Respir Care. 2013;58:1963–73.

Newman S. Principles of metered-dose inhaler design. Respir Care. 2005;50:1177–90.

Rottier B, Rubin B. Asthma medication delivery: mist and myths. Pediatr Respir Rev. 2013;14:112–8.

Rubin B. Pediatric aerosol therapy: new devices and new drugs. Respir Care. 2011;56:1411–21.

Smutney C, Grant M, Kincey P. Device factors affecting pulmonary delivery of dry powders. Ther Deliv. 2013;4:939–49.

Wong J, Chan H, Kwok P. Electrostatics in pharmaceutical aerosols for inhalation. Ther Deliv. 2013;4:981–1002.

Pulmonary Anti-Inflammatory Effects of Macrolides

62

Luis Enrique Vega-Briceño and Ignacio Sánchez

Contents

Introduction

The aim of this chapter is to present a brief update on the role of macrolides and their anti-inflammatory effect on the lungs, and their efficacy and safety regarding other specific respiratory conditions, such as cystic fibrosis (CF), bronchiectasis, asthma, obliterative bronchiolitis, and sinusitis.

L. E. Vega-Briceño (✉)
Faculty of Medicine, Universidad del Desarrollo, Santiago, Chile
e-mail: levega@udd.cl

I. Sánchez
Department of Pediatrics, School of Medicine, Pontificia Universidad Católica de Chile, Santiago, Chile

Macrolides

Macrolides are a complex and wide family of antibiotics derived from the *Streptomyces* family, discovered in the middle of last century, on Philippine soil. They are characterized by the presence of a lactonic ring with at least one amino sugar in their structure. Owing to their strong antibiotic effect on aerobic gram positive, anaerobic, and gram negative bacteria, there are an increasing number of studies revealing their immunomodulatory and anti-inflammatory properties both in children and adults. These drugs do not present a bacteriostatic or bactericide effect against *Pseudomona aeruginosa* almost at all, which is why the idea that there must be a different mechanism for its clinical effect to happen has been a point of discussion.

Macrolides' anti-inflammatory effect was first recorded during simple observations on patients with severe asthma in 1959, when

P. Bertrand, I. Sánchez (eds.), *Pediatric Respiratory Diseases*,
https://doi.org/10.1007/978-3-030-26961-6_62

Kaplan and Goldin reported that a group of patients with severe asthma—daily steroid users—required a smaller dose of steroids after being administered troleandomycin. Later, in the 1970s, Itkin et al. reported the benefit of administering macrolides, managing to reduce the steroid dose in patients with "infectious asthma." These two anecdotal experiences were the first published "evidence" suggesting a non-antibiotic property of macrolides.

The most convincing demonstration of the anti-inflammatory effect of macrolides on the lung was the treatment of diffuse panbronchiolitis (DBP) carried out in Japan. This disease of unknown origins was first reported by Homme in 1969 as generally initiating symptoms after the fourth decade of life with clinical characteristics similar to cystic fibrosis: Obstructive-restrictive ventilatory pattern, *Pseudomona aeruginosa* colonization, and development of bronchiectasis, and in individuals whose survival rate after 5 years was lower than 30%. A retrospective study of 498 adults suffering from diffuse panbronchiolitis showed that subjects who used erythromycin for different periods presented a significant increase in their survival rate over 10 years of up to 90%, along with reduction in morbidity and improvement in lung function. This effect was clearer in older patients colonized by *P. aeruginosa* who suffered from diffuse panbronchiolitis.

The effectiveness of macrolides as anti-inflammatory agents seems to be limited to members of the lactone 14 and 15 groups, such as erythromycin, clarithromycin, and azithromycin. These drugs have been shown to improve lung function and reduce morbidity and mortality in patients with diffuse panbronchiolitis and cystic fibrosis.

Physiopathology

Many studies have developed interesting hypotheses to explain the immunomodulatory effect displayed by macrolides in different respiratory conditions. There probably is no single mechanism for their action, given that these drugs act across the inflammatory cascade both in vitro and in vivo (Fig. 62.1).

- *Modulation of the inflammatory cascade.* Macrolides inhibit the production and discharge of pro-inflammatory cytokines (IL-1, IL-6, IL-9, and TNFα), both in vitro and in blood samples and bronchoalveolar lavage (BAL) in patients with diffuse panbronchiolitis. It is assumed that the cause of this effect is the inhibition of nuclear factor kappa B (NF-Kb), an essential protein for the transcription of the genes that encode pro-inflammatory molecules like IL-8. This molecule is released as a response to lipopolysaccharides, immune complexes, and other cytokines. IL-8 is a powerful chemotactic factor for neutrophils, eosinophils, and other inflammatory mediators. Generally speaking, macrolides inhibit the expression of the inducible nitric oxide synthase enzyme, reducing the formation of superoxide anions and free radicals, which may have a role in chronic lung conditions where the oxidative factor is prevalent, as in cystic fibrosis.
- *Effect on neutrophils.* Many studies have shown a reduction in neutrophil migration and chemotactic activity after being exposed to macrolides, as they inhibit the formation of cytokines, B4 leukotrienes, and other necessary macromolecules for the adhesion of these cells, such as ICAM. In vitro models show that erythromycin increases the levels of AMPc in neutrophils depending on dosage, accelerating cellular apoptosis with a marked reduction in the number of neutrophils in the sputum.
- *Biofilm.* Permanent (mucoid and non-mucoid) *P. aeruginosa* colonization occurs in around 70% of patients with diffuse panbronchiolitis and around 80% of patients with cystic fibrosis at some point during the disease. This colonization reduces the survival rate of patients as the number of polymorphonuclears and protease in the sputum increases, therefore increasing lung damage. Macrolides modify the virulence of *P. aeruginosa*, reducing the release of elastase, protease, phospholipase,

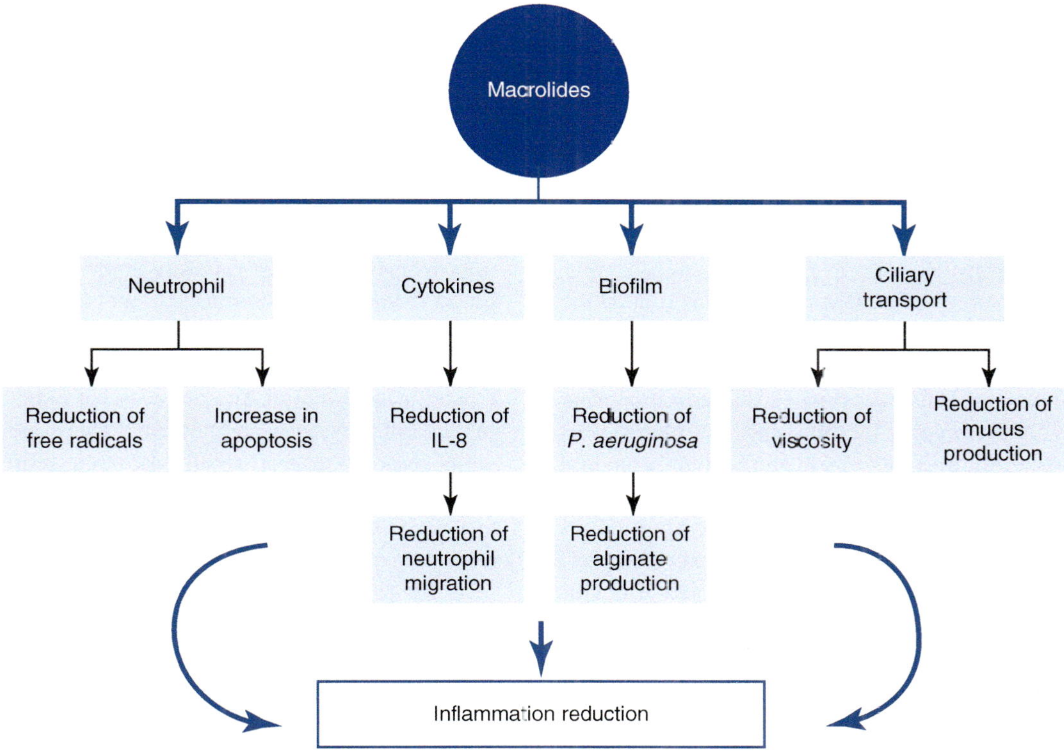

Fig. 62.1 Anti-inflammatory mechanisms of macrolides Macrolides act on neutrophils and reduce the production of free radicals while increasing cellular apoptosis. The stimulation of some cytokines inhibits the release of IL-8. In addition, they reduce the count of colonies of Pseudomona aeruginosa on the mucus biofilm or by increasing ciliary transport and reduction of its viscosity. All these effects together translate into a reduction of the inflammatory cascade in the airway

and exotoxins. Mucoid *P. aeruginosa* produces alginate, forming a biofilm that interferes with the elimination of this bacterium. It behaves like a specific antibody–antigen reaction, inducing antigen on the surface of the airway. Production of alginate has also been reported in other forms of *P. aeruginosa*. Azithromycin reduces serum immune complexes, secondary inflammation, and adherence of *P. aeruginosa* to the respiratory epithelium of the airway. Some randomized and controlled studies in patients with cystic fibrosis have shown that daily treatment with azithromycin for at least 3 months reduces the number of respiratory exacerbations without significantly altering the respiratory flora. This effect becomes clearer in patients infected by *P. aeruginosa*. The doses used are smaller than the minimal inhibitory concentration against this germ, suggesting that its antibacterial effect is not responsible and indicates the presence of a different mechanism. An in vitro study comparing the combination of ciprofloxacin and azithromycin versus ciprofloxacin showed that combined therapy increased the elimination of *P. aeruginosa*, suggesting a higher degree of penetration by the quinolone in the biofilm, favored by the action of the macrolide.

- *Aspects of the mucus*. Macrolides inhibit the expression of genes that produce mucin in the cells of the bronchial epithelium, therefore reducing the production of mucus by goblet cells. In patients with cystic fibrosis colonized by *P. aeruginosa*, macrolides reduce the viscosity of mucus in up to 80% compared to a placebo, perhaps related to the decrease in production of alginate. Rubin and company compared mucus discharges in healthy patients against those suffering from purulent rhinitis. After 2 weeks of therapy with clarithromycin, a reduction of mucus discharges was observed in both groups, but the group with purulent rhinitis also saw a reduction in viscosity.

- *Bronchoconstriction*. Macrolides reduce the expression of endothelin-1, a powerful natural vasoconstrictor and bronchoconstrictor. An in vitro study showed that administering erythromycin inhibits the contraction of smooth muscle cells of the human bronchial epithelium as a response to the electric stimulus. This action would happen when inhibiting the cholinergic response, because administering acetylcholine blocks this biological effect.

Clinical Effectiveness

- *Cystic fibrosis*. On the basis of the similarities between cystic fibrosis and diffuse panbronchiolitis, a pilot study on children with cystic fibrosis and *P. aeruginosa* infection showed a short-term improvement in lung function with the use of macrolides. Afterward, some controlled studies evaluated the effect of macrolides in the treatment of cystic fibrosis, showing an improvement in FEV_1 of 3.5–5.5% as well as a reduction in the use of antibiotics and the number of respiratory exacerbations. A trial of 185 patients with preliminary data suggested a substantial improvement in lung function in patients who received macrolides chronically. On the other hand, the Cochrane group concluded that the benefits of azithromycin in patients with cystic fibrosis are limited but significant. Similarly, administering nebulized deoxyribonuclease to patients suffering from cystic fibrosis has shown an increase in VEF_1, FVC, as well as a reduction in the number of acute exacerbations attributed to the reduction in the DNA levels of the bronchoalveolar lavage samples.
- *Bronchiectasis*. There is little evidence of the usefulness of macrolides in patients with bronchiectasis not associated with cystic fibrosis. A study did not find any differences in lung function tests when monitoring patients treated with roxithromycin for 12 weeks, but there was a reduction in bronchial hyperresponsiveness (BHR) and an improvement in mucus viscosity in the treated group. Many of these studies conclude that subjects with cystic fibrosis colonized by P. aeruginosa suffer from bronchiectasis, which is why it is hard to isolate the cause of either of the inflammatory components. There are valid reasons to test small-dose long-term plans in subjects able to undergo lung function tests that allow observing and monitoring the response, or, failing this, in those who do not respond to conventional treatments. Some countries in Europe recommend testing nebulized deoxyribonuclease for 2 months in patients who fail a macrolide test.
- *Asthma*. Asthma is the prototypical inflammatory airway disease. Some patients suffering from severe asthma who depend on systemic steroids and have received macrolides are capable of reducing or suppressing steroids without worsening their lung function. Using azithromycin has produced some benefits, despite the fact that it does not interact with the steroid metabolism, thus suggesting direct anti-inflammatory activity of macrolides, which would reduce bronchial hyperactivity. Patients with allergic asthma are able to reduce the levels of IL-8 released by eosinophils in a dose- and time-dependent manner. Low macrolide doses could be systemic steroid 'savers' in patients with more severe asthma, either because of lymphocyte proliferation inhibition, reduction in the accumulation of neutrophils, mucus, or contraction of the smooth muscle, because of its direct (inhibitory) action on nuclear factor NF-Kb or because of the induced reduction of eosinophils' apoptosis. Macrolides are effective in reducing bronchial hyperresponsiveness and eosinophilic inflammation. Amayasu et al. measured bronchoconstriction caused by inhaling methacholine in

17 patients suffering from asthma who received a placebo or 200 mg of clarithromycin twice a day for 8 weeks, with a significant decrease in all inflammatory indexes, symptoms, bronchial hyperresponsiveness, and eosinophil levels within the treated group. A possible explanation for the shown effects is the role that some infections by atypical germs play in the persistence of the airway inflammation. *M. pneumonia* can start or perpetuate an asthma attack in previously healthy or stable subjects. Also, it causes the expression of RANTES in cell cultures, an effect that becomes inhibited after the use of macrolides. The anti-inflammatory effect on asthma of macrolides is widely discussed because of its frequent association with *M. pneumoniae* and *C. pneumoniae*, not only because of the role they play in respiratory exacerbations but also as being responsible for prolonging the inflammatory process. Treatment with macrolides significantly improves FEV_1 in asthmatic patients with positive isolation for *M. pneumoniae* and *C. pneumoniae* through PCR techniques. There also was a reduction in inflammatory mediators, such as IL-5 and IL-12, and in neutrophil and IL-8 released by eosinophils in atopic patients. Most patients require at least 2 months of treatment before showing improvement, and the benefits disappear after suspending macrolide treatment for longer than 3 months. Lacking double-blind peer-reviewed studies it is not possible to recommend the use of macrolides for asthma treatment. Despite the complications in identifying and isolating inflammatory component vs. the infections component (cause-effect), the possibility of infection by atypical bacteria must be considered for patients with asthma who do not respond to the usual dose of inhaled steroids.

- *Obliterative bronchiolitis.* Since the 1980s, bronchiolitis obliterans (OB) has been recognized as a severe complication after lung transplant. Even though its pathogenesis is unknown, there are well identified risk conditions. Diagnosis is usually complex. Khalid et al. evaluated administering 500 mg. of azithromycin for 3 days, followed by 250 mg on alternate days for 12 weeks in 20 adults, observing in this way an improvement in FCV and FEV_1 of 20% and 22%, respectively. Another recent open and unreviewed study evaluated six lung transplant recipients who received azithromycin on alternate days, showing a considerable average improvement in FEV_1 of 17.1% over the base value before treatment. Even though its mechanisms are still unknown, there was good drug tolerance. However, more studies are required to determine the safety and benefit of these therapies.
- *Chronic sinusitis.* Since 1991, many, but mainly Japanese publications, have shown that macrolides, particularly clarithromycin on ~500 mg doses twice a day, produce better mucociliary clearance, a decreased discharge volume, and a reduction in inflammation markers on the mucus of chronic sinusitis patients. Sinus symptoms have been reduced at a rate of 50–100% according to a study using 600 mg/day doses of clarithromycin for 7 months. At the same time, patients suffering from chronic sinusitis and nasal polyposis saw a reduction in the size of their polyps correlated to the degree of IL-8 reduction. Clinical improvement was documented at 5%, 48%, 63%, and 71%, respectively after 2, 4, 8, and 12 weeks of treatment. The authors of the study speculated that the clinical effects they found were secondary to a circulating cytokine release control and their previously reported action on the nasal epithelium. Their long-term recurrence effects after suspending treatment have not been evaluated.

Adverse Effects

In general, new macrolides are well tolerated and most adverse effects are mild. The most common alterations are nausea and diarrhea (6%), dyspepsia, abdominal pain or headaches (1.6%). A minor, but typical, secondary effect of clarithromycin was altered taste in between 9% and 14% of patients. From 1% to 6% of patients have abandoned treatment because of their secondary effects, a similar rate to other antibiotics or placebos. Some aspects of distribution volume must be considered in patients with cystic fibrosis, as they usually receive higher doses at different intervals than known standards.

On the other hand, patients with cystic fibrosis do not usually metabolize macrolides, so in order to obtain beneficial effects, long treatments are required, which is why the correct dose for this patient subgroup is unknown. Despite the theoretical risk, overusing antibiotics may produce a dangerous increase in bacterial resistance, demanding constant monitoring. Still, the administered immunomodulating doses are small. Finally, yearly monitoring of liver enzymes must be considered for patients with cystic fibrosis who have been administered these drugs.

Limits of the Treatment

It is clear that some patients improve their condition after being exposed to macrolides. Yet, some patients do not. Currently, there is no way to predict the response to this treatment. Beyond sputum bacteriology or bronchoalveolar lavage, their usage must be suspended if there is no clear evidence of response to the treatment. Research is still in progress in this area, and "cut-off points" regarding their potential benefits are still necessary.

Sources

Brusselle GG, Vanderstichele C, Jordens P, et al. Azithromycin for prevention of exacerbations in severe asthma (AZISAST): a multicentre randomized double-blind placebo-controlled trial. Thorax. 2013;68(4):322–9.

Cameron EJ, McSharry C, Chaudhuri R, Farrow S, Thomson NC. Long-term macrolide treatment of chronic inflammatory airway diseases: risks, benefits and future developments. Clin Exp Allergy. 2012;42(9):1302–12.

Corris PA, Ryan VA, Small T, Lordan J, Fisher AJ, Meachery G, Johnson G, Ward C. A randomised controlled trial of azithromycin therapy in bronchiolitis obliterans syndrome (BOS) post lung transplantation. Thorax. 2015;70(5):442–50.

Essilfie AT, Horvat JC, Kim RY, Mayall JR, Pinkerton JW, Beckett EL, Starkey MR, Simpson JL, Foster PS, Gibson PG, Hansbro PM. Macrolide therapy suppresses key features of experimental steroid-sensitive and steroid-insensitive asthma. Thorax. 2015;70(5):458–67.

Feldman C. The use of antiinflammatory therapy and macrolides in bronchiectasis. Clin Chest Med. 2012;33(2):371–80.

Fouka E, Lamprianidou E, Arvanitidis K, Filidou E, Kolios G, Miltiades P, Paraskakis E, Antoniadis A, Kotsianidis I, Bouros D. Low-dose clarithromycin therapy modulates Th17 response in non-cystic fibrosis bronchiectasis patients. Lung. 2014;192(6):849–55.

Gielen V, Johnston SL, Edwards MR. Azithromycin induces anti-viral responses in bronchial epithelial cells. Eur Respir J. 2010;36(3):646–54.

Haworth CS, Bilton D, Elborn JS. Long-term macrolide maintenance therapy in non-CF bronchiectasis: evidence and questions. Respir Med. 2014;108(10):1397–408.

Koutsoubari I, Papaevangelou V, Konstantinou GN, Makrinioti H, Xepapadaki P, Kafetzis D, Papadopoulos NG. Effect of clarithromycin on acute asthma exacerbations in children: an open randomized study. Pediatr Allergy Immunol. 2012;23(4):385–90.

McCallum GB, Morris PS, Chang AB. Antibiotics for persistent cough or wheeze following acute bronchiolitis in children. Cochrane Database Syst Rev. 2012;(12):CD009834.

Parnham MJ, Erakovic Haber V, Giamarellos-Bourboulis EJ, Perletti G, Verleden GM, Vos R. Azithromycin: mechanisms of action and their relevance for clinical applications. Pharmacol Ther. 2014;143(2):225–45.

Rudmik L, Soler ZM. Medical therapies for adult chronic sinusitis: a systematic review. JAMA. 2015;314(9):926–39.

Shi ZL, Peng H, Hu XW, Hu JG. Effectiveness and safety of macrolides in bronchiectasis patients: a meta-analysis and systematic review. Pulm Pharmacol Ther. 2014;28(2):171–8.

Spagnolo P, Fabbri LM, Bush A. Long-term macrolide treatment for chronic respiratory disease. Eur Respir J. 2013;42(1):239–51.

Spurling GK, Doust J, del Mar CB, Eriksson L. Antibiotics for bronchiolitis in children. Cochrane Database Syst Rev. 2014;(10):CD005189.

Wong C, Jayaram L, Karalus N, Eaton T, Tong C, Hockey H, Milne D, Fergusson W, Tuffery C, Sexton P, Storey L, Ashton T. Azithromycin for prevention of exacerbations in non-cystic fibrosis bronchiectasis (EMBRACE): a randomised, double-blind, placebo-controlled trial. Lancet. 2012;380(9842):660–7.

Wong EH, Porter JD, Edwards MR, Johnston SL. The role of macrolides in asthma: current evidence and future directions. Lancet Respir Med. 2014;2(8):657–70.

Zarogoulidis P, Papanas N, Kioumis I, Chatzaki E, Maltezos E, Zarogoulidis K. Macrolides: from in vitro anti-inflam-matory and immunomodulatory properties to clinical practice in respiratory diseases. Eur J Clin Pharmacol. 2012;68(5):479–503.

Zeng M, Li ZY, Ma J, Cao PP, Wang H, Cui YH, Liu Z. Clarithromycin and dexamethasone show similar anti-inflammatory effects on distinct phenotypic chronic rhinosinusitis: an explant model study. BMC Immunol. 2015;16:37.

Chest Physiotherapy

63

Homero Puppo Gallardo
and Gonzalo Hidalgo Soler

Contents

Introduction

Respiratory physiotherapy has had a constant and sustained development thanks to a better understanding of the function of the natural defense mechanisms in the lung, the physiopathology of respiratory diseases, and the effect of non-pharmacological interventions on the respiratory system. This has resulted in the inclusion of the respiratory physiotherapist as a part of the team in respiratory care:

1. *Hospital level*: In mid and high complexity patients, their role is highlighted in the intensive care units performing respiratory physiotherapy and participating in the severely compromised patient's functional recovery, especially involved in inhalation therapy, medicinal gases, and mechanical ventilation.
2. *Primary health care*: In aspects of education, prevention, evaluation, and treatment of patients with severe chronic respiratory diseases and rehabilitation of all conditions with respiratory compromise.
3. *Home respiratory care*: Involved in follow-up and treatment of chronic respiratory patient on both invasive and non-invasive mechanical ventilation.

There are two approaches to respiratory physiotherapy management in children. An approach called conventional physiotherapy, used in Anglo-Saxon countries, and another branch

H. Puppo Gallardo (✉) · G. Hidalgo Soler
Respiratory Kinesiology, Faculty of Medicine,
Universidad de Chile, Santiago, Chile
e-mail: ghidalgo@med.uchile.cl

P. Bertrand, I. Sánchez (eds.), *Pediatric Respiratory Diseases*,
https://doi.org/10.1007/978-3-030-26961-6_63

called non-conventional physiotherapy, especially applied in French-speaking countries and Latin American countries. The conventional physiotherapy approach was initially applied in adults with surgery respiratory complications and chronic respiratory diseases, such as bronchiectasis and chronic obstructive pulmonary disease. Conventional kinetic respiratory techniques (postural drainage, percussions, vibrations, and forced expiration) were used in respiratory conditions without adequately considering the inherent characteristics of growth and development of the respiratory system in children, especially in infants. In these patients, the configuration of the thoracic cavity is trapezoidal, and the position of the fibers in the costal area of the diaphragm changes, losing the apposition zone, leaving the infant in mechanical disadvantage, especially in situations of greater breathing work. The infant presents a narrower airway, which increases the frictional resistance with even small decreases in radius. They also have higher susceptibility to fatigue of the respiratory musculature due to the composition of diaphragm having fewer type I fibers (fatigue resistant) than older children. In addition, infants have an inherent hyper reactivity of the airway, a higher thoracic *compliance* and lung elastance. All these factors determine that the session of respiratory physiotherapy has to be preceded by a careful evaluation, graded according to clinical and laboratory parameters, and performed with intensity and precision for brief periods in severe diseases.

Objectives

The goal of respiratory physiotherapy is to participate in the resolution of cases in which bronchial hygiene is compromised, resolution of collapsed lung zones (atelectasis) or alteration in which gas exchange or thoraco-pulmonary mechanic is compromised, contributing to optimize the ventilation/perfusion ratio and secretion draining, with the objective of decreasing airway resistance, thus decreasing the breathing work. On the other hand, in cases where bronchospasm or parenchymal compromise, respiratory physiotherapy has not had support from the literature that supports its prescription, because studies are too heterogeneous regarding sample size and baseline diagnosis included, investigation type in the application of techniques, and mainly the application of inadequate techniques for the age range. However, it is habitually prescribed in many health centers in cases where bronchial hypersecretion is present with—at least—moderate bronchoconstriction.

Bases

Mucociliary drainage participates in the protection of the respiratory system against harmful agents that enter with the inspired air. Under normal circumstances, the respiratory system produces daily between 10 and 100 ml of secretions that are eliminated by the permanent activity of the mucociliary system. The speed of the bronchial drainage depends on two interrelated factors: The viscoelastic capabilities of mucus and the frequency of cilliary movement. The viscoelastic properties are altered by illness (asthma, cystic fibrosis), dry air, tobacco, and other environmental pollutants. The ciliary shaking frequency decreases with age and during sleep, and conversely, increases during physical exercise, application of beta2-agonists, coughing, and vibration maneuvers. The imbalance between the viscoelastic qualities of mucus and cilliary movement will provoke a stasis of secretions. It is generally assumed that secretion stasis contributes to the obstruction of the lower airway and predisposes the development of lung infections.

In respiratory disease conditions, there is an exponential increase in the production of bronchial secretions. When the mucus gel coat is more than 5 μm thick, the action of the mucociliary chain will be surpassed (Fig. 63.1). Coughing is not effective beyond the seventh bronchial generation. Under these conditions, forced expiratory flows of turbulent characteristics are truly responsible for the draining secretions of the proximal airway. By performing a forced expiration, a point of equal pressure is produced in the airway, which suffers a dynamic compression, creating a choke point, which moves in the distal direction. This dynamic compression produces in

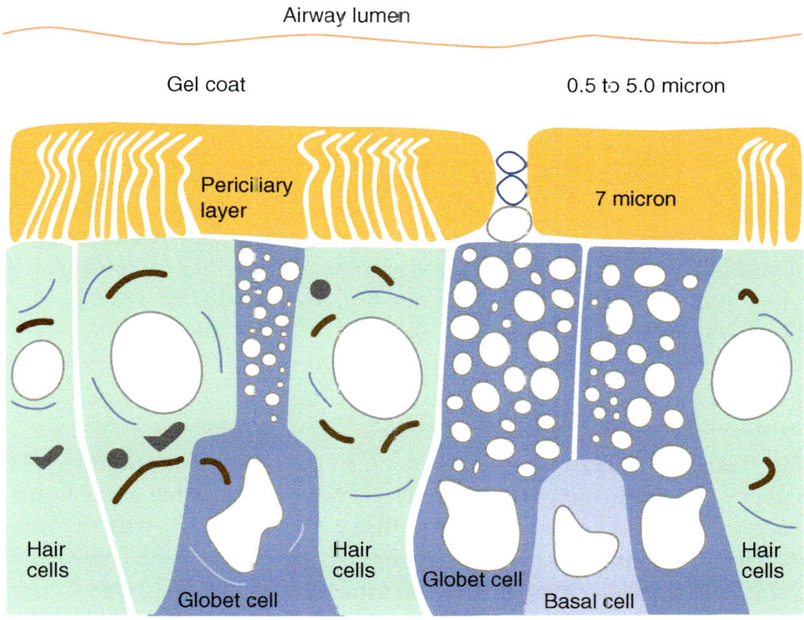

Fig. 63.1 Airway epithelium

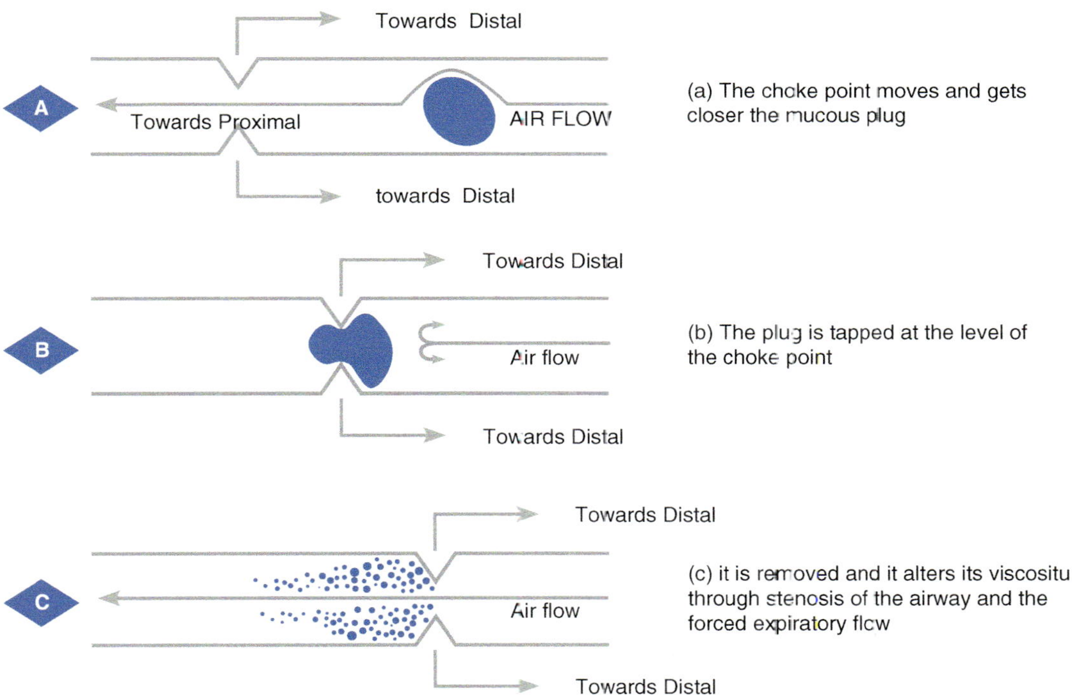

Fig. 63.2 Forced expiration and choke point. (**a**) The choke point moves and gets closer to the mucous plug. (**b**) The plug is tapped at the level of the choke point. (**c**) It is removed and it alters its viscosity through stenosis of the airway and the forced expiratory flow

turn an increase of the local expiratory flow that displaces in a proximal direction, favoring the closeness of the mucous plugs with the choke point, which will in the end allow the fragmented displacement of the bronchial secretions toward the central airways (Fig. 63.2).

At more distal levels, the two-phase flow (interaction between the airflow and the mucus layer over the ciliary epithelium) has a central role in the hygiene of the middle airways, and even the more peripheral ones. It has been described that at this level, slow and prolonged expiratory flows that aim to obtain flows with laminar characteristics enhance the natural action of the two-phase flow, producing a significant effect in the mobilization of secretions from the distal airways to the proximal airways.

Considering that airway compromise is not homogeneous, it is very important to focus on the compromised area by auscultation, as well as setting therapeutic objectives in proportion to the findings, to be able to choose the correct technique that results in the most benefit for the patient.

When there are areas with loss of air content (e.g., atelectasis), techniques that contribute to increase the inspired volume should be favored, to recruit collapsed zones. It is necessary to stress that lung recruitment will also favor the permeabilization of the middle airway and even the distal one, because there will be a higher lung volume that will allow an increment of the expired volume, which will favor the depurative action of the two-phase flow.

Therapeutic Intervention

In daily practice and as a sequential order to make decisions for choosing respiratory physical therapy techniques that apply to each patient, we propose the following action flow. This flow should be discerned after having evaluated the patient.

1. Determine the physiopathological disorder
2. Identify the degree of collaboration from the patient
3. Establish the level of compromise

1. *Physiopathological disorder*: Refers to the identification of a determined ventilation function syndrome (obstructive, restrictive or mixed) present at the moment of the evaluation of the patient. The obstructive physiopathological disorder is characterized by the decrease of the diameter of the central or peripheral airways, with an increment of the airflow resistance and flow decrease, especially expiratory flows, which will result in a significant increase in the work of breathing and the following hypoxemia (partial breathing insufficiency) and even hypercarbia (global breathing insufficiency) in some severe cases, such as in acute severe bronchiolitis.

   The restrictive physiopathological disorder encompasses a group of diseases in which the most important physiopathological disorder is a restriction of expansion that limits the pulmonary volumes, with the consequent possibility of losing recruited alveolar units, as in atelectasis.

   In any type of functional disorder there is a possibility of loss of effectiveness of coughing, which will result in higher secretion retention and the possibility of creating a feedback loop that will determine the recovery of the functional level of the child.

   Apart from determining the physiopathological disorder the patient presents, the severity of the compromise must be established, e.g., mild, moderate or severe obstruction.

2. *Level of cooperation*: It refers to the level of potential cooperation of the patient inasmuch as they can follow the instructions of the physiotherapist when a particular technique is being performed. One classification is the cooperative patient is able to follow instructions of the treating therapist, to cooperate, help and perform active and assisted-active techniques without problems. On the other hand, it is the uncooperative patient who doesn't have the physical, cognitive or psychomotor abilities to follow the instructions of the physiotherapist to perform a certain technique.
3. *Level of compromise*: It has to do with the zone of the respiratory system affected by the physiopathological or biomechanical disorder, which may be the thoracic cavity, respiratory musculature, lung parenchyma, or the proximal, mid or distal airway. Each one of

these levels has different functions regarding thoracic mobility, ventilation, conduction, and air conditioning.

Techniques of Respiratory Physical Therapy

The techniques of respiratory physical therapy can be classified into two main groups: manual and instrumented.

Manual Physical Therapy Techniques

- *Thoracic vibration*: Oscillatory movement produced by the isometric muscle contraction of the upper limbs which is transmitted by one or both hands of the therapist to the chest of the patient during expiration. The oscillation frequency must not be less than 3 Hz. The goal is to obtain a maximum expiratory flow at least 10% more than the maximum inspiratory flow, which would allow increasing the two-phase flow and loosen and decrease the viscosity of the secretions of the bronchial walls, allowing their mobilization to proximal airways.
- *Thoracic percussion (clapping)*: Rhythmic tapping performed with cupped hands on the ventral, dorsal, and lateral zones of the chest in both phases of breathing. It is generally applied while the patient maintains a specific position of postural drainage. It is contraindicated under clinical evidence of bronchospasm. Both vibrations and percussions have the goal of generating an oscillatory effect of the chest wall that will be transmitted to the lungs and airways, aimed at increasing ciliary activity and loosening and mobilizing secretions adhered to the bronchial wall, which would depend of the value of the oscillation frequency transmitted through the thorax. This frequency is close to 15–25 Hz, but it is limited in these manual techniques that only reach 2–8 Hz frequencies.
- *Postural drainage*: Consists in easing secretion transport through the action that gravity has on them. In order to obtain this, it is necessary to place the bronchial segment to drain as vertical as possible; placing the patient in different positions, many of them will be Trendelenburg positions. It is traditionally advised to simultaneously apply percussions and vibrations while the postures are sustained. One of its main limitations is the appearance of adverse effects associated with technique execution (gastroesophageal reflux, desaturation, or elevation of intracranial pressure).
- *Forced Expiration Technique*: The forced expiration technique (FET) consists in making forced expirations with open an open glottis starting with different lung volumes:

Low, mid, and high, interspersed with still breathing at tidal volume. The aim is to mobilize the bronchial secretions to the central airway where they can be swallowed or expectorated. In the specialized literature in English it is also known as the Huffing technique, and it is justified from the physiological concept of point of equal pressure and must be applied cautiously in chronic patients (e.g., cystic fibrosis) where stability of the bronchial walls is so altered that compression during the application of this technique results in the collapse of the airway and the following impact of secretions at a distal level of the collapse. This collapse warrants the avoidance of the forced expiration technique in these patients or its use only later in the bronchial hygiene process, when the secretions have been mobilized to the central airways.These four techniques are considered conventional chest physiotherapy. The techniques described below are considered nonconventional chest physiotherapy.

- *Prolonged slow expiration*: Passive technique of expiratory aid applied to the uncooperative patient (from infancy to 8 years), through slow manual thoraco-abdominal pressure that starts at the end of a spontaneous expiration and continues toward a residual volume. Its aim is to obtain a greater expiratory volume than in a normal expiration, to promote the two-phase low and thus contribute to the mobilization of secretions in the periphery of the respiratory tree to the central airway.

- *Autogenic draining*: This technique for the cooperative patient combines slow inspiratory and expiratory flows with forced expirations and coughs in a three-phase sequential cycle:
  - *First phase, loosening of secretions*: Slow inspirations/expirations must be performed, with breathing located in the diaphragm, mobilizing small volumes from the functional residual capacity to later gradually increase the inspiratory and expiratory volume, achieving a gradually increased pulmonary capacity, with the aim of unsticking and mobilizing secretions from the periphery to the central airway.
  - *Second phase, collection of secretions*: In higher volumes than the normal current volume, but maintaining slow expiratory flows, the secretions are accumulated in the central airways.
  - *Third phase, evacuation*: Three to four expirations are performed until the total pulmonary capacity is reached, to conclude with a forced expiration with open glottis or a voluntary cough.
- *Slow expiration with glottis opened in lateral posture* (*ELTGOL*): It is an active–assisted technique, in which the patient is in the lateral decubitus position with the lung to be treated specifically in the support plane (dependent) and thus making the superolateral lung and the mediastinum help with is maximum exsufflation during expiration. Owing to the position adopted, the pressure of the abdominal viscera will raise the diaphragm of the support lung. In this position, with an open mouth (or kept open by a cylindrical mouth accessory), the physiotherapist presses the abdomen with one hand at the level of the lung and eases the rise of the diaphragm, and applies pressure with the other hand on the superolateral chest wall, producing a pressure against the contralateral shoulder which will ease the reduction of the transversal diameter that favors a complete exsufflation of the inferolateral lung, always controlling that the expiration is slow and prolonged. Applying the maneuver in a slow manner avoids bronchial collapsing and allows a greater displacement of the inferolateral diaphragm toward the proximal end. The narrowing of the bronchial lumen in the inferolateral lung and the increase of its ventilation, due to the adopted position, creates a higher friction of particles of air over mucus (two-phase flow) and thus favors its movement toward the proximal end.

The aim of this technique is to loosen and move the bronchial secretions from the mid and distal zones of the respiratory tree to move them toward the proximal ways to be eliminated with the forced expiration technique. It is useful in patients of 8 years of age or older, since the child starts to present the inferolateral respiratory pattern that is preferred and characteristic in an adult.

- *Active respiratory cycle*: It is a technique that combines the voluntary ventilatory exercises with forced expiration techniques. Its aim is to mobilize and remove the bronchial secretions.

  It has three phases:
  - *First phase, breath control exercises*: It starts with soft respiratory cycles, at tidal volume that directs the movement to the lower part of the chest, relaxing the muscles of the upper thorax.
  - *Second phase, thoracic expansion exercises*: The patient performs deep nose inspirations with thorax elevation, followed by a slow and prolonged expiration. These respiratory movements are performed four to six consecutive times, taking care not to provoke hyperventilation that could generate respiratory alkalosis.
  - *Third phase, forced expiration technique*: Breath control exercises and forced expirations are performed again with low volumes and an open glottis, followed by deep inspiration followed by cough or a high volume forced expiration that enables one to swallow or expectorate secretions.

- *Controlled inspiratory flow exercise*: It is an active–passive technique, where the patient is in the lateral decubitus position, with the area to be treated in the superolateral position. Slow inspiratory exercises with a low flow and high volume, stopping when the inspiration ends. The exercises of controlled inspiratory flow in the lateral decubitus position take advantage of the effect of the passive expansion of the more peripheral air spaces that result from the relative hyperinflation of the superolateral lung and the increase of the transversal diameter of the chest, which results from the patient's position and profound and sustained inspiration.
- *Huffing*: Series of slow and tiered inspirations, starting from residual functional capacity until total lung capacity, including a pause at the end of the inspiration.
- *Thoracic compression*: Manual pressure on the chest during the inspiration phase. Its objective is to increase volume and exhaled volume.
- *Thoracic decompression*: Maneuver performed after an expiratory compression, which corresponds to the sudden removal of the hands of the therapist from the chest of the patient at the beginning of the inspiratory phase.
- *Thoracic blockage*: Manual pressure that is applied in a region of the chest attempting to restrict its expansion through several respiratory cycles, aiming to direct the air volume to the unblocked, affected contralateral zone.
- *Manual techniques to assist coughing*: The efficacy of coughing is related directly to the inspiratory volume before the expulsive maneuver is performed.
  - *Induced cough (TP):* It is performed in the uncooperative patient and it consists in the stimulation of the mechanic receptors of the cough reflex in the extrathoracic trachea, at the level of the sternal notch, to be able to increase the air volume expired when the cough is inefficient or it is not spontaneously produced.
  - *Assisted cough* (TA): It consists in placing the therapist's hands in the chest of the patient and asking for a deep inspiration followed by a forced expiration, and then asking for a cough. At the same time, abdominal pressure, or thoracic vibropressure that goes together with the acceleration of the expiratory flow generated by the cough.
  - *Glossopharyngeal breathing* (RGF): Described in 1951 by Clarence Dail, this technique acts on the inspiratory phase of the cough. It consists in taking multiple insufflations through movements of the mouth, cheeks, tongue and larynx to be able to "swallow air" that is sent to the lungs. The objective is substituting the weak respiratory musculature by the action of the oropharyngeal musculature. In order for the technique to be effective, glottis must be intact; patient must cooperate, and the patient must learn the maneuver well. To get a final volume over the tidal volume, each insufflation must consist of at least 80 ml.
  - *Air stacking* (AS): The classic technique describes a manual reanimation bag, a unidirectional bag, a 20–30 cm corrugated, and a nose pin if there is an air leakage. This technique acts during the inspiratory phase and it provides multiple inflations of air through a bag of manual reanimation, aiming to reach the maximum inspiratory capacity. This technique increases the inspired volume and replaces the periodic inflations (sighs), also contributing to improve thoracic mobility and to prevent atelectasis. It is reported as being most efficacious in patients with neuromuscular conditions and medullar lesions with certain degree of cooperation.

Instrumental Physical Therapy Techniques

They can be subdivided in mechanical devices of lung expansion, mechanical and electromechanical devices of bronchial hygiene, and mechanical devices to assist coughing.

Mechanical Lung Expansion Devices

- *Incentive Spirometers*: These are devices that, through slow and deep inspirations, aim to prevent or treat alterations in which the lung volume is compromised by using a visual incentive that gives feedback to the patient during the inspiratory effort which must be performed with a pause of at least 3 seconds at the end of the inspiration. Volume incentive spirometers are used (Voldyne® and Coach®) from 500 to 5000 ml or flow meters (Triflo II®, CliniFLO®) from 100 to 1200 ml/sec.

  Some models have a connection for additional oxygen. The main objective is to recover the functional residual capacity and re-expand the collapsed zones through the increase of the transpulmonary pressure, increase of the inspiratory capacity, and simulations of the effects of the physiological sigh that could contribute to the prevention or treatment of atelectasis caused by a diaphragmatic malfunction. They are normally indicated for thoracic and high abdomen surgeries, prolonged immobility, especially in patients with chronic respiratory disease and neuromuscular conditions.

Mechanical Devices for Bronchial Hygiene

- *Expiratory positive-pressure systems*: They are devices that, at the mouth level and during the active expiration of the patient, produce a stop in the expiration that generates a positive pressure that is transmitted to the airway and aims to avoid or delay the premature closure (collapsing) of the airway, which is a common occurrence in chronic diseases like cystic fibrosis and that we technically know as the dynamic compression of the airways. This early closure prevents an effective movement and elimination of the bronchial secretions, among other negative effects. With the application of positive expiratory pressure, the expiratory time is prolonged, the collateral ventilation increases and the early closure of the airways is minimized. There are mainly two types of expiratory positive-pressure instruments: The ones using continuous expiratory positive pressure, and the ones using oscillatory or discontinuous expiratory positive pressure.
- *Continuous expiratory positive-pressure systems*: As indicated by the name, the positive pressure that is produced in the airway is continued during the expiratory phase. They were initially developed in Denmark in the 1970s. There are many models in the market (PEPmask®; TheraPEP®; PiPEP®; PariPEP®; AeroPEP®) and all of them have a unidirectional valve connected to an adjustable piece, with many holes of different sizes where a resistance or stop to the expiration is generated. The smaller the hole, the higher the resistance and greater the positive expiratory pressure in the airway of the patient.

A pressure gauge in the system allows the monitoring of the pressure applied by each one of the holes and it is generally established between 10 and 20 cm H_2O. There is a small difference in the device ThresholdPEP® where the resistance is generated by the tension of an adjustable spring which is incorporated in the device.

- *Oscillatory or discontinuous expiratory positive pressure*: Initially developed in Switzerland, the devices with the most bibliographical support are Flutter®VRP1, Acapella®, and Cornet®, capable of producing an oscillating expiratory resistance that generates retrograde vibration waves in the airway. The aim is modifying the viscoelastic properties of the Bronchial mucus and maintaining the beneficial characteristics of the expiratory positive pressure described above. The Flutter®VRP1 is a pipe-shaped device formed by a mouthpiece, a plastic cone, a steel sphere, and a pierced lid. During expiration, the airway suffers internal vibrations provoked by the vibrations of the expired air and the changes in pressure inside the bronchi. The inclination angle of the Flutter®VRP1 will modify the resistance to the movement of the steel sphere and, with it, the generated expiratory pressure. The optimal work inclination is 30° to obtain an oscillatory pressure between 12 and 75 cm H_2O and an oscillation frequency between 15 and 32 Hz.

The *Acapella*® has in it a magnetized lever that intermittently closes a cone inside the dispositive during the expiration. This produces a positive expiratory pressure and makes an oscillating expiratory flow. On the other side of the device, a revolving part allows the regulation of the magnetized lever mechanism and thus the higher or lower resistance. There are four Acapella® models (Blue DM®, Green DH®, Choice®, and Duet®). The *Acapella*® models, unlike the Flutter®VRP1, have the advantage of being usable in any position (standing, sitting, lying down).

The RC Cornet® is a device with a horn shape, and it has a mouthpiece fixed to a curved tube that has rubber on the inside. The rubber on the inside of the horn produces the vibration in the airways when the patient blows through it.

The RC Cornet® offers less resistance than the Flutter®VRP1, and unlike it, it can be used in any position.

Bronchial Hygiene Electromechanical Devices

These are devices that use a source of electrical power to function.

- *High frequency oscillatory compression of the thoracic wall*: A generator of air pulses transmits compression/oscillation forces to an inflatable vest that is firmly adjusted over the thorax and offers externally oscillatory compressions to the thoracic wall with a frequency between 5 and 25 Hz. The mechanism of action can be explained by the increase of the airflow and the production of drag forces similar to the ones produced by coughing. The vibrations can also reduce the viscoelastic properties of the secretions. The manufacturers recommend 1–2 daily sessions of 20–30 minutes each. There are many models in the marked adapted to age (Vest Airway Clearance System®; Afllo Vest®; Respin 11® Bronchial Clearance System; SmartVest®; InCourage® System).
- *Intrapulmonary percussion–vibration*: The device is made up of a high-pressure flux generator, a valve to interrupt the flux and a breathing circuit with a nebulizer that can be connected simultaneously to the mouthpiece to inhale sprays. The device produces a two-phase vibration in the inspiration and expiration, with positive pressure that is overlapped by the breathing pattern of the individual. The small high frequency air pulses (50–150 cycles/min) that lead to an internal vibration of the airways, together with the oscillating expiatory pressure, aim to recruit collapsed units and increase the transport and elimination of proximal secretions. Their use must be avoided in patients with osteopenia or osteoporosis, uncontrolled chest pain, costal fractures, or coagulopathies, and it must not be used directly over implanted devices such as gastrostomies. There are many models in the market adapted to the age of the patient (Flimm- Fighter Percussor®; G5 Neocussor®; Fluid Flo 2500®; Electro Flo 5000®).

Mechanical Devices for Cough Assistance

Today there are many devices (Cough Assist In-exsufflator®, New Respironics T70 Cough Assist®, Pegaso® , and Nippy Clearway Cough Assistor®) that allow the mechanical improvement of the inspiratory or expiratory phases of coughing, either passively or with the collaboration of the patient.

- *Inflator–exsufflator*: A mechanical device provides a deep insufflation, followed by a forced exhalation, simulating a natural cough. This insufflation is generated by a device that provides positive pressure when inspiring and negative pressure when expiring (suction effect) of at least +40 to −40 cm H_2O. This mechanical device can be connected to the patient through an oral or nasobuccal interface or through a tracheotomy. Some authors have suggested that the use of mechanical cough assistance can diminish or avoid the need of secretion suctioning in patients with neuromuscular conditions, because the maximum coughing flow obtained is enough to eliminate them, avoiding the negative effects of repeated vacuuming in the airway mucosa. Finally, these devices are not available to all professionals, due to their high cost. However, it can be used with multiple patients if the strict circuit cleaning and sterilization standards are followed, in a similar way as is applied to the mechanical ventilation devices.

Conclusions

The physiotherapist who works in respiratory care must have a good knowledge of physiology, biomechanics, and physiopathology of the thoraco-pulmonary system, in addition to a thorough expertise in respiratory semiology. It must be noted that each patient has their own characteristics (genetic, anatomical-physiological, psycho-emotional, environmental, cultural influences, etc.), which will pose more than one goal and will require a combination of techniques regarding the condition and clinical evolution of the patient. The respiratory physical therapy techniques are adapted to the commitment level of the bronchial structure and lung parenchyma. To perform such techniques, it is vitally important to know and to correctly apply an optimal modulation of the inspiratory and expiratory flows and an adequate redistribution of the lung volumes.

Acknowledgement Acknowledgements to professors Jordi Vilaró C. (Universidad Blanquerna, Spain) and Rodrigo Torres-Castro (Universidad de Chile) for their valuable suggestions to the final writing of this chapter and to Rodrigo Gajardo R. for the drawings included in it.

Sources

Agostini P, Singh S. Incentive spirometry following thoracic surgery: what should we be doing? Physiotherapy. 2009;95(2):76–82.

Alves LA, Pitta F, Brunetto AF. Performance analysis of the Flutter VRP 1 under different flows and angles. Respir Care. 2008;53(3):316–23.

Bach JR. Mechanical insufflation-exsufflation. Comparison of peak expiratory flows with manually assisted and unassisted coughing techniques. Chest. 1993;104(5):1553–62.

Bach JR, Bianchi C, Vidigal-Lopes M, Turi S, Felisari G. Lung inflation by glossopharyngeal breathing and "air stacking" in Duchenne muscular dystrophy. Am J Phys Med Rehabil. 2007;86(4):295–300.

Del Corral T, Herrero B, Muñoz G, Ríos A. Técnicas manuales para el drenaje de secreciones bronquiales: técnicas espiratorias lentas. En: Manual de procedimientos SEPAR: técnicas manuales e instrumentales para el drenaje de secreciones bronquiales en el paciente adulto. Martí JD y Vendrell M, coords. Barcelona: Ed. Respira-Fundación Española del Pulmón-SEPAR; 2013.

Fahy JV, Dickey BF. Airway mucus function and dysfunction. N Engl J Med. 2010;363(23):2233–47.

Fink JB. Forced expiratory technique, directed cough, and autogenic drainage. Respir Care. 2007;52:1210–21.

Guía Clínica AUGE: infección respiratoria baja de manejo ambulatorio en menores de 5 años. Serie Guías Clínicas, Ministerio de Salud de Chile. 2013. https://www.minsal.cl/portal/url/item/7220fdc434124 4a9e04001011f0113b9.pdf

Gomes E, Postiaux G, Medeiros D, Monteiro K, Sampaio L, Costa D, et al. Rev Bras Fisioter. 2012;16(3):241–7.

Hidalgo G, Puppo H, Romero J. Kinesiterapia respiratoria. En: Enfermedades respiratorias en pediatría. Herrera O y Quezada A. Santiago/Buenos Aires: Ed. Mediterráneo; 2012.

Iñiguez F, Sánchez I. Desarrollo pulmonar: diferencias anatómicas y funcionales entre el lactante y el adulto. En: Enfoque clínico de las enfermedades respiratorias del niño. Santiago: Ed. Universidad Católica; 2007.

Kim CS, Iglesias AJ, Sackner MA. Mucus clearance by twophase gas–liquid flow mechanism: asymmetric periodic flow model. J Appl Physiol. 1987;62:959–71.

McCarren B, Alison JA. Phyiological effects of vibration in subjects with cystic fibrosis. Eur Respir J. 2006;27:1204–9.

Myers TR. Positive expiratory pressure and oscillatory positive expiratory pressure therapies. Respir Care. 2007;52(10):1308–26.

Oberwaldner B. Physiotherapy for airway clearance in paediatrics. Eur Respir J. 2000;15:196–204.

Postiaux G. Principales técnicas de fisioterapia de limpieza broncopulmonar en pediatría. En: Fisioterapia respiratoria del niño. Madrid: Ed. McGraw-Hill e Interamericana; 2000.

Postiaux G, Louis J, Labasse H, Gerroldt J, Kotik A, Lemuhot A, Patte C. Evaluation of an alternative chest physiotherapy method in infants with respiratory syncytial virus bronchiolitis. Respir Care. 2011;56(7):989–94.

Postiaux G, Zwaenepoel B, Louis J. Chest physical therapy in acute viral bronchiolitis: an update review. Respir Care. 2013;58(9):1541–5.

Pryor JA, Webber BA, Hodson ME, Batten JC. Evaluation of the forced expiration technique as an adjunct to

postural drainage in treatment of cystic fibrosis. Br Med J. 1979;2(6187):417–8.
Schechter MS. Airway clearance applications in infants and children. Respir Care. 2007;52(10):1382–90.
Torres-Castro R, Monge G, Vera R, Puppo H, Céspedes J, Vilaró J. Estrategias terapéuticas para aumentar la eficacia de la tos en pacientes con enfermedades neuromusculares. Rev Méd Chil. 2014;142(2):238–45.
Trebbia G, Lacombe M, Fermanian C, Falaize L, Lejaille M, Louis A, et al. Cough determinants in patients with neuromuscular disease. Respir Physiol Neurobiol. 2005;146(2–3):291–300.
Van der Schans CP. Bronchial mucus transport. Respir Care. 2007;52(9):1150–6.
Van der Schans CP. Conventional chest physical therapy for obstructive lung disease. Respir Care. 2007;52(9):1198–206.
Weibel ER. What makes a good lung? Swiss Med Wkly. 2009;139(27):375–86.

Pulmonary Rehabilitation in Children with Chronic Respiratory Diseases

64

Rodrigo Torres Castro, Homero Puppo Gallardo, and Daniel Zenteno Araos

Contents

Definition

Pulmonary rehabilitation is a comprehensive intervention based on a thorough evaluation of the patient followed by personalized therapies, which include muscle training, education, psychosocial intervention, and changes in life habits, in order to improve the physical and psychological condition of people with chronic respiratory disease, as well as promoting adherence to healthy behaviors that improve their quality of life in the long term.

R. Torres Castro · H. Puppo Gallardo
Respiratory Kinesiology, Faculty of Medicine, Universidad de Chile, Santiago, Chile

D. Zenteno Araos (✉)
Department of Pediatrics, Universidad de Concepción, Concepción, Chile

The team in charge of the pulmonary rehabilitation program should ideally be composed of a pediatric pulmonologist, chest physiotherapist, nurse, occupational therapist, nutritionist, psychologist, speech therapist, and a social worker. In addition, specialists, such as psychiatrist, neurologist, and others, that are necessary to meet the requirements of each child should also be included.

Goals of a Pulmonary Rehabilitation Program

The goals should be focused on reducing symptoms and exacerbations, increasing tolerance to exercise and increasing participation in educational, recreational, and social activities, with the corresponding increase in quality of life.

P. Bertrand, I. Sánchez (eds.), *Pediatric Respiratory Diseases*, https://doi.org/10.1007/978-3-030-26961-6_64

Parts of a Pulmonary Rehabilitation Program

To carry out a pulmonary rehabilitation program, the professional team needs to develop three components: evaluation, treatment, and education.

Assessment

General Physical Ability Assessment

Owing to the systemic nature of chronic respiratory diseases, it is necessary to assess the physical ability to perform daily activities. This assessment includes specific laboratory tests, which are less accessible, and field tests, which usually do not require large equipment and are easier to perform (Table 64.1).

Six-Minute Walk Test (6MWT)

This field test is used to assess the ability of a subject to perform physical exercise and is considered a submaximal exercise test, since it does not reach a maximum level of oxygen consumption. It has a wide acceptance by patients: well tolerated and easy to perform. It has been validated in children as well as in healthy people and people with chronic respiratory diseases.

To carry out the test, an ideally roofed place is needed, which must have a corridor of 30 meters long, with cones located 50 centimeters before each end, where the child can walk for 6 minutes. The circuit must have visible marks every 3 meters and at least 2 seats on the way in case the child wants to stop. In case the child stops, this should be recorded, but the test is completed when reaching 6 minutes. Before starting, the child should be at rest for at least 10 minutes and have proper clothing for physical exercise.

It is important to stress that for dyspnea assessment a Borg scale, especially modified for pediatric population, should be used (Fig. 64.1). One of the most important parameters to register is lower limbs fatigue, because chronic respiratory diseases condition a multisystemic compromise, so the cause of stops is not dyspnea but alteration

Table 64.1 Evaluation tests of a pulmonary rehabilitation program

General physical ability	Respiratory muscles
1. Exercise tolerance test	1. Respiratory muscle strength
Six-minute walk test Constant workload exercise test	Maximum inspiratory pressure Maximum expiratory pressure
2. Determining the training load or symptoms that limit exercise	2. Respiratory muscle endurance
Incremental shuttle walking test Maximal incremental exercise test	Sustained maximal inspiratory pressure Time limit

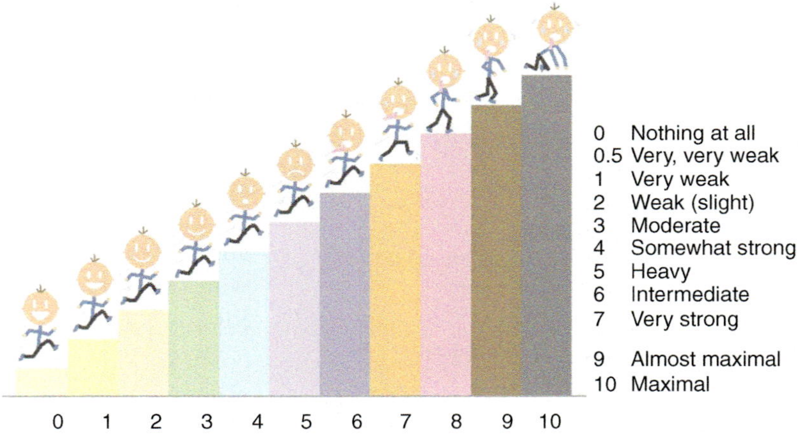

Fig. 64.1 Modified Borg scale for dyspnea

Table 64.2 Six-minute walk (6MWT) test reference values

	6 years	7 years	8 years	9 years	10 years	11 years	12 years	13 years	14 years
Women	562.5 ± 39.1	568.2 ± 31.6	556.5 ± 48.9[a]	575.7 ± 53.2	585.7 ± 28.7	605.7 ± 60.3	629.4 ± 20.3	631.4 ± 50.2[a]	638.5 ± 20.9
Man	562 ± 43.1	597.11 ± 33.6	605.8 ± 62.2[a]	611.4 ± 47	618.7 ± 67.5	608.7 ± 35.9	636.1 ± 47.3	673.9 ± 45[a]	674.3 ± 54.2
Total	562.3 ± 39.8	580.9 ± 34.7	580.1 ± 59.9	587.6 ± 52.8	603.7 ± 55	607.8 ± 47.3	633 ± 36.8	650.3 ± 51.8	657.2 ± 44.7

Source: Rev Med Chile 2012; 140: 1014 Creative Commons Licence 4.0
[a]$p < 0.05$

of glycolytic mechanisms that decrease the fatigability threshold.

The most important factor to be determined in the test is the distance walked, which must be compared with reference values. In Chile, for the pediatric population, we recommend the use of values of Gatica et al. (Table 64.2). The final report should consider the distance that was walked, the lower limit of the ideal distance, and the percentage of the distance that was walked over the lower limit of the ideal distance.

Shuttle Walking Test (SWT)

Described in 1992 by Singh et al. for chronic obstructive pulmonary disease, it is an incremental load test in which the participant must walk between two markers located in a corridor 10 meters long after an auditory signal. As time passes, speed increases, so the time between each sound stimulus is reduced.

It provides very useful information because, from the oxygen consumption standpoint, it creates a condition similar to an incremental load test with a cycle ergometer.

For its implementation, a 10-meter corridor, in which cones must be placed 50 centimeters from each end, is needed. The distance from one end to the other will be considered a shuttle. In addition, it is necessary to have standardized audio, which is divided into two types of signals. One beep is used to indicate the start of the walking and 3 beeps are used to indicate change in speed. The initial walking speed is 0.5 m/sec and it increases by 0.17 m/sec in each of the 12 levels until reaching a maximum speed of 2.37 m/sec. It presents a moderate correlation with 6MWT ($r = 0.68$). The test is finished when the participant is not able to complete the shuttle for a second consecutive time or when has fatigue symptoms or dyspnea that prevent him from continuing.

The values to be recorded are the walked distance and the last level of shuttle completed, which corresponds to the maximum speed reached.

Cardiopumonary Exercise Testing (CPET)

Cardiopulmonary exercise testing is a laboratory test that measures workload during exercise and analyzes the physiological components of oxygen consumption. In addition, it allows the identification of the mechanisms that limit the ability to exercise: respiratory, cardiovascular, or metabolic. Owing to its high reproducibility and repeatability, it is the gold standard of exercise tests. It can be performed on most children from 6 years old. Its utility lies in establishing the maximum training load and detecting which symptoms limit the maximum exercise.

Cardiopulmonary exercise testing must be performed in a pulmonary function lab and be carried out by trained personnel, with knowledge of exercise physiology and cardiopulmonary resuscitation. It can be done on a treadmill or cycle ergometer. The treadmill is mainly used in children with a size less than 120 cm who cannot reach the pedals of a traditional cycle ergometer.

There are several incremental protocols; among them, modified Balke or Harbord.

(a) *Constant load exercise test*

Another way to assess physical resistance of a patient with chronic respiratory disease is the constant load exercise test. This test consists of exposing the patient to a high and constant evaluation load (70–80%), and thus measuring the amount of time the patient is able to maintain the effort before stopping. In general, this is the most susceptible test to be modified after a pulmonary rehabilitation protocol that includes general physical training.

Assessment of the Respiratory Muscles

Respiratory muscles, as the skeletal muscles, from the standpoint of their morphology and functioning, are striated muscles, so they can be evaluated in both their strength and resistance.

Some children with chronic respiratory diseases have weak respiratory muscles. Although the diaphragm muscle is the main breathing motor, these children often resort to the use of accessory muscles to supplement the action of the diaphragm subjected to high respiratory workloads.

Therefore, an objective assessment of the strength and resistance of the respiratory muscles should be made, particularly in children with neuromuscular diseases in which the decrease in inspiratory muscle strength is the first indicator when there is compromise of the ventilatory pump, even before the reduction of forced vital capacity.

Assessment of the Inspiratory and Expiratory Muscle Strength

The assessment of the inspiratory and expiratory muscle strength can be done through measuring respiratory pressures at the mouth, which is a non-invasive method of assessment of strength, easy to perform and inexpensive. From this evaluation, maximum inspiratory pressure (MIP, through the Müller maneuver) and maximum expiratory pressure (MEP, through the Valsalva maneuver) can be determined.

To perform the maneuver, two operators are needed (Fig. 64.2), the main one with extensive experience. The assistant will stand behind the patient and will have to compress his cheeks to avoid the action of both buccinator muscles and any possible leak through the corners of the mouth. To perform the MIP maneuver, the child must be seated with both feet on the ground and the main operator in front of him. As it is not a familiar maneuver, a careful explanation must be

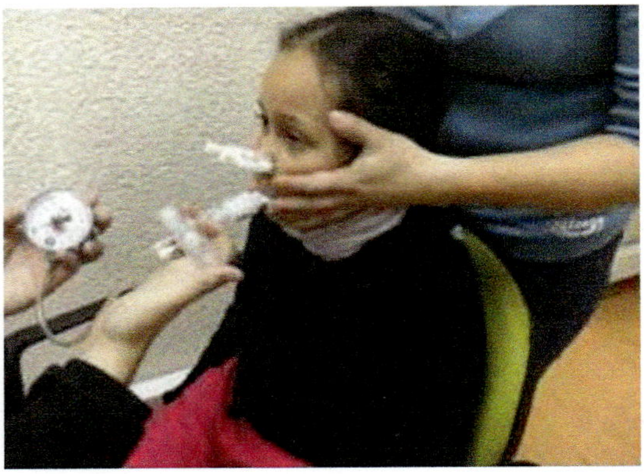

Fig. 64.2 Evaluation of Respiratory Muscle Strength (MIP/MEP)

given of what is sought and the characteristics of the orders that will be taught. A nozzle is then introduced into the mouth which is connected to a 3-way valve that has a 2 mm diameter hole (to avoid glottic closure during MIP and the involvement of the face muscles in MEP), which is attached to an aneroid manometer. The child is asked to breathe two or three times normally so that after starting from a maximum expiration, close to the residual volume, the main operator blocks the inspiratory branch of the 3-step valve and requests, with an energetic order, that the child make an inspiration as strong and maintained as possible (lasting at least 1–2 seconds). The child must be able to perform the maneuver in a repeatable way three times with a difference of less than 10%. If he does not get a good maneuver on the eighth try, he should be scheduled for another day. The MEP maneuver is performed in the same position (with the same connection but with a positive pressure gauge) and with similar initial orders of the MIP, although after an inspiration up to total lung capacity, requesting a maximum expiration of at least 2 seconds long.

The final report should consider: reference values used, values of the best MIP and MEP measured, average ideal values and lower limits to be reached, and percentage of MIP and MEP obtained concerning lower limits of the reference values used.

It is recommended to use the reference values of Szeinberg et al.,

(b) *Assessment of inspiratory muscle endurance*

Endurance of the inspiratory muscles can be evaluated through the ventilatory endurance test or the test based on the ability of these muscles to create sustained high-pressure levels.

- *Sustained maximal inspiratory pressure (SMIP)*: It is an incremental load test described by Nickerson and Keens, and has proven to be the most reproducible and best tolerated test. It is performed asking a child to breathe through an external threshold-type device, in which every 2 minutes the resistance increases between 5% and 10% (of the previously obtained MIP) until reaching the maximum load that the subject is capable of sustaining for two full minutes, and the maximal inspiratory pressure that is capable of being created during that period (sustained maximal inspiratory pressure, SMIP). Once the value of the SMIP is obtained, it must be related to the child's PIM. It has been established that a SMIP/MIP index must be higher than 65% to determine that the respiratory muscles have a proper resistance. Minor values may determine that the child is a candidate for specific training of his respiratory muscles.
- *Time limit test*: It is a constant load test in which the child must breathe as long as possible against a constant resistance that leads to fatigue. Use of high loads (over 60–80%) is recommended, although in patients with neuromuscular diseases (especially Duchenne muscular dystrophy) the use of low loads (35–40%) is recommended. The value to be recorded as result is the total time (in seconds) of the test duration.

Treatment

General Physical Training

Sustained activity of the skeletal muscles, with a set up intensity and duration, produces adaptive changes in their structure and in their performance. Physical training is a fundamental part of a pulmonary rehabilitation program. We define training as a process through which organs and systems are stimulated, periodically and systematically, in order to obtain a specific response dependent on the stimulus applied. The fundamental principles of muscle training are: progressive overload, specificity, and reversibility. In addition, the subject's initial physical capacity must always be taken into account. The professional who prescribes the exercise, supervises it, and applies it should be highly trained in exercise physiology, indications, and muscular training programming, knowing its beneficial and harmful effects.

In adults, there is ample evidence of the effectiveness of aerobic training programs. However, in pediatrics, only cystic fibrosis has produced an increasing number of publications with training protocols that have shown positive results for the different parameters evaluated. Vigorous physical activity increases exercise tolerance in children with cystic fibrosis, increases work capacity, improves cardiorespiratory fitness, respiratory and peripheral muscles endurance, and contributes to improve immune function. Recently, in a nine-year follow-up, it was demonstrated that high levels of physical activity in subjects with CF are associated with a lower decline in lung function measured through FEV1.

The best results have been obtained in supervised programs. Other programs that included swimming, cycling, and trampoline showed positive effects on exercise tolerance, work capacity, and improvement in physical capability, lower extremity strength, sputum production, dyspnea, and pulmonary function.

Among children with asthma, the vast majority should have a physical performance similar to normal subjects. The fact that asthma patients have physical deconditioning and a sedentary life would be given by the restriction to the realization of physical activity imposed mainly by his parents and the doctor, without a strong scientific basis.

There are several studies that show that general exercise programs, performed on a regular basis, improve aerobic physical capacity, work capacity, and VO2max in children with asthma. After reviewing 48 articles on physical activity of patients with asthma, Satta found: less need for medication, reduced number of visits to emergency rooms, less school absenteeism and, in addition, an improvement in spirometry parameters. Poor physical performance of these subjects could be related to their poor nutritional status, myopathy due to the use of corticosteroids or their physical deconditioning.

In neuromuscular diseases, the evidence of the benefit of physical activity is dissimilar regarding the intensity of exercise. In slowly progressive diseases, moderate endurance exercise programs have been shown to be effective, but high-load exercise programs have proven to be counterproductive.

There are several recommended protocols of physical training, which must be adapted to age, collaboration level, compromise degree, and available resources. In preschool, physical activity should be encouraged through games, according to the interests and motivations of their age. On the other hand, in schoolchildren and adolescents sports activities, especially in groups, will have a more important role. Regarding their degree of deterioration, attention should be paid to children who use supplemental oxygen. To avoid hypoxemia, associated with exercise should be evaluated increasing the fraction of inspired oxygen. In addition, training adaptations should be considered if it is conducted in a hospital environment, in primary care or in the community (Table 64.3).

Table 64.3 Physical training recommendations

Intensity	60–80% of the maximal work rate of the cardiopulmonary exercise test (cycle ergometer) 60–80% treadmill In primary care it is possible to use 60–80% of the average speed of the 6MWT or 60–80% of the heart rate reserve
Type	Intervallic/continuous
Frequency	3 times per week 8 sessions: 60% 8 sessions: 70% 8 sessions: 80%
Duration	24 sessions (at least 30 minutes)

Inspiratory Muscle Training (IMT)

Ventilatory muscles, as well as skeletal muscles, can change their strength and endurance in response to a specific training program.

The observable responses after a specific inspiratory muscles training process are:

(a) Improvement in strength and endurance of respiratory muscles
(b) Greater ability to perform exercises
(c) Decreased dyspnea
(d) Delays onset of muscle fatigue
(e) Restoration in the mechanical ventilation weaning process

Patients eligible to undergo inspiratory muscle training are:

(a) Restrictive diseases: kyphoscoliosis, neuromuscular symptoms, etc.
(b) Obliterative bronchiolitis
(c) Muscle weakness after prolonged mechanical ventilation
(d) Cystic fibrosis

The most used inspiratory muscle training system today is the threshold valve, which uses a 2 cm diameter valve with a spring that keeps it closed. To be able to inspire, the subject must create a certain pressure with their inspiratory muscles, such that it can overcome a preset load (30% of the MIP is usually recommended, combining efforts up to 70% of the MIP) allowing to open the valve and thus starting the inspiratory flow. This training system has the advantage that the load determined by the spring tension is independent of the flow that the patient uses.

In children, studies that apply specific inspiratory muscle training are scarce. Sawyer et al. indicate that 10 weeks of inspiratory muscle training in children with cystic fibrosis showed improvement in exercise tolerance and inspiratory muscle function parameters. In 1999, Gozal et al. demonstrated an improvement in the respiratory muscle function parameters of up to 30% of the MIP in a year in patients with Duchenne's disease and type III spinal muscular atrophy after specific ventilatory muscle training. They also noted that after stopping the training the patient returns to baseline values approximately 3 months after the end of the program. Topin applied a load of 30% of the MIP in subjects with Duchenne muscular dystrophy and found a significant improvement in inspiratory muscle endurance, showing that this load amount is effective and does not cause baseline MIP deterioration in these patients. It has also been established that, based on current knowledge, inspiratory muscle training should be applied along with general physical training to obtain maximum clinical and quality of life benefits.

In summary, specific training of the inspiratory muscles with appropriate equipment and with an inspiratory muscle training program that considers using low training loads of 30–40%, together with moderate loads of 50–60%, for at least 20 minutes a day, 3–5 times per week for a minimum of 8 weeks, will achieve positive results in multiple types of pediatric diseases, especially in aspects related to muscle endurance. However, based on current evidence, it should be taken into account that loads prescribed to children with Duchenne's disease do not exceed 30% of the MIP. For all the above, application of inspiratory muscle training should always be considered in rehabilitation programs of chronic respiratory patients, further studies being necessary for its systematic application in pediatrics.

Education

Education is a fundamental component in the success of a pulmonary rehabilitation program. It must be done by all the professional team and focused on improving therapeutic compliance and promoting a healthy lifestyle.

Among the educational interventions are:

- Supervision of the indicated treatment, in particular of the inhaled drugs, checking periodically their use and good execution.
- Recognition of early symptoms on the part of the patient for timely detection of exacerbations.
- Information about the benefits of physical activity and a balanced diet.

Final Comments

The scientific application of physical exercise for therapeutic purposes is the main component of a pulmonary rehabilitation program. At present, the World Health Organization recommends systematic physical activity as one of the main strategies in the prevention of the global increase of chronic noncommunicable diseases. However, pulmonary rehabilitation does not consist exclusively in physical training, but also in a series of components whose main objectives are to intervene in organic, functional, and social aspects that minimize the progression of the disease and improve the quality of life of chronic patients. It is essential that each health center be responsible for developing a comprehensive pulmonary rehabilitation program that involves a multidisciplinary team of professionals who are highly motivated and coordinated, maximize the benefits of each of the components of the program, always aiming to promote a healthy lifestyle to the patients.

The quality of pulmonary rehabilitation programs developed in centers of excellence should be ensured in such a way that their benefits can be transferred to less specialized health centers, in order to secure better accessibility for all patients.

Finally, we must not forget that "incurable is not the same as untreatable".

Sources

Berorza T, Cartagena C, Caviedes I, Céspedes J, Gutiérrez-Navas M, Oyarzún M, et al. Prueba de caminata de seis minutos. Rev Chil Enferm Respir. 2009;25(1):15–24.

Gatica D, Puppo H, Villarroel G, San Martín I, Lagos R, Montecino JJ, Lara C, Zenteno D. Valores de referencia del test de marcha de seis minutos en niños sanos. Rev Méd Chile. 2012;140(8):1014–21.

Güell R, Díaz Lobato S, Rodríguez-Trigo G, Morante F, San Miguel M, Cejudo P, et al. Normativa SEPAR Rehabilitación respiratoria. Arch Bronconeumol. 2014;50(8):322–44.

Matecki S, Topin N, Hayot M, Rivier F, Echenne B. Prefaut evaluation of respiratory muscle endurance in patients with Duchenne muscular dystrophy. Neuromuscul Disord. 2001;11:171–7.

Pianosi P, LeBlanc J, Almudevar A. Peak oxygen uptake and mortality in children with cystic fibrosis. Thorax. 2005;60:50–4.

Santuz P, Baraldi E, Filippone M, Zachello F. Exercise performance in children with asthma: is it different from that of healthy controls? Eur Respir J. 1997;10:1254–60.

Satta A. Exercise training in asthma. J Sports Med Phys Fitness. 2000;40:277–83.

Sawyer E, Clanton T. Improved pulmonary function and exercise tolerance with inspiratory muscle conditioning in children with cystic fibrosis. Chest. 1993;104:1490–7.

Schneiderman J, Wilkes D, Atenafu E, Nguyen T, Wells G, Alarie N, et al. Longitudinal relationship between physi-cal activity and lung health in patients with cystic fibro-sis. Eur Respir J. 2014;43:817–23.

Selvadurai HC, Cooper PJ, Meyers N, Blimkie CJ, Smith L, Mellis CM, Van Asperen PP. Validation of shuttle tests in children with cystic fibrosis. Pediatr Pulmonol. 2003;35(2):133–8.

Singh SJ, Morgan MD, Scott S, Walters D, Hardman AE. Development of a shuttle walking test of disability in patients with chronic airways obstruction. Thorax. 1992;47:1019–24.

Spruit MA, Singh SJ, Garvey C, Zuwallack R, Nici L, Rochester C, et al. An official American Thoracic Society/European Respiratory Society statement: key concepts and advances in pulmonary rehabilitation. Am J Respir Crit Care Med. 2013;188(8):e13–64.

Topin N, Matecki S, Hayot M, Le Bris S, Rivier F, Echenne B, et al. Dose-dependent effect of individualized respiratory muscle training in children with Duchenne muscu-Lar dystrophy. Neuromuscul Disord. 2002;12:576–83.

Zenteno D, Puppo H, Vera R, Torres R, Kuo CH, Salinas P, et al. Guías de Rehabilitación Pulmonar para Niños con Enfermedades Respiratorias Crónicas. Neumol Pediatr. 2008;3(Supl 1):25–33.

Prolonged Hospitalization Due to Chronic Respiratory Diseases

65

Mireya Méndez Raggi
and Claudia Astudillo Maggio

Contents

Introduction

The population with chronic respiratory disease is diverse, and it includes multiple congenital and acquired conditions. In the United States there is an estimated prevalence of 6–14 patients per 100,000 children. Taking into account that this population is at a higher risk of disease, hospitalization, and death, they entail a large economic and social cost for the country.

During the past few decades there has been a sustained improvement in different Chilean health indices due to the implementation of programs, such as pregnancy control, national immunization program, and national program for acute respiratory infections. In addition, great technological developments in neonatology and pediatric units have increased the sur-

M. Méndez Raggi · C. Astudillo Maggio (✉)
Pediatrics, Respiratory Diseases, Hospital Josefina Martínez, Puente Alto, Chile

Pontificia Universidad Católica de Chile, Santiago, Chile
e-mail: gestion@hjm.cl

P. Bertrand, I. Sánchez (eds.), *Pediatric Respiratory Diseases*,
https://doi.org/10.1007/978-3-030-26961-6_65

vival rate of very low weight preterm newborns or seriously ill children, thus generating patients with mainly respiratory and neurological sequelae.

Infants and children who suffer from chronic diseases are at the highest risk of physical, developmental, behavioral or emotional problems requiring special health care, adequate infrastructure, and management by qualified personnel. There is a particularly relevant group of critically ill chronic patients who depend on mechanical ventilation, patients who have undergone tracheotomy or those who are oxygen-dependent. They constitute a special challenge for the health care system. Most of these patients are hospitalized in pediatric intensive care and neonatal intensive care units, where even though they are a minority of admissions, their long stays consume a great amount of resources. This has made the existence of step-down units or long-stay hospitals much more necessary, so that these patients can continue their treatment and be discharged into a home hospitalization system. There have been national programs proposed in Chile to cover these needs, such as the ambulatory oxygen therapy program from 2003 and the domiciliary invasive and non-invasive mechanical ventilation program from 2006.

Definitions

It is not easy to find a pediatric definition for prolonged mechanical ventilation dependent patients, or for those who have had to use any other sort of technology. There is, however, a consensus on concepts, such as chronic mechanical ventilation and medically fragile patients or patients with special needs.

> *Prolonged mechanical ventilation.* Longer than 3 weeks with invasive or non-invasive ventilatory support.

> *Medically fragile or special needs population.* They depend on technology, including chronic oxygen therapy, invasive or non-invasive ventilatory support, periodic cardiorespiratory monitoring, chronic dialysis, tracheotomy, ventriculoperitoneal bypass valve, gastrotomy, or central venous catheter carrier; additionally, patients with severe delayed psychomotor development or suffering from three or more chronic conditions.

This type of patient would then be susceptible to chronic hospitalization. However, what would be the best scenario for these children? Their home, without a doubt. When this is not possible for different reasons, hospitalization must be done in an environment that allows their comprehensive development with the aim of home discharge. Ideally, this must be done outside of the intensive care unit.

Chronic Hospitalization Outside the Intensive Care Unit

The Josefina Martínez Hospital, founded in Santiago de Chile in 1945, is a pediatric center specialized in respiratory and integral care in children suffering from chronic respiratory diseases. It was created as a treatment center for children diagnosed with tuberculosis, later focusing on treating patients with mainly post-viral obliterative bronchiolitis, bronchopulmonary dysplasia, and cystic fibrosis in mechanical ventilation dependent patients. In 2006 the hospital started treating patients under both invasive and non-invasive mechanical ventilation. Currently, the hospital has 54 beds intended for patients suffering from chronic respiratory disease, neuromuscular diseases, or airway diseases, most of which have undergone tracheotomy and depend on mechanical ventilation. The average length of stay varies from months to years, with the most frequent prolongation cause being problems of a social nature (habitability, precarious family conditions) and neurological compromise of the patient.

Aims of Chronic Hospitalization

1. Receive care unavailable in outpatient programs.
2. Facilitate the transition from critical care units to home care, allowing the stabilization of the patient.
3. Educate the family, patients, and health care team about outpatient attention.
4. Evaluate, select equipment, choose ventilatory modality, and title the parameters for chronic mechanical ventilation.
5. Manage respiratory exacerbations.
6. Prevent caregiver fatigue. This last point has been raised in some countries with the aim of allowing parents to rest.

Centers that treat chronic respiratory patients must coordinate with the technical and human facilities to deliver respiratory and integral care in order to allow the harmonious development of children. Results will depend on a rigorous selection of qualifying patients (Table 65.1) and an initial evaluation by the multidisciplinary team in order to plan how the attention will be delivered and what the aims will be depending on each child's base condition and prognosis. At the same time, there must be a close interconnection between intensive care units, so that the patient can be transferred swiftly in case of a decompensation beyond the level of complexity the long term stay center can handle, and the home care service, in order to achieve an expeditious and safe transition to home care when conditions allow it.

Table 65.1 Admittance conditions

Clinic	Social-ethic
Hemodynamic stability during the past 2 weeks	Ethics committee if necessary
Stable ventilatory parameters for the past 3 weeks, with FiO_2 lower than 0.4. Last arterial blood gasses without acidosis	Agreement to transfer by parents or guardians
Permeable airway, mature tracheotomy	Updated psychosocial report
Negative viral respiratory study made during epidemic period	
Carriage of multi-resistant bacteria study (enterococcus, positive ESBL, MRSA) performed during the 7 days prior to transfer	

Goals of Chronic Hospitalization

1. Perform weaning, decannulation or programmed oxygen assistance removal when possible.
2. Restore swallowing, phonation, general and respiratory musculature.
3. Insert the patient in a preschool or school environment as applicable.
4. Collaborate both in the social and psychological recovery of the child and their family.
5. Transferring the patient home, ideally after overcoming the reasons for admittance.

In order to reach these goals, the hospital or unit must have a highly specialized multidisciplinary team with defined roles, monitoring teams and ventilatory support, while also having access to support diagnosis and therapeutical units.

Medical Team

The leader of the team must be a pediatric pulmonologist, coordinating diagnosis, treatment, and rehabilitation, designating the starting and end point of mechanical ventilation and oxygen, picking out the team and ventilatory strategy, organizing diagnostic and therapeutic procedures, while also performing, interpreting, and reporting tests on pulmonary function, bronchoscopy, polysomnography, oximetry, and continuous capnography.

The team's pediatrician is in charge of giving clinical attention, diagnosing, and treating respiratory exacerbations, coordinating health attention related to the general pathologies occurring from the child's developmental status.

The team's child neurologist must organize the neurorehabilitation team and evaluate, diagnose, and indicate pharmacological treatment of the neurological pathology.

The physiatrist is in charge of managing the rehabilitation team, performing diagnosis, indicating orthosis, and carrying out the necessary therapeutical procedures such as applying botox.

The nutritionist manages the clinical nutrition team and performs the nutritional evaluation and monitoring, diagnosing, as well as indicating the nutritional therapy to follow (energy intake and supplements). The dietitian is also in charge of defining the specifications and means of feeding.

Role of the Professional Team

It is of the utmost importance for comprehensive treatment to involve all professionals who constitute the health team. This team performs a complementary role and their functions are described as follows:

- *Nurse*: Manages care on the basis of models as the primary nurse and self-care, coordinates and supervises daily attention to the child, involving specific techniques and procedures. Trains professionals, technicians, and caregivers.
- *Respiratory physiotherapist*: Delivers respiratory care and ventilatory therapy, implements manual and assisted airway permeation techniques, performs pulmonary function tests, and assists in the rehabilitation of respiratory musculature. Performs and monitors weaning and decannulation.
- *Motor physiotherapist*: Determines motor diagnosis in the area of neurorehabilitation in order to develop the treatment plan. Intervenes in the case of a sensorimotor disfunction that limits patient functionality.
- *Occupational therapist*: Promotes the acquisition of daily life skills (independence and autonomy). Designs, elaborates, and applies technical assistance (orthosis). Promotes play, social participation, and schooling of the child.
- *Dietist*: Supervises the implementation of the diet as indicated by the nutritionist. Collaborates in diagnosis and prescription of nutritional therapy with the physician.
- *Speech-language pathologist*: Performs rehabilitation of swallowing and phonation with or without assistance devices (like phonation valves).
- *Psychologist*: Does psychological and social diagnoses. Gives psychological therapy to children in prolonged hospitalization. Comforts and supports parents and relatives of the patients.
- *Social worker*: Evaluates habitability through the use of instruments and support networks' management.

Infrastructure and Equipment

Adequate treatment requires non-invasive monitoring equipment, ventilators and flow generators that deliver invasive and non-invasive mechanical ventilation, exhalation systems, oxygen and vacuum network, drug and feeding infusion pumps, pulse oximetry and continuous capnography, and access to diagnosis support and therapy units, such as a lung function laboratory, sleep studies, bronchoscopy, radiology, and clinical laboratory.

Monitoring of Chronic Respiratory Ill Patient by Level of Complexity

From the time of admittance, children begin a dynamic and individualized process that takes into account their characteristics and potentials, going through their different levels of complexity (Table 65.2).

Table 65.2 Classification of most frequent diagnoses

Neuromuscular diseases	Spinal muscular atrophy, muscular dystrophy
Central nervous system diseases	Congenital central hypoventilation syndrome, Arnold Chiari
Airway diseases	Subglottic stenosis, malacias, Pierre Robin sequence and other genetic disorders causing the obstruction of the upper airway
Lung parenchyma diseases	Bronchopulmonary dysplasia, bronchiolitis obliterans, cystic fibrosis
Miscellaneous	Congenital scoliosis

The concept of health care safety is particularly relevant for such patients at high risk of adverse effects, such as accidental decannulation, obstruction of the airway, displacement of the gastrostomy tube or the cannula. This calls for permanent monitoring and continuous supervision, making sure of not interfering in the patient's psychomotor development. Therefore, the monitoring system must fit the therapeutic strategy and the risk level of each patient.

- *Patient with ventilatory support through tracheotomy*: Such a patient must have permanent non-invasive monitoring for cardiac frequency and hemoglobin saturation with or without capnography (particularly useful when changing parameters or managing exacerbations). Arterial blood gas to obtain instant information in case of decompensation or follow-up of the patient.
- *Patient with non-invasive ventilatory support*: Non-invasive cardiac frequency and saturation monitoring. Arterial blood gas if necessary.
- *Tracheotomized patient without ventilatory support*: Non-invasive monitoring at least during sleep. Arterial blood gas or capnography if necessary.
- *Oxygen assistance dependent patient*: Isolated monitoring of hemoglobin saturation except in unstable or exacerbated patients, who may require permanent monitoring.

It is important to note that any monitoring system must go hand in hand with direct control from a professional, a technician, or a well-trained caregiver who could interpret alarming signs.

Routine Monitoring to Avoid in-Hospital Infections

Prolonged hospitalization is not a linear process, because the patient may suffer from exacerbations or decompensation from their base condition that may delay or change the progression of the disease. Healthcare associated infections are still an important cause of morbidity and mortality. That is why it is so important to consider a monitoring system for multi-resistant or emergent pathogens, such as vancomycin-resistant enterococci or extended-spectrum beta-lactamase bacteria and a system to control associated infections to healthcare emphasizing hand sanitation in addition to the rational use of antimicrobial agents.

Additional Activities

The complete human development of the child requires other additional, but no less important, activities, such as play. There must be adequate spaces to develop therapeutic play activities guided by therapists, psychologists, technicians, and preschool educators, depending on the age of the patient. Many of these children have spent their whole lives under hospital care, which is why it is so important to be with them during their process of socializing and discovering the world beyond the hospital by visiting parks, the beach, the zoo, and by partaking in cultural and entertainment activities like the movies, circus, museum, etc. Every child has the right to receive an education. Some centers have created their own in-hospital classrooms, but it seems that the option of sending the child to a kindergarten or school beyond the hospital walls, despite coming at a higher physical and human cost, is an enriching experience within their integration process.

Progression

Progression and hospitalization time will be determined by the characteristics of the patient, underlying pathology and prognosis, as well as their rehabilitation potential. The patient may move from permanent invasive mechanical ventilation to partial or complete independence from the ventilator. A tracheotomized patient may also have to undergo corrective airway surgery, leading to a successful decannulation. There will invariably remain patients who depend on ventilation, but they may be able to use a wheelchair, improving their quality of life.

Discharge Planning

Discharge must be planned once the cause for hospitalization has been overcome or stabilized. In chronic patients, discharge is a process that starts the moment of admission and ends when the child is transferred back home. Discharge planning must be undertaken by the coordinated efforts of the medical team at the hospital center, the family or caregivers, and the health team that will tend to the patient at home. There is a home ventilation support program in Chile supported by the Ministry of Health. Networks formed by the treating team, the home care team, and the health team at the closest hospital to the patient's home are established much like they did before discharge.

When transferring the patient home is not an option, other alternatives must be offered, such as finding capable and willing relatives, hospitals close to the patient's home, or institutions that have the technology that the patient requires. Education of the health personnel and caregivers is perhaps the most critical factor regarding the safety and success of home care. That is why it deserves careful attention and planning. Training must be carried out in an organized manner without making assumptions about the education level of the health personnel, the tutors, or caregivers. A probe must be conducted to find out the skills that they have already acquired. It is recommended to have a structured training plan, including basic anatomy and physiology, learning, and skill acquisition. A successful transition to home care will require having all these factors in mind.

Sources

Carson S. Definitions and epidemiology of the chronically critically ill. Respir Care. 2012;57(6):848–56.

Dasgupta A, Rice R, Masha E, Litaker D, Stoller J. Four year experience with a unit for long term ventilation (respiratory special care unit) at the Cleveland Clinic Foundation. Chest. 1999;116(2):447–56.

Dursun O, Osel D. Early and long-term outcome after tracheostomy in children. Pediatr Int. 2011;53:202–6.

Escarravil J, Casolivé V. Terapias respiratorias y cuidados del paciente neuromuscular con afectación respiratoria. Manual SEPAR de Procedimientos 2012.

González-Cortés R, López-Herce-Cid J, García-Figueruelo A, Tesorero-Carcedo G, Botrán-Prieto M, Carrillo-Álvarez A. Ingreso prolongado en la unidad de cuidados intensivos pediátricos: mortalidad y consumo de recursos asistenciales. Med Intensiva. 2011;35(7):417–23.

Graf J, Montagnino B, Hueckel R, McPherson M. Pediatric tracheostomies: a recent experience from one academic center. Pediatr Crit Care Med. 2008;9(1):96–100.

Lenker C, Slayton D, Gutiérrez H. Planificación del alta en el niño con trastorno pulmonar crónico. En: Sánchez I y Prado F. Enfoque clínico de las enfermedades respiratorias del niño. Santiago de Chile: Ediciones Universidad Católica de Chile; 2007. p. 511–9.

Méndez M, Prado F, Navarro S, Sánchez I. Rol de un hospital especializado en los cuidados respiratorios de pacientes con enfermedades pulmonares crónicas. En: Sánchez I y Prado F. Enfoque clínico de las enfermedades respiratorias del niño. Santiago de Chile: Ediciones Universidad Católica de Chile; 2007. p. 521–8.

Monteverde E, Fernandez A, Poterala R, Vidal N, Siaba A, Castelani P, et al. Characterization of pediatric patients receiving prolonged mechanical ventilation. Pediatr Crit Care Med. 2011;12(6):287–91.

Paulides F, Plötz F, Verweij-van den Oudenrijn L, van Gestel J, Kampelmacher M. Thirty years of home mechanical ventilation in children: escalatin need for pediatric intensive care beds. Intensive Care Med. 2012;38:847–52.

Peterson-Carmichael S, Cheifetz I. The chronically critically III patient: pediatric considerations. Resp Care. 2012;57(6):993–1002.

Oxygen Therapy

66

Alejandra Zamorano Wittwer
and Claudia Astudillo Maggio

Contents

Introduction

Oxygen therapy is a therapeutic procedure designed to prevent and treat the symptoms of hypoxia, mainly hypoxemic, such as increased cardiovascular and respiratory work, depression of the central nervous system, cyanosis, and irritability. This is achieved by increasing the oxygen content in the arterial blood through the administration of additional oxygen in the air that the patient breathes, in sufficient quantity so that the arterial oxygen pressure and the hemoglobin saturation are maintained within normal ranges.

It is important to consider that low oxygen availability can have different etiologies, since it not only depends on oxygen delivery but also on ventilation, concentration and saturation of the hemoglobin, along with the cardiac output. This is why we can distinguish different hypoxia types: hypoxic hypoxia or hypoxemia with low PaO_2 and low hemoglobin saturation; anemic hypoxia with low concentration of hemoglobin; cardiac hypoxia due to low cardiac output; dissociative hypoxia with decreased capacity of hemoglobin saturation, increased affinity of hemoglobin (Hb) for oxygen. It is in hypoxemia where additional oxygen therapy is the most significant. In the other causes of hypoxia there is a secondary clinical benefit, but treatment of the underlying cause and disease is fundamental.

Administration of oxygen is indicated in the presence of acute or chronic hypoxemia with

A. Zamorano Wittwer (✉)
Department of Pediatrics, School of Medicine, Pontificia Universidad Católica de Chile, Santiago, Chile

C. Astudillo Maggio
Pediatrics, Respiratory Diseases, Hospital Josefina Martínez, Puente Alto, Chile

Pontificia Universidad Católica de Chile, Santiago, Chile

P. Bertrand, I. Sánchez (eds.), *Pediatric Respiratory Diseases*,
https://doi.org/10.1007/978-3-030-26961-6_66

PaO2 < 60 mmHg, where the affinity of Hb for O2 decreases rapidly, affecting the total content of O2 and the oxygenation of tissues.

Use of oxygen therapy dates back to the first decades of the twentieth century and is currently the fundamental therapeutic tool in treatment of patients with respiratory failure, both acute and chronic. In recent years, we have seen an increase in its indication as long-term therapy in pediatrics, explained by a rise in chronic respiratory diseases and by technological progress of neonatology and intensive care. In these cases, benefits, such as a shorter time of hospitalization, improved growth, better physical and neurological development of the child, increased tolerance to exercise, better sleep quality, and prevention of pulmonary hearth disease or *cor pulmonale,* have been demonstrated.

Physio Pathological Basis

Causes of Hypoxemia

It is essential to analyze which mechanism is responsible for hypoxemia, since it is closely related to the real benefit of oxygen therapy. These physiopathological mechanisms can coexist in the same patient simultaneously and in an evolutive form over time.

1. *Ventilation–perfusion mismatch.* Ventilation–perfusion mismatch occurs when ventilation and blood flow are unbalanced in different lung regions, making all gas transfer inefficient. It is the most common and frequent mechanism of hypoxemia in children. Its most prominent causes are obstructive pulmonary diseases, such as asthma and bronchiolitis, and restrictive disease, such as pneumonia and atelectasis. Other causes are interstitial lung disease and vascular disorders, such as pulmonary embolism. Under these circumstances, the administration of oxygen at low rate is usually very effective in improving arterial PaO2.
2. *Shunt.* A pulmonary shunt occurs when an important part of the blood reaches the arterial system without passing through the lung ventilated regions. This situation can be an extreme in the case of absence of ventilation, as in massive atelectasis or extended consolidated pneumonia, called intrapulmonary shunt. Intracardiac shunt or vascular shunt occur when the blood bypasses the pulmonary vessels by a cardiac defect or arteriovenous malformations. Shunts are a frequent cause of differential diagnosis in patients with hypoxemia in which a respiratory cause is not found. Oxygen administration, even 100%, only gives a small increase in arterial PaO2.
3. *Hypoventilation. Hypoventilation occurs when* the amount of fresh gas that reaches the alveoli per unit time (alveolar ventilation) is reduced. It always causes a concomitant elevation of the PaCO2 that allows differential diagnosis. It is usually caused by diseases outside the lungs, such as respiratory center depression secondary to drugs use; medulla oblongata diseases, such as encephalitis, hemorrhages and neoplasms; abnormalities of the spinal cord such as those related to upper cervical spine dislocations; anterior horn diseases such as poliomyelitis; nerve diseases that causes innervation in the respiratory muscles such as Guillain-Barré syndrome; neuromuscular junction diseases such as myasthenia gravis; respiratory muscles diseases, such as Duchenne muscular dystrophy, thoracic cage abnormalities, or upper airway obstruction.

The hypoxemia caused by hypoventilation, which is rarely severe, is easily reversed by adding a moderate oxygen supply to the inspired gas, but it does not reverse its main problem, hypoventilation and hypercarbia.

4. *Diffusion Limitation. Diffusion limitation occurs when the gases for interchange are dilated with inappropriate* balance between pulmonary capillary blood PCO2 and alveolar gas. At rest, capillary blood PCO2 reaches the balance of the alveolar gas after a third of the total contact time of three quarters of a second available in the capillary. In intense exercise, where the contact time is reduced to a quarter of a second, balance almost always occurs. In

some diseases where blood–air barrier is thickened, diffusion is so delayed that this balance is incomplete. Examples of diseases that can cause this disorder are: asbestosis, sarcoidosis, pulmonary fibrosis, interstitial pneumonia, and collagenopathies that compromise the lungs, such as scleroderma, rheumatoid arthritis, lupus erythematosus, Wegener's granulomatosis, Goodpasture syndrome, and alveolar cell carcinoma. A moderate increase of inspired oxygen concentration corrects the hypoxemia.

5. Diminished *Inspired PAO2. Alveolar PAO2 is decreased at high altitude* because atmospheric pressure is low and oxygen pressure decreases proportionally with lower basal oxygen saturation levels.

Oxygen Prescription

Acute Hypoxia

Respiratory Failure with Arterial Hypoxemia Oxygen therapy is prescribed if PaO2 < 60 mm Hg or Hb saturation is <93% according to national guidelines or ≤92% according to British and Canadian guidelines. Blood gases results are not needed to initiate oxygen therapy. When the patient presents with signs of possible hypoxemia, such as tachypnea, increased work of breathing or tachycardia, it is enough to start therapy with oxygen. It is important to evaluate the clinical response and titrate the oxygen amount according to clinical and saturation values.

Tissue Hypoxia without Hypoxemia May occur secondary to situations of low cardiac output, such as anemia, heart failure, hypovolemic shock, or carbon monoxide (CO) poisoning. Although PaO2 and hemoglobin saturation may be normal, there will be benefits in administering oxygen, improving tissue oxygenation. In the case of carbon monoxide poisoning, oxygen works against its binding to hemoglobin.

Chronic Hypoxemia Causes are related to chronic respiratory failure due to pulmonary and extrapulmonary problems. Table 66.1 lists the main causes of prescribing for long-term oxygen therapy.

Table 66.1 Oxygen therapy: chronic diseases

Lung diseases	
Intrinsic parenchymal disease	Restrictive lung disease
Chronic neonatal lung disease	Neuromuscular diseases
Pulmonary hypoplasia	Chest wall diseases
Congenital diaphragmatic hernia	Upper airway obstruction
Interstitial lung diseases	Primary pulmonary hypertension (PPH)
Idiopathic pulmonary fibrosis	PPH secondary to lung disease
Advanced cystic fibrosis	
Advanced bronchiolitis	
Bronchiectasis	
Heart disease with PPH	
Palliative care	

High Altitude The World Health Organization recommends the administration of additional oxygen in patients living at altitude >2500 meters above sea level with SpO2 ≤ 87%.

Air travel is a situation to consider in children with respiratory disease, as they could be at risk of developing hypoxemia events. Commercial flights are pressurized, so their altitude is equivalent to a range between 1525 and 2440 meters. In a normal child, compensation occurs with no distress, but in a child with respiratory disease, it may generate hypoxemia. General recommendations suggest waiting until newborns are older than a week before air travel; if they are preterm, they should have some oxygen management system in the plane if necessary; double oxygen administration during flight in oxygen-dependent patients; in case of pneumothorax, wait 2 weeks after resolution before flying. Perform the hypoxia altitude simulation test in patients with severe chronic respiratory disease.

Preterm and Newborns Infants Oxygen administration in newborns and particularly in preterm infants deserves special mention because of risks of toxicity with secondary lung injury and of producing retinopathy of prematurity, among other complications.

Current recommendations range from indication in the delivery room to patients who will require oxygen at home. In the delivery room it is suggested to immediately place a pulse oximeter sensor on the right wrist, maintain saturations between 85–92% the first 10 minutes of life and initiate oxygen with FiO2 30%, if required.

Regarding the early neonatal period, there are studies that show that with low levels of saturation, although the risk of severe retinopathy decreases, there is an increase in mortality. Current recommendations for this period suggest maintaining saturations between 91–95% up to 36 weeks of gestational age and 93–95% at later ages.

Devices for oxygen administration (Table 66.2) are the interfaces that will carry the oxygen to the patient. They will be chosen according to the needs of each patient individually, considering tolerance and compliance with therapy.

Prescription of Long-Term Oxygen Therapy

Titration

The oxygen flow titration required by the patient must be carried out when the patient is clinically stable. If possible, the infant should be evaluated during feeding and the schoolchildren during exercise or during sleep, when nocturnal desaturation events are suspected. Titration is carried out through continuous pulse oximetry for a minimum of 8 hours. Its interpretation will be carried out according to the technical standards of each country. In Chile, this means according to the regulations of the Department of Health and its home oxygen program.

Table 66.2 Oxygen administration devices

System type	Device	Advantages	Disadvantages
A. High-flow system: The Venturi system is used, where oxygen is mixed in a standardized way with ambient air through an opening of different diameter.	1. A Venturi mask delivers an exact concentration of oxygen, regardless of the patient's breathing pattern.	Provide specific FiO_2	
	2. Halo: It is a closed and compact bell used in infants.	Provides high oxygen concentrations It facilitates the breastfed contact with the environment Allows oral feeding Allows nebulized therapy	
	3. Face tent	It is useful in patients who cannot tolerate the mask or present facial trauma	
	4. Tracheostomy mask		High condensation
B. Low-flow systems: Use a lower flow of oxygen for the inspiratory flow of the patient	1. Nasal cannula: In children use flow of up to 3 L/min In newborns use a flow of no more than 2 L/min	Best accepted by the patient They are light They allow the patient to talk and feed They have a long lifespan	Different FiO2 according to the patient's body surface Decreased efficiency in mouth respirators
	2. Simple face mask	It allows the use of flows between 5 and 10 L/min, which provide FiO2 between 0.35 and 0.50	
	3. Mask with reservoir: It is a simple face mask with a bag or a reservoir at its lower end.		

Selection of an Oxygen Administration Source

According to the flow to be administered: If it is <2 liters per minute, prefer cylinders; if it is >2 liters per minute, prefer concentrators.

Sources of Oxygen Administration

Cylinders Cylinders contain pressurized gas and provide 100% oxygen. Its major limitation is its capacity, which makes it necessary to change them continuously. Its installation at home must be carried out by trained personnel, ensuring its fixation and minimizing the risks associated with manipulation.

- *Liquid oxygen*: Each liter of liquid oxygen produces 863 liters of oxygen gas. The capacity of a tank goes from 25 to 40 liters of liquid oxygen, so at a flow of 2 liters per minute it would last 11 days. Portable devices can give autonomy of up to 8 hours to the patient. They are the best option for those who ambulate, allowing them to develop their daily activities such as school attendance. There are new devices that release gas only during inspiration, reducing the loss that occurs with continuous release, but these are not recommended for young children due to a child's small flow in spontaneous breathing. The main disadvantage of these devices is their high cost.
- *Concentrators*: These electrical devices work by increasing the concentration of oxygen in the air by filtering the nitrogen. They take up little space and do not require recharging. Recently, more portable concentrator models have been developed. Their main disadvantage is that they require electricity, making treatment more expensive.

The selection of an oxygen delivery source at home will depend on several factors, such as age, current clinical condition, ambulation and patient autonomy, costs, and space at home or school.

Selection of the Method of Oxygen Administration

At home, a nasal cannula should be preferred and the use of masks should be optional. The nasal cannula can be changed every 1 or 2 weeks and the mask between 6 and 12 months. In children with tracheostomy, oxygen is delivered through filters designed for that purpose. Also, in all cases oxygen must be humidified.

Determine Oxygen Administration Period

The requirements will depend on each particular case: 24 hours, 12 hours, during feeding, during sleep, during exercise. At this point it is important to monitor the patient in a clinical and gasometric manner, and with their pulse oximetry record.

Other Material Needed

- *Manometer*: Indicates the amount of oxygen stored in a gas cylinder or a tank using a needle on a psi scale.
- *Flow meter*: Indicates the oxygen flow to be administered to the patient, in liters per minute, which is graduated using a floating ball.
- *Humidifier*: Because oxygen is compressed for storage, for its delivery it must be liquefied, cooled and dried. Before administering it, it must be humidified to protect the airway.

Training of Parents or Caregivers

They must be able to act in case of emergencies; therefore, they have to learn about the warning signs, cardiopulmonary resuscitation, the use of oxygen sources (cylinders, liquid oxygen backpacks, concentrators), transportation of the supply sources, need for recharging, security and prevention of accidents and infections.

Follow-Up and Monitoring

Depending on the clinical condition and location of the patient (hospital or home), follow-up and monitoring of oxygen therapy will be carried out through:

- *Clinical*

Parameters, such as respiratory rate, heart rate and respiratory distress, will be evaluated. The normalization of these parameters suggests the success of the therapy.

Regarding long-term therapy, the child's growth and development must be evaluated. Anthropometric parameters such as stagnant weight and height or psychomotor development problems compel us to review the oxygen prescription.

- *Arterial Blood Gases*

Arterial blood gas test is used to evaluate the respiratory function condition. It measures pH, partial pressure of CO2, partial pressure of O2 and HCO3. Among its advantages is the opportunity to evaluate the patient metabolic condition and knowing the PaCO2. Among its disadvantages, we can mention a painful examination, something important to consider especially in children. It is essential in the initial evaluation in patients with respiratory failure and subsequently in suspected hypoventilation.

In patients with chronic respiratory failure treated with home oxygen therapy, it is useful to evaluate mainly PaCO2, which allows making decisions concerning the ventilatory management. Its use is recommended in the event of changes in therapeutic behavior caused by changes in clinical situations such as exacerbations.

- *Pulse Oximeter*

Pulse oximeter allows estimating the arterial oxygen saturation in a non-invasive manner, using two LEDs and a receiver placed through a capillary bed. It is an easy-to-use method with which the patient can be monitored continuously. Among the disadvantages of this method, we can mention its dependence on the arterial pulse, so in situations in which the perfusion is altered, such as shock, fever, cold, or movement or decrease in the amount of hemoglobin, it could provide erroneous information. To determine indication, suspension or evaluation of a patient receiving long-term oxygen therapy, continuous pulse oximetry is used, which must be performed for periods of 8 hours, ideally including sleep, feeding, and activity with or without additional oxygen, based on the target of the evaluation in each patient. The information obtained is processed with different software, and its interpretation must be performed by a pediatric pulmonologist or a neonatologist.

Complications

Oxygen is a drug therapy that causes specific biochemical and physiological actions, a wide range in the effective dose and well-defined adverse effects in higher doses, so it must be administered in the right concentrations and time. The biochemical basis for the effects of hyperoxia is the formation of oxygen free radicals, which have one or several unpaired electrons that makes them very unstable. Peroxynitrite, the product of the reaction between superoxide and nitric oxide, acts with lipids, DNA, and proteins. These reactions trigger cellular responses ranging from subtle modulations of cellular signals to cell necrosis or apoptosis. When the time of exposure to oxygen is too long or when its concentration is too high, the cellular repair system is exceeded, which can cause damage and cell death.

The organism is affected in different ways depending on the type of exposure to oxygen. If it is a short time, high oxygen pressures can lead to central nervous system toxicity, for example, in hyperbaric oxygen therapy. Longer exposure times are required to cause pulmonary and ocular toxicity. This can lead to acute respiratory syndromes, such as adult respiratory syndrome, or chronic respiratory syndromes, such as bronchopulmonary dysplasia or retinopathy of prematurity, the latter in preterm infants. In patients with chronic hypercapnia, respiratory depression caused by high oxygen concentrations can be observed, so its administration should be restrained. Concentrations greater than or equal to 50% may favor the appearance of atelectasis due to displacement of the nitrogen that gives stability to the alveolus.

There may be other minor complications, such as dryness and irritation of the nasal mucosa, especially with flows greater than 3 L/min.

It is important to inform patients who use oxygen at home that it can speed up combustion, so it should be kept away from open flames and heat, avoid hitting the cylinder and the shut-off valve, do not smoke nearby, and close the oxygen source in case of fire.

Withdrawal of Long-Term Oxygen Therapy

In general, weaning of oxygen is carried out when chronic respiratory failure is overcome, this being common in diseases that affect preterm infants such as bronchopulmonary dysplasia. It is less likely in cases of interstitial diseases and obliterative bronchiolitis, and it depends on the age of the patient at the time of the injury, the possibility of recovery from their lung damage or if it is from progressive type diseases. In patients with bronchopulmonary dysplasia it is suggested to maintain saturations around 93–95% with <1% of the time under 85% and 5% under 90% measured with continuous pulse oximetry.

It should be considered to start weaning once the supplemental oxygen requirements reach 0.1 L/min. Oxygen is maintained during sleep and feeding. Finally, depending on the results of the monitoring, administration of supplemental oxygen is suspended.

Conclusions

Oxygen therapy is a fundamental tool in the treatment of acute and chronic respiratory failure. Its employment at home is an alternative after hospital discharge with proven benefits but not free of danger or complications. For this reason, it is important that specialists such as pediatric pulmonologists conduct it, maintaining periodic consensus about their indications, administration forms, and follow-up.

Sources

Addea F, Álvarez A, Barbisanc B, Guimarães B. Recommendations for long-term home oxygen therapy in children and adolescents. J Pediatr. 2013;89(1):6.

Aguerre V. Viaje en avión, riesgos y previsiones a considerar en los niños. Arch Argent Pediatr. 2012;110(1):66–9.

Cherian S, Morris I, Evans J, Kotecha S. Oxygen therapy in preterm infants. Paediatr Respir Rev. 2014;15(2):135–41.

De Lucas P. Oxigenoterapia aguda y crónica. En: Martin Ramos G y Sanchís J. Medicina respiratoria. 2ª ed. Madrid, España: Grupo Aula. Médica. 2006:349–60.

Harris M, Clark J, Coote N, et al. British Thoracic Society guidelines for the management of community acquired pneumonia in children: update 2011. Thorax. 2011;66(Suppl 2):iil–ii 23.

Ministerio de Salud. Guía Clínica Displasia Broncopulmonar del prematuro. MINSAL: Santiago; 2009.

Ministerio de Salud. Guía Clínica Auge Infección respiratoria baja de manejo ambulatorio en menores de 5 años: Serie de Guías Clínicas Minsal; 2013.

Sociedad Argentina de Pediatría, Subcomisiones, Comités y Grupos de Trabajo. Guías para el manejo de la oxigenoterapia domiciliaria en pediatría. Parte 1. Arch Argent Pediatr. 2013a;111(5):448–54.

Sociedad Argentina de Pediatría, Subcomisiones, Comités y Grupos de Trabajo. Guías para el manejo de la oxigenoterapia domiciliaria en pediatría. Parte 2. Arch Argent Pediatr. 2013b;111(6):549–55.

Sociedad Argentina de Pediatría, Subcomisiones, Comités y Grupos de Trabajo. Seguimiento neumológico de los niños con displasia broncopulmonar al alta de neonatología. Parte 2: Administración de oxígeno, tratamiento. Arch Argent Pediatr. 2013c;111(3):252–8.

SUPPORT Study Group of the Eunice Kennedy Shriver NICHD Neonatal Research Network. Target ranges of oxygen saturation in extremely preterm infants. N Engl J Med. 2010;362:1959–69.

The BOOST II United Kingdom, Australia, and New Zealand Collaborative Groups. Oxygen saturation and outcomes in preterm infants. N Engl J Med. 2013;368 2094–104.

Thomson L, Paton J. Oxygen toxicity. Paediatr Respir Rev. 2014;15(2):120–3.

West JB. Fisiopatología pulmonar. Sexta ed. Buenos Aires: Médica Panamericana; 2004; pp. 17–37; 163–176.

World Health Organization. Recommendations for management of common childhood conditions: evidence for technical update of pocket book recommendations: newborn conditions, dysentery, pneumonia, oxygen use and delivery, common causes of fever, severe acute malnutrition and supportive care. Geneva: World Health Organization; 2012. p. 69–76.

Acute Mechanical Ventilation

67

Andrés Castillo Moya

Contents

Historical Review of Mechanical Ventilation

Mechanical ventilation has been in the mind of humans since far before we might imagine. In 400 BC, Hippocrates had already mentioned the possibility of insufflating air into the lungs through the trachea. Many centuries later, Andreas Vesalius, famous physician and anatomy teacher of the sixteenth century, described in his treatise *De humanis corporis fabrica* the possibility of "restoring" the life of an animal by placing a tube in its trachea and blowing air through it. Despite this, it was not until the late 1800s that Alfred Woillez developed a tube-like ventilator that manually performed a process of changing internal pressures, which allowed an individual placed with their body inside this tube and their head outside to intake air into their lungs in a "noninvasive" way. Later, in 1931, John Emerson developed the "iron lungs", negative pressure devices that resulted in an improvement over the prototypes developed by Woillez, Drinker, and Shaw.

During the 1950s, and in connection with the polio epidemic, mechanical ventilation had a qualitative leap: the positive pressure ventilators were developed, which played an important role during this epidemic. In 1953, Henry Lassen

A. Castillo Moya (✉)
Department of Pediatrics, School of Medicine, Pontificia Universidad Católica de Chile, Santiago, Chile
e-mail: acastill@med.puc.cl

P. Bertrand, I. Sánchez (eds.), *Pediatric Respiratory Diseases*,
https://doi.org/10.1007/978-3-030-26961-6_67

published a report where he showed that the mere introduction of mechanical ventilation as therapy in polio determined a plummeting of mortality from rates over 80% to rates of less than 40% a few months after starting its use, becoming the basis for today's mechanical ventilation techniques in the serious patient.

Mechanical ventilation in the child has been developed from the principles and experience derived from mechanical ventilation in the adult, although its use in the pediatric population has had an increasing growth with a use of 20% of the patients admitted in the pediatric ICU, reaching numbers over 50% of the admissions in respiratory infection season. The decision to place a patient in mechanical ventilation is a combination of art and science, taking into consideration an appropriate and fair combination of clinical judgment, symptoms and signs of breathing insufficiency, and the incapability of the patient to maintain an adequate gas exchange or a permeable airway.

Mechanical Ventilation Physiology

Special Characteristics of the Child

Understanding that children are different from adults in anatomical and physiological terms is essential; thus, the most relevant aspects are analyzed. The form of the airway is different and children have a more prominent occiput, which makes the access to the airway more difficult, because in dorsal decubitus this involves bending of the neck, determining a potential obstruction of the airway. The tongue is disproportionately big in relation to the oral cavity, the larynx is higher related to its position in the neck and it has a funnel shape with its narrowest portion in the level of the cricoid cartilage, making a small edema in this zone a great increase in the resistance to the airflow. Not only is the larynx narrower but the rest of the breathing tree is much narrower, determining a high probability of obstruction as a result of small radius changes.

It is important to remember that the resistance in the airflow is inversely proportional to the radius to the fourth power for a laminar flow and to the fifth power for a turbulent flow; thus, small edemas can determine a great increase in the resistance and a high tendency of air trapping and insufflation. The thoracic wall in infants and children presents ribs in a horizontal shape, which hinders the generation of intrathoracic negative pressure.

On the other hand, the thoracic cavity is much more complacent; it is described as becoming more rigid only after 2 years of age. Since the thoracic wall is more complacent, it determines a minimal opposition to the natural tendency of the lung tissue to retract, which offers a lower residual functional capacity (RFC) and a clear lower functional reserve, adding to the fact that they require more breathing work to generate an adequate ventilation per minute. Thus, this functional residual capacity increases with the age of the patient, and it is increased with the total lung capacity and lung residual volume until puberty and adolescence, where it begins to have more stable levels until adult age.

Regarding lung tissue, children can maintain a continuous growth until adolescence. During that growth, the number of alveoli grows more than 10 times and the size of them increases close to four times. Children do not present an adequate development of collateral ventilation of alveolar units, a ventilation that plays an essential role in the presence of the obstruction of the distal airway, and given that the distal airways are proportionally smaller and their tidal volumes are closer to the closing capacity (lung volume under which the small airway collapses during breathing out), they have a greater tendency to develop atelectasis.

On top of this, the anatomical and functional differences described at the thoracic cavity and lung parenchyma level determine lung *compliance* or "distensibility", different time constants at different ages, and tidal volumes that vary related to weight and height, which are modified month by month and year by year.

Ventilation and Oxygenation

Mechanical ventilation corresponds to the ingress and egress of airflow into the lungs, produced by a machine external to the patient. This airflow is propelled by a pressure gradient created by the machine, thus determining the lung expansion. In most of the ventilators, the egress or expiration of the air that entered the lungs is produced passively due to the reversion of the pressure gradient created during inspiration. The main goals of mechanical ventilation are achieving an adequate ventilation and oxygenation of the patient, which are conditioned by their underlying physiopathological condition.

Oxygenation corresponds primarily to the gas exchange at the alveolar level, which allows an adequate PaO_2 and fundamentally depends on the mean airway pressure (mPaw). The main determining factors of mPaw are the tidal volume (Vc), the maximal inspiratory pressure (MIP), the inspiratory time (iT), and positive pressure end of expiration (PEEP). Any modification to these factors that results in an increase in mPaw will determine an increase in PaO_2.

The ventilation corresponds to the movement of gas inside and out of the lung. To achieve this airflow, airway resistance and lung *compliance* forces (Table 67.1) present in the respiratory system of the child must be overcome. This air movement will modify and optimize the movement of gas at the alveolar level (alveolar ventilation), the site where the equilibrium and elimination of CO_2 will take place. Thus, ventilation per minute can be divided in alveolar ventilation and dead space ventilation, which is constituted by the anatomical and physiological dead space. The dead space does not perform the exchange because it lacks alveolar epithelium, and it can be augmented by using very long endotracheal tubes or extensions between the TET and the ventilator. The physiological dead space corresponds to the alveolar volume that is due to overdistension in most cases or because of cessation of the lung blood flow; it transforms in a portion of the alveolar volume that does not participate in the exchange. The increase in the anatomical or physiological dead weight will determine a decrease in the alveolar ventilation and thus an increase in the CO_2 (Fig. 67.1).

Lung *compliance* (C) is defined as the change of volume in relation to the change of airway pressure (Fig. 67.2), meaning $\Delta V/\Delta P$, and it is determined by the elastic forces inside the lung in conjunction with the surface tension generated by the air–tissue interface inside the alveolus. The described curve is a sigmoid curve with a decrease of the slopes in the zones of low and high lung volume. Compliance can then be divided into dynamic compliance and static com-

Table 67.1 Normal values

	Newborn	1 year	7 years	Adult
Compliance (ml/cm H_2O)	5	15	50	60–100
Resistance (cm H_2O/l/s)	40	15	4	2

Fig. 67.1 Ventilation per minute and physiological dead space

Ventilation per minute = tidal volume (TV) × respiratory frequency (RF).

TV = Alveolar volume (AV) + dead space volume (DSV)

DSV = Anatomical + physiological

Alveolar ventilation = VA × FR

Patient with air trapping = ↑ physiological DSV and ↓ VA alveolar hypoventilation.

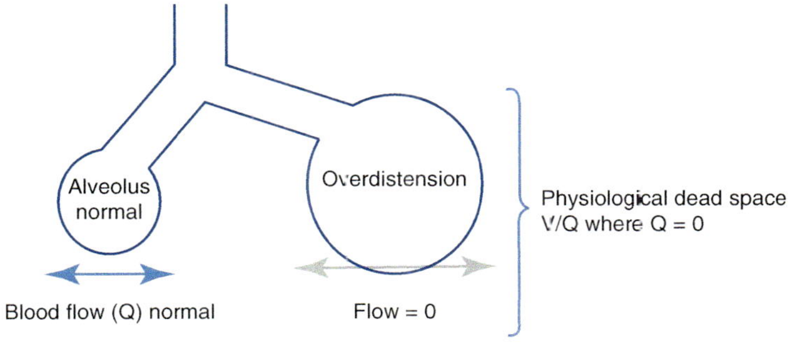

pliance. Static compliance provides an estimate of the total compliance of the lung system; it is calculated dividing the tidal volume by the difference between plateau pressure or static inflation pressure (Pplat) and PEEP. Dynamic compliance, on the other hand, includes and reflects the contribution of the airway resistance to the airflow, and it is calculated dividing the tidal volume by the difference between maximal inspiratory pressure (MIP) and PEEP.

The airway resistance is the pressure difference between the mouth and the alveolus needed to move air through the airway in a constant flow. It is determined by the flow rate, the length of the airway, the physical properties of the inhaled gas, and the radius of the airway, the latter being the most important variable.

The time constant (TC) corresponds to the measure of how fast an alveolar unit reaches a pressure equilibrium with the proximal airway, both in the filling as in the emptying phase. In operational terms, it is the product of C and R. In one CT, 63% of the equilibrium is reached: 85.5% in two, and 95% in 3-time constants (Fig. 67.3). Owing to this, according to age and the CT, inspiratory times that vary from 3 CT to a maximum of 5 CT are recommended, and it is important that the expiratory time has to have at least the same duration of inspiration. In a newborn, the CT can carry between 0.1 and 0.15 seconds, with an acceptable average inspiratory time (IT) of 3 CT. It must be noted that the CT in an older child is raised to 0.2 or 0.25, and thus the IT can reach 0.75.

All ventilation methods require that a pressure gradient is established between the alveoli and the airway (or atmospheric pressure) to produce a gas movement. Thus, adequate pressure must be generated to open the collapsed airway, so that any method that does not reach that critical pressure point during inspiration will determine the production of atelectasis and hypoxemia. The maximum pressure generated during the inspira-

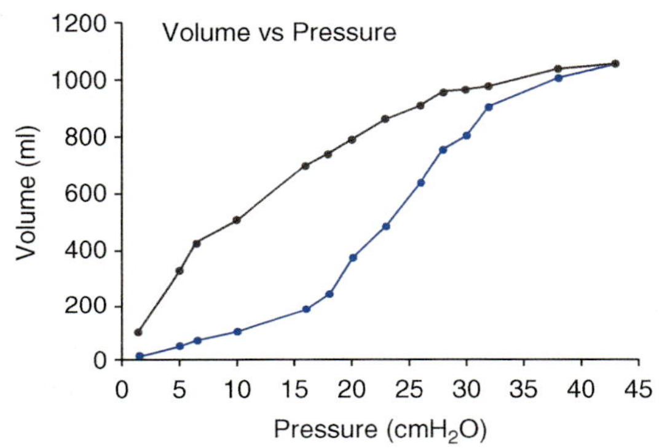

Fig. 67.2 Lung *compliance* and hysteresis curve

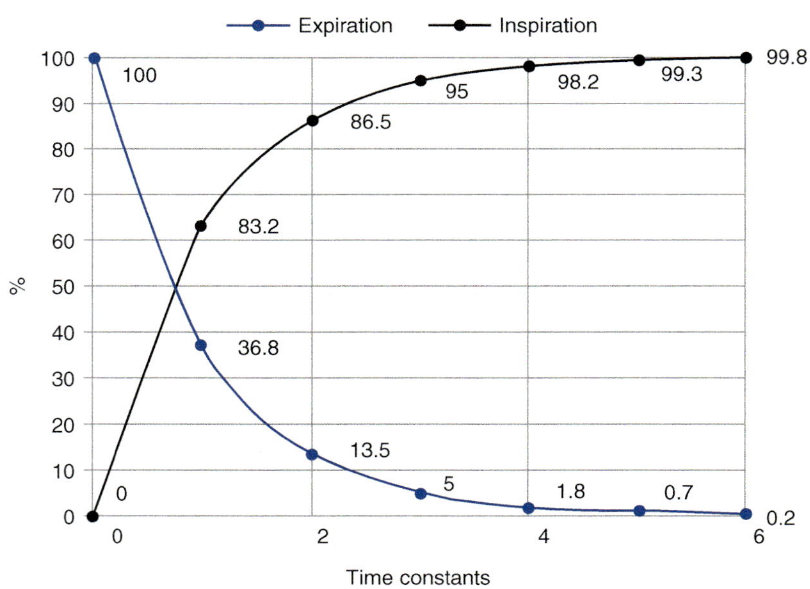

Fig. 67.3 Relationship between pressure equilibrium in the airway and the time constant

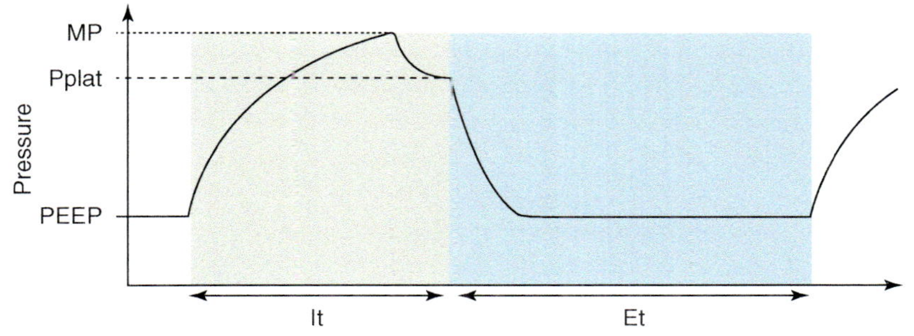

Fig. 67.4 Pressure/volume relationship in volume-control mode. *MIP* Maximal inspiratory pressure, *Pplat* plateau pressure, *PEEP* positive end expiratory pressure, *It* Inspiratory time, *Et* Expiratory time

tory phase of the mechanical ventilation that allows the airflow to overcome the airway resistance is known as maximum inspiratory pressure (MIP). This is proportional to the resistance and the tidal volume or mobilized volume during inspiration, and it is inversely proportional to lung compliance.

If one occludes the expiratory gate just before the expiration and pauses, a static inflation pressure or plateau pressure (Pplat) will be obtained, which, in practice, is considered as approximating the pressure that is reached in the distal alveoli. On the other hand, apart from the pressure generated by inspiration, an adequate level of pressure has to be maintained during expiration, in order to not reach a critical point in which the airway closes, generating atelectasis and hypoxemia again. This continuous positive pressure of the airway that avoids collapsing at the end of expiration is known as PEEP (Fig. 67.4).

Basic Elements of the Cardiopulmonary Interactions

During mechanical ventilation, a series of interactions are caused between the blood flow that enters and leaves the heart and the moments in which the lung is in inspiration or expiration as a consequence of the intrathoracic pressure variation. This intrathoracic pressure varies with the ventilatory maneuvers, and it affects the pressure gradient between the blood that returns to the heart (venous return) and the blood that leaves the thorax (stroke volume of the left ventricle).

In positive pressure ventilation, the increase of lung volume produces an increase in intrathoracic pressure, which is transmitted to all structures inside the thorax, affecting atria filling and ventricular ejection. During inspiration of positive pressure ventilation, the increase of intrathoracic pressure will determine an increase of pressure in the right atrium and a decrease of the venal return due to the decrease of the pressure gradient between the big veins and the atrium, thus determining a decrease of the preload of the right ventricle.

On the other hand, the positive pressure ventilation determined an increase of alveolar pressure and, consequently, an increase of the pressure of the alveolar vessels, determining a subsequent increase of the lung vascular resistance, meaning an increase in the afterload of the right ventricle and in consequence, a decrease of the lung blood flow. Despite an initial increase of the left atrium filling, after two to three cycles, a diminishing of the venous return appears, and, as a consequence, the preload of the left ventricle is reduced.

Finally, the afterload off the left ventricle that is related to the resistance to the left ventricle exit flow depends of the transmural pressure that exists in it; in other words, in the difference between the internal pressure of the left ventricle and the intrathoracic pressure. During positive pressure ventilation, the increase of intrathoracic pressure decreases the transmural pressure of the left ventricle, which determines a decrease of the afterload of the left ventricle and, in turn, an increase of its stroke volume (Fig. 67.5).

The understanding of cardiopulmonary interactions is essential when considering the mechanical ventilator as another therapeutic tool, for example, in heart failure, the use of invasive

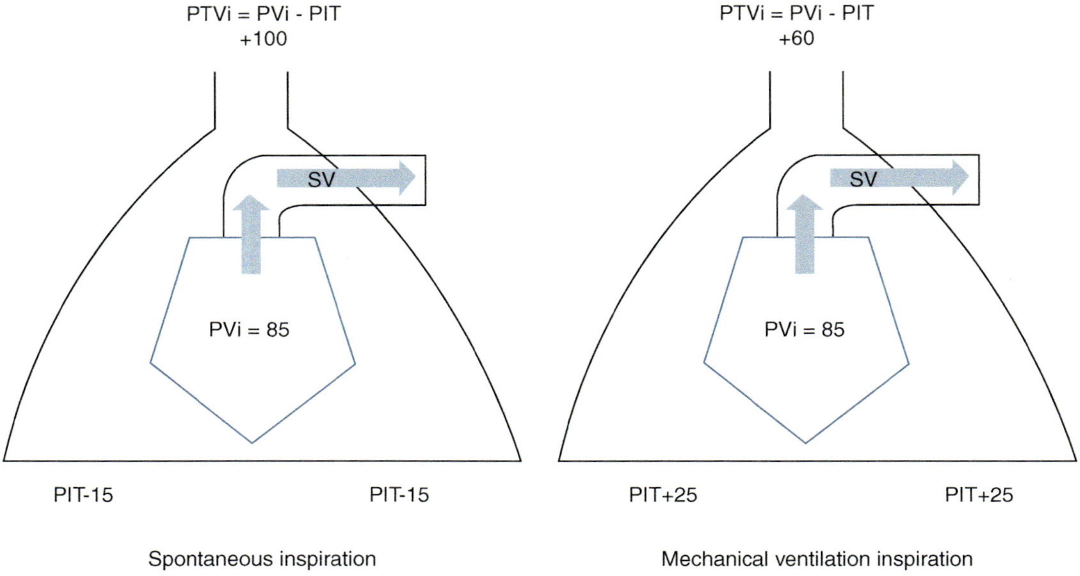

Fig. 67.5 Cardiopulmonary interaction in the left ventricle in positive pressure ventilation. *PTVi* left ventricular transmural pressure, *PVi* left ventricle peak pressure, *PIT* intrathoracic pressure, *SV* stroke volume

mechanical ventilation can be essential when diminishing the left ventricle afterload and improving cardiac output. The same considerations must be taken in patients with severe air trapping or a significant restrictive illness that could imply the use of mPaw that will deteriorate the output and worsen the prognosis of the patient.

Mechanical Ventilation Indications

The moment to start mechanical ventilation will depend of the desired clinical objective for the patient that needs connection. Before connecting the patient, the pediatrician must consider why the patient requires it: are they a patient with a severe lung disease? Is the lung disease obstructive, restrictive or mixed? Does the patient present neurological compromise? Does the patient have a serious ECT or signs of endocranial hypertension? Is the patient in septic shock or cardiogenic shock? Among other questions. All the previous questions allow defining which condition determines the indication of ventilating the patient invasively (Table 67.2).

Table 67.2 Indications to initiate mechanical ventilation

Alveolar hypoventilation: $PaCO_2 > 60$
Failure in arterial oxygenation ($PaO_2 < 70$ con $FiO_2 \geq 60$)
Severe obstructive symptoms
Apnea or respiratory arrest
Neuromuscular condition
Decrease of metabolic consumption: shock
Cardiogenic shock
Severe ECT
Complicated polytrauma
Substitution of breathing work
Thoracic wall stabilization
Surgery, ICU procedures

The most common cause of mechanical ventilation corresponds to the maintenance of gas exchange in the patient with respiratory failure, because an adequate arterial oxygenation was not achieved ($PaO_2 < 70$ with $FiO_2 > 60$) or an adequate alveolar ventilation was not achieved ($PaCO_2 > 55$–60 in the absence of chronic lung disease). Another indication of mechanical ventilation is in those situations that require a decrease or substitution of the breathing work, either because spontaneous breathing work is ineffective on its

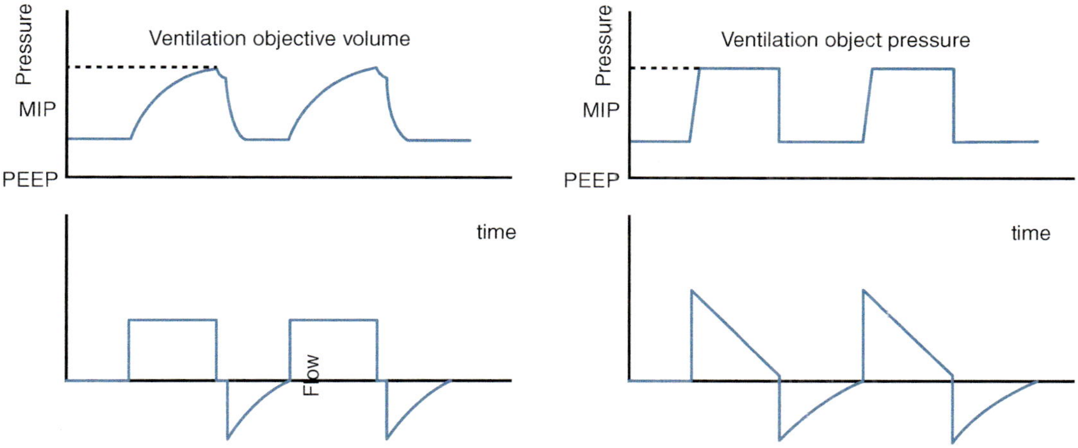

Fig. 67.6. Flow and pressure curves in invasive ventilation. *MIP* Maximal inspiratory pressure, *PEEP* Positive end-expiratory pressure

own, or because the respiratory system is incapable of performing its function due to a muscular or skeletal failure: scoliosis, trauma, thoracic cavity malformations, neuromuscular diseases, etc.

Decrease of the oxygen consumption (VO_2) constitutes another general indication of mechanical ventilation, because in pathological circumstances, oxygen consumption by the respiratory musculature can reach up to 50% of the total consumption. Thus, mechanical ventilation allows an oxygen reserve to be used by other tissues, which can be crucial in certain pathologies, such as septic shock, cardiogenic shock, endocranial hypertension, among others.

Finally, other indications of mechanical ventilation are the stabilization of the thoracic cavity in cases of polytrauma, flail thorax, thoracic surgery, or allowing sedation, analgesia, or muscle relaxation during the postoperative care of complex surgery, or in invasive procedures in critical pediatric care.

Most Used Ventilatory Modes and Initial Parameters of Ventilation in Pediatric Procedures

The ventilation offered by the mechanical ventilator is determined by an air flow provided to the patient whose only objective is usually to offer a determined volume or pressure (Fig. 67.6). The end of the inspiratory phase or cycle is reached at the moment that the objective of a determined volume, pressure, flow or time is reached according to the programming of the ventilator. The most commonly used modes will be detailed next (Fig. 67.7).

In *controlled ventilation*, all respirations are delivered by the ventilator, independently of the spontaneous effort of the patient, meaning that no spontaneous breathing is allowed, nor can the patient initiate an inspiratory cycle. In general, this ventilation mode is infrequently used, or used during general anesthesia.

Controlled-assisted ventilation consists in a preset volume or positive pressure delivered to the patient in a determined frequency, although each time the patient starts a spontaneous respiration with an inspiratory effort, the ventilator delivers an additional respiration similar to the preset ones. Despite the patient being able to increment the ventilation per minute according to their demands, they run the risk of suffering hyperventilation.

Intermittent mandatory ventilation allows the patient to breathe spontaneously and with their own effort in the mandatory ventilations.

Synchronized intermittent mandatory ventilation (SIMV) also allows the patient to breathe spontaneously between mandatory ventilations;

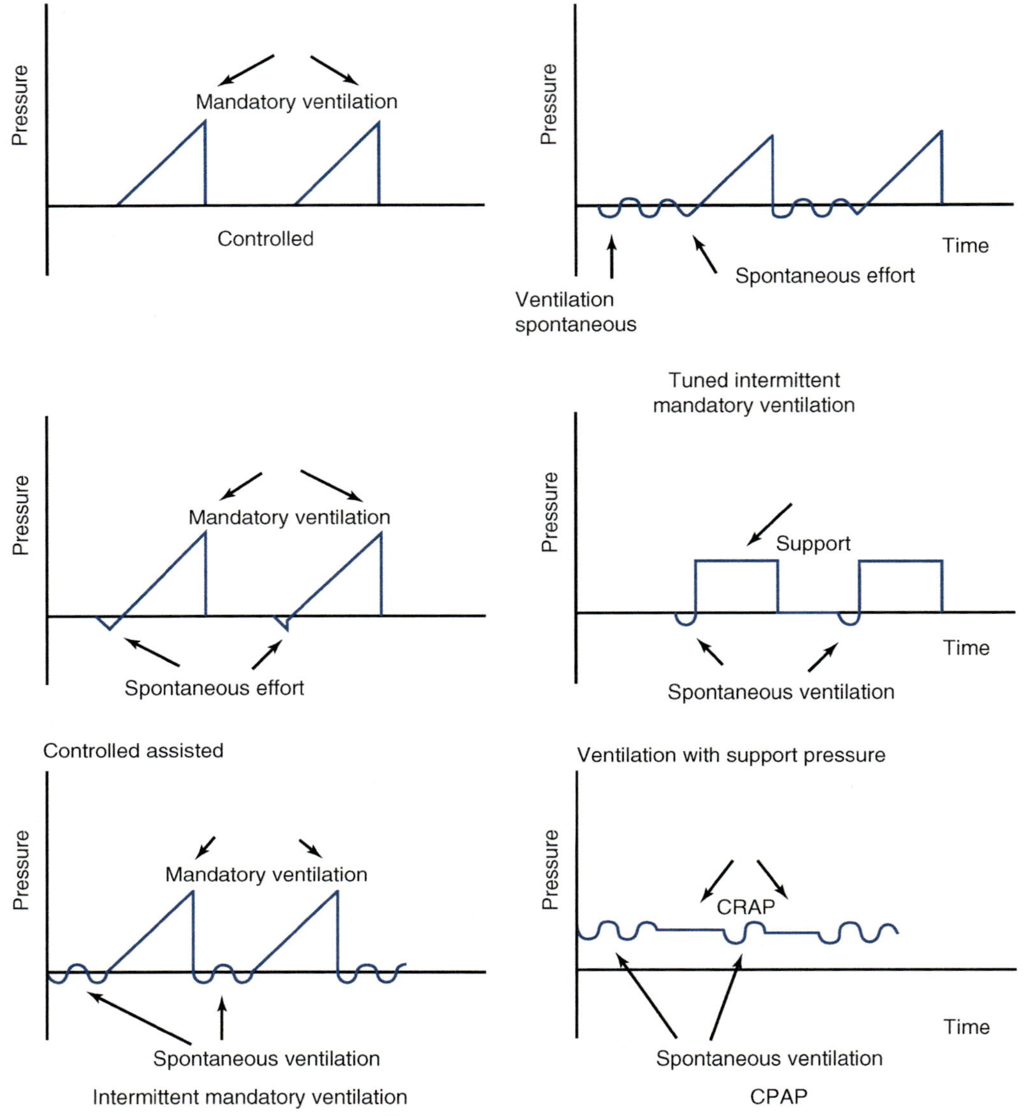

Fig. 67.7 Pressure/time curves on different ventilatory modes

however, this one allows synchronizing the mandatory ventilations with the effort of the patient, which affects the patient–ventilator interaction.

Ventilation with support pressure or assisted pressure is a form of positive pressure ventilation that provides preset pressure assistance with each voluntary inspiration the patient makes during the use of SIMV.

Pressure-regulated, volume-controlled ventilation corresponds to an increasingly common mode of use in which a determined tidal volume or minute volume is programmed, and this is delivered with a retardant flow that allows maintaining a constant volume, achieving the least pressure the system allows. In some ventilators, a maximum pressure limit can also be regulated, where the ventilator aims to provide the programmed volume with flow changes without exceeding the maximum determined pressure. This mode can be used in patients with restrictive lung disease, with risk of alveolar trauma or in those who present changes too frequently in the compliance due to their pathology.

Practical Parameters of Ventilatory Management

Once the decision to start the mechanical ventilation has been taken, the question is how to start, even though the ventilatory mode and the parameters that we use will depend on the interrelation between the patient condition (motive for the use of mechanical ventilation), equipment available, underlying pathologies of the patient, and the experience of the pediatrician or intensive care pediatrician that is treating the patient.

- *Ventilatory parameters in patients with lungs without a severe disease* (postoperative, post-procedure, neurological intubation cause, minor lung disease, etc.):

The objective is to maintain a SaO_2 and pCO_2 in physiological range. Mechanical ventilation always has to be started with FiO_2 100%, MIP between 20 and 25 (never more than 30), or tidal volumes between 5 and no more than 10 ml/kg, with PEEP from 4 to 5, and FR from 20 to 25 in infants, 15–20 in preschoolers and children in school, and between 10 and 20 in adolescents. The IT oscillates between 0.6 seconds for infants and 8.0 for adolescents, maintaining an inspiration: expiration ratio of approximately 1:2 for children and 1:3 for adolescents.

Lastly, the PEEP will have to be titrated in increments of 2 by 2 cm of H_2O, to increment the mPaw as much as necessary to achieve an adequate oxygenation according to the patient pathology and thus regulate and decrease the FiO_2 contribution, ideally reaching $FiO_2 \leq 40\%$ with saturations of ≥92–93%. These parameters intended to initiate mechanical ventilation in a normal lung or a lung without significant damage will have to be evaluated continually because they will require precise adjustments, according to the evolution of the patient and the degree of lung compromise.

- *Conventional ventilatory management in restrictive lung diseases* (ARDS, extensive pneumonia, etc.):

Severe restrictive lung disease is characterized by a heterogeneous lung compromise that varies in intensity, producing the general effect of significant decreasing of the functional residual capacity (FRC). The use of lung protection strategies is recommended for severe restrictive diseases to avoid lung damage due to overdistension and aperture, and cyclical collapse of the alveoli, also employing enough PEEP to achieve lung recruitment and improve the FRC.

As a practical matter, low tidal volumes are suggested (6 and no more than 8 ml/kg), with Pplat under 30 cm of H_2O, maintaining a sufficient PEEP to achieve and maintain an adequate lung recruitment and establish a difference between Pplat and PEEP (driving pressure) <20 cm of H_2O, ideally <15 cm H_2O. In severe lung failure, ventilatory management can be associated with a permissive management of the SaO_2 with target values ≥85%, as long as metabolic acidosis is not found and the patient does not have other hypoxia symptoms. In the same line, pCO_2 can be allowed to increase if the $pH \geq 7.2$ is kept constant. These strategies used in the severe lung failure are known as permissive hypoxemia and permissive hypercapnia, respectively, allowing management with a lower tidal volume and lower mPaw, in an effort to minimize the lung damage associated with mechanical ventilation.

- *Ventilatory management in obstructive diseases* (severe asthma, bronchiolitis, etc.):

Severe obstructive diseases are characterized by presenting significant air trapping secondary to expiratory flow obstruction. FRC is usually increased with hypercapnia secondary to the decrease of the alveolar ventilation produced by an increase of the dead space, especially the physiological space (Fig. 67.1). The recommendation in these patients is initial management with a sedated and paralyzed patient, in volume-controlled mode, with tidal volumes of 5–8 ml/kg and a per minute volume that maintains acceptable gases, even if they are not normal, with Pplat under 30 cm of H_2O. A ratio of I:E is to be maintained, ideally 1:3, because with the increase of resistance, these patients have a significant increase of the CT, which determines the need for adequate inspiratory times and long expiratory times to avoid the air trapping; this ratio can sometimes reach 1:4–1:6.

In these patients we should measure the intrinsic PEEP (PEEPi) or autoPEEP that is obtained after making a sustained expiratory pause maneuver, which will avoid the start of inspirations. This PEEPi is proportional to air trapping, so its magnitude will also determine the amount of extrinsic PEEP placed in the ventilator, which should not normally exceed the PEEPi and the sum of both should not be more than 10–15 cm H_2O, over which a hemodynamic compromise can be produced. In this way, the extrinsic PEEP should be established according to the degree of air trapping detected by the X-ray, the physical exam, and the autoPEEP or measured PEEPi. In these patients, sustained inspiratory pause maneuvers should also be realized, which will let us know the Pplat, by annulling the airway resistance, due to the 0-flow produced in the inspiratory pause. The gradient between MIP and Pplat is proportional to the severity of the obstruction and its measurement enables us to monitor the results to the treatment being applied.

Finally, in the ventilatory management of these patients, the strategies of permissive hypoxia and hypercapnia can also be applied, and will be determined by the severity of the respiratory failure.

Undesired Effects of Mechanical Ventilation

Mechanical ventilation is associated with a myriad of complications, including the need for sedation, the prolonged use of benzodiazepine, opioids, and muscle relaxants, the risk of subglottal stenosis, unscheduled extubation, and the lung damage induced by the mechanical ventilation, which we will mention below. The lung parenchyma can be affected because the mechanical ventilation is not a physiological process (Table 67.3). The lung lesion can be provoked due to biophysical factors, high pressures (barotrauma), high volumes (volutrauma), and the closing and opening process of the alveolar units.

Table 67.3 Lung damage associated with mechanical ventilation

Biophysical factors
Barotrauma:
Injury produced by high pressure
Volutrauma:
Injury induced by overdistension
Atelectrauma:
Injury induced by the repeated collapse-recruitment cycle
Biochemical factors
Biotrauma
Lung damage induced by the release of mediators at the lung tissue level

In general, the high maximum inspiratoy pressures damage the airway, added to the alveolar damage provoked by constant high Pplat and alveolar overdistension determined by an excessive volume. There are also biochemical factors that contribute to lung damage (biotrauma), due to the liberation of inflammation mediators by the airway and alveolar cells as a response to mechanical ventilation, which would increase the lung damage together with the exacerbation produced by the continuous production of atelectasis and new recruitment of the same alveolar units (atelectrauma).

At the hemodynamic level, mechanical ventilation can determine the decrease of the cardiac output due to the reduction of the venous return and the preload of both right and left ventricle. There is also an increase of the afterload of the right ventricle, which provokes a right ventricle disfunction. In the kidney, it is capable of reducing kidney blood flow and diuresis, and, on the other hand, it also provokes a decrease of the splanchnic and the pressure of cerebral perfusion. Another severe complication related to mechanical ventilation is respiratory infection that can oscillate between 6% and 26%, depending on the described series.

An increase of the risk after the fifth day of ventilation is described. The most common infections are pneumonia associated with mechanical ventilation, tracheobronchitis, and sinusitis. The associated risk factors are the loss of normal defense mechanisms of the respiratory tree provoked by the endotracheal tube overstepping these mechanisms and as a vehicle for the colonization of the lower airway, the supine position, the atelectasis, the deficient secretion clearance, and the underlying illness.

Ventilatory Weaning and Extubation

The weaning of the ventilatory support corresponds to the process that allows the movement of the patient from mechanical ventilation to spontaneous ventilation. Today's philosophy is that a gradual decrease of the ventilatory support of the patient is necessary once the cause that determined the connection to mechanical ventilation is controlled. This allows for progressive training of the respiratory musculature until the successful extubation is reached. There is no pediatric literature that supports the duration of this weaning, and the gradual process is increasingly questioned. Here, it is essential to establish what the clinical objectives will be to establish the rejection of the use of mechanical ventilation, which will depend on the relationship between the pathology or event that determined the intubation and the state of the patient. In general, it is considered that the process of *weaning* and extubation require the partial or total resolution of the problem that caused the intubation, which in global terms implies low levels of FiO_2 and mPaw (which implies low ventilatory parameters), hemodynamic stability (absence or decrease of vasoactive support), adequate neurological state that allows sustaining a permeable airway, and the correlation with the experience of the treating team.

Notwithstanding the duration of the weaning, the objective to be accomplished is successful extubation, without prolonging the mechanical ventilation if it is not necessary, because it is not without risks. This has to be considered alongside the risk that an extubated patient has of needing reintubation too early, which can be associated with both complications of the procedure and the lung and airway damage. The optimal duration of the *weaning* and the correct moment of extubation is the result of the balance between objective parameters, science, and the experience of the intensive care pediatric physicians in charge of the patient (Table 67.4).

Table 67.4 Adequate parameters to start ventilatory weaning

$FiO_2 \leq 50\%$
PEEP $\leq$5 cm H_2O
MIP $\leq$ 25–30 cm H_2O
Ventilatory frequency $\leq$20 per minute

The use of ventilatory weaning protocols in infants and children in some studies has shown a shortening of the mechanical ventilation days and lower rates of reintubation. Since there is no clear superiority of one protocol over another in the literature today, there are no standard recommendations regarding this; however, most of the patients are placed in modes with support pressure or volume, which consider the work of the patient by decreasing parameters with the additional support of their effort provided by the ventilator.

The prediction of a successful extubation in infants and children presents a great challenge in pediatrics, not only because of the weight differences but also because of the variability of pathologies that require ventilation. This is the reason that the failed extubation rates vary in the literature between 2% and 20%, depending on the population studied. In our experience, the pediatric population subject to congenital cardiopathy surgeries is 9.9%, with greater incidence on those who were exposed to deep hypothermic cardiac arrest, patients with Down syndrome and those under 6 months.

There are general accepted criteria of extubation that show evidence of adequate oxygenation and ventilation, when the cause of intubation has been overcome (Table 67.5).

Table 67.5 General criteria for extubation

Adequate oxygenation
$PaO_2 > 65–70$ or Saturation $\geq 94\%$ with $FiO_2 \leq 40$
PaFi > 180–200
Adequate ventilation
$PaCO_2 < 50$
Tidal volume >4–5 ml/kg
Negative maximum inspiratoy pressure. ≤ – 20 cm H_2O

Despite that there is not a single parameter validated as a predictor of successful extubation in the pediatric population, most of the studies coincide in using ventilometry, FiO_2, respiratory effort, and oxygenation parameters for the most important, alongside the performance of tests for spontaneous ventilation, where patients are subject to spontaneous ventilation connecting the endotracheal tube to a T tube or connecting the ventilator with low PEEP, with no frequency and with support pressure, and after a period (of at least 30 minutes), measuring physiological and clinical variables (FC, FR, PA, ventilatory effort), thus assessing the probability of extubation success.

Finally, despite what has been shown in today's literature there is no reliable and replicable method to predict the best moment to start the *weaning* or to predict the success of extubation, so the clinical judgment of an experienced treating physician has no replacement.

Conclusion

Today, ventilation has become a basic tool in the management of severe respiratory failure, and its use is increasingly frequent in pediatric intensive care units, especially high complexity units and in wintertime. The understanding of the physiological differences between pediatric and adult patients is a priority, which helps to understand the physiological processes that mechanical ventilation implies.

On the other hand, it is essential for the pediatrician working in intensive care to know not only about the physiopathology of the illness that caused the patient to connect to a respirator but also the interaction between this machine and the underlying pathology. In this way, the understanding of the functioning of the ventilator, the different modes, the different parameters to apply, the management of diverse pathologies, and secondary complications due to its use, will allow a proportionate management, with a decrease of the complications and a higher success in the treatment of the cause that motivated the connection.

Finally, the continuous evaluation of the patient will allow a process of retreat of the ventilation to be reached, followed by a successful extubation using clinical judgment and objective measurements.

Sources

Adewale L. Anatomy and assessment of the pediatric airway. Pediatr Anesth. 2009;19 (Suppl. 1:1–8.

Bronicki R, Anas N. Cardiopulmonary interaction. Pediatr Crit Care Med. 2009;10:313–22.

Carrillo A. Ventilación mecánica en pediatría (IV). Monitorización. Anales de Pediatría. 2003;59(3):252–85.

Cheifetz IM. Invasive and noninvasive pediatric mechanical ventilation. Respir Care. 2003;48(4):442–53; discussion 453–448.

Chernick V, Boat T, Wilmott R, Bush A. Kendig's disorders of the respiratory tract in children. 7th ed. Filadelfia, Pensilvania: Elsevier Saunders; 2006.

Farias JA, Alia I, Retta A, Olazarri F, Fernandez A, Esteban A, Palacios K, Di Nunzio L, Fernandez G, Bordon A, et al. An evaluation of extubation failure predictors in mechanically ventilated infants and children. Intensive Care Med. 2002;28(6):752–7.

Ferragut R. Ventilación mecánica en pediatría (II). Modalidades de ventilación. Anales de Pediatría. 2003;59(1):82–102.

Fontela PS, Piva JP, Garcia PC, Bered PL, Zilles K. Risk factors for extubation failure in mechanically ventilated pediatric patients. Pediatr Crit Care Med. 2005;6(2):166–70.

Foronda F, et al. The impact of daily evaluation and spontaneous breathing test on the duration of pediatric mechanical ventilation: A randomized controlled trial. Crit Care Med. 2011;39:2526–33.

Haitsma J. Physiology of mechanical ventilation. Crit Care Clin. 2007;23:117–34.

Kissoon N, Rimensberger P, Bohn D. Ventilatory strategies and adjuntive therapy in severe lung disease. Pediatr Clin North Am. 2008;55:709–33.

López-Herce J. Ventilación mecánica en pediatría: conceptos generales. Anales de Pediatría. 2003;59(1):59–81.

Mason RJ, Broaddus VC, Murray JF. In: Nadel JA, editor. Textbook of respiratory medicine. 4th ed. Filadelfia, Pensilvania: Elsevier Saunders; 2005.

Molini N, Ibiza E, Modesto V. Ventilación mecánica en pediatría (V). Ventilación en situaciones especiales. Anales de Pediatría. 2003;59(4):352–92.

Oddo M, et al. Management of mechanical ventilation in acute severe asthma: practical aspects. Intensive Care Med. 2006;32:501–10.

Prabhakaran P, Sasser W, Borasino S. Pediatric mechanical ventilation. Minerva Pediatr. 2011;63:411–24.

Prodhan P, Noviski N. Pediatric acute hypoxemic respiratory failure: management of oxygenation. J Intensive Care Med. 2004;19(3):140–53.

Ramírez JB. Ventilación mecánica en pediatría (III). Retirada de la ventilación, complicaciones y otros tipos de venti-lación. Anales de Pediatría. 2003;59(2):155–80.

Randolph AG, Wypij D, Venkataraman ST, Hanson JH, Gedeit RG, Meert KL, Luckett PM, Forbes P, Lilley M, Thompson J, et al. Effect of mechanical ventilator weaning protocols on respiratory outcomes in infants and children: a randomized controlled trial. JAMA. 2002;288(20):2561–8.

Rodríguez J, Ronco R, Castillo A, Guzmán G. Ventilación oscilatoria de alta frecuencia en niños con síndrome de dificultad respiratoria "del adulto". Rev Chil Pediatr. 1998;69(4):142–7.

Rogers ND. Textbook of pediatric intensive care. 4th ed. Filadelfia: Lippincot Williams & Wilkins; 2008.

Rubenfeld GD. Epidemiology of acute lung injury. Crit Care Med. 2003;31(4 Suppl):S276–84.

Slutsky AS. Ventilato-induced lung injury: from barotrauma to biotrauma. Respir Care. 2005;50(5):646–59.

Valle P, Ronco R, Clavería C, Carrasco J, Castillo A. Extubación fallida en pacientes pediátricos después de cirugía de cardiopatía congénita. Rev Chil Pediatr. 2005;76(5):479–84.

Vallejo-Manzur F, Perkins Y. Andreas vesalius, the concept of an artificial airway. Resuscitation. 2003;56:3–7.

Wheeler D, Wong H, et al. Children are not Small Adults. Open Inflamm J. 2011;4 (Suppl. 1–M2:4–15.

Chronic Invasive Ventilation

68

Claudia Astudillo Maggio, Patricio Barañao Garcés, and Mireya Méndez Raggi

Contents

Epidemiology

Even when the exact prevalence of chronic mechanical ventilation in children is unknown, some recent studies about patients under mechanical ventilation suggest a sustained increase of the need of this therapy in recent times. Indications of this therapy depend on ethical decisions, access to technologies, and diagnosis, leaving an undetermined number of patients with chronic respiratory insufficiency with no ventilation support.

In England, an increase from 141 children in chronic mechanical ventilation in 1998, to 933 children under the age of 17 years in 2008 has

C. Astudillo Maggio (✉) · M. Méndez Raggi
Pediatrics, Respiratory Diseases, Hospital Josefina Martínez, Puente Alto, Chile

Pontificia Universidad Católica de Chile, Santiago, Chile
e-mail: gestion@hjm.cl

P. Barañao Garcés
Respiratory Kinesiotherapy, Hospital Josefina Martínez, Puente Alto, Chile

Pontificia Universidad Católica de Chile, Santiago, Chile
e-mail: patricio.baranao@uc.cl

P. Bertrand, I. Sánchez (eds.), *Pediatric Respiratory Diseases*,
https://doi.org/10.1007/978-3-030-26961-6_68

been observed. Of the total patients, 91% were in their homes; the rest were in hospitals as critical patients or pediatric intensive care units. Most frequent pathologies that required the use of ventilation were: neuromuscular diseases (43%), lung diseases (39%), and conditions related to the central nervous system (18%). Of these patients, 71% had ventilation only while sleeping, and 22% had ventilation through tracheostomy. In 2002, in 46 Spanish intensive care units, 23.2% of patients had chronic mechanical ventilation through tracheostomy.

In Chile, according to data obtained at the Ministry of Health (Minsal), during 2003 and 2005 winter campaigns, between 20% and 30% of critical beds were used by patients with extended mechanical ventilation. In 2006, the national program of ventilatory support at home started, and in October of 2014, 734 patients under the age of 20 had joined this program. From these, 69% receive non-invasive ventilation support, and 31% invasive ventilation support through tracheostomy.

Josefina Martínez hospital, specialized in care of patients with child chronic respiratory diseases, formed a ventilation support unit in 2006. Currently, it counts with 40 of its beds for ventilation, 95% of its patients require invasive ventilation support through tracheostomy, and only 5% are patients with non-invasive ventilation support. These data reflect the increasing need of this kind of attention, both in home and in hospitals.

Chronic Respiratory Insufficiency Causes

We define chronic respiratory insufficiency (CRI) as that which persists for more than 3 weeks once the acute episode has been solved (Table 68.1).

Chronic respiratory insufficiency causes can be grouped according to:

Level of failure:

- *Respiratory*: Involving the lung parenchyma or airway.
- *Central nervous system*: The beginning of the ventilation is affected, especially during deep sleep.
- *Respiratory pump*: When nerve tracts, motoneurons, neuromuscular plate, musculature, or thoracic cavity are affected.
- *Mixed*: Involving more than one of the aforementioned causes.

Table 68.1 Chronic respiratory failure causes

SNC alterations	Congenital and acquired disorders of the control of the respiratory center	Myelomeningocele and Arnold-Chiari malformations	
Alterations in the ventilation pump	Congenital hypotonias	Myasthenia gravis	Phrenic and diaphragmatic paralysis
	Myopathy	Muscular dystrophy	Guillain-Barré syndrome
	Botulism	Diaphragmatic hernia	Spinal muscular atrophy
Skeletal alterations	Kyphoscoliosis	Thoracic walls deformities	
Alterations in the airway and respiratory parenchyma	Obstruction of the high airway: craniofacial malformative syndromes (Pierre Robin, Treacher Collins) Laryngotracheomalasia Tracheoesophageal fistula Subglottic stenosis Vocal chords paralysis	Bronchopulmonary alterations Bronchopulmonary dysplasia Cystic fibrosis Lung hypoplasia Obliterans bronchiolitis	
Others	Congenital and acquired cardiopathies	Metabolic diseases	

According to evolution or prognosis:
- *Susceptible to improvement*: Such as bronchopulmonary dysplasia, airway malacia, Guillain-Barré syndrome, obliterans bronchiolitis.
- *Stable or progressive*: Includes neuromuscular disease, hypoventilation syndrome.

Chronic Mechanical Ventilation Indications

The main indication of mechanical ventilation is to maintain gaseous exchange. Therefore, it is indicated in patients with chronic respiratory insufficiency, which include alterations of chest wall (severe scoliosis), alterations in breath control (central hypoventilation syndromes), serious alterations of the airway (malacia in trachea or bronchus), and alterations of lung parenchyma, such as obliterans bronchiolitis and bronchopulmonary dysplasia.

Must fulfill all physiological criteria and at least one clinical criterion:

Physiological criteria
- $PaCO_2 > 45$ mmHg $PaO_2 < 65$ mmHg

Clinical criteria
- Limited air intake
- Use of accessory musculature
- Decrease of physical activity
- Scarce weight gain

Objectives of Chronic Mechanical Ventilation

Patients requirements are different, as well as goals or objectives to achieve with each one.

In general, we may consider:

Respiratory ob.jectives
- Revert hypoxemia
- Revert respiratory acidosis
- Alleviate respiratory work
- Decrease systemic or myocardial oxygen consumption
- Stabilize chest wall
- Decrease the lung iatrogenic lesion and other ventilation complications

Systemic objectives
- Extend and improve life quality
- Provide an environment which increases each individual's potential
- Reduce morbidity
- Favor an appropriate child physical growth and psychosocial development

Selection of Ventilation Method

The selection of the method of mechanical ventilation, whether invasive or non-invasive, in the pediatric patient with chronic respiratory insufficiency, depends on some of the following factors:

- *Duration*: Quantity of hours per day of needing support. If more than 12 hours per day are required, the invasive way through tracheostomy is preferred. If the need is equal or less than 12 hours, non-invasive way, using the most appropriate interface for the patient.
- *Tolerance to interfaces*: This is an essential factor in the success or failure of non-invasive ventilation. Anatomical, psychological, and mental health factors may provoke intolerance to facial, nasal, or naso-buccal mask, and therefore the patient must be ventilated through tracheostomy.
- *Risk/benefit balance and ethical decisions*: The decision of using chronic ventilation and the method applied, force us to consider universal ethical principles. For instance, the case of limitation of therapeutic efforts.
- *Scenario*: Currently, chronic ventilation can occur in different scenarios, such as in a critical patient unit or in the pediatric room of a critical patients hospital, in a chronic patients hospital, or at home, depending on the degree of complexity of the patient and access to domiciliary programs.
- *Need for autonomy*: Patients with night exclusive ventilation have a greater autonomy for doing daily life activities such as attending school. In patients with total ventilation, this autonomy can be given through appropriate equipment selection.

Ventilation Modes

Most used modes for chronic mechanical ventilation in children are limited by pressure and time cycles. In Josefina Martínez hospital a working algorithm is used (Fig. 68.1) that allows choosing between modes from less to more complex:

- *CPAP*: It delivers continuous positive pressure in the airway during the whole respiratory cycle. It requires the patient to breathe spontaneously and be able to start an effective inhalation. It prevents the collapse of the upper and lower tract of the airway, as well as in the alveoli, improving oxygenation. It is used in patients with severe malacia and when removing the mechanical ventilation.
- *Spontaneous (S): Two leveled pressure (IPAP/EPAP):* It gives inspiratory and expiratory

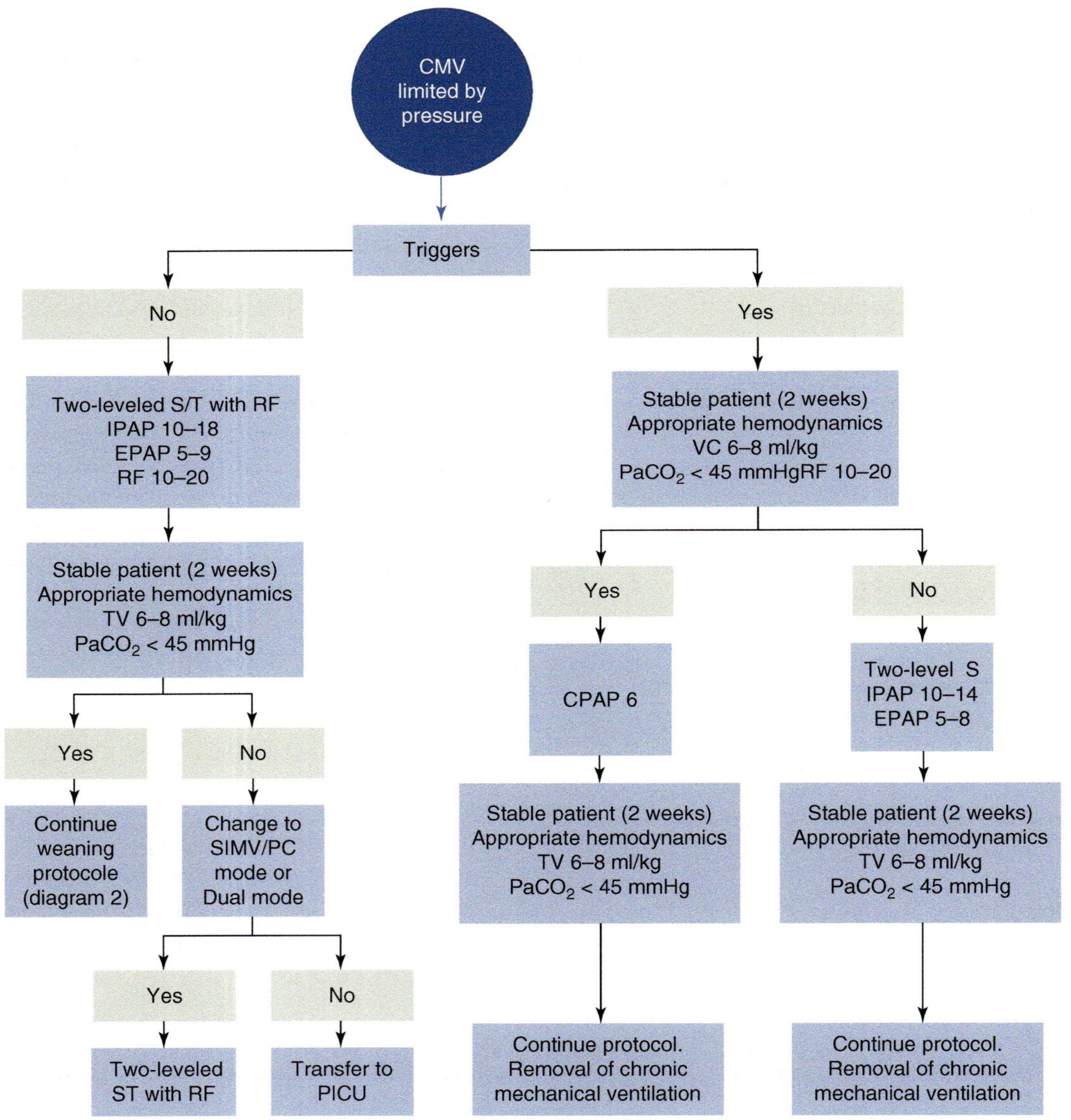

Fig. 68.1 Selection of method of ventilation

pressure, without the need for backup rate. It is used as a previous step at the employment of CPAP.

- *Spontaneous/cyclic (S/T)*: Two leveled pressure with respiratory frequency (RF).
- *Dual*: Two leveled inspiratory pressure (IPAP max/IPAP min). With assured tidal volume with or without respiratory frequency. Both are utilized for the treatment of patients with neuromuscular diseases or diseases of the lung parenchyma.
- *Intermittent synchronization (SIMV/PC):* It gives two leveled pressure (MIP/PEEP), backup respiratory rate, and programmable support pressure. In patients without ventilatory autonomy; for example, type I spinal atrophy, severe bronchopulmonary dysplasia, or obliterans bronchiolitis.

Equipment

When we choose the equipment for delivering chronic ventilation, we must know its technical specifications and which advantages are obtained compared to others (Table 68.2). Some of the most important elements are:

- *Registration*: Through cards, which are interpreted through a software, we can obtain information about hours of equipment use, percentage of respirations triggered by the patient, pressures and volume given by the ventilator in each respiration and for those generated by the patient, if present.
- *Autonomy*: It refers to the possibility of functioning without electric supply, in other words, whether the equipment possesses a battery or not. In this case, the internal battery duration is important, because it will enable us to use the equipment for transferences, or for going with the patient to school or other daily life activities.

In our hospital we've successfully utilized flow generators ventilators with turbines and two-leveled pressure (IPAP/EPAP-MIP/PEEP). This equipment was created for non-invasive ventilation, and because of their turbines, they do not require compressed air, so they can be implemented outside of hospital environments, in homes and transferences.

Monitoring

The monitoring level of the patient with invasive chronic ventilation will depend on the scenario in which the patient is in, the main objective being the patient's security.

Non-invasive monitoring through continuous measuring of pulse oximetry and heart frequency, immediately gives information and warning about complications, such as decannulation or cannula obstruction, which, if not

Table 68.2 Ventilation equipment

Equipment name	Trilogy 100 or 202®	Synchrony® Stellar 150	Harmony®, Stellar 100
Limited by	Pressure, volume or dual	Pressure or dual	Pressure
Modes	CPAP, S, S/T, T, Simv (PC, VC), AC	CPAP, S, S/T, T y PC	CPAP, S and S/T
Battery	2 internal per equipment	Only Stellar 150	Solo Stellar 100
Circuit type	Passive or active	Passive	Passive
Record system	SD Card	Encore Card/Pendrive	Encore Card/Pendrive
League compensation	Yes	Yes	Yes
Base with wheels	Yes	No	No
Air mixer/O_2 (FiO_2)	Only Trilogy 202	No	No
Humidification thermos (HT)	External	Built-in to equipment	Built-in to equipment
Electric consumption	165 Watts/h with HT	130 Watts/h with HT	130 Watts with HT

detected, could pose a risk to the life of the patient. This is the minimal monitoring that a child must have at home.

Besides, monitoring represents an important tool for tracking and clinical decision making in the case of exacerbations or the start of the removal of the mechanical ventilation.

In hospital environments, monitoring is made through:

- *Non invasive monitoring:* Pulse oximetry and permanent heart frequency. Vital signs control: Blood pressure, temperature, respiratory frequency.
- *Venous or arterial gases:* Are made routinely when the patient is admitted, and afterward are repeated with a frequency defined by the particular case. They are a vital tool in the management of exacerbations and decision making like parameters changes or ventilation removal.
- *Chest x ray*: Useful in the case of exacerbations or behavior changes, and the evaluation of the position of the cannula.
- *Capnography:* Not always available in every center, but very useful, because it prevents arterial puncture and the pain it provokes in the patient. It allows behavior changes and tracking in the case of respiratory exacerbations.
- *Polysomnography:* It allows defining the beginning of ventilatory, fixing or modifying parameters, and deciding the removal of ventilation support. In chronic mechanical ventilation, the examination musts have continuous capnography which allows measuring exhaled CO_2.

Sedation

It does not require the use of sedation, because one of our objectives with chronic mechanical ventilation is the patient's comfort and integral development. This is achieved by choosing the appropriate interface and ventilatory mode, which meets the needs of the patient.

Weaning or Removal of Invasive Chronic Mechanical Ventilation

Removal of mechanical ventilation, defined as the transition from assisted ventilation to autonomous ventilation, is possible when the cause that provoked the need of ventilatory support is overcome and, in consequence, is feasible to execute in the case of pathologies susceptible to improvement but not in stable or progressive ones.

The moment for starting the removal of ventilation is decided when it can be guaranteed:

- An appropriate neuromuscular function, with a ventilatory pump functioning that allows sustaining respiratory work during wakefulness and sleep.
- Minimal respiratory work.
- Clinical stability: no exacerbations in last month.

Parameters which correlate with better chance of success are:

- TV > 6.5 ml/kg
- Mid pressure of the airway <5 cm H_2O
- PIM < 10 cm H_2O and PEEP <6 cm H_2O
- $FiO_2 < 0.3$

Another necessary element for taking the decision of starting the removal is the airway and lung parenchyma structural and functional indemnity. This requires an evaluation through fibro bronchoscopy or thoracic images, such as X-rays or computed tomography.

The weaning or removal can be done following clinical criteria established by the treating doctor or through a ventilation removal protocol such as that presented hereunder:

Protocol of Removal of Chronic Mechanical Ventilation (Hospital Josefina Martínez)

1. Decrease to the point that maximum inspiratory pressure (MIP or IPAP), maintaining

PEEP or EPAP, and supporting with gases on awakening.
2. In parallel, evaluate the trigger of the patient using the registration cards that ventilation equipment possess, for starting the decreasing of back up frequency, to hit a spontaneous level.
3. Changes are executed slowly, every 2 weeks and one at a time (pressures or frequency), maintaining a differential pressure (IPAP-PEEP) of 4 cm of H_2O.
4. When IPAP hits 10 cm H_2O, with a PEEP of 6 cm of H_2O in spontaneous level, the next step is to let the patient just with PEEP of 6.
5. Decrease to a PEEP of 5.
6. After 2 weeks of clinical stability, ventilatory support is suspended.
7. Continue to protocol of decannulation.

Protocol of decannulation (Hospital Josefina Martínez)

1. Airway visualization, through fibro-bronchoscopy.
2. If there is no obstruction in the high airway, such as granulomas, laryngomalacia, craniofacial malformations, proceed to the next step.
3. Measuring of the expiratory pressure maintained in the airway (Villarroel et al.).
4. Use of phonation valve 24 hours a day.
5. Decrease the internal diameter of the TQT cannula, until reaching at least 3.5.
6. Use of cover of cannula throughout the day.
7. Cover cannula during sleep and execute night saturometry.

- If patient does not present saturations of less than 90, decannulation can be programmed.

Complications

Complications can be classified according to their cause, related to the use of tracheostomy, patient, or equipment.

Related to:

1. Tracheostomy:
   - Displacement
   - Obstruction
   - Infection — Granuloma — Bleeding
2. Patient
   - Use of positive pressure: pneumothorax, cardiopulmonary interactions
   - Patient/ventilator asynchrony
   - Infections (pneumonia associated with mechanical ventilation)
3. Equipment: including ventilator and circuits – technical malfunction
   - Disconnection

The frequency of major complications of tracheostomy in children, such as hemorrhage, pneumothorax, pneumomediastinum, emphysema, accidental decannulation, tracheoesophageal fistula, and cervical abscess, varies between 5% and 49%.

Congenital cardiopathies, prematurity, and age under 1 year, are characteristics associated with precocious mortality, before the 7 days after tracheostomy in children. Accidental decannulation is one of the most important causes of late mortality.

Accidental decannulation is a potentially lethal adverse event, and as well as pneumonia related to mechanical ventilation, it is an indicator of care quality. In Josefina Martínez hospital, accidental decannulation represents 30% of reported incidents between 2009 and 2014, having fatal consequences in one patient, and serious consequences, such as persistent vegetative state, in two patients. Rate of pneumonia associated with mechanical ventilation (PAMV) is of 1.4 per 1000 days of ventilation. This number is far below the ones reported in intensive care units.

Concerned about the increasing number of pediatric patients with tracheostomy dependent on technology, which potentially can present life-threatening complications, the American Heart Association, through their PALS continuous educational courses, spread the mnemonic rule DOPE (stands for displacement, obstruction, pulmonary, equipment), which allows a practical approach to the emergency.

Preventive protocols are necessary for preventing the frequency or severity of these complications. Among these, we can mention the protocol of management of tracheostomy, which includes the periodic inspection of the hold collar. In any case, very well-trained personnel are needed, and they should constantly improve their qualification.

Sources

Bach J. The use of mechanical ventilation is appropriate in children with genetically proven spinal muscular atrophy type 1: the motion for. Paediatr Respir Rev. 2008;9:45–50.

Bach JR, Saltstein K, Sinquee D, Weaver B, Komaroff E. Long-term survival in Werdnig–Hoffmann disease. Am J Phys Med Rehabil. 2007;86:339–45.

Bertrand P, Fehlmann B, Lizama M, Holmgren N, Silva MY, Sánchez I. Asistencia ventilatoria domiciliaria en niños chilenos: 12 años de experiencia. Arch Bronconeumol. 2006;42(4):165–70.

Graham R, Fleegler E, Robinson W. Chronic ventilator need in the community: A 2005 Pediatric Census of Massachusetts. Pediatrics. 2007;119:e1280.

Guzmán C. Ventilación mecánica en niños. In: Reyes M, Aristizábal G, Leal F, editors. Neumología pediátrica. 5th ed. Editorial Médica Panamericana: Bogotá; 2006. p. 713–20.

Harikumar G, Moxham J, Greenough A, Rafferty G. Measurement of maximal inspiratory pressure in ventilated children. Pediatr Pulmonol. 2008;43:1085–91.

MacIntyre N, Epstein S, Carson S, Scheinhorn D, Christopher K, Muldoon S. Management of patients requiring prolonged mechanical ventilation. Chest. 2005;128:3937–54.

Martin D, Smith B, Davenport P, Harman E, Gonzalez-Rothi R, Baz M, Layon J, et al. Inspiratory muscle strength training improves weaning outcome in failure to wean patients: a randomized trial. Crit Care. 2011;15:R84.

Méndez M, Prado F, Navarro S, Sánchez I. Rol de un hospital especializado en los cuidados respiratorios de pacientes con enfermedades pulmonares crónicas. In: Sánchez I, Prado F, editors. Enfoque clínico de las enfermedades respiratorias del niño. Santiago: Ediciones Universidad Católica de Chile; 2007. p. 521–8.

Monteverde F, Fernandez A, Poterala R, Vidal N, Siaba A, Castelani P, Albano I, Podesta F, Farias J. Characterization of pediatric patients receiving prolonged mechanical ventilation. Pediatr Crit Care Med. 2011;12(6):e287–91.

Nava S, Fasano L. Inspiratory muscle training in difficult to wean patients: work it harder, make it better, do it faster, makes us stronger. Crit Care. 2011;15:153.

Overman A, Liu M, Kurachek S, Shreve M, Maynard R, Mammel M, Moore B. Tracheostomy for infants requiring prolonged mechanical ventilation: 10 years' experience. Pediatrics. 2013;131:e1491.

Prado F, Salinas P, Astudillo P, Méndez M. Ventilación mecánica invasiva domiciliaria (VMI). Una propuesta para un nuevo programa. Rev Neumolog Pediátr. 2007;2:49–60.

Smith B, Bleiweis M, Neel C, Martin D. Inspiratory muscle strength training in infants with congenital heart disease and prolonged mechanical ventilation: a case report. Phys Ther. 2013;93:229–36.

The Cochrane Collaboration. Protocolized versus non-protocolized weaning for reducing the duration of invasive mechanical ventilation in critically ill paediatric patients. 2013.

Wallis C, Paton JY, Beaton S, Jardine E. Children on long-term ventilatory support: 10 years of progress. Arch Dis Child. 2011;96:998–1002.

Long-Term Non-invasive Ventilation

69

Francisco Prado Atlagic, Pamela Salinas Flores, and Gerardo Ferrero

Contents

Physiological Bases

Non-invasive ventilation (NIV) is a form of mechanical ventilation that is based on the application of cyclical or continuous positive pressure in the airway. It does not require an artificial airway, avoiding the complications generated by an endotracheal tube or tracheostomy. Accordingly, a nasal, nasolabial, or facial mask is used as an interface and can be implemented for managing acute and chronic respiratory insufficiency.

In adults and children, there is enough evidence to support its use in patients with chronic diseases that may present acute scenarios, especially in patients with neuromuscular diseases and also in pathologies with lung parenchyma and distal airways compromise, such as chronic obstructive pulmonary disease (COPD) and cystic fibrosis. In this scenario, when compared to invasive mechanical ventilation (IV), NIV shows

F. Prado Atlagic (✉)
Department of Pediatrics, Hospital Clínico San Borja Arriarán, Santiago, Chile

P. Salinas Flores
Pediatric Service, Clínica Las Lilas, Providencia, Chile

G. Ferrero
Respiratory Kinesiology and Physiatry, Hospital Rehabilitación Respiratoria María Ferrer, Buenos Aires, Argentina
e-mail: gerardo.ferrero@respironics.com

P. Bertrand, I. Sánchez (eds.), *Pediatric Respiratory Diseases*,
https://doi.org/10.1007/978-3-030-26961-6_69

lower mortality rates, fewer days of hospitalization, and fewer complications.

In addition, the evidence of its benefits as a prolonged mechanical ventilation strategy in patients with neuromuscular problems such as kyphoscoliosis has been established, relating its early onset, at the time of nocturnal hypoventilation, with a better prognosis, better health-related quality of life (HRQoL), and lower related costs.

Benefits of Non-invasive Ventilation in Chronic Patients

From physiological studies in adults, it has been demonstrated that non-invasive ventilation manages to diminish the electromyographic activity of the diaphragm, the transdiaphragmatic pressure, and the respiratory frequency. In addition, it increases tidal volume, which translates into less work of breathing and an increase in ventilation per minute, reversing chronic hypoventilation.

Among the main benefits of non-invasive ventilation in chronic patients it is possible to mention:

- Upper airway stability, which is especially important during sleep, as this allows a normal air flow with minimum resistance and achieves less work of breathing, which also adds to an improvement in sleep architecture. This justifies its use in patients with obstructive sleep apnea syndrome (OSAS) and in those with craniofacial syndromes.
- There is a lower O_2 consumption by decreasing the work of breathing, lower CO_2 production, and lower energy consumption by respiratory muscles. Added to these benefits is the increase of resistance to fatigue during the day when ventilatory support is used at night.
- Increased functional residual capacity (FRC) in patients with restrictive ventilatory defect, by providing support for transpulmonary pressure, which results in a lower predisposition to hypoxemia and lower O_2 requirements because it decreases the tendency to alveolar collapse (atelectasis) and improves ventilation/perfusion ratio. The increase in lung compliance optimizes the mechanics of the lung-chest system, improving gas exchange.
- Active assisted exercise to improve compliance of the developing thoracic cage, with tendency toward restriction due to weakness of inspiratory muscles in patients with neuromuscular pathology.

Positive pressure decreases thoracic deformity and helps its rectification and expansion.

Sustained use of this therapy improves respiratory center sensitivity to CO_2. This fact favors patients with chronic ventilatory insufficiency who receive non-invasive ventilation, presenting less acute exacerbations and hospitalizations. By lowering fatigability thresholds and mitigating respiratory work overload, the patient achieves a baseline condition, granting a better faces preparation for decompensation, leading to an improvement in health-related quality of life.

Non-invasive ventilation in chronic patients is delivered as the main strategy for long-term home mechanical ventilation. Indications and selection criteria for this are shown in Tables 69.1 and 69.2.

Table 69.1 Indications for home non-invasive ventilation

NIV indications
(a) Patients with chronic respiratory failure and sleep-related hypoventilation syndromes with at least one criterion:
Frequent SpO_2 <90% in continuous 8-hour observation
FVC <50%; PiMax <40 cm H_2O; Cough Peak Flow <150 L/min
$PaCO_2$ >50 mmHg; BE>4 mEq /L
(b) Patients with compromised control of ventilation and OSAS
Frequent SpO_2 <90% in continuous 8-hour observation
Apnea-Hypopnea Index>5; $TcCO_2$ >50 mmHg for more than 50%

Table 69.2 Selection criteria for home non-invasive ventilation

NIV selection criteria
Stable clinical condition that allows respiratory autonomy outside non-invasive ventilation
NIV requirements in less than 12 hours
Hypercapnia without respiratory acidosis; oxygen requirement <2 L/min to maintain SpO_2 >93%
Socioeconomic status that allows having appropriate facilities and basic amenities. Level of education that allows compliance with the indications
Caregivers committed to monitoring and controls

Equipment for NIV Delivery: Technical Considerations

Non-invasive ventilation uses pressure-controlled ventilation, which involves setting inspiratory and expiratory pressure limits. There are exclusive flow generators for this, less expensive than conventional positive pressure respirators. Among them the bi-level equipment stands out, which is transportable, electric, and of continuous flow, using a turbine connected to a compressor.

Bi-Level Positive Airway Pressure

It delivers a positive airway pressure in two levels with independent adjustment: inspiratory positive airway pressure (IPAP) and expiratory positive airway pressure (EPAP). The difference between the two is the pressure support level.

Inspiratory positive airway pressure (IPAP): Sets the inspiratory pressure limit and controls ventilation. The higher the IPAP is, the higher the tidal volume during inspiratory phase. The percentage of inspiratory time will determine the IPAP duration.

Expiratory positive airway pressure (EPAP): Sets the expiratory pressure limit above atmospheric pressure. It improves functional residual capacity and oxygenation.

Pressure support (IPAP–EPAP): The difference between IPAP and EPAP generates a pressure gradient called pressure support. Ventilation occurs as a consequence of the difference between these pressures.

Two pressure levels are useful in restrictive disorders that require increasing the functional residual capacity and decreasing the work of the respiratory muscles. For example, in patients with neuromuscular diseases (Duchenne muscular dystrophy, congenital muscular dystrophy, congenital myopathy, congenital spinal muscular atrophy), severe cases of kyphoscoliosis, and in diseases that compromise the central nervous system, such as myelomeningocele and type I and II Chiari malformations. It could also be used in alterations of the respiratory center (central hypoventilation syndromes).

Bi-level positive airway pressure can be used in different modes, with differences between available options by the different existing equipment.

Household equipment usually does not have an internal battery, which limits non-invasive ventilation in transport or in the event of a power outage. This can be solved with optional external batteries appropriate for the equipment which allows its operation, although this usually only works for the flow generator and not the associated humidifier. New equipment comes with lithium-ion batteries that deliver a minimum of 4 hours of autonomy.

Flow generators allow recognizing and compensating involuntary leaks in the system; more traditional equipment triggers inspiratory flow to deliver programmed IPAP when they sense in the system a flow generated by the patient of 40 ml/s for more than 30 ms. Inspiration ends when it lasts for more than 3 s or the flow has dropped to a quarter of the maximum flow. The VPAP II, III, Stellar 100 and 150, and VS III (Resmed) equipment can be programmed to deliver a minimum and maximum inspiratory time (Ti Control). Equipment, such as S/T-D 30, Vision, Harmony, Synchrony (Respironics), and currently Trilogy, A30 and A-40 (Philips), have a sensitivity algorithm defined as Auto-Trak, which detects patient flow pattern, automatically adjusting sensitivity thresholds through three algorithms: (1) Inspiratory trigger threshold of 6 ml/s in a period of 30 ms; (2) Triggering algorithm determined by the flow curve shape from IPAP to EPAP and EPAP to IPAP; (3) Trigger according to spontaneous expiratory threshold to cycle to EPAP.

Conventional microprocessor-based mechanical ventilators, which have a pressure support and built-in non-invasive mode (New Port Wave or New Port E500, Evita XL or Savina by Dräger, Vela and Aveas by Vyasis, I-Vent by Versamed, Servo I Maquet and Galileo, G1 and G5 of Hamilton, among others), can be used for non-invasive ventilation in patients in pediatric intensive care units. Its administration through a conventional ventilator allows to determine the inspired oxygen concentration (the new generation of hybrid equipment has internal oxygen mixers), to prevent rebreathing due to use of double tubing, and to use the ventilator monitors and alarms. The vast majority of these 'heavy' mechanical or institutional-use ventilators have non-invasive ventilation modes. For this, it is necessary to change the active exhalation option, through an exhalation valve, to passive exhalation (in the mask or in the proximal exhalation port), or to maintain the exhalation through the exhalation valve of the ventilator, requiring in these cases non-vented masks (they are indicated by their light blue elbow). The disadvantage of using these ventilators is that they do not produce good leak compensation, which creates a strong adjustment pressure of the mask to the face, causing discomfort, poor tolerance, and complications such as pressure ulcers.

The choice of the ventilator for the administration of non-invasive ventilation will depend on the variety and particular characteristics of the available equipment, the type of patient, the circumstances in which it is applied, and the operator experience.

Non-invasive Ventilation Modes with Bi-level Flow Generators

These devices regulate a constant flow of air and have the capacity to change that flow to achieve certain pressures chosen by an operator. The exhalation is usually established passively through the interface (masks with exhalation port) in the units that work with tubing for inspiration and exhalation, as is the case in the vast majority of flow generators marketed for home use. Regardless of the method to establish non-invasive ventilation, a device capable of correcting the leakage flow (Q leak) is required; some equipment even requires a minimum Q leak of 13 LPM. The turbine establishes accelerated flows that decline once the IPAP is achieved, with cycle times and inspiratory duration determined by the percentage of the total time of the chosen cycle for inspiration, by direct programming of the inspiratory time, and by the maximum fixed flow percentage; traditionally, this last parameter is established in a quarter of the maximum Q.

In sum, flow generators work with pressure programming and are usually limited by flow (to prevent undesirable prolongation of inspiration when there is a leak in the interface or an obstructive pathology) or by inspiratory time (to prevent short Ti in patients with decreased compliance). At present, there is equipment that, while cycling by pressure, deliver an "assured" tidal volume in the range of 2 IPAP, maximum and minimum. This feature decreases the risk of hypoventilation: these methods may have tidal volume targets (AVAPS™, Philips Respironics), or alveolar ventilation targets (iVAPS™, ResMed Inc).

Rise Time regulates the air entry speed during inspiratory time: the higher the Rise Time, the longer it will take to reach the set IPAP within a cycle, improving tolerance in some patients. This time should be minimal in patients with dyspnea due to restrictive lung diseases. The values oscillate between 0.1 and 0.9 s. It is important to note that Rise Time should not exceed 40% of the total inspiratory time, since it has a direct implication on the final tidal volume delivered.

Ramp time refers to a characteristic that some equipment has, in which there is a latency expressed in minutes for the pressures selected by an operator to be achieved. In general, the minimum EPAP to start ramp time is 4 cm H_2O and the time to reach planned pressures is 5–30 minutes. This method of progressive delivery of expiratory pressure in the airway is particularly useful and comfortable in patients with sleep apnea, giving them enough time to fall asleep.

Volume Assist-Control Ventilation (ACV)

Volume assist-control ventilation (ACV) is defined as a time or patient-triggered, flow-limited, and volume-cycled mode. A constant flow waveform is used, although a decelerating flow waveform can be used if the ventilator software allows it. The latter is recommended for the application of non-invasive ventilation (NIV), since it is the most comfortable one for the patient.

The ventilator delivers a predetermined tidal volume in response to the patient's inspiratory effort (assisted mechanical ventilation or AMV). If the patient does not trigger the respirator, it will give him the tidal volume added to a predetermined respiratory frequency (controlled mechanical ventilation or CMV) or the combination of both (ACMV). In the case of long-term home non-invasive ventilation, this method is the first choice in those patients with neuromuscular disorders with advanced symptoms, mainly for cough assistance (increase in inspiratory capacity and consequent increase in peak cough flow (PCF) or because there is no other ventilator available that offers more sophisticated or comfortable options for the patient (PSV, Bilevel, iVAPS)

Pressure-Control Ventilation (PCV)

In pressure-control ventilation (PCV) all breaths are time- or patient-triggered (in assisted mode), pressure-limited (inspiratory pressure), and time-cycled (inspiratory time). The flow waveform is decelerating.

The tidal volume will depend on the patient's thoraco-pulmonary impedance: the greater the latter, maximal inspiratory pressure will be obtained more quickly and with a smaller volume of alveolar ventilation.

With pressure ventilation, the maximal inspiratory pressure is the variable to be programmed instead of the Vt as in the volumetric mode. In addition, the operator must place a minimum respiratory rate, an inspiratory time (Ti) or I:E ratio, and the sensitivity level of the trigger.

The main differences between the pressure and the volumetric modes are the tidal volume consistency and the peak inspiratory pressure (PIP): the PIP is constant with the control pressure, but the tidal volume can vary. Its main advantage over NIV is that the flow is variable and can be adjusted to the patient's flow demand, within the framework of a pre-established pressure delta: the higher the delta, the greater the capacity to generate higher flows. This mode is chosen when the patient does not achieve an adequate ventilator adaptation in the pressure support ventilation (PSV) mode due to a leak around the mask: in PCV, since inspiratory time is fixed, the cycle to expiration will be according to the patient's demand, despite the system leak. Thus, the operator will determine the ventilator inspiratory time according to the patient inspiratory time (usually between 0.6 and 1.2 sec, depending on age and underlying pathology).

Interfaces

There are a wide variety of interfaces that adjust to the age and the morphology of the face of the patient. This choice is essential to achieve an adequate pressure transfer to the airway, which translates into proper ventilation and no unwanted side effects such as injuries where the pressure points are.

The interfaces must be made of soft, flexible, silicone material, transparent, with a smooth and padded adaptation surface (inflatable or gel-like material), and latex-free.

The nasal mask is the one that is better tolerated and is generally the choice for patients using home non-invasive ventilation. The naso-buccal mask is preferred in mouth breathers and in patients with acute respiratory failure and high ventilatory parameters. Full face mask is rarely used in pediatrics, although it is an alternative for children with craniofacial morphology variations or with lesions where the pressure points are. An alternative to masks is the high-flow nasal cannula. It is recommended for use at low pressures or for daytime use in patients with long-term non-invasive ventilation.

Interfaces must be fixed through elastic systems, minimizing involuntary leaks and at the same time allowing the patient to be as comfortable as possible, avoiding ocular occlusion, buccal movements, or excessive compression. It must be remembered that equipment designed for non-invasive ventilation compensates for leaks, and what matters is that they do not cause discomfort to patients.

To avoid lesions, it is recommended to install the interface on a clean face, do rotatory massages at the pressure points, and wash the interface daily.

Humidification Systems

Conditioning respiratory gas is essential to treat patients who need medical gases, oxygen therapy, invasive mechanical ventilation, and non-invasive ventilation.

Mucociliary clearance is probably the respiratory function most sensitive to changes in humidity and temperature of inspired gas. Dried up secretions can lead to alterations in ciliary activity, inflammatory changes, and respiratory epithelium necrosis, retained thick and adherent secretions with secondary impactation, bacterial colonization, atelectasis, and pneumonia.

In cases of acute respiratory failure, ineffective or insufficient humidification would be directly related to failed non-invasive ventilation. For this reason, in patients who require non-invasive ventilation for more than 12 consecutive hours, it is necessary to provide an efficient airway humidification, either with traditional systems as passover humidification or with those compatible with flow generators.

Use of passive humidification delivered by a heat and moisture exchanger (HME) is not recommended for non-invasive ventilation with a flow generator, because it increases system resistance and dead space, alters trigger response, and delivers insufficient conditioning of inspired air. It is reserved only for transportation.

Oxygen Therapy

In patients with motor neuron disease (MND) who present desaturation, oxygen administration is a mistake if there is not a proper management with assisted cough and proper ventilation protocols.

In patients with chronic lung damage, O_2 necessary for SpO_2 greater than or equal to 93% will be provided. Flow generators, except for most modern hybrid equipment, do not have an internal mixer. For this reason, the FiO_2 will vary depending on flows delivered by programmed pressures and on gas leak. The best alternative to deliver O_2 is by means of a T-connection placed at the exit of the BiPAP, prior to connection to the tubing, which can serve as a reservoir and determine a more stable FiO_2. This will depend on the mixture produced during the inspiratory and expiratory cycle between O_2 flow from its administration source (concentrator, cylinder, or network) and the flow created by the bi-level, with less than 3 L/min O_2 flows. In general, only a bubble type humidifier is required. In case of larger flows, it may be required to use traditional humidifiers, such as passover or those compatible with flow generators. Leaks through the interface are frequent causes of desaturation, which will not be corrected with an increase in O_2 concentration but repositioning and adapting the mask to the patient's face. It must also be ruled out that the desaturation cause is not excess of secretions, which are treated by applying assisted cough protocols.

The use of antibacterial filters is not recommended, since they increase resistance, affect the operation of triggers, and there is no evidence that these prevent infections associated with health care.

NIV as a 24 Hours per Day Prolonged Mechanical Ventilation Method

Patients with nocturnal non-invasive ventilation (NIV) who have dyspnea during daytime hours, respiratory infections despite assisted cough, and CO_2 >45 mmHg or SpO_2 <95% with room air, require daytime NIV. This happens naturally in children, adolescents, and adults with NMD.

Nocturnal and diurnal non-invasive ventilation is preferably performed with bi-level flow generators plus nasal masks. It is recommended to have two different mask models to vary the pressure points. The advantages offered by the bi-level in nocturnal hypoventilation prevention by using pressure-limited equipment (30 or 40 cm H_2O maximum delivery) with high differential pressure, not less than 7 cm H_2O, and that allow leak compensations and even average volume assured pressure support (AVAPS™, IVAPS™) are increased in patients who require continuous non-invasive ventilation due to a greater dependence.

Those patients with greater ventilatory demand, with little ventilatory autonomy and with NIV requirements greater than 16 hours per day should be evaluated for continuous assisted ventilation. Continuous NIV is defined as the use of it for more than 20 hours per day, as an alternative more effective than mechanical ventilation by TQT. This strategy is carried out with volume-controlled ventilators, with active exhalation valves in assist/control mode (S/T-PCV) and with pressure trigger to avoid auto-trigger. To avoid alarms, a minimum respiratory rate of 1–2 per minute is set and an angled 15 mm mouthpiece is used.

As there is always a leak flow around the nozzle, higher tidal volumes should be used than if a TQT was used, on 500 ml (700–1.200 ml) and inspiratory times of 1–1.5 s that generate inspiratory flows > at 40 L/m. When these flows pass through a system with specific resistance (angled mouthpiece), they generate an opposing pressure that prevents the activation of the low-pressure alarm. Currently, there are ventilators that include the option of a mouthpiece that allows delivering breathing cycles when they are needed and performing air-stacking maneuvers, optimizing complementary assisted cough protocols, impossible to achieve with continuous flow equipment such as bi-levels. To achieve efficient ventilation, it is necessary that the patient has sufficient control of the bulbar muscles and cervical mobility. This alternative is for daytime use. During sleep, conventional non-invasive ventilation with interfaces is used. Another alternative is volume-cycled ventilation via mask, as previously mentioned.

Indication of TQT should be reserved for patients without respiratory autonomy with subglottic stenosis, a vocal cord dysfunction due to severe bulbar involvement, which produces secretion or saliva aspiration that prevents maintaining a SpO_2 >95%.

Ethical Dilemmas

Survival of patients with NMD and technology dependent has improved, among other things, by specialized respiratory care, such as prolonged mechanical ventilation and assisted cough protocols. This also means an improvement in the HRQoL of the patient and their family environment. However, expected results are not always achieved, and psychological, social, and financial burdens constitute topics that require developing assessment criteria in the bioethics domain. The therapeutic challenges, which are possible thanks to the new applied technologies, require including bioethical principles considered as the sum of knowledge that orient in a rational sense the human action of promoting good and avoiding evil. These can be summarized as autonomy, beneficence, equity (justice), and non-maleficence.

The development of non-invasive ventilation has allowed improving the natural history of some NMD, especially DMD. However, in some neuromuscular diseases with progressive deterioration, such as spinal muscular atrophy type 1, characterized by its fatal evolution without ventilatory support, there is controversy about the technical feasibility of non-invasive ventilation support during the early stages of life (<6 months) and on the bioethical implications of the decision. This is especially true with infants with swallowing disorder due to bulbar compromise within the first 3 months of life that prevents holding SpO_2 stable above 95%. However, the rest of children whose bulbar involvement is not severe can benefit from non-invasive ventilation, assisted cough protocols, and gastrostomy feeding, regardless of their ventilatory autonomy level. Thus, without tracheostomy it is possible to maintain language and positively impact on HRQoL.

Bioethical aspects involved in managing patients with chronic, progressive, and potentially lethal diseases must be considered strongly when deciding together with patients and their families on mechanical ventilation therapies. It is essential to communicate all possible alternatives, such as non-invasive ventilation, ventilation through TQT or only accompaniment. Treatment decisions must consider not only technical feasibility aspects, but the aforementioned bioethical principles. Respecting the principle of justice, it is essential that healthcare systems understand the importance of addressing the necessary reimbursements for home care services that include such cost-effective and cost-efficient coverage.

Conclusions

Non-invasive ventilation is an alternative to invasive mechanical ventilation in patients who evolve with acute and chronic respiratory failure, who meet selection criteria. As the patient will be at home, it is necessary to organize activities there that include monitoring of clinical parameters, supervision of professionals, and continuing education to the patient and their family. Within the group of children with chronic respiratory diseases, it is useful in particular in NMD, kyphoscoliosis, obstructive sleep apnea syndrome, and cystic fibrosis, being able to alter the beginning of the natural history of the disease when identifying hypoventilation at night, without waiting until functional clinical deterioration is already obvious in wakefulness.

Respiratory compromise in neuromuscular diseases is a frequent cause of morbidity and mortality and ventilatory insufficiency of premature mortality. Over the past 10 years, we have gone from the consideration of the natural history of these diseases to both anticipatory and comprehensive recommendations in respiratory care.

The most substantial change in these recommendations is the routine inclusion of non-invasive ventilation and complementary protocols of assisted cough. Consequently, not only has the role of non-invasive ventilation been consolidated when it is initiated in a timely manner after confirming nocturnal hypoventilation but it has also been consolidated as the best strategy for delivering prolonged mechanical ventilation to those patients who require total ventilatory support or for more than 20 hours a day, reserving the indication of TQT exclusively for those who have a severe compromise of the bulbous muscles that prevent the SpO_2 from being continuously maintained over 95%. These strategies have allowed survival, with good HRQoL, in patients with DMD for more than 20 years and in patients with spinocerebellar ataxia type one for more than 10 years, avoiding tracheostomy.

Sources

Bach J, Goncalves M, Hon A, Ishikawa Y, Devito E, Prado F, Domínguez ME. Changing trends in the management of end-stage neuromuscular respiratory muscle failure. Am J Phys Med Rehabil. 2013;92(3):266–77.

Boitano LJ. Equipment options for cough augmentation, ventilation, and noninvasive interfaces in neuromuscular respiratory management. Pediatrics. 2009;123(Suppl 4):S226–30.

Dohna-Schwake C, Podlewski P, Voit T, Mellies U. Non-invasive ventilation reduces respiratory tract infections in children with neuromuscular disorders. Pediatr Pulmonol. 2008;43:67–71.

Fauroux B, Lofaso F. Non-invasive mechanical ventilation: when to start for what benefit? Thorax. 2005;60:979–80.

Fauroux B, Le Roux E, Ravilly S, Bellis G, Clément A. Long-term noninvasive ventilation in patients with cystic fibrosis. Respiration. 2008;76:168–74.

Ferrero G. Modos ventilatorios en ventilación no invasiva. Consenso 1 Chileno de ventilación no invasiva. Rev Chil Enf Respir. 2008;24:175–6.

González X, Salinas P, Farías A, Rodríguez C. Aspectos éticos de la ventilación mecánica domiciliaria. Neumol Pediatr. 2008;3:83–6.

Graham R, Fleegler E, Robinson W. Chronic ventilator need in the community: a 2005 pediatric census of Massachusetts. Pediatrics. 2007;119(6):e1280–7.

Hill NS. Saving face: better interfaces for noninvasive ventilation. Intensive Care Med. 2002;28:227–9.

Mellies U, Ragette R, Dohna Schwake C, Boehm H. Long-term noninvasive ventilation in children and adolescents with neuromuscular disorders. Eur Respir J. 2003;22:631–6.

Prado F, Salinas P. Asistencia ventilatoria no invasiva domiciliaria en niños: impacto inicial de un programa nacional en Chile. Rev Chil Pediatr. 2011;82(4):287–97.

Prado F, Salinas P, Pizarro G, Campos C, Zenteno D. Asistencia ventilatoria no invasiva: consideraciones teórico-prácticas en pediatría. Rev Chil Pediatr. 2008;6:580–92.

Prado F, Salinas P, Zenteno D, Vera R, Flores E, et al. Recomendaciones para los cuidados respiratorios del niño y adolescente con enfermedades neuromusculares. Rev Neumol Pediátr. 2010;5:74–88.

Simonds AK. Recent advances in respiratory care for neuro-muscular disease. Chest. 2006;130:1879–86.

Simonds AK. Respiratory support for the severely handicapped child with neuromuscular disease: ethics and practicality. Semin Respir Crit Care Med. 2007;28:342–54.

Toussaint M, Chatwin M, Soudon P. Mechanical ventilation in Duchenne patients with chronic respiratory insufficiency: clinical implications of 20 years published experience. Chron Respir Dis. 2007;4:167–77.

Wallgren-Petterssona C, Bushbyb K, Melliesc U, Simonds A. Ventilatory support in congenital neuromuscular disorders-congenital myopathies, congenital muscular dystrophies, congenital myotonic dystrophy and SMA (II). Neuromuscul Disord. 2004;14:56–69.

Ward S, Chatwin M, Heather S, Simonds AK. Randomised controlled trial of non-invasive ventilation (NIV) for nocturnal hypoventilation in neuromuscular and chest wall disease patients with daytime normocapnia. Thorax. 2005;60:1019–24.

Young HK, Lowe A, Fitzgerald DA, Seton C, Waters KA, Kenny E. et al. Outcome of noninvasive ventilation in children with neuromuscular disease. Neurology. 2007;68:198–201.

Tracheotomy

70

Bernardita Chateau Infante
and Constanza Beltrán Morales

Contents

Introduction

Tracheotomy is the communication between the trachea and the external environment, performed through a surgical procedure. The first references made to such a procedure date back to the year 1500 BC in India. In AD 1546, Musa performed the first successful tracheotomy, but it was not until 1620 that Habicot attempted to perform the first pediatric tracheotomy. At the beginning of

B. Chateau Infante (✉)
Department of Pediatrics, Clínica Los Andes, Santiago, Chile
e-mail: bchateau@clinicauandes.cl

C. Beltrán Morales
Department of Otorhinolaryngology, School of Medicine, Universidad de los Andes, Santiago, Chile
e-mail: cbeltran@clinicauandes.cl

P. Bertrand, I. Sánchez (eds.), *Pediatric Respiratory Diseases*,
https://doi.org/10.1007/978-3-030-26961-6_70

the twentieth century, American laryngologist Chevalier Jackson standardized the technique of the procedure, reducing morbidity and mortality associated with this intervention.

Anatomy

The pediatric airway anatomically differs from those of adults in important ways. They are of a smaller size and caliber, making them more susceptible to swelling-induced obstruction, mucus, or foreign bodies. In comparison with adults, its position is more cephalic and anterior, causing neck hyperextension to reduce the diameter of the airway.

In 2003, Litman studied the larynxes of 99 pediatric patients through nuclear magnetic resonance (NMR), determining that the smallest diameter is the transverse diameter of the glottis. After that, Dalal et al. verified these results through bronchoscopy, determining that the pediatric larynx presents a conical shape, rather than a cylindrical one. However, despite the fact that the glottis is the narrowest area of the larynx, the cricoid cartilage is the area with the highest risk of obstruction and injury, given its rigid structure that does not allow for distention and its elliptic aperture with a larger anteroposterior diameter.

Indications

Tracheotomy began to be considered a treatment as an emergency procedure for dealing with critical obstruction of the airway. The latest developments in this area have created two other indications: when prolonged invasive mechanical ventilation is needed and for lung hygiene.

Critical obstruction of the airway can be classified by origin: congenital or acquired (infection, injury, etc.); or by location: craniofacial, larynx, or trachea (Table 70.1).

The decision to perform a tracheotomy will depend on the degree of obstruction, possibility of spontaneous resolution within a reasonable amount of time, and the possibility of definitive corrective surgery. Currently, the main indications for tracheotomy in cases of airway obstruction are those that allow elective intervention, such as subglottic stenosis secondary to prolonged intubation during the neonatal stage, bilateral vocal cord paralysis, and injury to the high airway, such as burns and fractures, generally requiring temporary tracheotomy. Subglottic stenosis is one of the main indications for tracheotomy in children. Mature newborns have a lumen of at least 4 mm; a smaller lumen is considered stenosis. In older children, the reduction of subglottic caliber is determined by age and graded by percentage following the Myer–Cotton system (Table 70.2).

Most instances of stenosis in children happen as a result of endotracheal intubation, because the sub glottis, contained by the cricoid cartilage —a full ring that cannot dilate nor accommodate— becomes swollen at the epithelium by the mechanical injury of the tube, reducing the caliber of the airway. When these scars narrow, the result is subglottic stenosis. Grade IV stenosis by Myer–Cotton's system has an absolute indication of tracheotomy, but for grade II and III stenosis it will depend on the degree of respiratory compromise.

Table 70.1 Indications for tracheotomy by origin

1. High airway obstruction	
Congenital	Craniofacial dimorphism
	Paralysis of the vocal chords
	Subglottic hemangioma
	Subglottic membrane
	Upper subglottic or tracheal stenosis
	Pharyngeal collapse
	Severe laryngomalacia
Acquired	Secondary subglottic stenosis
	Severe obstructive sleep apneas
	Papillomatosis
	Burn injuries
	Tumors
2. Prolonged need of MV	
Congenital	Neuromuscular disorders
	Central hypoventilation
	Diaphragmatic hernia
	Severe bronchopulmonary dysplasia
Acquired	Traumatic chest injuries
	CNS tumors
	Severe chronic lungs damage
	Severe scoliosis
3. Lung hygiene	

Table 70.2 Classification of degree of subglottic obstruction

	From	To
I degree	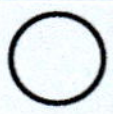 No obstruction	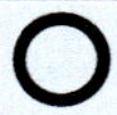 50% of lumen obstruction
II degree	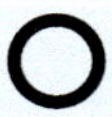 51% of lumen obstruction	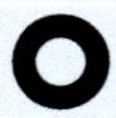 70% of lumen obstruction
III degree	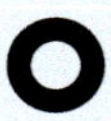 71% of lumen obstruction	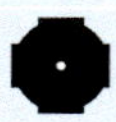 99% of lumen obstruction
IV degree	No detectable lumen	

For patients with respiratory failure caused by severe lung disease or by neuromuscular, neurological, or heart diseases, who also depend on mechanical ventilation for over 12 hours a day, tracheotomy is considered. In the case of acute respiratory failure requiring mechanical ventilation for over 21 days, tracheotomy may also be considered. The benefit of prolonged mechanical ventilation through tracheotomy lies in the reduction of laryngeal damage, improving the level of comfort for the patient, and improving their daily activities like mobility, speech, and oral feeding.

Tube Selection

Once the tracheotomy has been performed, it is necessary to insert a tube in order to keep the airway open and permeable. This tube is the tracheotomy cannula. There are different kinds of tubes designed to adjust to the appropriate needs of each patient.

By material:

- Metal (stainless steel, silver): rigid tubes
- PVC (polyvinyl chloride): may be rigid or flexible
- Polyurethane
- Silicone: these tubes are preferred for their flexibility, as they adapt to the size and shape of the patient's trachea

By structure:

- Simple or double tube
- With cuff or balloon: there is an inflatable device on the distal end of the tube. These tubes may be: high volume/low pressure, low volume/high pressure, and foam balloon. High volume/low pressure is the preferred option given their lower injury risk to the airway. Indications for using balloon are given mainly to lower the risk of aspiration, need of mechanical ventilation at high pressure, night ventilation, and for patients with chronic aspiration.
- Fenestrations: they improve trans-laryngeal flux and phonation, while also improving the handling of discharges. However, different studies have shown that these promote the emergence of granulomas on the fenestration area, so the use of the technique has been limited.
- Internal cannula: these tubes are indicated for patients with abundant thick discharges that stick to the walls of the tube. In this way, it is only necessary to remove the internal cannula during the cleaning procedure, thus avoiding frequent tracheotomy tube switching.

It is of the utmost importance to choose the precise cannula for each patient. The tracheotomy tube must be of the right size for the airway, with the exact shape and length to keep the tube secured to the airway without pressing the structures lying next to the trachea or the neck (Table 70.3). When choosing, the following parameters must be considered:

- Age: patients under 1 year must use cannulas that are specially designed for newborns.
- Reason for tracheotomy: in case of upper airway obstruction or if prolonged mechanical ventilation is needed.
- Diameter and curvature of the tube: the size of tracheotomy tubes is based on internal diameter, much like the selection of endotracheal tubes. When choosing the right diameter, many factors must be considered, including lung mechanics, upper airway resistance, need for ventilation/union, and procedure indications. The diameter must be wide enough to avoid damage to the wall of the trachea, minimize respiratory work, and promote laryngeal airflow. It should not exceed two thirds of the diameter of the trachea, thus avoiding damage to the wall of the trachea and allowing trans-laryngeal flow. Its curvature

Table 70.3 Characteristic of tracheotomy cannulas

	Age	PT-1 m	1–6 m	6–18 m	18 m -3a	3–6 a	6–9 a	9–12 a	12–14 a
Trachea	Diameter (mm)	5	5–6	6–7	7–8	8–9	9–10	10–13	13
Shiley	Size	3.0	3.5	4.0	4.5	5.0	5.5	6.0	6.5
	ID (mm)	3.0	3.5	4.0	4.5	5.0	5.5	6.0	6.5
	ED (mm)	4.5	5.2	5.9	6.5	7.1	7.7	8.3	9.0
	Length NB (mm)	30	32	34	36	–	–	–	–
	Length PED (mm)	39	40	41	42	44*	46*	–	–
	Length PDL (mm)	–	–	–	–	50*	52*	54*	56*
Portex	Size	2.5	3.0	3.5	4.0	4.5	5.0	5.5	–
	ID (mm)	2.5	3.0	3.5	4.0	4.5	5.0	5.5	–
	ED (mm)	4.5	5.2	5.8	6.5	7.1	7.7	8.3	–
	Length NB (mm)	30	32	34	36	–	–	–	–
	Length PED (mm)	30	36	40	44	48	50	52	–
Tracoe	Size	2.5–3.0	3.5	4.0	4.5	5.5	5.5	6.0	–
	ID (mm)	2.5–3.0	3.5	4.0	4.5	5.5	5.5	6.0	–
	ED (mm)	3.6–4.3	5.0	5.6	6.3	7.0	7.6	8.4	–
	Length NB (mm)	30 32	34	36	–	–	–	–	–
	Length PED (mm)	32 36	40	44	48	50	55	62	–
Rüsch	Size	–	3.0	4.0	–	5.0	–	6.0	–
	ID (mm)	–	3.0	4.0	–	5.0	–	6.0	–
	ED (mm)	–	4.8	6.0	–	7.0	–	8.2	–

m months, *y* years, *ID* internal diameter, *ED* external diameter, *NB* newborn, *PED* pediatric, *PDL* pediatric long
*with balloon

must be such that the distal portion of the cannula becomes aligned and concentric toward the trachea. It is recommended to confirm both position and adequate size of the cannula the first time it is placed in the larynx through a neck X-ray or a fibrobronchoscopy.

- Length of the cannula: the length of the cannula must be at least 2 cm beyond the stoma and remain 1–2 cm over the carina.

A commercial tube can be used for most patients. In limited cases, it may be necessary to use an individually customized tube. All tracheotomy cannulas must have a 15 mm universal terminal at their opening in order to connect to assisted ventilation when necessary.

Complications

Tracheotomy complications can be analyzed according to the moment they emerge during progression, considering early apparition during the first week after the procedure, and late apparition when it occurs at a later point.

Globally speaking, between 25% and 50% of pediatric tracheotomy patients will develop some form of complication. Children younger than 3 years of age usually have more problems than older children. When comparing emergency tracheotomy to an elective procedure, the former has a higher rate of complications: 75% versus 35%. Regarding newborns, premature children present a higher rate of complications with regard to full-term children, just like newborns weighing less than regular weight children (55% versus 34% in children who weight 2000 g. at birth). Complications are more common in children who suffer from obstruction of the upper airway (33%), followed by central nervous system disorders (22%).

Early Complications

- Hemorrhage. Bleeding of surgical wound. Infrequent. May represent a medical emergency. Depending on quantity, the patient must undergo medical ward examination and surgical resolution.
- Accidental decannulation, up to 5% of cases.

- Tube displacement or insertion of the tube in wrong path. It is suggested that the first time the cannula is swapped, the surgeon in charge of the procedure should perform the swapping in a safe environment.
- Acute obstruction of the tube caused by secretions or foreign body.
- Tracheoesophageal fistula. It is a rare complication and is caused by the erosion of the posterior wall in the trachea created by the inflated balloon or tube. It appears as discharges, dyspnea, gastric distention, or food aspiration through the cannula. Diagnosis is done through direct visualization through bronchoscopy or through an image contrast study leading to surgical resolution.
- Surgical wound infection. It is evidenced by local inflammatory signs.
- Acute occlusion of the tube caused by discharges or foreign bodies.
- Tracheoesophageal fistula. This is a rare complication that happens when the pressure exerted by the cannula or the inflated balloon erodes the posterior wall of the trachea. It is evidenced by an increase of local inflammatory signs.
- Laryngeal nerve damage. It is common during surgery. It is hard to diagnose. Since there is no laryngeal flow after the tracheotomy, the condition goes unnoticed. Common signs are dysphonia, bitonal voice, or stridor.
- Air leakage. Subcutaneous emphysema, pneumomediastinum, or pneumothorax because of interruption of the airway with adjacent spaces. It is detected by cutaneous crackles or progressive breathing complications. These are accompanied by compatible X-ray images.

Late Complications

There is a direct relation between the length of the tracheotomy and late postoperative complications. These are reported in 11% of tracheostomies that lasted less than 100 days; 55% in tracheostomies that lasted between 101 and 500 days; and in over 80% of tracheostomies that lasted over 500 days.

- Tracheal granulomas: This is the most frequent late complication, with granulomas being commonly seen on the rear wall of the trachea over the stoma. Distal granulomas may also be observed because of the contact between the distal end of the cannula and the anterior or rear wall of the trachea. Treatment depends on their size, with a conservative approach if they are small, or a surgical approach if these are large or symptomatic.
- Infections: Recurring infections are one of the most common complications. The direct contact between the airway and the environment, without regular defense mechanisms and given usual handling, bacterial colonization occurs and there is a higher risk of infection. Colonization is defined as the isolation of a pathogen within a tracheal culture for at least 4 weeks without clinical signs of acute infection. Moreover, in some cases bacterial biofilms may complicate antibiotic management, favoring recurring infections. The most commonly isolated agents are *Pseudomona aeruginosa, Streptococcus pneumoniae, Hemophilus influenzae, Moraxella catarrhalis*, gram negative enteric bacilli, and *Staphylococcus aureus*. Most infections tend to be local stomas and tracheitis. Microbiological surveillance with serial cultures is questioned, but it may guide the initial antibiotic treatment if necessary. Topical antibiotic treatment of the stoma may reduce colonization and infection in children, but there are no supporting studies to confirm this treatment.
- Decannulation/displacement of the cannula: Losing the artificial airway may lead to death. Safe fastening systems must be employed to avoid this complication, as well as monitoring of the patient in selected cases.
- Tube obstruction: Very frequent in children as shorter diameter cannulas may become easily obstructed by discharges.
- Tracheomalacia/tracheal stenosis: By using a medical instrument that is frequently manipulated in the airway, the structure of the trachea may be altered and cause stretching or malacia. It should be more common when positive pressure is applied (mechanical ventilation).

- Erosion of the tracheal wall or tracheoesophageal fistula.
- Persistent tracheocutaneous fistula: Persistence of the stoma will depend on technique and length of the tracheotomy. Surgical closure may be needed in some cases.
- Bleeding/hemorrhage: During late stages of the treatment, bleeding is unusual. When it does happen, it tends to be minimal, mainly caused by local infections. Treatment should deal with base infection. Hemorrhages are uncommon and are associated with traumatic vascular injuries.
- Tracheal fistula on the innominate artery: This is an uncommon, but severe complication. It happens because of contact and erosion of the anterior wall of the trachea and the innominate artery. It is generally caused by an excess manipulation of the tracheotomy tube, excessively pressured balloons or when the cannula reaches below the third tracheal ring. It requires urgency surgical management.

Care

The first step in tracheotomy care is knowledge. In most cases, patients are not capable of self-care as is the case with most adult patients, which is why people under medical care must be educated and trained. They must have basic anatomy knowledge as well as about care and emergency materials in case of clinical signs of respiratory distress and infection, and an easy and express means of communication in case of emergency. They must be trained in tracheotomy aspiration, cannula switching (when and how), and how to proceed in case of emergency.

Undergoing tracheotomy with a medical instrument in the airway is, in and of itself, a potential risk. Caregivers should recognize emergency situations and how to proceed with them. It is thus very useful and pertinent to establish protocols and flow diagrams on how to proceed.

When facing respiratory distress in a tracheotomy patient, a useful acronym to remember is DOPE:

- D for dislodgement: check the position of the cannula.
- O for obstruction: proceed to aspire the cannula and check if it is permeable; when in doubt, remove and change it.
- P for pulmonary: check if the respiratory distress is due to a different respiratory cause unrelated to the cannula.
- E for equipment: check that all the connections, drains and sensors are in the right position and in contact.

All the daily and emergency care materials must be available and close to the patient at all times:

- Humidifying equipment
- Discharge aspiration probes and equipment
- Tracheotomy cannulas: — One of the same number — One of a lower number Basic airway equipment: oxygen, self-inflating bag.
- Lubricating gel.
- Sterile gauzes, fixing tape, scissors, clean-up basin, physiological saline.
- Personal biosafety material: Sterile gloves, mask, coats, and safety goggles depending on specific needs.

Stoma and Skin Care

These are simple measures to prevent maceration and infection of the stoma. Use of the aseptic technique is related to a decrease in infection rates. It is recommended to wash the area of the neck with water and soap daily, clean the stoma from the medial border to the distal border with sterile gauze covered in physiological saline solution, and then cover the area with gauze to protect it from humidity and tracheal discharges. It is not recommended to make routine use of creams or similar items. Monitor for signs of infection (swelling, erythema, pain, discharges) or the emergence of friction-induced granulomas.

Changing the Cannula

The first scheduled cannula change must be done between the first 5–7 days on an empty stomach at the hospital, in a safe environment, and performed by the surgical team. Later on, the caregivers are allowed to do it under supervision as part of their training. The maneuver must be swift and accurate, with a round movement as the cannula enters, avoiding sharp angles in order to avoid eroding and later damage. How often and regularly the cannula must be replaced is a matter of discussion, and it depends on the composition of the cannula. On the one hand, having only brief periods between cannula swaps implies a higher degree of manipulation, carrying related complications with it (eroding, granulomas), while on the other hand, longer periods between swaps favor discharge-related obstructions and infection. Two to four weeks is considered a reasonable period of time. What matters is monitoring the good condition and permeability of the cannula.

Thermal Humidifying

Given that tracheotomy is a direct opening to the lower airway, air is not filtered and thermally humidified in a regular way, producing damage to the mucous membrane and altering mucociliary transport, thus increasing the risk of infection and obstruction. It is then essential to deliver humidity and warmth to the air inhaled by such patients.

Thermal humidifying may be active or passive. Active methods use equipment and tubes, making inhaled air pass through a hot water system before reaching the inspiratory part of the flow-volume loop. These methods are more effective, but they are also more expensive and usually require being connected to the electricity grid. Passive humidifiers include a filter installed on the cannula or between the ventilator and the cannula that collects the heat and humidity of the exhaled air for its use during inhaling. Ideally, the system allows the conditioning of inhaled air, reaching temperatures of 32°–34 °C and an absolute humidity of 36–40 mg/l at the level of the carina.

Inhaling Discharges

Scheduled and serial inhaling is not recommended in order to avoid unnecessary manipulation of the airway, and it is only indicated when there is evidence of discharges in the airway, suspicion of obstruction, or before cannula swap or balloon deflating.

The recommended adequate technique is:

- In a safe environment and with easy and working access to all the available material.
- Place the patient, ideally on an empty stomach and having previously aspirated the secretions, lying on their back.
- Keeping hands washed and wearing gloves. The technique must be performed under sterile conditions at the hospital due to the risk and control of in-hospital infections. However, when done at home, it is enough to use the clean technique (non-sterile gloves).
- Adjust inhaling pressure (pressure limits between 80 and 100 mmHg).
- Probe with an adequate size for the cannula (approximately half of the diameter of the cannula) and marked to the maximum introduction distance (not going beyond 0.5 cm from the distal end of the cannula).
- Avoid touching the distal end, lubricate the end of the probe with physiological saline solution, softly introduce it, occluding it in order to generate suction and administer inhaling both at the entry and at the end of the probe, and perform a circular movement of the catheter with the thumb and index fingers. Do not do it for longer than 5 seconds in order to avoid atelectasis.

Fixation

For tracheotomy patients, fixation is of vital relevance. There are multiple materials for the fixation system, such as cotton tapes with velcro, elastic tapes with hooks, and stainless-steel chains. Whatever the system, it must ensure the fixation of the cannula in its place. It is fundamentally important for the fixing to provide enough tension to avoid displacement of the cannula and accidental decannulation, but it must also allow for changes in neck size caused by crying, laughing, and feeding. It is recommended to fasten the fixation system with enough space to insert a finger between the neck and the system itself. In order to lessen the pressure on the stoma and to keep it dry, a dressing is applied between the cannula and the stoma. In the case of ventilation circuits connected to the cannula, they must be fastened in order to avoid producing more tension or movement on the cannula.

Phonation

Given the fact that there is a flow through the cannula of tracheotomy patients, the air flow is lost through the larynx, also taking away verbal language. This loss alters the psycho-social development of children. There are a number of options to allow the flow of air toward the glottis, such as using fenestrated cannulas or deflating the balloon in case there is one, but often this is not enough to allow phonation. There are devices that can connect to the cannula and are specifically designed to favor phonation. Its working principle is allowing airflow through the inhaling cannula, but applying resistance to exhalation, redirecting the airflow toward the vocal chords. It is therefore basic and fundamental to have space around the cannula (check free tracheal space on the X-ray and deflate the balloon) and a permeable upper airway. There are special models that may be employed when under mechanical ventilation.

As additional effects, phonation valves improve the efficiency of coughing by producing mucociliary clearance, and since there is a backward flow through the larynx, it would reduce the risk of inhaling in patients who feed orally while also optimizing olfaction.

There are phonation valve tolerance evaluation protocols for candidate patients. These protocols demonstrate that a registered pressure of 10–12 cm/H_2O at the moment of exhaling is associated with good tolerance.

Decannulation

When deciding on decannulating a pediatric patient, a number of criteria must be confirmed.

- Permeable upper airway. In the case of an earlier obstruction, this must be solved. Confirmation should be performed visually. Rigid or flexible laryngo-bronchoscopy.
- Independence from mechanical ventilation at least for the last 3 months, ideally including respiratory intercurrences.
- Regular swallowing, without clinical evidence or inhalation images. Must be confirmed by a video swallowing study.
- Adequate clearance of respiratory discharges.

There are a number of decannulation protocols for patients who fulfill the previous criteria. Most of them consider breathing and blocked cannula tolerance evaluations by hours and days, with sleep and activity tests, then reducing the size of the cannula for some days in order to finally decannulate in a safe environment under care and monitoring for 24–48 hours.

After successful decannulation, the stoma must be covered with gauze, waiting for closure by secondary intention. However, up to 40% of cases require surgical closure.

Sources

Al-Samri M, Mitchell I, Drummond D, Bjornson C. Tracheostomy in children: a population-based experience over 17 years. Pediatr Pulmonol. 2010;45(5):487–93.

Climent FJ, García M, Villalobos E. Manejo y cuidados del niño con traqueostomía. Actualizaciones SEPHO 2014.

Davis G. Tracheostomy in children. Paediatr Respir Rev. 2006;7(Suppl 1):S206–9.

Deutsch E. Tracheostomy: pediatric considerations. Respir Care. 2010;55(8):1082–90.

García R, Beltrán C, Chateau B. Infecciones respiratorias asociadas a traqueostomías en niños. Neumol Pediatr. 2011;6(3):134–7.

McGrath B, Bates L, Atkinson D, Moore JA. National Tracheostomy Safety Project. Multidisciplinary guidelines for the management of tracheostomy and

laryngectomy airway emergencies. Anaesthesia. 2012;67(9):1025–41.
Mitchell R, Hussey H, Setzen G, Jacobs I, Nussenbaum B, Dawson C, Brown C, Brandt C, Deakins K, Hartnick C, Merati A. Clinical consensus statement: tracheostomy care. Otolaryngol Head Neck Surg. 2013;148(1):6–20.
Paz F, Zamorano A, Paiva R, Hernández J, Mödinger P, Moscoso G. Cuidados de niños con traqueostomía. Neumol Pediatr. 2008;3(1):64–70.
Pérez-Ruiz E, Pérez-Frías FJ, Caro-Aguilera P. Cuidados del niño con traqueostomía. An Pediatr. 2010;72(Supl E1):41–9.
Trachsel D, Hammer J. Indications for tracheostomy in children. Paediatr Respir Rev. 2006;7(3):162–8.
Villarroel G, Jalil Y, Moscoso G, Barañao P, Astudillo C, Chateau B, Méndez M. Valores de presión espiratoria mantenida en la vía aérea como indicador de tolerancia al uso de válvula de fonación en pacientes traqueostomizados. Rev Chil Enf Respir. 2012;28:104–8.

71 Airway Surgery and Endoscopic Procedures

Patricio Varela Balbontín

Contents

Larynx Diseases

Diseases that affect the larynx and trachea can be classified according to their congenital and acquired nature (Table 71.1). The congenital forms are diverse and constitute a spectrum of possibilities in each of their types.

Congenital Laryngeal Anomalies

Laryngomalacia

It is the most frequent cause of stridor in newborns. More common in males, it constitutes 60% of the airway congenital anomalies, and it is usually a benign and self-limiting disease.

P. Varela Balbontín (✉)
Pediatric Surgery, Hospital Luis Calvo Mackenna, Universidad de Chile, Santiago, Chile

P. Bertrand, I. Sánchez (eds.), *Pediatric Respiratory Diseases*,
https://doi.org/10.1007/978-3-030-26961-6_71

Symptoms generally start between weeks 2 and 4, with progression until months 2 and 3. Most patients improve spontaneously after 12 and up to 24 months of age, if the treatment is conservative. Less than 15% correspond to severe cases. In them, supraglottoplasty is the method used, which is performed with microlaryngeal instruments or by using CO_2 laser. This surgery is performed endoscopically and requires general anesthesia. The patient remains intubated 24 hours and is extubated in an intensive care unit (Fig. 71.1).

Table 71.1 Congenital and acquired airway diseases

Congenital
Laryngomalacia
Vocal cord paralysis
Congenital subglottic stenosis
Subglottic hemangioma
Congenital laryngeal web
Laryngal atresia
Laryngotracheoesophageal cleft
Tracheomalacia
Bronchomalacia
Congenital tracheal stenosis
Tracheal agenesis
Acquired
Subglottic stenosis
Glottic stenosis
Tracheal stenosis
Bronchial stenosis

Congenital Subglottic Stenosis

It is a congenital narrowing of the subglottic space of less than 4 mm in term newborn infants and 3 mm in preterm newborn infants. It is the third larynx congenital malformation (10%), and it is a consequence of a recanalization failure of the laryngeal lumen during the embryonic period. In its embryological process, it is related to laryngeal atresia and congenital laryngeal diaphragms. Symptomatology is variable and is related to the degree of stenosis. It can appear as mild stridor at birth or severe obstructive symptomatology that requires an emergency tracheotomy (Fig. 71.2). In the case of severe stenosis, it is usually required to perform a tracheotomy to ensure proper ventilation. A final reconstructive surgery is performed at around 1 year of life and consists of a partial cricoid resection with trachea-thyroid anastomosis. The tracheotomy is removed. In cases of congenital subglottic stenosis the cricoid is malformed, with a narrower lumen and a characteristic elliptical shape.

Laryngeal Diaphragm or Webs

Diaphragms or congenital laryngeal webs are the result of an incomplete recanalization of the primitive larynx. They appear as an obstruction

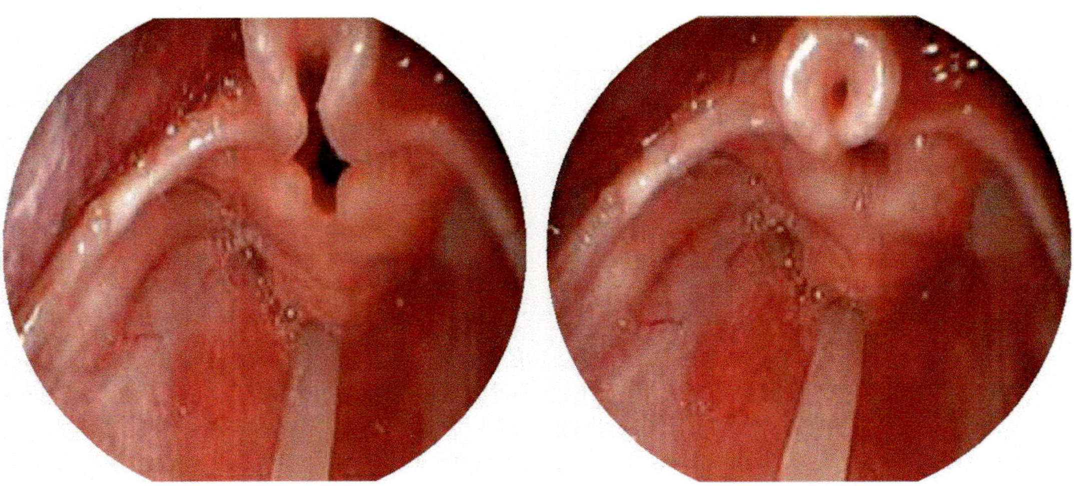

Fig. 71.1 Laryngomalacia. Omega shaped epiglottis, short aryepiglottic folds. (**a**) Expiration, (**b**) Inspiration

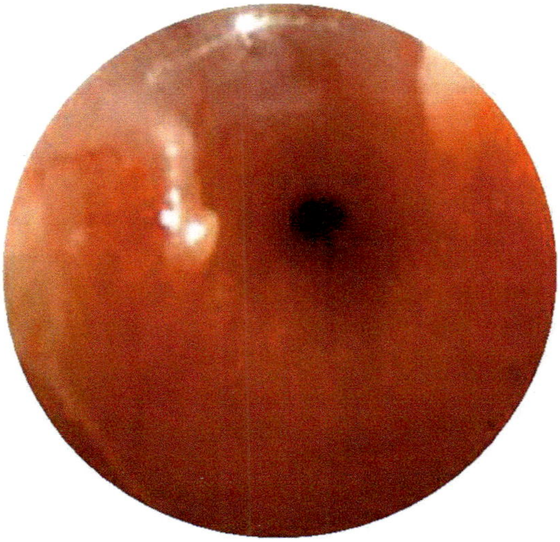

Fig. 71.2 Subglottic stenosis. Direct laryngoscopy shows a severe narrowing of less than 1 mm of the subglottic space in a newborn with respiratory distress

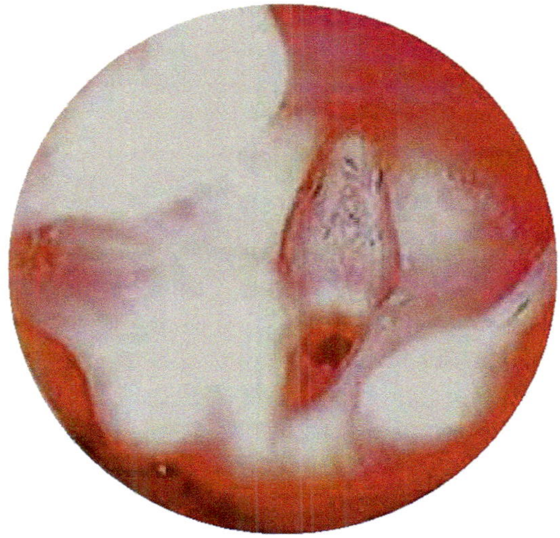

Fig. 71.3 Laryngeal web. Type III laryngeal web with 75% of lumen obstruction

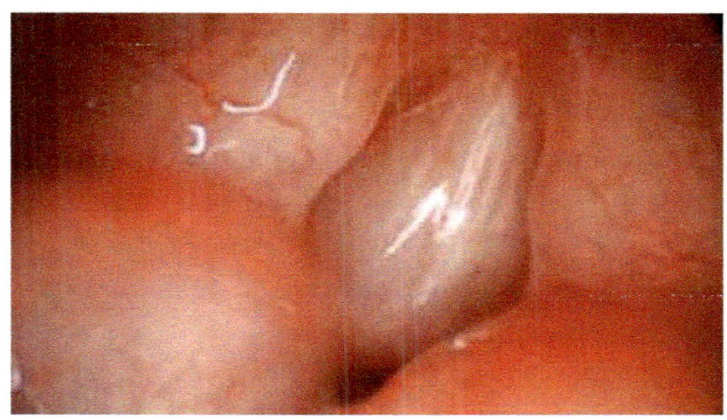

Fig. 71.4 Laryngeal web. Laryngoscopy performed in a newborn with laryngeal web that shows 95% glottis obstruction and reduction of interarytenoid space

of the upper airway, and characteristically with stridor. Newborn's crying is abnormal and can even cause aphonia. There are two types of congenital diaphragms: one is a thin web that is delimited to the glottis; the other is a thick diaphragm that extends into the subglottis. The latter is thought to correspond to a lower degree of laryngeal atresia rather than a real web. They are infrequent and constitute 5% of the congenital anomalies of the larynx. There is a genetic association with DiGeorge syndrome, which is characterized in some cases by a microdeletion of chromosome 22q11. The acquired webs are usually postintubation and produce a variable degree of synechia in the vocal cords. Most laryngeal diaphragms have associated subglottic stenosis and thickening of the cricoid cartilage, especially grades III and IV. According to Cohen's classification, they can be grouped into four types depending on the morphology and the degree of laryngeal obstruction they cause (Figs. 71.3 and 71.4).

Initial diagnosis is made with a nasolaryngoscopy conducted while the patient is awake, which will rule out other possible diagnoses, such as laryngomalacia or vocal cord paralysis. A final evaluation requires direct laryngoscopy. Different therapeutic options are available: a newborn with laryngeal diaphragm diagnosis and severe airway obstruction during the first hours of life characteristically corresponds to a case of diaphragm with severe obstruction of the glottic space, and in many cases emergency surgery is required to secure the airway (tracheotomy). In patients with thin and anterior diaphragms, an endoscopic cut can be performed. In thick diaphragms, with mild to moderate symptoms, later repair is suggested, because it is easier in technical terms. In children with more severe symptoms, the intervention must be done early. To relieve obstruction, tracheotomy is also endorsed as an option while the child grows, in order to repair at a later age.

In the majority of type III and IV diaphragms, open surgery involves a two-stage repair that includes the division of the diaphragm and enlargement of the subglottic space. The current recommended technique consists of performing anterior laryngofissure with a siliconized laryngeal stent placement plus a temporary tracheotomy. The purpose of this laryngeal prosthesis is to allow an adequate epithelization of the medial border of the cords that was congenitally adhered and thus prevent them from adhering again. Between 6 and 8 weeks later, the laryngeal prosthesis is removed endoscopically, and then it is possible to remove the tracheotomy. As mentioned, it is advisable to expand the airway using an anterior or posterior graft of costal cartilage due to the frequent association that this pathology has with subglottic space stenosis. In grade III patients, having to enlarge the subglottic space in the posterior plate and the anterior wall occurs frequently. In mild forms, the approach is endoscopic surgery conducted by experts, and requires cutting off the web using a laser, and also a mucosal flap in the cords to prevent posterior synechiae and recurrence. The insertion of a keel endoscopically, between the medial borders of the separated cords, is another endorsed alternative in older patients.

Subglottic Hemangioma

It is a benign vascular tumor located in the subglottic space, specifically in the left posterolateral region, close to the vocal cord on the same side. It corresponds to 1.5%–3% of all benign lesions of the larynx, and its evolution is self-limited, starting to remit after 18 months. Hemangiomas of posterior localization, left and bilateral, are less common. In our experience, we have evaluated eight subglottic hemangiomas, one of them posterior bilateral associated with congenital narrowing of the subglottic space. Because initial treatment with propranolol was not enough, surgery had to be done, resecting the hemangioma, removing the cricoid posterior mucosa, and performing a partial cricoid resection and a primary thyrotracheal anastomosis without tracheotomy.

Currently, the treatment of choice is the administration of propranolol; however, there are other treatment options that are second-line therapy that should be analyzed in each patient, considering the size of the lesion, age, degree of obstruction, and response to steroids and propranolol. Observation is appropriate for older patients, in whom there is little or minimal associated symptomatology of respiratory obstruction.

In cases where airway obstruction caused by hemangioma is less than 50% of the lumen and the symptoms are mild, the alternative to observe and re-evaluate is valid. Endoscopic techniques of intralesional steroids injection, submucosal dissection with microdebrider, and laser ablation can only achieve partial removal of the lesion and cause some degree of damage to the mucosa or cricoid cartilage, so currently there is controversy regarding these therapies. Temporary tracheotomy offers a stable airway during the growth and involution phase of the hemangioma. In case of opting for this alternative, the presence of the stoma should be considered for a period of approximately 10–30 months. The advantage of this option is that the involution of the lesion is achieved without a surgical intervention that may be associated with cord injury. However, it should also be considered that tracheotomy in infants has associated morbidity and mortality and requires special care. Open surgical resection is the treatment of choice in symptomatic patients with large hemangiomas that grow quickly. It would also be indicated in patients in whom the involution of the hemangioma has not occurred within 2 years (and where a tracheotomy or observation was chosen). Endoscopic excision with CO_2 laser, open resection, endoscopic resection with microdebrider, and tracheostomy are the main surgical alternatives. However, propranolol treatment currently prevails in most hemangiomas.

Congenital Tracheal Anomalies

Infrequent events, with an incidence of 1 per 60,000 live births. Most common congenital tracheal anomalies are tracheomalacia, bronchomalacia, tracheal cleft, and tracheal stenosis.

Tracheomalacia-bronchomalacia

Surgical alternatives, such as aortopexy, bronchopexy, intraluminal supports (stents), partial resections, and tracheotomy are reserved for severe cases: apneas, respiratory obstruction episodes during feeding, and recurrent respiratory infections.

Aortopexy Indicated when there is a collapse greater than 50% of the tracheal lumen. It consists of a suspension of the anterior wall of the aortic arch to the internal wall of the sternal manubrium in order to increase the space of the mediastinum, so that the malacic airway segment is free of compression by the vascular structures that surround it.

Stents Intraluminal supports that keep the airway lumen expanded (Figs. 71.5 and 71.6). Its effectivity has been confirmed. The insertion is done by endoscopy. The types of stents available are mainly metallic (Palmaz, nitinol, wallstents) and silicone (Dumon, Montgomery). Currently, self-expandable and heat-moldable stents are available, thus achieving a better resistance and effectiveness to solve a severe airway collapse. They can be inserted into the tracheal or bronchial lumen unilaterally or bilaterally as required.

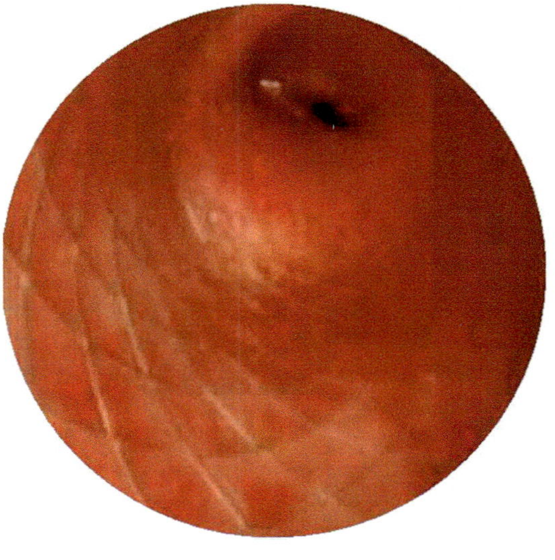

Fig. 71.5 Tracheomalacia. Inserted stent in the lower third of the trachea

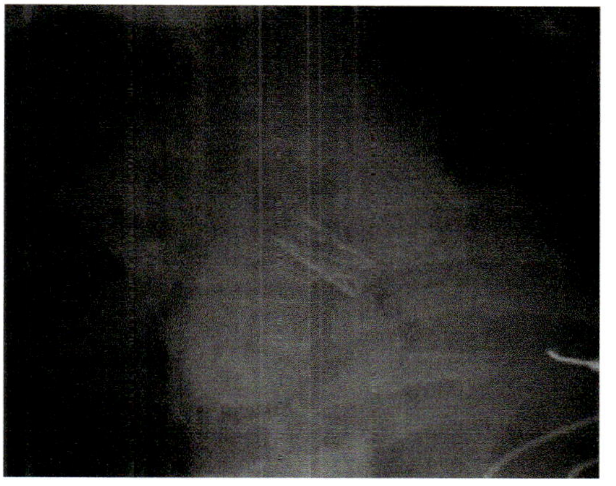

Fig. 71.6 Bronchomalacia. Patient with complete bronchial compression after cardiac surgery. The stent allowed reexpansion of the obstructed left main bronchus

Once in situ, it can remain for a long time or be removed as needed.

Congenital Tracheal Stenosis (Congenital Tracheal Rings)

It is a very infrequent malformation characterized by an anomaly of the tracheal skeleton, with presence of complete circular tracheal rings that are distributed along the stenosis and that determine a fixed narrowing of the tracheal lumen (Figs. 71.7. and 71.8).

The radiological study with chest X-ray can suggest the diagnosis. Bronchography is also a useful study tool (Figs. 71.9. and 71.10).

Symptomatology is variable and is related to the degree of the lumen narrowness; 50% are associated with vascular malformations, and the ring of the left pulmonary artery is the most frequent. There is a morphological classification of congenital tracheal stenosis that divides them into four groups:

Type I Long narrow segment. It is the most common morphology and usually the stenosis compromises 80% or more of the tracheal length.

Type II Funnel morphology.

Type III Short segment. Stenosis compromises less than 50% of the tracheal length.

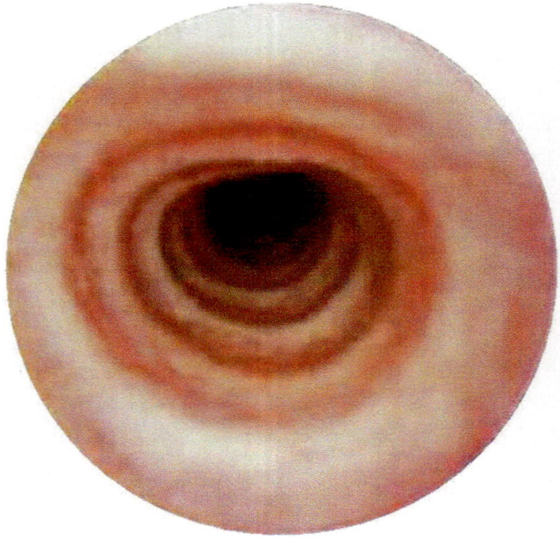

Fig. 71.7 Tracheal stenosis. Patient with complete bronchial compression after cardiac surgery. The stent allowed reexpansion of the obstructed left main bronchus

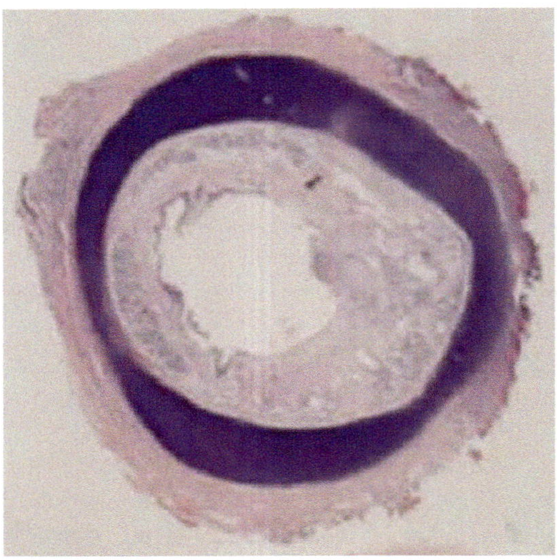

Fig. 71.8 Histology of a complete tracheal ring

Type IV It is characterized by the presence of an anomalous upper right bronchus and a long-left bronchus as a bridge, with presence of circular rings, which bifurcates to distal and originates main bronchus.

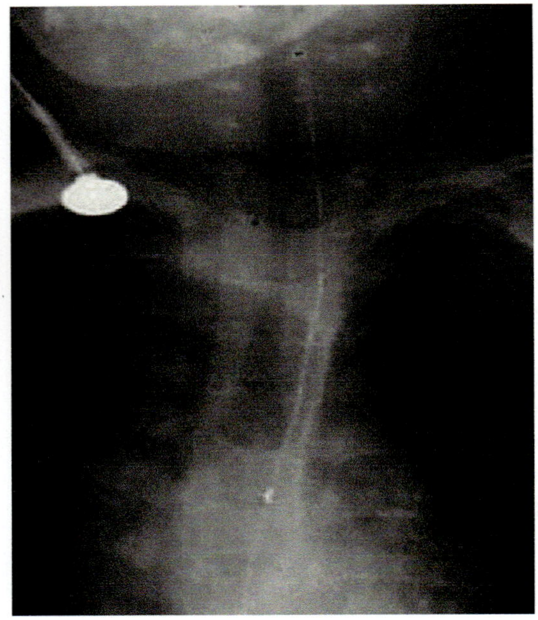

Fig. 71.9 Tracheal stenosis. 4-year-old child neck X-ray showing a trachea with an hourglass narrowing

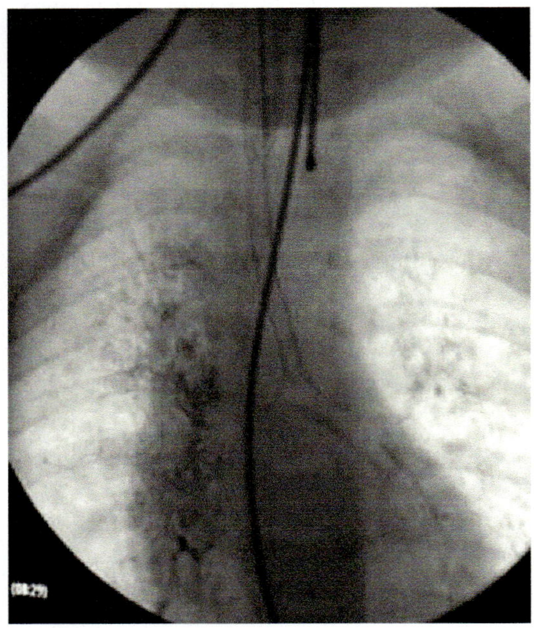

Fig. 71.10 Tracheal stenosis. Bronchography shows the morphology of trachea and bronchi in a 6-year-old child

Surgical indication depends more on the presence of associated respiratory symptomatology than on the morphology itself. Multiple surgical techniques have been devised to correct this complex airway abnormality. The most common ones involve resection and anastomosis for short stenosis cases. In longer stenosis, the extension of the tracheal lumen with pericardial graft or costal car-

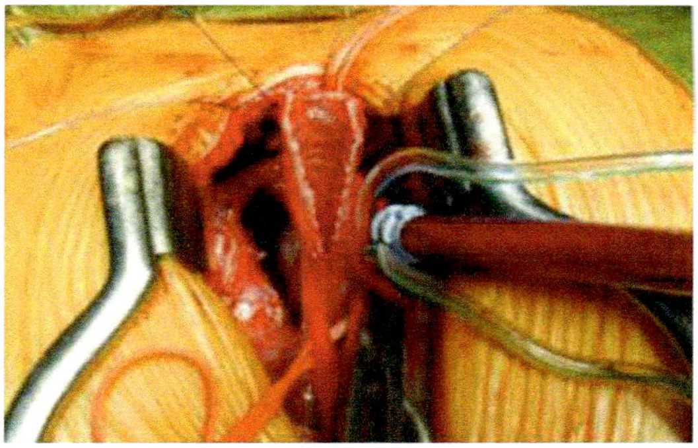

Fig. 71.11 Congenital tracheal stenosis repair. Patient with long segment tracheal stenosis undergoing extracorporeal circulation (ECC) repair

tilage was considered for many years. In the past decade, a tracheal enlargement technique called slide tracheoplasty has been predominant, which uses native tissue without graft, allowing a greater enlargement of the stenotic lumen. Corrective surgery can be performed through cervical or thoracic route, both techniques combined, or median sternotomy. Long segment tracheal stenosis usually requires repair with support of extracorporeal circulation (ECC) (Fig. 71.11) or extracorporeal membrane oxygenation (ECMO), ensuring adequate ventilation and oxygenation while the tracheal lumen remains open.

Laryngotracheal Cleft

Laryngotracheal cleft is an abnormal communication between the trachea and the esophagus. The extension of it is variable, from a cleft at larynx level exclusively to a wide abnormal communication between both conduits that can extend even to the bronchi. When the cleft goes beyond the cricoid cartilage, it is called a laryngotracheoesophageal cleft. Clefts are classified into five types (I-V), according to length (See Monnier)

Diagnosis is based on index of suspicion. Symptoms are sometimes vague, but most have typical associated respiratory manifestations as cough or drowning secondary to aspiration of food or gastric contents. Laryngomalacia and tracheomalacia are frequently associated. Definitive diagnosis must be made after endoscopic examination under anesthesia in the operation room. Grade I laryngeal cleft does not always have to be repaired. Some patients are asymptomatic and if there is no clinical, radiological, or lung evidence of aspiration, repair is not necessary. Grade II clefts and onward require surgical repair. In some cases, it will be necessary to perform a tracheotomy, gastrostomy, or anti-reflux surgery. A one stage cleft repair without tracheotomy is ideal. When a tracheotomy is performed, it should remain for at least 2–3 years. This is because the associated tracheomalacia that these patients present is further aggravated by the presence of the trachectomy, making it more difficult and delaying a successfully decannulation. Surgical repair can be done endoscopically or by cervical or thoracic surgery.

Technical Aspects

Endoscopic repair is indicated for grades I and II.

An anterior translaryngeal transtracheal is the choice approach and all types of clefts can be repaired in this way. A two layer repair is required, dividing the esophageal plane from the tracheal and closing both mucous membranes separately. After this, the posterior tracheal wall is closed. It is recommended to interpose synthetic fibrin between both layers. Then, the anterior tracheal wall is sutured with separate stitches (Fig. 71.12).

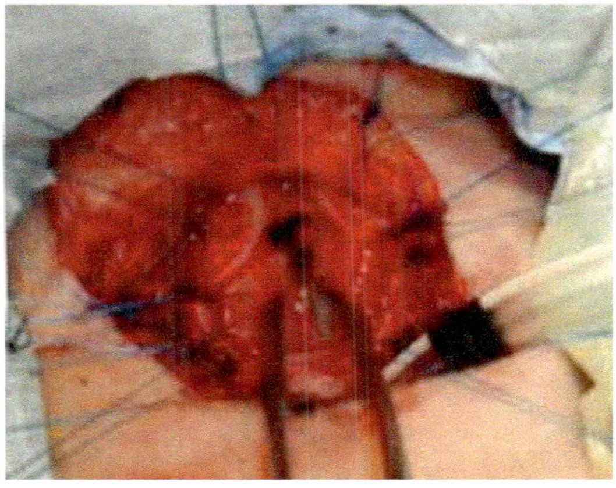

Fig. 71.12 Type III laryngotracheal cleft. Surgery through the neck. Communicated esophagus and trachea are observed. Nasogastric tube is seen in the esophagus

In more extensive clefts cases (IV–V), ventilatory assistance with ECMO is recommended.

Pediatric Airway Frequently Acquired Lesions

Acquired Subglottic Stenosis

Subglottic stenosis (Fig. 71.13) corresponds to a subglottic space narrowing and is usually associated with tracheal intubation. Other less common causes are trauma, tumors, and burns. It should be suspected in all patients who have stridor and who have history of a previous tracheal intubation. The most specific study to assess subglottic stenosis is endoscopic evaluation. Detailed evaluation of vocal cords should be obtained, verifying their mobility and eventual paralysis. Stenosis is assessed in its thickness, length, location, and maturity (acute, subacute, chronic, or fibrous).

The Cotton–Myer classification to define the narrowness degree is used, which is based on an objective graduation system of the subglottic space lumen, established by calibration with endotracheal tubes and that considers four grades according to subglottic lumen narrowness percentage:

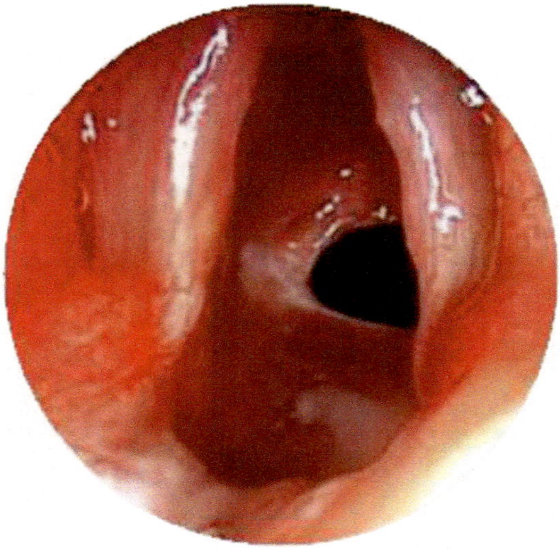

Fig. 71.13 Acquired subglottic stenosis. Surgery through the neck. Communicated esophagus and trachea are observed. Nasogastric tube is seen in the esophagus

Grade I Narrow lumen <50%

Grade II Narrow lumen between 50 and 75%

Grade III Narrow lumen between 75 and 99%

Grade IV Absence of lumen.

This grading system correlates directly with the prognosis of decannulation after surgery and is closely related to the surgical technique to be used. Philippe Monnier has modified this classification, adding subgroups depending on the presence of glottic compromise and comorbidities. According to this modification, it is now possible to define more accurately the prognosis of the injury and the most favorable surgical procedure.

Surgical Treatment

Endoscopic techniques using argon or CO_2 lasers are reserved for mild forms. Most severe forms have a higher success rate with open reconstructive surgery. In cases of acute or subacute injuries, endoscopic dilation with endotracheal tubes or balloon, plus topical use of mitomycin C, is an alternative with good results.

Open reconstructive surgery types:

A. *Extension without graft:* Indicated in newborns who have failed extubation on several occasions. It is an alternative to tracheotomy. The original technique considers opening the anterior wall of the cricoid cartilage, the lower third of the thyroid cartilage, and the first two tracheal rings without the need for grafting. The patient is then kept intubated for a period of 7–10 days in an intensive care unit. Sedation should avoid movement of the endotracheal tube as much as possible.

Criteria to perform this surgery are: failure in extubation at least on two occasions as a result of subglottic pathology, weight greater than 1500 grams, absence of ventilation requirements in the last 10 days, oxygen requirements less than 30%, and absence of respiratory infection at the time of evaluation.

B. *Enlargement with cartilage graft:* It consists in opening the anterior wall of thyroid cartilage lower third, cricoids, and first tracheal rings. This stenotic lumen enlargement can be combined with a cricoid section in its posterior lamina and lateral quadrants, depending on the degree of severity and morphology of the stenosis.

Costal cartilage graft is most commonly used (Fig. 71.14). Other alternatives consider hyoid, auricular, and thyroid cartilage.

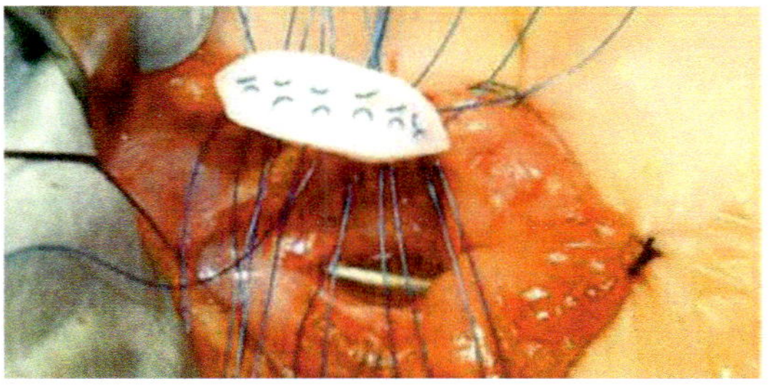

Fig. 71.14 Cartilage graft. Costal cartilage attachment in anterior laryngotracheal wall

C. *Stenotic zone resection (cricotracheal resection)*: Partial resection of the cricoid and first tracheal rings, with a primary anastomosis between the thyroid cartilage and trachea. It is a procedure indicated in patients with restenosis after failed laryngotracheal reconstruction and as a primary procedure for a selected group of patients with severe laryngotracheal stenosis (treatment of choice for grade II and IV stenosis). It is also useful in wide cricoid and tracheal resections for tumors (Figs. 71.15a, b).

Most procedures are performed in one stage, that is, stricture and closure of the stoma is resolved. In a smaller number of patients, surgery is performed in more than one stage, maintaining the tracheotomy temporarily. In cases where the subglottic stenosis also compromises the glottis (glotosubglottic stenosis), the recommended surgery is a partial cricotracheal resection extended in two stages, maintaining a transitory tracheostomy, with section of the interarytenoid muscle and placement of a siliconized laryngeal implant (LT Mold de Monnier), which is maintained for 6–8 weeks and subsequently removed by simple ambulatory endoscopic procedure (Fig. 71.16).

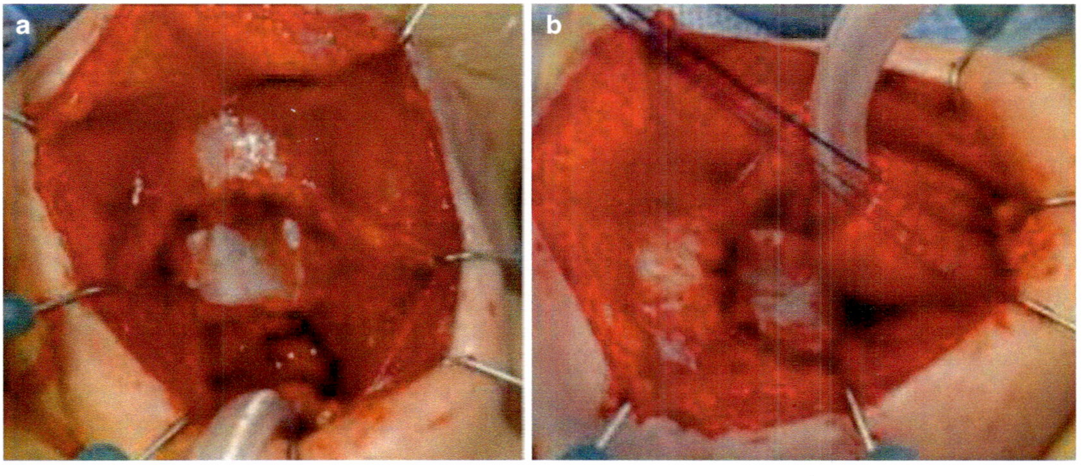

Fig. 71.15 (**a**) Cricoid resection. Thyroid cartilage and posterior cricoid lamina are observed. The anterior arch has been resected. (**b**) Tracheal cricoid resection. Trachea is ascended then anastomosed to the thyroid cartilage. Posterior cricoid is covered with posterior tracheal flap

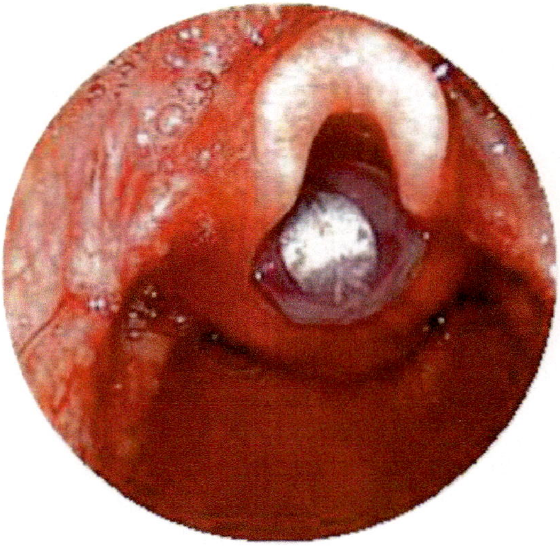

Fig. 71.16 Laryngeal stent. LT Mold Monnier's silicon stent is observed. Removal is done endoscopically 6–8 weeks after the procedure

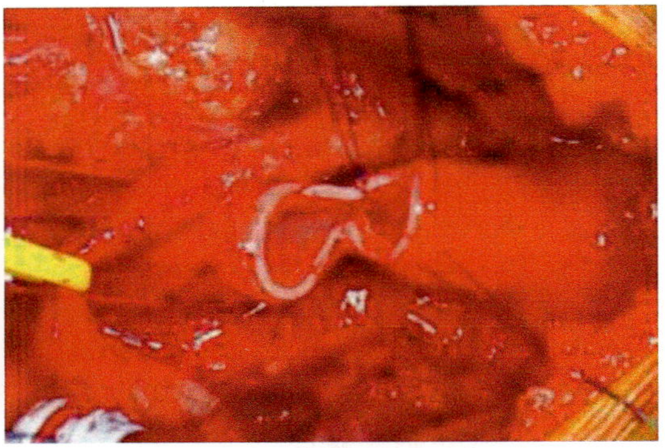

Fig. 71.17 Tracheal resection. End-to-end anastomosis in a patient undergoing tracheal resection for acquired stenosis

Postoperative management should be done in the intensive care unit. In this period, the patient is intubated with a nasotracheal tube. During the first hours, sedation is preferable. During the following days, sedation and analgesia without paralysis are preferable, depending on the patient's tolerance. In general, older children tolerate this period very well (intubated) with minimal administration of sedatives. Intubation time will depend mainly on the type of surgery. In patients older than 5 years and in whom reconstruction has required only a graft in the anterior wall, extubation can be performed in the immediate postoperative period and the patient can be transferred extubated to the intensive care unit. In case of maintaining intubation, time required is less than 5 days. In cases in which an extension is made with anterior and posterior graft, intubation is prolonged for 5–7 days, similarly for tracheal cricoid resections. A follow-up endoscopy is performed 4 weeks later to verify graft epithelization, chordal motility, and eventual development of granulomas in the suture areas, which must be removed.

Tracheal and Bronchial Stenosis Acquired After Intubation

In children, the main cause of tracheal stenosis is secondary to previous intubations. Initial treatment may consider a plan of periodic dilatations when stenosis is diagnosed early and there is no fibrous stenotic scar. Dilatations can be performed with endotracheal tubes or vascular balloons. The treatment of choice for critical and fibrous stenosis is surgical resection and primary anastomosis (Fig. 71.17).

The approach is mostly cervical anterior, which allows excellent access to a significant proportion of the trachea. In less frequent cases of distal stenosis or close to the carina, the cervical approach should consider an upper medial sternotomy or directly a lateral sternotomy at the third intercostal space. In cases of distal stenosis that compromise the carina, it is recommended to perform tracheal and bronchi reconstruction in extracorporeal circulation, ensuring adequate and safe oxygenation during the procedure. In cases of stenosis of one of the main stem bronchi, endoscopic repair using balloons is recommended. The procedure is performed through a rigid bronchoscope, which allows ventilating the patient while the procedure is performed, in addition to a direct visualization through Hopkins optics of 0° (Figs. 71.18a, b).

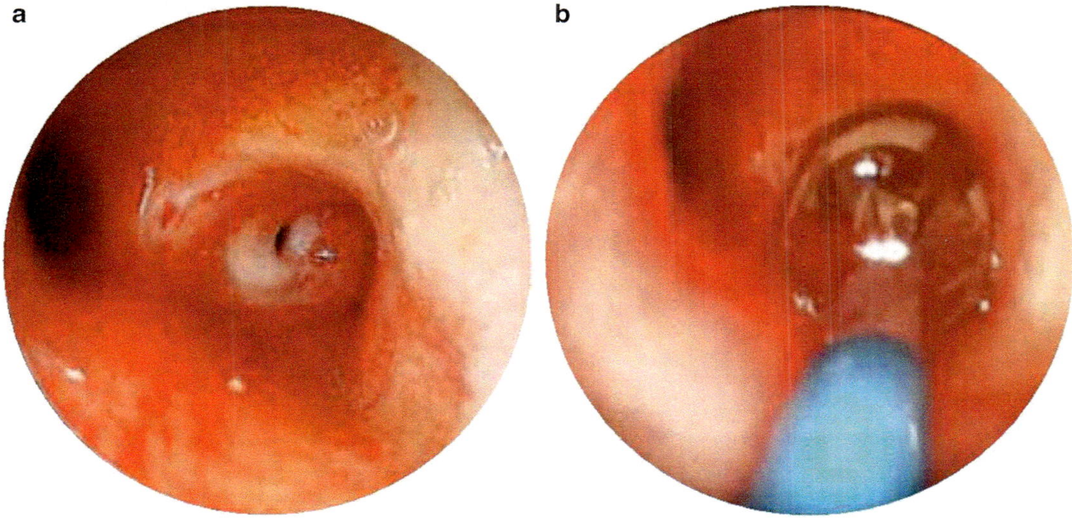

Fig. 71.18 (**a**) Bronchus intermedius stenosis. (**b**) Endoscopic balloon dilatation

Summary

Airway surgery requires tertiary health care centers, with professionals organized in airway units whose primary purposes are to diagnose and offer timely therapies for various congenital malformations and acquired injuries that affect the larynx, trachea, and bronchi.

The main congenital malformations that affect larynx and trachea are laryngomalacia, vocal cord paralysis, congenital subglottic stenosis, subglottic hemangioma, congenital laryngeal web, laryngotracheal cleft, congenital tracheal stenosis, tracheal and bronchomalacia, and tracheal agenesis. Acquired lesions that we most frequently diagnosed and treated are post-intubation stenotic lesions, mainly subglottic and tracheal stenosis. Bronchial lesions are less common and in those cases endoscopic therapy is used.

This chapter describes the main anomalies that affect adolescents and children's airway, emphasizing the importance of an early and accurate diagnosis as well as defining modern treatment alternatives that include complex reconstructive surgeries and endoscopic therapies.

The author illustrates this text with photographs of endoscopic and surgical records of a wide spectrum of anomalies, which he has compiled for more than a decade and are part of his personal experience as an airway surgeon.

Note All the photographies of surgery procedures and endoscopies were done by the author.

Sources

Alarcon A, Rutter MJ. Pediatric laryngotracheal reconstruction. Otolaryngol Clin N Am. 2008;41(5):959–80.

Donoso C, Varela P, Gómez N, Borel C, Herrera O. Estenosis traqueal congénita. Serie clínica. Rev Chil Pediatr. 2006;77(3):274–81.

Gustafson LM, Hartley BE, Liu JH, Link DT, Chadwell J, Koebbe C, Myer CM, Cotton RT. Single-stage laryngotracheal reconstruction in children: a review of 200 cases. Otolaryngol Head Neck Surg. 2000;123(4):430–4.

Hartnick CJ, Brigger MT, Willging JP, Cotton RT, Myer CM. Surgery for pediatric vocal cord paralysis: a retrospective review. Ann Otol Rhinol Laryngol. 2003;112(1):1–6.

Monnier P. Pediatric airway surgery. Ed. Berlin: Springer; 2011a.

Monnier P. Pediatric airway surgery. Berlín, Heidelberg: Springer-Verlag; 2011b.

Myer CM, O'Connor DM, Cotton RT. Proposed grading system for subglottic stenosis based on endotracheal tube sizes. Ann Otol Rhinol Laryngol. 1994;103(4 Pt 1):319–23.

Prado F, Varela P, Boza M, Koppmann A. Estenosis subglótica adquirida: tres años de experiencia. Rev Chil Enf Respir. 2003;19:71–7.

Rutter MJ, Cohen AP, de Alarcon A. Endoscopic airway management in children. Curr Opin Otolaryngol Head Neck Surg. 2008;16(6):525–9.

Torre M, Yankovic F, Herrera O, Borel C, Latorre JJ, Aguilar P, Varela P, Rutter MJ, Cotton RT, Azizkhan RG, Manning PB. Slide tracheoplasty for the management of complete tracheal rings. J Pediatr Surg. 2003;38(6):928–34.

Varela P, Haecker S, Herrera O, Fielbaum O, Osorio W. Estenosis traqueal congénita. Reparación con injerto de pericardio, en by pass cardiopulmonar. Reporte de caso clínico. Rev Chil Pediatr. 1999;70:4.

Vijayasekaran S, White DR, Hartley BE, Rutter MJ, Cotton RT. Open excision of subglottic hemangiomas to avoid tracheostomy. Ach Otolaryngol Head Neck Surg. 2006;132(2):159–63.

White DR, Cotton RT, Bean JA, Rutter MJ. Pediatric cricotracheal resection: surgical outcomes and risk factor analysis. Arch Otolaryngol Head Neck Surg. 2005;131(10):896–9.

White DR, Bravo M, Vijayasekaran S, Rutter MJ, Cotton RT, Elluru RG. Laryngotracheoplasty As an alternative to tracheotomy in infants younger than 6 months. Arch Otolaryngol Head Neck Surg. 2009;135(5):445–7.

Lung, Chest Cavity, and Dorsal Spine Surgery

72

Mauricio Campos Daziano, José Vuletin Solís, and Juan Carlos Pattillo Silva

Contents

Introduction

The subtle interaction between the chest and its contents is not only evidenced in the pathological states where restrictive ventilatory complications determine alterations in the chest. In particular, the critical periods of the developments of pathologies that affect the chest cavity or its components (e.g., dorsal spine or sternum) can provoke changes not only in ventilatory mechanics but also disturbances in the concomitant development of the lung parenchyma (e.g., alveolar multiplication) that could eventually cause permanent functional cardiopulmonary sequelae. In this chapter we address the eventual functional effects of the pathologies and the treatments that directly affect the chest or its components.

M. Campos Daziano
Pontificia Universidad Católica de Chile, Santiago, Chile
e-mail: macampos@med.puc.cl

J. Vuletin Solís (✉) · J. C. Pattillo Silva
Pediatric Surgery, Pontificia Universidad Católica de Chile, Santiago, Chile
e-mail: fvuletin@med.puc.cl; jpattill@med.puc.cl

Surgery of Congenital Malformations of the Chest Cavity

The thorax is composed by multiple independent bones (vertebrae, sternum, and ribs) that form the chest cavity along with several muscles that cover it. The chest cavity is often seen only as protection for intrathoracic organs, but the chest is a dynamic system that enables respiratory function.

P. Bertrand, I. Sánchez (eds.), *Pediatric Respiratory Diseases*
https://doi.org/10.1007/978-3-030-26961-6_72

Thus, any condition that results in its malfunction will significantly affect the respiratory system and the intrathoracic organs.

Malformation of the chest cavity means any abnormality that affects the normal structure and impairs chest function. These malformations can be divided into two main categories: congenital and acquired. The deformities of the chest cavity can be divided into two groups: the ones that have a depression or protrusion of the sternum and those that have different degrees of aplasia or dysplasia (Table 72.1). The most frequent malformations are pectus excavatum (88%) and pectus carinatum (5%), which we will describe in this chapter.

Pectus Excavatum

Pectus excavatum is the anterior depression of the costal wall. It is the most common malformation of the chest cavity, with an incidence of 1 in 400 births. It is more common in men than in women, with a ratio of 5:1. It is more common in the white race, and it is more frequently presented from the first year of life, progressing and becoming more noticeable during the puberty growing phase. The mechanism that provokes it is not completely identified. Some histological studies have shown a weakening in the components of the costal cartilages, which would allow for posterior sternal migration. There is no chromosomal defect, but it has been reported in conjunction with Marfan syndrome, Ehlers–Danlos syndrome, osteogenesis imperfecta, syndactyly, and Klippel–Feil syndrome. Also, a genetic predisposition of approximately 40% of the patients has been detected, who report having a family member with medical history of being a carrier of a malformation of the chest wall.

Table 72.1 Congenital malformations of the chest cavity

Funnel chest	Pigeon chest	Aplasia or dysplasia
Pectus excavatum	Pectus carinatum	Ectopia cordis
		Cleft sternum
		Poland's syndrome
		Asphyxiating thoracic dystrophy

Preoperative Evaluation

The objective of the preoperative evaluation is to define the morphology and seriousness of the deformation of the sternum, and its functional repercussions both in the lungs and the heart. It is also important to demonstrate that the subject is not allergic to the metallic compounds used when repairing the pectus excavatum, which is present in 2% of the cases.

Computerized tomography or magnetic resonance is used in the evaluation of the level of seriousness of the pectus excavatum when calculating the Haller index. This consists in the transverse diameter of the chest divided by the anteroposterior diameter of the point of the sternum with the greatest depression (Fig. 72.1).

In the lung evaluation, abnormalities in the lung function can be shown by measuring the forced vital capacity, forced expiratory volume in 1 second, and forced expiratory flow of 25–75% of the forced vital capacity.

Regarding the cardiac assessment, the echocardiographic assessment is important, which can show cardiac compression with alterations in the filling and emptying of the right ventricle, while showing deformations of the mitral ring, with prolapse and regurgitation of the mitral valve.

The symptoms produced in the patient are an important part of the preoperative evaluation. Symptoms, such as exercise intolerance, low endurance, and shortness of breath, are reported by the patients with pectus excavatum. Another important aspect is the cosmetic effect that this produces. It limits the normal life of some patients, because they avoid places where the

Haller Index = a/b

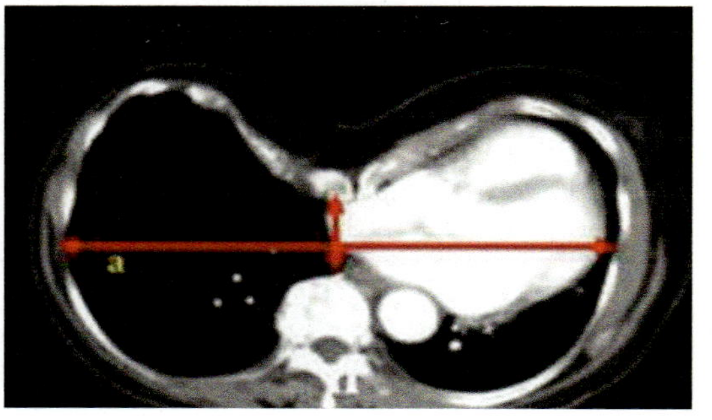

Fig. 72.1 Haller index (TAC)

chest deformity will have to be exposed, such as the beach or pools. It has been proven that patients with pectus excavatum have a lower quality of life and that the treatment statistically improves their bodily image.

Treatment

Surgical correction for pectus excavatum is recommended when the patient has one of the following criteria:

1. Computerized axial tomography or magnetic resonance that shows heart or lung compression with a Haller index of 3.25 or more.
2. Restrictive lung disease proven by a lung function test.
3. Heart compression with abnormalities in the mitral valve, either prolapse or regurgitation.
4. Exercise intolerance, decrease in endurance, and shortness of breath during exercise.
5. Recurrence after an open or minimally invasive surgery.
6. Cosmetic effect produced in patients.

The optimal correction age is between 10 and 14 years of age. In this period the chest cavity is more malleable, which allows for a lower rate of recurrence.

Today, the surgical treatments that are more widely used to correct pectus excavatum are the open technique or Ravitch procedure, and the minimally invasive repair technique or Nuss procedure. The Ravitch technique, described in 1949, consists in an open repair of the defect by a transverse inframammary incision, through which the malformed sternum and the costal cartilages are exposed. Through the anterior approach, costal cartilages are resected, preserving the perichondrium, and anterior sternal osteotomies are performed to correct the sternal depression defect. The wound is closed moving pectoral muscle flaps.

The minimally invasive surgery for pectus excavatum or Nuss procedure was described in 1998 by Dr. Donald Nuss. This technique allows the correction of the pectus excavatum without the need for a great incision in the skin or the resection of costal cartilages. In short, a lateral incision is performed in the thorax, through which, assisted by videothoracoscopy, a convex metal bar is inserted behind the sternum, which is exteriorized on the other side of the chest (Fig. 72.2). When the bar is flipped 180° the sternal defect pops up (Fig. 72.3). The bar is fixed to the ribs by stabilizers. This device is installed in the patient for 2–3 years.

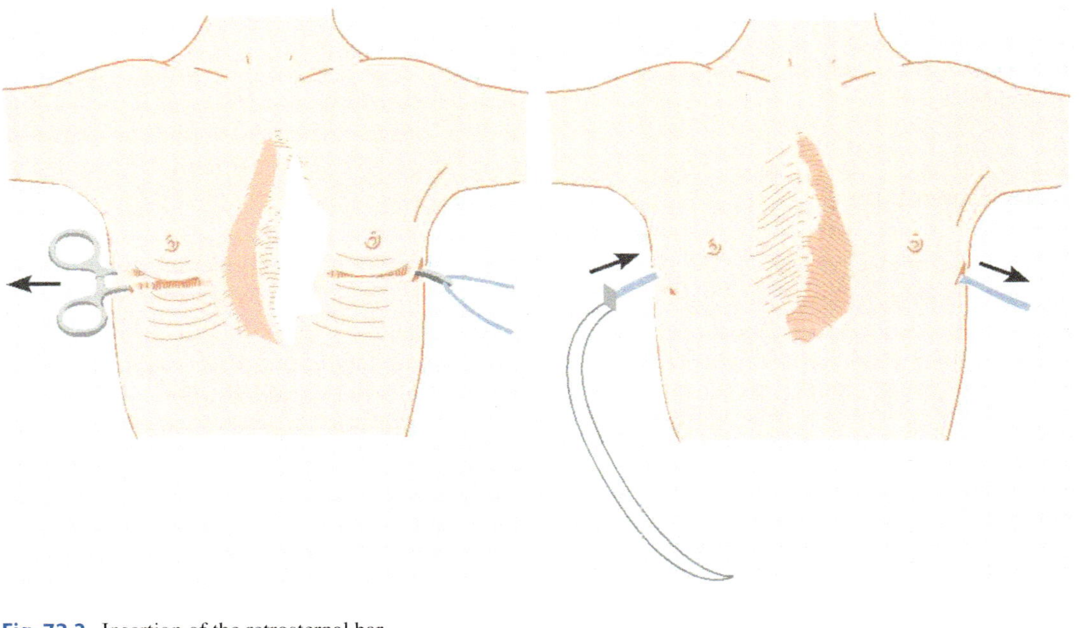

Fig. 72.2 Insertion of the retrosternal bar

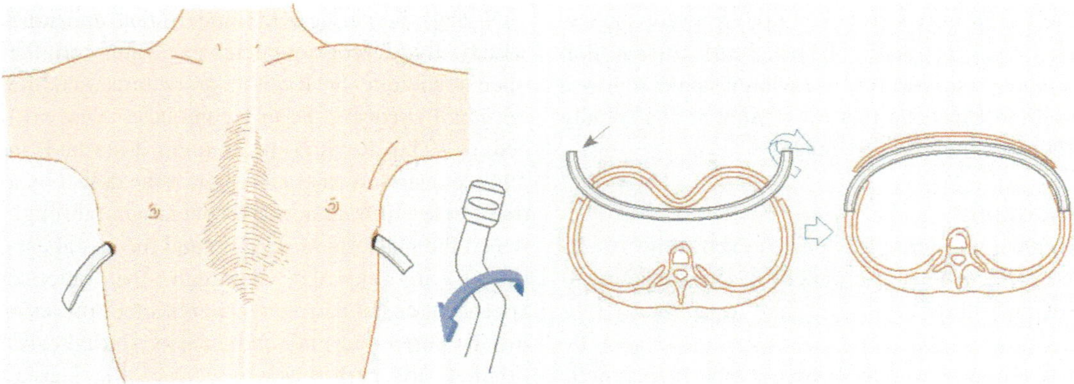

Fig. 72.3 Flipping of the retrosternal bar to pop out the sternal defect

Recently, a prospective, multicenter study was described in which the functional results were analyzed when correcting the pectus excavatum, whether by Ravitch technique or Nuss procedure. The results of this work show an important correction to Haller index and a significant improvement in the cardiac and pulmonary function tests (Table 72.2).

The complications of the surgical correction of pectus excavatum are uncommon, the most common being the displacement of the metallic devices, having to reoperate the patient to reposition the bar. Other more infrequent complications are wound infections, retrosternal hematomas, pneumothorax, hemothorax, myocardial lesions, and allergic reactions to metal. These complications tend to be more frequent after the Nuss procedure.

Table 72.2 Result of the surgical treatment of pectum excavatum

	Preoperative (average)	Postoperative (average)
Haller index	4.4	3.0
FVC (predicted %)	88.0	93.0
FEV 1 (predicted %)	87.0	90.0
TLC (predicted %)	94.0	100.0
VO_2 during exercise (l/min)	3.18	3.50
Pulse oximetry during exercise (VO_2/FC)	13.58	16.16

FVC forced vital capacity, *FEV1* forced expiratory volume in 1 second, *TLC* total lung capacity, *VO_2* oxygen consumption

Pectus Carinatum

Pectus carinatum is the second most frequent congenital malformation of the costal wall. Like pectus excavatum, it is more frequent in men than in women, with a ratio of 4:1. It is more frequent to have a late consultation, because it tends to appear after age 11, worsening during puberty.

Preoperative Evaluation

Medical history and complete physical examination are necessary. The protrusion of the sternum with different morphologies will allow the classification of the malformation in its different types. Type 1 or chondrogladiolar is the one that protrudes in the gladiolus or sternal body and lower cartilages. Type 2 or chondromanubrial is less common. Here the manubrium sterni and the higher cartilages protrude. Type 3 or lateral deformities are those in which there is a unilateral protrusion or sternal rotation. There are also mixed forms. Most of the patients will not present symptoms, being mainly a cosmetic problem, which significantly influences the development of a negative body image. Some patients may report musculoskeletal pain in the thorax and epigastrium.

The posteroanterior and lateral chest X-ray, and in some cases computerized tomography or magnetic resonance can be useful to have a surgical plan. Patients with a Haller index between 1.2 and 2.0 benefit from the correction of the deformity.

Treatment

Unlike pectus excavatum, the first line of treatment in pectus carinatum is the compressive therapy with orthosis according to the deformity type. In patients under 18 years of age, where the chest cavity is more malleable, the success rate varies between 65% and 80%. Dr. Marcelo Martínez-Ferro, a pediatric surgeon in Buenos Aires, developed a dynamic compression system that allows measuring the compression force electronically, with which he reports an 88% success rate (Fig. 72.4). Regarding the surgical treatment, it was initially described by Ravitch in 1952. The procedure is similar to the one for pectus excavatum, where the deformed costal cartilages are resected, keeping the perichondrium, and the sternal osteotomies are performed, depending on the type of information. Dr. Horacio Abramson, from Buenos Aires, published a paper in 2009 that described a minimally invasive technique to correct pectus carinatum. It is similar to the Nuss technique for pectus excavatum, but the bar goes through the sternum, allowing the retraction of the deformity (Fig. 72.5).

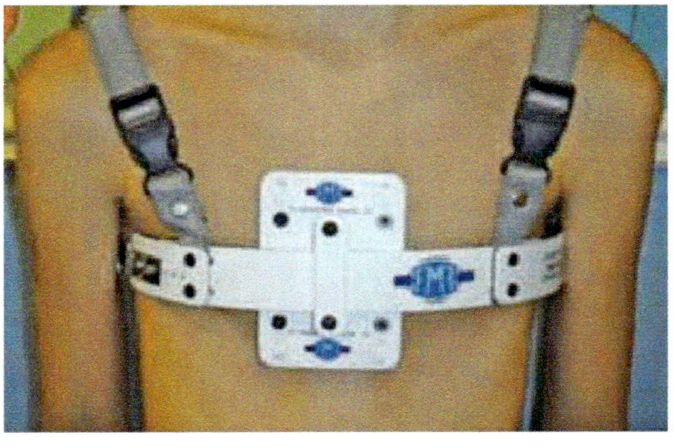

Fig. 72.4 Dynamic compression system. Dynamic compression system developed by Dr. Marcelo Martínez-Ferro

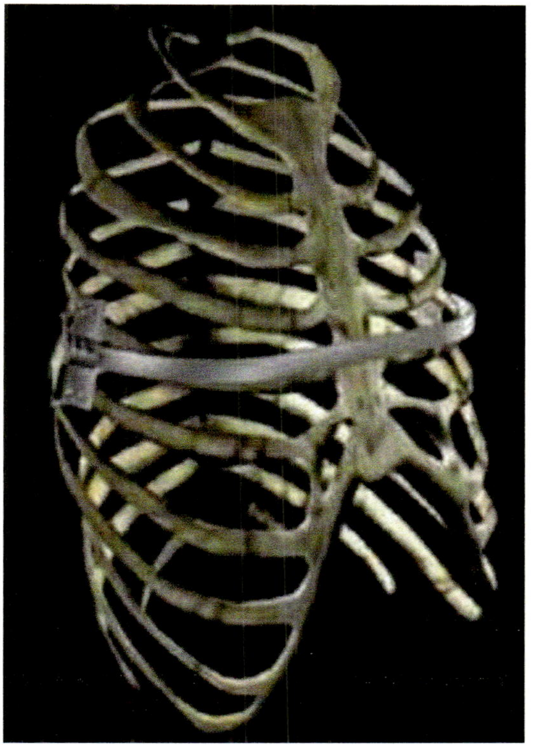

Fig. 72.5 Correction technique. Correction technique for pectus carinatum in a minimally invasive way developed by Dr. Horacio Abramson

Lung Surgery

Thoracotomy

Posterolateral thoracotomy is the classic way of accessing the thorax for the surgical treatment of lung lesions. The first lung lobectomy with anatomical dissection was performed in 1930. In 1941, Haight performed the first repair of an esophageal atresia in one stage through a left lateral thoracotomy. This kind of thoracotomy has an excellent access to the thorax, but to be able to perform it, the muscles of the costal wall (latissimus dorsi, trapezius, rhomboid, and serratus anterior) must be transected. It is associated with important adverse effects in the pediatric population, such as significant postoperative pain, winged scapula, alteration of the mobility of the shoulder, scoliosis and, cosmetically, a big scar.

Another technique for the open approach to the chest in the pediatric population is the thoracotomy with preservation of the muscle, described by Bianchi et al. in 1998. Kucukarslan et al. compared the results of the classic thoracotomy with that of muscle preservation. Regarding musculoskeletal deformities, the thoracotomy with preservation of the muscle significantly reduces the apparition of scoliosis (16% vs. 2.5%), shoulder elevation (30% vs. 7.5%), and winged scapula (38% vs. 12.5%). Besides, it significantly reduces the scale of pain and the hospitalization days.

Technique

The patient adopts the lateral decubitus position with a roll under the ribs to better open the intercostal spaces on the operation side. It is recommended to mark the important anatomical points before starting the surgery, as to have them as a reference during surgery (Fig. 72.6).

For the thoracotomy with preservation of the muscle, the place of the incision must be planned strategically to allow the most direct access to the pleural cavity. When the skin is opened, the latissimus dorsi and serratus anterior must be located. Then, the anterior edge of the latissimus dorsi is unlatched and retracted, exposing the serratus anterior, to which the posterior edge will be detached and retracted, exposing the intercostal space, accessing the pleural space through the fourth or fifth intercostal space. Once the surgery is finished, similar to the posterolateral thoracotomy, a pleural drainage is used; unlike the posterolateral thoracotomy, it is not necessary to close so many muscular planes.

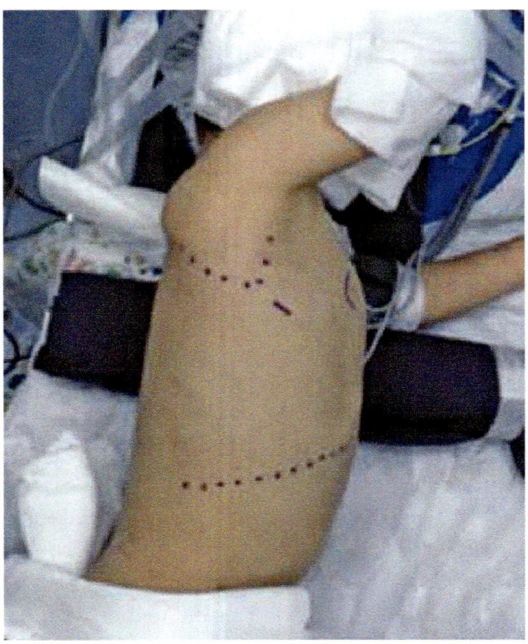

Fig. 72.6 Thoracotomy position

Videothoracoscopy

Introduction

Thoracoscopy has been used since the early twentieth century. However, the development and miniaturization of instruments, such as video cameras, optical devices, and surgical and hemostasis equipment, has caused its popularity to grow exponentially over the past decades.

Nowadays, all thoracic pathologies in children are treated with a thoracoscopy approach, which has reduced postsurgical pain, recovery periods, and morbidity rates, as well as the long-term sequelae of these procedures (Table 72.3).

In comparison with the open approach, thoracoscopy offers a superior exposure due to the visual magnification and closeness of the sur-

Table 72.3 Indications for pediatric thoracoscopy

Lung biopsy
Lung lobectomy
Cysts resection
Lung decortication
Resection of lung sequestration
Resection of intestinal duplication cysts
Esophageal myotomy
Anterior vertebral arthrodesis
Hernia repair or diaphragmatic plication
Patent ductus arteriosum ligation
Thoracic duct ligation (chylothorax)
Repair of esophageal atresia
Aortopexy
Resection and biopsy of mediastinal masses
Thymectomy
Sympathectomy
Pericardial window

geon's work area. Along with the lower morbidity rate of the minimally invasive procedures involved, this suggests that thoracoscopy should be the first-choice technique in virtually all thoracic procedures in children; however, we must recognize there is currently a lack of randomized studies supporting this proposal.

Preoperative Evaluation and Anesthetic Considerations

In general, both imaging studies, computerized axial tomography scan or magnetic resonance, provide guidance and can inform adequate planning for tackling most lesions.

The most important consideration when performing a thoracoscopy procedure in children is the creation of an actual space within the thorax which allows the surgeon to visualize and manipulate surgical instruments. This necessarily involves collapsing, at least partially, the ipsilateral lung. There is no specific preoperative test which may enable us to foresee if a child will tolerate mono-pulmonary ventilation. Nevertheless, most patients, even those with mechanical ventilation, will tolerate short periods of mono-pulmonary ventilation.

In order to achieve mono-pulmonary ventilation in children, patient size is a limiting factor. In patients over 30 kg, it is possible to use double lumen catheters in the same way as in adults. In smaller patients, it is possible to perform a selective bronchial blockage (Fig. 72.7). The bronchial blocker can even be used outside of the endotracheal tube and placed under bronchoscopy. In even smaller patients, when it is not possible to employ this technique, a selective mono-bronchial intubation can be performed, with a medium tube in a smaller size than the one advised for the patient. However, all these precautions may not be enough to obtain an adequate working space. In such cases, we can use a discrete CO_2 insufflation to the thorax, with low pressure and low current volumes, as a useful supplementary tool.

The positioning of the patient is key to achieve the best access to the lesion. In general, imaging techniques allow for an adequate planning for direct access, avoiding that any kind of tissue is interposed between the operator and the lesion.

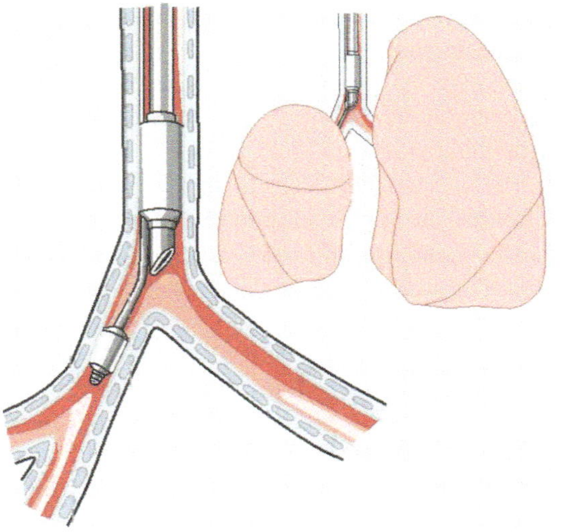

Fig. 72.7 Bronchial blocker

For example, a posterior mediastinum lesion is better faced with the patient in a semiprone position, making the lung fall forward. Similarly, when placing the patient and the trocars, care must be taken to maintain the eye-camera-monitor axis to facilitate the work of the surgeon. The same applies to the planning of a conversion to open surgery, if needed.

Finally, the postoperative care of these patients is not different from the usual handling of those with open thoracic surgery, having a better recovery due to the lower requirement of analgesics.

Dorsal Spine Surgery

Introduction

The pathological processes that can determine alterations in the child's spine can be many: congenital or neuromuscular anomalies, alterations of bone development, skeletal dysplasias, traumatic, infecticus, iatrogenic, or neoplastic pathologies, etc. It is basic to consider this heterogeneity regarding natural history, physiopathology, and comorbidities to formulate an adequate treatment. Additionally, regarding the child's spine, the growing and developing dynamics will modulate the types and opportunities of the treatment.

Normal Development and Growth of the Spine

During the first three or four weeks of gestation the organogenesis takes place in concomitance with the formation of somites, mesenchymal molds for the future vertebrae. The appearance of a noxa in this developmental stage explains the coexistence of malformations in other organs in up to 30% of the cases, such as the central nervous system, and renal or cardiac systems. This is why it is important that patients with spine malformations have a multidisciplinary evaluation to detect and eventually treat these comorbidities.

Notwithstanding the cause of the deformity, its prognosis will greatly depend on its seriousness at the moment of the diagnosis and the growth potential that the child has. This is why it is of the utmost importance to know the critical and accelerated growth periods of the axial skeleton: the first occurs between birth and 3–4 years of age, and the second during the pubertal growth spurt. In these lapses, a longitudinal growth of 1.75–2 cm/year is produced in the segments of the spine, and it coincides with periods in which the progression of the deformities can accelerate, meriting more frequent checks.

Also very importantly, there is a delicate interdependence between the development of the chest cavity and spine with the development of the lung parenchyma. This can affect the respiratory function of the child and shorten their survival. The most crucial stage for this is the first five years of life, especially the two first years when more than 80% of the alveoli are formed, together with the growth of the dorsal spine and wall. Thus, any alteration that affects the development of the spine or the chest cavity can potentially generate not only a severe spinal deformity in the future but it can also determine a decrease in the definitive lung function, beyond the thoracic restriction. Thus, Campbell et al. defined the term thoracic insufficiency syndrome as the inability of the thorax to support normal ventilatory mechanics and lung growth. This is generally present in the context of patients with vertebral malformations and a complex thoracic wall, for whom an early spinal fusion has no benefit, because the lung function remains below normal (Fig. 72.8).

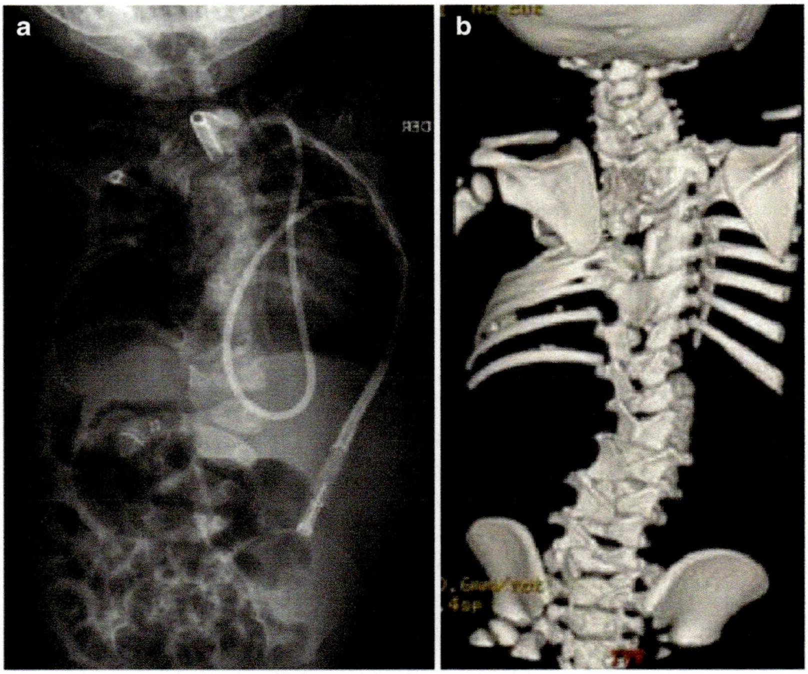

Fig. 72.8 Thoracic insufficiency syndrome. Patient of 2 years and 2 months of age, with multiple vertebral malformations and costal fusions, congenital left diaphragmatic hernia, without neurological or cognitive deficit, with recurring episodes of lung infection. (**a**) Total posteroanterior spine X-ray and (**b**) 3D reconstruction computerized axial tomography in posterior vision

Preoperative Evaluation

While it is not recommended to extrapolate the management between the different causes of spinal deformities, most of the indications of surgery in this age group are based on the projected risk, progression or worsening of the deformity, in the context of the natural history of its base pathology. This includes patients in whom the conservative corset management fails, and in whom a radiological progression is evident in the serialized monitoring. Even though it's controversial, avoiding the progression of thoracic curves in patients with potential restrictive pathologies (e.g., muscular dystrophy) would have a protective effect in the long run, decreasing the speed of degeneration of the lung function. The reach of this measure has to be evaluated in conjunction with the morbidity associated with surgery and the natural progression of the condition. Finally, in some congenital malformation cases, the risk of neurological compromise is up to 12%, which reinforces the indication of surgery.

As has been previously stated, many of these children have a multisystem condition of which the spine is just a part. Additionally, the severe and rigid deformities they can have require wider and more invasive surgery. Thus, many of these children are exposed to a higher rate of perioperative complications regarding wound infection, pneumonia, implant failure, non-union, pseudoartrhosis, augmented blood loss, respiratory postoperative failure, and even death.

Owing to multiple presentations, in complex cases, the planning and preoperative preparation must be multidisciplinary and individualized. Associated anomalies and comorbidities must be anticipated and evaluated, such as cardiac, renal, and central nervous system malformations. A renal ultrasound scan is a simple and effective exam to evaluate urogenital malformations. If there is clinical suspicion, a referral to cardiology and an echocardiogram could discover interauricular or ventricular septum alterations, persistent ductus arteriosum, transposition of great vessels, lung stenosis, etc., among 10% and 26% of the congenital scoliosis cases. In patients with evidence of neurological deficit, it is recommended to request a magnetic resonance to rule out an intraspinal pathology, such as diastematomyelia, syringomyelia, or tethered spinal cord. In other cases, where the base pathology presents a high prevalence of anomalies of the central nervous system, the resonance is indicated independent from the physical exam. In patients with idiopathic scoliosis of the adolescent with normal neurological exam, the preoperative resonance is not indicated, because its efficacy would be under 3%.

The lung function can be altered in many of these patients, due to the precocious formation of the curve or the seriousness of the restrictive phenomenon. In these cases, it is essential to involve anesthesia and pediatric bronchopulmonary specialists, anticipating an eventually difficult airway and prolonged postoperative mechanical ventilation needs. Moreover, it must be considered that some of these children have vertebral cervical malformations (for example Klippel–Feil syndrome) that might make intubation difficult. This includes considering early pre or postoperative tracheostomy in cases with marginal lung function, especially taking into account that up to a 60% decrease is reported in spirometry tests in the postoperative of scoliosis surgery in some series. However, the use of noninvasive mechanical ventilation has lowered this indication and has enabled the performance of surgery in patients that were previously considered outside the reach of surgery. In cases where a thoracic insufficiency syndrome is suspected, and given the difficulties for spirometry tests in younger patients, the evaluation of the chest volume by a computerized axial tomography can be considered. This has been well correlated in studies with spirometry tests. Additionally, Gollogly et al. have published the volumes of normal lung parenchyma for the different ages and genders.

Other important aspects in the preoperative planning of these patients are the nutritional aspects, because regularly these patients present symptoms of protein–calorie malnutrition, whose presence has been correlated with postoperative results. Some of these cases are carriers of clotting or immunity alterations, having to plan beforehand the availability of the blood elements needed in each situation with the anesthesia team and the blood bank. The multidiscipline management needed for these complex patients must be stressed. The implementation of management algorithms coordinated among multiple disciplines for these patients' preoperative stage has managed to diminish the general and ICU stay, along with a reduction in the rate of postoperative complications in some series.

Surgical Techniques

Traditionally, the most used technique to treat spinal deformities is the correction and instrumented spinal fusion. This was even applied for early start deformities (<5–10 years) under the precept that a short spine without a deformity was better than allowing the curve progression. However, it has recently been demonstrated that even early correction and fusion procedures that were considered successful result in the long term in a decrease of almost 50% of the FVC and FEV-1. Additionally, the frequent recurrence of deformities and the need of unplanned revision surgery have brought back the interest to develop systems that allow the correction of the curve but retain growth.

In generic terms these are called "growing" systems, and they are generally made through a posterior way of approach to the column. Owing to the enormous osteogenetic potential of children, the idea is not to touch the central zone with the instrumentation, latching only to the sides. Thus, the spontaneous fusion is avoided, placing the connective bars in subcutaneous or subfascial areas. These systems can be performed with a single bar or double bars connected with elongators. After the initial installation of the system, the periodic elongations only need to address this connective piece with the following minimization of surgery needed to produce growth (Fig. 72.9). The goal in general is to elongate until 10 years of age to later perform the defini-

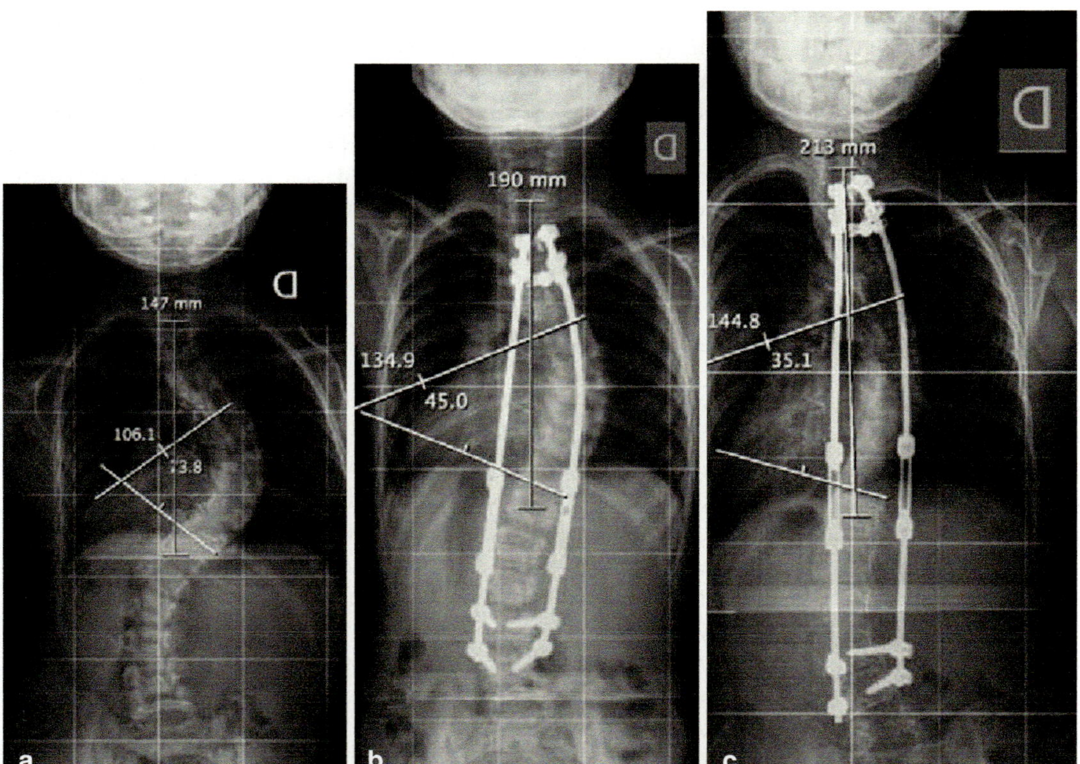

Fig. 72.9 Spinal fixation with growing bars. Patient with DiGeorge syndrome that presents progressive scoliosis despite treatment with orthosis. A preoperative X-ray is presented (**a**), after the first surgery with the dual "growing" bars was performed (**b**), and after seven elongations in the space of four years (**c**). Note the progressive correction of the deformity and the increase of the longitude T1–T12

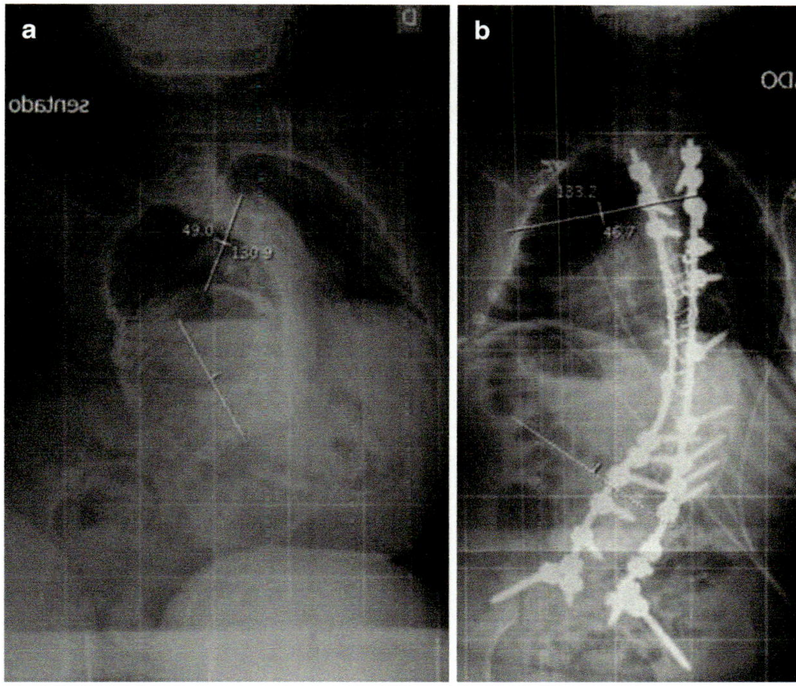

Fig. 72.10 Spinal fixation with fixed bars. Patient with type II spinal atrophy and severe neuromuscular scoliosis (Cob Index >100°). Preoperative (**a**) and postoperative (**b**) anteroposterior X-rays are shown. Note the typical pelvic obliqueness indicating neuromuscular scoliosis

tive fusion. Another parameter to follow is to manage a T1–T12 > 18 cm longitude toward skeletal maturity. Values below these are associated to FVC below 45%.

A separate mention has to be made for the VEPTR (*Vertical Expandable Prosthetic Titanium Rib*) used mainly for congenital spine deformities associated with costal malformations and fusions, provoking chest insufficiency. In these cases, the elongation of the spine would not provoke the expansion of the compromised hemithorax, so an expansive thoracotomy, together with costal instrumentation, is also subject to be progressively elongated. However, all these "growing" systems share the same kind of disadvantages: need for multiple surgery procedures to produce "growth", frequent complications, implant fractures, prominent instrumentation, considering that many of these patients are very small, the need to use a postoperative corset and the cost, among others. Although in general these complications are not serious, they happen in up to 48% of the cases, and they are more common when the surgeries start at a younger age. Given these factors, this group of patients is considered serious, and the controversy about the best treatment system persists.

In patients with severe progressive deformities around or after 10 years of age, the definitive correction and fusion is preferred. Although multiple ways to approach this exist (anterior, posterior, combined), the most used today is the instrumented (Fig. 72.10). With the development of modern column instrumentation and techniques, the ability to reduce and consolidate the deformities has increased up to 90%. The stability of definitive constructs has also eliminated the need for rest and postoperative orthosis. The morbidity derived from these procedures depends on the base pathology, being minimal for the adolescent idiopathic scoliosis and maximal for deformities in neuromuscular patients.

Sources

Abramson H, D'Agostino J, Wuscovi S. A 5-year experience with a minimally invasive technique for pectus carina-tum repair. J Pediatr Surg. 2009;44(1):118–23; discussion 123–114.

Campbell RM Jr, Smith MD, Mayes TC, et al. The characteristics of thoracic insufficiency syndrome associated with fused ribs and congenital scoliosis. J Bone Joint Surg Am. 2003;85-A(3):399–408.

Campos MA, Weinstein SL. Pediatric scoliosis and kyphosis. Neurosurg Clin N Am. 2007;18(3):515–29.
Fonkalsrud EW. Current management of pectus excavatum. World J Surg. 2003;27(5):502–8.
Gill I, Eagle M, Mehta JS, Gibson MJ, Bushby K, Bullock R. Correction of neuromuscular scoliosis in patients with preexisting respiratory failure. Spine (Phila Pa 1976). 2006;31(21):2478–83.
Gollogly S, Smith JT, White SK, Firth S, White K. The volume of lung parenchyma as a function of age: a review of 1050 normal CT scans of the chest with three-dimensional volumetric reconstruction of the pulmonary system. Spine (Phila Pa 1976). 2004;29(18):2061–6.
Hedequist D, Emans J. Congenital scoliosis. J Am Acad Orthop Surg. 2004;12(4):266–75.
Johnston CE. Preoperative medical and surgical planning for early onset scoliosis. Spine (Phila Pa 1976). 2010;35(25):2239–44.
Karol LA, Johnston C, Mladenov K, Schochet P, Walters P, Browne RH. Pulmonary function following early thoracic fusion in non-neuromuscular scoliosis. J Bone Joint Surg Am. 2008;90(6):1272–81.
Karpelowsky J. Paediatric thoracoscopic surgery. Paediatr Respir Rev. 2012;13(4):244–50; quiz 250–241.
Kelly RE Jr, Cash TF, Shamberger RC, et al. Surgical repair of pectus excavatum markedly improves body image and perceived ability for physical activity: multicenter study. Pediatrics. 2008;122(6):1218–22.
Kelly RE Jr, Mellins RB, Shamberger RC, et al. Multicenter study of pectus excavatum, final report: complications, static/exercise pulmonary function, and anatomic outcomes. J Am Coll Surg. 2013;217(6):1080–9.
Kucukarslan N, Kirilmaz A, Arslan Y, Sanioglu Y, Ozal E, Tatar H. Muscle sparing thoracotomy in pediatric age: a comparative study with standard posterolateral thoracotomy. Pediatr Surg Int. 2006;22(10):779–83.
Lam MW, Klassen AF, Montgomery CJ, LeBlanc JG, Skarsgard ED. Quality-of-life outcomes after surgical correction of pectus excavatum: a comparison of the Ravitch and Nuss procedures. J Pediatr Surg. 2008;43(5):819–25.
Martinez-Ferro M, Fraire C, Bernard S. Dynamic compression system for the correction of pectus carinatum. Semin Pediatr Surg. 2008;17(3):194–200.
McGuigan RM, Azarow KS. Congenital chest wall defects. Surg Clin North Am. 2006;86(2):353–70, ix.
Miller NH, Benefield E, Hasting L, Carry P, Pan Z, Erickson MA. Evaluation of high-risk patients undergoing spinal surgery: a matched case series. J Pediatr Orthop. 2010;30(5):496–502.
Obermeyer RJ, Goretsky MJ. Chest wall deformities in pediatric surgery. Surg Clin North Am. 2012;92(3):669–84, ix.
Parikh DH, Crabbe D, Auldist A, Rothenberg S. Pediatric thoracic surgery. Springer: London; 2009. https://doi.org/10.1007/B136543
Reames DL, Smith JS, Fu KM, et al. Complications in the surgical treatment of 19,360 cases of pediatric scoliosis: a review of the Scoliosis Research Society Morbidity and Mortality database. Spine (Phila Pa 1976). 2011;36(18):1484–91.
Velasco MV, Colin AA, Zurakowski D, Darras BT, Shapiro F. Posterior spinal fusion for scoliosis in duchenne muscular dystrophy diminishes the rate of respiratory decline. Spine (Phila Pa 1976). 2007;32(4):459–65.

Extracorporeal Circulation Membrane Oxygenation Therapy for Acute Respiratory Diseases

73

Javier Kattan Said, Álvaro González Morandé, and Andrés Castillo Moya

Contents

Introduction

Extracorporeal circulation membrane oxygenation (ECMO), or extracorporeal life support (ECLS), is a therapy that uses a modified partial cardiopulmonary bypass to give pulmonary or cardiac support over an extended period of time, generally ranging from 1 to 4 weeks. It is used on patients with reversible pulmonary failure caused by lung, heart, and other diseases. ECMO 'makes time' for resting the lungs or heart, thus creating a chance for recovery. Since ECMO therapy is invasive, there are potential risks associated with it, which is why there are criteria to choose patients with a prediction of mortality between 50% and 100%. The ideal candidate has a high value in their prediction of mortality but suffers from a potentially reversible lung or cardiovascular injury.

The first survivor of ECMO therapy was treated in 1971 by J. Donald Hill, who used a Bramson oxygenator on an adult patient with multiple injuries. This therapy was, however, abandoned because of its poor results. Years later, the therapy reemerged for newborn and

J. Kattan Said · A. Castillo Moya (✉)
Department of Pediatrics, School of Medicine, Pontificia Universidad Católica de Chile, Santiago, Chile
e-mail: kattan@med.puc.cl; acastill@med.puc.cl

Á. González Morandé
Pediatrics, Neonatology, Pontificia Universidad Católica de Chile, Santiago, Chile
e-mail: alvgonza@med.puc.cl

P. Bertrand, I. Sánchez (eds.), *Pediatric Respiratory Diseases*,
https://doi.org/10.1007/978-3-030-26961-6_73

pediatric patients due to Robert Bartlett's efforts, who in 1975, at Orange County Medical Center, treated his first newborn patient who survived this type of therapy, an abandoned newborn who suffered from respiratory distress syndrome. The use of this therapy on newborns increased during the late 1980s, with survival rates close to 80% in patients with a predicted mortality between 60% and 80%. Because of this increase in usage on newborn patients, a voluntary alliance between active ECMO centers was born in 1989, giving form to the Extracorporeal Life Support Organization (ELSO). Added to the good results in newborns since the 1990s, there has been a considerable increase in pediatric patients treated with ECMO, with over 14,000 registered cases, claiming a survival rate of up to 66% in pediatric patients suffering from respiratory conditions.

By the year 2009, around 80% of patients treated with ECMO were newborns or children. During the past few years, ECMO on adult patients suffering from respiratory conditions increased progressively by 1000%, and ECMO on pediatric patients suffering from respiratory conditions increased by 100%, which is partially explained by the influenza H1N1 pandemic and the new evidence emerged from controlled studies in adults.

During the 1990s, new therapies against cardiorespiratory diseases were developed, such as high-frequency oscillatory ventilation (HFOV), surfactant, or inhaled nitric oxide (iNO). These therapies, in association with ECMO centers, have managed to significantly lower morbidity in more developed countries.

During the past decade, ECMO has been used as a rescue therapy in almost 800 newborns reported to ELSO every year. These newborns did not respond to intensive care with HFOV or iNO. Currently, ECMO use rate for newborns suffering from respiratory failure in the United States sits at around 1 per every 6000 living newborns This therapy has shown a clear increase in global survival rate (Figs. 73.1 and 73.2), better long-term quality of life, and being more cost-effective for newborns with severe respiratory failure.

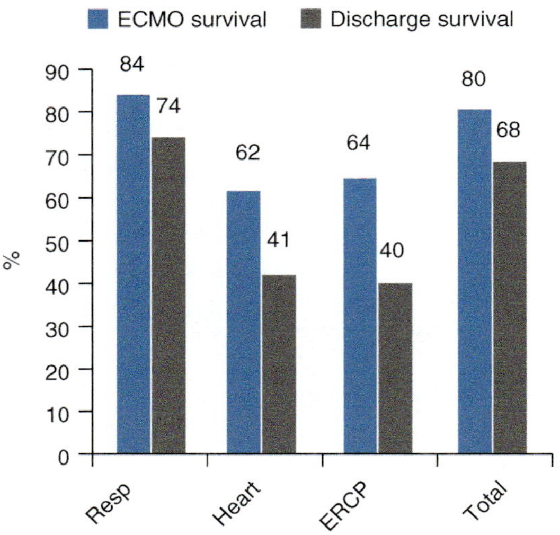

Fig. 73.1 Survival rate of newborns. Survival rate of 34,650 newborns after reported ECMO to the Extracorporeal Life Support Organization (ELSO), grouped by cause of admission to ECMO (*ERCP* Extracorporeal cardiopulmonary resuscitation)

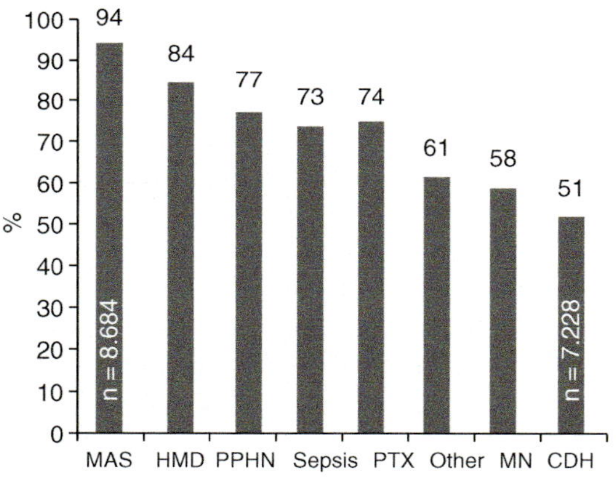

Fig. 73.2 Survival rate of Nnwborns. Survival rate to discharge of 27,728 newborns treated with ECMO, reported to ELSO by respiratory condition (*MAS* Meconium aspiration syndrome, *HMD* Hyaline membrane disease, *PPHN* Persistent pulmonary hypertension of the newborn, *PTX* Pneumothorax, *PN* Pneumonia, *CDH* Congenital diaphragmatic hernia)

For pediatric patients with respiratory conditions, the indications that lead to using ECMO are more diverse and harder to define than during the newborn stage, but during the past few years there has been an increase in the number of reported cases to ELSO, with close to 350 cases a year displaying a global survival rate of 57% at the discharge (Figs. 73.3 and 73.4).

It is worth noting that survival rate in pediatric patients varies according to the disease that determined the connection, with survival rates reported as high as 83% for severe asthma attack. Acute hypoxic respiratory failure is the most frequent pathophysiological mechanism leading to respiratory ECMO, of which viral pneumonia takes first place (22%), followed by respiratory failure (18%), bacterial pneumonia (10%), acute respiratory distress, and aspiration pneumonia. Acute viral pneumonia shows a survival rate of up to 70% as described for VRS, with an average of 64% for viral pneumonia. Survival rates are also high in the pediatric group for aspiration pneumonia and post-traumatic ARDS (Fig. 73.5). Patients are oftentimes admitted because of immunosuppression and suspected sepsis. These patients usually display multi-organ failure. Pediatric patients with the worst prognosis are those who have received bone marrow transplants, those who have suffered from *Bordetella pertussis* induced pneumonia and pulmonary hypertension, and those admitted to ECMO with multi-organ failure, as opposed to the positive prognosis for those who only show isolated lung involvement.

In 1972, Bartlett reported the first case of successful prolonged post-operative cardiac support in a 2-year-old patient who suffered from post-surgery heart failure after a Mustard procedure because of transposition of great arteries. At present, more than half of patients requiring perioperative heart ECMO are those suffering from complex cyanotic congenital heart diseases. The largest group of patients requiring ECMO sup-

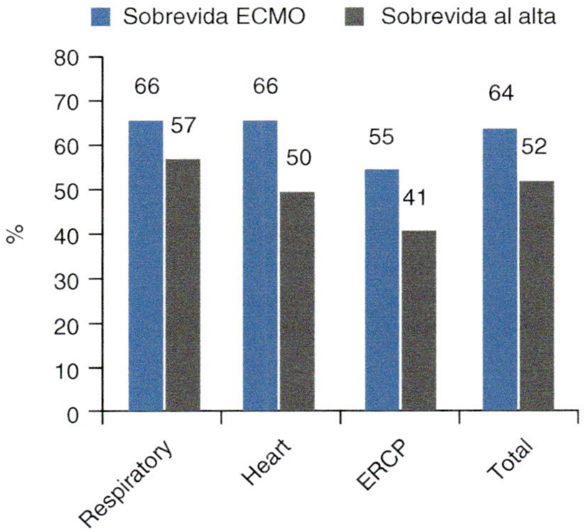

Fig. 73.3 Survival rate of pediatric patients. Survival rate of 16,253 pediatric patients after ECMO reported to the Extracorporeal Life Support Organization (ELSO), grouped by cause of admission to ECMO (*ERCP* Extracorporeal cardiopulmonary resuscitation)

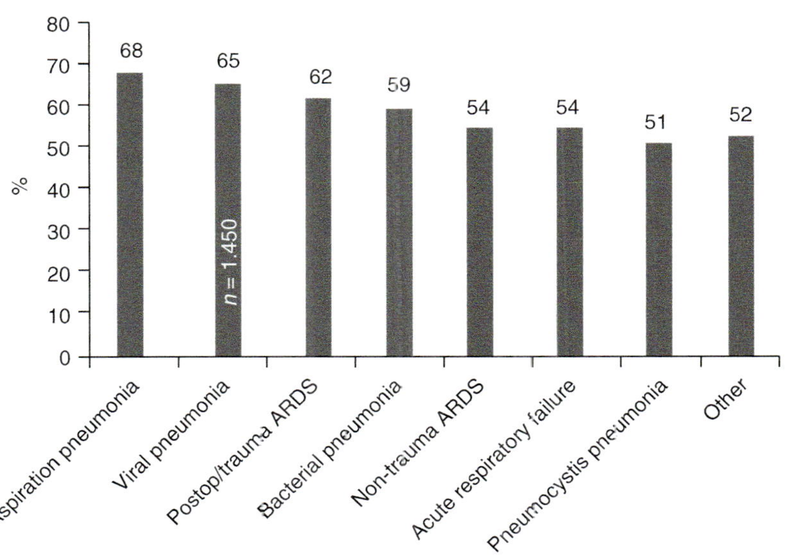

Fig. 73.4 Survival rate of pediatric patients. Survival rate of 6569 discharged pediatric patients treated with ECMO reported to ELSO by respiratory condition (*ARDS* Acute respiratory distress syndrome)

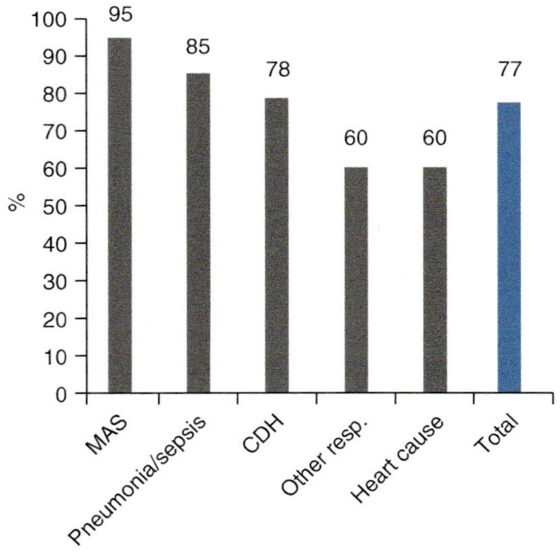

Fig. 73.5 Survival rate to discharge. Survival rate to discharge of 143 patients (123 newborns and 20 pediatric patients) treated in the Newborn-Pediatric ECMO Program at the Clinical Hospital of the Pontificia Universidad Católica de Chile (ECMO-UC) 2003–2014, reported to ELSO by main diagnosis (*MAS* Meconium aspiration syndrome; *CDH* Congenital diaphragmatic hernia)

port is those who, after cardiotomy, present complete AV canal (20%), complex single ventricle anomaly (17%), and tetralogy of Fallot (14%). Among the chief causes requiring perioperatory heart ECMO are hypoxia (36%), cardiac arrest (24%), and failure after leaving extracorporeal circulation support (14%).

ECMO Physiology

During extracorporeal circulation support, blood is drained from the patient to an outside pump (either a roller or a centrifugal pump), which is pushed through an exchange membrane (a silicone or a polymethylpentene oxygenator) for oxygenation and CO_2 removal. Then it passes through a heat exchanger and finally returns the blood to the patient's blood flow (Fig. 73.6). This therapy requires anticoagulation of the circuit and the patient through heparin administered to the ECMO circuit so as to avoid the activation of the coagulation cascade in the system. In addition to that, a variety of pressure, flow, bubble, and temperature monitors are used during therapy. It is of vital importance to continually monitor coagulation through the hourly measurement of activated clotting time (ACT) and the measurement of anti-factor Xa, fibrinogen, platelet count, PT, APTT and, in some patients, anti-thrombin III levels, and a thromboelastography.

There are in principle two different forms of ECMO:

(a) *Veno-arterial (VA)*: Blood is drained from the right atrium through a cannula inserted into the right internal jugular vein, the femoral vein, or directly to the right atrium; and it is picked back up at the thoracic aorta through a right carotid cannula, a femoral cannula or an aortic cannula. VA ECMO provides heart-lung support. It is common to use a transthoracic cannula (right ventricle and aortic cannula) in patients who have endured heart operations.

(b) *Veno-venous (VV)*: Blood is drained from the right atrium through the posterior and inferior orifices of a double-lumen cannula inserted into the right jugular vein and returned to the same right ventricle through the anterior orifices of the cannula, which are pointed toward the tricuspid valve. One of the limits of this method lies in the recirculation of already oxygenized blood through the double lumen cannula. This has been corrected with the new design for VV cannulas. VV ECMO may also be performed in older children through the use of two cannulas, draining blood from the jugular vein and returning it through the femoral vein. VV ECMO requires a well-functioning heart. This modality of ECMO prevents cannulation in the carotid or femoral arteries, thus reducing complications arising from cannulation or ligation of these arteries, as well as those arising from air entering the ECMO circuit. This method has seen an increase in usage during recent years, covering 40% and 50% of respiratory cases in newborn and pediatric patients, respectively. Oxygen is delivered during ECMO by the combination of blood oxygenation through the membrane,

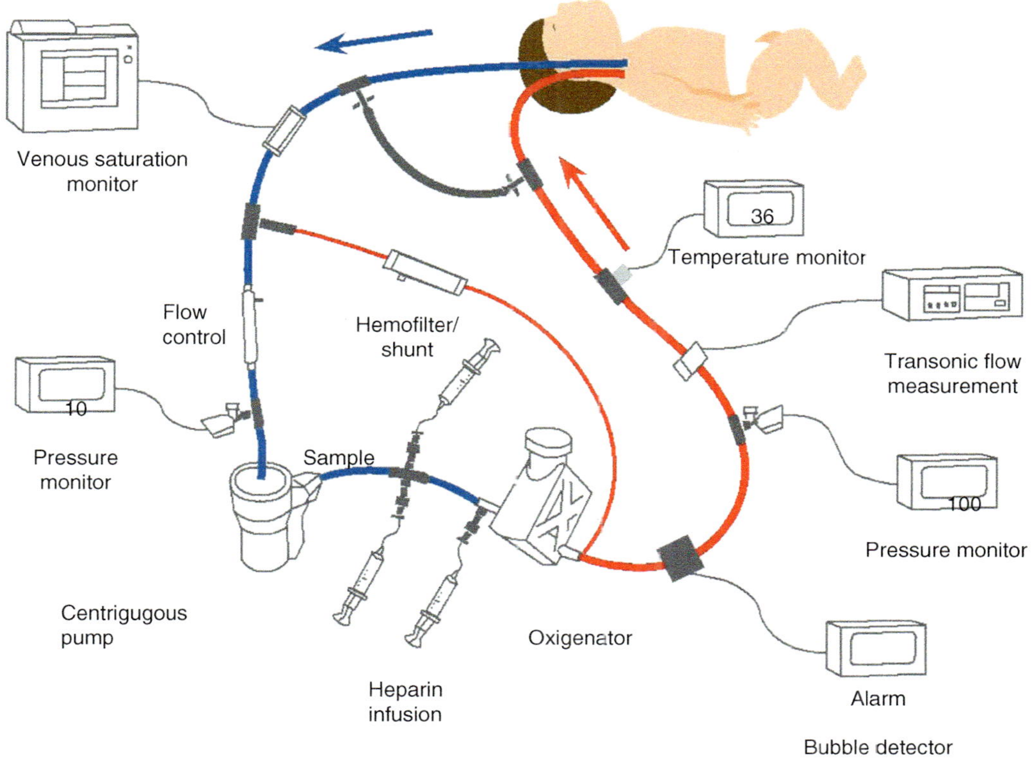

Fig. 73.6 Diagram of veno-arterial ECMO with pump and oxygenator. Venous blood is obtained from the right atrium through the right internal jugular vein. It is then pumped, oxygenized, heated and returned to the aorta through the right carotid artery. (Diagram used with permission from ECMO Manual of the Children's National Medical Center, George Washington University, Washington DC, 2010)

blood flowing through the extracorporeal circuit, native lung oxygenation, and native heart output. In turn, oxygenation at the ECMO membrane is a function of its geometry, material composition and thickness, blood and FiO_2 laminar thickness, time of permanence of red blood cells in the exchange area, hemoglobin concentration, and O_2 saturation. On the other hand, CO_2 removal during ECMO is a function of the geometry, materials, and surface area of the membrane, blood PCO_2 and, to a lesser extent, it depends on blood and gas flows through the membrane.

- In a VA ECMO, the bypass generates an essentially non-pulsatile blood flow. In this way, as the blood flow to the extracorporeal circuit increases, the pulse wave decreases, completely ceasing when it reaches a 100% bypass, except for occasional waves. However, it is normal for VA ECMO to only involve about an 80% bypass, allowing a blood flow of 20% or more through the left heart and lungs, resulting in a reduced but visible pulse wave. The kidney is without doubt the most affected organ by the absence of pulsatility, producing an antidiuretic effect because of juxtaglomerular stimulation. In addition, non-pulsatile flow has been linked to stimulation of the pressure receptors in the carotid sinus, causing a large release of catecholamines, with damaging effects to microcirculation.

Selection Criteria for Applying ECMO

Selection criteria differ for newborn (Table 73.1) or pediatric patients (Table 73.2), depending on

Table 73.1 Selection criteria for newborns

Gestational age ≥34 weeks
Weight at birth ≥2000 grams
Unresponsive to maximum medical care (including HFOV, iNO, surfactant)
Reversible cardiopulmonary condition
Mechanical ventilation ≤14 days
High pulmonary mortality (50–100%), considering:
Oxygenation index (OI) >35–40 for 4–6 hours (iNO, HFOV)
PaO_2 < 40 mmHg for 4 h (100% O_2)
OI ≥ 25 after 72 h with HFOV-iNO
Unmanageable metabolic acidosis (ph < 7.15 for 2 h)
Reduced cardiac output with reversible etiology
Impossibility to wean from cardiopulmonary bypass
As a bridge for heart transplant
No untreatable congenital cardiopathy or injuries after heart surgery
Absence of major intracranial hemorrhage (≥ III degree)
Absence of uncontrollable hemorrhage
No evidence of irreversible brain damage
No malformations or genetic syndromes with fatal prognosis

Table 73.2 Selection criteria for pediatric patients

OI > 40 for 4–6 h or PaO_2/FiO_2 < 60 during mechanical ventilation (MCV or HFOV)
OI > 35 for >12 h. High settings for mechanical ventilation, considering:
Pressure plateau >35 cm H_2O for 8–12 hours
PEEP >15
Average airway pressure >20–25 cm H_2O in MCV or >30–35 cm H_2O in HFOV
Hypercapnic respiratory failure with pH < 7.1 for 4–6 hours despite maximum medical care
Acute deterioration with optimal therapy

whether the primary cause of admission is cardiac or respiratory. These are general criteria and must be individualized for each patient, assessing the risks and benefits of applying ECMO. The basic selection criteria for pediatric patients with respiratory failure are similar to those for newborns, with particular emphasis on whether the patient faces a serious pulmonary condition with a high risk of death, or whether it is a process that can be reversed through respiratory, gasometrical, and hemodynamic rest. On the other hand, there are general exclusion criteria (Table 73.3), though none of them are absolute and must be

Table 73.3 General exclusion criteria in the pediatric population

Over 14 days with mechanical ventilation
Over 7 days of high ventilatory settings, given the possibility of iatrogenic lung damage
Acute or irreversible brain damage
Chronic acute or irreversible lung disease
Severe coagulopathy or uncontrolled bleeding
Untreatable congenital cardiopathy
Chromosomal syndrome with limited prognosis
Cardiopulmonary arrest unless there is an extracorporeal cardiopulmonary resuscitation program (post-arrest ECMO or E-RCP) at the ECMO center

discussed by the ECMO team. In summary, selection criteria have evolved and continue to do so as a result of discussion, debate, experience, and the emergence of new treatments and techniques. Currently, there are no unique or exclusive criteria, and not withstanding general inclusion criteria, the decision to exclude a patient must be discussed by the team, taking into account all possible points of view, without excluding any party from this discussion.

Managing ECMO

Before a patient is admitted to ECMO, both indications and exclusion criteria must always be assessed, making it essential to perform a patient evaluation prior to ECMO, including at least age and anthropometry, neurological status (general exam, pupillary reactivity, electroencephalogram, history of seizures, head ultrasound, and ideally a brain CT scan for pediatric patients); respiratory and cardiovascular evaluation (oxygenation index, vasoactive support and, if possible, an echocardiography), electrolytic and acid–base evaluation, coagulation and renal function evaluation, evaluation of infectious parameters, and an assessment of current or previous vascular accesses.

The initial ECMO parameters seek to achieve a bypass of at least 50% or more of estimated cardiac output (with cardiac output estimated at 200 mL/kg/min for newborns, 150 mL/kg/min for pediatric patients under 10 kg and 2400 mL/m2sc/min for patients over 10 kg), and are adjusted to maintain adequate oxygenation, arterial pressure, and acid–base state. In patients with heart failure, VA-ECMO is the preferred choice. At present, when proper cardiac function is preserved and the main pathology is pulmonary, VV-ECMO is considered to be of assistance in oxygenation and ventilation.

The main points of access will depend on the modality of ECMO being used. For VA-ECMO, the right internal jugular vein and the right common carotid artery may be used as well as the femoral veins and arteries. For VV-ECMO, either the right internal jugular vein and the femoral vein may be used, or a long unique double-lumen cannula inserted into the right internal jugular vein, reaching the right atrium. In post-operative cardiac patients, direct transthoracic cannulation is common.

At present, most oxygenators use polymethylpentene fibers. These have microscopic pores, making the exchange of gases easier and avoiding 'dripping'. They are quickly and easily primed, displaying low trans-membrane pressure. This avoids the loss of proteins and other components. In fact, by having a more homogenous surface they produce less hemolysis and preserve platelet activity.

The strength with which blood is pumped through the circuit depends on the pumps, which may be of the roller or centrifugal type. Centrifugal pumps are increasingly preferred given the advantage of not being occlusive, which causes less pressure on the circuit and less hemolysis. They do not need a reservoir, are primed faster, and help preserve the circuit for a longer period. Their man disadvantage lies in their high cost, which is why some units still use roller pumps.

ECMO treatment may vary between 1 and 3 weeks or even longer. In January 2014, pediatric respiratory ECMO lasted an average of 11.6 days, with a described maximum of 129 days. On the other hand, pediatric cardiac ECMO generally take less time, with an average of 6.7 days with a described maximum of 120 days. For respiratory patients, improvement is generally noticed after a few days or even weeks.

Meticulous attention to all aspects of the patient is essential. Frequent checks of blood gas are required for the patient and the ECMO circuit, as well as clotting and kidney function checks, and an ultrasound assessment of the brain to identify intracranial hemorrhage and cerebral infarction.

Both arterial and venal saturation of the patient must be continually monitored, taking into account saturation levels of the blood extracted from the patient before it enters the oxygenator (ideally over 70–75%). Saturation of the superior vena cava should also be monitored. However, something to keep in mind for these last two is that there should be no doubt that there is no unnoticed source of short circuit of oxygenated blood.

Anticoagulation is essential in managing patients, both for ensuring an adequate duration of the circuit and to avoid severe bleeding from excessive anticoagulation. In this regard, hourly managing of levels of ACT from 180 to 200 sec., with a platelet count of over 100,000 and fibrinogen levels of over 150 mg/dl is thought to be adequate.

At least during the first days, patients must receive adequate sedoanalgesia with continuous opiate infusions and benzodiazepines, considering the eventual use of muscle relaxants in some cases. There has been a current increase in considering the benefits of using a smaller amount of anesthesia, with some groups even keeping patients awake during the procedure. This particularly applies to older patients.

Once ECMO support is being used, the mechanic ventilator settings should be set to rest. Despite the lack of a proper definition for this, it is considered so for pediatric patients with PEEP of 6–8 in order to avoid unrecruited lung, tidal volumes that do not surpass 8 mL/kg, and an FR of 12–18 per minute with FiO2, usually at 21%. In addition, emergency settings must always be kept in mind in case of an ECMO malfunction, in which case FiO2 must be considered at 100%.

During ECMO, water balance and diuresis are needed as soon as possible, as well as volume overload prior to its commencement. Positive water balance and oligo-anuria must be avoided, because once hemodynamics is stable, water balance should become negative by using a proportional diuresis, and afterwards, neutral. If these objectives are not achieved, or if the patient develops an oligo-anuric kidney injury, continuous hemofiltration or hemodiafiltration should be considered for as long as diuretics are used and if adequate hemodynamics did not manage to restore an adequate kidney function to achieve the required balance.

Finally, prophylactic antibiotics are not generally considered for this treatment. Using antibiotics in most patients depends either on the underlying disease, which for a large percentage of patients corresponds to an infectious disease, or if there is a suspicion of superimposed infections and as the result of surveillance or secondary cultures under clinical suspicion of infection.

As the patient's condition improves, ECMO support is gradually reduced. The patient is decannulated when tolerance to minimal ECMO support is achieved (10% bypass in VA-ECMO) with low to moderate mechanical ventilation parameters. ECMO treatment generally lasts between 5 and 10 days for newborn patients with respiratory diseases, though this is extended in cases of congenial diaphragmatic hernia, bacterial pneumonia, and myocarditis (10–11 days in average).

Complications

The ECMO procedure presents varying complication risks as a consequence of the severity of the condition of the patient, the use of anticoagulants, and changes to the blood flow (lower pulsatility blood flow). Among the most common complications are hemorrhage (surgical site 6%, pulmonary 4%, gastrointestinal 2%), infarction or brain hemorrhage (9% and 5% respectively), convulsions (11%), cardiac dysfunction (myocardial stunning 6%, arrhythmia 4%), kidney failure (4%), sepsis (6%), hyperbilirubinemia (9%), arterial hypertension (12%), and hemolysis (13%). The most common complication with cardiac-based ECMO is, by far, the need for vasoactive drugs during extracorporeal support, followed by surgical site bleeding.

Intracranial hemorrhage is the primary cause of death during ECMO, and the appearance of convulsions is a sign of a poor prognosis. Additionally, there are complications arising from circuit failure either in the oxygenator or in the equipment used during ECMO.

Prognosis and ECMO Programs in Latin America

Post-ECMO survival in newborn patients varies depending on their underlying disease, though respiratory causes present the most positive outcome with a survival rate of close to 75% after discharge. ECMO treatment for meconium aspiration syndrome is usually of the veno-venous type, which is associated with a lower risk rate and fewer complications, such as cerebral infarction and convulsions, and to minor changes in blood flow patterns. During the past few years, ECMO has been used as a tool for cardiopulmonary resuscitation after cardiac arrest yielding mixed results, with a survival rate of close to 40%.

Newborns were the first age group for which ECMO therapy showed vast superiority over maximum conventional therapy, as shown by a controlled and randomized multicenter study with 185 newborns suffering from severe respiratory insufficiency in 55 hospitals in the United Kingdom. This study showed that mortality and severe disability assessed after 1, 4, and 7 years of life decreased significantly after ECMO therapy (59% for the conventional therapy group vs. 37% for the ECMO group). At the seventh year of follow-up, 76% of children presented normal cognitive development.

The most recent systematic reviews show that ECMO therapy used in close to term newborns with severe but potentially reversible respiratory failure significantly improves survival without increasing severe disability while also being cost-effective when compared to other intensive care therapies. Regarding ECMO as a rescue therapy for congenital diaphragmatic hernia with severe respiratory failure, evidence from controlled prospective studies only suggests a decrease in early mortality. However, a meta-analysis of retrospective studies and our own reported experience show a higher short- and long-term survival rate for congenital diaphragmatic hernia in units where ECMO is available.

Survival rate and neurological prognostic after 5 years in patients who underwent ECMO for non-cardiac causes is generally very positive, but it worsens for lower gestational age groups, lower weight at birth, and higher oxygenation index (OI) before ECMO. Patients with a septic shock diagnosis and congenital diaphragmatic hernia display the worst survival rate and neurological evolution outcomes. However, it is the pre-existent factors and the severity of the condition of the newborn when entering ECMO that apparently determines the long-term neurological prognosis.

Long-term respiratory prognosis depends on the base etiology, degree of barotrauma, and length of exposure to oxygen. Between 10% and 30% of patients suffering from congenital diaphragmatic hernia have episodes of wheezing by age 10, with close to 50 suffering from hyper insufflation and episodes of airway obstruction. Pediatric post-ECMO survival rate is lower than that of newborns, but the respiratory failure group presents a better prognosis, particularly for patients with aspiration pneumonia, viral pneumonia, and post-operative ARDS or ARDS developed after traumatic injury. Viral pneumonia is the most common condition leading to pediatric ECMO, and among its etiologies, respiratory syncytial virus presents the highest post-ECMO survival rate at 70%. On the other hand, patients suffering from pneumonia caused by other viruses and by Bordetella pertussis report lower survival rates of 56% and 39%, respectively.

Given the evidence that shows an increased survival rate and the cost-effectiveness relation of this therapy, the newborn intensive care unit at the Pontifical Catholic University established a newborn-pediatric ECMO program following the standards advocated by the Extracorporeal Life Support Organization (ELSO) for patients with severe but reversible cardiovascular or respiratory insufficiency refractory to maximum conventional treatment. Work began in 1999 with the formation of a multidisciplinary team (composed of neonatologists, intensive care pediatricians, cardiac and pediatric surgeons, nurses, perfusionists, respiratory therapists, and psychologists) that had undergone training in ECMO centers affiliated with ELSO in the United States. At the same time, ECMO equipment was procured in order to establish the first ECMO units according to ELSO recommendations. The main selection criteria applied were: reversibility of lung or heart condition, failure to respond to maximum conventional treatment, weight [3] of 2 kg, gestational age of 34 weeks, oxygenation index >40, mechanical ventilation <14 days, and absence of severe brain injury or multi-organ failure. This is the first ECMO program in Latin America to join ELSO. From May 2003 to December 2014, the program treated 143 patients for both severe respiratory and cardiac pathologies. Of these patients, 77% survived till hospital discharge and are currently being monitored. The 35 patients who died had as base diseases: CDH (n = 13), congenital heart disease operated with failure to wean from cardiopulmonary bypass or arrhythmias (n = 9), persistent pulmonary hypertension secondary to sepsis, pneumonia, meconium aspiration syndrome, SP-B or ABCA3 deficiency or without a defined cause (n = 12), and pneumonia due to Bordetella pertussis (n = 1). Among patients treated with ECMO, a relevant group of children treated with CDH stands out with a survival rate of 78% (45/48) at discharge.

In order to understand the impact of establishing a neonatal ECMO program on the survival rate of newborns with severe respiratory failure in a developing country such as Chile, we studied the data of newborns with severe respiratory failure and OI > 25 before and after ECMO treatment was available. ECMO was initiated for a newborn with acute refractory respiratory failure who did not respond to iNO or HVOF. Data compiled from treatment of 259 newborns were analyzed, resulting in a significant increase in survival rate, from 72% before ECMO to 89% during the ECMO period. During the ECMO period, 98 out of 159 patients with respiratory failure (62%) were rescued using iNO or HFOV, while 61 (38%) did not improve their condition; 52 out of these 61 patients underwent ECMO treatment. The survival rate at discharge after

ECMO was 85%. Severity of OI, late arrival to the referral center, presence of a pneumothorax, and a diagnosed CDH were associated with the need for ECMO treatment or death.

One hundred percent of the survivors from our program are currently undergoing a special ECMO follow-up program. Among neurological follow-up exams, Bayley II tests at 12–18 months show that over 90% of tested children had normal or slightly altered mental development indices (MDI), and over 70% of them had normal or slightly altered psychomotor development indices (PDI). In addition, no patient displayed disabling visual or auditive alterations

Regarding respiratory follow-up, 83% of patients had a normal or slightly altered clinical broncho-pulmonary evaluation at 12–18 months. During the first year of life, 30–40% of them required hospitalization because of acute respiratory syndrome. Close to one third of patients present bronchial hyperreactivity diagnosed through a methacholine test in the medium-term.

As happened in Chile, new neonatal-pediatric ECMO programs have been constituted during the past few years in high-complexity, high-volume centers in several countries in Latin America, such as Argentina, Colombia, Brazil, and Mexico, most of which have progressively joined ELSO, forming the Latin American chapter of ELSO in 2012. The mission of this new ELSO chapter is to contribute to the dissemination of ECMO therapy according to ELSO standards, practical and theoretical education through courses and workshops, as well as encouraging collaborative work between Latin American centers, of which 15 can be found across five different countries, with close to 200 newborns and 120 children as reported to ELSO by December 2014.

Conclusions and Future Considerations

ECMO therapy, or more broadly, extracorporeal life support (ECLS), is a standard therapy in neonatology and pediatrics with proven benefits in the short and long term. It can be incorporated to intensive therapy with positive results in developing countries, but it must be implemented by high-complexity neonatal and pediatric centers with trained personnel and a high level of commitment.

Future patients to be treated with ECLS will progressively present more complex conditions, which is why new ECLS modalities will be required. These will have to be simpler, automatic, and with a lower need for anticoagulants so as to minimize risks and make its extended use possible. In that way newborns and children with severe conditions can be submitted to ECLS while waiting for heart or lung transplant, or as a bridge for ventricular assistance devices. Even premature newborns with severe cardiopulmonary failure can benefit from partial umbilical ECLS in the future. New low-resistance micropore oxygenators will not require the use of a pump, with the umbilical artery and vein used as an arteriovenous shunt. Moreover, newborns with CDH could go through an early ECLS admission in order to minimize lung damage and promote lung growth, using, for instance, growth factors or liquid ventilation with perfluorocarbon associated with ECLS. Some centers, such as Boston Children's Hospital, have applied ex-utero intrapartum treatment (EXIT) to ECMO for patients either with CDH and prenatal markers of poor prognosis, or in order to ensure an effective ventilation of newborns who do not possess a safe airway or for whom it is expected suffer from severe respiratory failure at birth (CDH, cervical teratoma, airway pathologies, large pulmonary masses, bronchial cysts, etcetera).

The progressive increase of pediatric patients who benefit from the use of ECLS is worth noting, and it is something that has been increasingly determined by the growing number of pathologies that may indicate severe respiratory failure within this population. This has lead patients with sepsis, immunocompromised patients, patients suffering from heart failure and other complex pathologies, to be ECLS candidates. Continuous technical improvements have created a technique that is both safer and easier to perform, so it is expected that in the coming years we will witness a sustained increase in pediatric patients who can benefit from ECLS therapy.

In this way, we hope that ECLS will enable us to keep assisting pulmonary or cardiac functioning in a more rational way while severe but reversible cardiopulmonary processes are repaired.

Sources

Alvarado-Socarras JL, Gomez C, Gomez A, Cruz M, Diaz-Silva GA, Nino MA. Current state of neonatal extra-corporeal membrane oxygenation in Colombia: de-scription of the first cases. Arch Cardiol Mex. 2014;84:121–7.

Arens J, Schoberer M, Lohr A, Orlikowsky T, Seehase M, Jellema RK, et al. NeonatOx: a pumpless extracorporeal lung support for premature neonates. Artif Organs. 2011;35:997–1001.

Bartlett R. Physiology of ECLS. In: Annich GMLW, MacLaren G, Wilson JM, Bartlett RH, editors. ECMO: extracorporeal cardiopulmonar support in critical care. 4th ed. Ann Arbor, Michigan: ELSO; 2012. p. 11–31.

Bohn D. Acute hypoxic respiratory failure in children. In: Annich GMLW, MacLaren G, Wilson JM, Bartlett RH, editors. ECMO: extracorporeal cardiopulmonary sup-port in critical care. 4th ed. Ann Arbor, Michigan: ELSO; 2012. p. 41–72.

Dalton H, Butt W. Extracorporeal life support: An update of Rogers'textbook of pediatric intensive care. Pediatr Crit Care Med. 2012;13:461–71.

ELSO Data Registry. University of Michigan: Ann Arbor M. ECMO registry of the Extracorporeal Life Support Organization (ELSO). Ann Arbor Michigan: University of Michigan; 2015.

Fortenberry JD. The history and development of extracorporeal support. ECMO: extracorporeal cardiopulmonar support in critical care. 4th ed. Ann Arbor Michigan: ELSO; 2012. p. 1–10.

Hamutcu R, Nield TA, Garg M, Keens TG, Platzker AC. Long-term pulmonary sequelae in children who were treated with extracorporeal membrane oxygenation for neonatal respiratory failure. Pediatrics. 2004;114:1292–6.

Kattan J, Godoy L, Zavala A, Faunes M, Becker P, Estay A, et al. Improvement of survival in infants with congenital diaphragmatic hernia in recent years: effect of ECMO availability and associated factors. Pediatr Surg Int. 2010;26:671–6.

Kattan J, Gonzalez A, Becker P, Faunes M, Estay A, Toso P, et al. Survival of newborn infants with severe respiratory failure before and after establishing an extracorporeal membrane oxygenation program. Pediatr Crit Care Med. 2013;14:876–83.

Keller RL, Steinhorn RH. Extracorporeal membrane oxygenation in resource-limited countries. Pediatr Crit Care Med. 2013;14:900–2.

McNally H, Bennett CC, Elbourne D, Field DJ. United Kingdom collaborative randomized trial of neonatal extracorporeal membrane oxygenation: follow-up to age 7 years. Pediatrics. 2006;117:e845–54.

Moreno GE, Magliola R, Pilan ML, Althabe M, Balestrini M, Lenz AM, et al. Mechanical circulatory support in pediatrics. Experience at the hospital de Pediatria Dr. Juan P. Garrahan. Argentina. Arch Cardiol Mex. 2014;84(4):256–61.

Morini F, Goldman A, Pierro A. Extracorporeal membrane oxygenation in infants with congenital diaphragmatic hernia: a systematic review of the evidence. Eur J Pediatr Surg. 2006;16:385–91.

Mugford M, Elbourne D, Field D. Extracorporeal membrane oxygenation for severe respiratory failure in newborn infants. Cochrane Database Syst Rev 2008: CD001340.

Paden ML, Rycus PT, Thiagarajan RR. Update and outcomes in extracorporeal life support. Semin Perinatol. 2014;38:65–70.

Pawlik TD, Porta NF, Steinhorn RH, Ogata E, de Regnier RA. Medical and financial impact of a neonatal extracor-poreal membrane oxygenation referral center in the nitric oxide era. Pediatrics. 2009;123:e17–24.

Peek GJ, Mugford M, Tiruvoipati R, Wilson A, Allen E, Thalanany MM, et al. Efficacy and economic assessment of conventional ventilatory support versus extracorpor-eal membrane oxygenation for severe adult respiratory failure (CESAR): a multicentre randomised controlled trial. Lancet. 2009;374:1351–63.

Smalley N, MacLaren G, Best D, Paul E, Butt W. Outcomes in children with refractory pneumonia supported with extracorporeal membrane oxygenation. Intensive Care Med. 2012;38:1001–7.

Thiagarajan RY, Bratton V. SL. Cardiac failure: principles and physiology. In: Annich GMLW, MacLaren G, Wilson JM, Bartlett RH, editors. ECMO: extracorporeal cardio-pulmonar support in critical care. 4th ed. Ann Arbor, Michigan: ELSO; 2012. p. 33–9.

Zabrock LA, Brogan TV, Statler KD, Poss WB, Rollins MD, Bratton SL. Extracorporeal membrane oxygenation for pediatric respiratory failure: survival and predictors of mortality. Crit Care Med. 2011;39:364–70.

Pediatric Lung Transplantation

74

Anand Patel and Albert Faro

Contents

A. Patel · A. Faro (✉)
Washington University in St. Louis School of Medicine, St. Louis, MO, USA
e-mail: afaro@cff.org

P. Bertrand, I. Sánchez (eds.), *Pediatric Respiratory Diseases*,
https://doi.org/10.1007/978-3-030-26961-6_74

History

Dr. James Hardy performed the first lung transplant in 1963 at the University of Mississippi Medical Center in a 58 year old convict serving a life sentence. The patient succumbed to renal failure 18 days after the procedure. There were many subsequent attempts, but it was not until 1983 at the University of Toronto that Dr. Joel Cooper performed the first successful long-term lung transplant. Dr. Denton Cooley attempted the first heart-lung transplantation in a child in 1968. The patient was a 2 month old with pulmonary hypertension and a complete AV canal, but they only survived for 14 hours. The first successful isolated lung transplant in a child was performed at the University of Toronto in 1987 in a 16 year old boy with pulmonary fibrosis. The 1990s witnessed a rapid growth in the number of pediatric lung transplants performed annually. However, unlike lung transplantation in adults, that growth has not continued in the 2000s. At present, there are approximately 100 lung transplants done worldwide per year in children.

Indications

In general, lung transplantation should be considered in children suffering from life threatening end-stage lung disease or pulmonary vascular disease refractory to medical therapy. The indications in childhood vary by age. Pulmonary hypertension, secondary to congenital heart disease or other pulmonary vascular disorders, is the leading indication in infancy followed by interstitial lung disease, including surfactant protein abnormalities. For older children and adolescents cystic fibrosis (CF) accounts for half to three quarters of all lung transplant procedures. Although the most common diagnoses for children receiving lung transplants are listed in Table 74.1 determining which children may benefit from lung transplantation is often not as straightforward. In addition, determining the appropriate time to proceed is often challenging. Transplant physicians thoughtfully gage when a patient has entered the transplant window. This is the point in time where the patient is sick enough to warrant lung transplantation but not so sick that the odds of a good outcome have markedly deteriorated. Multiple variables must be carefully considered including the trajectory of the underlying disease. Lung transplantation is a procedure of last resort and, when performed, should provide the patient with not

Table 74.1 Common indications for pediatric lung transplantation by age group

Infants (<1 year of age)	
Congenital heart disease	16.7%
Surfactant protein B deficiency	16.7%
Idiopathic pulmonary hypertension	12.5%
Idiopathic pulmonary fibrosis	10.4%
Pulmonary vascular disease	8.3%
Other pulmonary fibrosis	7.3%
Preschool children (age 1–5 years)	
Idiopathic pulmonary hypertension	22.4%
Idiopathic pulmonary fibrosis	16.8%
Other pulmonary fibrosis	8.8%
Retransplantation	8.8%
Congenital heart disease	8.0%
Bronchiolitis obliterans (not retransplant)	8.0%
Pulmonary vascular disease	5.6%
School aged children (age 6–10 years)	
Cystic fibrosis	53.0%
Idiopathic pulmonary hypertension	8.7%
Bronchiolitis obliterans (not retransplant)	6.8%
Retransplantation	6.4%
Idiopathic pulmonary fibrosis	5.7%
Adolescents (age 11–17 years)	
Cystic fibrosis	70.6%
Idiopathic pulmonary hypertension	7.8%
Retransplantation	5.3%

only an improved likelihood of survival over their underlying disease but also an improvement in their quality of life.

Lung transplantation is a lifelong commitment to a complex and demanding regimen that includes daily immunosuppressive therapy, frequent physician visits, routine surveillance procedures, including bronchoscopy, transbronchial biopsy, radiographic examinations, and blood work. Therefore, the pediatric patient must have adequate family support and access to transplant services and medications as well as demonstrate a willingness and ability to adhere to this admittedly complex regimen.

For the referring center, the correct timing of the referral to a transplant center is at times difficult to determine. Even for CF, where many investigators have rigorously studied this question, the answer remains unclear. Therefore, it is best for the referring center to consider the possibility of lung transplantation in a child whose pulmonary disease has a well defined trajectory of continued decline and whose life expectancy is severely limited by the disease process.

Contraindications

Contraindications can be divided into two categories: absolute and relative (Table 74.2). These often vary from one transplant program and the difference is based on experience, expertise, and the center's view of the available data. In other words, an absolute contraindication at one center may be a relative contraindication at another. There is general agreement that multi-organ disorders, active malignancy, or certain types of active infection are absolute contraindications to transplant. At some centers multi-organ transplantation may be possible in select individuals. This may include heart-lung transplantation and in patients with CF combined liver–lung transplantation.

Table 74.2 Examples of contraindications to lung transplantation (varies by transplant center)

Absolute	Relative
Active malignancy	Poorly controlled diabetes
Multiorgan failure	Pleurodesis
HIV	Scoliosis
Sepsis	Markedly abnormal body mass index
Severe neuromuscular disease	Osteoporosis
Documented, refractory nonadherence	Prolonged mechanical ventilation
Hepatitis C	ECMO
Chronic airway infection with *Burkholderia cenocepacia* or *Mycobacterium abscessus*	Chronic airway infection with multi-drug resistant organisms
Active tuberculosis	Renal insufficiency

Disease Specific Indications and Contraindications

Cystic Fibrosis

Several different models have been developed over the years to predict survival in CF; however, none has demonstrated any greater accuracy than Kerem's criteria. This model found that a forced expiratory volume in 1 second (FEV1) of less than 30% predicted was associated with an increased risk of death within 2 years; associated factors include decreased arterial oxygen tension (PaO_2), an increase in arterial carbon dioxide tension ($PaCO_2$) on room air, younger age, and female gender.

Specific indications Progressive lung disease and worsening quality of life despite optimal medical therapy; FEV1 <30% predicted.

Specific contraindications Varies by individual transplant centers, but most commonly center around microbiologic concerns with *Burkholderia cenocepacia* constituting one of the more common absolute contraindications. Many centers now consider infection with *Mycobacterium abscessus* either an absolute or relative contraindication and this can vary from center to center based on whether the patient is only culture positive and smear negative or culture positive and smear positive. The data presently available suggest that outcomes for patients infected with other nontuberculous mycobacteria are not substantially different than for patients not infected with those organisms. Other potential relative contraindications may include malnutrition, poorly controlled diabetes, osteoporosis, previous pleurodesis (especially talc), and liver failure, if the center cannot perform a combined liver–lung transplant.

Surfactant Dysfunction Syndromes

Four distinct genetic surfactant deficiency syndromes have been identified and vary in their presentation. The diagnosis can be confirmed by genetic analysis. Lung biopsy may demonstrate diffuse alveolar type II cell hyperplasia, alveolar proteinosis, and septal thickening. Surfactant protein B deficiency is an autosomal recessive disorder. It presents in the newborn period with respiratory failure and is typically lethal within the first year of life. There is no effective medical therapy. Lung transplantation is the only intervention with the potential to sustain life.

Surfactant protein C deficiency has a more variable presentation and is inherited in autosomal dominant pattern. The age of disease onset spans from the newborn period to adulthood. In addition, even infants presenting with more severe findings such as respiratory failure can improve over time. This variability suggests that other genetic or environmental modifiers may influence the course. Corticosteroids, hydroxychloroquine, and azithromycin have been used in isolated cases, but the results are difficult to interpret.

Adenosine triphosphate binding cassette protein member A3 (ABCA3) deficiency has two distinct ways of presenting. It can be found in newborns with respiratory failure, but a milder form also exists that is found in older children presenting with interstitial lung disease. Dense lamellar bodies are seen by electron microscopy of lung tissue.

Mutations in the NKX2.1 gene, also known as the thyroid transcription factor gene, may cause findings similar to any of the previously mentioned surfactant abnormalities as NKX2.1 is important for the expression of SP-B, SP-C, and ABCA3. Mutations in the gene can lead to brain–thyroid–lung syndrome so that patients may present with hypothyroidism or benign chorea in addition to ILD.

Specific indications Once a decision to pursue transplant has been made, patients with SPB deficiency should be transferred as soon as a possible to the transplant center. For the other surfactant processing abnormalities, lung transplantation is indicated for refractory respiratory failure or progressive respiratory insufficiency unresponsive to medical interventions.

Specific contraindications Significant neurologic injury and, at some centers, VA-ECMO.

Pulmonary Vascular Disorders

In this broad group of disorders characterized by pulmonary hypertension, we will include idiopathic pulmonary hypertension (IPH), pulmonary vein anomalies, congenital heart disease (CHD), and patients with an inadequate pulmonary vascular bed. These patients may die from progressive right heart failure, arrhythmias, or massive hemoptysis. In general, a decreased cardiac index, elevated pulmonary vascular resistance, right atrial pressures >7.4 mm Hg, and right ventricular end diastolic pressure of >10.4 mm Hg predict mortality and are indications for transplant. Other factors that may impact survival include elevated von Willebrand factor, uric acid levels, and brain natriuretic peptide concentrations.

Advances in pharmacotherapy have dramatically changed the landscape for patients with IPH so that lung transplantation should only be considered in patients who have failed medical therapy. The same cannot be said for pulmonary venous anomalies, such as pulmonary vein stenosis (PVS) or pulmonary veno-occlusive disease (PVOD), which are not only poorly responsive to medical therapy but also poorly responsive to cardiac catheterization or surgical interventions.

The timing of transplantation in patients with pulmonary hypertension associated with CHD, including those with Eisenmenger syndrome, remains unclear. Many of these patients can live for years after diagnosis. An added decision that must be made for this group of patients is whether or not the cardiac defect can be repaired or if the patient will require a combined heart–lung transplant. Unfortunately, the need for two organs can markedly prolong the time on the waiting list. If the patient has an atrial septal defect, ventricular septal defect or patent ductus arteriosus, these are relatively simple repairs and can be performed at the time of lung transplantation.

For patients with an inadequate pulmonary vascular bed, such as those with pulmonary atresia, congenital diaphragmatic hernia, and ventricular septal defect with multiple aorto-pulmonary collaterals, lung transplantation is high risk, but it may be the sole life prolonging intervention.

Specific indications Idiopathic pulmonary hypertension – patients who have failed medical management

Pulmonary venous anomalies – upon making the diagnosis urgent referral is recommended

Congenital heart disease or inadequate pulmonary vascular bed – progressive severe hypoxia, syncope, massive hemoptysis

Specific contraindications Multiple prior thoracotomies associated with development of extensive collateral circulation and/or significant presence of preformed antibodies.

Donor Evaluation

Unfortunately, not only does there continue to be a shortage of donors but data from the OPTN/SRTR database in the United States shows that, in 2012, of the 8143 organ donors only 1708 donated lungs. In other words, only 21% of organ donors had lungs that were deemed suitable for procurement. The reasons are varied and include the mechanism of death, consequences of mechanical ventilation, and donor management, but they highlight the importance of understanding what characteristics make a donor acceptable. Beyond the basics of matching for size and blood type, the characteristics outlined in Table 74.3 may contribute to both short- and long-term outcomes and determine whether the donor lungs will be accepted by a transplant center.

Table 74.3 Ideal donor characteristics

1. Donor age	
Ideal donor	Less than 55 years old
Evidence	There is data to support poorer outcomes with older donors, especially if combined with ischemic times of greater than 6 hours.
2. Donor ABG	
Ideal donor	PaO_2 greater than 300 on FiO_2 1.0, PEEP of 5 cm H_2O
Evidence	Inadequate data to either support or refute this cutoff. Studies mainly focus on interventions to increase donor PaO_2 to over 300 and then procure them.
3. Radiographic findings	
Ideal donor	Clear CXR
Evidence	No data in regard to use of abnormal chest films. If finding is suggestive of atelectasis, aggressive airway clearance and use of the bronchoscope to remove mucus plugs may salvage an otherwise unusable lung.
4. Ischemic time	
Ideal donor	4–6 hours
Evidence	Reports describe successful outcomes with ischemic times from 6 to 11 hours. Poor outcomes clearly associated with older donors and prolonged ischemic times.
5. Size matching	
Ideal donor	Most centers use height and or predicted TLC. Accepted ranges are plus or minus 20%.
Evidence	Data demonstrates no adverse effect on outcome when using donor lungs within 75–125% of recipient TLC.
6. Airway secretions	
Ideal donor	No purulent secretions on bronchoscopy, negative gram stain
Evidence	Infection is a major source of early post-transplant morbidity and mortality. However, evidence suggests that a positive sputum gram stain does not correlate with the development of pneumonia. There is data to suggest that it is the amount of purulent secretions that may be of importance in predicting outcome post-transplant.

(continued)

Table 74.3 (continued)

7. Smoking	
Ideal donor	Less than 20 pack year history
Evidence	There is no data that either supports or refutes this criterion. Concerns include the development of malignancy post-transplant as well as the potential for increased risk for a poor peri-operative outcome.
8. Malignancy	
Ideal donor	No cancer history
Evidence	Little data, particularly in donors with a past history of a malignancy. The potential risk is likely based on histology, tumor stage, and length of cancer free survival. Primary CNS tumors rarely spread. Risk factors include medulloblastoma or glioblastoma, previous craniotomy, venticular shunt, tumor radiation. Renal cell carcinoma is the most common type of cancer that is transmitted from a donor.
9. Length of mechanical ventilation	
Ideal donor	Ventilated for less than 3 days
Evidence	Greater than 2 days of mechanical ventilation is a risk factor for the development of ventilator associated pneumonia. However, donors with prolonged courses and clear X-rays and good gas exchange may in fact be better donors since the sequelae of aspiration may not be evident within the first 24–48 hours.
10. Serologies	
Ideal donor	Seronegative for HIV and hepatitis A, B & C
Evidence	Higher risk of morbidity/mortality associated with immunosuppression.

Surgical Technique

The surgical technique used in children is similar to that used in adults with the following exceptions: (i) virtually all children will require cardiopulmonary bypass, (ii) in children bilateral, as opposed to single, lung transplantation is much more common. The typical approach is a bilateral sequential procedure with a transsternal bilateral anterior thoracotomy, referred to as the clamshell incision, which provides excellent access and visualization for the procedure. At our center, an end-to-end anastomosis is favored for the airway because of the higher incidence of stenosis seen with a telescopic anastomosis. Many centers will cover the anastomosis with peribronchial lymphatic tissue. It is important to note that the bronchial circulation, lymphatic system, and nervous system are not reanastomosed. However, a few centers do advocate direct bronchial revascularization.

If a cardiac repair is necessary, it is done after the pneumonectomies but prior to implantation as this provides the surgeon with a bloodless operative field. After the second lung has been implanted, they are inflated to expand all of the atelectatic portions. The patient is then weaned off of bypass. Two chest tubes are left in each pleural space. The pulmonary veins can be assessed at this time with transesophageal echocardiography, and the pulmonary artery anastomoses can be evaluated upon arrival to cardiac intensive care unit with a perfusion scan.

Living lobar transplantation has fallen out of favor in the United States because lungs are allocated on the basis of a disease severity score rather than just time spent on the list. This has obviated the most common reason for living lobar transplantation, presenting to a transplant center in extremis and not having accrued enough time on the list to realistically receive an organ in time. However, this procedure is commonly used in Japan with excellent outcomes reported.

Immunosuppression

Immunosuppressive regimens vary between transplant centers. About half of the lung transplant centers throughout the world use induction in the hopes of preventing early acute rejection. There is also a great deal of variability in the induction regimen of choice. Some centers will utilize an interleukin (IL)-2 receptor antagonist such as basiliximab. Other centers will use a lympholytic agent such as rabbit antithymocyte globulin (RATG) or equine antithymocyte globulin (ATGAM). These preparations are derived from animal serum and contain antibodies to human lymphocytes that can induce opsonization and phagocytosis of T lymphocytes, modulating their activation.

Table 74.4 Immunosupressive agents used in pediatric lung transplantation

Class of drug	Potential side effects
Calcineurin inhibitors	
Tacrolimus	Infection, hyperglycemia, hypertension, seizure, renal dysfunction, PTLD
Cyclosporine	infection, hirsutism, gingival hyperplasia, hypertension, seizures, renal dysfunction, PTLD
Cell cycle toxin inhibitors	
Mycophenolate mofetil	Infection, leukopenia, vomiting, diarrhea, hepatic dysfunction, PTLD
Azathioprine	Infection, leukopenia, PTLD
mTOR inhibitors	
Sirolimus	Infection, delayed wound healing, hypertriglyceridemia, interstial lung disease, PTLD
Everolimus	Infection, interstitial lung disease, renal dysfunction, stomatitis, leukopenia

Because of the relative high frequency of acute rejection among lung transplant recipients, a maintenance strategy of triple drug immunosuppression is commonly employed (Table 74.4). The three drugs will typically consist of a calcineurin inhibitor (CNI), a cell cycle toxin inhibitor, and systemic corticosteroids. In pediatrics especially, we attempt to minimize steroid exposure, and during the first post-transplant year we wean the steroid dose from 0.5 mg/kg to 0.2 mg/kg; at our center it typically remains at that dose.

Post-operative Monitoring and Management

After the procedure is completed, patients are transferred to the intensive care unit, still intubated and on mechanical ventilator support, with some patients still requiring ECMO. Monitoring must require at minimum cardiorespiratory monitoring, including pulse oximetry, careful measurement of fluid input and output, and measurement of arterial blood gases. While initial management of ventilator support and ECMO, if needed, is done by the intensivist, all aspects of care are best delivered through a team approach, where the intensivist, the cardiothoracic surgeon, and transplant pulmonologist discuss all important aspects and meet at least once if not twice daily to round as a group. Some key aspects of post-operative care are discussed below, as well as in the subsequent section on complications that occur both early and late after lung transplantation. More in-depth discussion of all aspects can be found in the references.

Fluids and Nutrition Management

Owing to both capillary leak and interrupted lymphatic drainage, the transplanted lungs are particularly fluid sensitive, and thus reaching a negative fluid balance within the first 48 hours post-operatively is important. Colloids and pressors should be used to reduce the amount of stress placed on the kidneys, as overly aggressive diuresis, when combined with CNI nephrotoxicity, can quickly lead to renal failure, resulting in fluid overload and subsequent pulmonary compromise. Thus, while one will always use diuretics in this setting, one must do so carefully. Enteral nutrition should be started as soon as is appropriate but may be delayed for anticipated extubation or other procedures.

Ventilator Management

Foremost, the goal is to wean off the ventilator rapidly with the goal of extubation. The former should be done per the general practice of the experienced intensivist. Pressure-controlled ventilation is recommended because it places limits on peak airway pressures that protect not only the parenchyma but also the healing airway anastomoses. At our center, a bronchoscopy is performed 1 day post-operatively to inspect the anastomoses, and to obtain BAL if infection is suspected. Airway clearance is important in the initial post-operative period, with appropriate limits in place to avoid anastomotic complications. Physiotherapy and mobilization are also important, as these will not only help mobilize secretions but will also enhance chest tube drainage and alveolar recruitment.

Surgical Complications

Airway anastomotic complications occur in ~13% of recipients. They primarily manifest as stenosis with resulting airflow obstruction. This can generally be managed with bronchoscopic interventions. As the bronchi of children grow with the recipient, stents are avoided if possible in favor of repeated balloon dilation. Partial or complete dehiscence of the anastomosis is rarely seen but can be catastrophic.

Vascular anastomotic complications are also rare. At our center, a perfusion lung scan is routinely performed within 24 hours of the transplantation to evaluate the vascular anastomoses. Any significant discrepancy between right- and left-sided perfusion should be immediately evaluated in consultation with the cardiothoracic surgeons.

Primary Graft Dysfunction

Primary Graft Dysfunction (PGD) occurs within 72 hours of transplant and is characterized by non-specific alveolar injury, non-cardiogenic pulmonary edema, and resulting decreased compliance and hypoxemia. It is caused by multiple factors, including ischemia–reperfusion injury, inflammation secondary to donor death, and other factors. In 2005, the ISHLT developed a classification system using chest X-ray infiltrates and PaO_2/FiO_2 ratio to grade PGD 0–3. On the basis of this classification, severe PGD (PaO_2/FiO_2 <200 at 48 hours post-transplant) occurs in 15% of recipients, which is concerning as severe PGD is associated with increased graft failure and mortality. Management of severe PGD is similar to the management of patients with acute respiratory distress syndrome (ARDS), including fluid restriction while maintaining perfusion to end organs, lung protective ventilator strategies, and nitric oxide. When the amount of oxygen and ventilator support is high and thus contributing to further lung injury, early ECMO is an important option to consider to both provide lung rest and minimize iatrogenic trauma to the graft.

Post-transplantation Monitoring

After the perioperative recovery period, recipients continue to require monitoring. Regular evaluation, initially at the transplant center, followed by close monitoring by a local physician with discussion with the transplant team, is necessary to identify and manage post-transplant complications. Routine monitoring includes measurement of CNI and antimetabolite levels, routine laboratory tests, pulmonary function testing, and chest imaging. While controversial, we believe that bronchoscopy with BAL and transbronchial biopsies by trained bronchoscopists an important part of post-transplant surveillance. Although scheduled surveillance bronchoscopy can detect asymptomatic acute rejection, allowing therapeutic interventions to occur sooner, a clear benefit in terms of outcomes has not been found. In infant lung transplant recipients, the use of surveillance bronchoscopy is more important as ambulatory lung function testing is not possible and patients are less able to report symptoms.

Post-transplantation Complications

Infections

Given the degree of immunosuppression needed to prevent acute rejection of the lung, infections are a predictable complication of lung transplantation. Selected infections are discussed in Table 74.5. However, virtually any pathogen, known and unknown, can present post-lung transplant. Clinicians must be vigilant and aggressive in managing these infections to preserve both graft function and the patient's well-being. A close working relationship with infectious disease specialists is extremely advantageous to lung transplant programs, with some programs including one on their transplant team.

Table 74.5 Infections

Pathogen/infection	Notes
Bacterial	
Bloodstream infections	Occur in 25% of recipients, usually early, when central lines are still in place.
Lower respiratory tract infections	Occur across the course of time post-transplant, seen in 80% of recipients.
Gram-negative bacteria (including multi-drug resistant isolates)	Cystic fibrosis recipients often have return of colonization from sinuses including resistant bacteria (P. aeruginosa, MRSA, etc.)
Burkholderia cenocepacia (genomvar III)	Absolute contraindication at nearly all centers due to poor post-transplant outcomes
Burkholderia gladioli	Associated with increased post-transplant mortality, relative contraindication
Burkholderia multivorans (Genomvar II)	No contraindication, no increased risk
Clostridium difficile	Occurs in 5–8% of recipients, most frequently within the first 6 months post-transplant, re-appearing as a late complication (>2 years post-transplant). Associated with significantly increased mortality, particularly when early post-transplant.
Viral	
CMV	The most important viral infection post-transplant, can promote rejection. Requires months of antiviral prophylaxis (length is center specific) if either donor or recipient with positive serology, started at time of transplant. All recipients monitored using blood PCR, frequency depends on pre-transplant status.
HSV	Can be reactive post-transplant, thus if not on antiviral prophylaxis for CMV, and recipient or donor with history of HSV, consider prophylaxis with acyclovir or valacyclovir.
VZV	Immunization pre-transplant strongly recommended. If exposed, treat with varicella zoster immune globulin or intravenous immunoglobulin immediately.
Respiratory viruses (including rhinovirus, influenza, parainfluenza, respiratory syncytial virus, and all other respiratory viruses)	Occur in more than half of recipients, often detected in the lower respiratory tract via bronchoscopy. Important to detect quickly and treat, as data suggest RSV can trigger rejection, data less clear for other viruses. Recommend recipients <2 years of age receive pavilizumab prophylaxis for RSV, all should get influenza vaccine yearly.
Mycobacteria	
Tuberculosis	Increased risk of active infection post-transplant, ~4% donor derived, others a combination of reactivation of latent TB and new infection. Tuberculin skin test and if ≥5 years of age, Interferon Gamma Release Assay (i.e., Quantiferon Gold) recommended pre-transplant. Active infection should prompt discussion of delaying transplant until infection cleared. Latent infection requires 9 months isoniazid, pre-transplant if possible. Donor screening recommended. Treatment post-transplant challenging due to drug-drug interactions and diagnostic difficulty due to immunosuppression causing anergy
Non-tuberculous mycobacteria	Mycobacterium avium-intracellulare is treatable; however, M. abscessus is a contraindication due to observed disseminated infection post-transplant, unless sputum can be cleared pre-transplant, chelonae is also treated this way.
Fungi	
Aspergillus & candida	Invasive fungal infections with Aspergillus and Candida can cause anastomotic complications, particularly early post-transplant, along with invasive pulmonary or disseminated disease. Detection requires vigilance; treatment requires aggressive approaches and consultation with infectious disease specialists. Antifungal azoles interact with calcineurin inhibitors and mTOR inhibitors, thus caution and close monitoring of drug levels must be used.
Pneumocystis jirovecii	Post-transplant prophylaxis with TMP/SMX started no later than 3 weeks post-transplant for the life of the recipient. Alternative agents include dapsone and pentamidine. TMP/SMX also provides prophylaxis for Nocardia spp., and Toxoplasma gondii.
Other fungi	Cryptococcus and other fungi have been seen post-transplant and are important considerations in any illness of an immunosuppressed recipient

Post-transplant Lymphoproliferative Disease (PTLD)

By 5 years post-transplant, 14% of pediatric recipients have had a malignancy of some type, nearly all of which are PTLD. The most common form of PTLD is caused by Epstein–Barr virus infection causing transformation of a CD20 cell, resulting in a B-cell lymphoma, most commonly polymorphic. Patients who develop primary EBV infection post-transplant are at greatest risk. For CD20 positive PTLD, anti-CD20 antibody (rituximab) therapy has revolutionized the management and allows successful treatment when combined with regimens of low-dose chemotherapy and reduced baseline immunosuppression. This approach causes far less toxicity than prior treatment options. Prognosis is substantially worse for CD20-negative PTLD, due to a combination of a lack of good therapeutic options and the toxicity of the available regimens. Overall, per the ISHLT registry (1/1992–6/2012), PTLD caused 3.3% of deaths in pediatric lung recipients, with other malignancies causing 0.8% of deaths.

The major challenge in PTLD is diagnosis, as it can present with anything from asymptomatic pulmonary nodules on CT scan, neurological or gastrointestinal symptoms, bone pain, or sinus pain. Further, although peak incidence is at 6 months post-transplant, it can be seen as a late complication as well. Thus, careful evaluation and assessment, including biopsies and imaging, are needed to make the diagnosis.

Gastrointestinal Complications

Gastrointestinal complications are seen in up to 50% of recipients. Clostriduim difficile is an important consideration, covered previously. Other GI issues seen include esophagitis, pancreatitis, gastroparesis, ileus, CMV infections of the gut and liver, cholecystitis, peptic ulcer disease, gastroesophageal reflux, and peptic ulcer disease. Patients with cystic fibrosis continue to be at risk for distal intestinal obstruction syndrome and must continue to take pancreatic enzyme supplements, along with bowel regimens (i.e., lactulose or Miralax), particularly in the early post-operative period to avoid obstruction. Gastroesophageal reflux deserves special mention, as data suggest that diagnosis and treatment of GER with anti-reflux surgery may prevent the development of bronchiolitis obliterans and ameliorate its progression if present, but these data have not been replicated in children. As mentioned above, PTLD can present as intussusception, obstruction, bowel perforation, feeding intolerance or abdominal pain. For GI complications, medical management for resolution is preferred. If this is not possible, elective surgical procedures are well tolerated, while data suggests that emergent surgical procedures carry a high morbidity and mortality risk.

Neurological Complications

Forty-seven percent of recipients have some neurological complications. The most common complication is seizures, generally felt to be related to calcineurin inhibitor induced cerebral vasoconstriction. Posterior reversible encephalopathy syndrome (PRES) can also be seen. PRES consists of seizure activity in 92% of cases, along with headaches, visual abnormalities, nausea/vomiting, other focal neurological signs, and varying degrees of impaired consciousness, ranging from confusion, somnolence, and lethargy to encephalopathy or coma. The diagnosis requires both symptoms and neuroimaging findings, with MRI being superior to CT scan for identifying PRES. Consultation with a neurologist is also recommended; however, long-term medication is not generally needed for seizures related to lung transplantation. Hypertension can be present and contributory, and should be managed accordingly. While calcineurin inhibitor toxicity is felt to contribute to both seizures and PRES, the correlation with levels and severity or incidence is incomplete. Although some patients respond to switching CNI (i.e., from tacrolimus to cyclosporine or vice versa) or alternative regimens, no general recommendation exists.

Diabetes

Diabetes is seen in 20% of recipients in 1 year, 30% at 5 years, and is seen most commonly in patients with cystic fibrosis and is thus likely related to pre-existing and ongoing pancreatic islet cell injury. Tacrolimus and corticosteroids both appear to increase the risk of diabetes.

Renal Dysfunction

Nearly all recipients develop hypomagnesemia post-transplant, with some developing renal tubular acidosis, and both are generally managed with oral supplements. Early renal failure suggests pre-transplant renal insufficiency. Thus, measurement of glomerular filtration rate is a mandatory aspect of pre-transplant evaluation, as patients with GFR <50 have a suspected risk for poor outcomes, and it thus represents a contraindication to transplant at some centers. Chronic effects of exposure to CNI and resulting renal vasoconsctriction contributes significantly to renal insufficiency and renovascular hypertension post-transplant. Generally, this is managed with calcium channel blockers. Five years of CNI based immunosuppression carries a 2.3% incidence of renal failure requiring dialysis, and 1% require renal transplantation at some point post-transplant.

Rejection

Acute Rejection

Acute cellular rejection is common in the first weeks to months post-transplant. While often asymptomatic, fever, hypoxemia, and dyspnea can be seen. CXR findings include infiltrates and bilateral pleural effusions. Similarly, a 10% decrease in either FEV1 or FVC on home spirometric monitoring should prompt further evaluation. Biopsies are graded per the 2007 Revision of the 1996 working formulation for the standardization of nomenclature in the diagnosis of lung rejection. The score consists of two components. The A score reflects the intensity and composition of infiltrating immune cells and the extent of parenchymal involvement (A0, no rejection, A1–4 minimal to severe acute rejection). The B score reflects airway involvement.

Only acute rejection episodes graded A2 or higher are treated, generally with 3–4 days of pulse IV methylprednisolone (10–20 mg/kg/day), with follow-up biopsy in 2–4 weeks. Persistent acute rejection is treated with additional pulse steroids, anti-T-cell antibody therapy, and augmented baseline immunosuppression. Acute rejection is infrequent after the first year post-transplant and is less common in infants than in older children.

Antibody Mediated Rejection

While hyperacute antibody-mediated rejection caused by pre-formed anti-donor antibodies present at the time of transplant is a well established cause of acute graft failure, it is rare. Antibody mediated rejection (AMR) outside that context is now recognized as an important complication in lung transplantation. As diagnostic criteria are still evolving, and retrospective evaluations in progress, the exact incidence of AMR in pediatric lung transplantation is as yet unknown. AMR can present as progressive worsening of lung function in the absence of acute or chronic rejection, and can rapidly result in death due to graft failure.

Currently, diagnosis of AMR requires three features be present, including evidence of allograft dysfunction, presence of circulating donor-specific antibodies, and histopathologic findings of AMR. However, this is complicated by the significant overlap of these patterns with pathology seen in other forms of lung injury, including high-grade or persistent acute cellular rejection, diffuse alveolar damage, high-grade or persistent lymphocytic bronchiolitis, obliterative bronchiolitis, arteritis without rejection, or other graft dysfunction without clear morphological explanation.

Treatment of antibody mediated rejection is still evolving. As such, the components of therapy, rather than specific regimens, will be discussed. Plasmapheresis or therapeutic plasma exchange is a process for removal of antibodies and other circulating proteins from the recipient's bloodstream by filtration and thus directly removes the responsible antibodies. Pulse corticosteroids are also generally used and have been found to impair T-cell and B-cell function, impair antibody and complement binding, and decrease levels of serum immunoglobulins. Rituximab, an anti-CD20 antibody used for PTLD, is also used in AMR, as it targets the B-cells that make antibody. Its use in AMR mirrors its successful use in antibody-mediated autoimmune diseases such as rheumatoid arthritis. Together, these three interventions make up the initial treatment of AMR.

In summary, while antibody mediated rejection is clearly an important process, the exact pathobiology, incidence, diagnostic approach, treatment, and understanding outcomes remain in evolution. Ongoing studies will help to determine how to best diagnose and treat this entity in pediatric lung recipients.

Chronic Lung Allograft Dysfunction

Chronic lung allograft dysfunction (CLAD) is a newer term used to define the varying patterns of long-term respiratory decline and failure seen in lung recipients. It encompasses both bronchiolitis obliterans and restrictive long-term allograft dysfunction.

Acute lung allograft dysfunction (ALAD) is defined as any acute cause of a drop in lung function, defined as a 10% drop from baseline in post-bronchodilator FEV1 and/or FVC, including acute rejection and infection. If this persists for more than 3 weeks, it is termed suspected CLAD, and evaluation should include bronchoscopy with biopsies. Should these prove nondiagnostic, and should lung function not recover, open lung biopsy is also an important consideration in pediatric recipients, particularly smaller children in which the diagnostic yield of transbronchial biopsies is limited by the use of small forceps. If there is evidence of persistent acute rejection, infection, anastomotic complication, diaphragm dysfunction, or other causes, CLAD is not diagnosed.

CLAD is divided into restrictive CLAD and obstructive CLAD. Restrictive CLAD, also called restrictive allograft syndrome, is named for the pulmonary function picture, which includes TLC ≤ 90% baseline and/or FEV1/FVC normal or increased, with FEV1 and/or FVC decline ≤ 80% of baseline. HRCT findings will include infiltrates, ground glass opacities, and upper lung zone fibrotic changes. Restrictive CLAD (R-CLAD) carries a significantly worse prognosis than BOS, with median survival of 541 days for patients with R-CLAD compared to 1421 for patients with BOS.

After 3 years post-transplant, obstructive CLAD or BOS becomes the major cause of death in pediatric recipients, and at 5 years, 50% of surviving recipients carry a diagnosis of BOS. In obstructive CLAD or BOS, the picture is dominated by the drop in FEV1, and FVC and TLC are stable or significantly less affected. HRCT findings will include air trapping.

In terms of diagnosing BOS, the new CLAD classification system overlaps with the prior definitions of bronchiolitis obliterans syndrome (BOS). For example, BOS 0p is defined as a ≥ 10 but <20% drop in post-bronchodilator FEV1 from baseline or FEF25–75 < 75% of baseline. In this group there appears to be a group of patients with what has been termed azithromycin-responsive allograft dysfunction (ARAD). Azithromycin entered use in bronchiolitis obliterans syndrome in the early 2000s, after it was noted that patients on thrice-weekly azithromycin, as used in cystic fibrosis, could have stabilization and even improvement of lung function in the setting of bronchiolitis obliterans, despite lack of a clear mechanism of action, though both anti-inflammatory and anti-fibrotic activities of azithromycin are posited as being responsible for this therapeutic efficacy.

Once pulmonary function testing suggests BOS, either by a drop in FEV1, or a drop in FEF25–75, which has been shown to be more sensitive and detects small airways dysfunction earlier, diagnosis requires biopsy to confirm the presence of small airway obliteration by a fibrotic process. Currently, open or thoracoscopic lung biopsy is used at our center when BOS is suspected but cannot be confirmed by transbronchial biopsies.

Treatment of BOS is varied, and over time has included use of augmented immunosuppression, change in baseline immunosuppression, azithromycin, extracorporeal photopheresis (ECP), and total lymphoid irradiation. Currently, our practice is to use pulse corticosteroids accompanied by 10 days of anti-thymocyte antibodies, along with initiation of azithromycin thrice-weekly. If this does not stabilize symptoms, ECP is initiated. This is consistent with the current best evidence. While inhaled cyclosporine and mTOR inhibitors have both been shown to be effective in small studies, larger trials have not found a consistent benefit in the use of either to prevent the development of BOS, or in its treatment. Surgical treatment of gastroesophageal reflux has been shown to be beneficial in adults in managing and preventing BOS, but this has not been replicated in children. Similarly, retrospective reviews suggest that statin therapy can prevent BOS and may be beneficial in treating BOS.

Outcomes

Outcomes in lung transplantation as a whole continue to lag behind those of other solid organ transplants, and this is also true in children. While 1-year survival rates have improved to ~85%, 3 year survival is ~65%, and median survival is 4.9 years, lower but not statistically significantly different than the 5.4 year median survival in adult recipients. As discussed previously, long-term survival is determined primarily by the development of BOS. While retransplantation continues to be offered at a small number of pediatric centers for allograft failure, outcomes are worse for retransplantation than primary transplantation (45% versus 58% survival at 3 years post-transplant), irrespective of whether or not re-transplantation was for BOS or other causes of graft failure. Data suggest that patients re-transplanted at least 1 year after their primary transplant had better outcomes, but the numbers of re-transplants are too small to make a definitive conclusion. Further, these outcomes have been relatively stable over the past 10 years, demonstrating the urgent need for new ways of managing recipients in order to preserve graft function and ultimately life.

Future Considerations

Several areas of active research offer the possibility of improved outcomes in lung transplantation. One such area is the expansion of donor lung availability using ex vivo lung perfusion. In this procedure, marginal donor lungs that are not accepted for transplant initially are ventilated and perfused ex vivo and allowed to recover. Lungs have been successfully transplanted this way, and expanding the donor pool provides the opportunity to save patients that still, at present, die waiting for organs. This procedure needs to be extended into children as soon as possible. Another such area is the use of pumpless oxygenators as a bridge to lung transplantation. In conventional ECMO, a pump takes blood from the patient, into the oxygenator then returns it. Recently, pumpless oxygenator systems have been used in candidates awaiting lung transplantation (i.e., NovaLung). While pediatric specific systems are still being developed, we have used a neonatal membrane oxygenator (Quadrox) to successfully bridge an infant suffering from alveolar capillary dysplasia to transplant. Both pumpless oxygenators and venovenous ECMO are being increasingly used as ways to less invasively bridge candidates to transplant for longer periods of time than conventional ECMO, which requires significant sedation, mechanical ventilation, and immobility, which while buying some time, also leads to progression of the primary lung disease, all of which limit the time a candidate can be bridged on conventional ECMO. Last, an array of anti-cytokine therapeutic antibodies being developed for other therapeutic indications (i.e., anti-IL-13, anti-IL-5R, anti-IL-17, and others) provide an opportunity to manipulate these mediators, all seen in different forms and stages of lung transplant rejection, in order to treat or prevent rejection, and potentially to promote engraftment.

In pediatrics, the small number of recipients worldwide limits performing adequately powered trials. While this is not the case in adult recipients, trials are generally done at single centers, and this has resulted in underpowered studies that have failed to show differences between therapies that have beneficial trends (i.e., everolimus compared to MMF, inhaled cyclosporine). Multicenter trials should become the standard in lung transplantation as they have in many other indications. In pediatrics, the International Pediatric Lung Transplant Collaborative works to make this a reality. As outcomes from BOS remain poor despite therapies, with BOS causing 40% of all mortality beyond the first year of transplant, such studies, along with work in recently established animal models of orthotopic lung transplantation, are desperately needed to improve outcomes in pediatric lung transplantation.

Sources

Belperio JA, Weigt SS, Fishbein MC, Lynch JP 3rd. Chronic lung allograft rejection: mechanisms and therapy. Proc Am Thorac Soc. 2009;6:108–21.

Benden C, Edwards LB, Kucheryavaya AY, Christie JD, Dipchand AI, Dobbels F, Kirk R, Lund LH, Rahmel AO, Yusen RD, Stehlik J. The Registry of the International Society for Heart and Lung Transplantation: sixteenth official pediatric lung and heart-lung transplantation report–2013; focus theme: age. International Society for Heart and Lung Transplantation. J Heart Lung Transplant. 2013;32(10):989–97.

Choong CK, Sweet SC, Guthrie TJ, Mendeloff EN, Haddad FJ, Schuler P, De La Morena M, Huddleston CB. Repair of congenital heart lesions combined with lung transplantation for the treatment of severe pulmonary hypertension: a 13-year experience. J Thorac Cardiovasc Surg. 2005;129(3):661–9.

Christie JD, Carby M, Bag R, Corris P, Hertz M, Weill D, ISHLT Working Group on Primary Lung Graft Dysfunction. Report of the ISHLT Working Group on Primary Lung Graft Dysfunction part II: definition. A consensus statement of the International Society for Heart and Lung Transplantation. J Heart Lung Transplant. 2005a;24:1454–9.

Christie JD, Van Raemdonck D, de Perrot M, Barr M, Keshavjee S, Arcasoy S, Orens J. ISHLT Working Group On Primary Lung Graft Dysfunction. Report of the ISHLT Working Group On Primary Lung Graft Dysfunction part I: introduction and methods. J Heart Lung Transplant. 2005b;24:1451–3.

Elizur A, Faro A, Huddleston CB, Gandhi SK, White D, Kuklinski CA, Sweet SC. Lung transplantation in infants and toddlers from 1990 to 2004 at St. Louis Children's Hospital. Am J Transplant. 2009;9(4):719–26.

Estenne M, Maurer JR, Boehler A, Egan JJ, Frost A, Hertz M, Mallory GB, Snell GI, Yousem S. Bronchiolitis obliterans syndrome 2001: an update of the diagnostic criteria. J Heart Lung Transplant. 2002;21:297–310.

Faro A, Hamvas A. Lung transplantation for inherited disorders of surfactant metabolism. NeoReviews. 2008;9:e468–76.

Faro A, Mallory GB, Visner GA, Elidemir O, Mogayzel PJ Jr, Danziger-Isakov L, Michaels M, Sweet S, Michelson P, Paranjape S, Conrad C, Waltz DA. American Society of Transplantation executive summary on pediatric lung transplantation. Am J Transplant. 2007;7(2):285–92.

Grady RM, Gandhi S, Sweet SC, Mao J, Huddleston CB. Dismal lung transplant outcomes in children with tetralogy of Fallot with pulmonary atresia compared to Eisenmenger syndrome or pulmonary vein stenosis. J Heart Lung Transplant. 2009;28(11):1221–5.

Gupta S, Fricker FJ, González-Peralta RP, Slayton WB, Schuler PM, Dharnidharka VR. Post-transplant lymphoproliferative disorder in children: recent outcomes and response to dual rituximab/low-dose chemotherapy combination. Pediatr Transplant. 2010;14:896–902.

Huddleston CB. Donor evaluation, surgical technique and perioperative management. In: Fine RN, Webber SA, Olthoff KM, Kelly DA, Harmon WE, editors. Pediatric solid organ transplantation. 2nd ed. Malden: Blackwell Publishing; 2007. p. 326–35.

Kerem E, Reisman J, Corey M, Canny GJ, Levison H. Prediction of mortality in patients with cystic fibrosis. N Engl J Med. 1992;326(18):1187–91.

Lim GY, Newman B, Kurland G, Webber SA. Posttransplantation lymphoproliferative disorder: manifestations in pediatric thoracic organ recipients. Radiology. 2002;222:699–708.

Liou TG, Adler FR, Cox DR, Cahill BC. Lung transplantation and survival in children with cystic fibrosis. N Engl J Med. 2007;357(21):2143–52.

Mendeloff E. Historical notes. In: Fine RN, Webber SA, Olthoff KM, Kelly DA, Harmon WE, editors. Pediatric solid organ transplantation. 2nd ed. Malden: Blackwell Publishing; 2007. p. 309–13.

Rivera-Spoljaric K, Faro A. Fibrosis quística: cuando referir para trasplante pulmonar pediatrico. Neumol Pediatr. 2007;2(2):84–9.

Schuurmans MM, Benden C, Inci I. Practical approach to early postoperative management of lung transplant recipients. Swiss Med Wkly. 2013;143:w13773.

Sharples LD, McNeil K, Stewart S, Wallwork J. Risk factors for bronchiolitis obliterans: a systematic review of recent publications. J Heart Lung Transplant. 2002;21:271–81.

Stegall MD, Gloor JM. Deciphering antibody-mediated rejection: new insights into mechanisms and treatment. Curr Opin Organ Transplant. 2010;15:8–10.

Stewart S, Fishbein MC, Snell GI, et al. Revision of the 1996 working formulation for the standardization of nomenclature in the diagnosis of lung rejection. J Heart Lung Transplant. 2007;26:1229–42.

Sweet SC, Aurora P, Benden C, Wong JY, Goldfarb SB, Elidemir O, Woo MS, Mallory GB, International Pediatric Lung Transplant Collaborative. Lung transplantation and survival in children with cystic fibrosis: solid statistics–flawed interpretation. Pediatr Transplant. 2008;12(2):129–36.

Yusen RD, Shearon TH, Qian Y, Kotloff R, Barr ML, Sweet S, Dyke DB, Murray S. Lung transplantation in the United States, 1999–2008. Am J Transplant. 2010;10(4:Pt 2):t-68.

Index

P. Bertrand, I. Sánchez (eds.), *Pediatric Respiratory Diseases*,
https://doi.org/10.1007/978-3-030-26961-6

F

G

J

K

L

M

O

Q

R

T

U

V

Printed by Printforce, the Netherlands